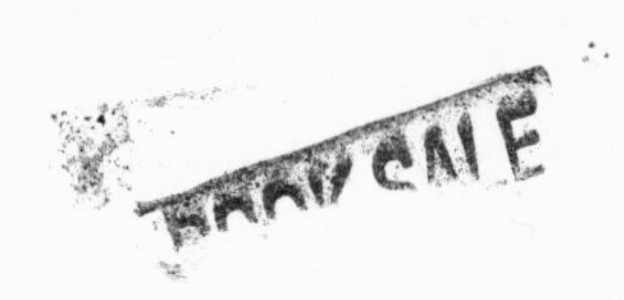
BOOK SALE

D1252470

SYSTEM OF OPHTHALMOLOGY

The scheme for the "System of Ophthalmology" is as follows.

Vol. I. THE EYE IN EVOLUTION

Vol. II. THE ANATOMY OF THE VISUAL SYSTEM

Vol. III. NORMAL AND ABNORMAL DEVELOPMENT
Pt. 1. Embryology
Pt. 2. Congenital Deformities

Vol. IV. THE PHYSIOLOGY OF THE EYE AND OF VISION

Vol. V. OPHTHALMIC OPTICS AND REFRACTION

Vol. VI. OCULAR MOTILITY AND STRABISMUS

Vol. VII. THE FOUNDATIONS OF OPHTHALMOLOGY
Heredity, Pathology, Methods of Diagnosis, General Therapeutics

Vol. VIII. DISEASES OF THE OUTER EYE
Pt. 1. Conjunctiva
Pt. 2. Cornea and Sclera

Vol. IX. DISEASES OF THE UVEAL TRACT

Vol. X. DISEASES OF THE RETINA

Vol. XI. DISEASES OF THE LENS AND VITREOUS; GLAUCOMA AND HYPOTONY

Vol. XII. NEURO-OPHTHALMOLOGY

Vol. XIII. THE OCULAR ADNEXA
Lids, Lacrimal Apparatus, Orbit and Para-orbital Structures

Vol. XIV. INJURIES
Pt. 1. Mechanical Injuries
Pt. 2. Non-mechanical Injuries

Vol. XV. INDEX OF GENERAL AND SYSTEMIC OPHTHALMOLOGY

SYSTEM OF OPHTHALMOLOGY

EDITED BY

SIR STEWART DUKE-ELDER

VOL. XIV

INJURIES

PART 1

MECHANICAL INJURIES

By

SIR STEWART DUKE-ELDER

G.C.V.O., F.R.S.

and

PETER A. MacFAUL

M.B., B.S., F.R.C.S.

Ophthalmic Surgeon, Middlesex Hospital, London;
Honorary Research Assistant, Institute of Ophthalmology,
University of London

WITH 690 ILLUSTRATIONS AND 26 COLOURED PLATES

ST. LOUIS

THE C. V. MOSBY COMPANY

1972

1972

MADE AND PRINTED IN GREAT BRITAIN

Published in London by
Henry Kimpton
134 Great Portland Street, W.1

PREFACE

TRAUMA is one of the Captains of the Men of Death. In war he was always so, and in our own generation with the multiplication of vehicles traversing the streets of our towns and the motorways of the country at ever-increasing speeds, and the growing tendency to violence in our society, his toll of damage continually augments. The subject of mechanical injuries to the eye is immense and embraces a vast variety of lesions in all its structures as well as in the orbits, the face, the skull and the brain.

With the rapid growth in the complexity of technology in industry, non-mechanical injuries are also increasing, a tendency which can be expected to augment in the future. This is nowhere more dramatically exemplified than in the chemical industry, for the many new materials and processes appearing as each year succeeds another carry with them dangers which are difficult to assess. This applies particularly to the pharmaceutical industry which continually deluges us with a flood of new drugs. To anticipate their effects is impossible, for even if experiments on animals or their short-term use in man shows no adverse results, many of their side-effects become apparent only after their prolonged administration to many patients or in peculiar circumstances such as damage to the unborn child when given to the pregnant mother. Toxicology is thus an ever-growing subject which shows no signs of contracting. Moreover, the addition of such physical agents as light-coagulation, lasers, ultrasonic energy and more concentrated ionizing radiation to our clinical armamentarium involves potentialities for harm.

Considered as a whole, the complex subject of injuries therefore embraces all aspects of ophthalmology and assumes a constantly growing importance in the practice of our specialty; and so it is that, to be reasonably complete, one volume in my *Text-Book* has necessarily been expanded to two in this *System*.

STEWART DUKE-ELDER

INSTITUTE OF OPHTHALMOLOGY,
UNIVERSITY OF LONDON,
1972.

ACKNOWLEDGEMENTS

THE writers of a text-book of this type, embracing a subject so large, must necessarily draw widely on the work of others. In a particular sense we must acknowledge with gratitude the valuable advice we have received in several subjects—from Professor George Dick of the Middlesex Hospital for help on immunological problems, Mr. M. A. Bedford on the ocular effects of radiation, Dr. David Cole for advice on the mechanism of chemical injuries, and Dr. M. D. Kipling of H.M. Factory Inspectorate for supplying us with much information on the incidence of industrial injuries in this country.

We have borrowed innumerable illustrations from ophthalmologists all over the world; these are all acknowledged as they appear in the text, but we are happy to thank them collectively. Special thanks, however, must be given to our greatest creditors—Professor Norman Ashton of the Institute of Ophthalmology and Dr. Helenor Wilder lately of the Armed Forces Institute of Pathology in Washington, for pathological illustrations; Dr. Glyn Lloyd of Moorfields Eye Hospital, Dr. W. Campbell of East Grinstead, and Dr. Stephen Trokel of New York, for radiographs; Dr. Stefan Jellinek for illustrations of electrical injuries from his book, *Elektrische Verletzungen* (Barth, Leipzig); and, as in other volumes of this series, Dr. F. N. L. Poynter of the Wellcome Institute of the History of Medicine for many of the photographs of illustrious pioneers which we have used to illustrate the text.

As in previous Volumes, we are very indebted to Sir Allen Goldsmith and Miss Mina H. T. Yuille for reading and correcting the proofs, and, most particularly, to Miss Rosamund Soley for her devoted work in preparing the manuscript and illustrations for publication, collecting and verifying the bibliographical references, and compiling the Index.

CONTENTS OF PART 1

INTRODUCTION

CHAPTER I

THE NATURE AND INCIDENCE OF OCULAR INJURIES

SECTION I

MECHANICAL INJURIES

CHAPTER II

CONCUSSIONS AND CONTUSIONS

CHAPTER III

INCISED WOUNDS

CHAPTER IV

RETAINED FOREIGN BODIES

CONTENTS OF PART 2

SECTION II

NON-MECHANICAL INJURIES

Chapter VII

Thermal Injuries

Chapter VIII

Ultrasonic Injuries

Chapter IX

Electrical Injuries

Chapter X

Radiational Injuries

CHAPTER XI

CHEMICAL INJURIES

SECTION III

TOXICOLOGY

CHAPTER XIII

INORGANIC AGENTS

CHAPTER XIV

ORGANIC AGENTS

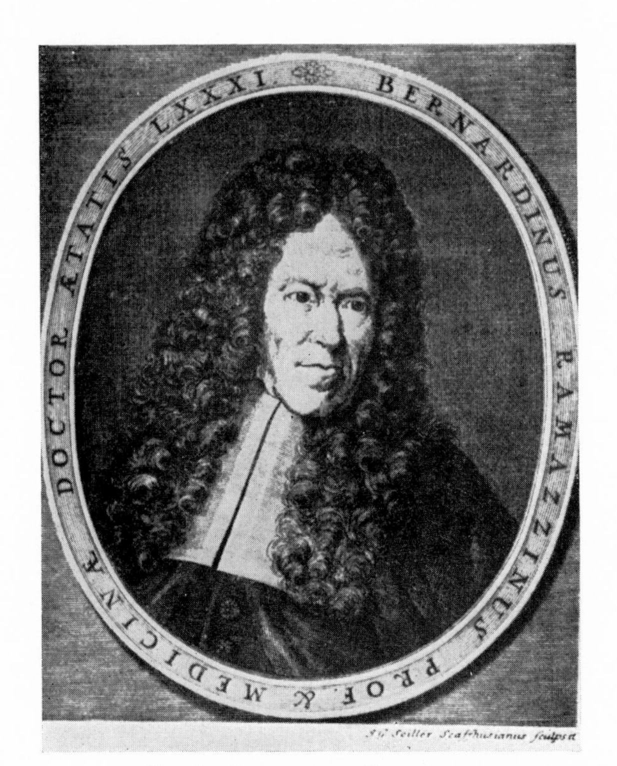

FIG. 1.—BERNARDINO RAMAZZINI
[1633–1714]
(From the *Opera omnia*, Geneva, 1717.)

INTRODUCTION

CHAPTER I

THE NATURE AND INCIDENCE OF OCULAR INJURIES

In mediæval Europe every city stank. The hundreds of tons of garbage thrown daily into the highways there to rot and the thousands of huge privy-vaults (" jakes ") used as lavatories, sometimes within the dwellings, sometimes adjacent to them where human excreta slowly accumulated, ensured that a city like Paris could be smelled, so it was said, 20 miles away on a summer day. Equally in Modena in Italy; but here a kindly but observant man, BERNARDINO RAMAZZINI [1633–1714] noted that the workman who came periodically to empty his jakes was working furiously. Questioning him as to the cause of his apparent eagerness, the man replied that a period of four hours in that place " was equally troublesome as to be struck blind ", and as he looked up Ramazzini noted that his eyes were red and sore. It was, indeed, the custom of the cleaners to return home immediately after their task was finished, remain in a dark room and wash their eyes with warm water to relieve the pain, symptoms known previously in classical Rome. Ramazzini was as curious as he was sympathetic and soon observed that the same ocular trouble affected many of those doing the same menial task and, significantly, that many of the blind or semi-blind beggars who swarmed in his city had been similarly employed, and he attributed the effect to the presence of a volatile acid arising from the excrement. Having unwittingly discovered the ocular effects of hydrogen sulphide kerato-conjunctivitis, he embarked on a long and extraordinarily elaborate series of researches on the ocular effects of a multitude of occupations of this period, all of which are discussed in his classical book *De morbis artificum diatriba* (Mutinae, 1700), in the 360 pages of which are many ophthalmological references; it immediately attracted much attention and enjoyed a wide circulation, the original Latin script being translated into English and German (1705), Italian (1745) and eventually French (1777).[1]

This, of course, is not the beginning of the history of ocular injuries. They doubtless began when one primitive man fought with another, when he first walked through the undergrowth of the forest or first chipped a piece of flint to make his primitive tool. At a much later date one was depicted on the tomb built by Rameses II at Thebes about the year 1200 B.C., wherein the artist painted the picture of the removal of a foreign body from the eye

[1] See translation by O. Cretton (Latin and French texts), *Les maladies des artisans*, Minerva, Torino (1933), and the English translation by W. C. Wright (Latin and English texts), *Diseases of Workers*, Univ. of Chicago Press (1940).

of a workman. But this classical book contained their first systematic and scientific integration and for this reason Ramazzini is justly known as the "Father of Industrial Medicine" and his portrait suitably forms the frontispiece of this Volume (Fig. 1). It is interesting how little change in habit there is with time: Ramazzini found that the chief risk to workmen was from flying particles, and his main difficulty lay in the impossibility of persuading the workers to take the simplest precautions to protect themselves. In his therapeutic suggestions he was most punctilious; he advised the cleaners of the jakes to change their occupation if possible or, alternatively, to place transparent masks over their faces while at work, and if the eyes became red to bathe them with Muscadine wine to induce the animal spirits to return from the brain and the optic nerve to the eyes whence "they had been driven by the sordid and penetrating damps".

Interpreted in its widest sense the subject of ocular injuries is indeed vast but some of it has already been dealt with in previous volumes of this *System*. This volume, therefore, will be confined to new matter and copious reference will be made to previous volumes wherein the relevant subject matter is fully discussed.

Despite the protection afforded the eye by nature—anatomically by its situation in the elastic fatty tissues of the orbital cavity overhung on all aspects except downwards and outwards by the sturdy bony projections of the orbital rim and the nose, and physiologically by the vigilance exercised by the blink reflex and the head-turning reflex on the approach of objects which can be seen, and the copious lacrimation which follows the intrusion of any irritant material—injuries to the eyes are common and may involve any tissue (Table I). Moreover, the effects of such injuries are much more

TABLE I

SITE OF INJURY IN 1,017 CASES OF ADULT OCULAR TRAUMA
(In Wolverhampton; Lambah, 1968)

SITE OF INJURY	NUMBER OF EYES AFFECTED
Lids and Conjunctiva	533
Cornea	841
Iris and Ciliary Body	410
Lens	151
Retina	146
Penetrating Injuries	307
Contusion of Globe	32
Others, including Orbit	57

severe than in any other part of the body, partly because of the delicacy of the ocular tissues and partly because a trauma which elsewhere would cause little and temporary inconvenience can readily result in permanent blindness. Ocular injuries therefore assume unusual social and economic importance involving a huge cost in human unhappiness, economic inefficiency and monetary loss. Even the aggregate sum of the trivial injuries which cause no permanent damage costs every industrialized community an amount in time and money which few would believe unless they had specifically looked into the matter.

General Incidence. The earlier statistics of the incidence of ocular injuries of all types among ophthalmic patients were first correlated by Zander and Geissler (1864), who found the estimates to vary from 1·8 to 9% of all eye diseases. In subsequent studies from many different countries the figures have varied according to the degree of industrialization of the area under review and to whether the incidence of superficial foreign bodies was included in the estimates. Thus Praun (1899), analysing the statistics of 45 clinics of different nationalities in Europe involving 444,819 ophthalmic cases subserving a mixed and largely peasant population, found a total incidence of 4·89%; in industrial regions this figure rose to 8%, while considering in-patients only, an average of 12% was obtained. Again, Weidmann (1888), among 30,000 ophthalmic patients at Zürich, found 10·41% injuries, of which more than half (56%) were due to foreign bodies. The statistics of the Tübingen clinic are extensive[1]—in the 16 years from 1896 to 1911, 90,652 ophthalmic patients were seen, 10·54% of whom were victims of ocular injury. In more recent times as industry has grown and become more complex, so also have these figures.

Thus in the industrialized community of modern London, Minton (1949) found that 30% of all acute ocular cases attending hospital were due to injury, while in the more highly industrialized city of Sheffield where metal industries preponderate, Cridland (1929) found that 39% of all cases attending hospital (including refraction cases) in 1909 and 53% in 1928 were the result of accident. In Birmingham, Roper-Hall (1959) noted that of 267 injuries admitted to hospital over an eight-year period almost 90% were the result of occupational and domestic accidents, while Holland (1965) found that industrial injuries accounted for 53% of 2,309 cases of ocular injury in Kiel between 1950 and 1963. From Sweden, Lindstedt (1966) reported 440 cases of injury representing 12% of all admissions, and at the Osaka University Hospital, over a three-year period, 2,484 ocular injuries were seen representing 7·8% of all new hospital cases (Yuasa *et al.*, 1967). Large numbers of cases have been reported by many writers including among others: Forsius and Nikupaavo (1964), over 27,000 cases in ten years, 40% of them corneal foreign bodies, representing about 3% of all occupational accidents; Maione (1967) 465 cases, and Lambah (1968), 1,017; Remky and his colleagues (1967) over 1,000 cases of perforating injuries representing 7·2% of all hospital admissions in Munich.

The incidence of trauma in causing bilateral (legal) blindness in England is seen in Table II.

The *sex incidence*, largely owing to the great preponderance of industrial injuries, is heavily weighted on the male side: on an average, indeed, statistics show that approximately 85 to 90% of such cases occur in men; thus in 1,017 cases seen in the industrial town of Wolverhampton there were 94·3% male and 5·7% female (Lambah, 1968). For the same reason the highest *age*

[1] Hartmann (1901), Rosenberg (1901), Schütz (1903), Braun (1907), Hescheler (1907), Pfeilsticker (1910), Jooss (1912), Huppenbauer (1912).

TABLE II

CAUSES OF BILATERAL BLINDNESS (1955–62)

MAJOR ÆTIOLOGICAL GROUP	1955–1960 (all ages)		1961 (0–60 years)		1962 (0–65 years)	
	M	F	M	F	M	F
Infectious Diseases	161	136	19	9	16	6
Trauma	208	45	15	6	25	4
Poisoning	112	86	6	7	4	10
Tumours (Ocular and Intracranial)	250	256	42	33	41	35
Systemic Diseases (Diabetes, Vascular, Neurological)	2,353	5,032	105	135	174	216
Prenatal Causes	1,682	1,440	210	163	231	203
Senile Cataract, Macular Degeneration and Myopic Degeneration	16,788	29,723	235	250	379	431
TOTALS	21,554	36,718	632	603	870	905

Figures taken from: Incidence and Causes of Blindness in England and Wales, 1948–62 (Sorsby), H.M.S.O., London (1966).

incidence is in adult life; but it is interesting that the frequency of injuries among children is remarkably high—and important, for in them the damage is frequently of a serious nature (Fig. 2).

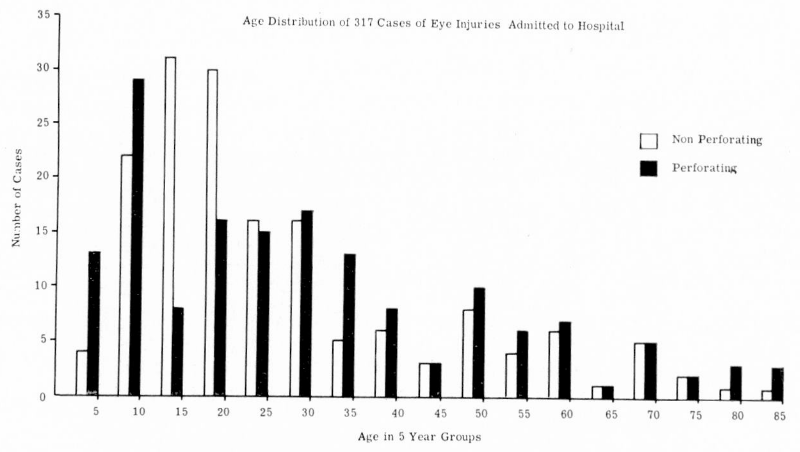

FIG. 2.—OCULAR INJURIES AT MOORFIELDS EYE HOSPITAL.
Note the high proportion of children.

Thus Seidelmann (1876), among his over-all figures, found children under 15 years of age in the proportion of 21·5%, Landesberg (1877) of 23·7% and Garrow (1923) of 14·5%. In Tübingen between 1896 and 1911, of 9,551 ocular injuries, 1,326 (13·9%) occurred in children under 14 (Huppenbauer, 1912). When non-industrial injuries alone are taken into account this proportion becomes much larger. Thus although the population with which he was dealing (over 2,000,000 persons) contained 82·3% above the age of 15 and only 17·7% below, Garrow (1923) found that out of 1,000 consecutive cases of injury 293 were non-industrial, among which the numbers of children and adults over 15 were almost equal (148 adults injured and 145 children). The figures of the Kiel clinic are extensive; between 1950 and 1963 non-industrial ocular injuries were most common in children who accounted for 20% of 2,309 hospital cases (Holland, 1965), and among 357 children under the age of 15 (282 males, 75 females) Holland (1961) found 140 penetrating wounds; traumatic cataract occurred in 49 and 33 eyes were enucleated. Bilateral injuries were rare and mostly in the nature of burns. It is interesting that the actual injury was self-inflicted in almost half of Holland's (1961) cases and that on three occasions the injury was caused by broken spectacles. In Sardinia between 1956 and 1966, Bertoni and Zedda (1967) noted 653 children, mostly boys under the age of 15, with ocular injuries of which 59·6% were perforating wounds. From various centres in Japan over a 15-year period 8,547 cases were collected by Söllner (1966), while Draeger and his colleagues (1967) reviewed 534 cases with particular reference to the mode of injury. Numerous other reports have stressed the large numbers of eye injuries in children, the high incidence of penetrating wounds, and the frequently serious nature of the resulting ocular damage which may lead to enucleation in from 20 to 30% of those cases in which ocular penetration has occurred.[1]

Apt and Sarin. *J. Amer. med. Ass.*, **181**, 948 (1962).
Bakurskaya and Kornilova. *Oftal. Zh.*, 144 (1963).
Bertoni and Zedda. *Rass. med. Sarda*, **70**, 453 (1967).
Braun. *Die Augenverletzungen in d. Tübinger Klinik in d. Jahren* 1903 *und* 1904 (Diss.), Tübingen (1907).
Cridland. *Brit. med. J.*, **2**, 615 (1929).
Draeger, Meves and Sichert. *Mschr. Kinderheilk.*, **115**, 77 (1967).
Forsius and Nikupaavo. *Ann. occup. Hyg.*, **7**, 373 (1964).
Garrow. *Brit. J. Ophthal.*, **7**, 65 (1923).
Gasteiger and Dietzsch. *Wien. klin. Wschr.*, **73**, 854 (1961).
Hartmann. *Die Augenverletzungen in d. Tübinger Klinik in Jahre* 1900 (Diss.), Tübingen (1901).
Hescheler. *Die Augenverletzungen in d. Tübinger Klinik in d. Jahren* 1905 *und* 1906 (Diss.), Tübingen (1907).
Holland. *Klin. Mbl. Augenheilk.*, **139**, 72 (1961); **145**, 915 (1965).
Huppenbauer. *Klinisch-statistische Mitteilungen ü. Augen-Verletzungen bei Kindern nach dem Material d. Tübinger Klinik* (Diss.), Tübingen (1912).
Jooss. *Die Augenverletzungen in d. Tübinger Klinik in d. Jahre* 1910 (Diss.), Tübingen (1912).
Khvatova. *Oftal. Zh.*, **22**, 433 (1967).
Kobor. *Klin. Mbl. Augenheilk.*, **146**, 740 (1965).
Kokriatskaya. *Oftal. Zh.*, 140 (1963).
Kovácik. *Cs. oftal.*, **23**, 54 (1967).
Lambah. *Lancet*, **2**, 1351 (1962).
Trans. ophthal. Soc. U.K., **88**, 661 (1968).
Landesberg. *Phila. med. surg. Rep.*, **38**, 308 (1877).
Lindstedt. *Acta ophthal.* (Kbh.), **44**, 590 (1966).
Maione. *Atti Soc. oftal. Lombarda*, **22**, 213 (1967).
Minton. *Occupational Eye Diseases and Injuries*, London (1949).
Pfeilsticker. *Die Augenverletzungen in d. Tübinger Klinik in d. Jahren* 1907 *und* 1908 (Diss.), Tübingen (1910).
Praun. *Die Verletzungen der Auges*, Wiesbaden (1899).
Remky, Kobor and Pfeiffer. *An. Inst. Barraquer*, **7**, 487 (1967).
Roper-Hall. *Trans. ophthal. Soc. U.K.*, **79**, 57 (1959).
Rosenberg. *Die Augenverletzungen in d. Tübinger Klinik in d. Jahren* 1896–99 (Diss.), Tübingen (1901).
Schütz. *Die Augenverletzungen in d. Tübinger Klinik in d. Jahren* 1901 *und* 1902 (Diss.), Tübingen (1903).
Seidelmann. *Zur Aetiologie u. Prophylaxis d. Erblindungen* (Diss.), Berlin (1876).
Söllner. *J. soc. Ophthal.*, 47 (1966).
Weidmann. *Ueber d. Verletzungen d. Auges durch Fremdkörper* (Diss.), Zürich (1888).
Yuasa, Bessyo, Ishibashi and Seguchi. *Folia ophthal. jap.*, **18**, 717 (1967).
Zander and Geissler. *Die Verletzungen des Auges*, Leipzig (1864).

THE TYPES OF OCULAR INJURY

From the ætiological point of view ocular injuries are difficult to classify since they occur from innumerable causes in every circumstance of life. It may be useful, however, to regard them as ætiologically divisible into seven

[1] Gasteiger and Dietzsch (1961), Lambah (1962), Apt and Sarin (1962), Bakurskaya and Kornilova (1963), Kokriatskaya (1963), Kobor (1965, 1024 cases), Khvatova (1967), Kovácik (1967), and others.

categories—intra-uterine injuries, birth injuries, domestic injuries, injuries due to travel and sport, agricultural injuries, industrial hazards, and war injuries.

INTRA-UTERINE INJURIES

Our knowledge of the effects of injuries sustained during fœtal life is still incomplete but the variety of potential damage is considerable; the whole question of teratogenesis by genetic and environmental influences has been fully discussed elsewhere in this *System*.[1]

It has long been known that MECHANICAL TRAUMA, whether taking the form of dissection, constriction, transplantation or mechanical agitation of the embryo, can produce developmental deformities sometimes of gross degree. *Amniotic bands* may be responsible for a variety of mutilations, varying from such gross defects as anophthalmos, microphthalmos, cyclopia and more or less complete destruction of the orbit and facial structures to smaller anomalies such as corneal opacities, colobomata of the lids and aberrations of the lacrimal passages (Ask and van der Hoeve, 1921). The role of variations in volume of the amniotic fluid in the production of ocular deformities is debatable but intra-uterine moulding, trauma (Born, 1897; Ochi, 1919) and mutilation of the embryo (Lewis, 1909; van der Hoeve, 1930) are clearly established as teratogenic agencies, and the Coulombres (1956–58) have shown that lowering the tension of the developing eye by puncture will impair its growth. Well protected although the human fœtus is during the period of its development, *mechanical trauma* may give rise to a congenital deformity. Such a case was reported by Achelis (1950) wherein after an attempted mechanical abortion in the second month a baby was born with anophthalmos, a small tumour on the upper and outer rim of the orbit and a large wound on the temporal side of the skull.

The principal PHYSICAL AGENTS which act as teratogens include ionizing radiation, ultrasonic energy, low temperatures and atmospheric changes. Of these the most important is *ionizing radiation* which has long been known to produce deformities such as cataract in the mammalian fœtus *in utero*[2] and, indeed, chromosomal changes induced by the same means may result in the transmission of ocular anomalies to the third generation (Bagg and Little, 1924). The variety of gross abnormalities in the fœtus produced by X-rays is considerable and depending on the time in gestation at which they are applied may include anophthalmos, microphthalmos, colobomata and cataract. Heterochromia (Lejeune *et al.*, 1960; Cheesemann and Walby, 1963) and an apparently benign pigmentary retinopathy in the newborn (François *et al.*, 1962) have also been observed. It follows, therefore, that diagnostic, therapeutic or industrial exposure to ionizing radiation in early pregnancy should be strictly limited.

[1] See Vol. III, p. 335.

[2] von Hippel (1907), Tribondeau and Belley (1907), Demel (1926), Desjardins (1931), Majima (1961), François *et al.* (1962), and others.

Ultrasonic energy, the effects of which will be discussed later in this Volume, may also be a cause of congenital cataract in man (Schenk, 1961).

Since the time of Virchow (1867) it has been recognized that *maternal infections* may be transferred to the fœtus either through the placental circulation or the amniotic fluid, and that the resultant diseases differ both in their clinical manifestations and in their sites of election from the typical pictures encountered in the adult; the most important of such infections are syphilis, toxoplasmosis and rubella. The evidence of experimental embryology has also shown that deformities ranging from anophthalmos and cyclopia to the formation of colobomata or cataract can be produced by subjecting the ovum to abnormal chemical influences.

The possible teratogenic effects of DRUGS AND CHEMICALS taken during pregnancy has attracted increasing attention in recent years, particularly since the thalidomide disaster. Thalidomide (Distaval), a non-barbiturate sedative drug, was responsible for gross and widespread congenital deformities, the most dramatic of these being complete aplasia or hypoplasia of the limbs and anomalies of the abdominal organs, eyes and ears. Ocular defects occurred in approximately 25% of thalidomide babies (Cullen, 1964–67), and were mostly of two types—firstly, lesions of a colobomatous nature affecting the iris, choroid and optic disc and occasionally gross defects, such as microphthalmos and anophthalmos; and secondly, disorders of the extra-ocular muscles. Apart from thalidomide many other drugs have from time to time been implicated in the causation of developmental defects in the fœtus, among them metals, growth inhibitors and cytotoxic agents, antibiotics, anticoagulants, sulphonamides and others (Leopold, 1967). Although it is true that the teratogenic significance of some of these substances is confined to laboratory conditions, nevertheless their use in pregnancy should be carefully controlled.

Achelis. *Med. Klin.*, **45**, 1214 (1950).
Ask and van der Hoeve. *v. Graefes Arch. Ophthal.*, **105**, 1157 (1921).
Bagg and Little. *J. exp. Zool.*, **41**, 45 (1924).
Born. *Arch. Entwickl.-Mech. Org.*, **4**, 349 (1897).
Cheesemann and Walby. *Ann. hum. Genet.*, **27**, 23 (1963).
Coulombre, A. J. *J. exp. Zool.*, **133**, 211 (1956).
Arch. Ophthal., **57**, 250 (1957).
Coulombre, A. J. and J. L. *Amer. J. Ophthal.*, **44**, 85 (1957).
Arch. Ophthal., **59**, 502 (1958).
Cullen. *Brit. J. Ophthal.*, **48**, 151 (1964).
Trans. ophthal. Soc. U.K., **86**, 101 (1966).
Brit. orthopt. J., **24**, 2 (1967).
Demel. *Strahlentherapie*, **22**, 333 (1926).
Desjardins. *Amer. J. Roentgenol.*, **26**, 639, 787 (1931).
François, Hooft, de Blond and de Loore. *Ophthalmologica*, **143**, 163 (1962).
von Hippel. *v. Graefes Arch. Ophthal.*, **65**, 326 (1907).
van der Hoeve. *Trans. ophthal. Soc. U.K.*, **50**, 237 (1930).
Lejeune, Turpin, Rethoré and Mayer. *Rev. franç. Ét. Clin. biol.*, **5**, 982 (1960).
Leopold. *Arch. Ophthal.*, **77**, 575 (1967).
Lewis. *Anat. Rec.*, **3**, 175 (1909).
Majima. *Jap. J. Ophthal.*, **5**, 104 (1961).
Ochi. *Brit. J. Ophthal.*, **3**, 433 (1919).
Schenk. *Öst. ophthal. Ges.*, **5**, 54 (1961).
Tribondeau and Belley. *C.R. Soc. Biol.* (Paris), **63**, 128 (1907).
Virchow. *Virchows Arch. path. Anat.*, **38**, 134 (1867).

BIRTH INJURIES

The mechanical strains and stresses of birth, particularly but by no means invariably when delivery is prolonged or aided by instrumental means, may lead to a wide variety of injuries involving the eye itself, the lids, the orbit, the skull and the visual neural apparatus. These injuries are probably much more common than is generally supposed or is indicated in the literature—particularly the obstetric literature. The generally accepted statement that ocular injuries during labour are rare is untrue; indeed, it would seem probable that some injury to the eyeball or its adnexa occurs in 20 to 25% of normal births, a percentage which may rise to 40 or 50% when the labour is protracted or difficult or when instrumental aid is necessary. Fortunately, practically all such injuries are mild and their effects transient; equally, they are difficult to diagnose unless specialist examination is available at an early stage; finally, in most cases no treatment is indicated nor, indeed, is possible so that the relative neglect of this type of case is of little moment. The vast majority is caused by compression either during the child's transit through the maternal passages in the normal way or with the aid of forceps or vacuum extraction; occasionally a direct trauma is caused by the fingers during injudicious vaginal examination undertaken for diagnostic purposes. Fortunately such an enormity as to mistake the orbit for the anus and to luxate the eye with the finger is an uncommon event (de Wecker, 1896; Polliot, 1914). In general terms, the only adequate method of dealing with the problem is prophylactically by ante-natal supervision so that difficulty in labour may be avoided so far as possible, a course which should be supplemented by care and discrimination when instrumental interference is necessary.

The literature dealing with birth injuries is considerable: general summaries will be found in the writings of Bloch (1891), Praun (1899), Wolff (1905), Berger and Loewy (1906), Wagenmann (1910) and Rintelen and his colleagues (1959).

The more common of these injuries will be discussed as they affect (*a*) the eyeball, (*b*) the ocular adnexa and (*c*) the central nervous system.

BIRTH INJURIES TO THE EYE

INJURIES TO THE GLOBE are caused by pressure, either directly on the eyeball or by its being forced against one of the orbital walls. The two most common sequels are intra-ocular hæmorrhages and corneal opacities.

Corneal opacities as a result of birth injury—fortunately usually uniocular—may be of two types which frequently occur together. The more common is a diffuse steamy opacity which is temporary and due to œdema, usually associated with bruising of the lids and subconjunctival ecchymoses. The state of the eye may appear serious at the time but in uncomplicated cases the cornea regains its transparency and the eye appears normal within 6 to 8 days (Fejer, 1904; Stephenson, 1905; Green, 1910; and others). Of considerably more importance are those cases wherein the compression of the globe leads to ruptures of Descemet's membrane. At the

FIGS. 3 to 6.—BIRTH INJURIES TO THE CORNEA.

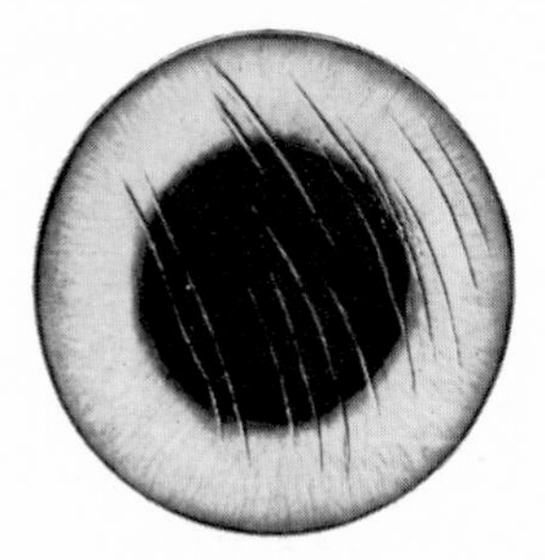

FIG. 3.

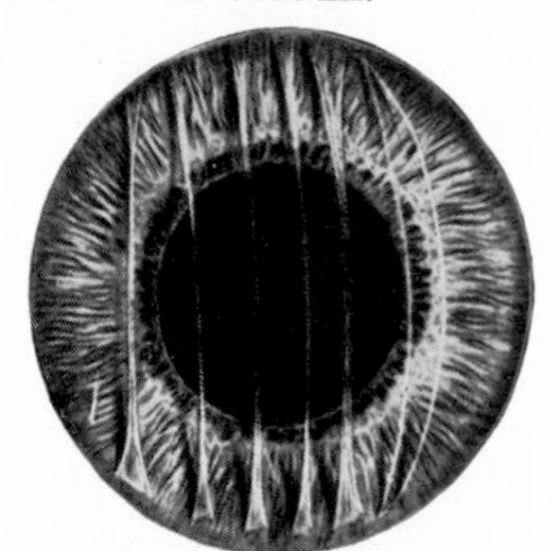

FIG. 4.

FIG. 3.—In a male, aged 23. The eye was injured by forceps at birth. There are numerous tears in Descemet's membrane, keratoglobus and a deep anterior chamber (R. I. Lloyd).

FIG. 4.—In a male, aged 18, who had a forceps delivery, showing the end-result of tears of Descemet's membrane. The deeper corneal layers are cloudy and across the anterior chamber run seven strands of hyaline material, the nasal six of which were free in the aqueous except for their attachment at each end to the posterior surface of the cornea, while the most temporal strand (on the left) was closely applied to the posterior corneal surface (R. I. Lloyd).

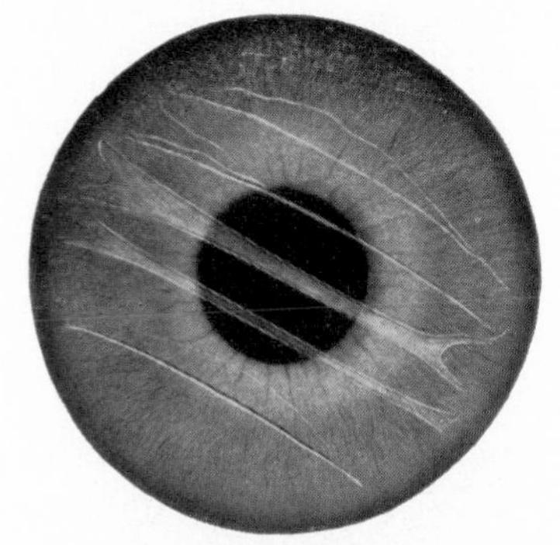

FIG. 5.

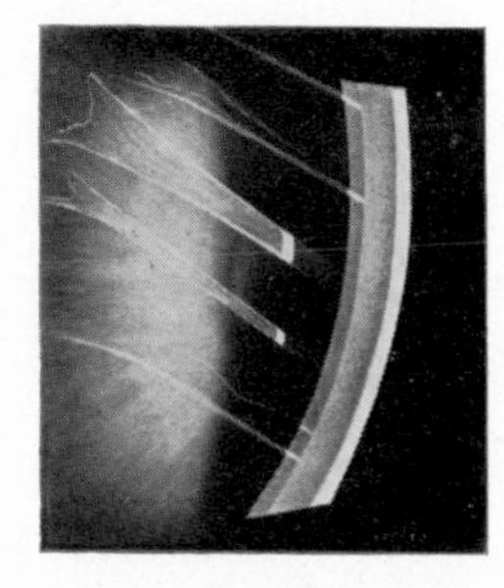

FIG. 6.

FIGS. 5 and 6.—Drawings of the cornea to show multiple ruptures in Descemet's membrane. Figure 6, the appearance as seen by the slit-lamp showing ruptures in Descemet's membrane and hyaline strands in the anterior chamber; some of these form ridges on the posterior surface of the cornea and the two central bands stretch ribbon-like across the anterior chamber attached to the cornea at their extremities where they are continuous with Descemet's membrane (C. A. Perera).

time of injury the cornea may again be uniformly milky and opaque due to interstitial œdema, but eventually as the tissue clears one or several linear, sinuous or crescentic opacities become evident, each associated with a discernible tear in Descemet's membrane, which is usually curled up at the edges or suffers extensive falciform detachments[1] (Figs. 3–6). Such leucomata resulting from birth injury were initially observed by de Wecker (1896), Truc (1898) and Thomson (1902) and were first histologically

[1] Vol. VIII, p. 709.

described by von Hippel (1898), but their true significance was first adequately presented by Thomson and Buchanan (1903–7) in a study of 22 cases; the subsequent literature is considerable.[1] The fate of such tears has been discussed previously,[2] but it is interesting that several records appear of the new formation by the endothelium of hyaline material spun into strands (Lloyd, 1938; Zanen and Rausin, 1949; Gasteiger, 1950), a spider's web arrangement (Hirose, 1932) or a retrocorneal membrane (Peyresblanques, 1967) after a birth trauma of this type (Figs. 5–6). The importance of these early corneal injuries lies in their liability to cause permanent visual defects such as amblyopia with consequent strabismus, high myopia (—14 D, Lloyd, 1938, —16 D, Straub, 1951), marked astigmatism or conical cornea.

Intra-ocular hæmorrhages are the most common result of the compression of the head which occurs at birth, and while they may follow the considerable congestion of the head and neck apparent at the termination of

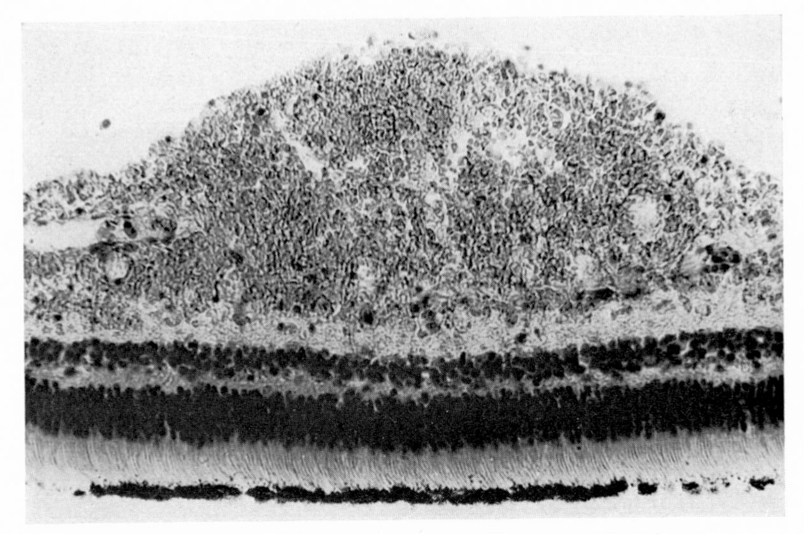

FIG. 7.—RETINAL HÆMORRHAGE IN THE NEWBORN (N. Ashton).

a prolonged but otherwise normal labour, they may be caused by constriction of the neck by the umbilical cord or after a difficult instrumental delivery, particularly where vacuum extraction is used (in 50 to 75% of such cases—Krauer-Mayer, 1965; Neuweiler and Onwudiwe, 1966; and others). They are also seen after an apparently easy birth, even in premature infants, and although extremely rare after Cæsarean section hæmorrhages have been observed in a few cases (3% of babies born by Cæsarean section—Neuweiler

[1] Seefelder (1905), Peters (1906), Rupprecht (1908), Fewell (1933), Lloyd (1938), Perera (1941), Montauffier *et al.* (1952), Boudon (1954) and others.

[2] Vol. VIII, p. 709.

and Onwudiwe, 1966). A hyphæma may be present (Wintersteiner, 1899; Thomson and Buchanan, 1903; and others) or a hæmorrhage into the vitreous (von Hippel, 1898; Stumpf and von Sicherer, 1909) but much the most frequent lesion is a retinal hæmorrhage: this, indeed, is the commonest of all birth injuries (Fig. 7). Estimates of the frequency of their occurrence vary from 2·6 to 50% of all births, depending on the time of the examination, and in about half of the cases they are bilateral. The hæmorrhages may be diffuse or isolated and circumscribed, and radial hæmorrhages around the optic disc are frequently observed. In most cases absorption takes place within 2 or 3 weeks leaving no sequelæ, but in a few cases damage to the macula may be responsible for the subsequent development of amblyopia and a squint.[1]

Other injuries to the globe due to the trauma of birth are more rare and their incidence more problematical. Œdema of the margins of the disc and commotio retinæ have been noted (McKeown, 1941). Injury to the lens producing a lamellar cataract subsequently overlaid by normal transparent tissue has been ascribed to a birth injury (Peck, 1898; Collins, 1916; Clegg and Renwick, 1921), as have iridodialysis (von Hippel, 1901) and choroidal tears (Schmidt-Rimpler, 1875); subluxation of the lens, leading to secondary glaucoma 6 years after birth, was recorded by Würdemann (1932); while the gross injury of retroversion of the ocular contents wherein the pars ciliaris retinæ was stripped from the ciliary body and the lens was dislocated to lie upon the optic nerve-head was described by Thomson and Buchanan (1903) as a result of the severe torsional pressure to which the eye was subjected in a case requiring craniotomy. Microphthalmos and more extensive intra-ocular changes are rare sequels of such gross injuries (Fisher, 1908; James, 1909; Henderson, 1910; and others).

BIRTH INJURIES TO THE OCULAR ADNEXA

Minor injuries to the lids and conjunctiva—œdema, chemosis, bruising, ecchymoses, hæmatomata and lacerations—are relatively common and unimportant; more dramatic are those affecting the orbit—orbital hæmorrhages frequently with proptosis, injuries to the extrinsic ocular muscles, fractures of the orbit with occasional injury to the optic nerve, and dislocation of the globe outside the palpebral aperture. A rare accident is a rupture of Tenon's capsule, resulting in a herniation of the orbital fat into the tissues of the eyelid (Franklin and Horner, 1922). Most of these lesions occur in difficult deliveries, but they are by no means absent when labour is normal (Levasseur and Chapuis, 1948).

[1] For a full description and bibliography of this subject see Vol. X, p. 139. Additional material has been reported by Neuweiler and Onwudiwe (1966) in a survey of 1,074 neonates, Krauer-Mayer (1966), Schenker *et al.* (1966), Gombos and Schenker (1967) and Takeda (1968); hæmorrhages have been reported in 17·8% of normal deliveries, none in 39 cases of Cæsarean section but in 50% of all vacuum extractions and in 40% of forceps deliveries by Jain and Gupta (1967) and many others.

Orbital hæmorrhages, sometimes of considerable dimensions and involving proptosis and exceptionally producing a dislocation of the globe (Hilding, 1948) have been reported following short and normal labour[1] (Figs. 8–9). Trauma following moulding of the head during birth is the common cause, giving rise to venous congestion and rupture sometimes, perhaps, associated with an orbital fracture. The hæmorrhage follows the usual course[2] and its effects, belying the immediate clinical appearance, are usually temporary (Fig. 9). Rarely, however, has the development of sepsis required enucleation of the eye (Veasey, 1904).

FIGS. 8 and 9.—ORBITAL HÆMORRHAGES AT BIRTH (K. F. Kundert).

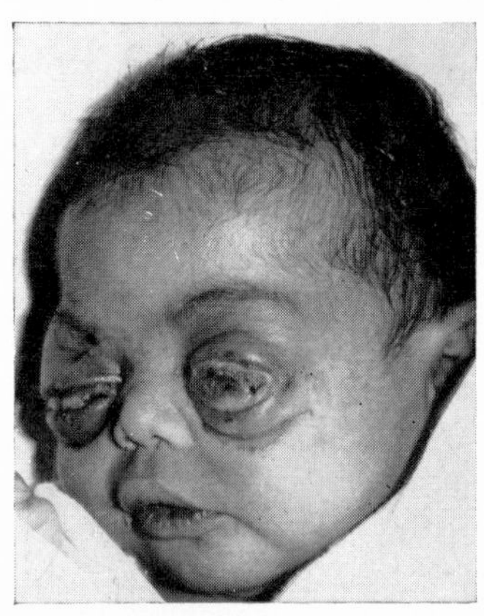

FIG. 8.—Extreme proptosis developing after birth. The figure shows the condition after 12 days. There was exposure keratitis with marked conjunctival chemosis probably due to orbital hæmatomata.

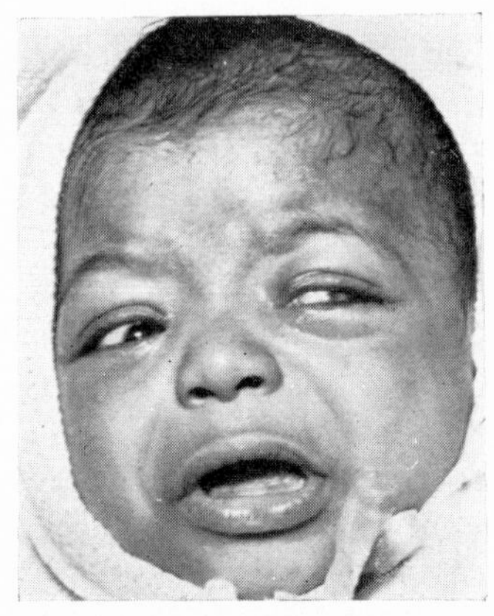

FIG. 9.—The same patient 6 weeks after the first photograph was taken (55 days after birth), showing complete resolution apart from slight diffuse corneal haze.

It is probable also that relatively minor *injuries to the extra-ocular muscles* owing to compression of the orbit may lead to tearing of their sheaths and the occurrence of hæmorrhages into their substance, resulting in permanent fibrosis and the consequent development of a squint—changes which occur most commonly in the lateral rectus.[3] Such a mechanism has been cited by Gallus (1920) as a cause of the retraction syndrome.[4] It is also likely that a pressure-anæmia lasting several hours may give a similar result, and Gifford (1926) concluded that the preponderance of left over right congenital ocular palsies was due to the usual orientation of the child's head in the left occipito-anterior presentation. It is interesting that, unlike retinal hæmorrhages, the occurrence of congenital strabismus seems to have little significant correlation with the difficulty of labour (Heinonen, 1947).

[1] Veasey (1904), Borland (1904), Crawford (1904), Velter and Mérigot de Treigny (1939), Windham (1942), Harley (1943), Kundert (1951) and others.

[2] p. 285. [3] Vol. XIII. [4] See Vol. III, p. 991.

Fractures of the orbit, on the other hand, may be of more serious import and are frequently associated with fractures of the base of the skull (Friedberg, 1864; and others). Such accidents may occur in a prolonged labour owing to excessive uterine contraction against the pelvic rim but are usually the result of trauma due to instrumental delivery, either directly by compression of the frontal portion of the orbit in antero-posterior application or indirectly in lateral application. The implications of such fractures will be discussed subsequently[1]; in the newborn they are always associated with œdema of the lids, almost always with orbital hæmorrhage, occasionally with damage to the lacrimal passages, muscular palsies owing to direct trauma to the muscles (particularly the lateral rectus) or the nerves, or optic atrophy (de Beck, 1889; Bloch, 1891; and others), and sometimes with more extensive cerebral complications and death.

Subluxation or luxation of the globe outside the palpebral aperture is fortunately rare and is due in most cases to the application of forceps which may squeeze the posterior part of the orbit or compress it from in front, acting like the backward thrust of a speculum; in 29 cases gathered from the literature, Friedenwald (1918) found that 4 occurred during spontaneous delivery while the remainder followed instrumental intervention. Such an accident during spontaneous delivery is well authenticated (Rao, 1927). Occasionally the globe has been gouged out by an injudicious exploratory finger (de Wecker, 1896; Polliot, 1914). As a rule the eyeball lies just outside the palpebral aperture, its position being maintained by spasmodic closure of the lids behind it; occasionally it lies loosely on the cheek with its muscular attachments torn and the optic nerve severed.[2] In the milder cases reduction of the globe leads to rapid recovery[3]; in the more severe cases when the optic nerve is torn and the cornea is usually gravely injured, enucleation may be the only possible course.

BIRTH INJURIES TO THE CENTRAL NERVOUS SYSTEM AND OCULAR NERVES

Traumata to the brain arise from three main causes: (1) fractures of the skull, either fissured or depressed, (2) hæmorrhages due to such fractures or caused by the tearing of the venous sinuses or vessels owing to overlapping of the bones of the skull, alterations of the cranial axes or lacerations of the tentorium, or (3) contusions and small hæmorrhages in the brain substance itself. Such hæmorrhages are common, even in infants born after easy and rapid labour without instrumental aid (Ehrenfest, 1922).

Thus among 200 average newborn children, Sharpe (1924) found blood in the cerebro-spinal fluid in 12%. Similarly in a series of 200 mature and 200 premature infants who came to early necropsy, Cruickshank (1923) found hæmorrhages of some

[1] p. 221.
[2] Snell (1903), Thomson and Buchanan (1903), Turnbull (1909), Griffith (1924) and others.
[3] Beaumont (1903), Fage (1907), Donaldson (1910), Friedenwald (1918) and others.

kind in 80% of the former and 66% of the latter; in 32% of all cases with hæmorrhage there were gross exudations into the cranium, and in 20% tears of the tentorium of the cerebrum or the cerebellum.

Such hæmorrhages are generally accepted as being the cause of some cases of spastic paraplegia in children although most of these cases are due to widespread degenerative changes occurring *in utero*. Meningeal lesions of the same type may give rise to arachnoid adhesions in the chiasmal region and optic atrophy (Buchanan, 1926); lesions in the parietal region may result in the occurrence of aphasia and word-blindness (Fisher, 1910; and

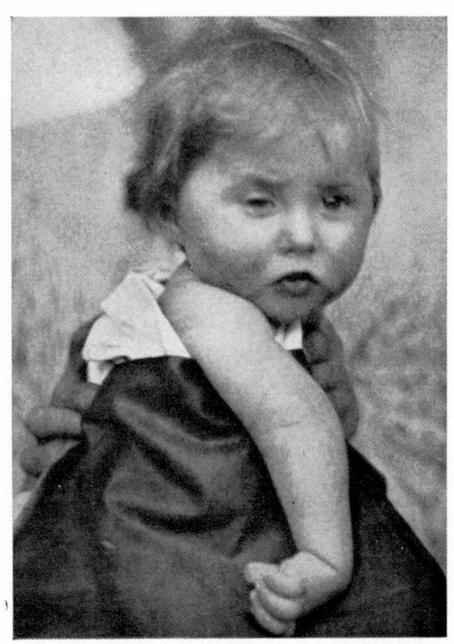

Fig. 10.—Traumatic Horner's Syndrome.
In Klumpke's paralysis from a birth injury (A. Franceschetti).

others). Similarly, small intrapontine hæmorrhages may give rise to ocular motor palsies and ptosis (Uhthoff, 1913), as also may meningeal hæmorrhages or the more direct trauma of fracture or compression of the skull upon the nerve roots at the base of the brain or at the apex of the orbit; a VIth nerve palsy is the most common result, but ptosis with other evidences of implication of the IIIrd nerve may occur while the subsequent development of a pseudo-Graefe phenomenon[1] has been recorded (Hinkel, 1902). A congenital nystagmus may have the same origin. A facial palsy with subsequent lagophthalmos may have a similar ætiology or arise from direct compression (usually by forceps) of the petrous bone (Nettleship, 1903; Sidler-Huguenin,

[1] See Vol. III, p. 900.

1903; Peters, 1906; and others); a Marcus Gunn phenomenon[1] has been reported as a sequel (Gasteiger, 1950). Finally, injury to the sympathetic may follow compression of the neck by forceps producing Horner's syndrome of ptosis, pseudo-enophthalmos, miosis with failure of dilatation of the pupil with cocaine, heterochromia of the iris and unilateral facial anhidrosis (Mayou, 1910–16; Burrows, 1915; Rosetti and Roi, 1948; Gasteiger, 1950) (Fig. 10).

It has been suggested that damage incurred at birth may be responsible for the occurrence of facial hemiatrophy with its concomitants of underdevelopment of the orbit and hypoplasia of the skin and its appendages on the affected side[2] (Penfield and Robertson, 1943; Calnan, 1949).

The reader of this section may gather the impression that entering this world is a difficult and dangerous adventure—almost as dangerous as living in it. It is; but it is to be remembered that most of the scars thus sustained are transient; most of us arrive safely, few of us are permanently maimed.

Beaumont. *Trans. ophthal. Soc. U.K.*, **23,** 282 (1903).
de Beck. *France Méd.*, **2,** 1229 (1889).
Berger and Loewy. *Ueber Augenerkr. sexuellen Ursprungs bei Frauen,* Wiesbaden, 116 (1906).
Bloch. *Zbl. prakt. Augenheilk.*, **15,** 134 (1891).
Borland. *Lancet,* **2,** 1344 (1904).
Boudon. *Arch. Ophtal.*, **14,** 787 (1954).
Buchanan. *Trans. ophthal. Soc. U.K.*, **46,** 32 (1926).
Burrows. *Ophthalmoscope,* **13,** 13 (1915).
Calnan. *Brit. med. J.*, **2,** 56 (1949).
Clegg and Renwick. *Trans. ophthal. Soc. U.K.*, **41,** 230 (1921).
Collins. *Trans. ophthal. Soc. U.K.*, **36,** 403 (1916).
Crawford. *Lancet,* **2,** 1450 (1904).
Cruickshank. *Lancet,* **1,** 836 (1923).
Donaldson. *Brit. med. J.*, **1,** 200 (1910).
Ehrenfest. *Birth Injuries of the Child,* N.Y. (1922).
Fage. *Arch. Ophtal.*, **27,** 516 (1907).
Fejer. *Zbl. prakt. Augenheilk.*, **28,** 235 (1904).
Fewell. *Trans. Amer. ophthal. Soc.*, **31,** 329 (1933).
Fisher. *Trans. ophthal. Soc. U.K.*, **28,** 158 (1908); **30,** 216 (1910).
Franklin and Horner. *Amer. J. Ophthal.*, **5,** 601 (1922).
Friedberg. *Virchows Arch. path. Anat.*, **31,** 344, 357 (1864).
Friedenwald. *Amer. J. Ophthal.*, **1,** 9 (1918).
Gallus. *Arch. Augenheilk.*, **87,** 35 (1920).
Gasteiger. *Dtsch. Gesundh.-Wes.*, **5,** 616 (1950).
Gifford. *Amer. J. Ophthal.*, **9,** 3 (1926).
Gombos and Schenker. *Harefuah,* **72,** 229 (1967).
Green. *Ophthal. Rec.*, **19,** 344 (1910).
Griffith. *Amer. J. Ophthal.*, **7,** 472 (1924).
Harley. *Amer. J. Ophthal.*, **26,** 1314 (1943).
Heinonen. *Acta ophthal.* (Kbh.), **25,** 19 (1947).
Henderson. *Trans. ophthal. Soc. U.K.*, **30,** 154 (1910).
Hilding. *Amer. J. Ophthal.*, **31,** 1484 (1948).
Hinkel. *Ueber das Pseudo-Graefe'sche Symptom im Anschluss an Lähmungen d. Augenmuskeln* (Diss.), Jena (1902).
von Hippel. *v. Graefes Arch. Ophthal.*, **45,** 31 (1898); **52,** 467 (1901).
Hirose. *Acta Soc. ophthal. jap.*, **36,** 121 (1932).
Jain and Gupta. *Proc. All India ophthal. Soc.*, **22,** 119 (1967).
James. *Trans. ophthal. Soc. U.K.*, **29,** 33 (1909).
Krauer-Mayer. *Ann. paediat.* (Basel), **204,** 168 (1965).
Gynéc. et Obstét., **65,** 77 (1966).
Kundert. *Amer. J. Ophthal.*, **34,** 1173 (1951).
Levasseur and Chapuis. *J. Prat.* (Paris), **32,** 281 (1948).
Lloyd. *Amer. J. Ophthal.*, **21,** 359 (1938).
McKeown. *Arch. Ophthal.*, **26,** 25 (1941).
Mayou. *Trans. ophthal. Soc. U.K.*, **30,** 196 (1910).
Ophthalmoscope, **14,** 421 (1916).
Montauffier, de la Bernardie and Devilla. *Arch. Ophtal.*, **12,** 605 (1952).
Nettleship. *Trans. ophthal. Soc. U.K.*, **23,** 287 (1903).
Neuweiler and Onwudiwe. *Gynaecologia* (Basel), **162,** 308 (1966).
Peck. *Med. News* (N.Y.), **73,** 689 (1898).
Penfield and Robertson. *Arch. Neurol. Psychiat.*, **50,** 405 (1943).
Peters. *Arch. Augenheilk.*, **56,** 311 (1906).
Perera. *Arch. Ophthal.*, **25,** 75 (1941).
Peyresblanques. *Bull. Soc. Ophtal. Fr.*, **67,** 1058 (1967).

[1] See Vol. III, p. 900.
[2] Vol. III, p. 1026.

Polliot. *Clin. Ophtal.*, **6,** 296 (1914).
Praun. *Die Verletzungen des Auges*, Wiesbaden (1899).
Rao. *Brit. J. Ophthal.*, **11,** 79 (1927).
Rintelen, Berger and Stauffenegger. *Schweiz. med. Wschr.*, **89,** 427 (1959).
Rosetti and Roi. *Atti Soc. med. chir. Padova*, **26,** 19 (1948).
Rupprecht. *Klin. Mbl. Augenheilk.*, **46** (1), 134 (1908).
Schenker *et al.* *Obstet. and Gynec.*, **27,** 521 (1966).
Schmidt-Rimpler. *Klin. Mbl. Augenheilk.*, **13,** 418 (1875).
Seefelder. *Klin. Mbl. Augenheilk.*, **43** (2), 321 (1905).
Sharpe. *Illinois med. J.*, **45,** 264 (1924).
Sidler-Huguenin. *Korresp.-Bl. schweiz Aerz.*, **33,** 205 (1903).
Snell. *Trans. ophthal. Soc. U.K.*, **23,** 294 (1903).
Stephenson. *Ophthalmoscope*, **3,** 12 (1905).
Straub. *Ophthalmologica*, **122,** 239 (1951).
Stumpf and von Sicherer. *Beitr. Geburtsch. Gynäk.*, **13,** 408 (1909).
Takeda. *Rinsho Ganka*, **22,** 217 (1968).
Thomson. *Trans. ophthal. Soc. U.K.*, **22,** 240 (1902).
Thomson and Buchanan. *Trans. ophthal. Soc. U.K.*, **23,** 296 (1903).
Ophthalmoscope, **3,** 267 (1905); **5,** 186, 415 (1907).
Truc. *Ann. Oculist.* (Paris), **119,** 161 (1898).
Turnbull. *Brit. med. J.*, **2,** 1529 (1909).
Uhthoff. *Klin. Mbl. Augenheilk.*, **51** (2), 344 (1913).
Veasey. *Ophthal. Rec.*, **13,** 201 (1904).
Velter and Mérigot de Treigny. *Bull. Soc. Ophtal. Paris*, 569 (1939).
Wagenmann. *Die Verletzungen d. Auges: Graefe-Saemisch Hb. d. ges. Augenheilk.*, 2nd ed., Leipzig, **9** (5), 813 (1910).
de Wecker. *Ann. Oculist.* (Paris), **116,** 40 (1896).
Windham. *Amer. J. Ophthal.*, **25,** 1236 (1942).
Wintersteiner. *Z. Augenheilk.*, **2,** 443 (1899).
Wolff. *Beitr. Augenheilk.*, *Fest. J. Hirschberg*, 311 (1905).
Würdemann. *Injuries of the Eye*, Chicago (1911); 2nd ed., London, 208 (1932).
Zanen and Rausin. *Bull. Soc. belge Ophtal.*, No. 93, 508 (1949).

NON-OCCUPATIONAL DOMESTIC INJURIES

NON-OCCUPATIONAL DOMESTIC INJURIES—comprising the multitude of accidents that constantly occur in everyday life outside the place of work—although they excite little attention owing to their local and individual significance, are nevertheless numerous and quite frequently severe.[1] Many of them are trivial and are not recorded; but although significant statistics are few, of all cases of ocular injury reporting to hospital there seems to be general accord that some 70% to 80% are incurred in occupational pursuits and 20% to 30% in non-occupational circumstances (Praun, 1899; Garrow, 1923; Roper-Hall, 1959; Holland, 1965; and others).

The types of injury thus sustained are legion. The most common is certainly a foreign body in the eye—usually a trivial affair; almost as frequent are abrasions by a finger-nail, a cosmetic utensil or the hundred and one things of everyday life varying from the bristles of a brush to the claw of a cat. Of the serious injuries probably some 75% in adults are contusions by a blunt object such as are sustained in falling or by being hit (by the fist, an implement, a piece of chopped wood, a stone, and so on); for the rest, perforating injuries by a sharp object (a knife, scissors, corkscrew, fork, needle, nail, hat-pin, broken spectacle lenses, glass or earthenware) contribute their share, while burns by fire, hot irons, ammonia, lime, acids, match-heads or cigarette ash account for a considerable number (Table III). The injuries thus produced vary from lacerations of the lids and abrasions of the cornea to wounds or ruptures of the sclera, intra-ocular hæmorrhages,

[1] In the U.S.A., accidents at home account for 28,000 deaths, 100,000 permanent and 4,000,000 temporary disablements each year—*U.S. Statistical Bull.*, **34,** 6 (1953).

dislocation of the lens and detachment of the retina; in a considerable percentage of cases (almost 25% of those seen in hospital, Garrow, 1923) these may necessitate enucleation either immediately or after some time, and in a greater percentage may entail grave damage to, or loss of vision. Although Garrow found that such non-occupational injuries formed only 29·3% of all ocular injuries in Scotland, his figures show that they were responsible for 42·9% of all enucleations, a proportion due to the frequency of extensive ruptures of the sclera and the gross nature of the penetrating wounds so frequently characteristic of this type of case. Similarly, in the United States it was computed for the years 1935–36 that some 18% of uniocular blindness

TABLE III

THE CAUSES OF NON-INDUSTRIAL INJURIES

(A. Garrow)

		ADULTS		CHILDREN	
		Injuries	Enucleations	Injuries	Enucleations
Blows from blunt instruments—					
In fights	35	121	27	55	9
In falls	17				
Chopping wood	17				
In sport	7				
Other blunt instruments	23				
Unrecorded contusions	22				
Sharp instruments		12	1	31	9
Glass and earthenware		10	4	23	7
Spectacle glass		1	0	0	0
Dust		5	0	0	0
Coal fragments		3	0	0	0
Burns		4	2	8	0
Ammonia		1	0	0	0
Toys, explosions and firearms		7	1	11	0
Not recorded		4	2	16	4
TOTAL		168	37	144	29

due to all causes and 36% of uniocular blindness from accidental causes, and 5% of bilateral blindness due to all causes and 25% of bilateral blindness from accidental causes were the result of accidents in the home.[1]

Children are the victims of a surprisingly high percentage of domestic injuries, probably some 20%.[2] Blunt objects are the most common cause (pieces of metal, wood and stone or falls, kicks and blows), while penetration of the globe by sharp instruments (scissors, knives, forks, sticks, pin-points, air-gun projectiles, arrows and other toys; broken glass and earthenware) makes up a considerable proportion: burns and explosions, as in fireworks, contribute a share which is apt to assume tragic proportions in such national festivals as Guy Fawkes's Day in England or Independence Day in America (Table IV). Practically all such injuries are due to over-exuberance or lack of

[1] Nat. Health Survey, 1935–36; U.S. Pub. Health Services, Bull. No. 10, 1938.

[2] p. 6.

controlling influences, the result of carelessness in playing, the use of dangerous articles or a bout of temper. An interesting point in this connection observed by Holland (1961) concerning his series of 357 children under 15 (282 boys, 75 girls) was that in 160 cases the injury was self-inflicted; in 184 cases another child was involved. Dangerous toys were implicated in over two-thirds of another large series (Pisano and Castellazo, 1967). Unfortunately, many of these injuries in children are serious and extensive and, in the young, damage to the lens, the effects of a quiet cyclitis and the

TABLE IV

OCULAR INJURIES IN CHILDREN UNDER 15 YEARS OF AGE

(Adapted from Lambah, 1962)

CAUSE OF INJURY	NUMBER OF CASES TOTAL	PENETRATING	
THROWN MISSILES			
Stones, pieces of brick, conkers, marbles	137	14	6–10 year age-group, mostly at risk, usually thrown by older boy at more helpless junior
ASSAULTS			
Sticks, pieces of wood, rulers, steel bars, etc.	82	17	Compared with adults, fist and finger injuries rare
ARROWS . . .	57	26	Commonest cause of blind eye, almost 50% penetrating wounds: "Cowboys and Indians"
GAMES OR PLAY . .	49	5	
CATAPULTED MISSILES .	47	3 }	Mostly in older children
FIREWORKS . . .	39	3 }	1 case of bilateral blindness from fireworks
FALL	39	13	
AIRGUN PELLETS . .	39	12	
MISHAP . . .	34	13	
POINTED OBJECTS . .	32	26 }	40% in children under 5 years
Knives . . .	16	15 }	
CHOPPING WOOD			
Hammering . .	15	10	Note 2/3 penetrating
ANIMALS . . .	12	0	
MISCELLANEOUS . .	12	6	
TOTAL . . .	610	163	27% penetrating injuries

Chief causes of blindness: Arrows, Airgun Pellets, Assaults and Pointed Objects.

incidence of sympathetic ophthalmitis provide problems more pressing and difficult to control than in the case of adults.

The seriousness of these accidents is shown in the figures of numerous authors; thus, Werner (1952) found among 215 cases of ocular trauma in children (79% boys) 161 perforating wounds involving the loss of 53 eyes; Gasteiger and Dietzsch (1961) 227 cases, more than one-third being perforating wounds with enucleation in 16%; Holland (1961) 357 cases with perforating wounds in 140, of which 49 developed traumatic cataract and 37 eyes were enucleated; Lambah (1962) among 614 cases over a 10-year period, 167 penetrating wounds leading to enucleation in 54; Kokriatskaya (1963) 237 cases, loss of sight in 27·5% due to secondary glaucoma, optic atrophy or lens-induced uveitis; Bakurskaya and Kornilova (1963) 470 injuries, 65 eyes enucleated, all with retinal detachment; Kobor (1965) 19% of all ocular injuries to occur in children under the age of 15, among which an unfavourable outcome resulted in 20%; Khvatova (1967) 273 eyes lost after penetrating injuries; Kovácik (1967) 409 cases, enucleation required in 21% of all perforating wounds, 1·3% of contusion injuries and 3·4% of chemical injuries; Apt and Sarin (1962), reviewing the reasons for enucleation in children up to the age of 15 years, found that trauma was responsible in more than half. Many others have reported similar experiences.

Injuries due to the use or abuse of *fireworks* are common and while most are relatively minor cases of superficial foreign bodies or corneal burns leaving no permanent sequelæ, many serious injuries occur, usually as a result of explosions near the face or due to flying particles from disintegrating projectiles (May, 1956).

In England the majority of such injuries occur in the period around Guy Fawkes's day but occasional tragedies are the result of misguided chemical experiments by boys trying to construct their own fireworks or bombs, such as by placing a mixture of sodium chlorate and sugar in a metal pipe.[1] The figures in Table V, compiled from the

TABLE V

ANALYSIS OF INJURIES DUE TO FIREWORKS—1962–66

Year	1962	1963	1964	1965	1966
Total number of accidents	2,832	2,461	2,220	2,339	2,302
Age: 15 years and over	682	620	610	654	654
Under 15 years	2,150	1,841	1,610	1,685	1,648
Cases admitted to hospital	483	332	241	213	259
Site of injury:					
EYE	1,038	916	749	797	831
FACE	642	493	481	543	482
HAND	978	827	707	816	723
ELSEWHERE	687	518	518	505	494

reports of the Home Office Inspector of Explosives, show the number of persons who received hospital treatment for injuries caused by fireworks over the Guy Fawkes celebrations in the years 1962–66. During the whole of this period there were two fatalities and although the figures for 1967 showed a slight decline in the total number of accidents, perhaps because of propaganda and restrictions on the sale of fireworks, the figures for 1968 showed a disappointing reversal of this trend, with not only an increase in the total number of accidents (2,537 cases, 604 ocular injuries) but a higher proportion of serious injuries; thus of the 392 cases classified in this way, ocular injuries accounted for 168 (43%). In 1969 and 1970, however, as a result of further intensive publicity, a significant reduction occurred in the number of these injuries. It is clear from the Table that the vast majority of the casualties occurs in children under the age of fifteen and that the eye is involved more frequently than any other part of the body, followed closely by injuries to the hands.

Injuries, dangers and nuisances from fireworks are not entirely contemporary events; Macaulay tells us that after the Peace of Ryswick in 1697 fireworks to the value of £12,000 were let off and a similar sum was expended in celebration of the peace with Russia in May, 1856. In October, 1770, on market day at Milborne Port the grandfather

[1] For a graphic description of the appalling consequences to life and limb from such experiments and for detailed statistics relating to firework injuries see the reports of H.M. Inspector of Explosives, H.M.S.O., London, No. 91, 1967, and 92, 1968.

of C. P. Scott, the famous newspaper editor, lost an eye due to injury from a lighted squib. In 1697 Parliament foreshadowed more recent legislation by the limitation of the manufacture of fireworks to those required for military purposes, the preamble to the Act[1] including the following: " whereas much mischief hath lately happened by throwing, casting and firing of squibs, serpents, rockets and other fireworks, some persons having thereby lost their lives, others their eyes, others have had their lives in great danger and several other damages have been sustained by many persons and much more may happen if not speedily prevented . . ."[2]

It is interesting that serious injuries resulting from *broken spectacles* are rare.[3] Among children Buchanan (1921) found that of 61 eyes enucleated after trauma only 2 cases were of this type and in both of these the accident was caused by the direct blow of a stone of such force that the eye would have been destroyed if spectacles had not been worn, and in a series of 357 cases of injuries in children Holland (1961) found only three instances in which the injury resulted from splintered spectacles. Among adults the incidence is similarly low considering the vast numbers of people wearing spectacles.[4] Of 36 injuries due to broken spectacles, 10 of which resulted in legal blindness, Keeney (1960) found that 14 were caused by flying objects such as nails, stones and baseballs, in 4 cases the lenses were smashed by the lead weights used by fishermen, 3 were the results of blows by the fist and others followed car accidents and falls. Among 1,099 industrial ocular accidents Kaufmann (1956) recorded 11 cases of injury due to fragments of glass, 9 of which were caused by flying objects striking ordinary spectacle lenses which shattered under the impact with serious results in 2 cases; and in the very large series of over 1,000 perforating injuries reported by Remky and his colleagues (1967), 139 (13·5%) were caused by fragments of glass, among which spectacles accounted for 17. Fragmentation of a concave lens is the usual cause of injury which is not often serious, but penetration of the globe by fragments of glass may occur with consequent laceration of the intra-ocular tissues. Such wounds, however, are not usually infected, possibly because the smooth surface of the glass is not an ideal place for the harbouring of organisms. In addition to ocular injuries, severe lacerations of the lids may occur, even after the breakage of underwater goggles (Fig. 11). The question of safety glass in spectacles will be discussed subsequently.[5] We should mention here the possible risks from the use of spectacle frames made of inflammable material, such as cellulose nitrate which has a low ignition temperature and burns rapidly: Schultz (1967) reported a case in which severe eyelid and facial burns resulted in an elderly man when an old pair of cellulose nitrate spectacles were accidentally ignited by a cigarette

[1] 1697, 9 Wm. III C.7.

[2] A historical account concerning the legislation relating to the manufacture and sale of fireworks can be found in *Brit. med. J.*, **2**, 1132, 1965.

[3] Bourgeois (1901), Mitchell (1903), Hirschberg (1906), Vogt (1912), Lauber (1914), and others.

[4] Stephenson (1915); 5 cases in 150,000 ocular accidents, Lauber (1923); 11 out of 133 consecutive incised wounds of the globe, Moncreiff and Scheribel (1945).

[5] p. 43.

lighter. Cellulose acetate with a slow burning rate and resistance to temperature up to 180° Centigrade has now replaced the nitrate form in the manufacture of spectacle frames, but such frames may still be in use.

The wearing of *contact lenses* sometimes leads to ocular complications, the most common being abrasions of the corneal epithelium which, as a rule, heal rapidly with simple measures, such as antibiotic ointment and padding until the affected area no longer stains with fluorescein; such accidents occur mostly when the lenses are being used for the first time, or following excessively long periods of wear. Cases have been recorded in which a contact

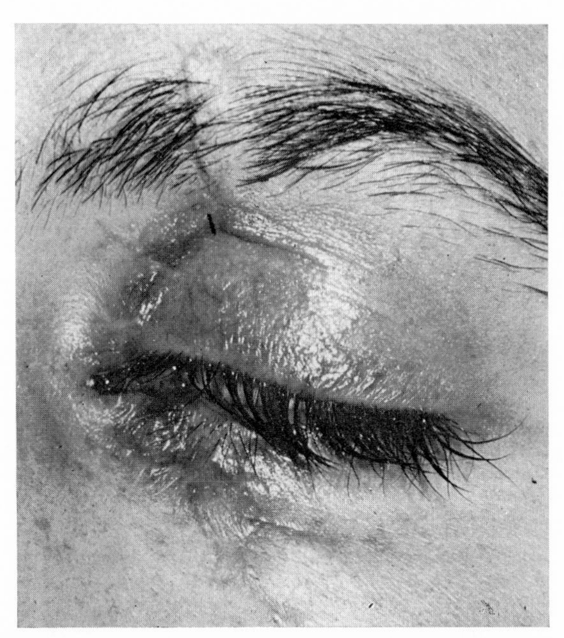

Fig. 11.—Injury from Swimming Goggles.
Affecting the upper lid; the lower canaliculus has gone.

lens, supposedly lost, has subsequently been found embedded in the palpebral conjunctiva, necessitating surgical removal, or tucked away in the recesses of the superior fornix (Green, 1963; Shenken, 1969). More serious results, however, may follow such as corneal vascularization, particularly in cases of keratoconus with œdema (Dixon, 1963; Dixon and Lawaczeck, 1963) or endophthalmitis after trauma to a filtering bleb (Wild, 1962; Ashline and Ellis, 1968).

An extensive survey of the incidence of ocular complications in contact-lens wearers in the United States of America was made by Dixon and his colleagues (1966); thus among nearly 50,000 patients over a period of 1 year the following incidents were reported: 14 eyes removed or blinded, and 157 reports of permanent corneal scarring and opacification attributed to contact lenses or associated factors. Less serious

262,396 injured as a result of road accidents, whereas in 1965 these figures had risen to 7,952 killed and 389,985 injured; the figures for the United States of America over the same period were 37,437 killed in 1955 and 48,050 in 1965,[1] to which must be added many hundreds of thousands with non-fatal injuries, some resulting in permanent incapacity.

The true significance of the situation can be seen from another angle; thus in the Korean War the United States Army lost more personnel from

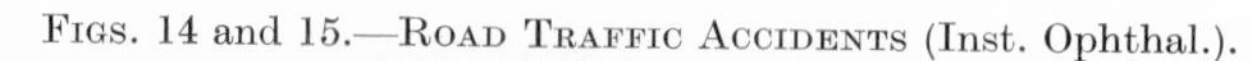
FIGS. 14 and 15.—ROAD TRAFFIC ACCIDENTS (Inst. Ophthal.).

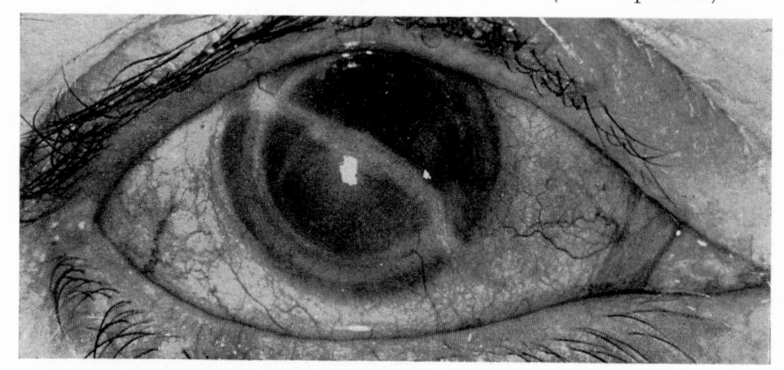

FIG. 14.—Perforating wound of the cornea caused by the windscreen. The injury was bilateral (see Fig. 278).

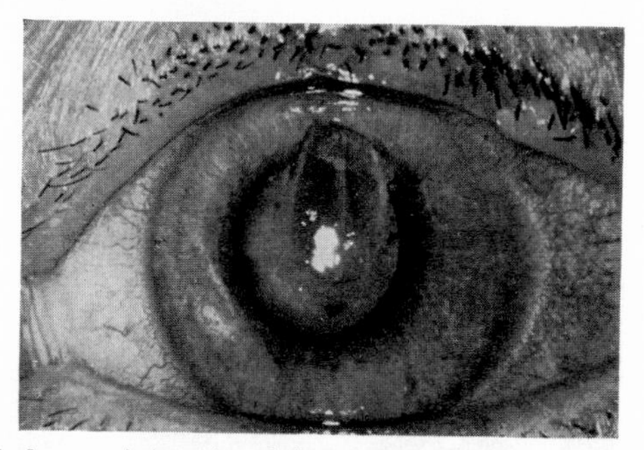

FIG. 15.—A windscreen injury involving a perforating wound of the cornea with a large piece of glass in the anterior chamber and a traumatic cataract.

motor accidents than from combat injuries and the figures in the study at Cornell University on automobile trauma showed that eye injuries are five times more frequent in relation to all road traffic injuries than is ocular cancer in relation to all forms of body cancer (Keeney, 1964).

The implication of all this for the ophthalmologist is clear from numerous accounts in the literature: thus, in the Cornell University study (Keeney, 1964) 4,506 persons (9·8%) out of a total of 27,697 passengers in traffic accidents sustained ocular or orbital injuries, and according to Braunstein (1957) head injuries occur in approximately 75% of the victims of road accidents.

[1] W.H.O. *Stat. Reports*, **21,** 5 (1968).

Entering and leaving the vehicle produce their toll of traumata, but injury usually results from collisions when on the road. In all travelling accidents whether incurred in trains, aeroplanes or cars the injury tends to be severe, as a rule a contusion leading to fracture of the orbit and concussion or rupture of the globe or perforating injuries due to glass, and quite frequently the ocular injury is associated with considerable facial damage, particularly lacerations of the eyelids and cheek.[1]

In the majority of cases the actual damage is inflicted by fragments of glass from a windscreen shattered by the impact of the head of the victim, frequently the front-seat passenger,[2] injuries which in many instances might have been prevented by the presence of a laminated windscreen or the use of safety seat-belts (Nahum, 1965); even with the former, however, eyes have been perforated and lost (Halbron and Vignaud, 1969) (Fig. 17). Usually the eye is severely damaged and perforation of the globe is

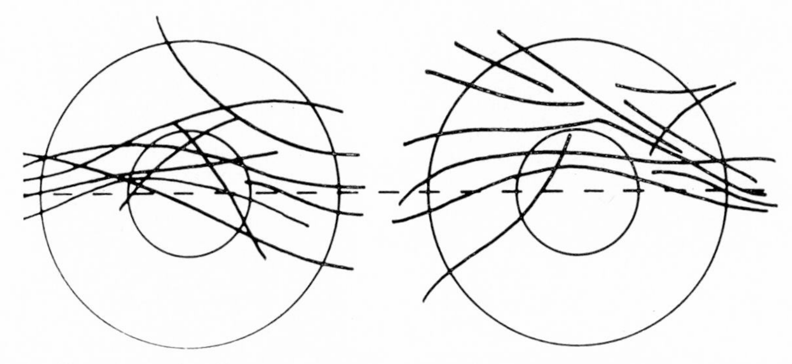

FIG. 16.—DIAGRAMMATIC REPRESENTATION OF THE POSITION OF CORNEAL LACERATIONS.
In 8 cases of bilateral injury sustained in road accidents (after H. Friedrich).

common (Figs. 12 to 15); thus in 133 cases, Müller-Jensen and Allmaras (1968) found perforation in 65% (bilateral in over one-third) with retention of a glass fragment within the eye in 17% or in the orbit (Figs. 15 and 18); perforating injuries have been reported in 19 of 20 eyes (Rasmussen, 1966) and in 16 of 36 cases seen by Meyerratken (1967). It appears that horizontal perforating wounds of both corneæ with associated damage to the nasal root are characteristic of windscreen traumata: such was the situation in 5 out of 6 cases reported by Thorkilgaard (1966), in 8 cases by Friedrich (1968) (Fig. 16), and in 34% of the large series reported by Müller-Jensen and Allmaras (1968), who also found severe injuries to the lids in 95% of their patients. Luxation of the globe is a rare event (Remler and Hadlund, 1970). In all such injuries the outlook for vision is poor since to the effect of concussion on the globe is added the damage resulting from penetration and laceration of the ocular tissues and the not unusual retention of a glass fragment within the eye, while in those eyes predisposed to retinal detachment this may follow at any time after the injury. An unusual complication was the development of diplopia in a case described by Surugue (1968) wherein a piece of glass almost completely transected the superior oblique muscle.

[1] Detailed accounts of eyes damaged in this way have been made by Holland (1967), 75 cases; Tanaka and Akiyama (1967), 36 cases; Junghannss (1967), 47 cases; Müller-Jensen and Allmaras (1968), 133 cases; Hollwich and Huismans (1969); Ivendíc (1969); and others.

[2] Junghannss (1967), Holland (1967), Pouliquen and Defoug (1969).

Injuries to the orbit are commonly found after road accidents; indeed, something like 50 to 60% of orbital fractures are caused in this way (Macdonald, 1964; Obear, 1967; and others).

Finally, mention may be made of the controversial condition of *whiplash injury*, in which various disturbances of accommodation and increased pupillary diameter leading to difficulty in reading and near vision, may be the result of hyperextension of the spine followed immediately by acute flexion such as may occur when a standing car is rammed from behind, in a frontal crash or with other causes of rapid deceleration (Billig, 1953; Wiesinger and Guerry, 1961). A temporary paralysis of the VIth nerve may also occur. In some cases these signs represent the effects of an injury to the cervical

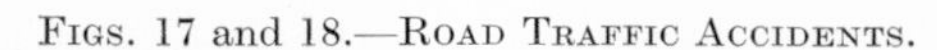

FIGS. 17 and 18.—ROAD TRAFFIC ACCIDENTS.

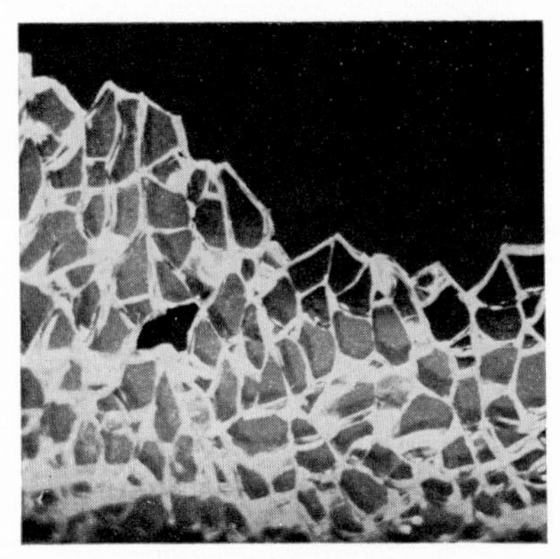

FIG. 17.—The shattered windscreen of safety glass (H. Friedrich).

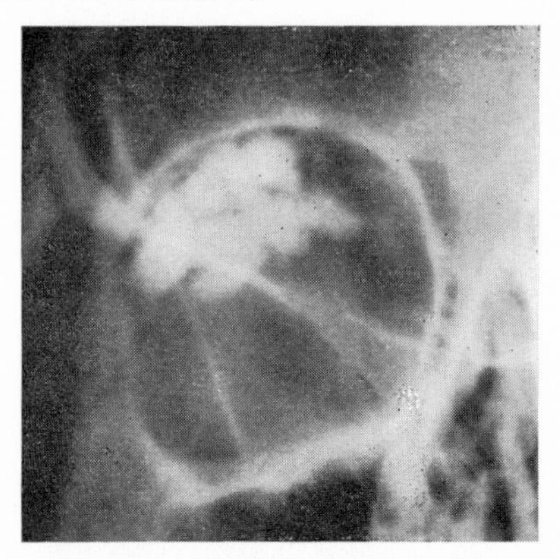

FIG. 18.—Particles of glass from a shattered windscreen in the orbit (K. Müller-Jensen and W. Allmaras).

sympathetic nerve leading to a Horner's syndrome, but in others the visual disturbance may well be a manifestation of the post-concussional syndrome or of a post-traumatic neurosis.

The hazards to the eye and vision associated with high-speed flight and underwater exploration will be considered at a later stage in this Volume.

Injuries sustained in *sport* are usually in the nature of a severe contusion of the globe from the impact of a blunt object—a ball, club, stick or racquet, the fist or the foot—to which may be added lacerations of the soft tissues and occasionally fractures of the orbit. Such accidents are relatively common in football, rugby, cricket, hockey, baseball, tennis, squash, lacrosse, golf and so on (Boshoff and Jokl, 1948; Favory and Sédan, 1951). The various activities of winter sports provide a number of similar and sometimes serious injuries with the additional hazard of ultra-violet injury to the cornea if protective glasses are not worn (81 cases in 10 years—Heider, 1967). Although injury to the eye is relatively rare compared with the number of broken bones sustained in skiing accidents, nevertheless such injuries usually caused by ski sticks tend to be severe. Thus in addition to perforating corneo-scleral wounds and contusion injuries and the later hazard of retinal detachment, Durand and Sourdille (1967) have seen avulsion of the intact eye following tearing of the optic nerve by a ski stick.

General reviews of the frequency of sporting injuries can be found in the papers of Kaplan (1961), ocular injuries in 3% of 20,000 sporting accidents; Sunada (1967), 842 cases, eye injuries in 63 (7·5%); Burstein (1963); Frey (1969), and others.

Ocular injuries from *boxing* have caused concern to a number of ophthalmic surgeons, for it is to be remembered that visual disability in boxers may result not only from contusion of the globe and injuries to the extra-ocular tissues but also from lesions of the visual pathway and other parts of the brain, the effects of which may be delayed in onset and are probably due to numerous repeated blows about the head resulting in a traumatic encephalopathy.[1] Damage to the eyelids or brows is a commonplace in boxing and many a contest has been terminated by hæmorrhage from a lacerated lid; severance of the lacrimal canaliculi has also occurred (Stallard, 1951). Diplopia resulting from injury to the extra-ocular muscles, especially the superior oblique when the trochlea has been damaged or displaced, or to the bony orbit, or the more common and less obvious muscular imbalance may present considerable problems for the boxer and may even lead to premature retirement from the ring.[2] Subconjunctival hæmorrhages which may conceal a scleral rupture, corneal abrasions and stromal scarring, intra-ocular hæmorrhage, displacement of the lens and choroidal rupture can all follow a contusion of the globe—in fact, the whole range of contusion injuries may occur. But the most dreaded ocular complication of boxing is detachment of the retina, the prognosis in such cases being poor because of the associated ocular damage and the likelihood of recurrence; indeed, bilateral cases have occurred.[3] Because of the serious risk of retinal detachment it is probably unwise for myopes and others with prominent eyes to take up boxing.[4]

In *golf*, apart from the risk of contusion from a ball or the back-swing of a club, there is an additional hazard from the occasional rupture of the golf-ball with explosive projection into the eye of material from the central filling. Such an event was described by Johnson and Zimmerman (1965) in which two children succeeded in cutting into a golf-ball which then exploded

[1] Carroll (1936), Winterstein (1937), Symonds (1941), Doggart (1951–55).

[2] In a lighter vein can be mentioned the case recalled by Whiting (1951) of the boxer Bill Softly who certainly was handicapped by double vision: " Yes," he said. " I see two chaps in the ring and I hit the one that isn't there and the one that is there hits me ".

[3] A case in which retinal detachment occurred during the course of a fight is described by Venco *et al.* (1966).

[4] Albaugh (1952), Löhlein (1954), Glees (1954), Alajmo (1957), Paul (1966), Venco *et al.* (1966).

and crystalline material composed of barium sulphate and zinc sulphide was subsequently found in the eyelid, conjunctival sac and orbital tissues; other similar cases have occurred, some with more serious consequences mainly due to the explosive nature of the injury (Penner, 1966; Millar, 1967; Slusher *et al.*, 1967; Taylor and Greer, 1969; Nelson, 1970).

Injuries to the eye among *fishermen* are rare but penetrating wounds with all their potential complications have occurred as a result of the engagement of a fish-hook in the cornea (Lugli and Vallavanti, 1967) and from the breakage of spectacles caused by the impact of lead weights (Keeney, 1960, 4 cases). An extraordinary case was described by Tanton and Elliott (1967) in which a fishing spear traversed the orbit, inferior orbital fissure and petrous temporal bone; complete recovery resulted.

Swimming also has its own peculiar hazards including the breakage of under-water goggles (Fig. 11): in 4 cases reported by Mitchell (1962) an extremely painful and indolent corneal lesion resulted from the sting of a jelly fish (*Cyanea annaskala*).

In this category should be included injuries from *sporting guns* and small arms—a not unusual occurrence. The injury from pellets of small shot varies considerably with the force with which they strike; if the marksman is far away and the impact light they remain in the skin of the lids or lie under the conjunctiva or imbed themselves in the sclera, doing little harm; severe contusions may lead to considerable intra-ocular damage (hyphæma, mydriasis, traumatic cataract, rupture of the choroid or detachment of the retina), while penetration of the globe, a through-and-through wound (Kutschera and Kosmath, 1968—16 cases) or injury to the brain may occur. Such injuries may occasionally be the result of a badly locked breech which discharges into the eye of the victim unhappily (accidentally or with suicidal intent) looking down the barrel at the moment the trigger goes off (Viallefont *et al.*, 1967—7 cases). Since the shot is aseptic the damage is usually limited to mechanical effects (Ovio, 1895; Tornatola, 1896) but binocular incapacity or blindness may result. Air-gun injuries are usually penetrating in type and frequently disastrous (Fig. 618), while the effects of bullet wounds are comparable to those incurred in war.[1]

Although hardly a form of sporting activity (except to a few individuals) and perhaps more correctly considered under the heading of domestic injuries, it is convenient to conclude this section with a note on the ocular hazards associated with *drinking*. The explosions of bottles containing sparkling drinks may have disastrous consequences, as Leydhecker (1963) found in 17 cases, 14 of which sustained perforating wounds, 2 eyes being lost; while the impact of a champagne cork may inflict a severe concussion, such as occurred in 9 cases reported by Tiburtius (1962), 4 of which developed traumatic cataract with a subsequent retinal detachment in 2 cases, whereas in the 9 cases described by Archer and Galloway (1967) the eyes returned to normal with the exception of the development in two cases of residual changes in the angle of the anterior chamber.

[1] p. 49.

Alajmo. *Arch. Ottal.*, **61**, 73 (1957).
Albaugh. *J. int. Coll. Surg.*, **17**, 191 (1952).
Archer and Galloway. *Lancet*, **2**, 487 (1967).
Billig. *J. int. Coll. Surg.*, **20**, 558 (1953).
Boshoff and Jokl. *Arch. Ophthal.*, **39**, 643 (1948).
Braunstein. *J. Amer. med. Ass.*, **163**, 249 (1957).
Burstein. *J. sport. Med.*, **3**, 25 (1963).
Carroll. *Amer. J. med. Sci.*, **191**, 706 (1936).
Doggart. *Trans. ophthal. Soc. U.K.*, **71**, 53 (1951).
Arch. Ophthal., **54**, 161 (1955).
Durand and Sourdille. *J. Méd. Lyon*, **48**, 1773 (1967).
Favory and Sédan. *Arch. Ophtal.*, **11**, 429 (1951).
Frey. *Proc. roy. Soc. Med.*, **62**, 917 (1969).
Friedrich. *Klin. Mbl. Augenheilk.*, **153**, 798 (1968).
Glees. *Klin. Mbl. Augenheilk.*, **124**, 101 (1954).
Halbron and Vignaud. *Bull. Soc. Ophtal. Fr.*, **69**, 517 (1969).
Heider. *Öst. ophthal. Ges.*, **9**, 187 (1967).
Holland. *Klin. Mbl. Augenheilk.*, **151**, 415 (1967).
Hollwich and Huismans. *Klin. Mbl. Augenheilk.*, **155**, 877 (1969).
Ivendíc. *Klin. Mbl. Augenheilk.*, **155**, 863 (1969).
Johnson and Zimmerman. *Amer. J. clin. Path.*, **44**, 533 (1965).
Junghannss. *Med. Mschr.*, **21**, 325 (1967).
Kaplan. *Vestn. oftal.*, No. 4, 51 (1961).
Keeney. *Surv. Ophthal.*, **5**, 405 (1960).
Industrial and Traumatic Ophthalmology (Symp. New Orleans Acad. Ophthal.), St. Louis, 51 (1964).
Kutschera and Kosmath. *Klin. Mbl. Augenheilk.*, **153**, 808 (1968).
Leydhecker. *Klin. Mbl. Augenheilk.*, **142**, 929 (1963).
Löhlein. *Klin. Mbl. Augenheilk.*, **124**, 570 (1954).
Lugli and Vallavanti. *Atti Soc. oftal. Lombarda*, **22**, 365 (1967).
Macdonald. *Industrial and Traumatic Ophthalmology* (Symp. New Orleans Acad. Ophthal.), St. Louis, 82 (1964).
Meyerratken. *Fortschr. Med.*, **85**, 979 (1967).
Millar. *Amer. J. Ophthal.*, **64**, 741 (1967).
Mitchell. *Med. J. Aust.*, **2**, 303 (1962).
Müller-Jensen and Allmaras. *Klin. Mbl. Augenheilk.*, **153**, 803 (1968).
Nahum. *Trans. Amer. Acad. Ophthal.*, **69**, 396 (1965).
Nelson. *Brit. J. Ophthal.*, **54**, 670 (1970).
Obear. *Proc. II int. Symp. plastic reconstr. Surg. Eye and Adnexa* (ed. Smith and Converse), St. Louis, 237 (1967).
Ovio. *Ann. Ottal.*, **24**, Supp., 14 (1895).
Paul. *Dtsch. Gesundh.-Wes.*, **21**, 2002 (1966).
Penner. *Arch. Ophthal.*, **75**, 68 (1966).
Pouliquen and Defoug. *Arch. Ophtal.*, **29**, 41 (1969).
Rasmussen. *Ugeskr. Laeg.*, **128**, 615 (1966).
Remler and Hadlund. *Eye, Ear, Nose, Thr. Monthly*, **49**, 129 (1970).
Slusher, Jaegers and Annesley. *Amer. J. Ophthal.*, **64**, 736 (1967).
Stallard. *Trans. ophthal. Soc. U.K.*, **71**, 58 (1951).
Sunada. *Folia ophthal. jap.*, **18**, 754 (1967).
Surugue. *Bull. Soc. Ophtal. Fr.*, **68**, 21 (1968).
Symonds. *Proc. roy. Soc. Med.*, **34**, 289 (1941).
Lancet, **1**, 1 (1962).
Tanton and Elliott. *Amer. J. Ophthal.*, **64**, 973 (1967).
Tanaka and Akiyama. *Folia ophthal. jap.*, **18**, 743 (1967).
Taylor and Greer. *Med. J. Aust.*, **1**, 632 (1969).
Thorkilgaard. *Ugeskr. Laeg.*, **128**, 617 (1966).
Tiburtius. *Klin. Mbl. Augenheilk.*, **141**, 602 (1962).
Tornatola. *Arch. Ottal.*, **3**, 350 (1896).
Venco, Rigamonti and Boschetti. *Minerva oftal.*, **8**, 161 (1966).
Viallefont, Boudet and Phillipot. *Bull. Soc. franç. Ophtal.*, **80**, 601 (1967).
Whiting. *Trans. ophthal. Soc. U.K.*, **71**, 57 (1951).
Wiesinger and Guerry. *Klin. Mbl. Augenheilk.*, **139**, 841 (1961).
Winterstein. *Lancet*, **2**, 719 (1937).

INJURIES IN AGRICULTURE

Although the comparative quietude of the life of the farmer, the gardener or the game-keeper might suggest a relative immunity from ocular trauma, such is by no means the case, and unfortunately many of the injuries sustained in rural surroundings result in serious visual loss, partly because of the gross nature of many of them, partly owing to the prevalence of superimposed infection, and partly because of the frequent difficulty in obtaining adequate and timely expert assistance (G. and R. Kunde, 1970).

In countries where the economy is predominantly agricultural rather than industrial, injuries sustained in the course of farming, husbandry, horticulture, lumbering and so on account for a high proportion of all accidents; thus, in Finland for the years 1955–57, 11·4% of all permanently damaging ocular injuries occurred amongst agricultural workers compared with an incidence of 9·9% of such injuries in constructional workers and 7·6% among industrial workers, and whereas in the last group perforating wounds and corneal foreign bodies were predominant, amongst agricultural workers contusion injuries were more common (19·8% of all such injuries, Forsius and Nikupaavo, 1964). The frequency with which even apparently slight corneal abrasions become infected and develop into hypopyon ulcers has often been remarked in agricultural and cattle zones (Perez Toril, 1949; Cerveira, 1950; and many others). Thus Garrow (1923) found that in all accidents of this type, enucleation was required in 14·2% of cases, and Smith (1940) that 14·8% lost the eye or perception of light, while a further 25% retained no useful vision—a very high proportion.[1]

The commonest typical accidents are abrasions or even perforation of the eye by thorns and twigs, occurring sometimes in walking and frequently in hedge-trimming and bush-cutting (Blake, 1969); the entry of straw or irritating chaff into the eye particularly while stacking or feeding threshing machines is also common. A different and more severe type of trauma is that sustained by a blow from an animal's head, horn or hoof, a swish from its tail, or an injury from a pitchfork or similar implement. Dust, lime-wash and chemical injuries from fertilizers provide their quota, while the ordinary pursuits of agricultural life are associated with the usual hazards from the sharp and blunt instruments that are encountered elsewhere. Abrasions and perforations which readily become infected and severe contusions are therefore the most formidable hazards.

Table VI gives statistics of the typical causes of agricultural accidents. Compilations in ophthalmological literature are found in the writings of Eschenauer (1903) (1,409 cases in Central Europe), Garrow (1923) (42 cases in Scotland), Smith (1940) (259 cases in Ireland), Blake (1969) (416 cases in Ireland) and G. and R. Kunde (1970) (101 cases in Germany).

The progressive mechanization of agricultural processes has added the hazards of the engineering industries to those typical of rural surroundings. The development, for instance, of the rotary lawn-mower has created a source of ocular injury among gardeners and workers on estates. Small objects such as stones, nails and sometimes metallic fragments from the blades, which revolve at something like 3,000 to 4,000 r.p.m., may be thrown up into the eyes of the operator with a velocity of approximately 300 feet per second, thereby causing considerable damage through contusion or penetration of the globe (White, 1957). Among 200 cases of traumatic hyphæma, Ferguson and Poole (1968) found that in 19% the injury was caused in this way, and

[1] For an analysis of fatal and non-fatal industrial diseases and accidents in agriculture in Great Britain for the years 1966 and 1967, see *The Report on Safety, Health and Welfare in Agriculture*, H.M.S.O., London, 1968.

in 99 cases of injury resulting from rotary mowers the eyes were involved in 10% (Kenny and Everding, 1966). Reports of penetrating wounds in such cases have been made by Barsky (1960), Fenton (1965) and others, while damage to the feet and hands from amputations or lacerations by the blades, or injuries due to the impact of high-velocity missiles elsewhere in the body, have been described by Butterworth (1957) and White (1957).

Finally the tremendous increase in the horticultural application of chemicals as pesticides, weed-killers and growth-regulators has resulted in a number of accidents and cases of industrial disease; indeed, fatalities have occurred. In such cases the eyes may be damaged either through direct local contamination with the chemical in the form of aerosols, liquids[1] or powders, or indirectly by the toxic effects on the visual apparatus of these substances absorbed systemically via the skin, lungs or alimentary tract.

TABLE VI

CAUSES OF AGRICULTURAL ACCIDENTS

England* (1922) (238 cases)	%	Ireland (Smith, 1940, 259 cases)	%
Hedge cutting, etc.	20·0	Twigs, thorns, sticks, etc.	66·8
Blows from animals	6·3	Blows from animals	9·2
Working with straw, etc.	4·6	Tools, machinery	8·8
Whitewashing, chemicals, etc.	3·8	Stones	3·8
Chopping wood	3·0	Fertilizers, chemicals, etc.	2·3
Threshing	2·5	Lime	1·9
Miscellaneous	59·8	Miscellaneous	7·2

Smith (1940) found the end-result in 250 cases to be: loss of the eye or of perception of light, 14·8%; vision less than 6/60, 24·8%; 6/60 to 6/18, 25·2%; 6/12 or better, 35·2%. It will be seen that these injuries have a more than usually bad prognosis.

* Causes and Prevention of Blindness, *Min. of Health Department Comm. Rep.*, H.M.S.O., London, 1922.

Many insecticides are based on compounds of phosphorus such as cholinesterase inhibitors the ocular toxic manifestations of which may include conjunctival hyperæmia, twitching of the lids, ptosis, constriction of the pupil and blurred vision. The whole question of the toxicology of these substances and related matters such as treatment and measures for the protection of those concerned in their manufacture and use in the field will be considered at a later stage in this Volume.[2]

In passing, mention may be made of an ocular inflammation which has been observed among workers in rice fields. Such cases have been attributed to the use of Blasticidin powder to suppress disease among the plants (Ojima, 1964); this substance sprayed into the eyes of rabbits has produced a severe pseudo-membranous conjunctivitis and a keratitis.[3] Rice threshing with sticks may lead to corneal injury through paddy grains being thrown up into the eyes, the resulting corneal abrasion usually showing multiple spiky hairs projecting from the lesion (Joseph, 1968; 277 cases), a

[1] A case in which severe conjunctival damage with a tendency to the formation of symblepharon followed a splash of weed-killer containing Paraquat and Diquat was recorded by Cant and Lewis (1968), and another wherein a corneal opacity occurred by Joyce (1969).

[2] Chapter XIII.

[3] p. 1194.

condition in some respects resembling that known as ophthalmia nodosa caused by the hairs of certain caterpillars (Watson and Sevel, 1966).

Barsky. *Arch. Ophthal.*, **64**, 385 (1960).
Blake. *Proc. III Cong. europ. Soc. Ophthal.*, Amsterdam, 125 (1969).
Butterworth. *Amer. Surgeon*, **23**, 815 (1957).
Cant and Lewis. *Brit. med. J.*, **2**, 224 (1968).
Cerveira. *Bol. Liga port. Profil. Ceg.*, **1**, 245 (1950).
Eschenauer. *Ueber die Unfallverletzungen d. Auges im landwirtschaftlichen Betriebe* (Diss.), Giessen (1903).
Ferguson and Poole. *Trans. ophthal. Soc. N.Z.*, **20**, 54 (1968).
Fenton. *Amer. J. Ophthal.*, **59**, 312 (1965).
Forsius and Nikupaavo. *Ann. occup. Hyg.*, **7**, 373 (1964).
Garrow. *Brit. J. Ophthal.*, **7**, 65 (1923).
Joseph. *Brit. J. Ophthal.*, **52**, 191 (1968).
Joyce. *Brit. J. Ophthal.*, **53**, 688 (1969).
Kenny and Everding. *Med. J. Aust.*, **2**, 547 (1966).
Kunde, G. and R. *Klin. Mbl. Augenheilk.*, **157**, 39 (1970).
Ojima. *Rinsho Ganka*, **18**, 813 (1964).
Perez Toril. *Arch. Soc. oftal. hisp.-amer.*, **9**, 534 (1949).
Smith. *Trans. ophthal. Soc. U.K.*, **60**, 252 (1940).
Watson and Sevel. *Brit. J. Ophthal.*, **50**, 209 (1966).
White. *Amer. J. Surg.*, **93**, 674 (1957).

INDUSTRIAL HAZARDS

The immense number of ocular hazards which occur in industry, their toll in human suffering, wasted time and monetary loss, and the realization that most of them are preventable, have focused attention particularly on this type of injury. Of necessity such accidents were known from the earliest times and reference was made to them in papyri and classical writings. The father of Demosthenes, for example, was an armourer who suffered from chronic blepharitis owing to the heat of his forge; not wishing his son to be similarly afflicted, he took him from the forge and sent him to practice rhetoric.[1] Fear of an industrial hazard thus provided Greece with her greatest orator. Such references, however, as the description by Paracelsus[2] of the ocular damage associated with work in mines and at furnaces, were scanty,[3] and it was not until the work of Ramazzini (1700) of Modena (Fig. 1) that the widespread intricacies of the subject were correlated and its importance adequately stressed. At the beginning of this chapter we have already pointed out that his attention was initially drawn to these problems by noticing inflammation of the eyes of workmen clearing the sewers of his native town and learning that many of them eventually lost their sight and became beggars, and from this starting point his researches and observations covered the entire field of industrial activity known at that time. For the first time in history this " Father of Industrial Medicine " correlated the subject in his classical book, *De morbis artificum diatriba* (1700), which immediately attracted much attention; the title page of the first edition is reproduced in Fig. 19.

Although started so early under auspices so good, it must be said that the science and particularly the practical applications of industrial medicine —and industrial ophthalmology—progressed very slowly. But as the industrial revolution spread throughout the world from its starting-point in England, as the speed of machines and consequently their danger increased, and particularly within more recent times as the ramifications of the chemical

[1] Juvenal, *Sat.*, x, 130.
[2] *Opera omnia, medico-chemico-chirurgica*, Genevae, 1658.
[3] Non-ocular industrial diseases also received little mention in the old literature—poisoning by lead (Hippocrates), mercuric sulphide (Pliny the Elder) or the " ulceration of the lungs " among miners of the Carpathian mountains, whose wives married as many as seven successive husbands, each of whom succumbed in turn to the disease (Agricola, *De re metallica*).

industries expanded to provide a bewildering and ever-increasing array of toxic hazards, interest has quickened so that today the subject is served by a considerable periodical literature, is fostered by active societies in most industrialized countries, supervised by governmental legislation in many, and is sustained by the International Labour Office. In Great Britain, the first legislation of this type was passed in 1891–95 when the Factories Acts laid down safety regulations for the bottling of aerated waters, and today the

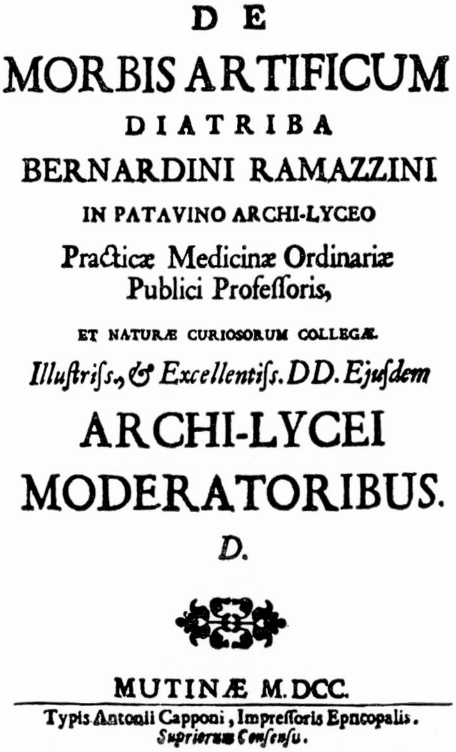

D E

MORBIS ARTIFICUM

DIATRIBA

BERNARDINI RAMAZZINI

IN PATAVINO ARCHI-LYCEO

Practicæ Medicinæ Ordinariæ
Publici Professoris,

ET NATURÆ CURIOSORUM COLLEGÆ.

Illustriss., & Excellentiss. DD. Ejusdem

ARCHI-LYCEI

MODERATORIBUS.

D.

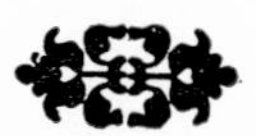

MUTINÆ M.DCC.

Typis Antonii Capponi, Impressoris Episcopalis.
Superiorum Consensu.

FIG. 19.—THE TITLE PAGE OF THE FIRST EDITION OF RAMAZZINI'S *De morbis artificum diatriba* (1700).

dangers are (theoretically) controlled by the immense powers of the Factories Acts of 1937 and the situation is watched by a staff of Factory Inspectors. In the United States with its millions of workers, the hazards of industry have also excited much interest and the situation is closely controlled. A considerable literature has now accumulated on the subject.[1]

[1] The most important works of the previous century are those of White Cooper (1859), Lawson (1867), Arlt (1875), Yvert (1880), Bergmeister (1880) and Praun (1899), and of the present century those of Ramsay (1907), Beaumont (1907), Oblath (1917), Resnick and Carris (1924), Würdemann (1932), Stassen (1933), Langelez (1936), Junius (1937), Coutela (1939), Resnick (1941), W. B. Clark (1943), C. P. Clark (1944), Sherman (1944), Kuhn (1944–50), Tisher (1945), and Hunter (1969).

The Incidence of Industrial Injuries

The general incidence of industrial injuries varies greatly with the industrial development of the region involved; their occurrence, therefore, differs widely in different countries and in most tends to increase with time. Elschnig (1925) of Prague found that 8·53% of all ocular conditions treated in his clinic from 1907 to 1924 were of industrial origin, Fuchs (1926) found 8% in Vienna, while Minton (1949) found that occupational eye injuries and diseases (7,000 cases) accounted for 30% of all acute ocular cases attending a typical London hospital. In more highly industrialized cities this proportion is higher: thus, in the steel centre of Sheffield injuries accounted for

TABLE VII

ANALYSIS OF 1099 INDUSTRIAL OCULAR INJURIES
(Kaufmann, 1956)

NATURE OF INJURY		NUMBER OF CASES
EYELIDS	Burns	3
	Lacerations	4
	Subtarsal Foreign Bodies	15
CONJUNCTIVA	Foreign Bodies	13
	Hæmorrhages	6
	Lacerations	14
	Acute Conjunctivitis	25
	Ultra-violet Conjunctivitis	9
CORNEA	Foreign Bodies	839
	Burns	25
	Chemical Injuries	17
	Abrasions	95
	Lacerations	4
SCLERA	Foreign Bodies	2
Ocular Contusions		4
Glass Foreign Bodies		11
Intra-ocular Foreign Bodies		6
Mechanical Irritation		44

52% of all eye cases (Cridland, 1929) and of 555 cases of intra-ocular foreign body in Birmingham 91% were fragments derived from the use of hammers or drills (Roper-Hall, 1954).[1] Considering traumata of all kinds to the eye in a mixed industrial community such as Glasgow, Garrow (1923) found that occupational injuries formed 70% of the total of all types of accident involving the eyes.

In general, however, the figures of the last 20 years have shown that injuries to the eyes account for something like 3 to 5% of all accidental occupational injuries with a higher proportion in the more industrial communities; thus, in Sweden they constituted 10% (von Bahr, 1946), in France 18% (Laignier and Dubreule, 1957) and in Switzerland 18·5% of all insured cases, mostly corneal foreign bodies (Zollinger, quoted by Forsius and Nikupaavo, 1964). In Germany between 1950 and 1963, of 2,309

[1] Of course, not all hammering accidents occur at work but the vast majority certainly does arise in this way.

injuries admitted to Kiel University Eye Clinic 53·5% were due to occupational hazards (Holland, 1965); on the other hand in Finland ocular injuries accounted for about 3·2% of all industrial accidents, the majority of serious cases being in agricultural workers (Forsius and Nikupaavo, 1964).

In the United States of America it has been computed that more than 300,000 ocular accidents necessitating cessation of work for one day or more occur annually—that is, one accident every 30 seconds of the working day (Resnick, 1941). In 1950 such injuries were reported to represent 2·9% of all occupational accidental injuries, whereas in 1958 this figure had risen to 5% (Kuhn, 1950; Mattos, 1958).

In Great Britain government statistics for 1950 showed that in factories during that year 9,366 ocular accidents occurred which disabled the workman for more than three days, representing 5% of all industrial accidents, the majority being due to flying particles. In 1966 a total of 296,610 industrial

TABLE VIII

TRADE INCIDENCE OF INDUSTRIAL OCULAR ACCIDENTS IN 1966
(From the Report of H.M. Inspector of Factories for 1966, H.M.S.O. 1967)

TRADE	NUMBER OF OCULAR INJURIES	FOREIGN BODIES	BURNS
Food, Drink and Tobacco	345	146	65
Chemicals	522	206	197
Metal Extraction and Processing	1,478	836	314
Engineering (heavy and light)	2,429	1,564	288
Motor Vehicles (manufacture and repair)	1,246	813	129
Nuts, Bolts, Screws, Wire, Cutlery, etc.	715	416	102
Textiles	277	103	47
Leather	28	10	9
Clothing and Shoe Manufacture	73	38	8
Building Materials, Pottery, Glass	379	215	47
Timber and Furniture	204	106	8
Paper and Printing	206	88	26
Rubber, Plastics and Toys	235	133	34
Construction and Building	1,599	1,007	92
Miscellaneous Services	368	199	37
Unspecified	331	168	50

accidents of all types were reported to the Factory Inspectorate, of which 10,824 (about 3·7%) involved the eyes; of these foreign bodies accounted for 6,250 cases, and burns due to chemicals or molten metal occurred in 1,474.[1] In assessing these figures it is to be remembered that by no means all industrial injuries find their way to hospitals, the great majority of trivial injuries being dealt with on the spot by the medical and nursing staff in the factories.[2]

The trade-distribution of industrial accidents varies with the activities of the community studied; indeed, no industry is entirely immune from ocular hazards, but in general they fall into five main groups (Tables VII to IX).

(1) ENGINEERING WORKERS liable to injury with cold metal, notably iron

[1] Figures taken from the reports of H.M. Inspector of Factories, H.M.S.O., London, 1967.

[2] Amongst many important regulations, the Factories Act 1961 states that " accidents causing loss of life or disabling a worker for more than three days from earning full wages at the work at which he was employed must be reported to the District Inspector and entered on his register ".

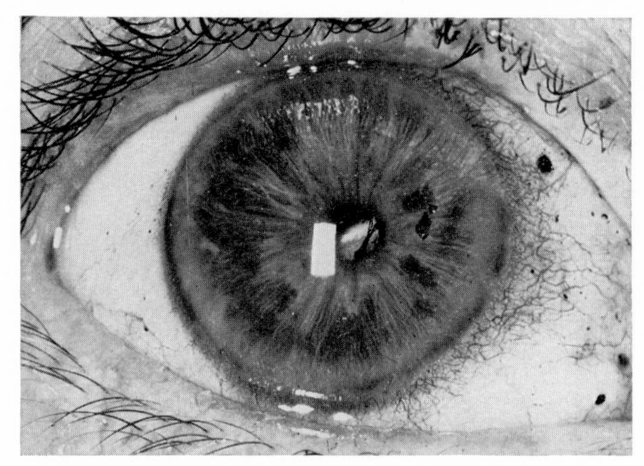

Fig. 20.—Multiple Superficial Foreign Bodies.
Many small metallic foreign bodies are embedded in the cornea and conjunctiva (Inst. Ophthal.).

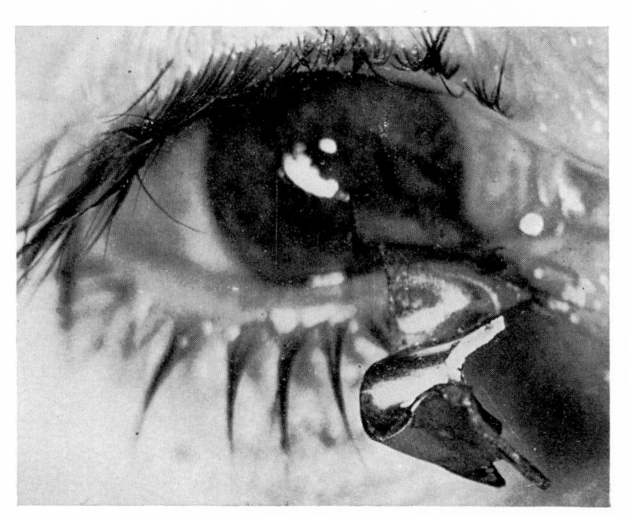

Fig. 21.—A Perforating Injury due to a Metal Swarf.
Sustained in machine-turning (Inst. Ophthal.).

and steel, are the commonest sufferers—steel and iron dressers and turners, drillers, platers, riveters and blacksmiths such as are found in the engineering, machine and tool-making, ship-building and kindred trades. The most frequent agents—as well as the most dangerous—are small chips of flying metal producing an infected abrasion or a perforating wound, while larger pieces of metal cause contusions which produce a varying degree of intra-ocular damage, and laceration and penetration of the cornea frequently result from the sharp end of metal wire springing up into the eye (Figs. 20–21). Corneal foreign bodies are by far the most common of all such industrial injuries; thus during the years 1912–26, 4,865 corneal foreign bodies were removed at the Helsinki University Eye Clinic (Werner, 1933) and between 1951 and 1960 at the same clinic the number had risen to 12,060, of which 71% were occupational in origin, mostly in those engaged in metal working (Forsius and Nikupaavo, 1964). This type of injury, indeed, constitutes a proportion ranging from 25 to 80% of the total of all types of industrial injury to the eye. The opportunities for such accidents are innumerable and occur constantly in all branches of work, both in the lighter industries and in the heavy branches where armour plating and castings are made. Particularly exposed to such accidents are tool-grinders and those who use abrasive wheels and dress and chip castings and ingots. It has to be remembered, also, that the danger does not arise only from the metal worked on, but that splinters are continually sparking off the hammer-head, the chisel-head or the chisel-point, particularly if these tools are well worn or of poor quality (Figs. 454–5). The use of hand-tools giving rise to flying

TABLE IX

THE MAIN CAUSES OF BLINDNESS AND LOSS OF WORK IN 1,017 INDUSTRIAL INJURIES
(Adapted from Lambah, 1968)

CAUSES OF INJURY	NO. OF CASES	PENETRATING WOUNDS	NO. OF EYES BLINDED	% TOTAL BLINDED	WORKING DAYS LOST
Hammering	140	87	36	23·3	3,303
Hot Metal	130	11	13	8·4	1,312
Construction and Decorating	85	1	1	0·1	976
Chemicals	52	4	2	1·3	648
Mining	60	8	4	2·6	690
Light Industry	125	72	30	20	2,616

particles was responsible for 44% of all compensatable eye injuries in Wisconsin in 1921 (Würdemann, 1932), for 91% of 555 cases of intra-ocular foreign body in Birmingham (Roper-Hall, 1954), for 24 of 47 consecutive cases of metallic intra-ocular foreign body in Manchester (Stevens, 1956), and in the industrial area of Wolverhampton 23% of all eyes blinded as a result of injury were due to this cause (Lambah, 1968).

(2) Workers liable to injury with MOLTEN METAL provide a less but considerable proportion of injuries in industrial communities; thus in Sheffield, Snell (1899) found that this type of trauma constituted 11·9% while metal splinters made up 48·1% of all ocular injuries; Garrow's (1923) corresponding figures from Glasgow are 8·3% and 26%; in 1950 an average of one ocular accident with molten metal occurred every day throughout the year in the factories of England. At the Birmingham and Midland Eye Hospital between 1962 and 1964, 46 cases of thermal injuries required admission, of which 17 were due to hot metal. The splashing of molten metal produces a burn of the lids, conjunctiva or cornea, which in the slighter cases leads to an erosion but may well result in corneal opacification or even necrosis, conjunctival scarring and the formation of symblepharon (Fig. 22). Among such

workers, also, a different type of injury may be caused by the radiant heat of molten metal, producing typically a radiational cataract.

(3) MINERS AND QUARRYMEN constitute a third class with a high incidence of ocular injuries, particularly coal miners in whom a chip of coal or a " spark " from the pick readily causes an abrasion which frequently becomes virulently infected, while a large piece of coal may cause a mutilating contusion; here also explosions account for accidents frequently of a more dramatic type. In Great Britain between 1920 and 1933 the incidence of accidents involving the eyes in mines, necessitating absence from work for

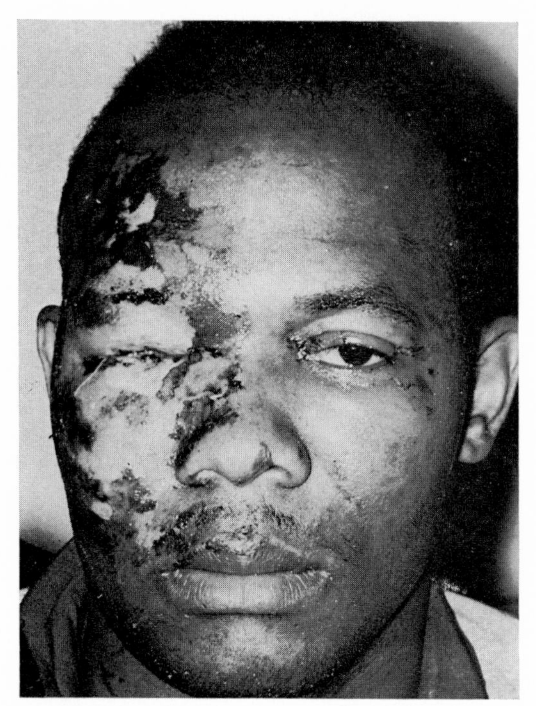

FIG. 22.—THE RESULTS OF A SPLASH OF MOLTEN METAL.

Showing the extensive heat burn over the face and eyelids caused by a splash with molten aluminium (Inst. Ophthal.).

more than seven days, rose from 3·71 to 5·73 per 1,000 persons employed, a rise perhaps coinciding with increasing mechanization, while in quarries raising igneous rocks the accident-rate in 1933 was as high as 8·9 per 1,000 workers (MacNalty, 1942). In this country in 1950 mining produced more ocular accidents of sufficient severity to require official notification than all other industries added together (11,058 out of a total 20,424 notified accidents), but since the recent decline in the importance of the coal industry and the closure of many pits the number of such injuries has considerably decreased.

(4) While these three categories make up the great mass of the total of industrial accidents, it is to be remembered that the increasing ramifications of the CHEMICAL INDUSTRY are responsible for a steadily growing number of toxic hazards; the implications of most of these are disabling and some are serious and permanent. The number of such poisons is legion and increases each year as new chemical or pharmaceutical processes are evolved. Their action includes direct chemical irritation of the cornea, conjunctiva and lids by vapour, droplets or dust, splashes of vesicant or corrosive material into the eye, or absorption through the lungs or skin through continuous handling which may lead to optic neuritis and visual failure.[1]

In the chemical industry the general accident-rate is low, but the ocular hazard and in particular the incidence of chemical burns are greater than in most other occupations. In the majority of cases these injuries are treated entirely in the medical departments of the works and only a very few lose working time; of 1,163 industrial injuries, 129 were due to chemical splashes, of which 8 were serious (Whitehead, 1965), and in 1962 at the Birmingham and Midland Eye Hospital 203 cases of chemical burns were treated, only 10 of which required in-patient treatment (Roper-Hall, 1965).

(5) Finally a number of injuries may result from the effects of RADIATION, whether it be infra-red, ultra-violet or ionizing in type, or due to microwaves absorbed during the course of some industrial process or research (Cogan, 1950–58; Krokowski and Ehling, 1962; Newell, 1964; Merté, 1967; and others). Among steel-workers and others concerned with molten metal or in glass-workers, the radiant heat can produce a typical form of cataract but this is now very rare and largely a matter of historical interest.[2] The experience of a very painful kerato-conjunctivitis due to the action of ultra-violet radiation is well known to welders; between 1959 and 1961, 452 cases of "arc eye" involving absence from work for more than three days were reported in Great Britain, and probably many more of a minor nature occurred.[3] Ionizing radiation has numerous applications throughout industry; indeed, well over 300 have been listed (Packman, 1968), the more important being industrial radiography for the detection of flaws in metal and the integrity of welds, the measurement of weight and density, the elimination of static electricity, the sterilization of food and medical equipment, chemical processing and quality control, prospecting and various forms of chemical analysis, the luminizing of clocks and watches, and so on. A further risk

[1] Some examples of liquids known to have caused accidents to the eyes at work: hot sugar, caustic potash and caustic soda, hydrochloric acid and vitriol, soap solution, hot tar, dichlorphenol, formaldehyde, potassium cyanide, ammonia, paint-thinners and petrol. Such a variety of substances emphasizes the difficulty in providing simple and uniformly effective protective measures which should prevent the majority of ocular accidents resulting from liquid splashes.

[2] p. 878.

[3] For a detailed account of the safety aspects of arc-welding see Booklet No. 38, Dept. of Employment and Productivity, H.M.S.O., London, 1968.

arises from the problems associated with the disposal of radio-active waste, but the whole subject is controlled by legislation and regulations exist concerning protective measures and the maximum permitted exposures. Microwaves have long been used in television, radar and telecommunications and their applications have now extended even into the field of cooking, sterilization and so on; changes in the lens thought to be due to the action of such radiation have been described in a number of workers in these fields (Kurz and Einaugler, 1968; and others).

High-intensity visible light, as in the case of the *laser* which is being used extensively in industry and research, represents another source of radiational injury to the eye and, indeed, ocular accidents from this cause have occurred either from direct exposure or as a result of reflection from smooth surfaces (Zweng, 1967; Geeraets and Berry, 1968; Curtin and Boyden, 1968).

The *cost of this holocaust* which goes on quietly and persistently year after year is, of course, appalling. The toll of human suffering and distress is great, the loss of efficiency and working time in a competitive industrial community is serious and the financial cost is hardly credible. Comparative figures of the position in different countries are of interest. In the United States some 300,000 reported accidental injuries to the eyes occur each year, corresponding to almost 1,000 for each working day, the loss in financial terms to society in general being of the order of at least 100,000,000 dollars or the equivalent of more than 53,000,000 working hours, not including the colossal cost of medical care, compensation and so on (Resnick, 1941; Mattos, 1958; and others). In Great Britain, as we have already seen, there occur each year over 10,000 registered ocular accidents in factories and elsewhere, the majority mechanical or chemical in origin, severe enough to disable the worker for more than three days, to which must be added a large number sustained in the operations of mining[1] and many more of a trivial nature that involve only short periods away from work. In 1953 official Government statistics showed the average number of days off work for 998 out of 1,048 cases was 16·5 days, whereas a period of up to three months may be required if permanent visual loss has occurred; in general, however, in about 70% of ocular injuries recovery is complete within two weeks (Noro, 1953; and others). In Sweden in the decade up to 1946 the cost of eye injuries was reckoned at 2·25 million Swedish crowns annually (von Bahr, 1946), in Czechoslovakia a similar sum was estimated (König, 1962), while in Finland where agricultural injuries predominate something like 170,000 working days are lost each year from this cause alone (Forsius and Nikupaavo, 1964).

On the relative role of accidental injuries among the causes of blindness the following figures are of interest: in the United States between 1935 and 1936 almost 20% of all cases of uniocular blindness and 8% of all binocular blindness were caused by occupational injuries, in Finland in 1934 13·8% of

[1] 11,000 cases; Royal Commonwealth Society for the Blind, 1962.

unilateral and 2·5% of bilateral loss of sight were due to industrial accidents (Vannas, 1935), but by 1963 these figures had risen to 35% and 22·8% respectively (Vannas and Raivio, 1964). On the other hand, in the big industrial countries such as the U.S.A., Great Britain and Germany accidental injuries do not rank quite so high in the general causation of blindness. The statistics of bilateral blindness as set out in Table II show that most of these cases are caused by senile changes such as cataract and macular degeneration, myopic degeneration and the end-results of diabetes and vascular disease; trauma assumes significant proportions only in the young age-groups and mainly in men: it was responsible for 6·1% of all cases in males aged 15–29 years and for 3·1% aged 30–49 years between 1950–62. On the other hand, trauma is a leading cause of uniocular blindness (Sorsby, 1966)

TABLE X
UNILATERAL BLINDNESS DUE TO TRAUMA
(1955–60)
(A. Sorsby)

NUMBER OF EYES BLINDED BY TRAUMA	MALES 966	FEMALES 406
	% of all causes	
Occupational Activities	8·6	0·5
Household Activities	0·7	1·4
Play or Sport	3·8	2·2
Travel and Traffic	0·4	0·2
Military Operations	2·3	0·5
Sympathetic Ophthalmitis	2·0	2·0
Other Activities	7·4	3·7
	25·2	10·5
All Other Causes of Blindness	74·8	89·5
	100·0	100·0

(Table X). The real tragedy of these figures is that it is probable that with a modicum of reasonable care some 90% of these injuries are preventable.

The PREVENTION of industrial injuries is therefore a matter of first-class social significance, and although it is gradually forcing itself into public notice particularly in recent years, largely through the activities of voluntary societies in many countries, the efforts of medical officers of health and governmental inspection, the practical effect of this endeavour is strangely handicapped by the ignorance of the industrial community, the spirit of *laissez-faire* and the lure of short-term economy on the part of the employers, and carelessness and the tendency to take risks among employees; both parties forget that the eyes of the workman are the choicest of his working tools and the most deserving of care, even if the assessment is made at the lowest denominator—merely in terms of cash. A programme for such prevention must be comprehensive if it is to be adequate. It should include the preliminary screening of employees so that their visual and ocular motor capacity is suitable for their work and the correction of visual defects when necessary, the adequate illumination of the place of work so that the worker can see what he is doing, and the adequate design and painting of the workshop and the machines so that dangerous moving machinery stands out clearly. To this general background should be added immediate protection against particular hazards—the fitting of guards on machines from which flying particles are to be expected and the use of adequate goggles which are comfortable to wear and through which vision is easy for men exposed to this risk or to splashes of hot or corrosive material, the wearing of adequate protection, by goggles or otherwise, by those exposed to glare or radiant energy, the elimination of noxious fumes or dusts and protection against toxic hazards by suitably adapted exhaust ventilation, screens, masks and

FIGS. 23 and 24.—SAFETY GOGGLES.

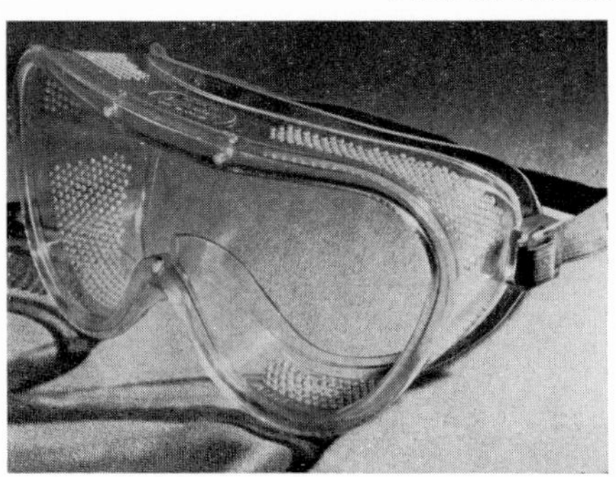

FIG. 23.

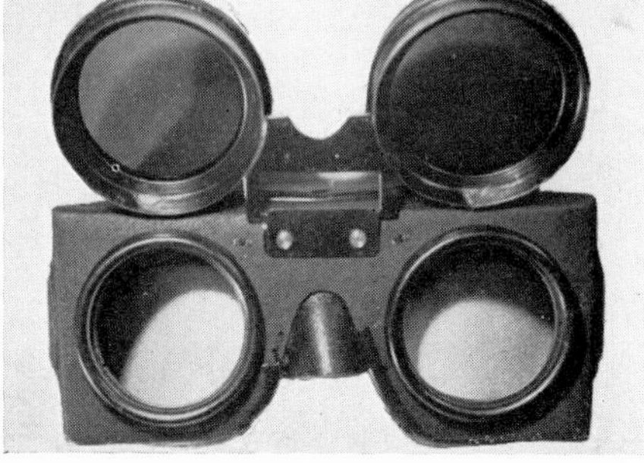

FIG. 24.

Fig. 23.—Vistamax safety goggles; they are light, well-ventilated and comfortable. Fig. 24.—Welders' goggles, made of fibre-cups carrying metal frames, glazed with clear glass. The protective filter glasses are carried in a second pair of frames hinged to the top of the goggles and can be raised when welding is not going on (H. C. Weston).

other protective devices (Figs. 23–4). In extreme cases in some chemical processes the protection of the entire body must be complete and that of the eye forms part of the over-all device (Figs. 25–6). The protection of employees with defective vision is particularly important (Hughes and Cooke, 1967). Finally, the seriousness of such accidents as may occur can be greatly diminished by the provision of adequate first aid by trained personnel in the workshop and early reference to a doctor or a hospital whenever such a course is indicated[1] (Fig. 27).

Several accounts in the literature demonstrate the value of well-organized schemes involving protective measures and discipline in the prevention of ocular injuries among industrial workers. Among these three examples of interest may be noted here: at a steel-works in Great Britain the management were concerned at the large and ever-increasing number of ocular accidents and the legal complications arising therefrom.

[1] Snell (1899), Resnick and Carris (1924), Heinrich (1931), Resnick (1941), Kuhn (1944), Ryan (1964), Whitehead (1965), and many others.

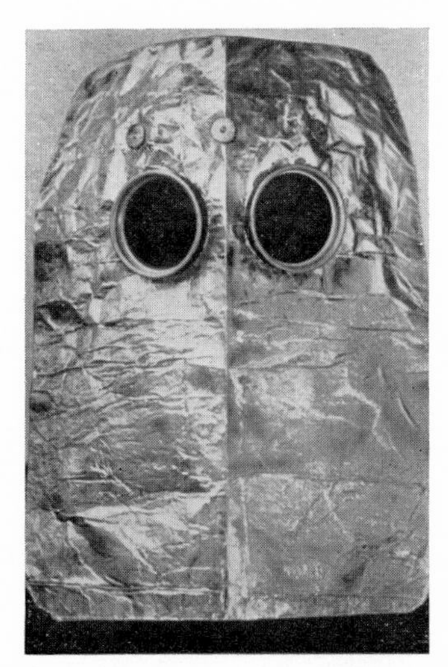

FIG. 25.—ALUMINIUM-FOIL FACE SHIELD GIVING PROTECTION FROM INFRA-RED RADIATION.

Made of asbestos, covered with aluminium-foil—a highly efficient reflector of radiant heat. The eye-pieces are fitted with heat-absorbing glass (H. C. Weston).

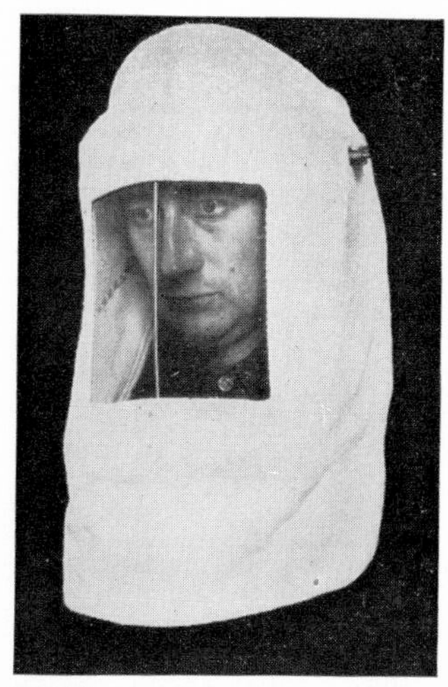

FIG. 26.—FACE-MASK GIVING PROTECTION FROM SPLASHES OF CORROSIVE LIQUIDS.

The mask is made of asbestos supported on an adjustable head-band. The window is of non-flame celluloid and the whole front can, if necessary, be raised from the supporting band (H. C. Weston).

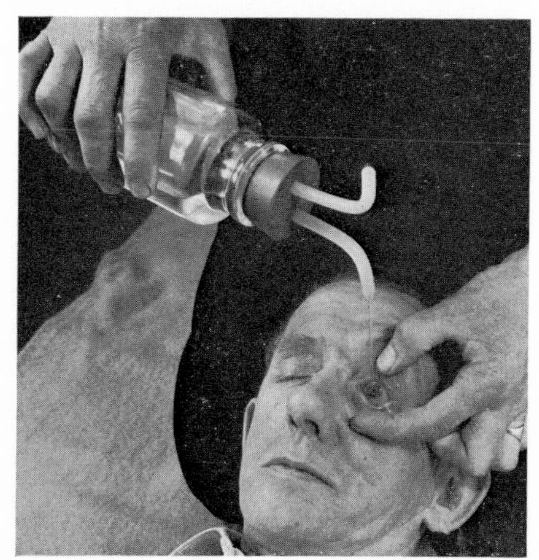

FIG. 27.—EMERGENCY TREATMENT FOR INDUSTRIAL CHEMICAL INJURIES.

The important immediate procedure is a thorough wash-out (Imperial Chemical Industries).

A scheme of wholesale ocular protection for all employees was instituted including the provision of some 8,000 pairs of goggles. In the succeeding three months only two reportable eye accidents occurred at this factory, one of which concerned an office-cleaner disposing of rubbish outside the building.[1] In the United States of America at the

[1] H.M. Inspector of Factories Report, H.M.S.O., London, 1953.

Sperry plant over a period of 10 years following the introduction of a comprehensive eye-care programme, no eyes were lost (Sager, 1956); and at the massive establishment of Kaiser Steel where in 1958 ocular injuries cost 48,622 dollars, injuries which had been at the rate of 149 per million man-hours of working time in 1959 dropped after the introduction of a similar eye-protection scheme to only 27 in 1962 (Tudor, 1963).

The question of protection of the eyes by goggles has always been difficult, for most are heavy and uncomfortable, restrict the visual field and frequently become steamed and misted, so that workmen tend to risk what they consider an unlikely hazard rather than endure their obvious disadvantages. The qualities required in goggles and other appliances to

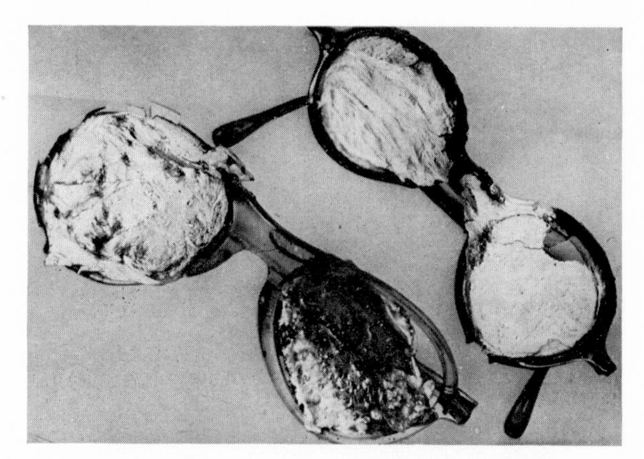

Fig. 28.—The Protection given by Goggles.

Although the lenses are destroyed the goggles are intact and have protected both eyes from an explosion incurred when pouring molten aluminium (H.M.S.O.).

ensure adequate ocular protection include resistance to the impact of high velocity missiles or molten metal and to the action of corrosive chemicals, and the ability to absorb various types of radiation such as ultra-violet, infra-red and intense visible light (Figs. 28–9). In addition, such appliances should be light in weight, comfortable in use, well ventilated to avoid misting, able to transmit sufficient light to permit comfortable vision and to be sufficiently strong to withstand the usual wear and tear. For many purposes simple (plano) spectacles offer adequate protection, and when flying particles travelling at a high velocity might splinter glass, shatter-proof lenses can be provided. These take three forms:

(1) *Case-hardened lenses* (whether plano or made to prescription) are prepared in the ordinary manner so that there is a minimum central thickness of 3 mm. The lens is then heated to 1330° F in an oven and rapidly cooled by an air-draught or oil-immersion. This temperature is just not sufficient to distort the glass, but yet adequate to anneal it so that when it is rapidly cooled the outer shell hardens more quickly than the inner mass. The resulting compression generated within the lens makes the outer layer crumble on an impact without the lens fracturing or breaking into pieces.

(2) *Reinforced* or *laminated glass* may be employed wherein two thin lenses have an inset of cellulose acetate between them to prevent splinters flying when they are shattered. It is to be remembered, however, that the cellulose tends to become discoloured after prolonged exposure to daylight, a change which cuts down visibility considerably after some time.

(3) *Plastic lenses*, which may be moulded into optical form, are both light and unbreakable by ordinary forces; their softness, however, allows ready scratching so that in industrial conditions they are rapidly perishable. This handicap, however, has been largely overcome by the use of a hard thermosetting resin, allyl diglycol carbonate, which compares well with glass in resistance to scratching and is, indeed, superior to it in resisting pitting (as when used at a grinding wheel or when welding or sand-blasting)

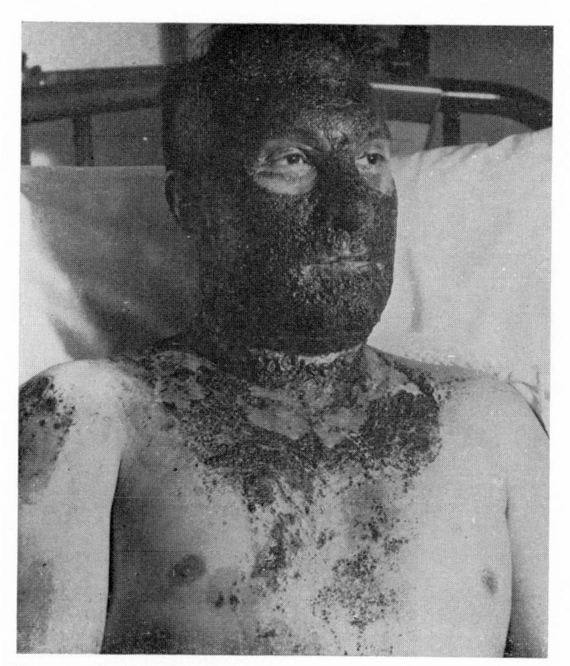

FIG. 29.—AN EXTENSIVE BURN FROM A SPLASH OF MOLTEN METAL.
The man was wearing protective goggles and the eyes are unscathed (R. Vaughan-Jones).

because of a difference in impact-resistance; it does not fog up so quickly as glass in changing temperatures since it warms up more rapidly. Such lenses can also be dyed to reduce their transmission of light and surface-coated to reduce annoying reflections (Nugent and Graham, 1950; Keeney, 1956).

Extensive research into this whole field has shown that the best material for the manufacture of goggles, visors and face-screens is a plastic substance known as " polycarbonate " BS2092/62, which can withstand the impact not only of molten metal but also of a quarter-inch-diameter steel ball moving at velocities of up to 500 feet per second; it is also non-inflammable. Unfortunately, plastic materials do not give protection against infra-red radiation whereas certain types of glass will do so; for use in circumstances where both types of protection are required goggles containing both polycarbonate and glass lenses have been developed, the plastic lens always being nearer the eye to prevent ocular damage should the glass lens be shattered. In the case of welders and others who may be exposed to high-intensity visible light or to infra-red or particularly ultra-violet radiation, goggles which reduce the radiation reaching the eye and at the same time protect against flying particles are available. Suitable filters for this purpose have been evolved.[1]

Arlt. *Ueber d. Verletzungen d. Auges*, Wien (1875).

von Bahr. *Acta ophthal.* (Kbh.), **24,** 217 (1946).

Beaumont. *Injuries of the Eyes*, London (1907).

Bergmeister. *Die Verletzungen d. Auges u. seiner Annexe*, Wien (1880).

Clark, C. P. *J. Amer. med. Ass.*, **124,** 157 (1944).

Clark, W. B. *Amer. J. Ophthal.*, **26,** 1054 (1943).

Cogan. *J. Amer. med. Ass.*, **142,** 145 (1950). *New Engl. J. Med.*, **259,** 517 (1958).

Cooper. *Wounds and Injuries of the Eye*, London (1859).

Coutela. *L'oeil et les maladies professionelles*, Paris (1939).

Cridland. *Brit. med. J.*, **2,** 615 (1929).

Curtin and Boyden. *Amer. J. Ophthal.*, **65,** 188 (1968).

Elschnig. *Münch. med. Wschr.*, **72,** 2219 (1925).

Forsius and Nikupaavo. *Ann. occup. Hyg.*, **7,** 373 (1964).

Fuchs. *Wien. med. Wschr.*, **76,** 307 (1926).

Garrow. *Brit. J. Ophthal.*, **7,** 65 (1923).

Geeraets and Berry. *Amer. J. Ophthal.*, **66,** 15 (1968).

Heinrich. *Industrial Accident Prevention*, N.Y. (1931).

Holland. *Klin. Mbl. Augenheilk*, **145,** 915 (1965).

Hughes and Cooke. *Brit. J. indust. Med.*, **24,** 240 (1967).

Hunter. *The Diseases of Occupations*, London (1969).

Junius. *Die entschädigungspflichtiger Berufskrank. d. Auges*, Stuttgart (1937).

Kaufmann. *Canad. med. Ass. J.*, **75,** 284 (1956).

Keeney. *Trans. Amer. ophthal. Soc.*, **54,** 521 (1956). *Surv. Ophthal.*, **5,** 405 (1960).

König. *Cs. oftal.*, **18,** 306 (1962).

Krokowski and Ehling. *Dtsch. med. Wschr.*, **87,** 2081 (1962).

Kuhn. *Industrial Ophthalmology*, St. Louis (1944). *Eyes and Industry*, St. Louis (1950).

Kurz and Einaugler. *Amer. J. Ophthal.*, **66,** 866 (1968).

Laignier and Dubreule. *J. Ophtal. soc.*, No. 21, 7 (1957).

Lambah. *Trans. ophthal. Soc. U.K.*, **88,** 661 (1968).

Langelez. *Les maladies professionelles*, Paris (1936).

Lawson. *Injuries of the Eye, Orbit and Eyelids*, London (1867).

MacNalty. *Brit. med. J.*, **1,** 173 (1942).

Mattos. *J. Ophtal. soc.*, No. 22, 7 (1958).

Merté. *Münch. med. Wschr.*, **109,** 501 (1967).

Minton. *Occupational Eye Diseases and Injuries*, London (1949).

Newell. *Industrial and Traumatic Ophthalmology* (Symp. New Orleans Acad. Ophthal.), St. Louis, 158 (1964).

Noro. *Duodecim* (Helsinki), **69,** 712 (1953).

Nugent and Graham. *Amer. J. Ophthal.*, **33,** 1763 (1950).

Oblath. *Le malattie professionali dell'occhio*, Rome (1917).

Packman. *A Guide to Industrial Safety and Health*, London (1968).

Praun. *Die Verletzungen d. Auges*, Wiesbaden (1899).

Ramsay. *Injuries of the Eye and their Treatment*, London (1907).

Resnick. *Eye Hazards in Industry*, N.Y. (1941).

Resnick and Carris. *Eye Hazards in Industrial Occupations*, N.Y. (1924).

Roper-Hall. *Brit. J. Ophthal.*, **38,** 65 (1954). *Trans. ophthal. Soc. U.K.*, **85,** 631 (1965).

Ryan. *Industrial and Traumatic Ophthalmology* (Symp. New Orleans Acad. Ophthal.), St. Louis, 131 (1964).

Sager. *Sight-sav. Rev.*, **26,** 27 (1956).

Sherman. *Arch. Ophthal.*, **32,** 33 (1944).

Snell. *On the Prevention of Eye Injuries occurring in Trades*, London (1899).

Sorsby. *Incidence and Causes of Blindness in England and Wales*, London (1966).

Stassen. *Les maladies professionelles*, Paris (1933).

Stevens. *Brit. J. Ophthal.*, **40,** 622 (1956).

Tisher. *Arch. Ophthal.*, **33,** 152 (1945).

Tudor. *Indust. Med. Surg.*, **32,** 478 (1963).

Vannas. *Duodecim* (Helsinki), **51,** 195 (1935).

Vannas and Raivio. *Acta ophthal.* (Kbh.), **42,** 307 (1964).

Werner. *Finska Läk.-Sällsk. Handl.*, **75,** 1125 (1933).

Whitehead. *Trans. ophthal. Soc. U.K.*, **85,** 617 (1965).

Würdemann. *Injuries of the Eye*, 2nd ed., London (1932).

Yvert. *Traité pratique et clinique des blessures du globe de l'oeil*, Paris (1880).

Zweng. *Arch. Ophthal.*, **78,** 596 (1967).

[1] British Standard No. 679, 1959; filters for use during welding and similar industrial operations. For a comprehensive review of this subject see Keeney (1956–60) and the report of the Joint Advisory Committee on Foundry Goggles, H.M.S.O. London (1964), and Electric Arc-Welding, H.M.S.O. London (1968).

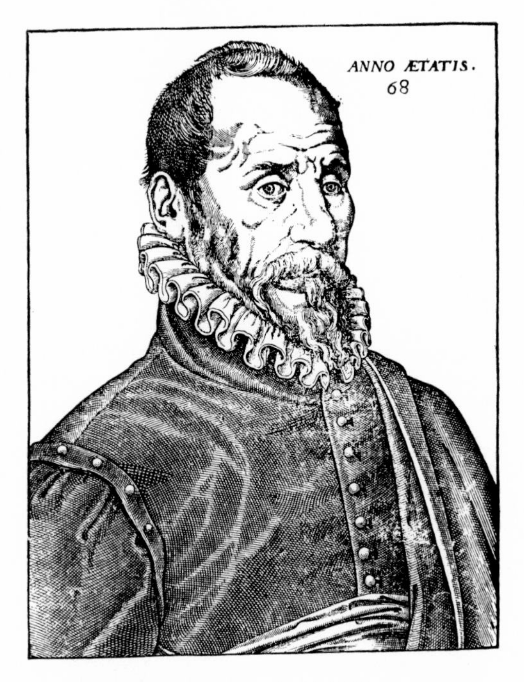

IN EFFIGIEM A. PARÆI.

Humanam AMBROSII *verè hæc pictura* PARÆI
Effigiem, ſed opus continet ἀμβροσίην.
IO. HEROALDVS.

FIG. 30.—AMBROISE PARÉ [1510–1590].
(From *Opera* . . ., Paris, 1582; courtesy of the Wellcome Trustees.)

WAR INJURIES

Ever since man evolved it would seem probable that he quarrelled and fought in his struggle for existence; it follows that such injuries must have been known throughout his long history. Certainly the records we have of the earliest surviving civilizations in the valleys of the Tigris and the Nile recorded them and Homer sang of them and annotated their treatment. The classical treatment of these wounds remained much as it was advocated in the Hippocratic writings: " diseases not curable by iron are curable by fire ", and the first dressing was boiling oil to drive out the " poison "—a somewhat savage and crude approach to antiseptic surgery. AMBROISE PARÉ [1510–1590] (Fig. 30) changed this; and this great French surgeon must be acknowledged as the first traumatic surgeon and the greatest exponent of surgery of his time.

The apprentice of a rustic barber, he went to Paris to become a dresser in the Hôtel Dieu (1529); thereafter he was constantly employed in wars, usually in the front of the field of battle. Beloved by the soldiers, he was carried in triumph by them through the streets of Metz and he was the only Protestant to be spared by royal mandate in the massacre of St. Bartholomew. Fortunately one day in battle his supply of boiling oil ran out so he discontinued it and, seeing the result, abandoned it to rely on aseptic methods of treatment in which the danger of flies in the spread of infection was stressed, sometimes supplemented by the soothing application of the fat of puppy-dogs, much to the soldiers' comfort: " I dressed him and God cured him ". The innovations he introduced into surgery are too numerous to mention, and were not by any means confined to military surgery: he invented a host of instruments, he employed ligatures for amputations, discarded since the time of Celsus, introduced massage, artificial limbs and eyes, made the first exarticulation of the elbow, described fractures of the neck of the femur, abolished castration and popularized the truss in hernia, described strangury from prostatic hypertrophy and was the first to draw attention to the occurrence of aneurysms in syphilis; all these and many more, in addition to practical and original contributions to obstetrics and dentistry. He performed the first judicial necropsy in France in 1562. A garrulous and prolific writer in the vernacular French instead of Latin, his greatest works were his treatise on gunshot wounds (*La manière de traieter les playes*, Paris, 1545) and his classical book on surgery (Paris, 1564), but others appeared from his pen such as a book on monsters (1573) and on mummies and the unicorn, disposing therein of ancient therapeutic superstitions (1582). Truly a great figure.

The injuries sustained in war are extremely varied in type and differ in succeeding wars as the techniques of combat change and man's ingenuity in bringing about his own and his fellows' destruction increases. Before the general use of explosives, ocular injuries were usually due to the gross effects of hand weapons, but as long-range fighting developed, bullets and shells assumed pride of place. Until comparatively recent times, however, few of the wounded survived the universal ravages of sepsis and the consequences of inadequate treatment.[1] By the time of the first World War the survival-rate reached more reasonable proportions but the unprecedented mass of men deployed resulted in an increase in the number of the injured, while the previous pattern of casualties was complicated by the increased concentration of machine-gun fire, the greater explosive power of artillery with its blast-effects, and the immense toll of injuries due to war-gases; in the second World War the extensive use of mines and tanks added considerably to the number of ocular casualties, the indiscriminate bombing of cities extended their incidence yet again over a much wider population, while towards its end the use of atomic bombs added an entirely new category to a total already sufficiently appalling. As the use of aircraft became more common, burns in flying personnel involving the face, and indirectly the eyes, increased proportionately. At the same time, with each successive war the progressive mechanization and motorization of the armies have resulted in an increase of injuries of the industrial type and those incurred in accidents with vehicles, until these have equalled or exceeded the casualties sustained in battle; thus while the incidence of ocular wounds in combat was approximately the same in the two World Wars in the armies of the United States, that of non-combat injuries to the eyes increased in the second approximately four-fold (from 0·5 to 2% of all non-combat injuries, Stone, 1950).

[1] Thus at the British Base Hospital of Scutari in the Crimean War (1854–56) the intake of patients over two months was 2,349 and the number who died was 2,315. Compare these dreadful figures with those at the beginning of the Korean War (1950): of 18,000 men admitted to an American Base Hospital, 40 died.

BATTLE CASUALTIES

The incidence of ocular battle casualties is high proportionately to other parts of the body. It is true that the eye presents an exposed area of 1/375 of the surface of the body, but it must be remembered that in open warfare in trenches or in tanks the head is apt to be preferentially exposed; moreover, the vulnerability of the eye to flying particles which would excite little or no attention elsewhere accounts for the undue preponderance of ocular casualties arising from this type of injury. The figures derived from the records of various wars are of interest but it is to be remembered that most of them are inaccurate, and as a rule they do not include fatal injuries, maxillo-facial wounds wherein the ocular injury was an incident in more widespread damage, and cranial injuries wherein visual defects, some of them gross and incapacitating, were incidental.

It may be said that direct ocular injuries constitute some 2 to 2·5% of all modern battle casualties, although in the British Liberation Army in north-west Europe in 1944 there were occasions when they rose to 3·8% and in the Korean War the number of ocular casualties reached the unprecedented proportion of 8·1% of all combat casualties (Lowrey and Shaffer, 1954). To the more usual figure of around 2·5% must be added the involvement of the eyes and their adnexa in approximately one-third of maxillo-facial wounds (6% of all battle casualties, Stone, 1950), while the visual apparatus is seriously implicated in a large proportion of all head-injuries involving the skull and brain (Calvert, 1947). Towards the end of the war of 1914–18 ophthalmic injuries were grouped with neurosurgical and maxillo-facial injuries and this arrangement, which came to be known as "the Trinity", worked well in the war of 1939–45, the combined injuries amounting to about 10% of the whole[1].

The following figures have been reported (Reich, 1879; Oguchi, 1912; Gombos, 1969; Treister, 1969 and official sources):

Crimean War (English) (1854–56) ocular casualties		0·65%	of all casualties
American Civil War (1861–65) ocular casualties		0·57%	,, ,,
Franco-Prussian War (1870–71) ocular casualties—			
German		0·86%	,, ,,
French		0·81%	,, ,,
Russo-Turkish War (1877–78) ocular casualties		2·5%	,, ,,
Sino-Jap War (1894) ocular casualties		1·2%	,, ,,
Russo-Jap War (1904–5) ocular casualties		2·22%	,, ,,
First World War (1914–18) ocular casualties		2·14%	,, ,,
Second World War (1939–45) ocular casualties		2·0 to 2·5%	,, ,,
Korean War (1950–53) ocular casualties		8·1%	,, ,,
Israeli-Arab War (1967)	Gombos (1969)	10·0%	,, ,,
	Treister (1969)	5·6%	,, ,,

[1] See *History of the Second World War: Surgery*, H.M.S.O., London, 1953, p. 393 for orbito-cranial injuries and p. 615 for ophthalmology in war, and also *Surgery in World War II, Ophthalmology and Otolaryngology*, Dept. of the Army, Washington D.C., 1957.

The origin of the injuries received in battle has also varied with the evolution of military techniques. During the half century before the first World War, the statistics gathered by Praun (1899) show that the following incidence was approximately true: firearms, 92·2%; sword and bayonet, 3·8%. In the first World War (1914–18) average British statistics for battle casualties were: shell and trench mortars, 70·67%; bullets 16·9%; bombs and grenades, 12·5%. To these must be added an immense number of casualties from war gases which in the main caused temporary disability to be followed 20 years later by more permanent damage. For the second World War (1939–45) the samples shown in Table XI are typical of the more open types of warfare and also of those encountered in jungle fighting.

In aerial warfare to the effects of missiles must be added those of aeroplane crashes and burns; in naval warfare those of burns and exposure; and in all of them the concussive damage caused by blast from high explosives.

TABLE XI

CAUSES OF BATTLE CASUALTIES IN GROUND WARFARE IN WORLD WAR II

	BRITISH		AMERICAN
	African Desert Campaign (Scott and Michaelson, 1946)	Burma Campaign (Somerville-Large, 1946)	(Greear, 1950)
	%	%	%
Shells and mortars	31·3	16·32	42·4
Grenades	25·0	63·51	3·3
Gunshot wounds	11·3	12·17	15·0
Mines and traps	12·3	6·82	30·0
Aerial bombs	5·3	0	3·0
Miscellaneous	14·8	1·18	6·3

The types of injury sustained in the first and second Great Wars are indicated in Tables XII and XIII. A great many of the injuries were gross, necessitating immediate or early excision of the eye either from the gravity of the damage inflicted at the time of the wound, persistent pain, panophthalmitis, or from the fear of sympathetic inflammation. Many of the casualties resulted from the retention of small foreign bodies which did not immediately disorganize the eye, while a large number resulted from concussions and contusions. As time went on, however, the percentage of enucleations and the

TABLE XII

TYPES OF OCULAR WAR INJURY (FIRST WORLD WAR)

Analysis of Ophthalmic War Casualties admitted to a Military Hospital (1914–19) (Ormond, 1920)

Number blinded (mainly perforating or penetrating injuries by shells, bullets and bombs)	1,008
Enucleations (mainly gross direct injuries and foreign bodies)	
Bilateral	250
Unilateral	780
Perforating injuries and foreign bodies with retention of the eye	294
Indirect injury (contusion, concussion)	405
Conjunctivitis and keratitis due to gas	83
Traumatic keratitis	162
Traumatic cataract	162
Intra-ocular hæmorrhage	140
Retinal detachment (?traumatic)	31
Lid injuries	104

final proportion of blindness resulting from injuries sustained in battle steadily diminished, partly because of the increasing efficiency of the medical services in the early treatment of the wounded, partly because of the gradual improvement in surgical techniques in dealing with such problems as intra-ocular foreign bodies, and partly because of the possibility of almost completely eliminating sepsis by the early exhibition of antibiotic drugs. Retinal detachments were more frequently noted than in previous wars but it was generally held that only 20% of such cases were due purely to military trauma. In the wars waged prior to the present century the usual fate of the injured eye was enucleation or neglect which frequently resulted in total blindness from the development of sympathetic ophthalmitis. Thus in the American Civil War, 1,190 gunshot wounds involving the eye were recorded,

TABLE XIII

TYPES OF OCULAR WAR INJURY (SECOND WORLD WAR)

	BRITISH	AMERICAN
	Cases (Scott and Michaelson 1946)	Cases (Bellows 1947)
Gross injuries requiring immediate enucleation	56	104
Non-perforating foreign bodies	52	–
Perforating foreign bodies	138	102
Contusions	52	54
Blast and concussion	26	13
Direct injuries to lids, orbit, etc.	–	30
Indirect injuries	–	40
Burns	–	9

In the Israeli-Arab War of 1967, Gombos (1969) reported 54 direct, 4 indirect injuries and 1 miscellaneous injury with 2 injuries of the orbit and adnexa out of a total of 61 ocular injuries. There were 7 cases of contusion, 26 perforations with 17 intra-ocular foreign bodies and 28 penetrating injuries; 2 eyes required primary enucleation.

91 of which developed sympathetic ophthalmitis or decreased vision in the remaining eye,[1] while in the Franco-Prussian War 56·5% of patients injured by projectiles developed sympathetic disease (Steindorff, 1914). In the second World War, on the other hand, sympathetic ophthalmitis was practically unknown in the British and American armies, and in comparing the two World Wars separated by the short space of 20 years, although the proportion of ocular injuries in both was approximately equal, in the British army the percentage of enucleations in the second was approximately half that in the first.

Although the circumstances of war hampered the detailed collection of statistics concerning combat injuries, the figures of Stallard (1944–47) are of considerable interest. In the Western Desert Campaign 328 intra-orbital injuries were seen including 102 retained intra-ocular foreign bodies and, in addition, 110 cases of intracranial wounds involving the visual pathways, some of these being orbito-cranial in continuity; in the latter part of the war in the British Liberation Army in north-west Europe 72 cases of

[1] *The Medical and Surgical History of the War of the Rebellion.* Govt. Printing Office, Washington. Surg. Vol. II (1), 325, 1870.

retained intra-ocular foreign body were dealt with among 335 battle-casualties and 62 accidental ocular injuries. Almost 70% of the foreign bodies were successfully removed, mostly by the posterior route; panophthalmitis and gross post-operative intra-ocular inflammation were not encountered. Figures quoted by Stallard (1947) dealing with work done in the 21st Army Group in the four months following the Allied invasion of north-west Europe showed 2,188 ocular casualties, of which 1,440 were sustained in combat, 480 were penetrating ocular wounds and 157 intra-ocular foreign bodies. It is noteworthy that many injuries are not directly due to enemy action but rather to the type of accidents that occur in civil and industrial circumstances or as a result of road traffic accidents, some of which might have been prevented by adequate ocular protection; indeed, the commonest single cause of accidental intra-ocular foreign bodies was the ubiquitous " hammer and chisel ".

Between Pearl Harbor and the end of the war almost 4,000 eyes were enucleated in U.S. army hospitals, subsequent histopathological examination being carried out at the Armed Forces Institute of Pathology in Washington: Rones and Wilder (1947) reported the findings in 104 cases of non-perforating injury and Wilder (1948) described 731 cases of intra-ocular foreign body—37% magnetic, 63% non-magnetic (copper and brass)—and drew attention to the not unusual finding of small particles within the eye and collections of other foreign material, such as vegetable matter or pieces of clothing or skin carried into the eye by the projectile, sometimes associated with the development of abscesses.

In the Korean War 8·1% of the wounded were ocular casualties, a higher proportion than in previous major conflicts, and of all those with head wounds 40% had ocular injuries; sympathetic ophthalmitis occurred in 2% of those with ocular perforation (Lowrey and Shaffer, 1954). The figures for the Vietnam War are not yet available but Hoefle (1968) has described the arrangements on board the *U.S.S. Repose*, one of two hospital ships located near the combat zone; in 1966, 119 ocular injuries sustained in combat received their initial treatment on board this ship, including 18 intra-ocular foreign bodies, 33 surface foreign bodies, 37 perforating wounds, 13 palpebral lacerations, 8 burns and 12 contusion injuries. Enucleation was required in 24 cases, all of them with perforating wounds, and no case of sympathetic ophthalmitis was seen among this group.

Following the six-day Israeli-Arab War (1967), Treister (1969) analysed the records of all ocular combat casualties apart from those associated with otherwise fatal injuries; of 2,500 combat casualties ocular injuries occurred in 140 (5·6%), shell fragments were responsible for 62% of these and one-quarter of the victims were members of tank-crews; the nature of the injury was a corneal foreign body in 30%, perforation of the globe in 20%, bilateral injury in 26·1%; no case of sympathetic ophthalmitis was reported.

AERIAL BOMBING

The aerial bombing of military and civil populations by high explosive and incendiary bombs provides problems of its own. In such conditions the ocular casualties may be very high, but much the commonest injuries—fortunately, many of them trivial—are due to foreign bodies derived from the disintegration of burning buildings; the type of injury, however, which results from the embedding of multiple foreign bodies of dust and debris in the cornea in an explosion may be very incapacitating. The more serious injuries are due to flying objects—particularly glass—and to the effects of blast. The great majority is made up of lacerations and perforating wounds of the globe, lids and orbit, contusions, concussion due to blast, intra-ocular foreign bodies and burns of varying severity. In atomic bombing, in addition to these effects of blast and indirect injury due to flying debris and burning buildings, there are added the hazards of radiational flash-burns due to the thermal effect of infra-red, visible and short-waved light, the abiotic effect of ultra-violet rays and the delayed effects, either incapacitating or lethal, of ionizing radiation. Most of the immediate casualties are due to the thermal effect, for the kinetic energy liberated in the process of nuclear fission involves temperatures greater than 100,000,000° C, a temperature sufficient to vaporize steel in the immediate vicinity and to cause serious burns up to a distance of 4,000 m. or ignite clothing at 3,500 m. from the hypocentre of the explosion. The effects on the eye of radiation and flash from nuclear explosions will be described later in this Volume.

In view of the fact that some 50% of ocular injuries in modern warfare are due to small flying particles not in themselves lethal, suggestions have been made for the protection of the eyes by a steel gauze or meshwork or a perforated shield attached to the steel helmet commonly worn in battle (Morax and Moreau, 1916; Cruise, 1917–44) or by an eye-shield of plastic material some 2 or 2·5 mm. thick (Parsons, 1941). The dislike of extra equipment by the soldier, however, and his desire at all costs to maintain the visual alertness and mobility so necessary for his survival, have made these appliances unpopular in war; moreover, the visual field, perception of depth and dark adaptation are all impaired by metal visors or shields even when worn in the best conditions (Parsons, 1941), and the difficulties are much increased when their apertures or perforations become obscured by rain or mud. There is, however, undoubtedly a place for the lighter, transparent and almost as stout plastic visor for the soldier in circumstances wherein multiple flying particles are to be expected, as in negotiating a minefield, and for the civilian in air-raids when he is exposed to injuries from flying glass and the cloud of disintegrating brick-dust and other debris which account for the great majority of the numerous ocular catastrophes associated with these melancholy events.

The literature on war injuries is large. For summaries dealing with early wars see Praun (1899) and Wagenmann (1910); for the Franco-Prussian war, Cohn (1872) and von Oettingen (1897); the Russo-Turkish war, Reich (1879) and von Oettingen (1897); and the Russo-Japanese war, von Merz (1907), Inouye (1909) and Oguchi (1912). The literature analysing the casualties of the first World War is enormous: see the official Medical History (Great Britain), Lister (1918), Ormond (1920) and others in English literature; Mills (1917), Greenwood (1924) and de Schweinitz (1924) in the United States official History; Moreau (1916), Morax and Moreau (1916), Lagrange (1917–18), Valois (1918), Guillain and Barré (1918) in French literature; Dimmer (1916), von Szily (1916) and Hertel (1922) in German; and Angelucci (1922) in Italian. The literature dealing with the second World War is even more extensive; it has been well and conveniently summarized up to 1945 by Struble and Kreft (1945); and Masters (1946–48); subsequent papers of note are those of Bellows (1947), Stallard (1947), Marshall

(1947), Gundersen (1947), Thomson (1947), Bellecci (1949), Greear (1950). Ocular casualties in the Korean War were annotated by Hull (1951), Lowrey and Shaffer (1954); and in the Vietnam War by Hoefle (1968). Blast injuries seen during the Algerian War have been reviewed by Quere and his colleagues (1969), and the ocular injuries dealt with during the six-day Israeli-Arab War of June 1967 by Gombos (1969) and Treister (1969).

Angelucci. *Arch. Ottal.*, **29,** 193 (1922).
Bellecci. *Ann. Med.*, **54,** 49 (1949).
Bellows. *Amer. J. Ophthal.*, **30,** 309 (1947).
Calvert. *Brit. J. Surg., War Surg. Suppl.*, No. 1, 119 (1947).
Cohn. *Schussverletzungen des Auges*, Erlangen (1872).
Cruise. *Trans. ophthal. Soc. U.K.*, **37,** 176 (1917); **64,** 165 (1944).
Dimmer. *Klin. Mbl. Augenheilk.*, **57,** 257 (1916).
Gombos. *Amer. J. Ophthal.*, **68,** 474 (1969).
Greear. *Blindness* (ed. Zale), Princeton, 568 (1950).
Greenwood. *Med. Dept. of the U.S. Army in World War*, **11,** 556 (1924).
Guillain and Barré. *Travaux neurologiques de la guerre*, Paris (1918).
Gundersen. *Trans. Amer. Acad. Ophthal.*, **52,** 604 (1947).
Hertel. *Hb. des ärtzl. Erfahrungen im Weltkrieg 1914–18*, Leipzig, **5** (1922).
Hoefle. *Arch. Ophthal.*, **79,** 33 (1968).
Hull. *Trans. Amer. Acad. Ophthal.*, **55,** 885 (1951).
Inouye. *Die Sehstörungen bei Schussverletzungen*, Leipzig (1909).
Lagrange. *Fractures de l'orbite par les projectiles de guerre*, Paris (1917).
Atlas d'ophtalmoscopie de guerre, Paris (1918).
Lister. *Lancet*, **2,** 67 (1918).
Lowrey and Shaffer. *Trans. Pac. Cst. oto-ophthal. Soc.*, **35,** 39 (1954).
Marshall. *Trans. Amer. Acad. Ophthal.*, **52,** 237 (1947).
Masters. *Ophthalmology in the War Years*, Chicago, **1,** 480 (1946); **2,** 359 (1948).
von Merz. *Klin. Mbl. Augenheilk*, **45,** Beil., 238 (1907).
Mills. *Amer. Encycl. Ophthal.*, **10,** 7706 (1917).
Morax and Moreau. *Ann. Oculist.* (Paris), **153,** 321 (1916).
Moreau. *Clin Ophtal.*, **7,** 364 (1916).
von Oettingen. *Die indireckten Schussläsionen des Auges*, Stuttgart (1897).
Oguchi. *v. Graefes Arch. Ophthal.*, **80,** 353 (1912).
Ormond. *Med. Res. Counc. Stat. Rep.*, No. 6 (1920).
Parsons. *Trans. ophthal. Soc. U.K.*, **61,** 157 (1941).
Praun. *Die Verletzungen des Auges*, Wiesbaden (1899).
Quere, Bouchat and Cornand. *Amer. J. Ophthal.*, **67,** 64 (1969).
Reich. *Klin. Mbl. Augenheilk.*, **17,** 96 (1879).
Rones and Wilder. *Amer. J. Ophthal.*, **30,** 1143 (1947).
de Schweinitz. *Med. Dept. U.S. Army in World War*, **11,** 659 (1924).
Scott and Michaelson. *Brit. J. Ophthal.*, **30,** 42 (1946).
Somerville-Large. *Trans. ophthal. Soc. U.K.*, **66,** 647 (1946).
Stallard. *Brit. J. Ophthal.*, **28,** 105 (1944); **31,** 12 (1947).
Steindorff. *Berl. klin. Wschr.*, **51,** 1787 (1914).
Stone. *J. Amer. med. Ass.*, **142,** 151 (1950).
Struble and Kreft. *War Med.* (Chicago), **8,** 290 (1945).
von Szily. *Atlas der Kriegsaugenheilk.*, Stuttgart (1916).
Thomson. *Trans. ophthal. Soc. U.K.*, **67,** 245 (1947).
Treister. *Amer. J. Ophthal.*, **68,** 669 (1969).
Valois. *Les borgnes de la guerre*, Paris (1918).
Wagenmann. *Verletzungen d. Auges: Graefe-Saemisch Hb. d. ges Augenheilk.*, 2nd ed., Leipzig, **9** (5), 45 (1910).
Wilder. *Amer. J. Ophthal.*, **31,** 57 (1948).

Before bringing this chapter to a close two other types of injury should be mentioned—self-inflicted injuries and those resulting from malpractice.

SELF-INFLICTED INJURIES are relatively rare and while they are often mild they may occasionally be serious. Such cases fall readily into three groups. The most common is the *malingerer* who, in order to evade an unwanted task such as military service or to prolong a disability in the expectation of greater compensation, inserts irritative substances into the conjunctival sac.[1]

[1] Typical of such cases is that of the miner injured in an explosion who developed a traumatic kerato-conjunctivitis refractory to all forms of treatment until, after the lapse of

The immense variety of irritant materials which have been used for this purpose and their harmful and sometimes disastrous effects on the eye, are considered elsewhere.

A second type of case is the *psychopath*. The neurote will similarly produce an irritant kerato-conjunctivitis to attract attention or to excite sympathy (Fig. 31). Rarely extreme domestic stress may precipitate severe self-injury as in the case described by Riebel and his colleagues (1961) in which carbide of lime was used to burn both eyes following which penetrating wounds of the cornea and lens were inflicted with a needle. It is interesting that self-mutilation may occur in epidemics; thus Segal and his team (1963) noted this feature in a group of 22 young male prisoners all with personality disorders who between them achieved a total of 166 injuries to 43 eyes. On

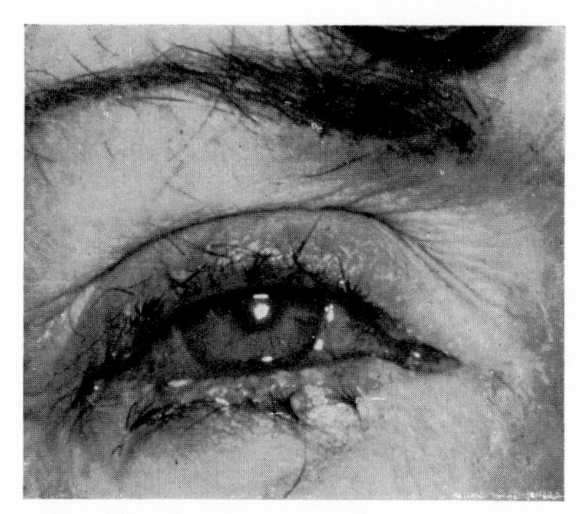

Fig. 31.—Self-inflicted Conjunctivitis.
In a nurse combating many personal problems(B. R. Jones).

148 occasions chemical means were employed (aniline pencil in 119, chloride of lime in 17), in 29 mechanical means such as ground glass, metal or wood-splinters, and in 3 cases burns resulted from lighted cigarettes inserted into the open eye. As a rule such patients do not seek medical aid at an early stage and many may actively resist treatment. Furthermore, the search for the responsible agent may be time-consuming and fruitless since the ingenuity of the patient usually exceeds the diligence of those concerned in his care. Persistent rubbing of the eyes with the finger represents an unusual form of mechanical trauma which in the case of a young psychotic woman resulted after two years in ruptures of Descemet's membrane and ectatic leucomata of the corneæ; psychotherapy cured the patient of her habit but not of her blindness (Arouh, 1957).

21 months and the expenditure of over £1,000 by an insurance company, it was established that the inflammation had been self-perpetuated by the deliberate introduction of dust and beard shavings into the conjunctival sac (Blum, 1965).

Visual damage has also resulted from self-inflicted solar retinopathy against a background of mental illness or the use of drugs (Eigner, 1966; Gilkes, 1968; MacFaul, 1969; Ewald and Ritchey, 1970), and Bulanda (1958) has reported the case of a young man who rubbed his corneæ with permanganate crystals in an attempt to blot out the unpleasant visual hallucinations resulting from his addiction to cocaine.

Finally in *maniacal or depressive states* self-mutilation may go to the extreme of attempted or actual gouging out of one (Axenfeld, 1899; Poulard and Veil, 1923) or both eyes (Zamkowsky, 1934; Byrnes and Shier, 1949) with the finger or some implement like the handle of a spoon.[1] Reviewing the literature up to 1962, Davidson (1962) found eight cases in which both

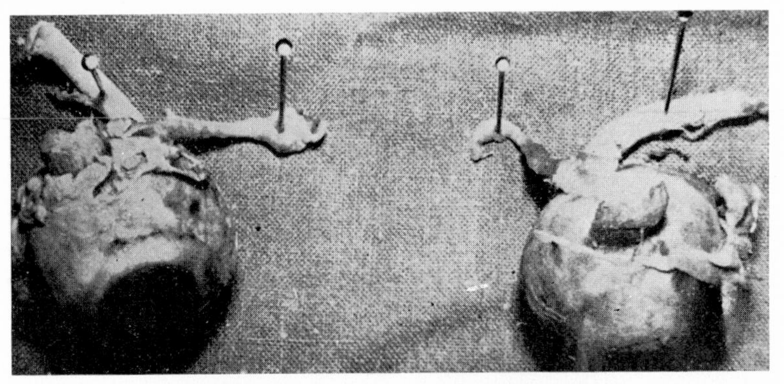

FIG. 32.—SELF-INFLICTED BILATERAL ENUCLEATION.

By a Negro aged 25 with schizophrenia. The patient in a psychiatric hospital performed a bilateral enucleation on himself with his hands. He was being checked by a nurse every 15 minutes, and she found him not uttering a sound and with an eye clutched in each hand. On healing the sockets were markedly contracted (M. Gorin).

eyes had been torn out; all the patients were psychotic or had evidence of organic brain disease. Perforation and evisceration of both eyes were achieved by a young epileptic in a state of stupor, leaving Saebø (1948) to enucleate what remained, and Gorin (1964) recorded the discovery of a 25-year-old psychiatric patient clutching an eye in each hand following bilateral manual enucleation (Fig. 32). Occasionally the eye may be involved in a suicidal attempt as in the case of a young psychotic who thrust a pencil through his upper lid and orbit into the posterior cranial fossa, thereby causing a complete unilateral ophthalmoplegia and blindness (Albert *et al.*, 1965) (Fig. 33).

[1] In this connection can be recalled the story of Œdipus, son of Laius, King of Thebes, and Jocasta; not knowing his parentage, he unwittingly murdered his own father and later took his mother as his wife by whom he had two sons and two daughters. Subsequently when he discovered the true facts, in horror at his crimes and in a state of deep remorse, Œdipus put out his own eyes. The tragedy was dramatized by Sophocles in *Œdipus Rex*.

INJURIES DUE TO MALPRACTICE, CARELESSNESS OR ACCIDENT on the part of a medical attendant or ignorance or carelessness on the part of the patient are by no means unknown; idiosyncrasies or allergies cannot properly be included in this list. Into this category come the effects of the injudicious or accidental use of drugs, as the formation of corneal leucomata from the use of too strong solutions of silver nitrate in the eyes of the newborn (Hornberg, 1883; Sie-Boen-Lien, 1949), as well as the kerato-conjunctivitis which may follow the accidental introduction of irritant applications such as chrysarobin into the eye; cocaine keratopathy comes into the same category[1]. Corneal damage owing to exposure or abrasion under anæsthesia should be

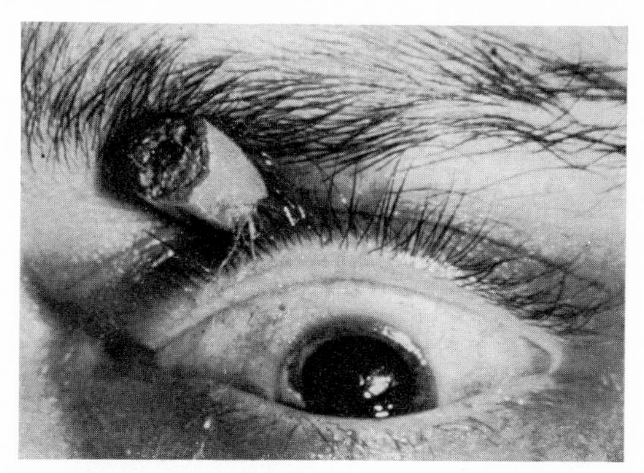

FIG. 33.—SELF-INFLICTED ORBITO-CRANIAL PERFORATING INJURY.

The patient, a man aged 27, pushed a 6-in. pencil through his orbit into the posterior fossa in an attempted suicide. The tip of the pencil was removed through a right fronto-temporal craniotomy and the pencil itself withdrawn through the orbit. The lesion was followed by optic atrophy with no perception of light and complete ophthalmoplegia. Otherwise the patient recovered and was transferred to a psychiatric hospital (D. M. Albert *et al.*).

remembered, while surgical traumata, such as perforation of the globe in strabismus surgery (Gottlieb and Castro, 1970) and severance of the optic nerve during operations on the nasal sinuses, have occurred on more than one occasion. Even over-enthusiastic packing of the nose for epistaxis has led to temporary blindness and ophthalmoplegia (Giammanco and Binns, 1970). Few have had the courage to publish these incidents (Freudenthal, 1905; Laas, 1907; Onodi, 1907; Purtscher, 1910; and others). Finally, it should be noted that foreign bodies in the eyes of the patient undergoing dental treatment are by no means unknown (Hales, 1970), as well as paralysis of the VIth nerve and transient amaurosis after blockage of the mandibular nerve (Cooper, 1962; Blaxter and Britten, 1967).

Albert, Burns and Scheie. *Amer. J. Ophthal.*, **60,** 1109 (1965).
Arouh. *Arch. Oftal. B. Aires*, **32,** 5 (1957).
Axenfeld. *Z. Augenheilk.*, **1,** 128 (1899).
Blaxter and Britten. *Brit. med. J.*, **1,** 681 (1967).

[1] p. 1178.

Blum. *Klin. Mbl. Augenheilk.*, **145,** 913 (1965).
Bulanda. *Klin. oczna*, **28,** 109 (1958).
Byrnes and Shier. *Amer. J. Ophthal.*, **32,** 268 (1949).
Cooper. *J. oral. Surg.*, **20,** 151 (1962).
Davidson. *Acta psychother.* (Basel), **10,** 286 (1962).
Eigner. *Amer. J. Ophthal.*, **61,** 1546 (1966).
Ewald and Ritchey. *Amer. J. Ophthal.*, **70,** 491 (1970).
Freudenthal. *Arch. int. Laryngol.*, **20,** 761 (1905).
Giammanco and Binns. *J. Laryngol. Otol.*, **84,** 631 (1970).
Gilkes. *Brit. med. J.*, **3,** 678 (1968).
Gorin. *Arch. Ophthal.*, **72,** 225 (1964).
Gottlieb and Castro. *Arch. Ophthal.*, **84,** 151 (1970).
Hales. *Amer. J. Ophthal.*, **70,** 221 (1970).
Hornberg. *Beitrag z. Casuistik u. Statistik d. Augenverletzungen* (Diss.), Berlin (1883).
Laas. *Zbl. prakt. Augenheilk.*, **31,** 78 (1907).
MacFaul. *Brit. J. Ophthal.*, **53,** 534 (1969).
Onodi. *Klin. Mbl. Augenheilk.*, **45** (2), 276 (1907).
Poulard and Veil. *Bull. Soc. Ophtal. Paris*, 127 (1923).
Purtscher. *Aerztl. Standeszeitung*, No. 9, 1 (1910).
Riebel, Anton and Kumstát. *Cs. oftal.*, **17,** 396 (1961).
Saebø. *Acta ophthal.* (Kbh.), **26,** 451 (1948).
Segal, Mrzyglod, Czaplicka *et al.* *Amer. J. Ophthal.*, **55,** 349 (1963).
Sie-Boen-Lian. *Chin. med. J.*, **67,** 328 (1949).
Zamkowsky. *Bull. Instit. opt. Ukraine*, 127 (1934).

SECTION I

MECHANICAL INJURIES

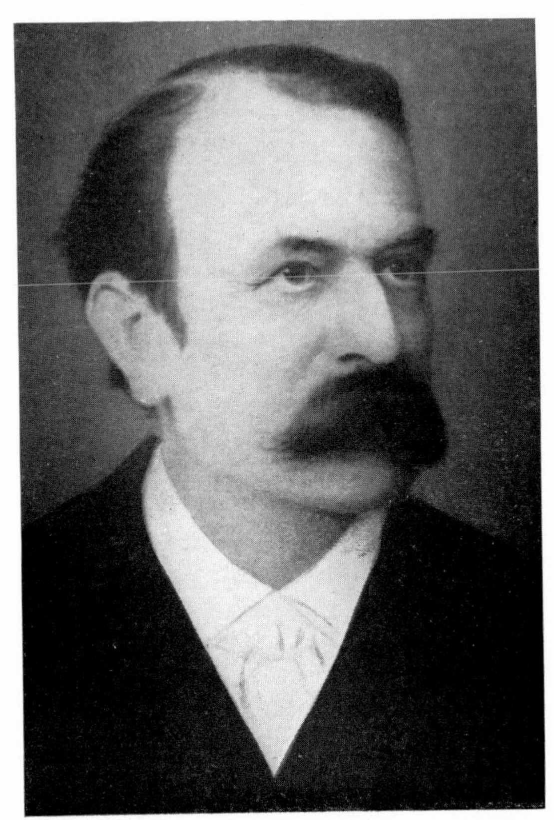

FIG. 34.—RUDOLF BERLIN
[1833–1897].

CHAPTER II

CONCUSSIONS AND CONTUSIONS

Mechanical injuries can best be discussed under three main headings: (1) *concussions* and *contusions* caused by blunt objects, jarring or blast, (2) *wounds* and *perforating injuries* caused by sharp objects, blunt objects endowed with great momentum, or small bodies travelling with a high velocity, and (3) the effects of *retained foreign bodies*. Two further types of injury should be noted which have features peculiar to themselves—*explosion injuries* wherein the concussive effects of blast are combined with the impaction of multiple small foreign bodies onto and into the eyes, and *gunshot wounds* wherein the effects of a foreign body, usually of some size, are augmented and their character changed by the explosive forces generated by the velocity of its impact.

CONCUSSIONS AND CONTUSIONS OF THE GLOBE

Many ophthalmologists of note have contributed lavishly to our knowledge and appreciation of the effects of concussion injuries of the eye, but there is little doubt that the most appropriate of the early workers to introduce this chapter is Rudolf Berlin [1833–1897], Professor of Ophthalmology at Rostock (Fig. 34). We have chosen him before all others because he was the first to interpret the significance of clinical observations, which had been many, through the crucial test of experiments, which had been few; he found more satisfaction in verified facts than in theories, and applied with effect the advice of John Hunter's famous aphorism—"Do not think. Try. Be patient. Be accurate." The sudden blindness, for example, following a frontal blow which had been generally accepted since the time of Hippocrates to be due to concussion of the frontal nerve, was proved by Berlin to be due to bony injury to the optic nerve at the apex of the orbit; and his name is immortalized in "Berlin's œdema", the dramatic changes that appear in the retina following concussion, the true nature of which he elucidated by an elaborate series of experiments whereby he induced graduated concussion effects in animals by striking their eyes with elastic rods. He was, indeed, the first to put our knowledge of these injuries on a firm and logical basis.

In contradistinction to the wounds caused by sharp objects or blunt objects travelling at a high velocity or endowed with great momentum, concussions are the result of the sudden acceleration (or deceleration) imparted by the impact of a blunt force such as is sustained by a blow from a large object or in a collision or fall.

The wounding capacity of an impact depends on the kinetic energy involved. This depends on the weight and velocity of the object, which in the case of simple forward motion is computed from the formula $mv^2/2g$, where m is the weight in pounds, v the velocity in feet per second, and g the acceleration of gravity (32 ft./sec.). Thus the kinetic energy of a moving body increases arithmetically with regard to its weight and geometrically in relation to its velocity. If two bodies, one twice the weight of the other, are travelling at the same rate, the kinetic energy of the first will be twice that of the second: but if they both have the same weight and one travels at twice the speed of the other, the kinetic energy will be four times as great. The damage done, of course, is not proportional to the kinetic energy of the mass in motion, but varies with the amount expended in changing the state of rest or uniform motion of the tissue struck. Thus the force of impact which may be utilized to induce uniform motion of the tissues is not injurious; hence the advisability of prolonging the duration of the impact in order to diminish the force expended in disrupting the tissues, as is seen in the tumbler who rolls with his fall or the ball-player who moves his hand with the caught ball.

If the term CONCUSSION were used strictly definitively it would refer to changes which are in large part, at any rate, reversible; when the force of the impact transmitted through the integument is of sufficient intensity to disrupt the walls of the small vessels so that the tissues are bruised and disorganized by perivascular hæmorrhages which are usually visible macroscopically without the solution of the continuity of the surface layers, the term CONTUSION is more appropriately employed; and when they are disrupted or torn a LACERATION may be said to have occurred. It is to be remembered that an external impact may cause an internal laceration, at the same time leaving the surface layers intact. The total effects upon the eyeball may be due to several factors, all of which, of course, are usually in some degree combined—the *direct impact* of the force upon the globe with its maximum effects at the point where the blow is received; *transmitted force* appearing as a wave of pressure when the eye is suddenly compressed travelling throughout its fluid contents in all directions sometimes with explosive force, in which case the maximum damage may be at a point distant from the actual place of impact (*contre-coup*); and *indirect force* whereby the globe is suddenly hurled against the elastic contents of the orbit and its resistant bony walls.

Such effects are seen not only when a blunt force impinges directly upon the globe; somewhat similar injuries are seen when the shock of a mechanical catastrophe affecting neighbouring structures primarily, such as a fall on the head or the traversal of the orbit by a missile, jars the structures of the eye indirectly: intra-ocular hæmorrhages, a subluxation of the lens, a traumatic cataract, a macular lesion, a rupture of the choroid or a detachment of the retina are among the commoner types of damage thus caused.

The type of concussive injury thus indirectly sustained varies considerably with the structures receiving the primary impact (Lagrange, 1917–18). A blow striking the upper orbital arch communicates its force through the internal and external orbital processes of the frontal bone and dissipates itself in the facial mass; a blow on the frontal bone above the orbit therefore tends to leave the eye unharmed but, apart from cerebral injury, produces fractures of the thin orbital vault at the level of the optic foramen and sphenoidal fissure injuring the optic, sensory and motor nerves crowded in this area. On the other hand, a force striking the face below the orbit is largely dissipated over the cranial vault through the orbital processes of the frontal bone. The rim of the orbit is relatively solid, but in stirring up the soft tissues of the face and retro-maxillary region the impact produces waves of force which are transmitted through the semi-fluid fatty tissue into the orbit through the pterygo-maxillary fissure so that concussion effects are produced at the posterior pole of the eye and the macula is readily damaged.

When the force fractures the orbital wall and crushes it in without actually touching the eyeball, serious injuries are liable to occur, prominent among which is an intra-ocular lesion situated on the aspect of the globe opposite the fracture of the orbital wall. Sometimes this may result from a contact lesion caused by the fractured orbital wall being driven temporarily against the globe, and on other occasions it may be due to a wave of pressure which starts from the site of the fracture, traverses the orbital tissues and impinges on the eye. Such a force tends to cause lesions in the globe anterior to the site of the fracture, but macular lesions may also result. If, in addition to fracturing the bony wall, the object passes through the orbit, to this damage must be added lacerations of the orbital contents, including the severance or avulsion of the optic nerve.

Finally, when the object grazes but does not rupture or perforate the eyeball or when the wall of the orbit is driven onto it, traumatic reactions and lacerations occur particularly at the point of impact; macular and other lesions may be caused in addition, but in such a case the macula is not damaged alone.

BLAST INJURIES due to atmospheric concussions, such as result from explosions occurring either industrially as in mining and quarrying, or in war either in combat by the bursting of a shell, grenade or mine, or in aerial bombing, are of the same type, the force in this case being the impact of an atmospheric wave of high pressure, the effects of which are magnified by the succeeding wave of low pressure. The sudden release of compressed air at close range produces a similar effect. The subsequent injuries are due to the establishment of sharp pressure-gradients within the body, for differences between tissues in inertia, compressibility, cohesion and fixation result in a response to the displacing force so varied that widespread disruptive effects may occur. The forces involved may be quite considerable: the primary compression-wave may travel at a velocity of the order of 25,000 feet per second with a pressure component up to 200 atmospheres (3,000 lb.) per square inch, and the succeeding phase of rarefaction is never less than 15 lb. per square inch. Both of these components are capable of producing considerable trauma, the first by direct compression, the second by suction which, indeed, may be so violent that it has been reported as causing gross disorganization and even complete avulsion of the globe (Stoewer, 1907, in the explosion of a munition factory; Ormond, 1917, and Lagrange, 1918, in war). Although on the evidence of animal experiments any gross injury from this cause, apart from retrobulbar hæmorrhage, has been denied unless gross lethal damage has been caused (Zuckerman, 1941), the clinical evidence of such injuries is overwhelming.

In this type of injury the structures of the anterior segment are commonly affected (extensive subconjunctival and intra-ocular hæmorrhages, tears in Descemet's membrane with deep corneal opacities, iridoplegia and impairment of accommodation, tearing of the iris, acute traumatic iritis with secondary glaucoma, luxation of the lens or traumatic cataract), but lesions at the posterior pole (retinal œdema, ruptures of the choroid near the disc, macular lesions, large areas of choroidal degeneration and diffuse pigmentary disturbances) are more characteristic, while considerable hæmorrhages may occur into the retrobulbar tissues. In the worst cases a rupture of one or both globes may occur (Cross, 1941; Zorab, 1945). Similar effects are also caused by the force of an under-water explosion during immersion in the sea, a not uncommon occurrence in modern naval warfare (*immersion blast*).

In assessing the results of concussions, whether due to direct or indirect force and particularly those due to blast, the cerebral and mental effects of the " post-concussion state " must be remembered.[1] The essential features of this syndrome, the effects of which may be of considerable duration, are headache, dizziness, impairment of memory and concentration, liability to fatigue, particularly in finely coordinated activities such as using the eyes for reading, together with psychiatric complications such as emotional instability and changes in the personality. It is sometimes difficult to differentiate the effects of the damage to the peripheral and central mechanisms; thus a deficiency in accommodation may sometimes result from the ready development of ciliary fatigue (Smith, 1949) and sometimes from a disturbance of the higher cortical centres without significant change in the amplitude of accommodation (Wescott, 1943). Considerable clinical judgment is thus required in the evaluation of each particular case.

The literature on the effects of concussions and contusions on the eye is vast and special treatises devoted to the subject date back for a century (White Cooper, 1859; Arlt, 1875; and others): the earlier observations were conveniently summarized by Praun (1899) and Wagenmann (1915). During the last 50 years the slit-lamp has given facilities for the elaboration of the clinical effects of trauma of this type in much greater detail, the most important descriptions of which are still to be found in the monumental work of Vogt (1921–41). The literature on the ocular effects of blast is less extensive; nevertheless, since the time of Stoewer (1907) who described the effects of an explosion in a munition factory, much knowledge has accumulated, most of it derived from experiences in war. The first World War stimulated the writings of Lister (1918), Tooke (1918), de Schweinitz (1919), Anderson (1919) and McKee (1923), and the second of Stallard (1940), Zuckerman (1941), Campbell (1941), Travers (1942), Wakeley (1943), Pugh (1943), Dean (1943), Schenk *et al.* (1944), Barrow and Rhoads (1944), Rones and Wilder (1945), Shapland (1946), and a large number of others. Experimental studies

[1] Wittenbrook (1941), Symonds (1941–62), Fulton (1942), Paterson (1942–44), Symonds and Ritchie Russell (1943), Denny-Brown (1943), Pollock (1943), Denker (1944), Pflugfelder (1949), Le Grand (1963), Johnson (1969) and others.

with a useful r v of the literature were contributed by Clemedson (1949) and Weidenthal (1964), wl he *contre-coup* mechanism of ocular injuries has been reviewed by Wolter (1963) a lenbrander (1965). Peripheral fundus changes following contusions have been studi perimentally in the eye of the pig by Weidenthal and Schepens (1966).

The precise *anism of concussive injuries* to the eye is not yet completely understoo The classical explanation propounded by Arlt (1875) attributed much o damage to the effect of an impinging force, usually acting antero-poster in forcibly expanding the globe around the equator to the line of impact, f being sought in circumferential lateral distension to compensate for the lden antero-posterior compression (Fig. 35). To this concept Förster (1 added the effect of the impact of the wave of pressure traversing the contents of the eye by which, when the cornea

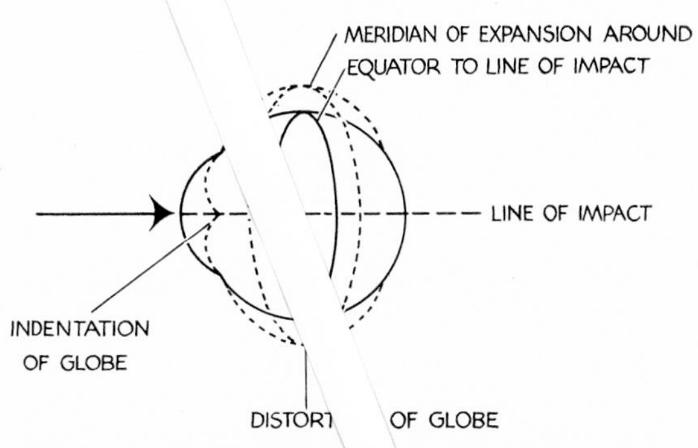

FIG. 35.—THE EFFECT OF A CUSSION ON THE GLOBE.

The effect of a force striking the eye in direction of the arrow is illustrated exaggeratedly. The cornea is indented at th e of impact as shown by the dotted line. A compensatory expansion occurs aroun he equator to the line of impact, the deformation being again indicated by dotted l

was driven in, the aqueous was forced back rds, driving in front of it the lens and iris and hurling the vitreous again the posterior pole. Ogilvie (1900) put forward a detailed theory to exp n the mechanism of foveal damage in contusion injuries of the globe; the was compared to a fluid-filled elastic sphere in which vibration waves ld be reflected from the point of impact to a corresponding point oppos it where the maximum stress was felt. For the reflection theory to be rue explanation of the macular damage following a blow on the front of t eye, however, the eye would have to be a complicated paraboloid shape an t also fails to account for damage to the lens in these cases (Wolter, 1963). is to be remembered that if the intra-ocular contents are considered as an in mpressible fluid, an impinging blow will act not only in the direction of pact but with explosive force in all directions from the centre towards th eriphery, hurling the ocular contents against their outer envelope (Figs. and 37). This general concept is certainly true, but to it must also be added the complicating effects of the sudden movements of the various tissues in relation with each other, and the impact of more firmly fixed tissues against more mobile or of heavier against lighter—the spasmodic contraction of the pupil, the rush of aqueous peripherally as the anterior chamber is compressed, the backward thrust and rebound of the lens, the sudden mass movements of the vitreous, the forcing of the choroid and retina against the sclera—all of these complications acting and reacting with each other produce a picture much more complicated than can easily be explained by the simple hydrodynamic concept of an incompressible fluid transmitting in all directions the pressure applied to it.

A reasonable explanation of *contre-coup* damage in the eye can be derived from the views of Courville (1942–62) concerning the same phenomenon in the brain. Cerebral damage at a point opposite to the impact of a

Figs. 36 and 37.—The Mechanism of Ocular Injuries (modified from J. R. Wolter).

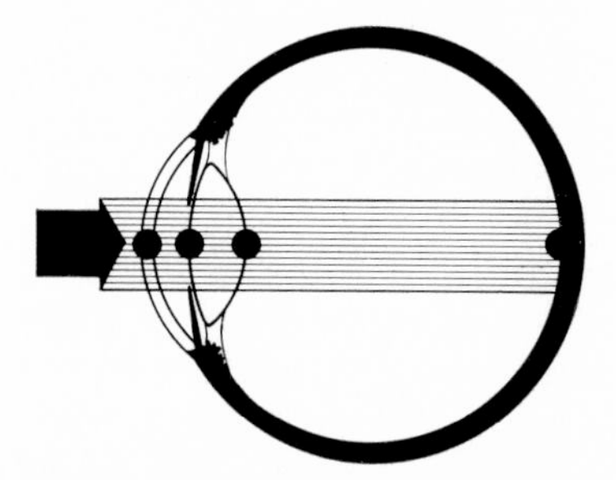

Fig. 36.—To show how a force is thought to traverse the eye. The areas of direct coup and contre coup injuries are indicated by black circles.

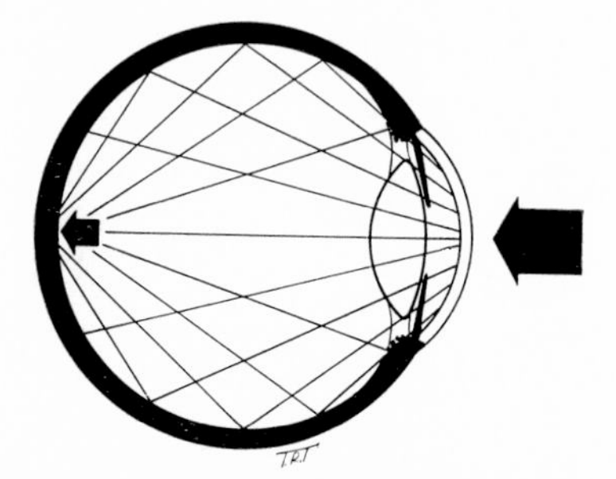

Fig. 37.—To illustrate the concentration of waves of force at the posterior wall by reflection from the coats of the eye.

blow on the head was first observed by Fallopius in the latter part of the 16th century and then by Valsalva in 1700; subsequently the term *contre-coup* was applied to such brain injuries by a group of French surgeons in the 18th century. The original explanation of this type of cerebral damage was that oscillations of the brain starting at the point of impact traversed the head and injured the brain by local vibrations against the inner table of the skull. Subsequent authors, however, confused the issue by adding the factors of deformation of the whole head and complicated reflections of concussion-waves within the skull. Courville divided *contre-coup* injuries of the head into two groups, (1) those cases in which the head is in motion and in which the brain gets damaged by a sudden stop of this motion, and (2) those cases in which a moving object strikes the head while stationary. In this second group the direct blow to the resting head usually produces some local " coup " damage such as a fracture, and a direct line of force traverses the brain to the opposite wall of the skull (Fig. 38). In the brain foci of damage are found along the direct line of force at all interfaces due to differences in density of the brain-tissue, dura, skull and ventricles. The interface with the greatest difference in density is that between brain and skull and the most severe damage to the brain is found at this interface opposite to the site of the blow. Courville spoke of a block of force moving straight through the brain with no evidence of the reflection of waves of force causing damage in his cases. According to Wolter (1963) *contre-coup* injuries of the eye can be compared with Courville's second group of brain injuries. Thus a line of force traversing the eye causes damage at all interfaces, the extent of such damage depending on the force applied, the most posterior interface between the retina-choroid and sclera being most commonly involved (Figs. 36, 39 and 40).

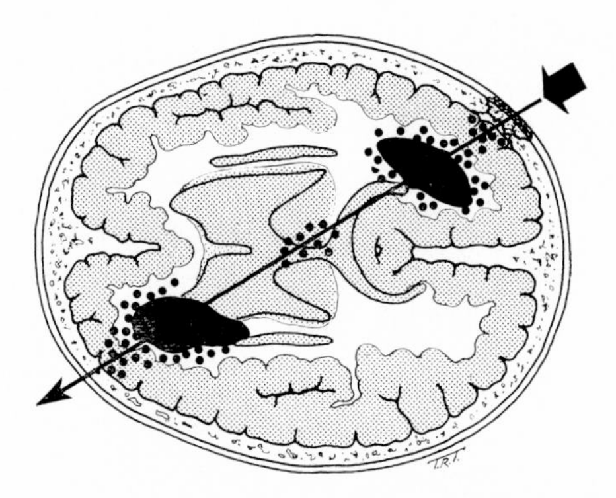

FIG. 38.—THE MECHANISM OF CRANIAL INJURIES.

To illustrate Courville's observation of direct damage at the site of impact and the contre-coup damage at all the interfaces along the line of force that traverses the brain in cases wherein a moving object hits the resting head (J. R. Wolter).

The injuries thus caused tend to be diffuse and multiple and vary widely in severity from a small intra-ocular hæmorrhage to the rupture and complete disorganization of the globe. In general they are due to three causes: (1) immediate damage to the tissue-cells sufficient to cause a disruption of their physiological activity, (2) the more remote effects of the accompanying vascular reactions, and (3) the more gross effects of mechanical tearing and laceration of the tissues.

The question of how far subtle *molecular disturbances in the protoplasmic structure of the cells* themselves contribute to the total disability in concussion is as yet not fully elucidated; it has received most attention in injuries of this type to the brain and spinal cord.[1] Most of the changes observable by histological techniques are associated with œdema of the tissues and other extracellular changes but disturbances of the structural integrity within the cell are by no means ruled out: thus Windle and his co-workers (1944) found

[1] Wilson (1917), Holmes (1918), Brunner (1925), Denny-Brown and Russell (1941), Walker *et al.* (1944), Windle and his associates (1944–46) and others.

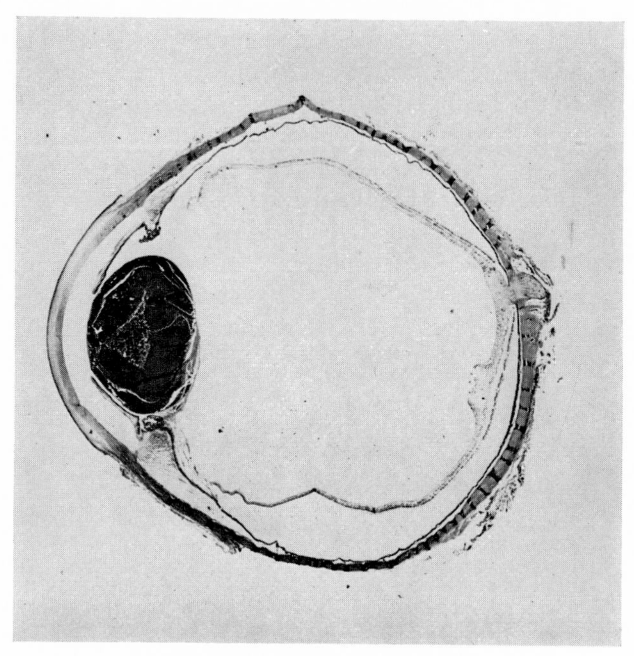

FIG. 39.—CONTRE-COUP DAMAGE.

In a boy aged 12 whose left eye had been struck with the end of a whip. There is a scar of corneal perforation, cataract, a rupture of the posterior lens capsule and central cystic degeneration of the retina (see also Figs. 40, 49, 140–1) (J. R. Wolter).

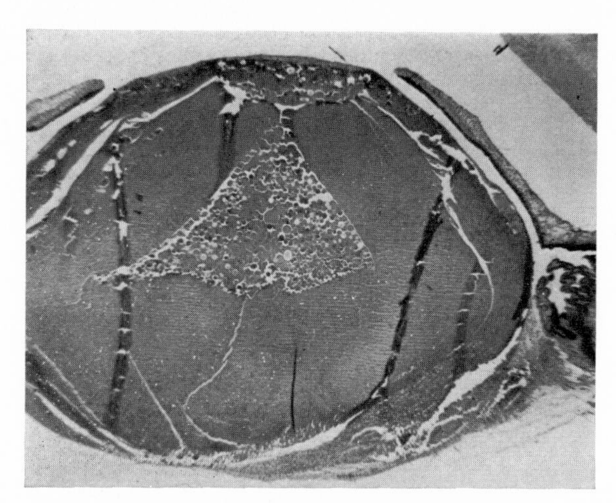

FIG. 40.—CONTRE-COUP INJURY TO THE LENS.

There is thickening of the anterior capsule, a central cortical and nuclear cataract and a membranous scar on the ruptured posterior lens capsule (J. R. Wolter).

—extreme vasodilatation with œdema and hæmorrhage and consequent disruption of the tissues.

How far these vascular effects are determined locally by mechanical factors depending on the passage through the endothelial cells of lines of force, and how far these may be aided by nervous reflexes have been disputed. The initial reaction to trauma is a vasoconstriction of the peripheral arteries—essentially a protective mechanism and occasionally life-saving; it is well and very dramatically seen, for example, in the reflex constriction of the vessels of the iris, which is usually sufficient to control hæmorrhage completely in an iridectomy.

The traumatic arterial spasm whereby a contraction of the muscular coats of arteries occurs as a response to injury was first studied and described by John Hunter.[1] For long it was widely accepted that this reaction was due to a nervous reflex mediated by the sympathetic supply (see Barnes and Trueta, 1942; Trueta *et al.*, 1947). It is interesting, however, that one of Hunter's original observations concerned the placenta and he showed that the blood vessels therein retained the power of contraction until the 4th day, even after separation from the body. Later experimental research has confirmed this independence of the reaction from the activity of the sympathetic and it may now be accepted as a working hypothesis that the phenomenon is due to direct mechanical stimulation of the vessel wall resulting in a sustained contraction of smooth muscle, in the maintenance of which nervous factors do not play a demonstrable part, and is not relieved by sympathectomy (Kinmonth *et al.*, 1949; Kinmonth, 1952; Kinmonth and Simeone, 1952).

Often this vasoconstriction is so transient and slight after a concussion as to produce few if any symptoms; thus a spasmodic constriction of the retinal arteries has been observed to occur and disappear within a quarter of an hour after a knock-out blow sustained at football (Sédan and Alliès, 1951). Sometimes it is sufficiently severe to lead to an ischæmia resulting in local necrosis of the tissues, and the occasional long duration of its effects may be evident in the attenuation of a retinal artery sometimes persisting long after a contusion to the eye (Thomson, 1947). In the ordinary course of events, however, the disturbance of cellular metabolism caused by the anoxia liberates histamine-like substances in the tissues so that the initial phase of vasoconstriction is followed by a subsequent phase of reactive hyperæmia associated with capillary dilatation and greatly increased permeability of the small vessels.

These vascular changes are obviously followed by profound disturbances in the tissues. Initially the escape of fluid results in œdema and swelling (*concussion œdema*), and the escape of corpuscular elements results in the formation of petechial hæmorrhages (*contusion effects*). But these changes themselves tend to set in motion a vicious circle for it seems probable that enzymes which flourish in the acid medium created in the state of anoxæmia break down first the more highly differentiated cells and later the interstitial elements, a process which culminates in autolysis and liquefaction and

[1] *Works of John Hunter*, edited by J. F. Palmer, London, i, 538; iii, 127, 158 (1835).

terminates in necrosis. In the first stage—that of œdematous tumefaction —the œdema and the hæmorrhages may be absorbed, the affected area may shrink and function be restored, but if the stage of necrosis and liquefaction has been reached, permanent atrophy and loss of function result.

Such changes have been demonstrated and minutely studied in the brain by Scheinker (1947) and are very obvious in almost all the tissues of the eye. Complete necrosis of an entire tissue such as the iris and ciliary body may occur: the stroma of the iris loses its normal structure partially or entirely, the cells become pale, shrunken and disintegrated, and the entire tissue may stain uniformly with eosin or disappear altogether, and the ciliary body may similarly degenerate (Tillema, 1937; Kilgore, 1942) (Fig. 44).

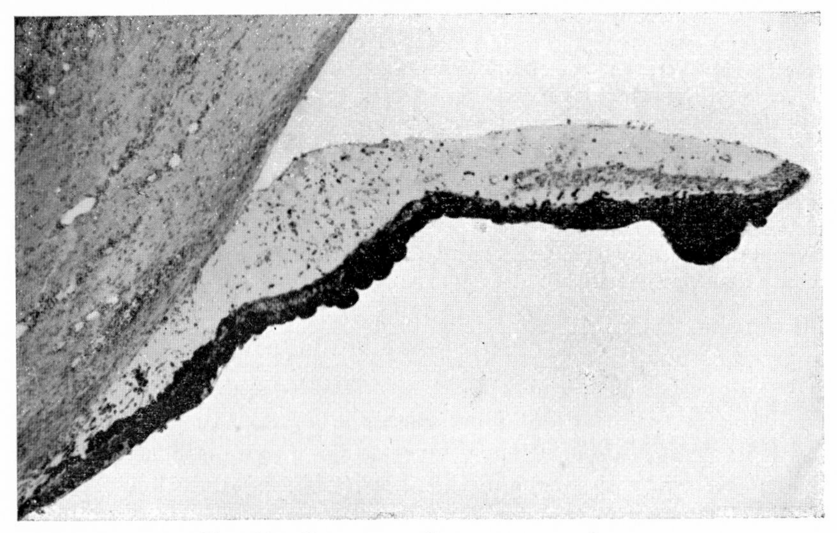

Fig. 44.—Concussion Changes in the Iris.

Showing widespread necrosis of the iris stroma with loss of its structure and peppering with pigment granules. The angle of the anterior chamber is closed (A. Tillema).

Similar gross disintegrative changes are also typically seen in the choroid and particularly in the retina where, on the one hand, a transient and reversible tumefaction and œdema may appear or, on the other, acute necrosis on a large scale may be marked by the dissolution of the tissue into structureless globules or undefined masses of uniformly staining material (A. Fuchs, 1923–27; Lister, 1924; Tillema, 1937; and others).

The third element in the damage from a concussion is mechanical tearing of the tissues (*laceration effect*). When a relatively light force is involved the intercellular substance and the perivascular tissues give way, assisting the development of œdema, but in the more severe injuries the blood vessels and the tissues may suffer a complete solution of their continuity so that hæmorrhages and tissue destruction on a large scale or considerable ruptures may occur. Again, these effects may be seen in dramatic form in the eye: tears in the iris, ciliary body, choroid or retina or ruptures in the lens capsule are common events, of which the culmination is seen in a complete rupture of the globe itself.

All these influences—the actual solution, protoplasmic or gross, of the tissues, vascular damage involving acute ischæmia followed by an œdematous flooding or hæmorrhages, to which may perhaps be added trophic changes caused by disturbance of the nerve supply (Fig. 42)—set the stage for a variety of effects varying from a transient loss of function to necrosis and permanent disorganization of the tissues; these effects, although fundamentally similar, make themselves evident in characteristic fashion in the various ocular structures. Each of these may be thus involved; the resulting lesions which may occur may be summarized as follows:

OCULAR CONCUSSION INJURIES

1. *Lesions of the Conjunctiva*
   - (*a*) Hæmorrhages, œdema, chemosis.
   - (*b*) Bruising and lacerations.

2. *Lesions of the Cornea*
   - (*a*) Œdematous and hæmorrhagic changes.
     - (i) Epithelial opacities and erosions.
     - (ii) Interstitial œdematous opacities.
     - (iii) Blood-staining of the cornea.
     - (iv) Hæmorrhage into the corneal tissues.
     - (v) Folding of the corneal tissues.
       - (α) Folds of Bowman's membrane, lattice-like opacities.
       - (β) Folds of Descemet's membrane, striate keratopathy.
   - (*b*) Pigmentary deposits.
   - (*c*) Corneal lacerations.
     - (i) Partial lacerations.
     - (ii) Tears in Descemet's membrane.
     - (iii) Complete rupture of the cornea.

3. *Lesions of the Iris and Ciliary Body*
   - (*a*) Changes in the pupil and accommodation.
     - (i) Traumatic miosis and accommodative spasm.
     - (ii) Traumatic iridoplegia and cycloplegia.
   - (*b*) Vascular changes.
     - (i) Reactive hyperæmia and exudation.
     - (ii) Hæmorrhages (α) into the tissue of the iris and ciliary body.
       (β) traumatic hyphæma.
   - (*c*) Lacerations of the iris and ciliary body
     - (i) Interstitial tears of the sphincter.
     - (ii) Tears at the pupillary border, partial or complete.
     - (iii) Tears in the iris stroma.
     - (iv) Dehiscences of the pigmentary layer.
     - (v) Iridodialysis.

(vi) Irideremia (traumatic aniridia).
(vii) Iridoschisis.
(viii) Traumatic cyclodialysis; tears in the ciliary muscle; recession of the angle.
(ix) Retroflexion (inversion) of the iris.

(*d*) Inflammatory and atrophic changes
(i) Traumatic iridocyclitis.
(ii) Post-traumatic atrophy of the iris and ciliary body.
(iii) Acute necrosis of the iris and ciliary body.
(iv) Pigmentary changes; traumatic heterochromia.

4. *Lesions of the Lens and Zonule*

(*a*) Lenticular opacities.
(i) Vossius's ring opacity.
(ii) Discrete subepithelial opacities.
(α) Subepithelial disseminated opacities.
(β) Cobweb subcapsular opacities.
(iii) Traumatic rosette-shaped opacities.
(iv) Traumatic zonular cataract.
(v) Pre-senile and senile changes following concussion.
(vi) Diffuse concussion cataract.

(*b*) Subluxation and dislocation of the lens.

5. *Lesions of the Choroid*

(*a*) Vascular changes.
(i) Choroidal hæmorrhage.
(ii) Choroidal detachment.

(*b*) Choroidal lacerations.
(i) Direct and indirect choroidal rupture.
(ii) Rupture of the pigmentary epithelium.
(iii) Chorioretinal rupture.

(*c*) Traumatic choroiditis.

6. *Lesions of the Retina*

(*a*) Œdematous and atrophic changes.
(i) Concussion œdema.
(ii) Concussion necrosis.
(iii) Concussion changes at the macula.
(α) Macular œdema.
(β) Macular cysts and holes.
(γ) Traumatic macular atrophy of Haab.
(δ) Acute concussion necrosis.
(iv) Peripheral atrophic retinal changes.

(*b*) Vascular changes in the retina.
(i) Traumatic hæmorrhages.
(ii) Embolism and thrombosis.
(iii) Traumatic aneurysm.

(*c*) Retinal tears.

(*d*) Traumatic retinal detachment.

7. *Lesions at the Optic Disc*

(*a*) Papillitis and atrophy.

(*b*) Rupture and avulsion of the nerve.

8. *Effects on the Vitreous*
   (*a*) Vitreous liquefaction and opacification.
   (*b*) Vitreous hæmorrhages.
   (*c*) Vitreous detachment and herniation.

9. *Ruptures of the Sclera*
   (*a*) Contusion rupture.
      (i) Complete rupture, direct and indirect, typical and atypical.
      (ii) Incomplete rupture, direct and indirect, typical and atypical.
   (*b*) Rupture due to indirect force.

10. *Changes in Refraction*
   (*a*) Traumatic hypermetropia.
   (*b*) Traumatic myopia.

11. *Changes in the Ocular Tension*
   (*a*) Traumatic instability of the tension.
   (*b*) Traumatic glaucoma.
   (*c*) Traumatic hypotony.

This list seems long and formidable, but in fact it is essentially simple and integrated, illustrating the varied pictures formed by a consistent pathology on tissues which, because of the difference in their structure and physiology, vary greatly in their response to a common stimulus and, because of their delicacy, react thereto with unusual drama. No better example could be given of the unique interest of ophthalmic pathology, for in the minute microcosm of the eye and its adnexa there are enacted all the events with their manifold variations which may occur throughout the body in response to a single cause—here the reaction of highly vascularized tissues, there that of avascular tissue, elsewhere that of nervous tissue. Moreover, the interest of the pathology is heightened by the intriguing problems of the mechanics presented by the effects of an explosive force striking a number of structures so differently constituted, encased in a tough and resistant shell —some of them frail and delicate, others firm and solid, some fixed and others floating in a medium half-fluid, half-gel, none of them without vital importance and all of them readily liable to changes which can be accurately studied.

From the clinical point of view the various individual lesions habitually occur in groups. A severe contusion may, of course, disorganize and burst the eye; but in the case of milder lesions wherein a differentiation can be made, the anterior or the posterior part of the eye tends to be preferentially affected. The first to recognize the clinical significance of this was the French ophthalmologist Frenkel (1916–32), who gave so much thought to these injuries. The group of lesions commonly seen in the anterior segment of the globe is often known eponymously as the *anterior traumatic syndrome of Frenkel*: it usually comprises a traumatic mydriasis, a hyphæma, small tears near the pupillary margin of the iris, discrete punctate opacities of the lens, often a subluxation of this tissue and occasionally iridodialysis. The most common lesions occurring in the posterior segment of the globe are retinal œdema and sometimes hæmorrhages, a migration of retinal pigment into the vitreous, macular changes and sometimes tears in the choroid.

Clinically, the most dramatic lesions which are seen immediately after a severe concussion are intra-ocular hæmorrhage, cataract, tearing of the iris and gross detachment of the choroid and retina. The most common pathological findings in eyes which require excision, as indicated in a series of 104 cases reported by Rones and Wilder (1947), are as follows:

Cataract	29	Hæmorrhage: organized	8
Cataract, calcified	17	Detachment of retina	36
Dislocated lens	5	Detachment of choroid and ciliary body	6
Chronic endophthalmitis	48	Phthisis bulbi	6
Secondary glaucoma	32	Ossification of choroid	15
Staphyloma	6		
Hæmorrhage: recent	13		

These authors also found that the clinical diagnoses determining enucleation had the following incidence:

Secondary glaucoma	34
Recurrent inflammation	16
Recurrent hæmorrhage	4
Phthisis bulbi	3

The *clinical picture* appearing after such an injury varies greatly. A mild contusion may excite little ocular reaction apart from a transitory perilimbal injection, perhaps a slight aqueous flare, perhaps a traumatic iridoplegia with a vague feeling of irritability and discomfort. In this type of case the anterior segment of the eye is particularly affected and minor lesions such as a mild degree of iridoplegia, small tears and dehiscences of the iris, subluxation and subcapsular opacities of the lens, or a transient hyphæma may easily be missed unless early or minute examination of the eye is undertaken. It is probable that they are more often missed than not. It is interesting that Davidson (1936) found that small iridic lesions were seen in 50% of minor contusional traumata if sufficiently careful examination were made.

A moderately severe contusion, on the other hand, presents a characteristic immediate picture which is frequently difficult to assess accurately for some time after the accident owing to the swelling of the lids from œdema or hæmorrhage which may occur almost instantaneously. In such cases both the anterior and posterior segments of the globe are prone to suffer damage. In addition to suffusions of blood in the lids and perhaps some proptosis from an orbital hæmorrhage, the more gross and readily recognizable injuries may include conjunctival petechiæ and chemosis, an interstitial corneal opacity with considerable pericorneal injection denoting an irritative iridocyclitis, a dilated immobile pupil, a hyphæma in the anterior chamber, an absence of the fundus reflex if the vitreous is full of blood, while the tension may be low; an increase or variability in the depth of the anterior chamber or the presence of iridodonesis will indicate a displacement of the lens. There is usually some pain with considerable photophobia and lacrimation, while the vision is reduced sometimes to the mere perception of light, the projection of which may not be accurate.

In the assessment of the effects of these injuries it is to be noted that resolution may be delayed for long periods sometimes measured in years (vitreous hæmorrhage, blood-staining of the cornea), many of the sequelæ are permanent (ruptures, etc.), others are progressive (cataract) and some not amenable to treatment (macular changes, atrophy of the globe), while the onset of others may be delayed until some time after the accident (secondary glaucoma, infection, traumatic cyclitis, cataract, retinal detachment, shrinkage of the globe). It should always be remembered that an eye which may appear initially to have been lightly hurt—so slightly as to have attracted little attention at the time or even to be neglected both by the patient and his medical attendant—may develop major complications after some days or weeks (such as glaucoma, iridocyclitis or retinal detachment), and that in many cases the full effects of the accident may not be known for years when perhaps a cataract may develop. It follows that in general in such cases a *guarded prognosis should always be given*, for in addition to the more dramatic complications which may arise an eye which appears to be convalescing well may develop a recalcitrant traumatic iridocyclitis associated with a rise of tension which may destroy its function, or a persistent hypotony which may end in shrinkage, atrophy and blindness, while the the spectre of sympathetic disease occasionally arises to give cause for further anxiety.

The *treatment* of such injuries is usually expectant, calling for little action and much patience on the part of both surgeon and patient. At first —fortunately in those cases wherein early examination is difficult—little is usually required except rest with sedation if necessary, simple cleansing and bandaging; cool compresses which should not be overdone frequently give most relief. Atropine is usually unnecessary and may sometimes be inadvisable. This regime should be continued until the immediate effects of the injury clear sufficiently to allow full examination, when further treatment will depend on the nature of the damage sustained.

The more important lesions which may thus be caused will now be discussed *seriatim*.

Anderson. *Brit. J. Ophthal.*, **3,** 15 (1919).
Arlt. *Ueber d. Verletzungen des Auges,* Wien (1875).
Barnes and Trueta. *Brit. J. Surg.*, **30,** 74 (1942).
Barrow and Rhoads. *J. Amer. med. Ass.*, **125,** 900 (1944).
Berner. *Virchows Arch. path. Anat.*, **277,** 386 (1930).
Brunner. *Mschr. Ohrenheilk.*, **59,** 697, 763 (1925).
Campbell. *Brit. med. J.*, **1,** 966 (1941).
Cattaneo. *Ann. Ottal.*, **62,** 81, 161 (1934).
Clemedson. *Acta physiol. scand.*, **18,** Supp. 61 (1949).
Colenbrander. *Ophthalmologica,* **149,** 142 (1965).

Cooper. *On Wounds and Injuries of the Eye*, London (1859).
Courville. *Arch. Surg.*, **45**, 19 (1942).
J. forens. Sci., **7**, 1 (1962).
Cross. *Proc. roy. Soc. Med.*, **34**, 730 (1941).
Davidson. *Amer. J. Ophthal.*, **19**, 757 (1936).
Dean. *Kentucky med. J.*, **41**, 203 (1943).
Denker. *N.Y. St. J. Med.*, **44**, 379 (1944).
Denny-Brown. *Ann. intern. Med.*, **19**, 427 (1943).
Denny-Brown and Russell. *Brain*, **64**, 93 (1941).
Evans and Scheinker. *Arch. Neurol. Psychiat.*, **50**, 258 (1943).
J. Neurosurg., **1**, 306 (1944); **2**, 306 (1945); **3**, 101 (1946).
Förster. *Klin. Mbl. Augenheilk.*, **25**, Beil., 143 (1887).
Frenkel. *Ann. Oculist.* (Paris), **153**, 233 (1916); **155**, 78 (1918).
Arch. Ophtal., **48**, 5 (1931); **49**, 431 (1932).
Fuchs. *Atlas d. Histopathologie des Auges*, Wien (1923–27).
Fulton. *New Engl. J. Med.*, **226**, 1 (1942).
Holmes. *Brit. J. Ophthal.*, **2**, 353, 449, 506 (1918).
Brit. med. J., **2**, 193 (1919).
Jakob. *Histol. und histopath. Arbeiten ü. d. Grosshirnrinde*, (ed. Nissl and Alzheimer), Jena, **5**, 182 (1913).
Johnson. *Brit. J. Psychiat.*, **115**, 45 (1969).
Kilgore. *Amer. J. Ophthal.*, **25**, 1095 (1942).
Kinmonth. *Brit. med. J.*, **1**, 59 (1952).
Kinmonth and Simeone. *Brit. J. Surg.*, **39**, 333 (1952).
Kinmonth, Simeone and Perlow. *Surgery*, **26**, 452 (1949).
Lagrange. *Les fractures de l'orbite par les projectiles de guerre*, Paris (1917).
Atlas d'ophtalmoscopie de guerre, Paris (1918).
Le Grand. *Bull. Soc. belge Ophtal.*, No. 133, 222 (1963).
Lister. *Lancet*, **2**, 67 (1918).
Brit. J. Ophthal., **8**, 305 (1924).
McKee. *Amer. J. Ophthal.*, **6**, 725 (1923).
Ogilvie. *Trans. ophthal. Soc. U.K.*, **20**, 202 (1900).
Ormond. *Trans. ophthal. Soc. U.K.*, **37**, 60 (1917).
Paterson. *Lancet*, **2**, 717 (1942).
Proc. roy. Soc. Med., **37**, 556 (1944).
Pflugfelder. *Mschr. Psychiat. Neurol.*, **118**, 288, 379 (1949).
Pollock. *Illinois med. J.*, **83**, 165 (1943).
Praun. *Die Verletzungen des Auges*, Wiesbaden (1899).
Pugh. *Surg. Clin. N. Amer.*, **23**, 1589 (1943).
Rones and Wilder. *Amer. J. Ophthal.*, **28**, 1112 (1945); **30**, 1143 (1947).
Roscin. *v. Graefes Arch. Ophthal.*, **127**, 401 (1931).
Schaller, Tamaki and Newman. *Arch. Neurol. Psychiat.*, **37**, 1048 (1937); **45**, 1 (1941).
Scheinker. *J. Neurosurg.*, **4**, 255 (1947).
Schenk, Silcox and Godfrey. *U.S. Navy med. Bull.*, **42**, 802 (1944).
de Schweinitz. *Amer. J. Ophthal.*, **2**, 313 (1919).
Sédan and Alliès. *Rev. Oto-neuro-ophtal.*, **23**, 374 (1951).
Shapland. *Trans. ophthal. Soc. U.K.*, **66**, 376 (1946).
Smith. *Amer. J. Ophthal.*, **32**, 959 (1949).
Stallard. *Postgrad. med. J.*, **16**, 179 (1940).
Stoewer. *Klin. Mbl. Augenheilk.*, **45** (1), 347 (1907).
Symonds. *Proc. roy. Soc. Med.*, **34**, 289 (1941).
Lancet, **1**, 1 (1962).
Symonds and Ritchie Russell. *Lancet*, **1**, 7 (1943).
Thomson. *Trans. ophthal. Soc. U.K.*, **67**, 245 (1947).
Tillema. *Arch. Ophthal.*, **17**, 586 (1937).
Tooke. *Amer. J. Ophthal.*, **1**, 223 (1918).
Canad. med. Ass. J., **8**, 308 (1918).
Travers. *Aust. New Zealand J. Surg.*, **12**, 74 (1942).
Trueta, Barclay, Daniel *et al.* *Studies of Renal Circulation*, Oxford (1947).
Vogt. *Lhb. u. Atlas d. Spaltlampenmikroskopie d. lebenden Auges*, Berlin, 1st ed. (1921); 2nd ed. (1930–41).
Wagenmann. *Die Verletzungen des Auges, Graefe-Saemisch Hb. d. gest Augenheilk.*, 3rd ed., Leipzig, **1**, 397 (1915).
Wakeley. *Glasg. med. J.*, **139**, 91 (1943).
Walker, Kollros and Case. *J. Neurosurg.*, **1**, 103 (1944).
Weidenthal. *Arch. Ophthal.*, **71**, 77 (1964).
Weidenthal and Schepens. *Amer. J. Ophthal.*, **62**, 465 (1966).
Wescott. *Illinois med. J.*, **83**, 170 (1943).
Wilson. *Trans. ophthal. Soc. U.K.*, **33**, 92 (1917).
Windle, Groat and Fox. *Surg. Gyn. Obstet.*, **79**, 561 (1944).
Windle, Rambach, de Arellano, *et al.* *J. Neurosurg.*, **3**, 157 (1946).
Wittenbrook. *J. nerv. ment. Dis.*, **94**, 170 (1941).
Wolter. *Amer. J. Ophthal.*, **56**, 785 (1963).
Zorab. *Brit. J. Ophthal.*, **29**, 579 (1945).
Zuckerman. *Trans. ophthal. Soc. U.K.*, **61**, 45 (1941).

Contusion Effects on the Conjunctiva

In the conjunctiva contusions may produce hæmorrhages which may vary from small petechiæ to extravasations of considerable size. These of themselves are of little moment if produced by local injury but a SUB-

PLATE I

SUBCONJUNCTIVAL HÆMORRHAGES.

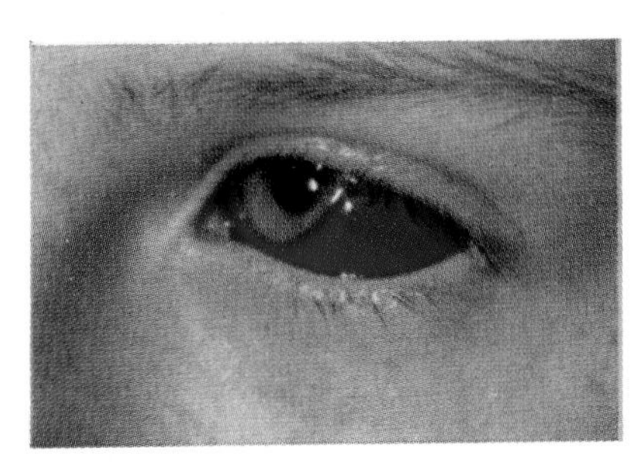

FIG. 1.

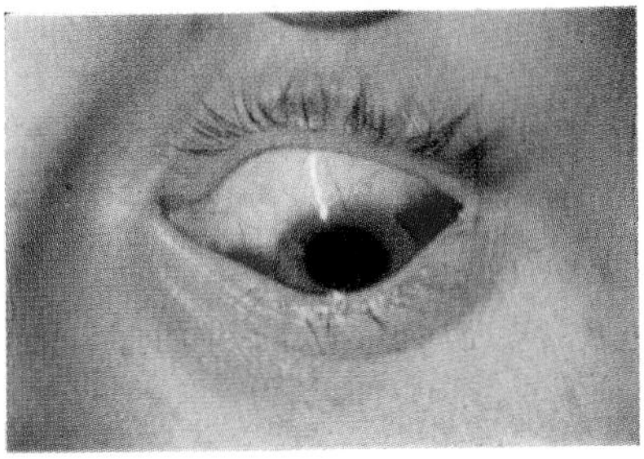

FIG. 2.

FIGS. 1 AND 2.—Subconjunctival hæmorrhage following a blow from a stick.

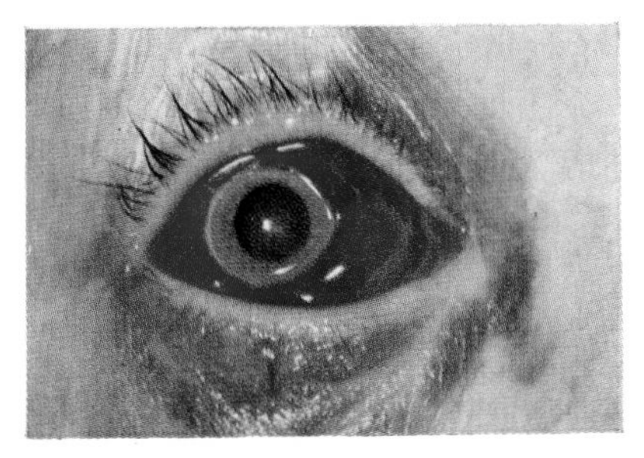

FIG. 3.

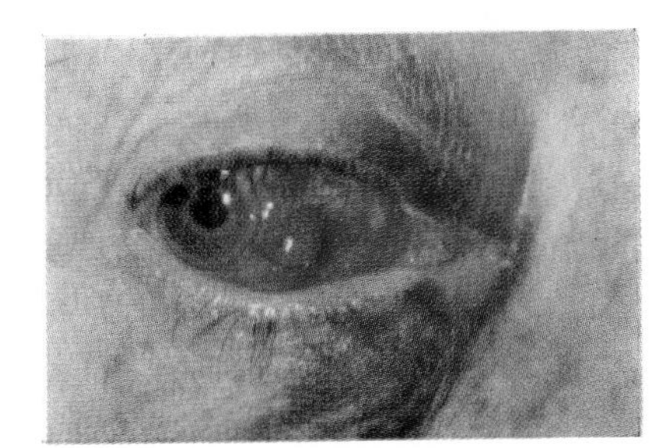

FIG. 4.

FIGS. 3 AND 4.—Massive hæmorrhage following a blow in a patient with defective blood clotting associated with cirrhosis and portal hypertension. Fig. 4 is at a later stage than Fig. 3.

[*To face p.* 80.

CONJUNCTIVAL HÆMORRHAGE may be due to the tracking forwards of blood from the orbit following a fracture of the orbital walls or the base of the skull. The diagnostic importance of these will be discussed subsequently,[1] but as a general rule they can be differentiated from local bleeding by the fact that, when a fracture is the cause, the densest and most extensive part of the hæmorrhage is posteriorly where no edge is usually apparent, while anteriorly it may not reach the limbus; in the case of local bleeding, on the other hand, unless it is very extensive, the densest area is usually on the anterior part of the globe and it can be seen to fade away or disappear towards the equator (Plate I, Figs. 1–4). Moreover, in bleeding from a distant fracture the local blood is purplish in colour from the commencement (not bright red) and subconjunctival in site (rather than intraconjunctival, moving with this membrane). The clinical evolution and management of such cases have already been described.[2]

CONJUNCTIVAL ŒDEMA and perhaps CHEMOSIS may occur; in the absence of a perforating wound this is of no consequence. The clinical appearance which has already been described[3] should be distinguished from that due to traumatic emphysema.

BRUISING AND LACERATIONS of the conjunctiva may occur owing to the direct impact but they are rarely extensive owing to the thinness and the extreme mobility of this membrane: their treatment will be discussed subsequently.

As a late complication the occurrence of thickened EPITHELIAL PLAQUES has been noted some years after a contusion (Lister and Hancock, 1903). They consist of several layers of cells forming a well-defined and localized hyperplasia somewhat resembling the epithelial plaques which may occur in the cornea of injured eyes subject to continued irritation; it is uncertain, however, if these can be considered a direct sequel to a concussion injury.[4]

Concussion Effects on the Cornea

The effects of injuries from concussions on the corneal tissues form, in the main, two pathological types. The corneal tissues may be primarily damaged and a concussion-necrosis occurs, a change seen particularly in the endothelium, while severe injuries may involve lacerations of its substance in all degrees up to complete rupture. More commonly, however, these changes are secondary, the substance of the cornea being invaded by œdematous fluid or hæmorrhagic products either through the damaged endothelium or from the dilated perilimbal plexus; the resulting infiltrations frequently present dramatic clinical pictures.

ŒDEMATOUS AND HÆMORRHAGIC CHANGES

EPITHELIAL LESIONS

The impact of a blunt body may damage the corneal epithelium directly, causing a superficial œdematous opacity or an abrasion: these will be discussed under the heading of Wounds. It is probable, however, that

[1] See pp. 268, 287
[2] Vol. VIII, p. 34.
[3] Vol. VIII, p. 42.
[4] Vol. VIII, p. 1148.

such a condition may arise secondarily for a sudden and forceful contusion on the cornea may damage the endothelium, the ensuing œdema from which may appear as a localized collection of fluid among the epithelial cells of the corresponding area, giving the appearance of an erosion (Chandler, 1945).

INTERSTITIAL ŒDEMATOUS OPACITIES

Shortly after a severe concussion œdematous changes may be evident in the substantia propria, forming typically a disc-shaped opacity 2 to 3 mm. in diameter but occasionally taking the form of ring-shaped opacities of a similar size; the latter, however, are more often seen in injuries due to explosions wherein the effects of concussion are complicated by the lodgement in the cornea of minute foreign bodies. The lesion is caused by œdema and the affected area of the interstitial portion of the cornea is hazy, mottled and swollen, staining diffusely with fluorescein, particularly in its deeper layers (Plate II, Figs. 1 and 2); the separation and swelling of the corneal lamellæ by fluid may give the œdematous area a criss-cross striated appearance, which may be accentuated by folds in Bowman's (the LATTICE-LIKE OPACITY of Caspar, 1903–16) and Descemet's membranes (the THREAD-LIKE OPACITY of Schirmer, 1896; Fuchs, 1902). Although the epithelium, Descemet's membrane and the endothelium may remain structurally intact, the condition seems usually to be associated with and is probably due to a temporary disturbance of the cells of the corneal endothelium, their permeability being altered so that aqueous gets free access to the corneal tissue, a change presumably due to the direct effect of the concussion. Such appearances have been described by several writers.[1] The lesion is associated with some pericorneal injection and subjective irritation, but it clears up without specific treatment, frequently in a few days, although its final disappearance may be delayed for some weeks.

A more diffuse and massive œdematous lesion is associated with tears in Descemet's membrane accompanied by a complete solution of the continuity of the endothelium. Here again the opacity tends to clear up after the endothelium has re-clothed the torn area on the inner surface of the cornea, but in more severe cases wherein the laceration of the tissues has been more extensive and tearing of the corneal fibres has also occurred, permanent cicatricial opacities may result.

The mechanism of the occurrence of such an œdema has already been discussed at length.[2] Normally, apart from the controlled metabolic interchange, the corneal endothelium is waterproof, but if this layer becomes freely permeable either by damage to the cells or owing to an actual solution of its continuity by a tear, the corneal tissues imbibe fluid from the aqueous, becoming cloudy and opaque, the effect produced being comparable to the cloudy swelling seen at the lips of a corneal wound or at the edges of

[1] Blaauw (1911), Meller (1913–17), Caspar (1916), Pichler (1916), Palich-Szántó (1917), Lampert (1924), Löwenstein (1931), and others.

[2] See Vol. VIII, p. 661 and p. 666 for a summary of the causes of secondary corneal œdema.

PLATE II

Concussion Changes in the Cornea.

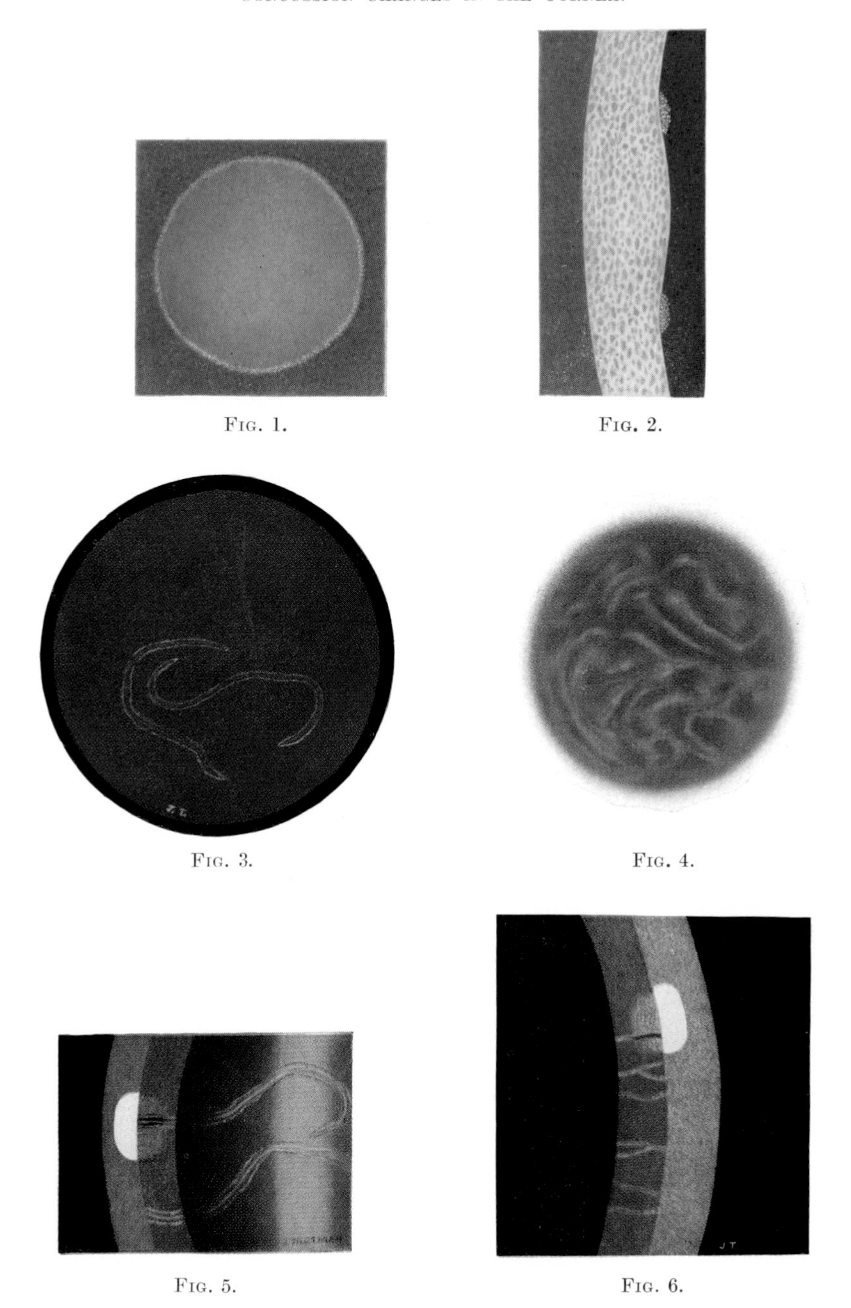

Fig. 1. Fig. 2.

Fig. 3. Fig. 4.

Fig. 5. Fig. 6.

Figs. 1 and 2.—Contusion œdema of the cornea, showing the swelling of the tissue in the central area and a ring of golden pigment on the endothelium surrounding it (A. Loewenstein).

Figs. 3 and 5.—Ruptures of Descemet's membrane (J. H. Doggart).

Figs. 4 and 6.—Folds in Descemet's membrane.

an ulcer.[1] Such an opacity tends to remain until the imperviousness of the endothelium is restored when the condition rapidly resolves unless the corneal lamellæ have themselves been damaged or lacerated.

An unusual result of a contusion was reported by Muller (1949). After a blow by the branch of a tree a keratitis with hypopyon developed leading eventually to a mosaic degeneration of Bowman's membrane (" crocodile skin " degeneration of Vogt).

As a rare delayed complication EPITHELIAL PLAQUES, similar to those occurring in the conjunctiva, have been noted on the corneæ of eyes which have suffered injury and have been subjected to continued irritation (Hocquart, 1881).[2]

BLOOD-STAINING OF THE CORNEA

Staining of the cornea by the decomposition products of blood pigment absorbed from the anterior chamber is a somewhat uncommon result of a *contusion which is associated with a massive hyphæma and raised intra-ocular pressure*; as a rule to produce this effect the anterior chamber must be completely filled with blood, whether the hæmorrhage has occurred as a direct result of the injury or has appeared after some days as a secondary hæmorrhage, and a raised ocular tension seems to be a usual accompaniment. Bilateral cases are uncommon but have been reported when both eyes have been involved in the same trauma (Gradle, 1922; Norris, 1949). The clinical appearance and pathology of this condition have been fully described in a previous volume.[3] It is still a moot point whether the granular products of hæmoglobin found in the interstitial tissues of the cornea are absorbed through a damaged endothelium (Parsons, 1904; Elschnig, 1919) or enter this tissue from the periphery (Wood, 1935); both routes may be taken, the first being the more important.

The opacity, which is formed by innumerable highly refractile granules scattered throughout the lamellæ, and pigmented particles in the corneal corpuscles derived from decomposition products of hæmoglobin together with phagocytic cells, usually occupies the greater part of the cornea in the initial stages (Figs. 45–7); sometimes a disciform central area only is involved (Schousboë and Morard, 1935) (Plate III, Fig. 3). At first a red rusty brown, it gradually changes colour to a greenish yellow or white and disappears with extreme slowness, the process frequently involving a period of two years or more. Although the periphery of the cornea may become vascularized, the tissues eventually become clear, probably owing to the scavenging action of phagocytic cells; good visual acuity may be obtained eventually and the eye may ultimately settle down (history of seven years in a bilateral case injured by the branch of a tree—Norris, 1949). Such functional recovery, however, is unusual owing to damage to the other structures of the eye; thus in a series of 9 cases Rychener (1944) reported no instance of the recovery of useful vision even although the cornea cleared, while 5 of the 9 eyes had to be

[1] Leber (1873), Panas (1878), Elschnig (1894), Fuchs (1917), Juler (1930), and others.
[2] See p. 81 and Vol. VIII, p. 1148.
[3] See Vol. VIII, p. 982.

in contusions sustained as birth injuries (Figs. 3 to 6), and a similar rupture is liable to occur in the absence of injury when the cornea is stretched or strained, as in buphthalmos or conical cornea.

At the time of the injury the rupture is usually obscured by coincident œdema of the corneal tissues, but as the endothelium repairs the defect by laying down a new membrane, this generalized opacity tends to clear up; in this event the site of the rupture may eventually be seen only with difficulty, appearing optically as bright double contour lines with the slit-lamp (Plate II, Figs. 3 and 5). At other times the trauma and œdema cause permanent damage to the corneal lamellæ so that the formation of fibrous tissues leaves a permanent interstitial opacity; frequently a high degree of myopia or irregular astigmatism results (—14 D, Lloyd, 1938) with occasionally the development of a deformity resembling keratoglobus (—16 D, Straub, 1951); sometimes overactivity of the endothelium gives rise to the formation of duplications in Descemet's membrane (Coats, 1907),[1] or the development of hyalin-like strands forming ridges on the posterior corneal surface or spanning the concavity of the cornea in the anterior chamber, where delicate lattice-like networks may be formed (Lloyd, 1938; Zanen and Rausin, 1949; Gasteiger, 1950)[2]; exceptionally, the endothelium and its underlying glass-membrane may grow over the angle of the anterior chamber and spread across the surface of the iris (Wagenmann, 1889–96).

COMPLETE RUPTURE OF THE CORNEA is a rare event which occurs only on the impact of severe force directly upon this tissue; on the application of a broad-based force the sclera usually bursts at its weakest point near the corneo-scleral margin. If, however, the cornea is pushed quickly into the globe the pressure so generated within the eye may be such that this tissue has to give way; the presence of an old cicatrix derived, perhaps, from an ulcer, may increase the tendency. The direct blow from a fist, the horn of a cow or a blunt implement on the cornea itself, therefore, or even a blast injury as by the compression-wave from an air-gun (Callaert, 1912), may rupture this tissue, particularly in children in whom the cornea is weaker; thus among 17 cases reported by Müller (1895) only 4 were above 20 years of age. Usually the rupture is linear, small and near the limbus, perhaps 2 to 4 mm. in length; but extensive flap-shaped wounds may occur extending over a large arc of the limbus and running towards the apex of the cornea, while in extreme cases this tissue may be almost completely detached round the periphery.

The force involved in such injuries and the enormous intra-ocular pressure suddenly generated make prolapse of the intra-ocular tissues invariable. The smaller ruptures near the limbus are associated with a prolapse of the iris, while in the case of larger ruptures the lens, the vitreous and a varying proportion of the uveal tract may be extruded. If such

[1] Vol. VIII, p. 711. [2] Vol. VIII, p. 726.

an ulcer.[1] Such an opacity tends to remain until the imperviousness of the endothelium is restored when the condition rapidly resolves unless the corneal lamellæ have themselves been damaged or lacerated.

An unusual result of a contusion was reported by Muller (1949). After a blow by the branch of a tree a keratitis with hypopyon developed leading eventually to a mosaic degeneration of Bowman's membrane (" crocodile skin " degeneration of Vogt).

As a rare delayed complication EPITHELIAL PLAQUES, similar to those occurring in the conjunctiva, have been noted on the corneæ of eyes which have suffered injury and have been subjected to continued irritation (Hocquart, 1881).[2]

BLOOD-STAINING OF THE CORNEA

Staining of the cornea by the decomposition products of blood pigment absorbed from the anterior chamber is a somewhat uncommon result of a *contusion which is associated with a massive hyphæma and raised intra-ocular pressure*; as a rule to produce this effect the anterior chamber must be completely filled with blood, whether the hæmorrhage has occurred as a direct result of the injury or has appeared after some days as a secondary hæmorrhage, and a raised ocular tension seems to be a usual accompaniment. Bilateral cases are uncommon but have been reported when both eyes have been involved in the same trauma (Gradle, 1922; Norris, 1949). The clinical appearance and pathology of this condition have been fully described in a previous volume.[3] It is still a moot point whether the granular products of hæmoglobin found in the interstitial tissues of the cornea are absorbed through a damaged endothelium (Parsons, 1904; Elschnig, 1919) or enter this tissue from the periphery (Wood, 1935); both routes may be taken, the first being the more important.

The opacity, which is formed by innumerable highly refractile granules scattered throughout the lamellæ, and pigmented particles in the corneal corpuscles derived from decomposition products of hæmoglobin together with phagocytic cells, usually occupies the greater part of the cornea in the initial stages (Figs. 45–7); sometimes a disciform central area only is involved (Schousboë and Morard, 1935) (Plate III, Fig. 3). At first a red rusty brown, it gradually changes colour to a greenish yellow or white and disappears with extreme slowness, the process frequently involving a period of two years or more. Although the periphery of the cornea may become vascularized, the tissues eventually become clear, probably owing to the scavenging action of phagocytic cells; good visual acuity may be obtained eventually and the eye may ultimately settle down (history of seven years in a bilateral case injured by the branch of a tree—Norris, 1949). Such functional recovery, however, is unusual owing to damage to the other structures of the eye; thus in a series of 9 cases Rychener (1944) reported no instance of the recovery of useful vision even although the cornea cleared, while 5 of the 9 eyes had to be

[1] Leber (1873), Panas (1878), Elschnig (1894), Fuchs (1917), Juler (1930), and others.
[2] See p. 81 and Vol. VIII, p. 1148.
[3] See Vol. VIII, p. 982.

FIGS. 45–7.—BLOOD-STAINING OF THE CORNEA.

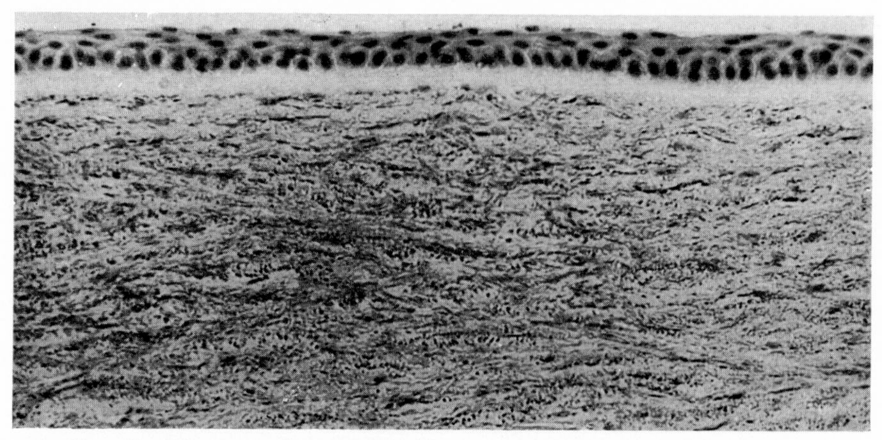

FIG. 45.—The stroma is peppered with crystals of hæmosiderin (N. Ashton).

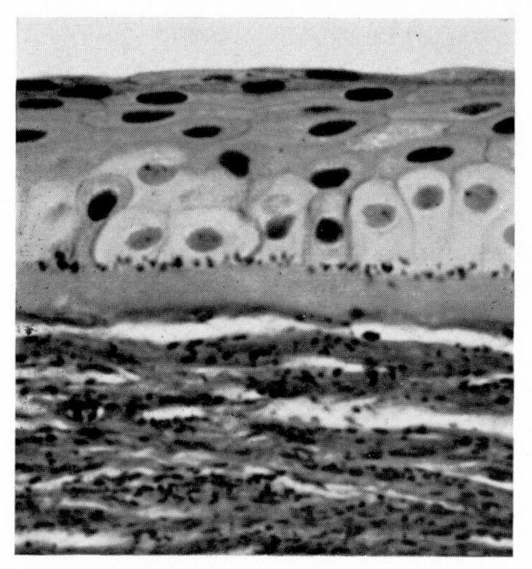

FIG. 46.—Minute refractile bodies packing the corneal lamellæ and lying between Bowman's membrane and the epithelium (W. A. Manschot).

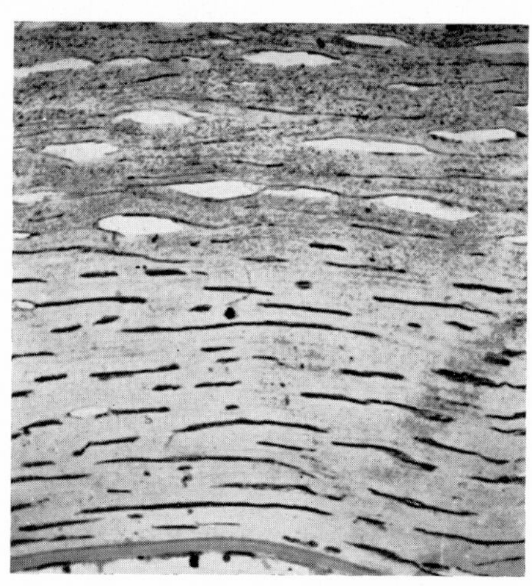

FIG. 47.—The two types of corneal staining. Below, large accumulations of pigment between the lamellæ; above, the minute refractile granules lying within the lamellæ. In a narrow intermediate zone both types of deposition are seen (W. A. Manschot).

excised mainly because of the intractable pain of the associated glaucoma, a disappointing outcome which is by no means unique (Fig. 48) (Leoz Ortin, 1943; Thygeson and Beard, 1952; and others).

Treatment is unavailing for once blood-staining has developed in the cornea the only remedy is time. Prophylactic measures to prevent its occurrence are therefore of the utmost urgency, the aim being both to evacuate the blood and to control the rise of tension, which appears to be an important factor in the development of the corneal infiltration; these will be discussed subsequently in the section on traumatic hyphæma.[1]

Blood-staining of the cornea is to be distinguished from an occasional HÆMORRHAGE INTO THE CORNEAL TISSUE, which usually takes the form of a migration of blood corpuscles into the peripheral parts of the cornea from a hyphæma or a subconjunctival hæmorrhage following a contusion, or it may arise from newly formed blood vessels as in interstitial keratitis or mustard-gas keratitis. Sometimes the hæmorrhage stains the peripheral parts of the corneal parenchyma a brownish-yellow colour, sometimes the staining is concentrated in Descemet's zone, while at other times a linear migration of blood corpuscles may be observed on the surface of Bowman's membrane.

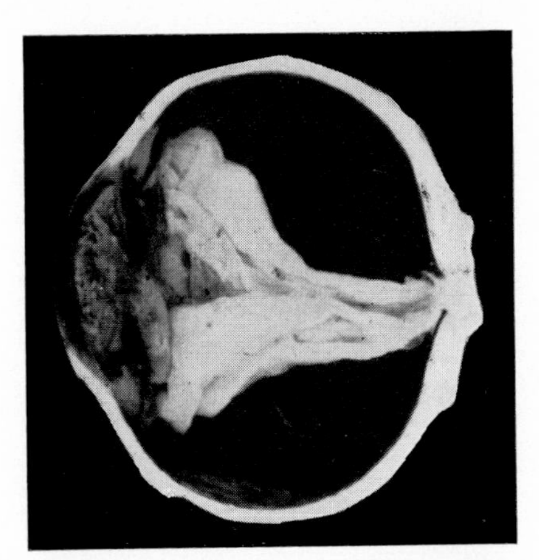

FIG. 48.—OCULAR CONTUSION DUE TO A BLOW.

The anterior chamber is filled with blood and the substance of the cornea is deeply stained. The lens is missing, the retina is totally detached and degenerate (Museum, Inst. Ophthal.).

FOLDING OF THE CORNEAL TISSUES

FOLDS OF BOWMAN'S MEMBRANE are an occasional result of concussions when a force impinges directly on the cornea, particularly when hypotony and inflammatory changes supervene. The appearance is that of grey ridges with a double optical contour sometimes assuming complex geometrical shapes (the LATTICE-LIKE OPACITIES of Caspar, 1903). This condition has already been described and illustrated[2]; no specific treatment is indicated.

FOLDS OF DESCEMET'S MEMBRANE are much more common, producing a deep striate opacity (TRAUMATIC STRIATE KERATOPATHY); they occur after injuries associated with hypotony but are more typical of perforating wounds than of contusions (Plate II, Figs. 4 and 6). The delicate grey striæ with their double optical contour, sometimes producing a lattice-like pattern and at other times associated with a diffuse œdematous opacity of the parenchyma, have already been described.[3] A somewhat similar appearance may result from prolonged tight bandaging. Treatment is expectant.

[1] p. 96. [2] Vol. VIII, p. 701. [3] Vol. VIII, p. 705.

PIGMENTARY DEPOSITS on the posterior surface of the cornea, which usually appear golden on oblique illumination (Plate II, Figs. 2 and 6), are occasionally seen after a concussion. These are derived from the iris and are usually scattered diffusely and irregularly over a wide area; the migration of iris pigment into the anterior chamber may be an immediate effect of the injury or be due to a consequent traumatic iritis. Occasionally, however, the deposition takes on an annular form corresponding to the pupillary margin, the appearance resembling Vossius's ring on the anterior lens capsule; such an occurrence may be due to the cornea being momentarily forced into apposition with the iris at the time of the impact of the blow (Alajmo, 1927). It is to be remembered that a concussion injury may temporarily abolish the anterior chamber so that contact of the cornea with the iris is possible (Knapp, 1883; Fromaget, 1911; Brons, 1931).

LACERATIONS OF THE CORNEA

When considerable force is involved in the concussion, the cornea may be forcibly indented so that INTERSTITIAL FRACTURES OF ITS TISSUE occur; Bowman's membrane and some of the corneal lamellæ may be torn or

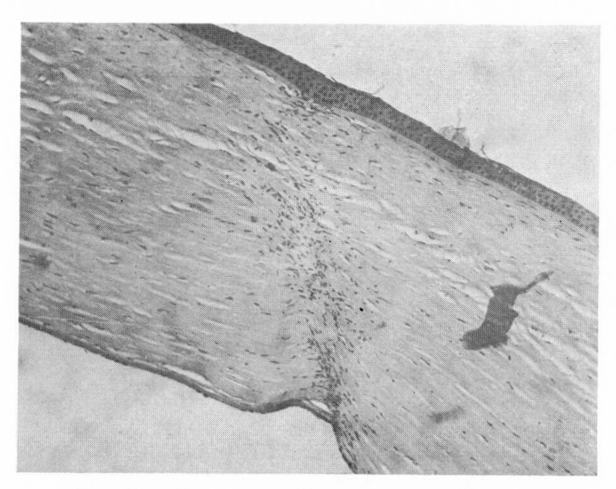

FIG. 49.—CONCUSSION INJURY TO THE CORNEA.
A 12-year-old boy was struck in the left eye by the end of a whip. The same case as Fig. 39 (J. R. Wolter).

fibrillated (Pascheff, 1918), while a fracture extending across the cornea involving the substantia propria but leaving the epithelium intact has resulted from the sudden and forceful application of direct pressure[1] (Fig. 49). It is probable that Bowman's membrane and the epithelium survive in these cases because of their elasticity, while the fibres of the substantia propria give way, sometimes in company with Descemet's membrane. The lesion is associated with a circumcorneal injection, miosis and often intra-ocular damage (iridodialysis and subluxation of the lens—Herrmann, 1906), and there is always much pain, photophobia, lacrimation and blepharospasm.

[1] Herrmann (1906), Majewski (1907), Gallenga (1928), Toselli (1950), Wolter (1963).

Initially the fracture, which can take on various forms (linear, V-shaped, and so on), may be largely hidden by a cloudy swelling and œdema of the corneal tissues, and ultimately such a lesion, of course, leaves a permanent opacity.

TEARS IN DESCEMET'S MEMBRANE are more common and are a typical result of sudden compression of the globe, for when the cornea is thus forcibly

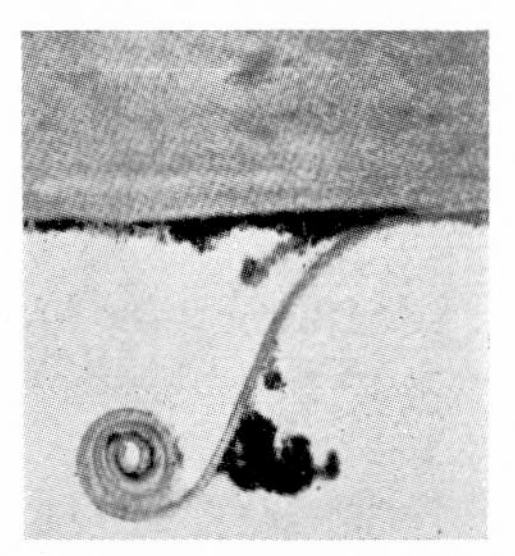

FIG. 50.—RUPTURE OF DESCEMET'S MEMBRANE.

Occurring as a birth injury during labour. A section of the posterior part of the cornea, showing separation and curling of Descemet's membrane with massing of pigment upon it (W. E. Thomson and L. Buchanan).

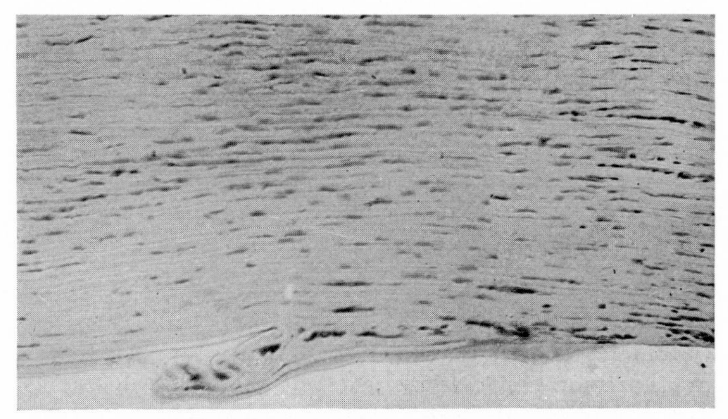

FIG. 51.—RUPTURE AND FOLDING OF DESCEMET'S MEMBRANE (N. Ashton).

indented this membrane with its slight elasticity readily gives way. Usually a few long, sinuous or crescentic tears are formed, sometimes as multiple short dehiscences, while occasionally the membrane curls up at its torn edges or forms falciform detachments floating in the anterior chamber (Figs. 50–51). The clinical appearance of these ruptures has already been fully described[1] and need not detain us further; the rupture usually leaves a gap in Descemet's endothelium, a circumstance which distinguishes such a lesion from a fold in the membrane wherein the endothelium is intact; but a subendothelial rupture with tearing of the deeper lamellæ has been recorded as a rarity (Gallenga, 1928). We have already seen that such tears are sometimes found

[1] Vol. VIII, p. 707.

in contusions sustained as birth injuries (Figs. 3 to 6), and a similar rupture is liable to occur in the absence of injury when the cornea is stretched or strained, as in buphthalmos or conical cornea.

At the time of the injury the rupture is usually obscured by coincident œdema of the corneal tissues, but as the endothelium repairs the defect by laying down a new membrane, this generalized opacity tends to clear up; in this event the site of the rupture may eventually be seen only with difficulty, appearing optically as bright double contour lines with the slit-lamp (Plate II, Figs. 3 and 5). At other times the trauma and œdema cause permanent damage to the corneal lamellæ so that the formation of fibrous tissues leaves a permanent interstitial opacity; frequently a high degree of myopia or irregular astigmatism results (—14 D, Lloyd, 1938) with occasionally the development of a deformity resembling keratoglobus (—16 D, Straub, 1951); sometimes overactivity of the endothelium gives rise to the formation of duplications in Descemet's membrane (Coats, 1907),[1] or the development of hyalin-like strands forming ridges on the posterior corneal surface or spanning the concavity of the cornea in the anterior chamber, where delicate lattice-like networks may be formed (Lloyd, 1938; Zanen and Rausin, 1949; Gasteiger, 1950)[2]; exceptionally, the endothelium and its underlying glass-membrane may grow over the angle of the anterior chamber and spread across the surface of the iris (Wagenmann, 1889–96).

COMPLETE RUPTURE OF THE CORNEA is a rare event which occurs only on the impact of severe force directly upon this tissue; on the application of a broad-based force the sclera usually bursts at its weakest point near the corneo-scleral margin. If, however, the cornea is pushed quickly into the globe the pressure so generated within the eye may be such that this tissue has to give way; the presence of an old cicatrix derived, perhaps, from an ulcer, may increase the tendency. The direct blow from a fist, the horn of a cow or a blunt implement on the cornea itself, therefore, or even a blast injury as by the compression-wave from an air-gun (Callaert, 1912), may rupture this tissue, particularly in children in whom the cornea is weaker; thus among 17 cases reported by Müller (1895) only 4 were above 20 years of age. Usually the rupture is linear, small and near the limbus, perhaps 2 to 4 mm. in length; but extensive flap-shaped wounds may occur extending over a large arc of the limbus and running towards the apex of the cornea, while in extreme cases this tissue may be almost completely detached round the periphery.

The force involved in such injuries and the enormous intra-ocular pressure suddenly generated make prolapse of the intra-ocular tissues invariable. The smaller ruptures near the limbus are associated with a prolapse of the iris, while in the case of larger ruptures the lens, the vitreous and a varying proportion of the uveal tract may be extruded. If such

[1] Vol. VIII, p. 711. [2] Vol. VIII, p. 726.

PLATES III AND IV

CONCUSSION EFFECTS ON THE ANTERIOR SEGMENT

[To face p. 88.

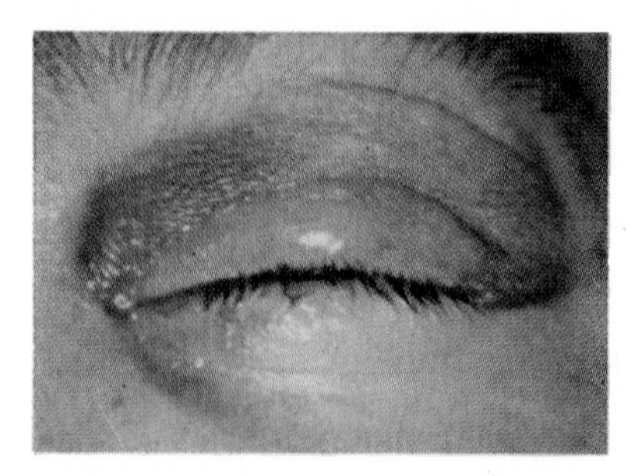

FIG. 1.—Black eye due to orbital hæmorrhage resulting from an air-gun pellet.

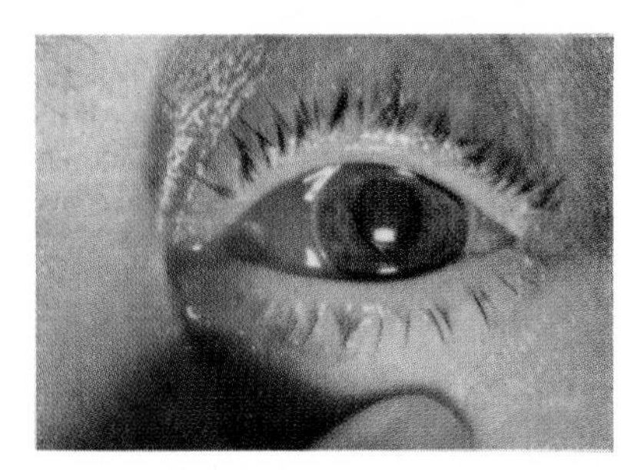

FIG. 2.—The same case as Fig. 1, showing a conjunctival wound on the nasal side and traumatic mydriasis.

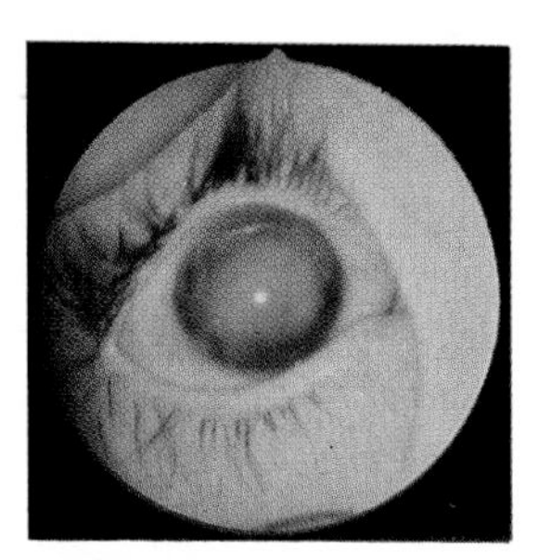

FIG. 3.—Blood-staining of the cornea, following a traumatic hyphæma due to a cricket ball.

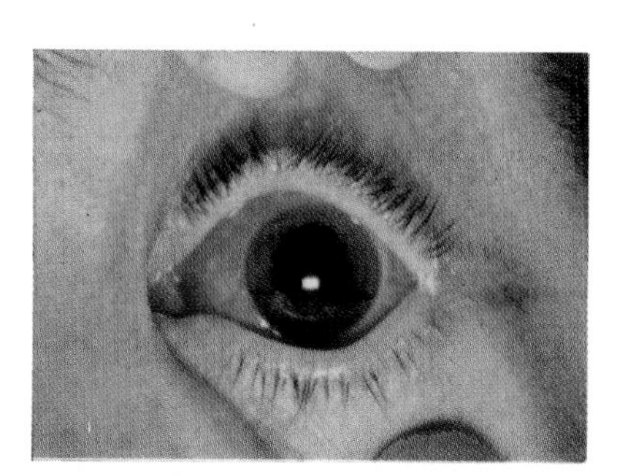

FIG. 4.—The same case as Figs. 1 and 2; the injured eye after five days showing a traumatic hyphæma.

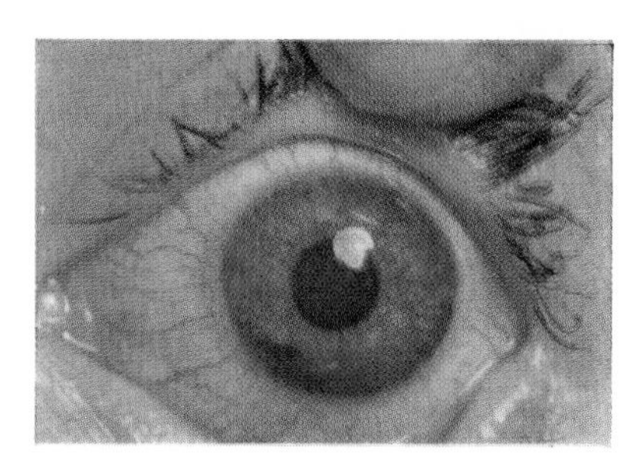

FIG. 5.—Traumatic hyphæma.

PLATE IV

CONTUSION EFFECTS ON THE IRIS.

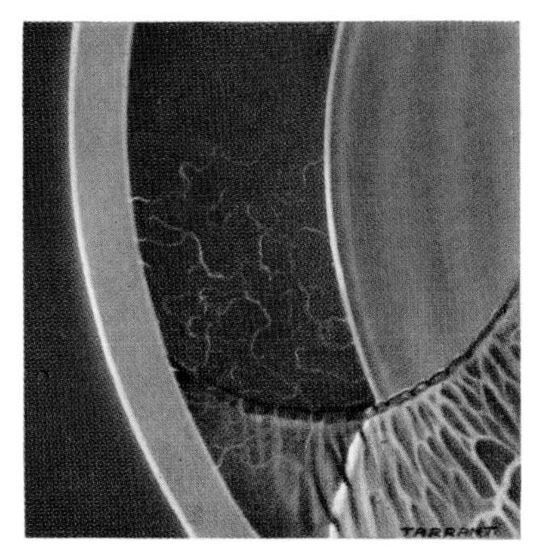

FIG. 1.—Fibrinous exudate into the anterior chamber.

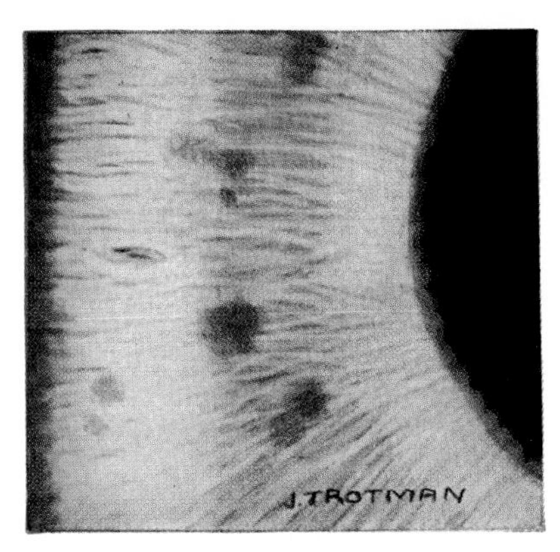

FIG. 2.—Hæmorrhages in the iris (J. H. Doggart).

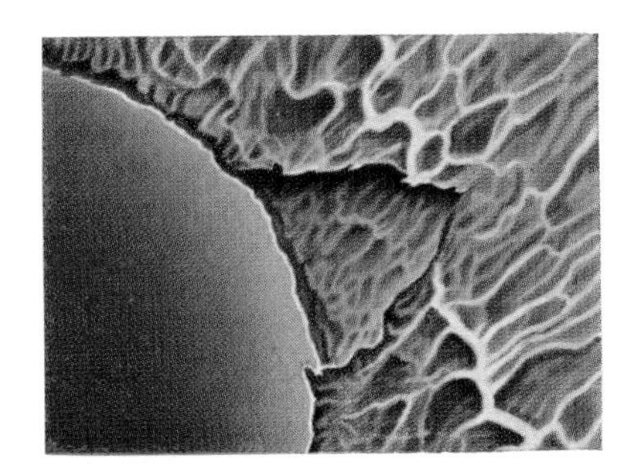

FIG. 3.—Rupture of the stroma.

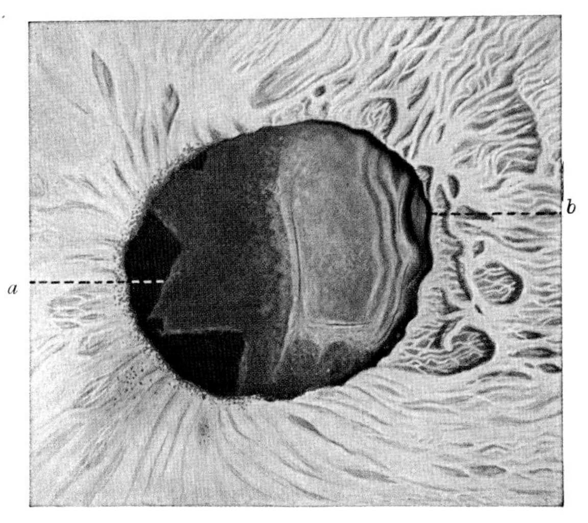

FIG. 4.—Rupture of the sphincter: *a*, traumatic rosette; *b*, blood-tinged prolapse of vitreous (A. Vogt).

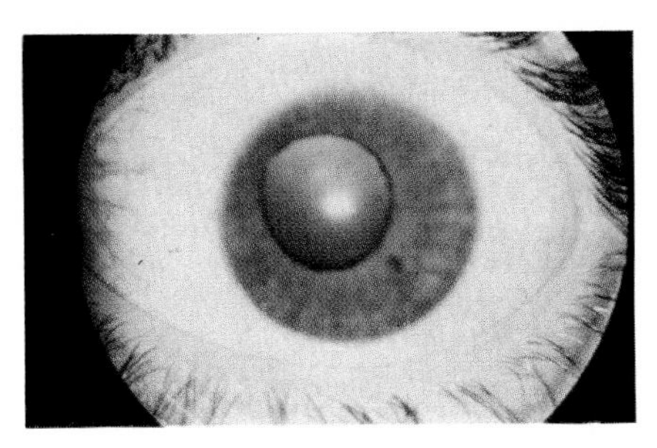

FIG. 5.—Traumatic mydriasis with rupture of the pupillary margin following contusion by a stone.

extensive damage has not been caused, however, the prognosis may be good, for excision of the prolapsed iris tissue and accurate suturing of the corneal wound usually result in good healing. The whole subject of rupture of the globe will be considered more fully at a later stage.[1]

Alajmo. *Boll. Oculist.*, **6,** 578 (1927).
Blaauw. *Ophthal. Rec.*, **20,** 59 (1911).
Brons. *Danish ophthal. Soc.* (1930). See *Zbl. ges. Ophthal.*, **25,** 534 (1931).
Callaert. *Klin. Mbl. Augenheilk.*, **50** (2), 382 (1912).
Caspar. *Klin. Mbl. Augenheilk.*, **41** (2), 289 (1903); **57,** 385 (1916).
Chandler. *Amer. J. Ophthal.*, **28,** 355 (1945).
Coats. *Trans. ophthal. Soc. U.K.*, **27,** 48 (1907).
Elschnig. *Klin. Mbl. Augenheilk.*, **32,** 25 (1894); **63,** 10 (1919).
Fromaget. *Bull. Soc. franç. Ophtal.*, **28,** 346 (1911).
Fuchs. *Trans. ophthal. Soc. U.K.*, **22,** 15 (1902).
v. Graefes Arch. Ophthal., **92,** 145 (1917).
Gallenga. *Boll. Oculist.*, **7,** 1089 (1928).
Gasteiger. *Dtsch. Gesundh.-Wes.*, **5,** 616 (1950).
Gradle. *Amer. J. Ophthal.*, **5,** 638 (1922).
Herrmann. *Die Kontusionsverletzungen d. Auges in klin. u. path.-anat. Beziehung* (Diss.), Leipzig (1906).
Hocquart. *Arch. Ophtal.*, **1,** 289 (1881).
Juler. *Trans. ophthal. Soc. U.K.*, **50,** 118 (1930).
Knapp. *Arch. Augenheilk.*, **12,** 85 (1883).
Lampert. *Arch. Ophtal.*, **41,** 567 (1924).
Leber. *v. Graefes Arch. Ophthal.*, **19** (2), 87 (1873).
Leoz Ortin. *Arch. Soc. oftal. hisp.-amer.*, **2,** 45 (1943).
Lister and Hancock. *Roy. Lond. ophthal. Hosp. Rep.*, **15,** 346 (1903).
Lloyd. *Amer. J. Ophthal.*, **21,** 359 (1938).
Löwenstein. *v. Graefes Arch. Ophthal.*, **127,** 598 (1931).
Majewski. *Ophthal. Klin.*, **11,** 129 (1907).
Meller. *v. Graefes Arch. Ophthal.*, **85,** 172 (1913).
Klin. Mbl. Augenheilk., **59,** 62 (1917).
Müller. *Ueber Ruptur der Corneo-Skleralgrenze durch stumpfe Verletzung*, Wien (1895).
Muller. *Ann. Oculist.* (Paris), **182,** 122 (1949).
Norris. *Amer. J. Ophthal.*, **32,** 259 (1949).
Palich-Szántó. *Klin. Mbl. Augenheilk.*, **59,** 425 (1917).
Panas. *Gaz. Méd. Paris*, **7,** 318 (1878).
Parsons. *Pathology of the Eye*, London, **1,** 249 (1904).
Pascheff. *Klin. Mbl. Augenheilk.*, **61,** 678 (1918).
Pichler. *Z. Augenheilk.*, **36,** 311 (1916).
Rychener. *J. Amer. med. Ass.*, **126,** 763 (1944).
Schirmer. *v. Graefes Arch. Ophthal.*, **42** (3), 1 (1896).
Schousboë and Morard. *Bull. Soc. Ophtal. Paris*, 17 (1935).
Straub. *Ophthalmologica*, **122,** 239 (1951).
Thygeson and Beard. *Amer. J. Ophthal.*, **35,** 977 (1952).
Toselli. *Rass. ital. Ottal.*, **19,** 46 (1950).
Wagenmann. *v. Graefes Arch. Ophthal.*, **25** (1), 172 (1889); **37** (2), 21 (1891); **38** (2), 91 (1892); **42** (2), 1 (1896).
Wolter. *Amer. J. Ophthal.*, **56,** 785 (1963).
Wood. *Sth Afr. med. J.*, **9,** 142 (1935).
Zanen and Rausin. *Bull. Soc. belge Ophtal.*, No. 93, 508 (1949).

Concussion Effects on the Iris and Ciliary Body

Most injuries of the iris due to concussions probably result from the sudden impact of a pressure-wave of aqueous driven backwards by the in-curving of the cornea, which forces the iris against the relatively unyielding lens (Franke, 1886–87; Förster, 1887; Schirmer, 1890). As with all highly vascularized tissues the essential pathology comprises the three elements we have already discussed—the vascular reaction characteristic of concussion, the essential feature of which is a paretic vasodilatation associated with œdema and hæmorrhage, necrosis of the tissues and, finally, their actual disintegration. The peculiar structure of the anterior segment of the uveal tract, its great vascularity and the delicacy of its tissues endow these re-actions with highly individual characteristics. When a slight amount of force is involved, hyperæmia and perhaps small hæmorrhages appearing

[1] p. 198.

clinically and an irritative iritis may be the only result; more severe force usually leads to damage to the nerves, massive hæmorrhages, displacement and laceration of the tissues in various degrees, and even their complete necrosis and atrophy, while any concussion injury, slight or severe, may be followed by pigmentary and atrophic anomalies or a traumatic iridocyclitis with its enigmatic and sometimes disastrous course.

CHANGES IN THE PUPIL AND ACCOMMODATION

TRAUMATIC MIOSIS AND SPASM OF ACCOMMODATION

A SPASTIC MIOSIS is a constant immediate sequel to trauma to the globe, a reaction which was shown experimentally by Caillet (1869) to occur immediately on the receipt of blunt trauma to the cornea whether or not a post-traumatic mydriasis subsequently developed (Förster, 1887); a similar spastic miosis follows an injury which involves perforation of the globe. The constriction of the pupil is intense and is usually transient, to be followed frequently by an iridoplegia. Occasionally, however, it may last a considerable period, but even then is usually of temporary duration and is abolished by atropine. It is generally associated with a SPASM OF ACCOMMODATION, also transient in duration unless perpetuated by a functional element (Tange, 1913–14; Morgan, 1940). The symptoms and diagnosis of this condition have been fully discussed[1]; no treatment is necessary, but if inconvenience is caused the instillation of atropine may give relief.

It may be that in some cases the miosis and accommodative spasm following an accident may be due to a sympathetic paralysis resulting from an injury to the skull or the neck, which abolishes the normal antagonistic action to the parasympathetic nerve to the pupil and ciliary muscle; in this event the miosis is found to be paralytic in nature rather than irritative (Bolotte, 1934; Dejean and Guignot, 1938; and others).[2] It is also to be remembered from the diagnostic point of view that an accommodative spasm occurring after trauma may be due to functional causes or to an irritative lesion in the central nervous system,[3] while a spastic miosis may follow a pontine hæmorrhage.[4]

TRAUMATIC IRIDOPLEGIA AND CYCLOPLEGIA

A dilatation of the pupil is a very common sequel of a concussion of the globe and it is usually associated with a paralysis of accommodation coming on after the preliminary intense miosis has passed. Both the sphincter and dilatator muscles are usually involved and thus the classical descriptive term, *traumatic (paralytic) mydriasis*, is somewhat misleading in so far as it suggests a paretic injury to the sphincter only. The functions of the iris and ciliary muscle are usually simultaneously affected (Cosmettatos, 1905), but occasionally iridoplegia may occur with unimpaired accommodation (Würdemann, 1932). The pupil is moderately but not maximally dilated and often

[1] Vol. V, p. 469. [2] Vol. XII, p. 632.
[3] Vol. XII, p. 706. [4] Vol. XII, p. 631.

eccentric, sometimes with absent, usually with diminished reactions to light and accommodation, both direct and consensual (Fig. 52; Plate IV, Fig. 5); further slow dilatation may occur with atropine and some constriction with eserine, but at other times miotics have no effect. Although the condition may resolve in a few weeks, as a rule the deformity is permanent.

The mechanism of these reactions is disputed and is probably varied. The frequent absence of discoverable pathological change has suggested that the effect may be due to injury to the nerves, which may be damaged or torn in their passage through the ocular tissues by the wave of pressure which traverses the eye; in other cases tears in the iris are visible or transillumination reveals ruptures in the sphincter muscle, the presence of either of

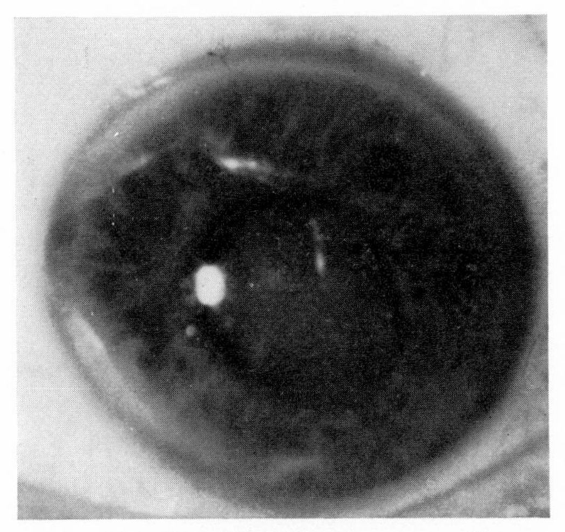

FIG. 52.—CONCUSSION EFFECTS ON THE IRIS.
The pupil is dilated and eccentric (A. J. B. Goldsmith).

which may be betrayed by a D-shaped pupillary aperture wherein a chord may replace the arc in a sector; similar minute traumata may occur in the ciliary muscle. Indeed, Kilgore (1942) has shown experimentally that sometimes after relatively slight injury in the monkey, cyclitic changes followed by the replacement of muscle by fibrous tissue and subsequent atrophy were frequent sequels. Events such as this may be of more common occurrence than is supposed and correspond in their ætiology and pathology to the changes generally associated with concussion injuries.

In the diagnosis of such cases a mydriasis due to orbital or cranial injury must be remembered, as also must accommodative failure due to injury to the zonule. Moreover, after an injury due to concussion or blast, while a deficiency in the amplitude of accommodation may be demonstrated in some cases (Smith, **1949**), in others the power of the ciliary muscle may be found to be within normal limits and the functional disability may be due to a disturbance in the higher cortical centres (Wescott, **1943**; Grove, **1943**).

The *symptoms* following a lesion of this type are largely confined to the results of impairment of the function of the ciliary muscle. Attempts to read precipitate discomfort and sometimes pain with the early onset of fatigue, while the subnormal amplitude of accommodation may be periodically replaced by periods of a compensatory spasm. The prognosis is somewhat uncertain, and several months may elapse before recovery ensues; indeed, some permanent disability may remain.

Treatment of the accommodative failure due to ocular injury is probably best by cycloplegia and the constant wearing of the full optical correction for distant and near vision. So far as the mydriasis is concerned, no treatment is of value, but miotics may improve the cosmetic appearance of the eye and diminish the discomfort due to dazzling.

VASCULAR CHANGES

REACTIVE HYPERÆMIA AND EXUDATION

Most concussions, no matter how small, produce the usual vascular effects on the uveal vessels, comprising initially an ischæmic spasm followed by a prolonged reactive vasodilatation. This involves a widespread REACTIVE HYPERÆMIA of the anterior segment of the uveal tract. Clinically the condition is made evident by a circumcorneal injection and the vascular dilatation is associated with the characteristic œdema of the tissues. This effect becomes apparent in the aqueous wherein slit-lamp examination undertaken shortly after the injury always reveals a flare due to the presence of increased protein in the anterior chamber. Occasionally this effect is sufficiently gross to lead to the formation of macroscopically visible masses of fibrin which

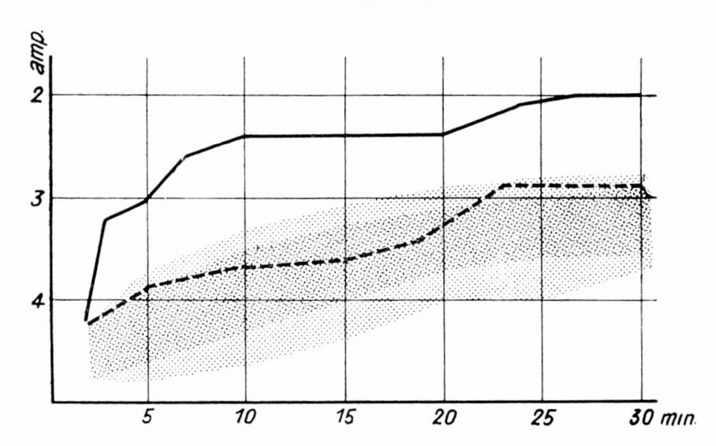

FIG. 53.—THE FLUORESCEIN TEST AFTER CONCUSSION.

The increased permeability after a contusion (continuous line) and in the sound eye (dotted line). The limits of normal are indicated in the shaded area. It is seen that the permeability in the sound fellow eye is in the upper limits of normal (M. Amsler and A. Huber).

traverse the anterior chamber in tangled networks, the threads adhering by thickened footplates to the anterior surface of the iris, the capsule of the lens and the posterior surface of the cornea[1] (Plate IV, Fig. 1). The rapidity with which the aqueous flare and even those more striking manifestations of the same reaction sometimes disappear is remarkable; all traces may have gone within an hour of the injury so that their occurrence is frequently missed.

This increased permeability of the capillaries after a contusion is clearly demonstrated by the fluorescein test by which this dye is injected intravenously and its rate of appearance observed across the blood-aqueous barrier into the anterior chamber. A rapid rise in the permeability of the capillaries occurs soon after a concussion; and it is interesting that the fellow eye, although apparently normal, shows a slight increase in permeability, the curve in this case following faithfully the fluctuations in the injured eye (Amsler, 1946–48; Amsler and Huber, 1946–49) (Fig. 53). This observation finds a correlation with the changes in intra-ocular pressure which occur in both eyes after a concussion to one of them.

HÆMORRHAGES INTO THE IRIS TISSUE

Not infrequently, small hæmorrhages, usually lying deeply in the interstitial tissue of the iris, are a transient sequel of contusion injuries (Plate IV, Fig. 2); they are merely a further extension of the hyperæmia and exudative reaction just described. They are often difficult to see since they are usually invisible in direct or oblique examination. They appear, however, as red-brown flakes or as a red glow in indirect light and are best discovered by the slit-lamp when the focal beam is moved across the iris, in which event the hæmorrhage stands out clearly in the unilluminated tissue on either side of the beam and disappears when the light falls directly upon it. Such hæmorrhages are of no special importance and are absorbed within a few days, although darkened areas in the iris stroma due to hæmatogenous pigmentation may remain as a permanent legacy.

Kilgore (1942) has shown experimentally in animals that similar hæmorrhages also occur in the ciliary body; these may be followed by atrophic changes wherein the muscle is replaced by fibrous tissue with permanent effects on the accommodative power.

TRAUMATIC HYPHÆMA

An accumulation of free blood in the anterior chamber is a logical sequence of the same process and is a common result of mild contusions, and an almost invariable sequel of more serious injuries of this type (Plate III; Tables XIV and XV). Particularly in the case of children, a *primary hyphæma* appears at the time of the accident and, as it settles gravitationally, varies in size from a small sediment 1 or 2 mm. in height at the bottom of the anterior chamber to a large mass of blood which may almost or completely fill the chamber. Most hyphæmata are small and the bleeding even from a vessel

[1] Nagel (1873), Schmidt-Rimpler (1883), Bäck (1899), Sala (1904), Cordes and Horner (1932), and many others.

of arteriolar size is usually transient, partly owing to an equilibration between the vascular and the intra-ocular pressures and partly because of the immediate contraction and recession of the wall of the lacerated vessel; the potency of this latter effect is seen in the usual absence of bleeding after an iridectomy even when the globe is open. The larger hæmorrhages usually denote a rupture of an arterial vessel of some size, particularly near the root of the iris or in the ciliary body. Such hæmorrhages usually absorb rapidly but the picture may be complicated by the occurrence of a *secondary hæmorrhage* usually on the second or third, sometimes on the fourth or fifth post-traumatic day, a complication which may ensue while the patient is at rest in bed apparently recovering satisfactorily and the primary hæmorrhage is absorbing. While primary hæmorrhages are most common in children, the

TABLE XIV

CAUSES OF INJURY IN 200 CASES OF TRAUMATIC HYPHÆMA
(Ferguson and Poole, 1968)

NATURE OF INJURY			NUMBER OF CASES
MISSILES:	THROWN.	Stones	62
		Balls, etc.	21
	SHOT.	Guns	4
		Arrows and Darts	7
		Sling Shot	8
BLOWS:		Fists and Boots	10
		Flexible Objects	18
		Sticks and Wood	26
MISCELLANEOUS:		Corks	9
		Occupational	21
		Toys and Fireworks	14
		TOTAL	200

secondary type is seen most frequently in older patients. On rare occasions these continue to recur at periodic intervals for weeks or even months (Duane, 1926). Such secondary hæmorrhages tend to be more profuse than the primary bleeding; they usually fill the entire anterior chamber and are a serious complication (Fig. 48) (Table XV).

When a hyphæma develops the blood settles in the lower part of the chamber, and over it the aqueous shows a typical Tyndall flare caused by a suspension of yellow-red cells; as a rarity hæmatogenous pigment may rapidly diffuse all over the anterior chamber, so that the aqueous is uniformly coloured and the iris is seen as it were through a ruby-red glass. If repeated hæmorrhages occur the hyphæma becomes stratified, the lower and older layers of blood assuming a darker hue, and occasionally a dull gelatinous appearance results, suggesting that the blood is heavily mixed with a richly albuminous clot.

The great majority of traumatic hyphæmata absorb rapidly and permanently in from 1 to 7 days, leaving no trace; Ferguson and Poole (1968) found that in 134 out of 197 cases absorption occurred within five days. Absorption is probably mainly through the anterior surface of the iris, and multitudes of erythrocytes have been seen on histological examination entering the crypts 24 hours after injury (Wolff, 1935). Using radio-active 51 chromium Hørven (1964) and Jocson and his team (1965) found that the labelled erythrocytes were absorbed by the trabecular endothelium and the histiocytes within the meshwork of the angle as well as by the stromal cells in the iris; free red cells in the anterior chamber disappear rapidly in this way but when they become enmeshed in a clot of fibrin they remain over a period of some 10 days while this is absorbed. Before this is effected, however, an iridocyclitis may develop with the formation of anterior and posterior synechiæ, and eventually the trabeculæ at the angle of the anterior chamber may become impregnated with hæmatogenous products (Vannas, 1960), while at a later stage stratified layers of collagenous tissue may be laid down. If the pupillary aperture has been covered by the hyphæma, however, absorption

Table XV

Incidence of Secondary Hæmorrhage

AUTHORS	NUMBER OF CASES	INCIDENCE OF SECONDARY HÆMORRHAGE
Loring (1958)	56	29·0%
Henry (1960)	204	17·0%
Gregersen (1962)	200	5·5%
Spaeth and Levy (1966)	85	24·0%
Geeraets, Liu and Guerry (1967)	198	7·0%
Oksala (1967)	128	10·0%
Ferguson and Poole (1968)	200	17·5%

from the anterior capsule of the lens may be much delayed and thereon a ring-shaped deposit corresponding to the pupillary aperture may remain for a long time; similarly a powdering of blood cells may linger on the posterior surface of the cornea.

Complications may arise, particularly when the hæmorrhage is massive and usually when it is delayed. The most important of these is the occurrence of a *secondary glaucoma*, a frequent result of a secondary hæmorrhage, due usually to the vasodilatation, the increased colloid content of the aqueous and embarrassment of the drainage channels. Such a rise of tension, of course, may be aided by other concomitant effects of the injury; too often it presents grave problems in its treatment and the visual prognosis is, in general, poor. A second complication is the *invasion of the corneal substance by blood corpuscles*, usually in linear streaks—a matter of little moment[1]—but a more serious event occurring usually when the hyphæma is associated with a rise in tension is the development of *blood-staining of the cornea*—unfortunately a cause of long and perhaps permanent disability.[2] Particularly when inflammatory complications supervene, the presence of a

[1] p. 85. [2] p. 83.

hyphæma may also accentuate the formation of exudates in the pupillary area, leading to the seclusion of the pupil.

Long-term complications are by no means unknown. An occasional occurrence is the development of hæmatogenous pigmentation of the iris causing a *heterochromia iridum* wherein the iris of the injured eye becomes darker. Some considerable time after the contusion the aqueous humour may be seen to contain cholesterol crystals and may be xanthochromic in its reaction, giving positive tests for the break-down products of blood pigment (Appelmans and Michiels, 1950); while chronic degenerative changes may spread throughout the globe, frequently associated with the formation of granulomatous masses densely packed with crystals of cholesterol and multi-nucleated giant cells located particularly in the iris, the ciliary region and the angle of the anterior chamber. Such a condition of *hæmophthalmitis*, characterized by chronic irritation with the occurrence of frequent subacute relapses and often leading in the end to the enucleation of a useless and painful globe, will be studied more fully in the section on perforating wounds.[1] Finally, organization of the blood may lead to the formation of peripheral and posterior synechiæ (Figs. 54–6).

The cause of the secondary hæmorrhages which create so serious a therapeutic problem is unknown. They bear little resemblance to the hyphæmata following a cataract operation, wherein the blood is usually derived from the sectioned limbal vessels, the rupture of which is presumably due to a slight separation of the lips of the wound; these occur later, from the 5th to the 7th day, are relatively benign, rarely fill the anterior chamber but may eventually cause glaucoma. The secondary hæmorrhages after an ocular contusion resemble more closely those derived from the spleen in abdominal contusions which, arising from the 2nd day onwards, often prove fatal.

Gonioscopic studies of the angle of the anterior chamber following ocular contusions have been made by several investigators[2] and, as we shall see in a subsequent section[3] where these lesions are discussed more fully, the commonest result of such an injury is a tear into the face of the ciliary body, separating the circular from the longitudinal muscle fibres, while traumatic cyclodialysis and iridodialysis may also be seen. It will be recalled that the major arterial circle of the iris lies in this area and that it is fed not only by the two long posterior ciliary arteries but also by the branches of the anterior ciliary arteries which have reached the anterior part of the ciliary body after penetrating the sclera. In the normal angle with the gonioscope it is usually possible to see loops of this arterial system and presumably it is from these vessels torn apart by the concussion injury that bleeding occurs. It may be that the absence of fibroblastic repair which is a characteristic of injuries of the iris and premature lysis of blood clot in the injured vessels, the ends of which are not able to retract effectively, are factors in the causation of recurrent hæmorrhage.

Treatment

In most cases a traumatic hyphæma absorbs satisfactorily with no treatment other than keeping the patient relatively quiet with rest in bed if

[1] p. 390.

[2] Alper (1963), Pettit and Keates (1963), Rodman (1963), Blanton (1964), Howard *et al.* (1965), Britten (1965), Litvinova (1967), Thorkilgaard and Moestrup (1967), Tonjum (1969), and others.

[3] p. 111.

FIGS. 54 to 56.—THE IMMEDIATE AND END-RESULTS OF A TRAUMATIC HYPHÆMA (B. Rones and H. C. Wilder).

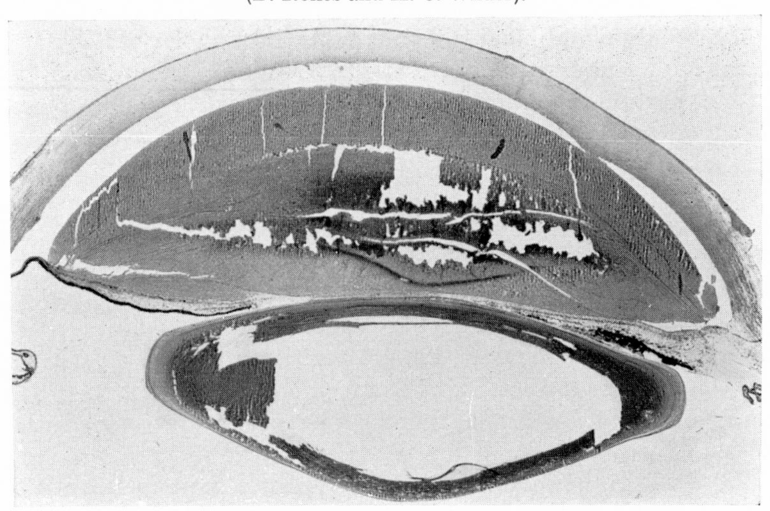

FIG. 54.—A fresh hyphæma after a contusion.

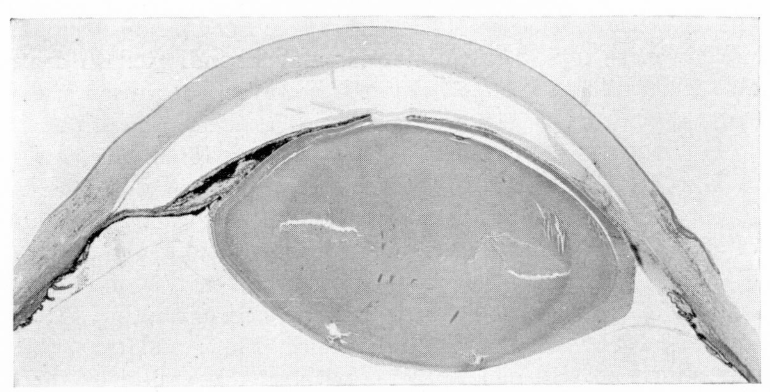

FIG. 55.—The hæmorrhage in the anterior chamber which resulted from a traumatic iridodialysis has become organized. There is marked atrophy of the iris and ciliary body with extensive peripheral anterior synechiæ and posterior synechiæ. The lens is cataractous and misplaced.

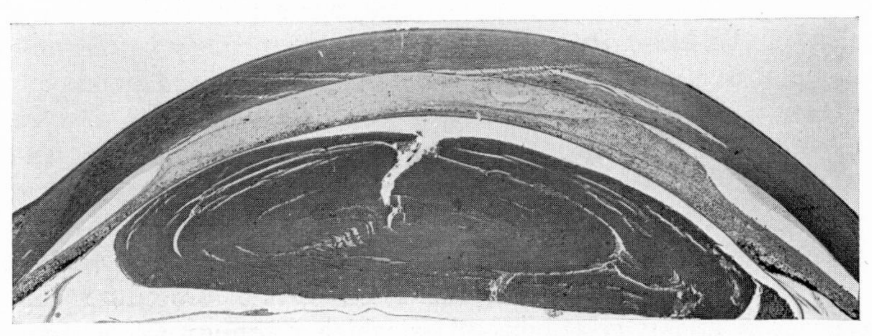

FIG. 56.—The blood in the anterior chamber has become organized, totally occluding the pupil. There is anterior displacement of the lens with the formation of cataract.

necessary, sedation and bandaging or the use of pinhole spectacles. In any case if the hyphæma is sufficiently large to preclude examination of the inner eye such expectant treatment is essential until an adequate assessment of the effects of the injury has been made. Miotics used at an early stage were recommended by Rychener (1944), Smith (1949) and O'Neill (1952). The question of the instillation of atropine has given rise to some controversy. Some authors advocate its use (Laughlin, 1948), others have suggested homatropine (Thygeson and Beard, 1952). On the whole any mydriatic is usually unnecessary and may be dangerous and, indeed, is contra-indicated if a gross hyphæma is present since absorption of the blood is partly through the anterior surface of the iris; the greater the available surface, the more rapid is this process and mydriatics may embarrass this action still further. In the presence of a hyphæma, therefore, expectant treatment without the instillation of atropine is probably the safest course so long as the tension is normal or low. If, however, any anxiety is felt regarding a raised tension, the use of miotics rather than mydriatics at an early stage is the sounder method of treatment and may forestall the complications of a hyphæma and avoid the necessity for surgery (Rychener, 1944; Lock, 1950). Subsequently atropine as well as topical corticosteroids may be indicated to control the inevitable iridocyclitis; it is to be noted, however, that when given at an early stage steroids have been said to inhibit the absorption of blood (Benedict and Hollenhorst, 1953; Podos *et al.*, 1965; Liu, 1967).

If, however, the entire anterior chamber becomes filled with blood, as in a secondary hæmorrhage which sometimes occurs 4 to 5 days or more after the injury, measures to prevent intractable glaucoma, corneal blood-staining and possible loss of the eye are urgently required, although there is still controversy as to the most suitable form of treatment (Rychener, 1944; Stokes, 1958; Loring, 1958; Kushner, 1959; and others). If the hyphæma shows no sign of absorption within 24 hours, or at the earliest possible time if the ocular tension is raised, every effort should be made to control this complication, as by the use of carbonic anhydrase inhibitors (acetazoleamide, etc.) or osmotherapy by intravenous urea or mannitol, or oral glycerol. It frequently happens that when the tension returns to a normal level the blood tends rapidly and spontaneously to disappear. If these hypotensive measures are not effective the standard practice used to be to perform a paracentesis, which was reopened or repeated on subsequent days to control the pressure. An extraction of the clot with forceps through a linear corneal incision has been advocated (Callahan and Zubero, 1962) or even its manual expression (Sears, 1970), while removal of the clot with a cryogenic probe has also proved successful (Hill, 1968), but this is a difficult and sometimes impossible procedure since the blood forms a sticky gelatinous mass which often cannot easily be dislodged (Tillema, 1937). For this reason lavage with saline achieves little result: a much more effective method is to wash out the anterior chamber with proteolytic enzymes through a relatively small incision. For this purpose streptokinase (fibrinolysin) (5,000 units in 1 ml. of saline) was advocated by Scheie and his colleagues (1961), Liebman (1963), Morton and Turnbull (1964), and Podos *et al.* (1964). A marked irritation, however, may follow the intracameral injection of this enzyme (Jukofsky, 1951; Friedman, 1952). A safer product is urokinase (5,000 units in 5 ml. saline) which, being an enzyme of human origin, eliminates the likelihood of antigenic reactions (Pierse and LeGrice, 1963; Pierse, 1964; Heath, 1966). With the use of these fibrinolytic enzymes the blood rapidly disappears within a few minutes while the lavage is being performed. The subsequent instillation of miotics and the introduction of an air-bubble into the anterior chamber tends to prevent the formation of peripheral anterior synechiæ (Friedenwald, 1950). Although the measures just described may succeed in liquefaction and removal of the blood clot, they are unlikely, perhaps with the exception of air injection (Wilson *et al.*, 1954), to prevent further bleeding or lead to the arrest of the hæmorrhage; indeed, further bleeding may be provoked by the manipulations within the anterior chamber. Hypotensive therapy utilizing ganglion-blocking drugs and other agents to reduce the systolic blood pressure combined with elevation of the head during the removal of the clot and the use of tranquillizers such as chlorpromazine and promethazine post-operatively have been advocated by Kenny (1959), Werner (1959) and Hill (1968); two cases of traumatic hyphæma with secondary glaucoma in small boys were successfully treated in this way by Moore and Youngman (1968).

Apart from the therapeutic measures outlined above, other forms of treatment have been recommended. The use of œstrogens was suggested by Goldberg (1960) and Gillan (1961), but in a controlled trial Spaeth and Levy (1966) found that they were of little value in reducing the incidence of secondary hæmorrhages. Anti-inflammatory drugs, such as hydroxyphenylbutazone (Tanderil) (Restrepo Córdoba, 1967) have also been employed; the use of laser energy to accelerate absorption of hyphæmata was explored in rabbits by Kecik and his colleagues (1967); and the concept of phacoemulsification introduced by Kelman (1967) using low frequency sonic-ultrasonic energy to dissolve and emulsify a cataractous lens which is then removed by aspiration has recently been applied in the treatment of traumatic hyphæmata; in four such cases with intractable glaucoma, Kelman (1969) succeeded in emulsifying and aspirating the blood clot through a small corneal incision with satisfactory control of the intra-ocular pressure and the prevention of further hæmorrhage.

The literature dealing with traumatic hyphæmata is extensive. A series of cases treated with proteolytic enzymes together with an extensive review of the literature is given by Oosterhuis (1968). A report of interest is that of Henry (1960) dealing with 204 cases of which 49% developed complications such as secondary hæmorrhage, glaucoma, dislocation of the lens and cataract; good vision resulted in about 80% after being treated with bed-rest and binocular occluding spectacles; the age group 5 to

15 years was most frequently affected. Gregersen (1962) summarized the treatment of 200 patients of which 123 were children under 15 years of age treated by rest in bed and pinhole spectacles, local mydriatics and cortisone in some cases after 10 days because of iritis. Other reports are those of Kushner (1959) 100 patients, 82 under 15 years of age; Cole and Byron (1964); Geeraets and his colleagues (1967) treated 198 cases without drops, in which secondary hæmorrhage occurred in 7% and of these 40% developed secondary glaucoma; Darr and Passmore (1967) 109 cases wherein secondary hæmorrhage occurred in 32% of those treated with drops, but only in 5·3% of those in which drops were not used. In 128 cases treated by Oksala (1967) with partial bed-rest for 3 to 4 days without occluding spectacles but with strong mydriatics and corticosteroid drops, the greater mobility permitted did not increase the number of complications seen. In Shea's (1957) series of 113 cases in children most commonly due to injuries by airgun pellets, glaucoma occurred after a primary hæmorrhage in 2% and after a secondary hæmorrhage in 25%. In Liu's (1967) series of 121 cases, 81 treated with steroids cleared in five days, and 40 cases treated without steroids cleared in three days; Ferguson and Poole (1968) also reported 200 cases.

When the hæmorrhage has cleared from the anterior chamber detailed examination is required for the detection of residual serious ocular damage such as cataract or displacement of the lens or injury to the retina such as a peripheral disinsertion, and the subsequent treatment will depend on the nature of any damage found. The gonioscopic appearance of the angle of the anterior chamber in cases of traumatic hyphæma has been described in several reports, among others those of Thorkilgaard and Moestrup (1967): of 44 cases observed from 1 to 22 months after injury, 45% showed cleavage of the angle while in 30% a variety of changes was seen including disruption of the pectinate ligament, a localized iridoschisis, iridodialysis, stromal tears of the iris and pigment accumulation. Litvinova (1967) recorded 125 cases ranging from 7 to 90 years of age; among these gonioscopy showed blood in the trabeculæ, excess pigmentation, tears of the root of the iris and broadening of the angle of the anterior chamber in 50%; while Wolff and Zimmerman (1962) described the histopathological changes associated with concussion glaucoma.[1]

Alper. *Arch. Ophthal.*, **69**, 455 (1963).
Amsler. *Bull. Soc. franç. Ophtal.*, **59**, 304 (1946).
Trans. ophthal. Soc. U.K., **68**, 45 (1948).
Amsler and Huber. *Ophthalmologica*, **111**, 155 (1946).
v. Graefes Arch. Ophthal., **149**, 578 (1949).
Appelmans and Michiels. *Acta XVI int. Cong. Ophthal.*, London, **2**, 702 (1950).
Bäck. *v. Graefes Arch. Ophthal.*, **47** (1), 82 (1899).
Benedict and Hollenhorst. *Amer. J. Ophthal.*, **36**, 247 (1953).
Blanton. *Arch. Ophthal.*, **72**, 39 (1964).
Bolotte. *Arch. Ophtal.*, **51**, 662 (1934).
Britten. *Brit. J. Ophthal.*, **49**, 120 (1965).
Caillet. *Des ruptures isolées de la choroide* (Thèse), Strasbourg (1869).
Callahan and Zubero. *Amer. J. Ophthal.*, **53**, 522 (1962).
Cole and Byron. *Arch. Ophthal.*, **71**, 35 (1964).
Cordes and Horner. *Amer. J. Ophthal.*, **15**, 942 (1932).
Cosmettatos. *Arch. Ophtal.*, **25**, 664 (1905).
Darr and Passmore. *Amer. J. Ophthal.*, **63**, 134 (1967).
Dejean and Guignot. *Arch. Soc. Sci. méd. biol.*, Montpellier, **19**, 73 (1938).
Duane. *Amer. J. Ophthal.*, **9**, 531 (1926).
Ferguson and Poole. *Trans. ophthal. Soc. N.Z.*, **20**, 54 (1968).
Förster. *Klin. Mbl. Augenheilk.*, **25**, 143 (1887).
Franke. *v. Graefes Arch. Ophthal.*, **32** (2), 261 (1886); **33** (1), 245 (1887).

[1] Vol. XI, p. 705.

Friedenwald. *Amer. J. Ophthal.*, **33,** 1523 (1950).
Friedman. *Amer. J. Ophthal.*, **35,** 1184 (1952).
Geeraets, Liu and Guerry. *Med. Coll. Va. Quart.*, **3,** 20 (1967).
Gillan. *Trans. Canad. ophthal. Soc.*, **24,** 217 (1961).
Goldberg. *Arch. Ophthal.*, **63,** 1001 (1960).
Gregersen. *Acta ophthal.* (Kbh.), **40,** 192, 200 (1962).
Grove. *Wisconsin med. J.*, **42,** 210 (1943).
Heath. *Trans. ophthal. Soc. U.K.*, **86,** 843 (1966).
Henry. *Amer. J. Ophthal.*, **49,** 1298 (1960).
Hill. *Arch. Ophthal.*, **80,** 368 (1968).
Hørven. *Erythrocyte Resorption from the Rabbit and Human Eye*, Oslo (1964).
Howard, Hutchinson and Frederick. *Trans. Amer. Acad. Ophthal.*, **69,** 294 (1965).
Jocson, Tabowitz and Kara. *Amer. J. Ophthal.*, **59,** 392 (1965).
Jukofsky. *Amer. J. Ophthal.*, **34,** 1692 (1951).
Kecik, Falkowska, Malinowska and Szretter. *Klin. oczna*, **37,** 467 (1967).
Kelman. *Amer. J. Ophthal.*, **64,** 23 (1967); **67,** 464 (1969).
Kenny. *Amer. J. Ophthal.*, **47,** 697 (1959).
Kilgore. *Amer. J. Ophthal.*, **25,** 1095 (1942).
Kushner. *Survey Ophthal.*, **4,** 2 (1959).
Laughlin. *Trans. Pac. Cst. oto-ophthal. Soc.*, 133 (1948).
Liebman. *Trans. Amer. ophthal. Soc.*, **61,** 638 (1963).
Litvinova. *Oftal. Zh.*, **22,** 166 (1967).
Liu. *Chin. med. J.*, **14,** 270 (1967).
Lock. *Brit. J. Ophthal.*, **34,** 193 (1950).
Loring. *Amer. J. Ophthal.*, **46,** 873 (1958).
Moore and Youngman. *Brit. J. Ophthal.*, **52,** 172 (1968).
Morgan. *Brit. J. Ophthal.*, **24,** 403 (1940).
Morton and Turnbull. *Amer. J. Ophthal.*, **57,** 280 (1964).
Nagel. *Jber. Ophthal.*, **4,** 342 (1873).
Oksala. *Brit. J. Ophthal.*, **51,** 315 (1967).
O'Neill. *Eye, Ear, Nose Thr. Mthly.*, **31,** 481 (1952).
Oosterhuis. *Ophthalmologica*, **155,** 357 (1968).
Pettit and Keates. *Arch. Ophthal.*, **69,** 438 (1963).
Pierse. *Trans. ophthal. Soc. U.K.*, **84,** 271 (1964).
Pierse and LeGrice. *Lancet*, **2,** 1143 (1963).
Podos, Fingerman and Becker. *Invest. Ophthal.*, **4,** 76 (1965).
Podos, Liebman and Pollen. *Arch. Ophthal.*, **71,** 537 (1964).
Restrepo Córdoba. *Arch. Soc. oftal. hisp.-amer.*, **27,** 1013 (1967).
Rodman. *Arch. Ophthal.*, **69,** 445 (1963).
Rychener. *J. Amer. med. Ass.*, **126,** 763 (1944).
Sala. *Klin. Mbl. Augenheilk.*, **42** (1), 316 (1904).
Scheie, Ashley and Weiner. *Arch. Ophthal.*, **66,** 226 (1961).
Schirmer. *Klin. Mbl. Augenheilk.*, **28,** 161 (1890).
Schmidt-Rimpler. *Arch. Augenheilk.*, **12,** 135 (1883).
Sears. *Trans. Amer. Acad. Ophthal.*, **74,** 820 (1970).
Shea. *Canad. med. Ass. J.*, **76,** 466 (1957).
Smith, H. *Amer. J. Ophthal.*, **32,** 959 (1949).
Spaeth and Levy. *Amer. J. Ophthal.*, **62,** 1098 (1966).
Stokes. *Sth. med. J.*, **51,** 1476 (1958).
Tange. *Ned. T. Geneesk.*, **1,** 1305 (1913). *Arch. Ophtal.*, **34,** 463 (1914).
Thorkilgaard and Moestrup. *Acta ophthal.* (Kbh.), **45,** 51 (1967).
Thygeson and Beard. *Amer. J. Ophthal.*, **35,** 977 (1952).
Tillema. *Arch. Ophthal.*, **17,** 586 (1937).
Tonjum. *Proc. III Cong. Europ. Soc. Ophthal.*, Amsterdam, 49 (1969).
Vannas. *Acta ophthal.* (Kbh.), **38,** 461 (1960).
Werner. *Trans. ophthal. Soc. U.K.*, **79,** 81 (1959).
Wescott. *Illinois med. J.*, **83,** 170 (1943).
Wilson, McKee, Campbell and Miller. *Amer. J. Ophthal.*, **37,** 409 (1954).
Wolff, E. *Pathology of the Eye*, London (1935).
Wolff, S. M., and Zimmerman. *Amer. J. Ophthal.*, **54,** 547 (1962).
Würdemann. *Injuries of the Eye*, London (1932).

LACERATIONS OF THE IRIS AND CILIARY BODY

Gross TEARS AND LACERATIONS OF THE TISSUES of the anterior uvea are relatively common sequels of severe contusions, but the occurrence of smaller and less obvious dehiscences after comparatively slight injuries are much more common than is realized. The mechanism of the production of these lesions has caused some controversy, but several factors are undoubtedly concerned. The most important of these are (*a*) a dilatation of the corneo-scleral ring occurring in compensation for the antero-posterior compression of the globe (Arlt, 1875); (*b*) the prompt and marked contraction of the sphincter of the iris which occurs immediately on the application of blunt trauma to the cornea whether or not a post-traumatic mydriasis develops (Förster, 1887); (*c*) the impact of the compression-wave of aqueous which forces the iris onto the lens and the lateral displacement of the aqueous; and possibly (*d*) a rebound of the lens from the vitreous against which it is thrust, an action which may distend the iris " as a fœtus distends the uterine cervix " (Frenkel, 1931–32). It is possible that some or all of these forces acting simultaneously and momentarily may produce different end-results depending on the relative effectivity of each in a particular case. If the peripheral pull on the iris by the dilatation of the corneo-scleral ring, for example, is greater than the pull exerted by the contraction of the sphincter, ruptures will tend to occur near the pupillary margin of the iris; if the opposite relationship obtains, tearing will tend to occur at the root of the iris or, perhaps, at the anterior insertion of the ciliary body; when both forces are balanced it is more probable that the pressure-wave of the aqueous will cause dehiscences in the body of the iris itself or damage the zonule. It is also probable that weakness either congenital or acquired in the structure of the iris will determine which particular region will give way. It is important to remember, however, that whatever the cause of the tearing of the tissues, there is no subsequent attempt at healing; *a tear in the iris, no matter how minute, remains permanently* and is a perpetual witness of the occurrence of the accident, a fact which may be of considerable medico-legal importance.

INTERSTITIAL TEARS OF THE SPHINCTER

Tears of the sphincter muscle without external involvement of the tissues of the iris are usually small and may be multiple. They are difficult to see clinically but are made most obvious by transillumination, in which case the torn area appears as a reddish glow. Their presence, however, may be noted on careful examination with the slit-lamp by the occurrence of delicate, corkscrew-like pleats or twists in the radial strands of the iris due to torsion caused by the defective action of the muscle at the point where it has given way (Vogt, 1923) (Plate IV, Fig. 4). There may also be changes in the contour of the pupil involving a minimal amount of notching and a local embarrassment of dilatation.

TEARS AT THE PUPILLARY BORDER

These injuries are also common and are more obvious, although in many cases they may be extremely minute. The laceration may involve the anterior layers of the stroma of the iris and leave the sphincter intact; alternatively, the posterior pigmented layer and the sphincter may be implicated, while the anterior stroma may remain unscathed; but much more commonly the whole depth of the tissue—anterior stroma, sphincter muscle and pigmentary epithelium—is torn. In the first type, the superficial tears involving the stroma of the iris, the fibrils of the tissue of the iris are usually torn and reflected in a triangular area (Fig. 57), sometimes showing short, loose ends, the appearance resembling the perforation of a finely woven piece of basket-work. At the base of the torn area the sphincter muscle may appear as a carpet of solid tissue and the pupillary border is usually intact; even although a mydriasis may occur, the shape and reactions of the pupil may eventually become normal. Such an injury is rarely complicated by a hyphæma but it may be followed by atrophic changes in the part of the iris involved.

If the tear involves the posterior pigmentary epithelium, the sphincter muscle is usually also implicated. A hyphæma is a common accompaniment owing to hæmorrhage from the capillaries of the muscle, but the injury may be difficult to detect clinically unless by transillumination when the defect in the pigmented layer becomes apparent. Such an injury usually causes a permanent defect manifested by pupillary dilatation.

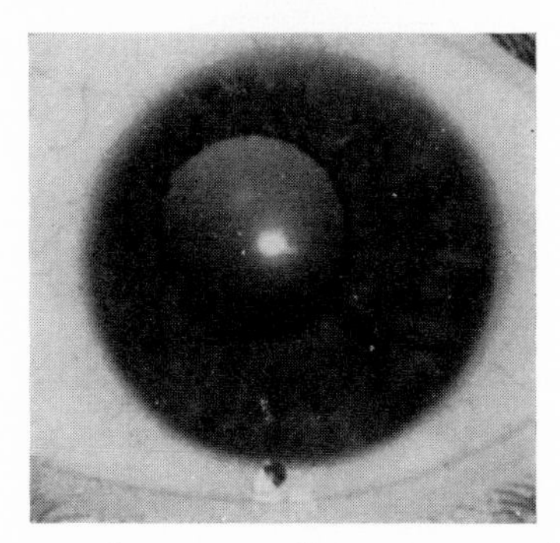

Fig. 57.—Concussion Changes in the Iris.
With multiple tears of the sphincter pupillæ, due to a blow by a stone.

A complete tear, involving all the layers of the iris, is the most common occurrence and, in contradistinction to the other two injuries, is usually multiple, one large rent being typically associated with several smaller tears (Fig. 58). Thus Weiss and Klingelhöffer (1899) annotated 31 cases, Eisenhuth (1899) saw 27 cases in eight years, and Herrmann (1906) 47 cases (or 6·9% of all concussions), 18 being single tears and 29 multiple. The laceration rarely extends more than a millimetre into the substance of the iris but on occasion a radiating tear may extend far down towards the periphery[1]; all the tissues are torn through cleanly and the subsequent irregularity of the pupil associated with some degree of immobility is obvious and permanent.

Only when the sphincter itself is torn is there a permanent functional disability, and even when such a laceration has occurred the unruptured portion of the sphincter regains its action after a few months so that eventually there is pupillary play in all but the ruptured area. It is interesting that in these cases there is usually some associated weakness of accommo-

[1] Reid (1850), Sweet (1901), Praun (1902), Ayres (1905), Herrmann (1906), and others.

dation (Gradle, 1934), a failure probably due in most cases to coincident and similar injury to the ciliary muscle. In such lesions no treatment is of value.

TEARS IN THE STROMA OF THE IRIS

Radial tears of considerable dimensions in the stroma of the iris are not uncommon, sometimes commencing at the pupillary border, sometimes occurring in the body of the iris and leaving the pupillary border intact; as a rule, the sphincter muscle is torn in the same direction as a radial tear in the stroma. Such tears are frequently multiple and they result in the permanent formation of large ragged areas in the iris over which tags of stroma sometimes wave loosely (Plate IV, Fig. 3).

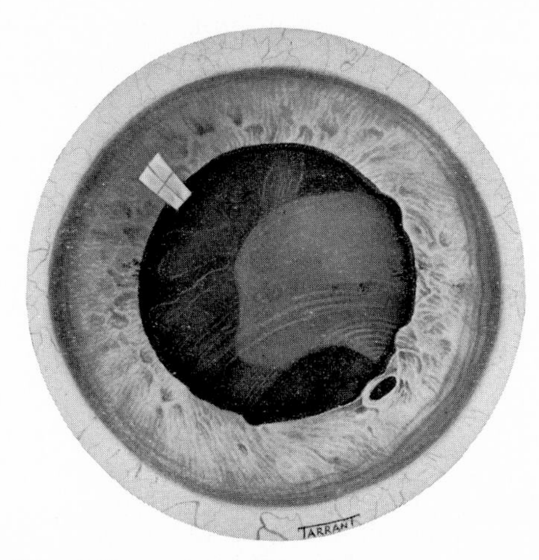

FIG. 58.—A HOLE IN THE IRIS FOLLOWING CONCUSSION.

In a boy aged 9 hit in the eye by a marble fired from a catapult. A hyphæma formed and on its absorption the outer and inferior quadrants of the stroma of the iris were distorted and atrophic and there were multiple ruptures of the pupillary margin. A red reflex was obtained through the oval hole at 4 o'clock (J. D. Abrams).

DEHISCENCES OF THE PIGMENTARY LAYER OF THE IRIS

These are common sequels of concussion injuries which are frequently overlooked since they are not visible ophthalmoscopically or by direct observation but only by retro-illumination when they appear as bright red areas. Their frequent occurrence, however, has been attested by many observers from the time of Pohlenz (1891).[1] Graves (1929) called the condition *epidialysis* and Vannas (1932) *diastasis* of the pigment layers. The dehiscences are either single or multiple, round, oval or irregular, and occur preferentially near the root of the iris where this tissue is thinnest, although they may extend far inwards towards the pupillary margin. When of any size, pupillary dilatation may be impaired, a circumstance which suggests that the dilatator muscle is usually involved along with its parent cells;

[1] Koby (1926), Mawas (1928), Cattaneo (1930), Vannas (1932), Schenk and Papapanos (1958), and others.

apart from this, however, no symptoms are apparent and no treatment is indicated.

IRIDODIALYSIS

When the trauma is of considerable severity as from the direct blow of a stone, a ball or other flying object or from an explosion, the *iris may be torn away from its insertion into the ciliary body to a greater or less extent.* The expansion of the corneo-scleral ring is opposed by the contraction of the sphincter, and the pressure-wave of aqueous impinging on the stretched iris finds this tissue supported centrally by the lens and peripherally by its attachment so that it gives way and is torn where support is lacking opposite the deepest part of the posterior chamber, a region where, in addition, the iris

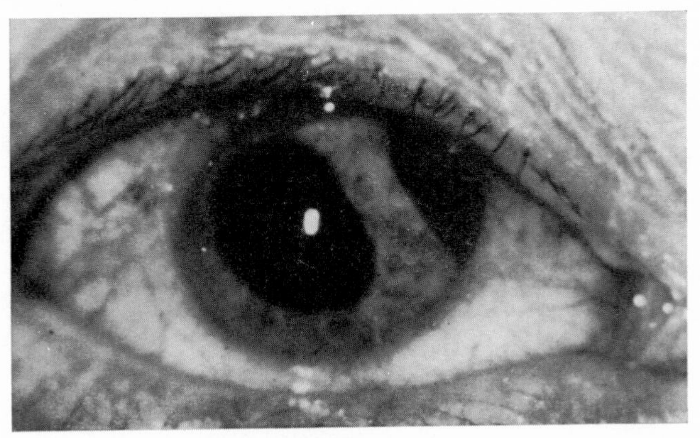

FIG. 59.—IRIDODIALYSIS.
From an injury by an airgun pellet. The remainder of the eye was intact.

itself is thinnest. As a rule the tear is small in extent (IRIDODIALYSIS) occurring preferentially at the outer aspect of the globe (10 out of 18 cases, Herrmann, 1906), but occasionally multiple lesions occur at various points around the circumference[1] (Figs. 59–62).

In milder degrees of injury a black, linear, crescentic slit at the periphery of the iris may be seen only with difficulty and requires gonioscopic examination for its appreciation. More usually, however, a black crescentic gap is obvious through which the zonule and even the periphery of the lens and ciliary processes may be visible and through which the vitreous may occasionally herniate. As a rule such an injury is accompanied by a hyphæma of considerable size owing to rupture of the large vessels supplying the iris, and consequently the lesion first becomes apparent some time after the accident on the absorption of the blood in the anterior chamber. Depending on the size of the tear, the pupillary margin is deformed, becoming flat or

[1] Wintersteiner (1894), Müller (1895), Praun (1899), Würdemann (1909), and others.

FIGS. 60 to 62.—TRAUMATIC IRIDODIALYSIS (B. Rones and H. C. Wilder).

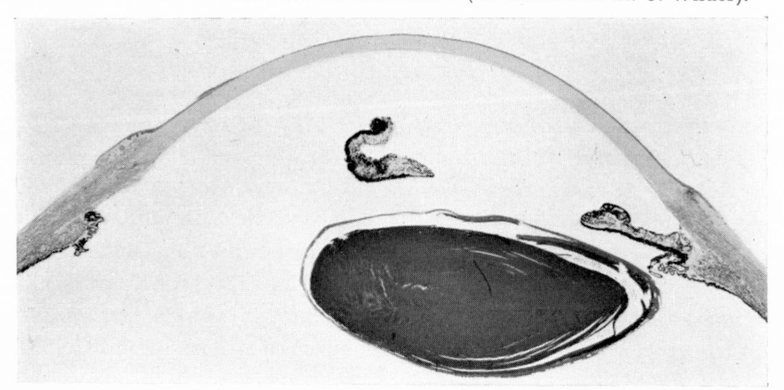

FIG. 60.—A recent case showing the iris completely torn from the ciliary body on the left.

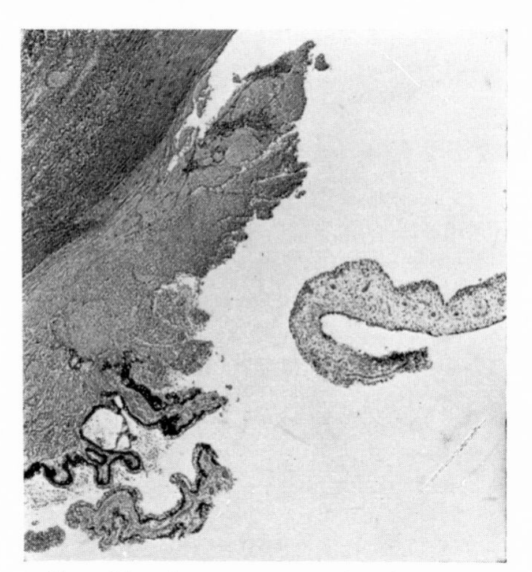

FIG. 61.—A recent case showing the iris torn from its root with hæmorrhage into the anterior and posterior chambers.

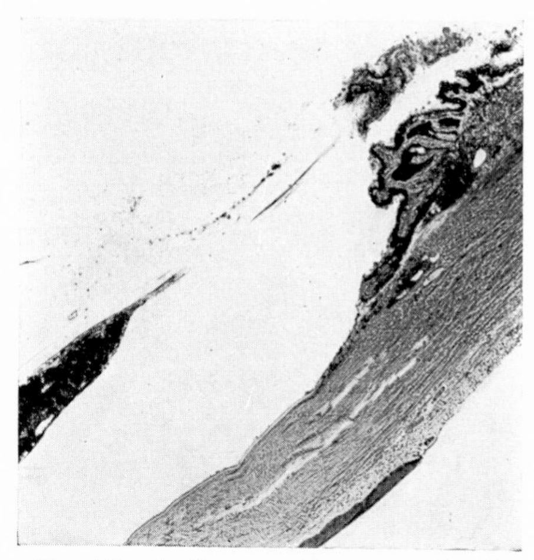

FIG. 62.—In the organizing stage, showing the beginning of the closure of the coloboma by organizing hæmorrhage between the torn part of the iris and the ciliary body.

even convex opposite the lesion. The deformity is usually permanent and the ciliary region atrophies (Fig. 63), but rare cases have been reported in which, with expectant treatment and full mydriasis, spontaneous restitution of the defect has occurred owing to the gap being bridged over by the organization of fibrin and blood clot liberated by the associated hæmorrhage and traumatic iritis (Fig. 64).[1] The subjective symptoms are unimportant unless the dialysis is of sufficient size to cause visual confusion owing to the irregular diffusion of light or, acting as a second pupil, allows the formation of a second image with the development of uniocular diplopia.

In most cases of iridodialysis *treatment*, after the initial period of rest and

[1] Werner (1887), Wicherkiewicz (1904), Shedlov (1924), Brown (1924), Duane (1926).

mon as an age-change or as a degenerative sequel of conditions such as long-standing glaucoma (Loewenstein and Foster, 1945). In some of the traumatic cases the history after injury has been long and it may well be that the element of atrophy is also involved. Gala (1941) recorded a similar appearance in a man with glass-workers' cataract. The causal injury is usually diffuse as is sustained in high diving (Schoenberg, 1927) or a fall (Loewenstein *et al.*, 1948) and it is possible that the lesion is due to the forcible entry of the aqueous into the substance of the iris through the crypts and the consequent separation of the insecurely soldered layers along a line of presumably least resistance.

The detached portion may float forwards in the anterior chamber and may even simulate an anterior synechia; if it is massive it remains rigid and does not follow the movements of the pupil. At other times large dehiscences occur where the anterior layer of the iris has sprung away and the tissue is broken up into strands floating in the anterior chamber as if teased by a crochet needle (Plate V, Figs. 1 and 3); Loewenstein and Foster (1945) and Moffatt (1950) found that some of these strands could adhere to the cornea. On removing a portion by iridectomy these authors found the sphincteric portion of the iris to be intact and the dilatator well preserved but that the entire anterior leaf of the mesodermal layer was absent.

A less common sequel is a *detachment of the entire stroma of the iris from the pigmented epithelium.* A case of this type was described by Mawas (1928) wherein a partial separation occurred in front of the pigmentary epithelium, the exposed surface of which resembled a melanotic tumour. A still more dramatic case of complete separation was described by Veirs (1949) in an aphakic eye following an injury in a hurricane many years previously; the split occurred between the pigmented epithelium and the mesodermal stroma which was intact, so that when the anterior layer was dilated with atropine a brown pigmented sheet remained behind in which a small pupillary aperture and two adventitious rents were visible (Plate V, Fig. 2).

A TRAUMATIC CYCLODIALYSIS may occur as a rare event after severe contusional trauma such as a direct and powerful blow from the horn of a cow; it is usually but by no means invariably associated with a rupture of the globe. In less severe degrees of injury the pectinate ligament is stretched, some of its fibres are torn and the trabeculæ are filled with blood and later with hæmatogenous pigment (Tillema, 1937; Rones and Wilder, 1947) (Fig. 68). In more severe injuries the ciliary body is completely torn from its anterior scleral attachment and with the iris is displaced backwards sometimes to the equator, while the anterior chamber and the suprachoroidal space become continuous resulting in a choroidal detachment, an injury which may give the appearance of aniridia[1] (Fig. 69).

[1] Collins (1892), Buchanan (1903), Mayou (1909), Stephenson (1916), Lister (1924), and others.

are clear the red reflex corresponds to the margin of the limbus. The iris may remain attached to the ciliary body by a small pedicle and gonioscopic observation may show that it is retracted far into the filtration angle (Legrand and Dubois-Poulsen, 1949); alternatively, it is completely detached and lies curled up into a little ball at the bottom of the anterior chamber where it eventually shrinks into a nondescript grey body (Würdemann, 1932); dislocation into the vitreous or beneath a detached retina has been reported (Mauthner, 1872; Tvyl, 1900; Fejer, 1903), and if the globe is ruptured the iris may be extruded or lie underneath the conjunctiva sometimes together with the lens (Gangoso, 1948). In the differential diagnosis

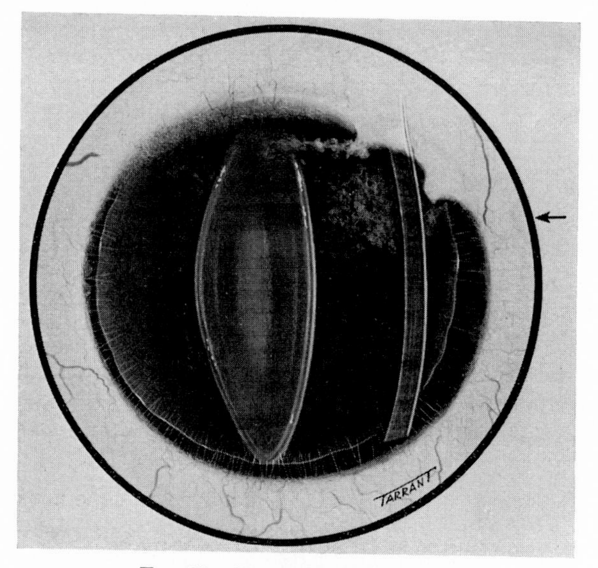

Fig. 67.—Traumatic Aniridia.

In a man wearing spectacles who was hit by a cricket ball. There was a penetrating wound at 2 o'clock, traumatic aniridia and cataract.

the only lesion with which confusion can occur is total retroflexion of the iris.[1] An eye thus injured, of course, rarely survives with any useful vision, but exceptions have occurred when useful or even normal sight has been retained (Rogers, 1924; Agnello, 1925; Montanelli, 1925; Cashell, 1948). Traumatic aniridia also occurs after a perforating injury (Fig. 67).

IRIDOSCHISIS

A detachment of the anterior leaf of the mesodermal stroma of the iris from the deeper layers is a rare result of severe trauma[2]; the lesion is more com-

[1] p. 114.

[2] Bailliart (1924), Koby (1926), Schoenberg (1927), Loewenstein *et al.* (1948) and Berliner (1949).

(1866) originally brought the periphery of the iris into a corneal section but the most satisfactory technique is a modification of the suggestion made by Smith (1891) whereby the central area of the detached portion of the iris is incarcerated in a scleral section underneath a conjunctival flap in the manner of an iridencleisis. The iris may be drawn out if necessary by a hook (Goldfeder, 1932) and anchored by sutures[1] or incorporated in the scar by the light application of diathermy[2] (Figs. 65–6).

If the iridodialysis is very extensive the detached portion sometimes becomes completely rotated, possibly by the pressure-wave of aqueous, so that the pigmented back of the iris faces forward; such an appearance—*anteflexion of the iris*—is rare.

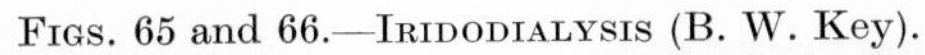

FIGS. 65 and 66.—IRIDODIALYSIS (B. W. Key).

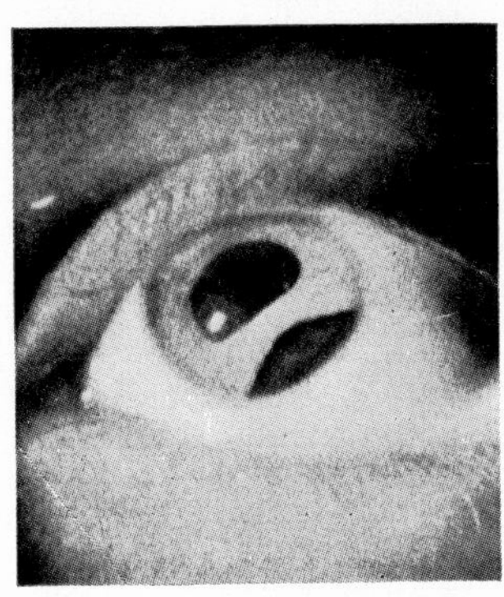

FIG. 65.

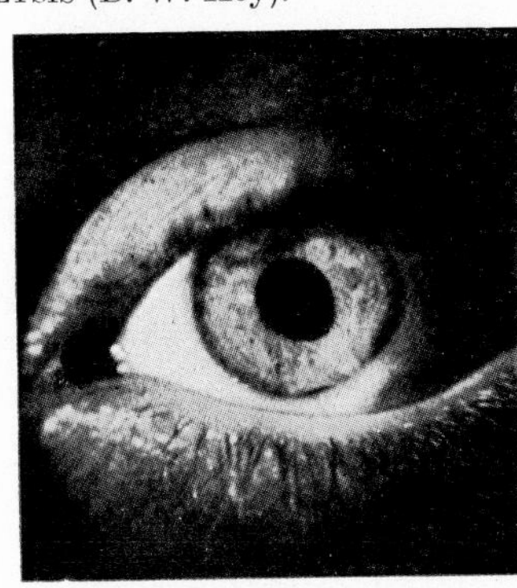

FIG. 66.

FIG. 65.—Showing the extent of the tear at the root of the iris, in a boy aged 16 who had been struck in the left eye by a BB shot 9 years previously. The dialysis measured one quarter of the circumference of the base of the iris and the pupil is oval.

FIG. 66.—The appearance after operative re-attachment.

IRIDEREMIA

If the *root of the iris is wholly torn from its attachment* to the ciliary body, that is if the dialysis is complete, the condition of IRIDEREMIA or TRAUMATIC ANIRIDIA results.[3] Such a lesion, of course, results only from a gross injury, always causing severe damage to the other ocular tissues, usually but not invariably one which involves the rupture of the globe. A complete hyphæma is the rule, usually accompanied by a massive vitreous hæmorrhage as well as a dislocation of the lens and detachment of the retina entailing ultimate blindness. In some cases, however, the other ocular tissues may suffer surprisingly little damage.

The clinical picture is dramatic (Fig. 67). When the hyphæma is absorbed the whole of the interior of the eye appears black, and if the media

[1] Jameson (1909), Bulson (1920), Key (1932–34), Barlow and Weiner (1945).

[2] Safar (1947), Arruga (1950), García Miranda (1951).

[3] Mauthner (1872), Wintersteiner (1894), Pischel (1900), Purtscher (1905), Oguchi (1913).

FIGS. 63 and 64.—THE FATE OF IRIDODIALYSIS (B. W. Key).

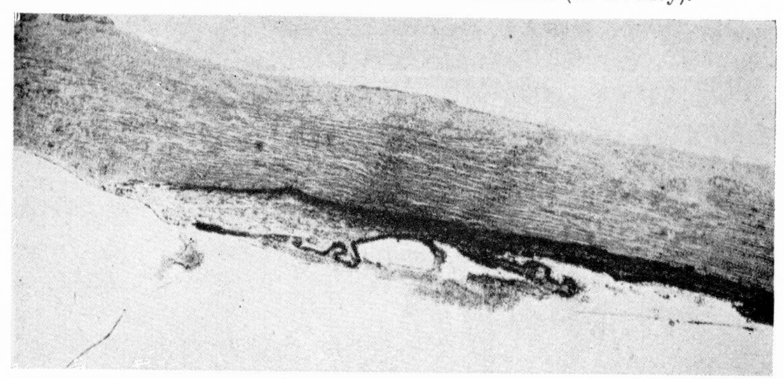

FIG. 63.—The more common event, atrophy. The part of the ciliary body from which the iris was torn is atrophic and partially destroyed.

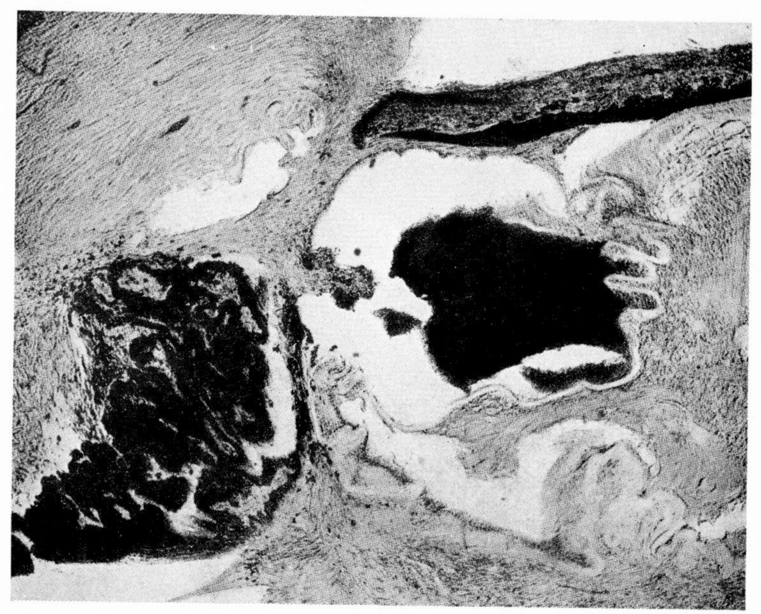

FIG. 64.—The more rare event, re-attachment. A section showing the repair of iridodialysis at a late stage. At the base of the iris there is a considerable amount of organization of fibrous tissue which has resulted in re-anchoring the iris.

expectancy, is usually not required. However, if visual confusion and diplopia distress the patient, operative measures may be indicated; the suggestion of wearing stenopæic glasses is rarely successful in practice. The simplest operative procedure is to convert the iridodialysis into a complete coloboma by an iridectomy, but if the defect is large, an alternative is to make a scleral section opposite the tear in the root of the iris and anchor the periphery in the wound. This is a somewhat tricky procedure. Amédée

PLATE V

Iridoschisis.

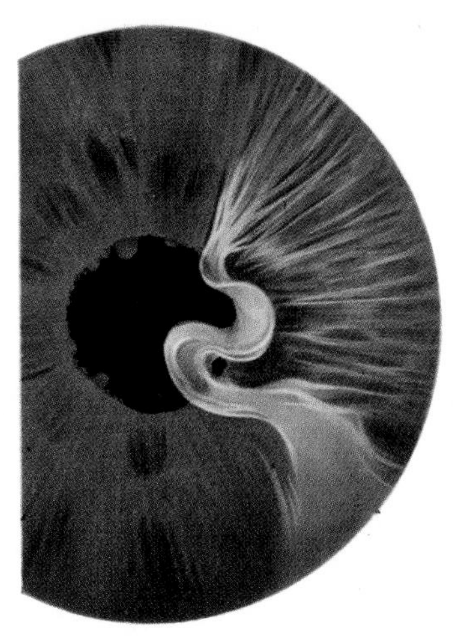

Fig. 1.—Massive traumatic separation of the anterior leaf of the iris (M. Berliner).

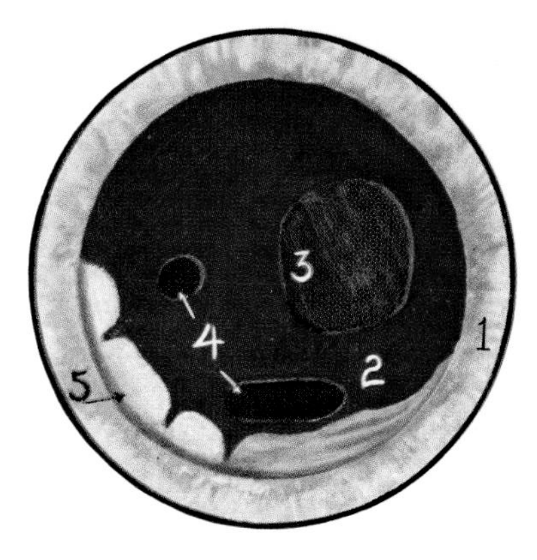

Fig. 2.—Complete separation between the stroma and the pigment epithelium.

1, Dilated anterior layer of iris; 2, pigmented layer; 3, pupil; 4, rents in pigmented layer; 5, ridges of white tissue (E. R. Veirs).

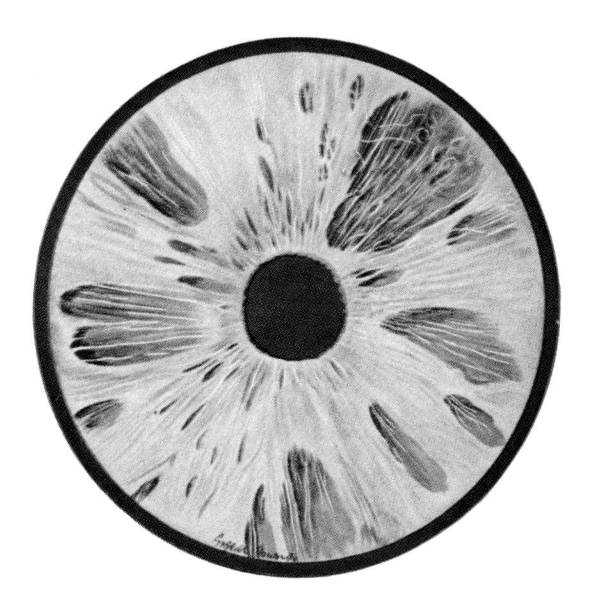

Fig. 3.—Atrophy of the anterior layers of the iris with persistence of floating strands of tissue. Through the atrophic areas the deep pigmented layer is apparent (A. Loewenstein *et al.*).

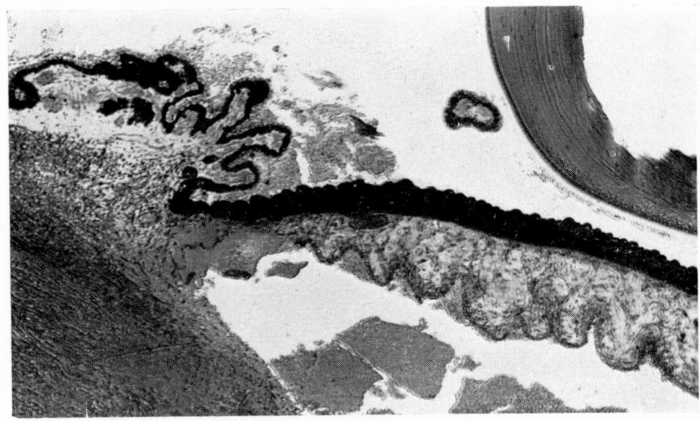

FIG. 68.—TEARING OF THE PECTINATE LIGAMENT.

After a contusion the pectinate ligament is torn with a rupture extending into the filtration angle. There is a considerable amount of hæmorrhage into the anterior and posterior chambers (B. Rones and H. C. Wilder).

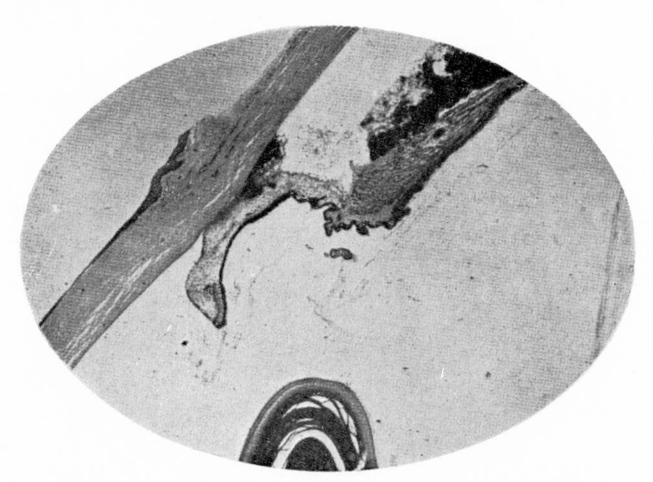

FIG. 69.—TRAUMATIC CYCLODIALYSIS AFTER A CONTUSION.

The rent has occurred at the attachment of the ciliary body to the sclera (W. Lister).

While the significance of iridodialysis and the less common cyclodialysis as evidence of injury is well recognized, there is, in addition, a more subtle change that may easily be overlooked or be confused with a cyclodialysis. This lesion, generally known as *recession of the angle of the anterior chamber*, is produced by a concussive force which tears into the face of the ciliary body resulting in a separation of the circular and radial fibres from the longitudinal muscles (Figs. 70 and 71). Such injuries are usually but not always accompanied by severe hæmorrhage into the anterior chamber, the consequences of which have already been discussed. The longitudinal fibres remain intact

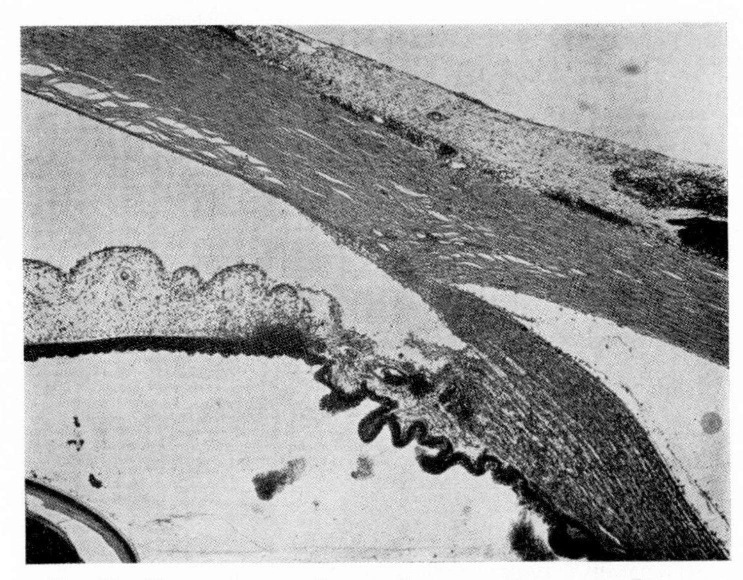

Fig. 70.—Tearing of the Ciliary Body in a Concussion Injury.

The rent runs deeply into the ciliary body from the angle of the anterior chamber, separating the circular from the longitudinal muscle fibres (W. Lister).

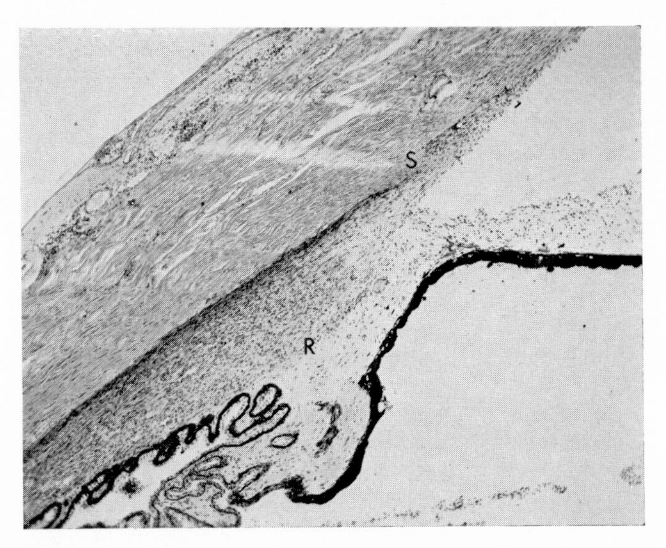

Fig. 71.—Recession of the Angle of the Anterior Chamber.

The recessed iris has become adherent to the longitudinal ciliary muscle giving the illusion that the angle is not recessed. R, root of the iris; S, scleral spur (M. E. Smith and L. E. Zimmerman).

attached to the scleral spur, while the separated circular and radial fibres and the root of the iris tend to retract posteriorly thereby giving the appearance of an abnormal depth to the anterior chamber, the recess of which on gonioscopy appears to be well behind the scleral spur. The deformity was first recognized by Treacher Collins (1892–1916) and has since received much attention.[1]

Such a recession of the angle is not infrequently seen in association with unilateral simple glaucoma which may not become apparent until some considerable time after the original injury, all other signs of which may have disappeared. On the other hand, recession may be observed after contusions without clinical or tonographic evidence of glaucoma. In general, however, it is true that the greater the extent of the recession the more likely is interference with the function of the outflow passages of the aqueous.[2]

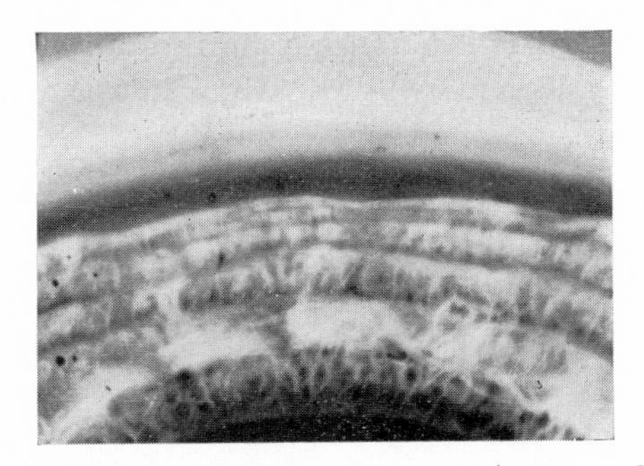

Fig. 72.—Recession of the Angle of the Anterior Chamber.

Gonioscopic view showing the traumatic cleft of the angle of the anterior chamber with a tear into the face of the ciliary body. Note the clumps of pigment scattered in the angle (T. H. Pettit and E. U. Keates).

Another result of contusion in this region is rupture of the trabecular meshwork which, together with subsequent degeneration and hyalinization, may contribute to the later development of post-traumatic glaucoma (Zimmerman, 1964).

The early recognition of recession of the angle of the anterior chamber is important because of the possibility that a sequential chronic glaucoma may develop in eyes showing this lesion. A positive diagnosis can only be made by gonioscopy, which should be done when any hyphæma that may be present has completely dispersed, and the appearances compared with those of the other eye. With the gonioscope any or all of the following signs may be observed (Fig. 72): (1) a broad, deep groove at the location of the ciliary face, (2) deepening of the angle of the anterior chamber in the periphery, (3) a more posterior insertion of uveal tissue into the angle, (4) tags of iris

[1] Lister (1924), Lamb (1927), Wolff and Zimmerman (1962), Pettit and Keates (1963), Alper (1963), Rodman (1963), Zimmerman (1964), Makabe (1970), and others.

[2] Vol. XI, p. 707.

forming a ruff at the site of their original insertion, and (5) lighter coloured tissue deep in the cleft which may give the appearance of sclera showing through where the ciliary body has been torn away or in other areas resembling newly formed fibrous tissue or exposed non-pigmented uveal tissue (Pettit and Keates, 1963). If recession of the angle or other lesions such as iridodialysis or cyclodialysis are found, the patient should be kept under observation from time to time so that ocular hypertension can be detected before the vision becomes impaired.

The whole question of the pathology, diagnosis and treatment of traumatic glaucoma including the angle-recession syndrome is discussed fully elsewhere in this *System*.[1]

RETROFLEXION OF THE IRIS

In a severe concussion as from spent shot or an explosion, as a rare event the iris may be pushed back so as to lie horizontally upon the ciliary body (Fig. 73) (Schmidt, 1805; v. Ammon, 1855; Samelson, 1872; Lister, 1924;

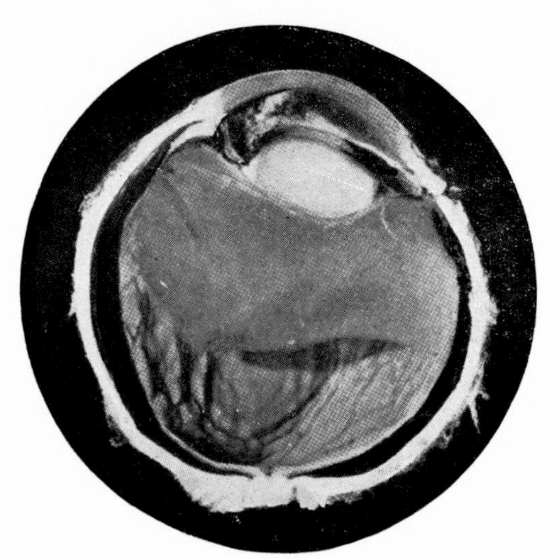

FIG. 73.—RETROFLEXION OF THE IRIS AFTER CONCUSSION.

The iris (on the left) has been bent back and caught between the ciliary body and the lens (W. Lister).

and many others). The mechanism of such an injury is probably the forceful impingement of the aqueous pushing this tissue backwards; supported at either end by its ciliary attachment and the lens, the middle portion of the iris is thrust backwards into the posterior chamber where there is least resistance and, if the miosis is not maintained or if the sphincter muscle is torn, the iris is forced backwards onto the zonule or into the vitreous if this

[1] Vol. XI, p. 712.

structure gives way. In these circumstances, of course, the firm contraction of the sphincter usually prevents the iris slipping around the lens and an iridodialysis results. A retroflexion may also be found if the globe is ruptured (Praun, 1899).

The displacement is usually *partial* involving a segment of the iris so that the pupillary edge is folded over; in such cases the clinical appearance is that of a partial coloboma except that the pupillary margin and the pattern of the iris pass uninterruptedly right up to the coloboma. More rarely the retroflexion is *complete* and the appearance of irideremia is simulated, but the ciliary processes are found to be covered over by the iris. Other lesions are invariable accompaniments, particularly traumatic cataract and a violent iridocyclitis so that the iris usually becomes rapidly attached to the ciliary body by organized exudate (Erdmann, 1901; Alt, 1902; Young, 1911).

No *treatment* is indicated in such cases and miotics are ineffective in righting the deformity; but in a partial inversion the removal of a cataractous lens has resulted in the spontaneous restitution of the iris (Würdemann, 1932).

INFLAMMATORY AND ATROPHIC CHANGES

TRAUMATIC IRIDOCYCLITIS AND ENDOPHTHALMITIS

The invariable presence of an aqueous flare of all degrees of intensity up to the outpouring of a profuse albuminous and fibrinous exudate after a concussion is an indication of the constant occurrence of a vasodilatation and an inflammatory reaction in the anterior uveal tract after a trauma of this type; we have already discussed its pathological basis—a spasmodic and temporary ischæmia followed by a prolonged paretic vasodilatation associated with much endothelial damage. The reaction may be transient and of little consequence; on the other hand, it may be of considerable severity and resistant to treatment, sometimes involving necrosis of the tissues, while the irritation may be prolonged by such extra-uveal complications as a dislocation of or injury to the lens with the development of a cataract, a retinal detachment or by such factors as an allergic response to the presence of extraneous protein material. In animal experiments Kilgore (1942) showed that extensive changes of this type may occur in the ciliary body even after comparatively trivial concussions—œdema and inflammatory infiltration, the subsequent development of fibrous tissue which replaces the muscle fibres and eventually atrophy. After more severe injury a plastic iridocyclitis may develop with the formation of exudative pupillary and cyclitic membranes which ultimately show all degrees of degeneration up to ossification (Fig. 74). In these cases the inflammation may excite a secondary glaucoma or, particularly if it is plastic in type involving the formation of posterior synechiæ, it may eventually result in a persistent hypotony and the development of atrophic changes in which neurotrophic influences may play a part. A chronic iridocyclitis of this type may be a source of great anxiety for the disease may be extremely persistent and recalcitrant and the inflammation may progress slowly and inexorably until the eye is lost. The prognosis of such cases should, therefore, be guarded, particularly when a raised or a lowered tension is a feature of the condition. *Treatment* is on general lines[1] but too frequently the response is feeble or absent and recourse must eventually be made to excision of the globe.

Where bleeding has been profuse and recurrent, the degenerative products of the hæmorrhage and the chronic granulomatous infiltration to which they may give rise not infrequently set up a relapsing uveitis which may persist for an indefinite period, sometimes for years and frequently until

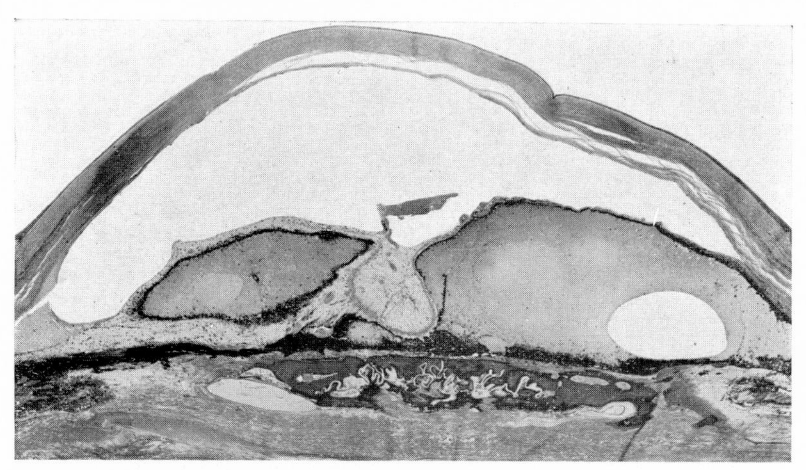

FIG. 74.—POST-CONCUSSIONAL CHRONIC ENDOPHTHALMITIS.

The end-result of the condition showing ossification of a cyclitic membrane around the incarcerated lens capsule (B. Rones and H. C. Wilder).

the eye is excised. This condition of CHRONIC HÆMOPHTHALMITIS will be described more fully in the section dealing with perforating wounds, of which it forms a more characteristic sequel.[2]

POST-TRAUMATIC ATROPHY

ATROPHY of the post-inflammatory type, sometimes of very marked degree, may follow a concussion and affect the entire anterior region of the uveal tract including not only the iris but also the ciliary body and the anterior portion of the choroid (Velhagen, 1927), a condition which may be particularly marked in association with a dislocated or subluxated lens (Santori, 1929) (Figs. 75–7). Such a condition has the usual clinical and histological characteristics of post-inflammatory atrophy,[3] and usually results in shrinkage of the globe. Occasionally, however, a typical POST-

[1] Vol. IX, p. 167. [2] p. 390. [3] Vol. IX, p. 676.

FIGS. 75 to 77.—POST-CONCUSSIONAL ATROPHY (B. Rones and H. C. Wilder).

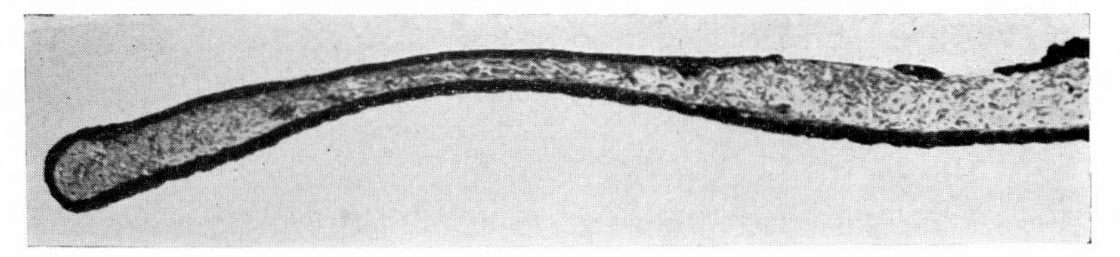

FIG. 75.—Showing marked ectropion of the uveal pigment.

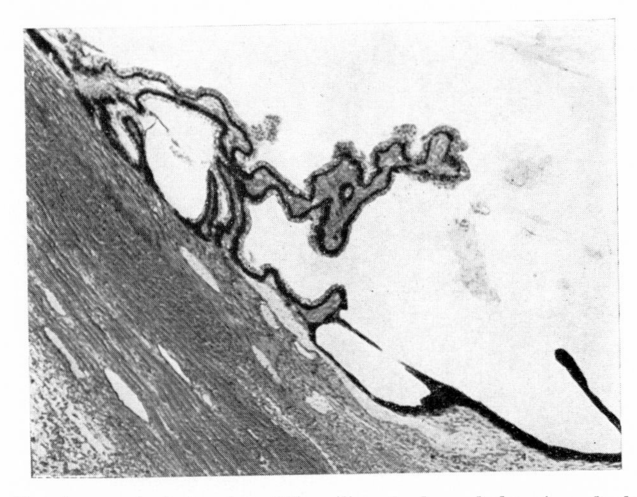

FIG. 76.—Showing marked atrophy of the ciliary body and chronic endophthalmitis.

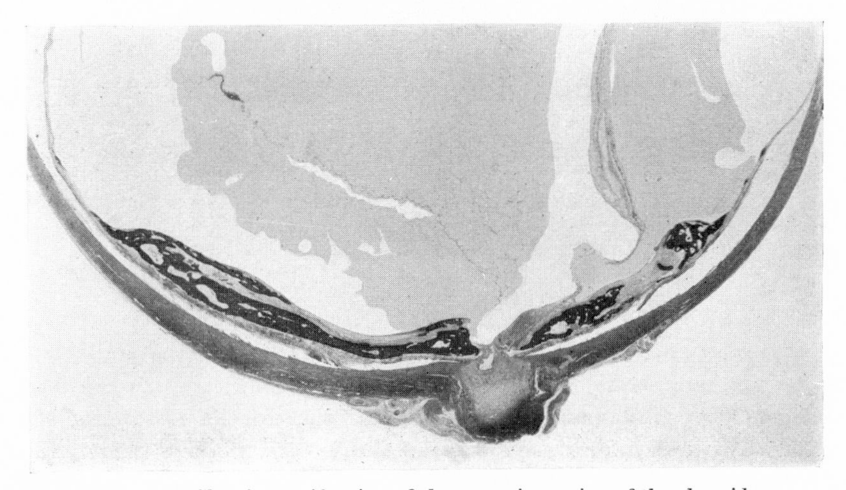

FIG. 77.—Showing ossification of the posterior region of the choroid.

CONCUSSION ATROPHY occurs due presumably to acute necrosis of the tissues, the pathology of which we have already discussed.[1] The clinical picture may be that of a generalized atrophy with loss of the delicate structure of the iris stroma and pigmentary changes; occasionally, however, it may be more dramatic. Localized patches of extreme atrophy of the stroma of the iris may occur wherein the mesodermal tissue disappears so that the pigmentary epithelium shines through (Goldberg, 1910); exceptionally complete atrophy of the iris may develop wherein the entire tissue suffers necrosis (Tillema, 1937) (Fig. 78).

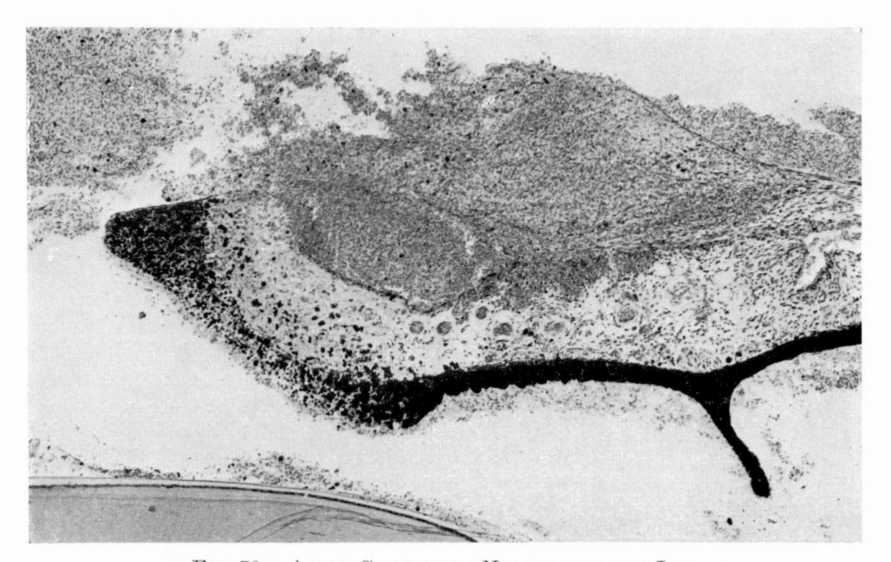

FIG. 78.—ACUTE CONCUSSION NECROSIS OF THE IRIS.

The stroma is necrotic, there is a considerable scattering of pigment and an extensive hæmorrhage on the surface of the iris (N. Ashton).

A dramatic case of this type was reported by Rychener (1944) in a child of 11 in whom a hyphæma with blood-staining of the cornea developed; as the cornea slowly cleared the iris was seen to be atrophic in patches which gradually enlarged and coalesced until eventually the entire iris was absorbed.

PIGMENTARY CHANGES

PIGMENTARY CHANGES are an almost constant accompaniment and an equally common sequel of ocular concussions. Shortly after the injury a powdering of uveal pigment on the surface of the iris, the posterior surface of the cornea and the anterior capsule of the lens is the rule, while granular deposits are frequently seen in the vitreous; the corneal pigmentation is usually transient particularly when inflammatory sequelæ are not obvious,

[1] p. 74.

but the deposits on the lens capsule and in the vitreous tend to be permanent. A generalized pigmentary peppering is usual, but the deposition may be localized. On the iris the region near the pupil may be particularly affected, or the contraction folds on the anterior surface may be loaded with pigment giving rise to the appearance of curved pigmented lines; at other times, following an atrophy of the iris, the pigmentary layer may show an extensive ectropion, spreading widely over the anterior surface of this structure (Fig. 79). On the posterior surface of the cornea an endothelial area of dystrophy may be powdered over or be surrounded by a halo of golden pigment, while the forcible contact of the cornea or the lens capsule

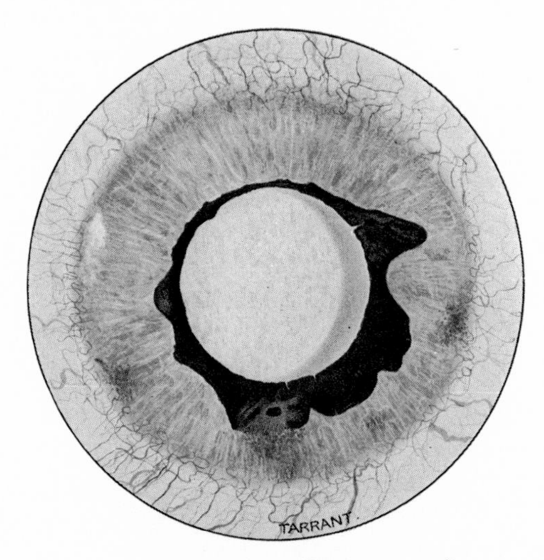

Fig. 79.—Ectropion of Pigmentary Layer.
The extensive ectropion developed after a concussion injury.

with the iris may leave imprinted on either tissue a ring of pigment corresponding to the pupillary margin. These changes may be associated with a patchy depigmentation of the posterior pigmentary layer of the iris wherein lacunæ are formed rendered clinically apparent by transillumination, and a similar pigmentary degeneration and migration may occur in the pigmentary epithelium of the retina.

Further pigmentary changes may occur as a long-term result of concussion injuries whereby, sometimes 10, sometimes 30 years afterwards, partly owing to the migration of pigment and possibly owing also to the new formation of pigment as a result of the trauma or the consequent iritis (Vogt, 1941), the injured iris becomes darker than its fellow so that it resembles that of a normal but very dark brown eye—an appearance of *inverse* (*hyperchromic*) *heterochromia* which is particularly evident in lightly coloured eyes. The superficial layers of the stroma are most markedly affected whereon nævoid-like clumps of dense pigmentation may be very prominent; some degree of atrophy is usually associated with the hyperpigmentation. Owing to the length of time taken for such changes to develop, they are seen most typically after an injury in youth; they are, however, more characteristic of perforating injuries than concussions and have also been seen after a discission operation for congenital cataract (Koby, 1930).

Traumatic hyperchromic heterochromia developed in 11 cases described by Sugar (1965–68) in each of which the causative injury occurred before the age of 10 years; the area of hyperchromia appeared to be the result of hypertrophy of the superficial layers of the stroma of the iris. Apart from siderotic hyperchromia which was specifically excluded from his group, Sugar (1968) considered that these changes might be due to an increased blood supply associated with temporary inflammation or to the migration of chromatophores from the normal tissue bordering the injured area, a phenomenon which was demonstrated experimentally in rabbits by Heydenreich (1958).

HÆMATOGENOUS PIGMENTATION is a more rare sequel, whereby a circumscribed area around a hæmorrhage into the iris stroma or the whole iris in cases of massive hyphæma may assume a yellowish appearance.

Agnello. *Lettura oftal.*, **2,** 171 (1925).
Alper. *Arch. Ophthal.*, **69,** 455 (1963).
Alt. *Amer. J. Ophthal.*, **19,** 4 (1902).
Amédée. *Gaz. Hôp. Paris*, **39,** 39 (1866).
von Ammon. *v. Graefes Arch. Ophthal.*, **1** (2), 119 (1855).
Arlt. *Ueber d. Verletzungen des Auges*, Wien (1875).
Arruga. *Chirurgie oculaire*, Barcelona (1950).
Ayres. *Amer. J. Ophthal.*, **22,** 138 (1905).
Bailliart. *Bull. Soc. Ophtal. Paris*, 308 (1924).
Barlow and Weiner. *Arch. Ophthal.*, **34,** 292 (1945).
Berliner. *Biomicroscopy of the Eye*, N.Y., **2,** 916 (1949).
Brown. *J. Amer. med. Ass.*, **83,** 1865 (1924).
Buchanan. *Trans. ophthal. Soc. U.K.*, **23,** 283 (1903).
Bulson. *Amer. J. Ophthal.*, **3,** 357 (1920).
Cashell. *Trans. ophthal. Soc. U.K.*, **68,** 241 (1948).
Cattaneo. *Ann. Ottal.*, **58,** 11 (1930).
Collins. *Trans. ophthal. Soc. U.K.*, **12,** 180 (1892); **36,** 204 (1916).
Duane. *Amer. J. Ophthal.*, **9,** 531 (1926).
Eisenhuth. *Bericht ü. d. bei Contusionsverletzungen beobachteten Veränderungen d. Uvealtractus* (Diss.), Giessen (1899).
Erdmann. *Ueber d. wahre u. scheinbare Luxation d. Linse in d. vordere Kammer* (Diss.), Freiburg (1901).
Fejer. *Arch. Augenheilk.*, **48,** 267 (1903).
Förster. *Klin. Mbl. Augenheilk.*, **25,** Beil., 143 (1887).
Frenkel. *Arch. Ophtal.*, **48,** 5 (1931); **49,** 431 (1932).
Gala. *Wien. med. Wschr.*, **91,** 355 (1941).
Gangoso. *Arch. Soc. oftal. hisp.-amer.*, **8,** 402 (1948).
García Miranda. *Arch. Soc. oftal. hisp.-amer.*, **11,** 513 (1951).
Goldberg. *Ann. Ophthal.*, **19,** 457 (1910).
Goldfeder. *Klin. Mbl. Augenheilk.*, **89,** 229 (1932).
Gradle. *Arch. Ophthal.*, **11,** 92 (1934).
Graves. *Proc. roy. Soc. Med.*, **22,** 962 (1929).
Herrmann. *Die Kontusionsverletzungen d. Auges in klin. u. path.-anat. Beziehung* (Diss.), Leipzig (1906).
Heydenreich. *v. Graefes Arch. Ophthal.*, **160,** 236 (1958).
Jameson. *Arch. Ophthal.*, **38,** 391 (1909).
Key. *Arch. Ophthal.*, **7,** 748 (1932).
Amer. J. Ophthal., **17,** 301 (1934).
Kilgore. *Amer. J. Ophthal.*, **25,** 1095 (1942).
Koby. *Biomicroscopie de l'oeil vivant*, Paris (1926).
Slit-lamp Microscopy of the Living Eye, London (1930).
Lamb. *Arch. Ophthal.*, **56,** 332 (1927).
Legrand and Dubois-Poulsen. *Bull. Soc. Ophtal. Fr.*, 937 (1949).
Lister. *Brit. J. Ophthal.*, **8,** 305 (1924).
Loewenstein and Foster. *Brit. J. Ophthal.*, **29,** 277 (1945).
Loewenstein, Foster and Sledge. *Brit. J. Ophthal.*, **32,** 129 (1948).
Makabe. *Klin. Mbl. Augenheilk.*, **157,** 79 (1970).
Mauthner. *Ber. nat.-med. Vereins in Innsbruck.*, **2,** 197 (1872).
Mawas. *Biomicroscopie de la chambre antérieure*, Paris (1928).
Mayou. *Trans. ophthal. Soc. U.K.*, **29,** 254 (1909).
Moffatt. *Proc. roy. Soc. Med.*, **43,** 1011 (1950)
Montanelli. *Lettura oftal.*, **2,** 370 (1925).
Müller. *Ueber d. Ruptur d. Corneo-Skleralgrenze durch stumpfe Verletzung*, Wien (1895).
Oguchi. *Beitr. Augenheilk.*, **9** (83), 75 (1913).

Pettit and Keates. *Arch. Ophthal.*, **69,** 438 (1963).
Pischel. *Arch. Augenheilk.*, **40,** 357 (1900).
Pohlenz. *Ueber Risse d. Sphincter iridis u. d. Chorioidea* (Diss.), Halle (1891).
Praun. *Die Verletzungen des Auges*, Wiesbaden, 270, 283, 284 (1899).
Zbl. prakt. Augenheilk., **26,** 268 (1902).
Purtscher. *Beitr. Augenheilk., Festschr. für Hirschberg*, 227 (1905).
Reid. *Ann. Phys. Med.*, Jena, **1,** 83 (1850).
Rodman. *Arch. Ophthal.*, **69,** 445 (1963).
Rogers. *Amer. J. Ophthal.*, **7,** 950 (1924).
Rones and Wilder. *Amer. J. Ophthal.*, **30,** 1143 (1947).
Rychener. *J. Amer. med. Ass.*, **126,** 763 (1944).
Safar. *Ophthalmologica*, **114,** 77 (1947).
Samelson. *Brit. med. J.*, **2,** 351 (1872).
Santori. *Boll. Oculist.*, **8,** 31 (1929).
Schenk and Papapanos. *Klin. Mbl. Augenheilk.*, **133,** 212 (1958).
Schmidt. *Ophthal. Bib.*, Jena, **3** (1), 171 (1805)
Schoenberg. *Arch. Ophthal.*, **56,** 538 (1927).
Shedlov. *J. Amer. med. Ass.*, **83,** 1507 (1924).
Smith, E. *J. Amer. med. Ass.*, **17,** 445 (1891).
Stephenson. *Trans. ophthal. Soc. U.K.*, **36,** 202 (1916).
Sugar. *Amer. J. Ophthal.*, **60,** 1 (1965); **66,** 710 (1968).
Sweet. *Ophthal. Rec.*, **10,** 345 (1901).
Tillema. *Arch. Ophthal.*, **17,** 586 (1937).
Tvyl. *Z. Augenheilk.*, **3,** 149 (1900).
Vannas. *Arch. Augenheilk.*, **106,** 1 (1932).
Veirs. *Amer. J. Ophthal.*, **32,** 261 (1949).
Velhagen. *Klin. Mbl. Augenheilk.*, **78,** Beil., 156 (1927).
Vogt. *v. Graefes Arch. Ophthal.*, **112,** 89 (1923).
Lhb. u. Atlas d. Spaltlampenmikroskopie d. lebenden Auges, 2nd ed., Zurich, **3,** 906 (1941).
Weiss and Klingelhöffer. *Arch. Augenheilk.*, **39,** 237 (1899).
Werner. *Ophthal. Rev.*, **6,** 103 (1887).
Wicherkiewicz. *Klin. Mbl. Augenheilk.*, **42** (1), 363 (1904).
Wintersteiner. *v. Graefes Arch. Ophthal.*, **40** (2), 1 (1894).
Wolff and Zimmerman. *Amer. J. Ophthal.*, **54,** 547 (1962).
Würdemann. *Northwest. Med.*, **7,** 55, 87 (1909).
Injuries of the Eye, London (1932).
Young. *Ophthal. Rec.*, **20,** 215 (1911).
Zimmerman. *Industrial and Traumatic Ophthalmology* (ed. Allen), St. Louis, 227 (1964).

Concussion Effects on the Lens and Zonule

Injuries to the lens and its supporting mechanism from concussions are common and are frequently seen after direct blows on the eyeball or as a result of force applied to the skull or the passage of a bullet through the orbit. They develop with unexpected frequency even after minor concussions of the globe (60% of cases, Davidson, 1936); after severe injuries they almost invariably occur; and indeed, apart from paresis or tearing of the iris, lenticular damage is the commonest sequel of injuries of this type.

POSTERIOR LENTICONUS. While the common result of a concussion is the formation of one or other type of lenticular opacity, a posterior lenticonus, presumably due to the occurrence of a capsular tear in the region of the posterior pole, has been noted (Rosen, 1945; Bégué, 1949; Tipshus, 1969).

LENTICULAR OPACITIES AND CONCUSSION CATARACT

The earliest record of changes in the lens following concussion is somewhat curious: Ezra Dyer (1867) reported to the American Ophthalmological Society the appearance of a " fracture " of the lens and the anterior capsule in a man who was hanged, and in a spirit of true scientific ardour he confirmed the ætiological relationship by observing the same effects in three dogs hanged as an experiment. Subsequent observations multiplied rapidly until Wagenmann (1915) collected some 200 cases from the world literature. The early clinical descriptions, however, were somewhat vague and general agreement on the precise ætiology was lacking until the advent of the slit-lamp offered abundant opportunities for detailed and exact observation. In this the work of Vogt (1921–31) was fundamental; he first described the many morphological forms these lens changes may assume, a large number of them hitherto unrecognized because of their minuteness; he traced their life-history and established their prognostic significance. Several observers have expanded his observations, among whom Koby (1930), Lugli (1935) and Davidson (1940) deserve special mention.

A considerable amount of experimental work on animals has confirmed the occurrence of cataractous changes after concussions of the eye since Dyer's (1867) enthusiastic interest in the subject; of particular note are the publications of Berlin (1873), Schlösser (1887), Bäck (1898), Bonnefon (1912) and Cattaneo (1934). The observations of early workers on the effects of direct massage of the lens in inducing opacities is also germane to the subject, a procedure at one time advocated to hasten the maturation of a senile cataract.

The *mechanism of the damage to the lens* in concussions has excited considerable interest; in this tissue, however, the vascular reaction and therefore contusion effects are absent so that only the concussion effects on the cells themselves and lacerations of the tissues become evident. The pathogenesis is therefore relatively simple. When a sudden force strikes the eye, a wave of pressure thrusts the aqueous and iris forcibly against the lens and pushes it backwards onto the vitreous; on its rebound the lens hurls itself back against the iris. Moreover, in the fluid contents of the globe the force is transmitted in all directions so that the capsule and its epithelium as well as the lenticular substance itself are concussed; this may damage the protoplasmic structure of lens fibres (Hudson, 1910), and necrosis of the capsular epithelium as well as the ciliary epithelium may result (d'Oswaldo, 1925). In addition, the lens substance may be torn from the capsule, the tissues suffering, as it were, an intracapsular subluxation involving epithelial injury and a severance of the physiological connection between the mass of the lens and its capsule (zur Nedden, 1904; Law, 1932; Cattaneo, 1934). Similar mechanical disturbances may occur among the fibres; it is interesting that Bellows and Chinn (1941) found experimentally that after digital manipulation *in vitro*, even when the capsule was not torn, the slightly traumatized lens imbibed twice as much water as controls, a significant increase which these workers attributed to a separation of the normal contiguity of the fibres. Finally, the damage to the capsule due to concussion may impair its semi-permeability, allowing the imbibition of aqueous by the lens substance and disturbing the active transport of metabolites, and in more severe traumata the mechanical forces involved—the forcible to-and-fro movement of the lens, the distortion of its shape, and the strain put on the zonule by the sudden antero-posterior contraction and the associated circumferential expansion of the equatorial region of the globe—may cause tears in the capsule (Weidenthal and Schepens, 1966). Not infrequently these occur at the thinnest part of the capsule at the posterior pole where it may give way as an alternative to (and sometimes in association with) a rupture of the zonule (Schirmer, 1890).

The question of the frequency of capsular tears and their importance in the genesis of lenticular opacities has excited much interest and considerable controversy. That gross tears in the capsule do occur after a concussion has long been known and was noted by early writers both in the anterior capsule[1] and in the posterior region[2] (Fig. 113); similarly, although less frequently, tears near the equator have been observed in cases of iridodialysis (Fuchs, 1888; Gründgens, 1902). In more recent years delicate tears in the posterior capsule have been seen with the aid of the slit-lamp when they have not been suspected (Gscheidel, 1939).

It has been the general custom to divide concussion cataracts into two categories—those associated with a capsular tear and those in which no tear was observed; the opacification in the first type was generally agreed to be due to the free entry of aqueous into the lens, in the second to a derangement of the normal semi-permeability of the capsule leading to a similar but less dramatic imbibition of fluid; the mechanism of the first type was taken to be exactly parallel to that of the traumatic cataract which follows a wound of the lens in a perforating injury. It has also been argued that the differentiation may not be valid, since failure to see a tear clinically does not necessarily exclude its presence, particularly if it is small and equatorial in site so that it is hidden by the iris. Moreover, the clinical appearances of the two types of cataract, that occurring with and that occurring without a visible capsular tear, are frequently very akin; the same or similar morphological pictures are observed in both as well as after perforating wounds, and in either type the opacification may be diffuse or remain segmental or local. Even in the observable presence of a tear in the anterior capsule the opacification may remain localized or a preliminary local clouding of the lens may disappear so that normal vision results, the tear itself being rapidly sealed off by fibrin while the imbibition of fluid is still reversible (Landesberg, 1886; Stern, 1945). Moreover, in perforating wounds wherein the lens capsule is directly injured, a large proportion of the cases shows not rapid and generalized opacification but the localized and morphologically distinctive opacities characteristic of concussion injuries (Davidson, 1940).

The *healing of experimental tears in the capsule* was originally studied by Schlösser (1887) and Schirmer (1889). Histologically a cap of fibrin is formed over the rent and in the immediate region the epithelial cells rapidly degenerate. Shortly thereafter the neighbouring subcapsular epithelium grows over the defect, at first as flattened cells which subsequently take on a spindle shape. These cells eventually decrease in size and become replaced by a homogeneous matrix which in turn becomes covered by normal epithelium which secretes a hyaline membrane both in front of it and behind it. If the tear occurs in the region of the iris the reconstitution of the injured area is reinforced by fibroblasts from this tissue and sometimes pigment from the iris is incorporated in the scar. In this way the tear may be completely and rapidly closed, in which case the damage to the lens is localized, the disintegrated fibres in the neighbourhood are absorbed, and new fibres are laid down, at first disposed irregularly but later assuming the normal configuration.

[1] Dyer (1867), Bresgen (1881), Landesberg (1886), Hosch (1889), Liebrecht (1895), and many others.

[2] Knapp (1869), Aub (1871), Collins (1891).

This unpredictable behaviour of the lens after a capsular rupture is well known and is most dramatically seen in the occasional failure of a discission operation to induce a lenticular opacity of more than local extent, a disappointing surgical result typically seen in a subluxated lens; it may be that the lack of zonular and capsular tension in these cases prevents the tear from gaping. The difficulty in inducing a widespread opacity in the lenses of such animals as the rabbit by discission is also well known, and it is possible that this failure is due to the association of poor accommodation in these animals with a slight zonular tension.

For these reasons Vogt (1931) suggested that after contusions wherein a capsular tear was seen or suspected, atropine should be avoided and relaxation of the zonule ensured by the use of miotics in order that the rent might be more readily sealed.

It would appear probable, therefore, that an alteration in the semi-permeability of the capsule so that it can no longer control the normal interchange of fluid between the aqueous and the lens, brought about either by direct concussive injury to the epithelial cells or by an internal tearing away of the subcapsular epithelium, may cause a temporary disturbance resulting in a localized opacity; the same effect may be produced by a small capsular tear which rapidly becomes occluded. A more generalized concussive effect or a larger gaping tear will lead to a more widespread or a complete opacification; but it is possible that the essential mechanism in each case is the same. Traumatic capsular rupture associated with simple penetrating wounds or the passage of an intra-ocular foreign body or as an inadvertent or intentional result of ocular surgery will be discussed subsequently.[1]

A great variety of lenticular changes may follow concussions. In the vast majority of cases the opacity is localized and stationary, with morphological appearances so characteristic as to be diagnostic of previous injury even in the absence of a definite history of trauma: this is of obvious medico-legal importance. Such lesions are typically seen in the young; both experimentally and clinically they invariably commence in the subcapsular zone and they frequently retain a segmental distribution. Some of these changes are transient, in which case they are probably due to the presence of fluid between the cellular elements accompanied by cytoplasmic changes so slight as to be reversible. The more permanent changes are associated with the interstitial appearance of granules, fluid clefts and vacuoles as well as intracytoplasmic structural changes (observed ultra-microscopically in his experiments by Cattaneo, 1934) leading eventually to necrosis and fragmentation of the cells and fibres. As time goes on these subcapsular lesions tend to be buried by the new formation of clear lens fibres, so that eventually they lie deeply in the lens with a zonular distribution, separated from the

[1] p. 352.

capsule by an optically clear band. Finally, in less severe lesions no immediate pathological changes may be evident but, although the lens may remain apparently normal for a considerable time, sufficient damage may have been done to determine the development of opacities at a later date; this again is of obvious prognostic and medico-legal importance.

In persons above 40 or 45 years of age, however, the case is somewhat different. Initially the same or similar opacities may appear but these tend to be followed by progressive changes, either pre-senile changes of the coronary type or those typical of senile cataract; it would seem that the injury serves to activate these degenerative processes which gradually obliterate the specific morphology of the concussion opacities. The difference in the reaction of the young and the old lens may be partly due to the greater resilience of the iris and the softer and more readily moulded consistency of the youthful lens, and partly to the tendency already present in the ageing lens to develop senile changes. Apart, therefore, from the rapid development of a diffuse cataract in the presence of a large capsular tear, the prognosis of concussion opacities in a lens under the age of 40 is on the whole good, while after this age it should be guarded.

The lenticular opacities which may follow concussion are thus protean in their morphology. They comprise:

1. *Vossius's ring opacity*, the most striking feature of which is the epicapsular deposition of pigment.

2. Localized opacities due to subcapsular changes; these opacities may be discrete, punctate and scattered (*disseminated subepithelial opacities*), film-like in their distribution (*cobweb opacities*) or sufficiently numerous to develop into a *zonular* (*lamellar*) *cataract*. On the other hand, a diffuse subepithelial œdema may give rise to a *rosette-shaped opacity*. These localized changes may eventually give rise to an atrophic condition of the lens or may precipitate the development of pre-senile or senile changes.

3. *Diffuse cataractous changes* may result, usually associated with a capsular tear of some dimensions, and these may lead to total absorption of the lens in the young and its ultimate degeneration in the aged.

A unique case was reported by Rychener (1945) wherein an area of violaceous blood-staining or hæmorrhage developed in the cataractous lens apparently after the rupture of the posterior capsule in the presence of a large vitreous hæmorrhage.

VOSSIUS'S RING OPACITY

A ring corresponding to the pupillary aperture composed of myriads of reddish-brown or bronze amorphous granules of pigment disposed flatly on the anterior lens capsule following a concussion was first described by Vossius (1903) (Plate VI). The ring is typically about 1 mm. in breadth and the pigment lies in a single layer on the surface of the capsule, but the concentration of granules lessens and becomes more irregular axially and equatorially; the ring is also usually segmented in shape with constrictions or gaps in its contour, an appearance which seems to correspond to the ridges and folds on the posterior surface of the iris. This annular deposition of pigment appears only in the young (Purtscher, 1913; Vogt, 1931) and tends to disappear slowly and gradually in the course of several weeks or months. Sometimes from the beginning but more frequently at a later stage after the pigment has largely been absorbed, very fine discrete punctiform opacities are seen in the same annular arrangement immediately under the capsule; initially these tend to increase, they may persist for several years but eventually also tend to disappear.

Occasionally the deposition of pigment may be continued beyond the ring almost up to the equator of the lens (Vogt, 1931), and the imprint of a " negative photograph " of the iris on the capsule has been recorded (Anderson, 1919).

The cause of this ring of pigment has been disputed, but the original explanation advanced by Vossius (1903) is generally accepted, that it is an imprint of the pupillary border of the iris upon the capsule caused after the manner of a rubber stamp, its size corresponding to the extreme miosis which develops on receipt of the injury; this may be followed by the development of degenerative changes of a concussive type in the capsular epithelium, resulting in the appearance of transient opacities in these cells. It may be that the pigment is made to adhere to the surface of the capsule by a simultaneous fibrinous exudate from the iris. The imprint occurs at the time of injury and may be due to the iris being suddenly forced against the lens (Vossius, 1903) or to the lens in its rebound engaging the pupillary aperture (Frenkel, 1931); the occasional occurrence of a duplicated ring may be explained by a combination of both mechanisms, while its appearance after a concussion injury at the back of the orbit (as by a bullet) may be a result of the latter alone (Steiner, 1910; Purtscher, 1913). In favour of this hypothesis is the fact that the ring assumes an eccentric form if the pupil is deformed (Caspar, 1909; Purtscher, 1913) and that the corresponding region of the posterior surface of the iris is depigmented, the degree of depigmentation varying with the density and extent of the ring (Alajmo, 1929). The fact that it appears only in the young suggests that the iris must possess considerable elasticity to deposit the imprint.

It has been suggested that the annular deposit is composed of blood pigment and that it may develop after a hyphæma which is not necessarily traumatic in origin (Hesse, 1919; Zentmayer, 1924; Gundersen, 1946). It is true that a ring-shaped deposit of blood pigment may be found on the capsule after a hyphæma whether traumatic or not in origin, or after iridocyclitis, but this is to be differentiated from a true Vossius's ring by its comparative narrowness, its coarser clumps of pigment, its aggregation in heaps, the presence of isolated particles axial to the main ring, and the frequent presence of fibrous whitish exudates associated with the pigment. It is to be noted that whether it occurs in the presence or absence of a hyphæma, a true Vossius's ring is always most dense immediately after the trauma and tends to disappear gradually even although blood remains in the anterior chamber.

PLATE VI

A VOSSIUS RING OPACITY (J. H. Doggart).

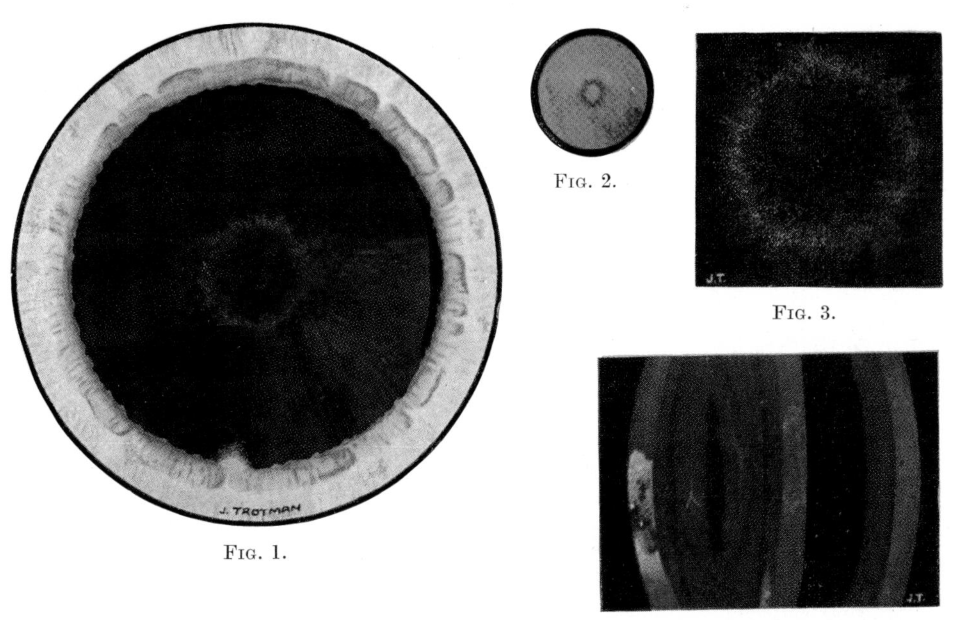

FIG. 2.

FIG. 3.

FIG. 1.

FIG. 4.

FIG. 1.—As seen by oblique illumination.

FIG. 2.—Ophthalmoscopic appearance.

FIG. 3.—A magnified surface view.

FIG. 4.—Optical section. On the right of the lens two segments of the Vossius ring are seen; on the left, changes in the posterior capsule with deposition of blood.

PLATE VII

CONCUSSION CATARACT.

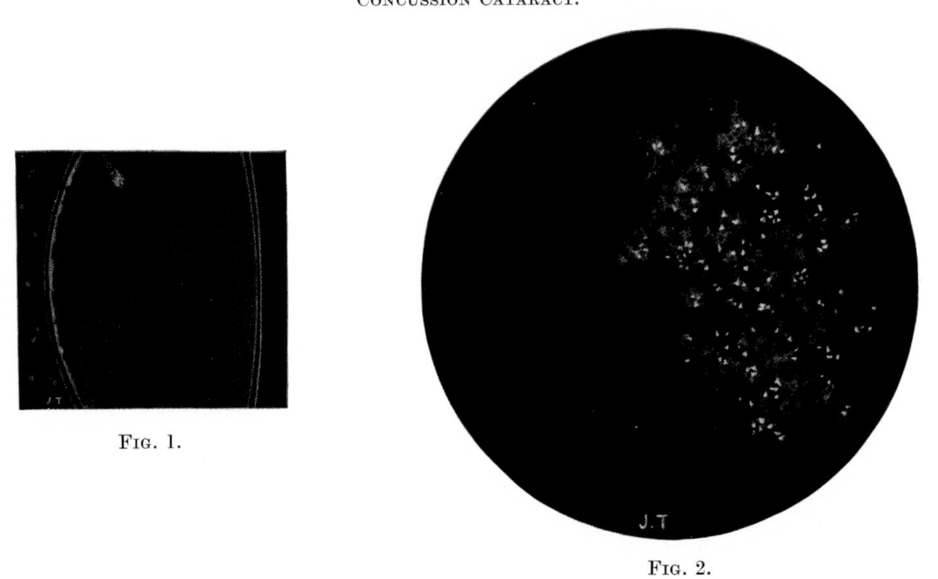

FIG. 1.

FIG. 2.

FIGS. 1 AND 2.—Stationary punctate opacities at a late stage (J. H. Doggart).

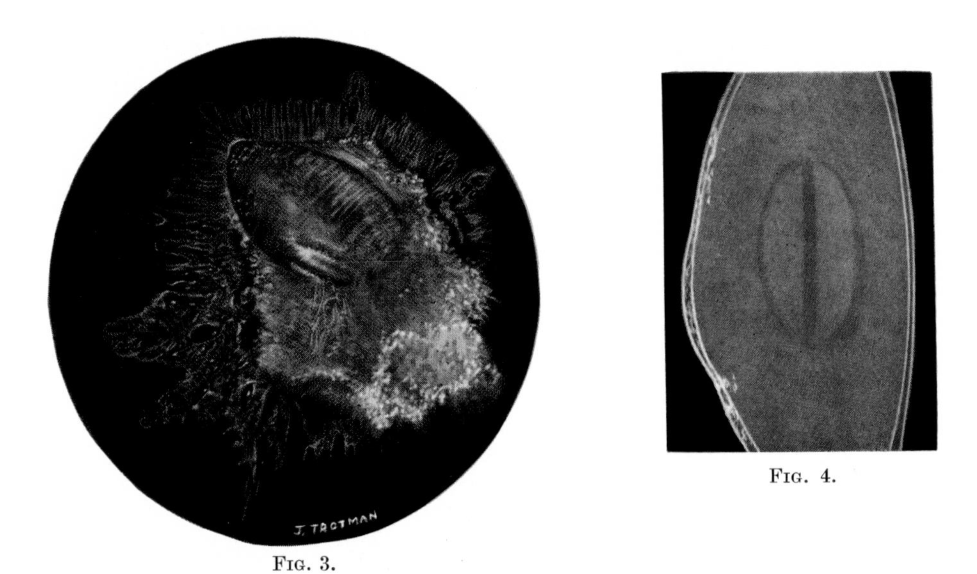

FIG. 4.

FIG. 3.

FIGS. 3 AND 4.—Diffuse subcapsular opacities at a late stage.

An annular ring of opacity on the posterior capsule analogous to the ring of Vossius has been observed by Disler (1938), Davidson (1940) and Papagno (1950), formed presumably by retinal pigment liberated into the vitreous.

DISCRETE SUBEPITHELIAL OPACITIES

We have seen that concussion damage to the capsule so that its permeability is impaired, or mechanical injury to the epithelial cells, may determine the formation of subcapsular opacities. Depending on the extent of the damage, few and localized or more widespread opacities may result and, depending on the degree of force involved, these opacities will tend to be transient or permanent. Upon this common basis a great variety of clinical pictures can be built, differing little in their ætiology and pathology.

SUBEPITHELIAL DISSEMINATED TRAUMATIC OPACITIES

The occurrence of small, discrete punctate or flattened flake-like opacities lying underneath the anterior epithelium following concussions to the eye was first adequately studied by Vogt (1922), and the observations of Davidson (1940) have shown their great frequency even after the milder types of injury (Figs. 80–81; Plate VII); it is interesting that somewhat similar punctate opacities are also seen after an acute attack of glaucoma.[1] Such opacities may be axial or equatorial in distribution and, although they may

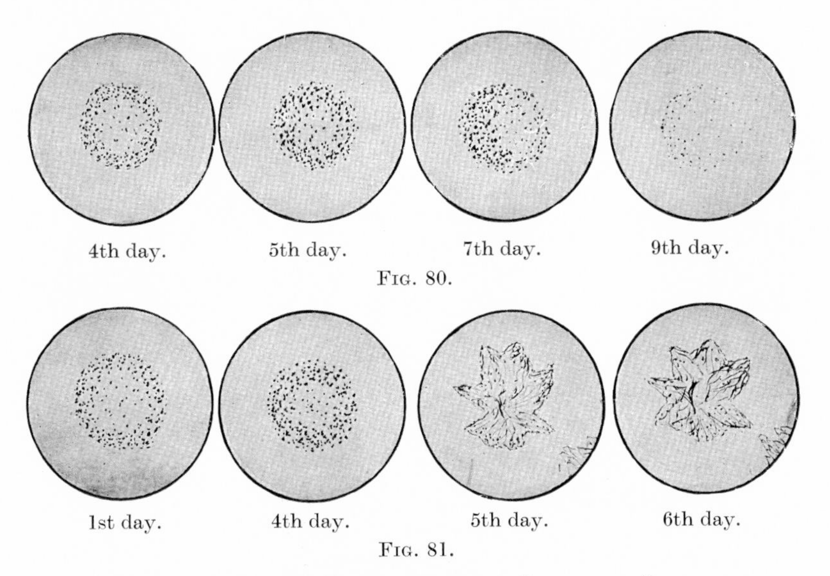

4th day. 5th day. 7th day. 9th day.

Fig. 80.

1st day. 4th day. 5th day. 6th day.

Fig. 81.

Figs. 80 and 81.—The Disappearance of Concussion Changes.

To show the changes in the opacities of the lens. The changes present in each lens on the days subsequent to a concussion are shown as they appear in each eye. All the opacities were in the anterior cortex. The right lens (Fig. 80) became clear on the 13th day and the left (Fig. 81) on the 9th day after the injury (M. H. Whiting).

[1] Vol. XI, p. 40.

be scattered irregularly over a large area in the axial region of the lens, they have a predilection for a segmental distribution; an orderly radial arrangement has been observed (Foster, 1938). Sometimes such opacities tend to disappear within a few days or weeks after the injury, their behaviour resembling the subcapsular opacities associated with a Vossius's ring (Whiting, 1916) (Figs. 80–81); they may be superseded by a stellate opacity which itself may be transient but they are usually stationary and permanent. In the last event they gradually become separated from the subepithelial zone as the lens grows and new fibres are laid down peripherally, so that they remain as a permanent imprint of the injury, the age of which is roughly determined by the depth in the lens at which they lie. Occasionally,

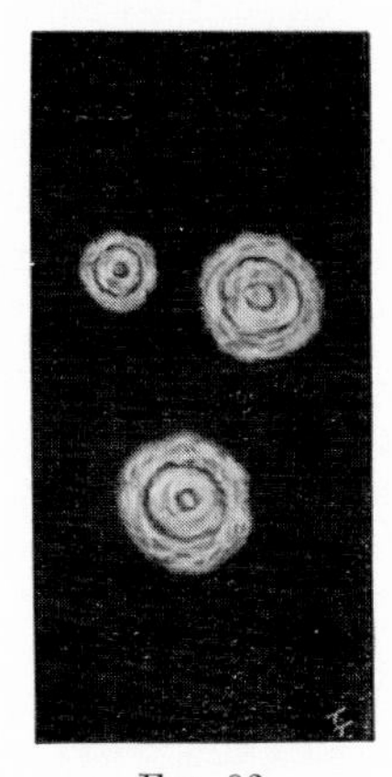

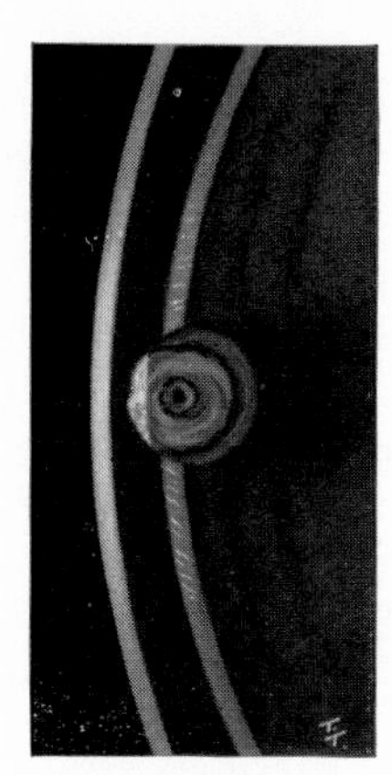

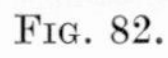

Fig. 82. Fig. 83.

Figs. 82 and 83.—Cataracta Nodiformis of Vogt.
As seen by diffuse illumination (Fig. 82); in the beam of the slit-lamp (Fig. 83).

as the opacities sink more deeply into the growing lens, small " tags " remain adherent to the capsular epithelium (Berliner, 1949).

The delayed formation of these subepithelial opacities so that they were first apparent two years after the injury has been recorded by Vogt (1922).

More rarely the subepithelial opacities are of considerable size, discrete, dense and round with a layered structure somewhat like a small anterior polar cataract (cataracta nodiformis, Vogt, 1922) (Figs. 82–83).

A more diffuse cobweb subcapsular opacity with a filmy structure supporting fine dust-like opacities is a more rare occurrence affecting young people after injuries, both concussive and perforating. Such changes have been described by Rolett (1940) usually in association with the anterior, less frequently with the posterior capsule (Plate VII; Figs. 84–88). They are permanent and, occurring in the apparent absence of a capsular rupture, may be due to mechanical damage to the epithelium resulting from changes in the shape of the lens following a sudden and violent concussion, or to an

FIGS. 84 to 88.—CONCUSSION CATARACT.

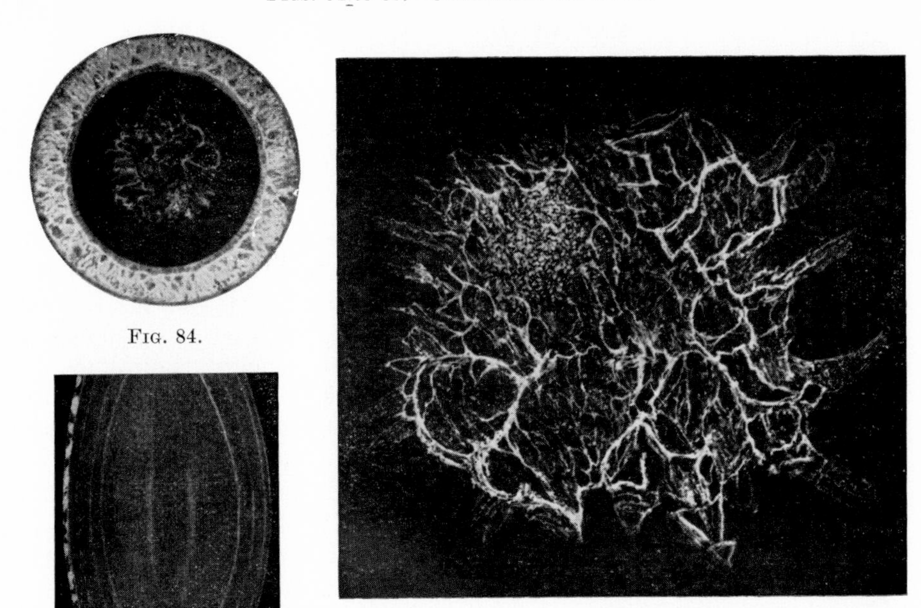

FIG. 84.

FIG. 85.

FIG. 86.

FIGS. 84 to 86.—COBWEB SUBCAPSULAR OPACITY (D. M. Rolett).

FIG. 84.—The condition as seen by oblique illumination.

FIG. 85.—The lens in the beam of the slit-lamp shows the opacity lying on the surface immediately under the capsule.

FIG. 86.—Enlargement of the opacity shows that it consists of a delicate framework supporting dust-like spots which, towards the periphery, end in sharply pointed processes.

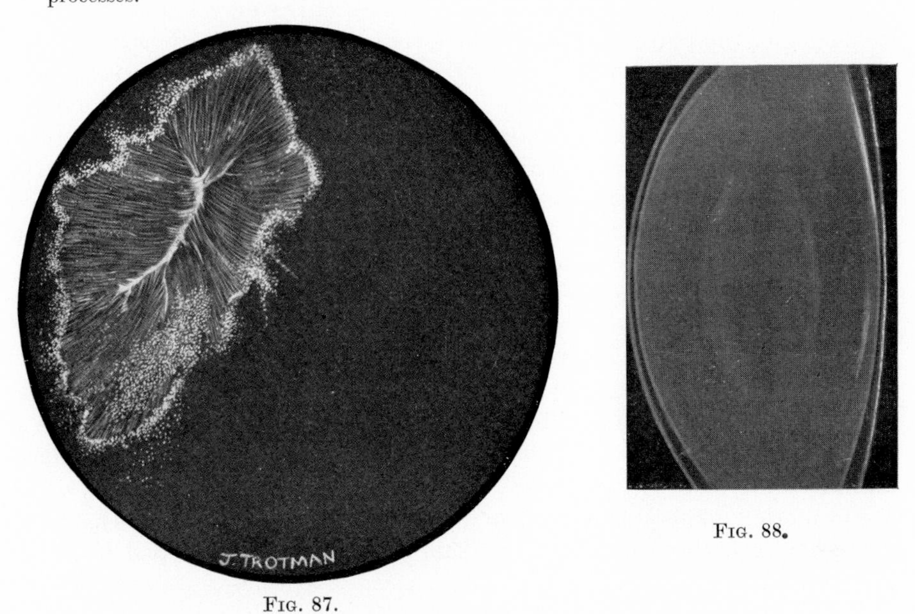

FIG. 87.

FIG. 88.

FIGS. 87 and 88.—CHANGES IN THE ANTERIOR SUBCAPSULAR REGION FOLLOWING A BLOW ON THE EYE WITH A STONE 3 MONTHS PREVIOUSLY.

The drawing was made with full dilatation of the pupil.

FIG. 87.—With oblique illumination.

FIG. 88.—Slit-lamp section showing the localization of the opacity.

interference with the permeability caused by an outpouring of exudate on the surface of the lens at the time of the accident; in the latter case the fine subcapsular opacities are analogous to those associated with a Vossius ring.

TRAUMATIC ROSETTE-SHAPED OPACITY

A TRAUMATIC ROSETTE-SHAPED OPACITY (STELLATE CATARACT; FOLIAFORM CATARACT, Rauh, 1930; RADIATING SUBCAPSULAR CATARACT, Cattaneo, 1934) is the result of a more acute and diffuse change than the punctate opacities just described and constitutes the most typical clinical picture following both concussive and perforating injuries; it occurs either in the presence or presumed absence of a tear in the capsule. The opacities originally described by Dyer (1867) in the lenses of a hanged criminal[1] were of this type; Schlösser (1887), Fuchs (1888) and zur Nedden (1904) made careful studies of the changes; Hudson (1910) made the most important contribution in the pre-slit-lamp era, and Vogt (1922), Lugli (1935) and Haldimann (1942) established the minute picture as seen with this instrument.

Two types of opacity are generally recognized—those occurring very shortly after the injury and those appearing after some time (late rosette).

The FRESH TYPE OF ROSETTE OPACITY may appear sometimes in the anterior, sometimes in the posterior subcapsular region and sometimes in both simultaneously in which case the two layers are connected at any rate in one segment at the equator. There is some controversy as to the relative frequency of the two types, but after a concussive injury anterior opacities are probably more common; after a perforating injury the posterior rosette is perhaps more frequently seen (Figs. 89–97). These may be evident within a few hours after the injury (Hudson, 1910) or their appearance may be delayed for some weeks (Alajmo, 1929) or months (Nordmann, 1931). Initially the first change is the appearance of a carpet of fine fluid droplets lying between the radiating lens fibres immediately under the capsular epithelium so that their architecture is traced out in feathery parallel rays running outwards from the dark suture-lines which the opacity renders clearly conspicuous. In this way a rosette-shaped figure is formed, determined by the arrangement of the sutures branching out from the axial region towards the equator (Fig. 92); in experimental lesions in animals in which the structure of the lens is different, the picture is not therefore the same as that seen in man. Sometimes the entire suture-system is thus defined, forming a complete rosette figure; at other times the rosette is only partial, one or more " petals " appearing in a quadrant of the lens (Fig. 91). In all cases, however, the opacity lies in a thin delimited layer of equal thickness throughout.

[1] p. 121.

FIGS. 89 to 91.—CONCUSSION ROSETTE CATARACTS.

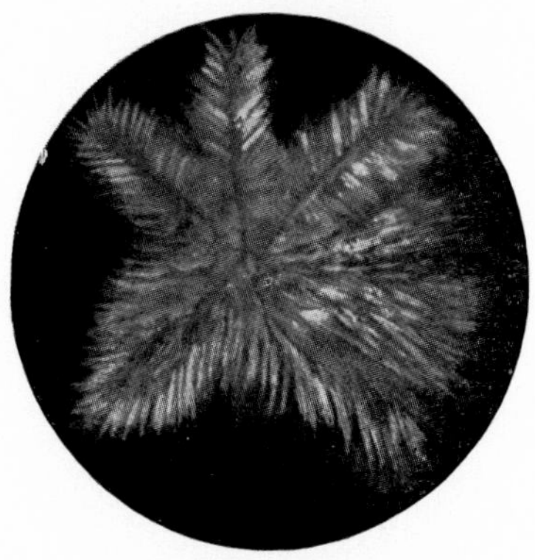

FIG. 89.

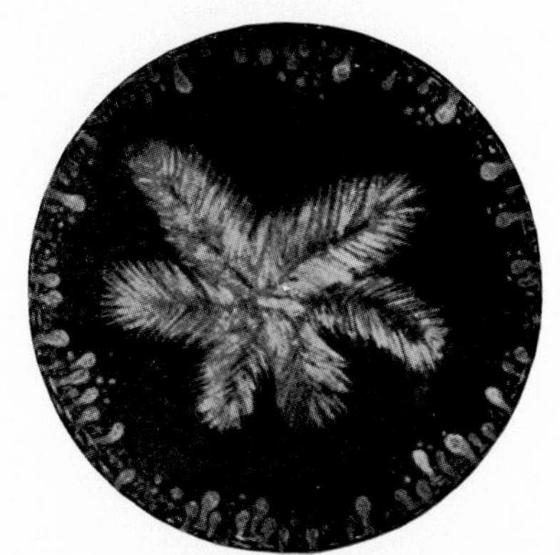

FIG. 90.

FIGS. 89 to 90.—THE OPACITIES LIE IN THE SUPERFICIAL LAYER OF THE POSTERIOR CORTEX (D. Cattaneo).

FIG. 89.—Two days after injury.
FIG. 90.—Three days after injury.

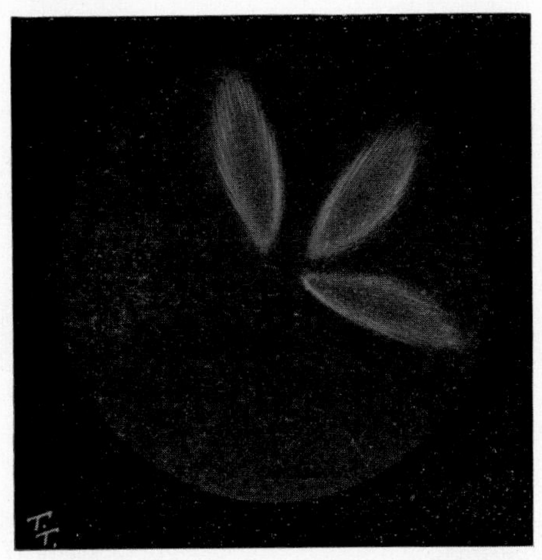

FIG. 91.—Partial concussion rosette cataract situated in the adult nucleus; 6 years after a concussion injury.

Small, dust-like opacities may appear immediately under the capsule itself, lying anteriorly and peripherally to the main rosette under the zone of discontinuity. Lugli (1935) suggested that they corresponded to the formation of new fibres, but Haldimann (1942) observed that they were formed at the time of the injury simultaneously with the main rosette-shaped opacity. In the course of a few months both are pushed inwards, the subcapsular opacities tending to become absorbed while the subepithelial rosette generally becomes more distinct.

In mild injuries these opacities may be very translucent and they have been known to clear up within a few days or weeks leaving no trace (Avizonis, 1923; and others); presumably in such cases the fluid droplets become

FIGS. 92 to 97.—THE LATER STAGES OF EARLY CONCUSSION CATARACT (D. Cattaneo).

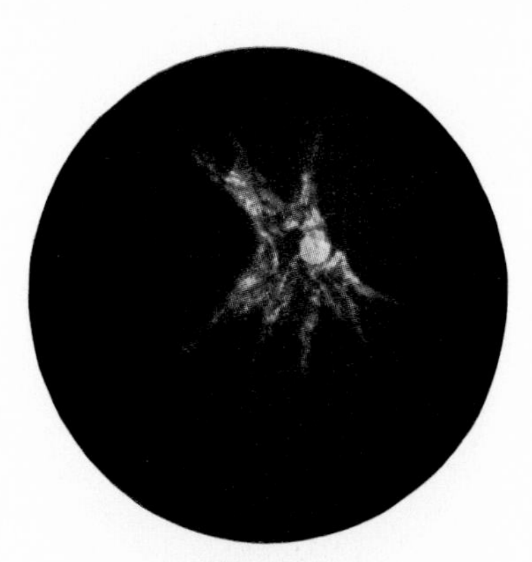

FIG. 92.

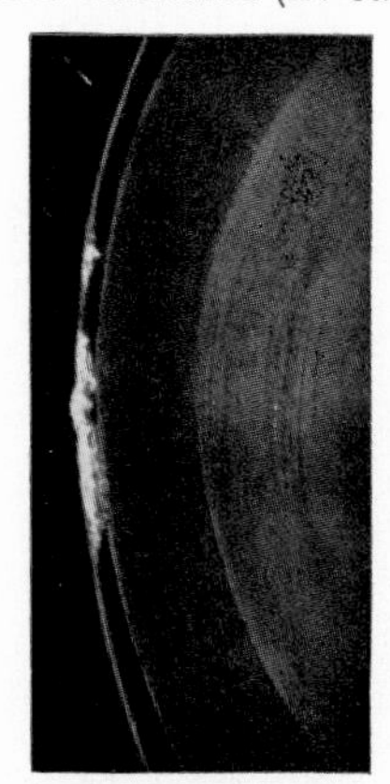

FIG. 93.

FIGS. 92 and 93.—Three days after injury. Punctate opacities with a general stellate form in the superficial layers of the anterior cortex with a dense discoid opacity in the capsule.

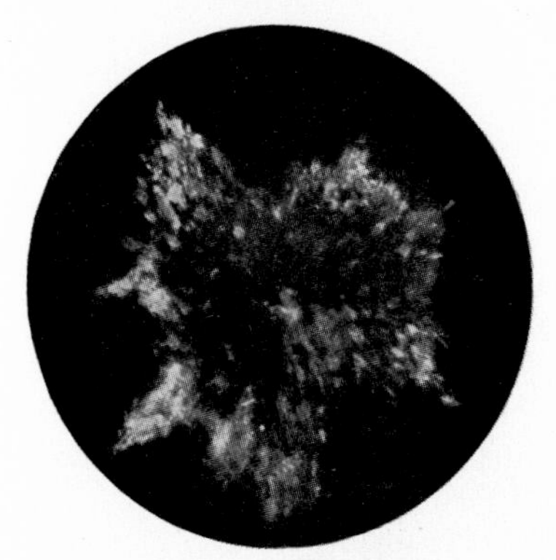

FIG. 94.

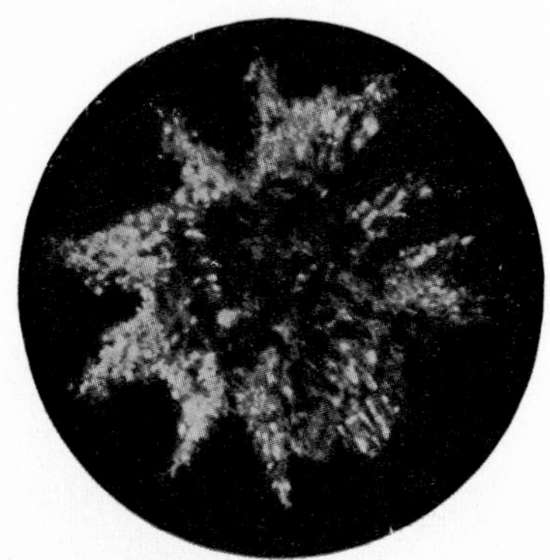

FIG. 95.

FIGS. 94 and 95.—Eight days after injury, showing the evolution of the rosette into irregular mottling and striations. Fig. 94, in the anterior cortex. Fig. 95, in the posterior cortex.

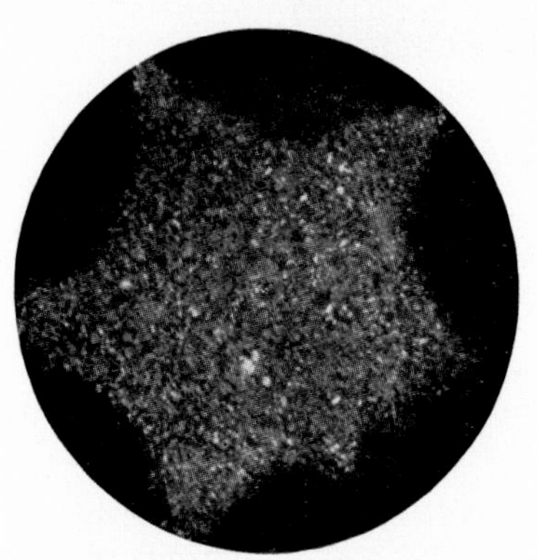

FIG. 96.

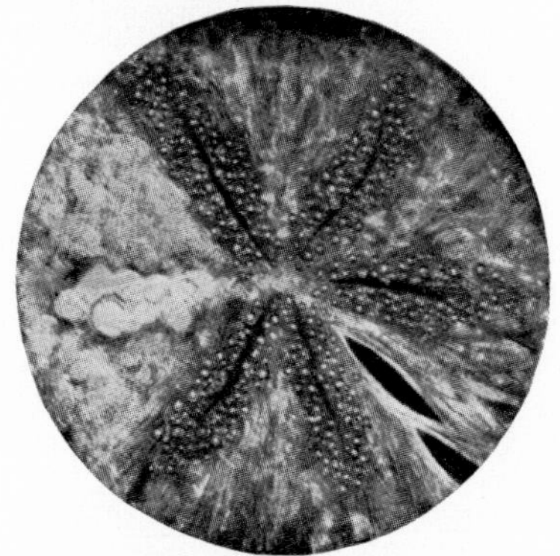

FIG. 97.

FIG. 96.—Five days after trauma showing punctiform opacification with a general suggestion of a stellate appearance in the posterior cortex.

FIG. 97.—Two months after trauma, showing subcapsular vacuoles and opacities in a radiating arrangement in the anterior cortex, with a small hole out of which protrudes lens substance (to the left).

Figs. 98 to 103.—Late Stages of Concussion Cataract (D. Cattaneo).

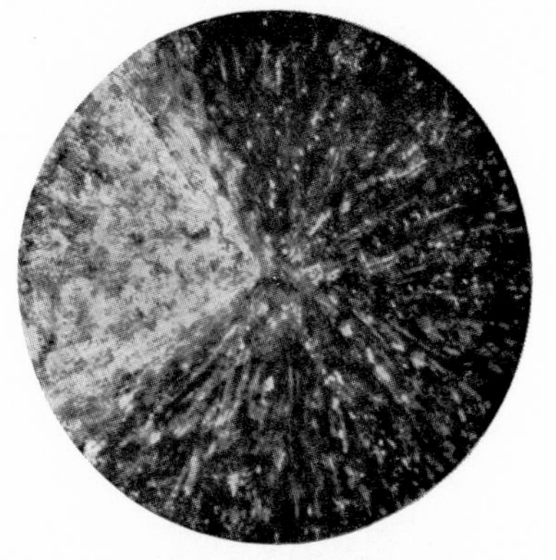

Fig. 98.—Diffuse mottling intensified in the nasal sector of the anterior cortex, one year after trauma.

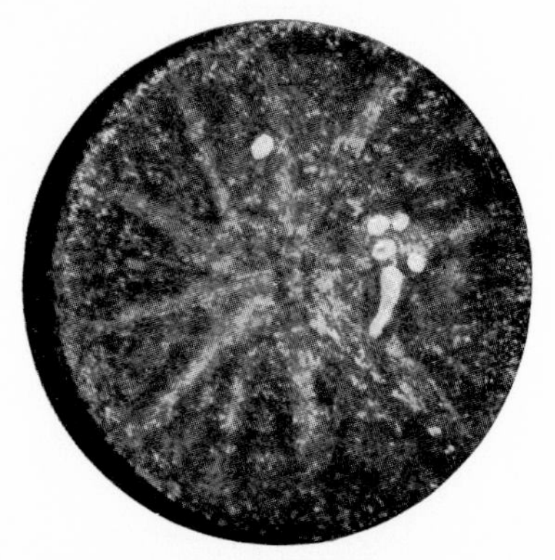

Fig. 99.—The general outline of the stellate opacity in the deeper layers of the cortex, separated from the equator by a clear zone, making a zonular configuration. One year after injury.

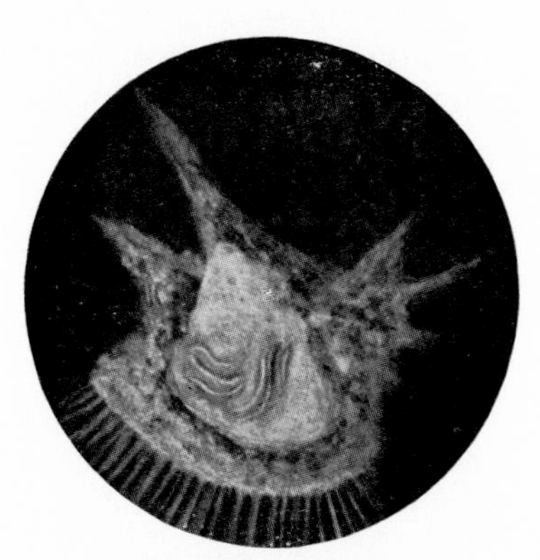

Fig. 100.

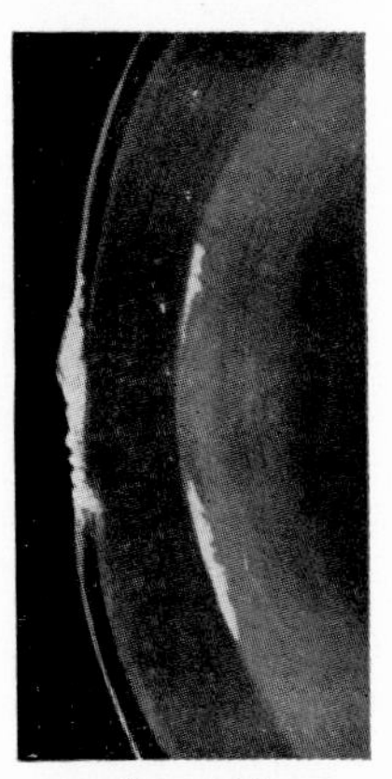

Fig. 101.

Fig. 100.—Twelve years after injury. There is a dense anterior segmental capsular opacity with radial striæ running towards the equator. The two opacities are seen to be separated by a clear zone of cortex (Fig. 101).

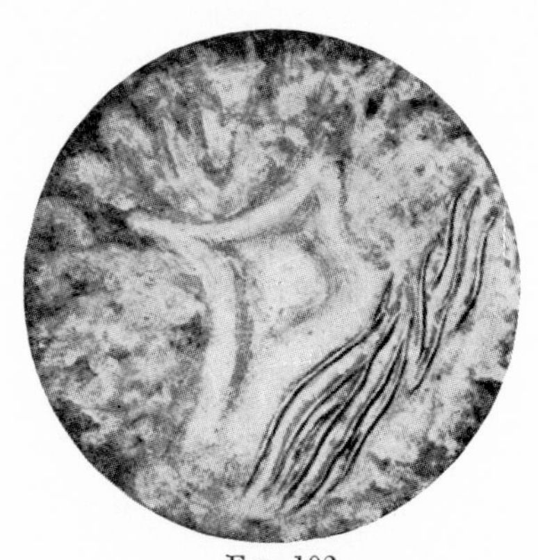

Fig. 102.

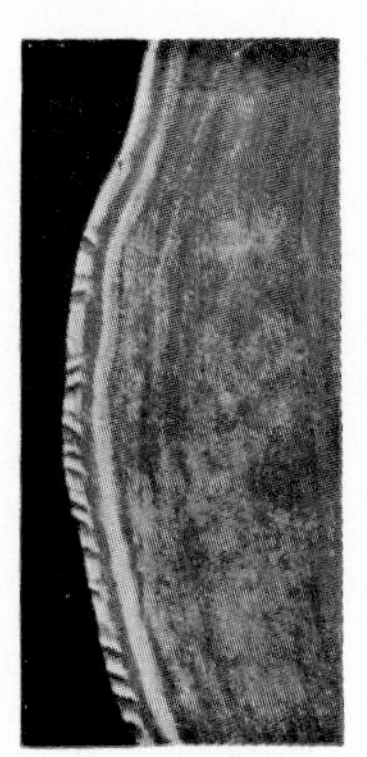

Fig. 103.

Fig. 102.—Forty-nine years after injury. Diffuse opacity of the anterior cortex especially at the anterior pole. Fig. 103 shows the extent of post-traumatic atrophy with irregularity of the superficial layers of the lens.

absorbed while the lens fibres themselves have not been irreversibly damaged (Fig. 80). More usually the opacities are permanent and stationary and if they are not unusually dense they may cause little impairment of vision; it is important, however, that after the age of 45 their presence may determine the early development of senile opacities (Vogt, 1922; Davidson, 1940). In other cases after more severe injuries disintegrative changes may appear after some time wherein vacuoles form in the midribs of the feathery opacities and between the rays and these may be associated with vacuoles in the equatorial region, either discrete or arranged as a palisade in conformity with the axes of the lens fibres. Sometimes within a few days this vacuolation progresses until the striate appearance of the rosette gives way to a lace-like pattern in which the vacuoles become gradually smaller, and finally all that remains is a collection of fine granules lying in a solid, thin porcelain-like layer which in their arrangement give some suggestion of the antecedent stellar design (Figs. 98–101). Alternatively, a fine punctate residual opacity may develop (Fig. 96). Even when these changes occur the opacity remains stationary. In all cases in the youthful lens the progressive formation of new fibres interposes clear lens material between the capsule and the opacity and the rosette figure is gradually buried as the growth of the lens proceeds so that, depending on the age at which the injury was sustained, this eventually lies somewhere between the infantile nucleus and the deeper cortex (Figs. 101, 104 and 105).

LATE ROSETTE OPACITIES are seen some years after the trauma and are usually found lying deep in the cortex or in the adult nucleus, separated from the capsule by a clear zone of varying thickness[1] (Figs. 104–107). Such an opacity appears to be invariably the result of a concussion, sometimes an incident forgotten by the patient; and in view of the fact that the design of the rosette formation corresponds to the arrangement of the fibres in the subcapsular zone and that it is frequently associated with some residual opacities lying subcapsularly, Vogt (1922) concluded that it is due to a minimal degree of damage to the subcapsular fibres sustained at the time of injury, which does not become clinically apparent until a later date. In such an opacity the relationship of the sutures to the rays is the reverse of that found in fresh cases, for whereas in the latter the sutures run up the centre of the petals and the rays of opacity run from them as from a midriff, in the late type the sutures run between the petals which are formed by the outcrop of rays from two neighbouring sutures (compare Figs. 89, 106, 108 and 109). In the late rosette the rays may reach out much further peripherally and, indeed, all or only a few of them in one segment may extend outwards to the equator and then turn backwards to form a second posterior rosette in the posterior cortex.

It is interesting that these rosette opacities, if they are tenuous and

[1] Vogt (1922), Graves (1925), Bücklers (1934), Lugli (1935), Geller (1943), and others.

FIGS. 104 to 107.—LATE CONCUSSION ROSETTE OPACITIES.

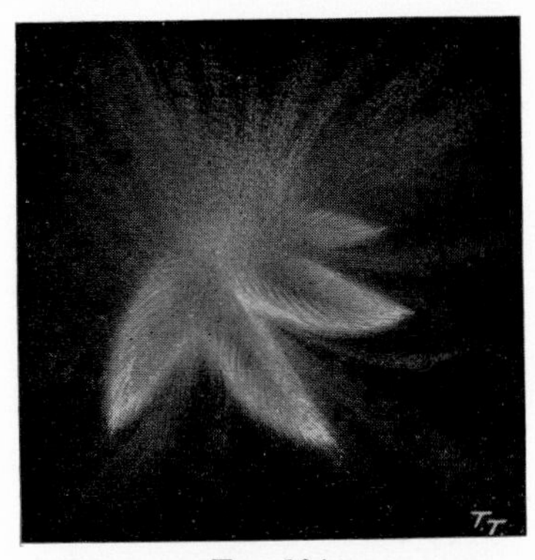

FIG. 104.

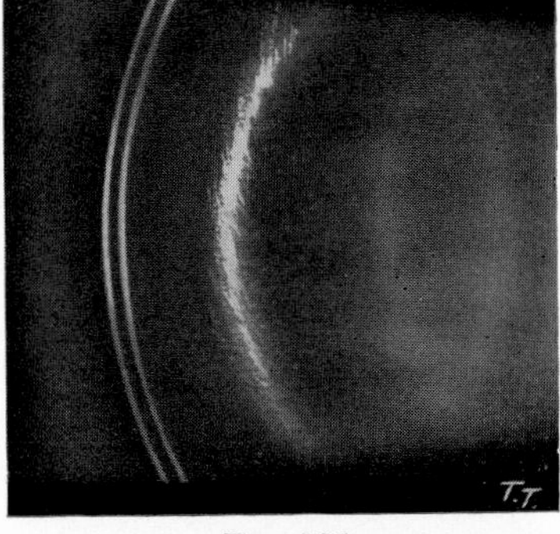

FIG. 105.

FIG. 104.—Appearing in a young man of 30, 12 years after a concussion injury.
FIG. 105.—The optical section shows the location of the cataract deep in the adult nucleus.

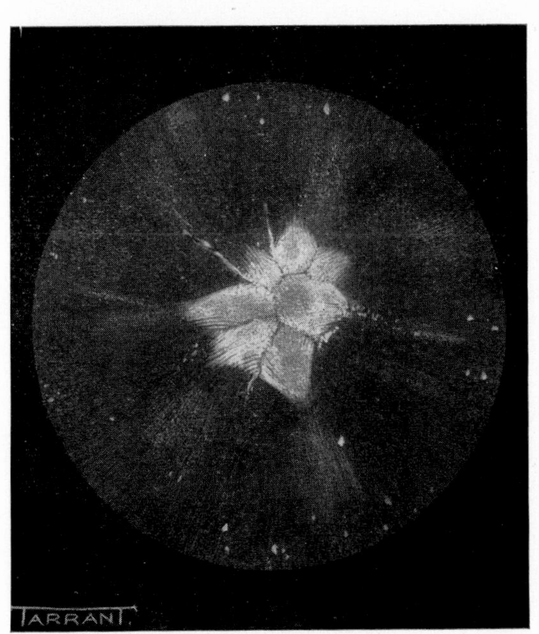

FIG. 106.

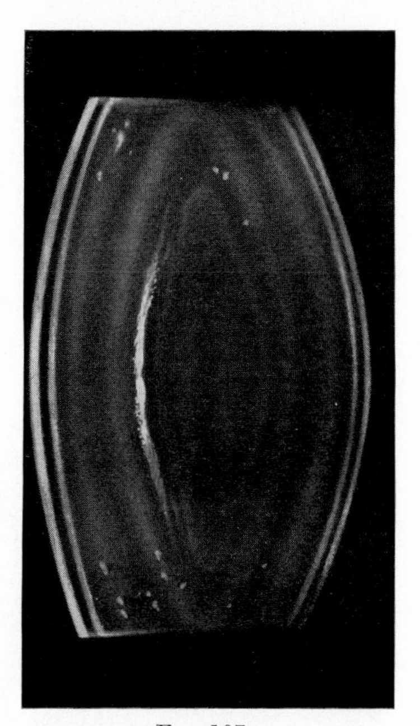

FIG. 107.

FIGS. 106 and 107.—Lying deeply in the adult nucleus, 12 years after injury.

particularly if they are situated in the anterior portion of the lens, may cause little functional inconvenience and may leave the visual acuity so slightly impaired that the patient may be unaware of their presence (Handmann, 1927; and others); if they are dense, of course, the visual loss may be considerable.

FIGS. 108 and 109.—THE DIAGRAMMATIC RECONSTRUCTION OF TRAUMATIC ROSETTE CATARACT.

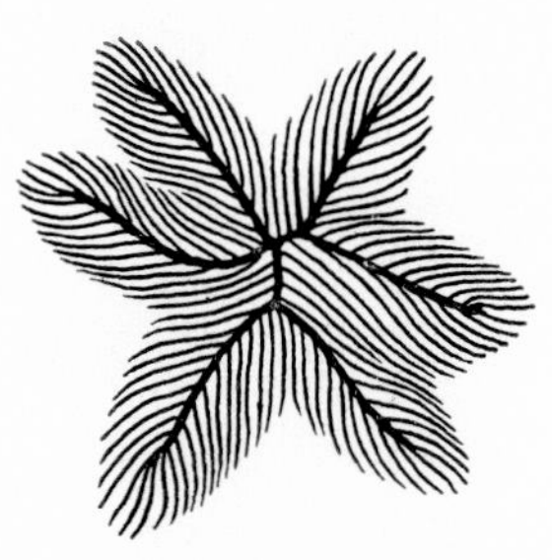

FIG. 108.—Represents an early concussion rosette or a perforation rosette where the lines of opacity feather out from the sutures which themselves lie in the centre of each petal.

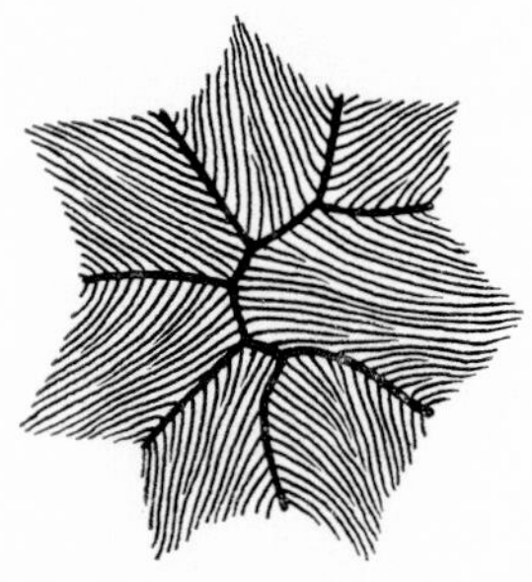

FIG. 109.—Late concussion rosette where the lines of opacity feather out from the sutures in such a way that the petals are formed from adjacent sutures which themselves lie between the petals.

The *differential diagnosis* of traumatic rosette opacities must take into consideration a complicated cataract after uveitis; this latter, however, is not sharply limited to one zone but extends centrally, especially in the axial region; it remains subcapsular and is not buried as the lens grows, and its polychromatic lustre in the early stages and the irregular breadcrumb appearance in its later evolution are usually quite distinct from the sharply demarcated, thin, traumatic opacity.[1] Occasionally cortical senile changes may resemble a traumatic rosette, but the lamellar separation and water clefts in the former are usually readily distinguishable from the pathognomonic appearance of the latter.

A TRAUMATIC ZONULAR (LAMELLAR) CATARACT is probably the end-result of disseminated opacities occurring extensively over the lens or a rosette opacity following an injury received in early youth. Such cases of uniocular zonular cataract with a precedent history of concussive injury are rare but

FIGS. 110 and 111.—CONCUSSION CATARACT.

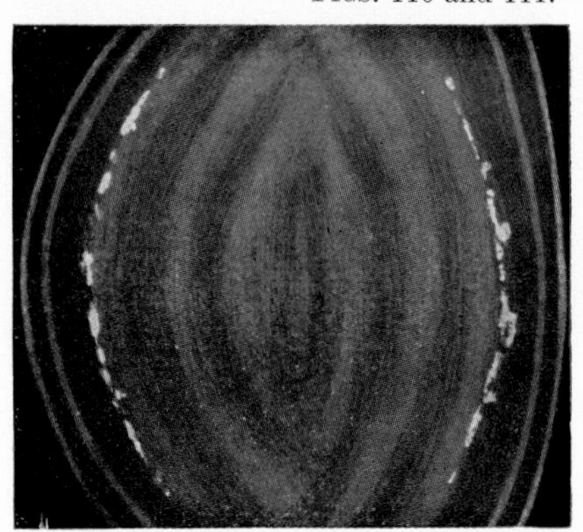

FIG. 110.—Optical section of the lens 3 years after trauma, showing the burying of the original subcapsular opacity in the anterior and posterior cortices (D. Cattaneo).

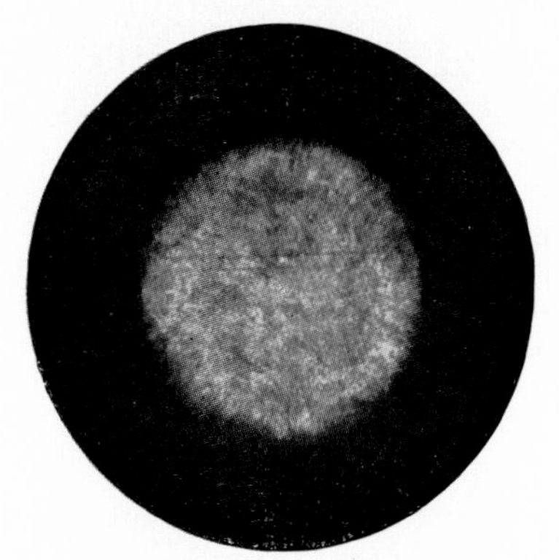

FIG. 111.—Disc-shaped type of punctate opacity in the posterior cortex 19 months after trauma.

[1] See Vol. XI, p. 20.

have excited interest since the time of von Graefe (1857)[1]; the literature has been summarized by Walter (1917) and Law (1932) (22 cases). The opacity is similar to that of other lamellar cataracts,[2] its depth and size being determined by the age of the trauma; it usually follows an injury sustained before the age of 12 years but occasionally has followed a blow received up to the age of 20. The opacity may be vague and cloudy or dense and sufficiently opaque to abolish useful vision; the density may vary in different sectors while the outline may be irregular and typical riders may be evident, but the periphery of the lens and its centre are clear (Figs. 101, 110 and 111).

POST-TRAUMATIC ATROPHY OF THE LENS may be evident some years after a severe concussion wherein no opening in the capsule is found; the condition is characterized by a thinning of its substance so that the sagittal diameter may be reduced by as much as a third (Vogt, 1931). After concussions the shrinkage tends to be symmetrical but it is not necessarily so since, even when the capsule is apparently intact, one part of the lens may shrink much more than the other so that the whole architecture becomes deformed. Dust-like opacities are characteristically seen under the anterior capsule which is flatter than normal, while the band of the adult nucleus is similarly flat and relucent with extensive opacification; unlike the comparable atrophic condition following perforating wounds, folds in the capsule are not seen. The shrinkage in the lens may be attributed partly to the absorption of some of its substance and partly to a disturbance of the growth of new fibres owing to epithelial damage (Fig. 103).

PRE-SENILE and SENILE LENS CHANGES FOLLOWING A CONCUSSION are not unusual and have frequently been remarked—coronary cataract, water clefts, punctate cortical opacities and sclerotic nuclear opacities. The intensive studies of Vogt (1922–31) have demonstrated this causal relationship, largely by comparing the difference in development of such changes in the two eyes of the same individual, one of which has been injured; while Davidson (1940) has stressed the prognostic importance of the rapid and premature progression of such changes long after the time of the injury when the patient reaches the age of 40 to 45 years. Ocular concussions are common in the early years of life and it is probable that many unilateral lens opacities which are commonly labelled "congenital" or "adolescent" are in reality the result of trauma, as well as some of those similarly considered "senile" which happen to be noticed first in adult life.

DIFFUSE CONCUSSION CATARACT

A diffuse opacification of the lens substance is a rare result of concussions unless these are associated with a rupture of the capsule. In such cases a

[1] Marcus Gunn (1895), Merz-Weigandt (1900), Weiss (1902), Stein (1904), Cattaneo (1934), and others.

[2] Vol. XI, p. 136.

rapidly spreading milkiness appears owing to the imbibition of aqueous in quantity, producing an opacity resembling that following perforating wounds of the lens (Fig. 112). Occasionally, as we have seen, such an effect may be localized and transient, and it may be that in these cases the tear in the capsule is rapidly sealed with fibrin and later becomes epithelialized. If, however, the tear is extensive, the opacification is rapidly progressive and the swollen fibres may herniate out from the opening protruding either into the anterior chamber or the vitreous, in which situation they finally become granular and necrotic (Fig. 113). In this event the lenticular epithelium may proliferate and, spreading round the rent in an endeavour to enclose the protruding lens substance, may grow exuberantly and eventually cover the

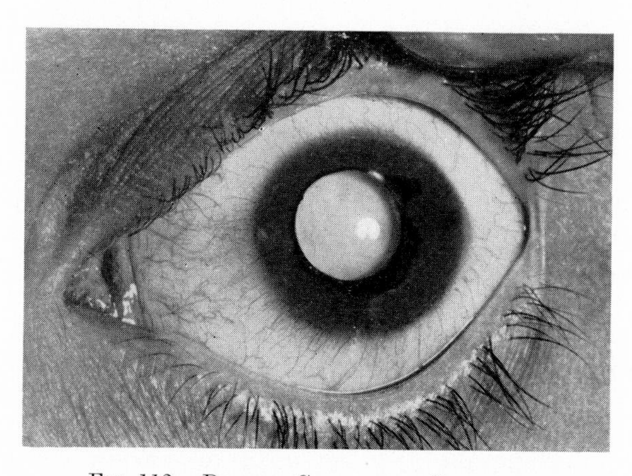

Fig. 112.—Diffuse Concussion Cataract.

Three months after a concussion injury the lens is uniformly milky white. There is a considerable amount of atrophy of the iris (Inst. Ophthal.).

anterior surface of the vitreous and the zonule (Fig. 114) (Tillema, 1937). In the young, slow and total absorption of the cataract may occur, leaving only the lens capsule; in the old, iritis and secondary glaucoma may develop, and long-term degenerative changes such as calcification and ossification occasionally occur (Hager and Ebel, 1964; Finkelstein and Boniuk, 1969) (Figs. 115 and 134).

Such diffuse changes do not, however, always occur and the localization of what appears immediately to be a destructive injury may occasionally be dramatic and unexpected. An unusual sequence was reported by Stern (1945) in a man of 25 after an injury by a stone: although a white mass of lens substance mushroomed into the anterior chamber through a rent in the anterior capsule, this was rapidly absorbed and the continuity of the capsule was restored, leaving the lens eventually clear and little damaged apart from a few fine capsular opacities. A posterior rosette opacity similarly disappeared and normal vision and an emmetropic refraction was regained. Such a happy ending, however, is unusual.

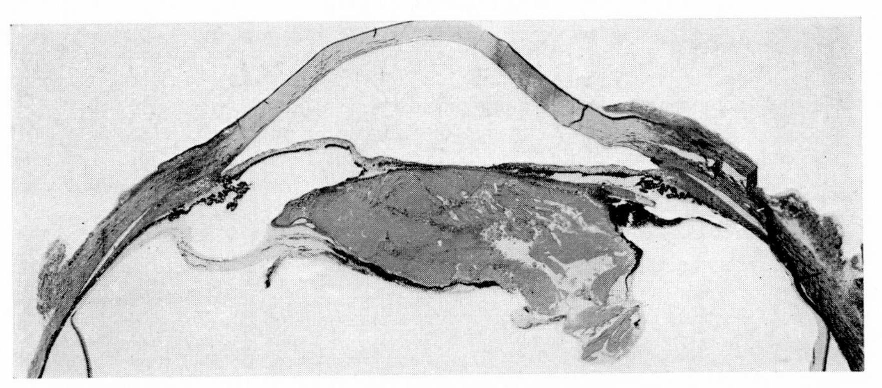

FIG. 113.—CONCUSSION CATARACT.

After a blow there was a complete concussion cataract, the iris was adherent to the anterior surface of the lens and the lens capsule was ruptured posteriorly (N. Ashton).

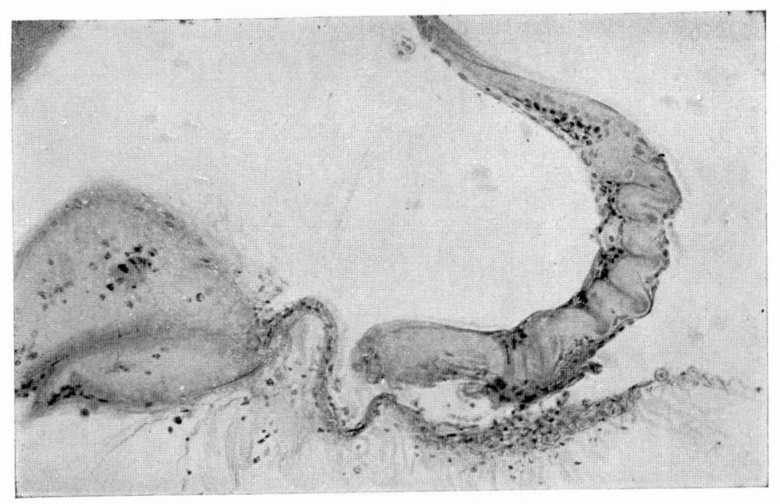

FIG. 114.—CONCUSSION CATARACT.

The capsule of the lens has ruptured; both it and the anterior part of the vitreous are covered by cells derived from the epithelium of the lens (A. Tillema).

MASSAGE CATARACT

It has long been known that cataractous changes in the lens can be induced by simulating the effects of a concussion by the mechanical massage of the anterior capsule; in this way Förster (1881) demonstrated that the maturation of an early cataract could be hastened, for which purpose the procedure used to be employed. A considerable amount of experimental work has been done on this question wherein it has been found that, depending on the age of the animal and the duration and force of the manipulation, changes varying from the formation of fine subcapsular opacities, which may regress, to total clouding of the entire lens may be induced (Hess, 1887; Schirmer, 1888; Demaria 1904). These gross changes are associated with degeneration of the subcapsular epithelium and an enormous and rapid swelling of the lens owing to the imbibition of fluid: thus Salffner (1904) found that the lens increased 22·5% in weight and 24·3% in volume within 24 hours, and Bellows and Chinn (1941) that, after manipulation in this way, the lens *in vitro* imbibed twice as much water as control lenses. It is probable that this imbibition of fluid is due partly to the increased permeability of the capsule following damage to the epithelium (Leber, 1880; Hess, 1887; Peters, 1901), possibly aided by the ease of diffusion throughout the lens afforded by the mechanical separation of its fibres (Guaita, 1890; Bellows and Chinn, 1941), and partly to the osmotic effect of the products of disintegration of the lens substance (Busacca, 1926).

It is interesting that the occurrence of transitory superficial lenticular opacities has been noted in the case of recurrent dislocation of the lens into the anterior chamber[1] (Schmid, 1946): these were presumably caused by repeated contact between the lens and the posterior surface of the cornea.

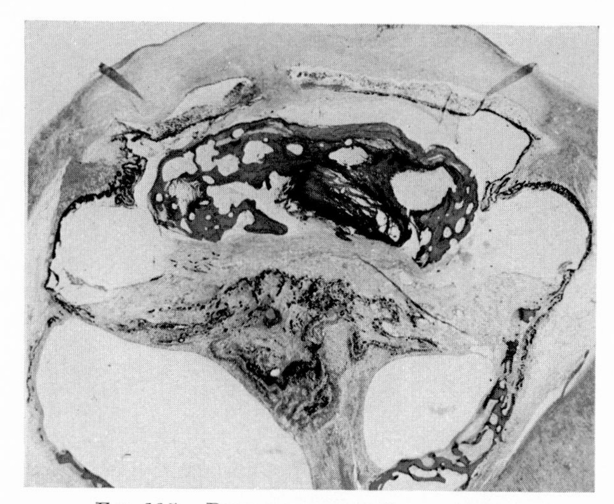

Fig. 115.—Post-traumatic Ossification.

In a woman aged 49 whose eye suffered trauma of an unknown type 46 years prior to enucleation. The lens fibres have been replaced by calcified lamellar bone with fatty marrow and cholesterol slits. There is also ossification along the inner surface of the choroid (H. & E.) (E. M. Finkelstein and M. Boniuk).

Treatment. The great majority of cases of concussive opacities, being stationary and having little deleterious effect on vision, requires no treatment; this is indicated only when the opacity is dense as in zonular cataracts or is diffuse. In all cases, in the absence of complications the most urgent of which is a raised tension, a conservative attitude is indicated, if possible until the associated iritis has quietened and the eye has become white. Particularly *if the tension is subnormal operation should be avoided*, since hypotony usually indicates a quiet iridocyclitis or a tendency thereto which operative interference may light up with disastrous results. If, however, the eye is white and the tension good and if surgery is desired, general surgical principles should be followed: discission may be practised in the young, linear extraction in the third decade and either an intracapsular or

[1] Vol. XI, p. 304.

extracapsular extraction in older people, while removal of the lens by aspiration may be the most satisfactory form of treatment in some cases. It is to be remembered that the zonule is often damaged, and even if not partially ruptured it frequently degenerates after the accident so that intracapsular extraction is usually easy. This problem will be further discussed subsequently in connection with perforating wounds of the lens. If, however, the lens is subluxated or dislocated the surgical problems become greater; these will be discussed immediately.

Alajmo. *Boll. Oculist.*, **8,** 1, 103 (1929).
Anderson. *Brit. J. Ophthal.*, **3,** 15 (1919).
Aub. *Arch. Augenheilk.*, **2,** 256 (1871).
Avizonis. *Z. Augenheilk.*, **50,** 113 (1923).
Bäck. *v. Graefes Arch. Ophthal.*, **47** (1), 82 (1898).
Bégué. *Bull. Soc. Ophtal. Fr.*, 738 (1949).
Bellows and Chinn. *Amer. J. Ophthal.*, **24,** 979 (1941).
Berlin. *Klin. Mbl. Augenheilk.*, **11,** 42 (1873).
Berliner. *Biomicroscopy of the Eye*, N.Y., **2,** 1249 (1949).
Bonnefon. *Arch. Ophtal.*, **32,** 748 (1912).
Bresgen. *Arch. Augenheilk.*, **10,** 265 (1881).
Bücklers. *Ber. dtsch. ophthal. Ges.*, **50,** 172 (1934).
Busacca. *Boll. Oculist.*, **5,** 70 (1926).
Caspar. *Klin. Mbl. Augenheilk.*, **47** (1), 606 (1909).
Cattaneo. *Ann. Ottal.*, **62,** 81, 161 (1934).
Collins. *Trans. ophthal. Soc. U.K.*, **11,** 126 (1891); **36,** 204 (1916).
Davidson. *Amer. J. Ophthal.*, **19,** 757 (1936); **23,** 252, 1358 (1940).
Demaria. *v. Graefes Arch. Ophthal.*, **59,** 568 (1904).
Disler. *Vestn. oftal.*, **13,** 5 (1938).
Dyer. *Trans. Amer. ophthal. Soc.*, **1** (2), 13 (1867).
Finkelstein and Boniuk. *Amer. J. Ophthal.*, **68,** 683 (1969).
Förster. *Ber. dtsch. ophthal. Ges.*, **13,** 133 (1881).
Foster. *Trans. ophthal. Soc. U.K.*, **58,** 436 (1938).
Frenkel. *Arch. Ophtal.*, **48,** 205 (1931).
Fuchs. *Wien. klin. Wschr.*, **1,** 53, 86 (1888).
Geller. *Klin. Mbl. Augenheilk.*, **109,** 105 (1943).
von Graefe. *v. Graefes Arch. Ophthal.*, **3** (2), 372 (1857).
Graves. *Amer. J. Ophthal.*, **8,** 904 (1925).
Gründgens. *Ueber Katarakt nach Kontusion ohne Bulbusruptur* (Diss.), Jena (1902).
Gscheidel. *Klin. Mbl. Augenheilk.*, **102,** 142 (1939).
Guaita. *Ann. Ottal.*, **19,** 517 (1890).
Gundersen. *Amer. J. Ophthal.*, **29,** 837 (1946).
Gunn. *Trans. ophthal. Soc. U.K.*, **15,** 121 (1895).
Hager and Ebel. *Klin. Mbl. Augenheilk.*, **144,** 513 (1964).
Haldimann. *Ophthalmologica*, **103,** 302 (1942).
Handmann. *Klin. Mbl. Augenheilk.*, **78,** 31 (1927).
Hess. *Ber. dtsch. ophthal. Ges.*, **19,** 54 (1887).
Hesse. *Z. Augenheilk.*, **41,** 226 (1919).
Hosch. *Arch. Augenheilk.*, **20,** 54 (1889).
Hudson. *Roy. Lond. ophthal. Hosp. Rep.*, **18,** 112 (1910).
Knapp. *Arch. Augenheilk.*, **1,** 20 (1869).
Koby. *Slitlamp Microscopy*, London (1930).
Landesberg. *Klin. Mbl. Augenheilk.*, **24,** 320 (1886).
Law. *Brit. J. Ophthal.*, **16,** 385 (1932).
Leber. *v. Graefes Arch. Ophthal.*, **26** (1), 283 (1880).
Liebrecht. *Beitr. Augenheilk.*, **2,** 693 (1895).
Lugli. *Arch. Ophthal.*, **14,** 392 (1935).
Merz-Weigandt. *Zbl. prakt. Augenheilk.*, **24,** 353 (1900).
zur Nedden. *Z. Augenheilk.*, **11,** 389 (1904).
Nordmann. *Arch. Ophtal.*, **48,** 392 (1931).
d'Oswaldo. *Z. Augenheilk.*, **54,** 60 (1925).
Papagno. *Boll. Oculist.*, **29,** 178 (1950).
Peters. *Klin. Mbl. Augenheilk.*, **39** (1), 351 (1901).
Purtscher. *Zbl. prakt. Augenheilk.*, **37,** 282 (1913).
Rauh. *Klin. Mbl. Augenheilk.*, **84,** 766 (1930).
Rolett. *Arch. Ophthal.*, **24,** 1244 (1940).
Rosen. *Brit. J. Ophthal.*, **29,** 370, 373 (1945).
Rychener. *Amer. J. Ophthal.*, **28,** 534 (1945).
Salffner. *v. Graefes Arch. Ophthal.*, **59,** 520 (1904).
Schirmer. *v. Graefes Arch. Ophthal.*, **34** (1), 131 (1888); **35** (3), 147 (1889).
Klin. Mbl. Augenheilk., **28,** 161 (1890).
Schlösser. *Exp. Studien über traumatische Katarakt*, München (1887).
Schmid. *Ophthalmologica*, **111,** 365 (1946).
Stein. *Beitr. Augenheilk.*, **7** (63), 158 (1904).
Steiner. *Klin. Mbl. Augenheilk.*, **48** (1), 60 (1910).
Stern. *Brit. J. Ophthal.*, **29,** 48 (1945).
Tillema. *Arch. Ophthal.*, **17,** 586 (1937).
Tipshus. *Arch. Ophthal.*, **82,** 548 (1969).
Vogt. *Lhb. u. Atlas d. Spaltlampenmikroskopie d. lebenden Auges*, Berlin, 1st ed. (1921); 2nd ed. (1931).
v. Graefes Arch. Ophthal., **107,** 196; **109,** 154 (1922).
Klin. Mbl. Augenheilk., **85,** 586 (1930).
Vossius. *XV int. Cong. Med.*, Lisbon (1903).
Arch. Ophthal., **35,** 566 (1906).

Wagenmann. *Verletzungen des Auges: Graefe-Saemisch Hb. d. ges. Augenheilk.*, 3rd ed., Leipzig, **1,** 486 (1915).
Walter. *Ueber traumatischen Schichtstar* (Diss.), Rostock (1917).
Weidenthal and Schepens. *Amer. J. Ophthal.*, **62,** 465 (1966).
Weiss. *Z. Augenheilk.*, **8,** 37 (1902).
Whiting. *Trans. ophthal. Soc. U.K.*, **36,** 167 (1916).
Zentmayer. *Amer. J. Ophthal.*, **7,** 676 (1924).

SUBLUXATION AND DISLOCATION OF THE LENS

The whole problem concerning displacements of the lens including the clinical symptoms and signs and the question of treatment has already been discussed at length elsewhere in this *System.*[1] It will be recalled that normally the lens remains suspended by the fibres of the suspensory ligament[2] so that its axis corresponds approximately to the visual line; it may become displaced owing to a congenital defect in the zonule or through disease or as a result of injury whereby the suspensory apparatus becomes weakened so that the lens becomes tremulous or subluxated, or it is ruptured so that a complete dislocation occurs. The latter is a serious condition frequently leading to grave complications such as uveitis, glaucoma and retinal detachment, the treatment of which may be very difficult.[3]

Injury to the suspensory mechanism of the lens is a common sequel to a concussion; indeed, Frenkel (1916–31) believed that minimal subluxations of the lens, whether or not they are clinically demonstrable, occur almost constantly after such injuries. The forces involved are readily understandable and have received considerable study both from the experimental (Zoldan, 1924) and clinical points of view[4]—the backward thrust and rebounding of the lens, the pressure-wave of the aqueous which forces the root of the iris backwards and, probably more important, the forcible recoil of the vitreous body which wells forward around the lens and, particularly in antero-

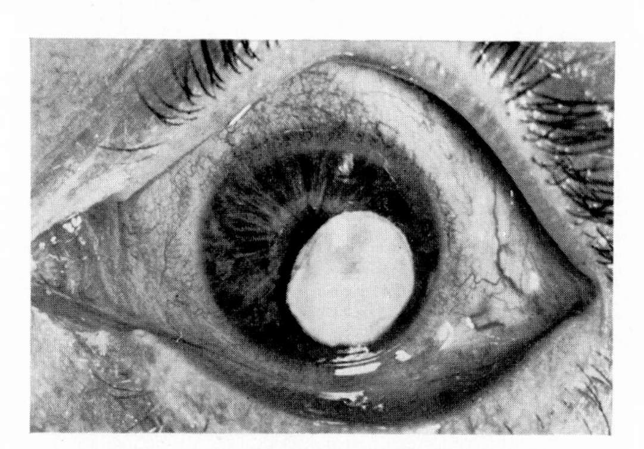

Fig. 116.—Concussion Cataract.
The lens suffered a spontaneous dislocation.

[1] Vol. XI, p. 295.
[2] For the detailed anatomy of this structure see Vol. II, p. 325.
[3] For figures relating to the relative frequency of congenital, traumatic and consecutive or secondary lens displacements and for the literature dealing with the complications resulting therefrom, see Vol. XI, p. 295.
[4] Parisotti (1891), Peretti (1899), Beauvieux and Monod (1924), Ringelhan and Elschnig (1931), and others.

posterior compressions of the globe, the compensatory sudden enlargement of the corneo-scleral ring—all these factors combine to strain and stretch a structure the delicacy and fragility of which are obvious. Moreover, it is understandable that, if the zonule is already degenerate or atrophic as occurs in mature cataract, high myopia and old uveitis, an injury so slight as to escape attention (rubbing the eyes, stooping suddenly, sneezing) may produce the same result, the subsequent dislocation of the lens being apparently spontaneous (Fig. 116). In the case of a cataractous lens, of course, such an accident may suddenly (and apparently happily) restore the vision (Heinz, 1947; and others). Such cases (for example, of high myopia) provide the rare examples of bilateral traumatic dislocation of the lens (Badal, 1878; Peretti, 1899; and others), and in the case reported by Lambros and Cinotti (1967) bilateral subluxation due to trauma in childhood was followed at the age of fifty-six by bilateral dislocation after repeated blows about the head and face.

Syphilis is present in a surprisingly high proportion of cases of traumatic lens displacement: thus Jarrett (1967) found positive serology in 23 (27%) of 85 cases and in 21 of 29 cases with known syphilis trauma was the precipitating cause; whether these figures reflect the ability of the spirochæte to weaken the zonule or the increased susceptibility to ocular trauma of the patient with acquired syphilis remains open to speculation.

As a rule the zonule itself is injured, tearing most readily at its attachment to the lens; rupture at its ciliary insertion is rare, so that in most cases the equator of the lens is bare of zonular fibres. If observation by the slit-lamp is possible through a coloboma or dialysis of the iris, the zonular bundles may be seen to be stretched or torn, curled upon themselves or entirely absent, the anterior fibres being usually most severely affected so that the posterior may be the sole survivors. In such cases these surviving fibres are stretched and deformed and may be powdered with deposits of pigment or blood with herniations of vitreous appearing between them. Alternatively, the zonular lamella becomes detached and this is seen to float as a fine, crinkled membrane drawn behind the iris by its attached fibres, leaving the equator of the lens evenly rounded and its capsule intact.[1]

SUBLUXATION. Once the zonular attachment has been damaged or ruptured the lens may remain in the posterior fossa retained by its attachment to the vitreous (the ligamentum hyaloideo-capsularis), becoming tremulous, perhaps, and sinking downwards somewhat owing to the action of gravity. In such cases the lens itself becomes more spherical, and if the zonular damage is partial, in young people in whom the lens is plastic, its edge may become undulated and deformed after the manner of a smooth and shallow coloboma at the site where tension has been released; myopia, some-

[1] Meesmann (1922), Maggiore (1924), Stein (1926), Jess (1926), Busacca (1927), Ringelhan and Elschnig (1931), and others.

times with astigmatism and impairment of accommodation, is the visual result (Schoeler, 1875; Pflüger, 1875; and others). In such cases the vitreous may be seen to herniate through the pupil or to exude into the anterior chamber (Plate IV, Fig. 4). If the subluxation is greater, the lens may slip from its axial position and its equatorial edge may appear as a crescent in the pupillary aperture, dividing it into a phakic and aphakic part (*lateral subluxation*). Such lateral displacement may be combined with some rotatory displacement so that the lens lies obliquely (*axial subluxation*); in both types iridodonesis results and the anterior chamber becomes of unequal depth round its circumference. In its most extreme form the axial subluxation may involve a rotation through 90°, so that the equator of the lens presents through the pupil into the anterior chamber. It is possible that in these cases a total dislocation has been prevented by the spasmodic irritative contraction of the pupil at the moment of luxation (Veasey, 1901; Ask, 1913).

The clinical appearances, signs and symptoms of such a subluxated lens have already been discussed and need not detain us here.[1] Occasionally, but only occasionally, the eye may remain quiet indefinitely with good vision (after $10\frac{1}{2}$ years with normal vision in the aphakic part of the pupil, Maxwell, 1951). More usually less fortunate events occur—traumatic opacities are a very frequent accompaniment and a progressive total opacity may develop (32% of 144 cases, Kutschera and Ebner, 1964) to which must be added the effect of severe uveitis either irritative or phaco-anaphylactic in origin,[2] and secondary glaucoma, a common sequel due to a number of causes[3] among which should be noted the insidious rise in ocular tension associated with damage to the structures in the angle of the anterior chamber resulting from the original contusion.[4] Finally, retinal detachment may follow in a considerable proportion of eyes harbouring a displaced lens either following its surgical removal or while the lens is still *in situ* (38 eyes in 34 patients, Jarrett, 1967); the problems involved in treating such patients are considerable since observation of the retina and localization of the holes may be rendered difficult owing to the abnormal position of the lens and its prior removal to facilitate these essential diagnostic procedures may result in loss of the eye (vitreous loss in 47 of 114 cases, Jarrett, 1967).

In COMPLETE TRAUMATIC LUXATION the lens may follow different routes —into the anterior chamber, the vitreous, the inter-retinal space, the subscleral region, or outside the eye if the globe is ruptured so that it lies impacted in the rupture itself, comes to rest in the subconjunctival or Tenon's space or is extruded altogether.

Dorsch (1900), analysing the literature, found the following incidence: dislocation into the anterior chamber, 28 cases; into the vitreous, 21; under the conjunctiva, 59;

[1] Vol. XI, p. 300. [2] Vol. IX, p. 501. [3] Vol. XI, p. 307.
[4] Hegner (1915), Maggiore (1924), Ringelhan and Elschnig (1931), Rodman (1963), Chandler (1964), Kutschera and Ebner (1964, 44% of 144 cases).

into Tenon's space, 3; while in 7 cases the lens was extruded entirely and lost. 188 cases of traumatic lens displacement reported by Kutschera and Ebner (1964) showed the following distribution: subluxation in 144; complete dislocation into the vitreous in 31; and 11 into the anterior chamber.

The pathological changes which occur in dislocated lenses and the damage caused to the globe have been studied by several observers.[1] Degenerative changes are the rule, setting in slowly after 3 or 4 months—a disintegration of the epithelium and cleft formation in the cortical layers (Ritter, 1898) followed by the appearance of amorphous masses resembling morgagnian changes[2] under the cortex with eventually the formation of calcareous deposits and shrinkage (Habben, 1897); partial or total absorption is a rare event (Pagani, 1926, in the anterior chamber; Snell, 1882; Augstein and Ginsberg, 1896, in the vitreous) (Figs. 117–118).

Figs. 117 and 118.—Traumatic Dislocation of the Lens.

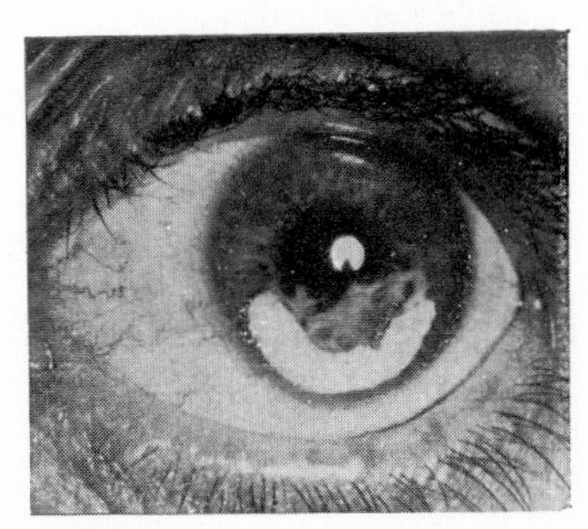

Fig. 117.—The remains of the lens in the anterior chamber after a traumatic dislocation (Inst. Ophthal.).

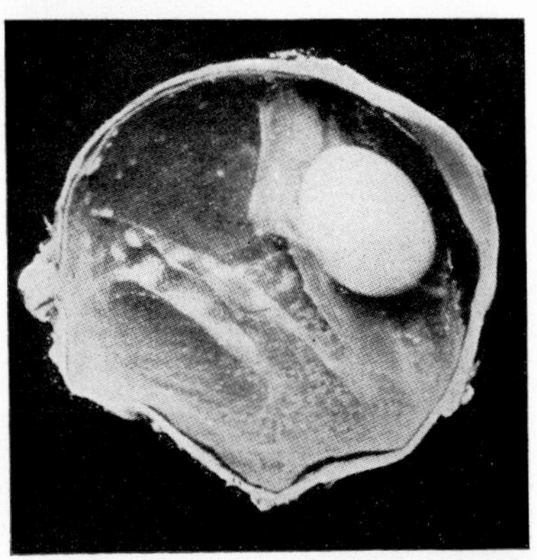

Fig. 118.—A large morgagnian cataract lies embedded in inflammatory exudate; in the exudate are many white inflammatory foci (R. H. Elliot).

Dislocation into the anterior chamber,[3] sometimes associated with a rotation of the lens through 180° so that its posterior surface is next to the cornea (Saunders, 1889; Ask, 1913; Stein, 1926), is an unfortunate accident (Fig. 119). The lens lies in front of the iris as a transparent body sometimes almost filling the anterior chamber, sometimes lying in its lower part with its rim showing a golden lustre so that it resembles a large globule of oil in the aqueous. Through its substance the iris is seen pushed backwards with the pupil spasmodically contracted. Occasionally the condition appears to be well tolerated with the retention of normal (aphakic) vision for long periods (Rampoldi, 1882; 25 years, Ayberk, 1939), but almost invariably an

[1] Davey (1882), Lawford (1887), Wagenhäuser (1912), Burk (1912), Ask (1913), and many others.

[2] Vol. XI, p. 136.

[3] Vol. XI, p. 302.

intractable iridocyclitis supervenes and a fulminating glaucoma follows (14 out of 15 cases, Hegner, 1915; 90% of cases, Maggiore, 1924; Ringelhan and Elschnig, 1931). Sympathetic ophthalmitis has also been reported as a sequel (Walker, 1892), although this is exceptional (Dor and Paufique, 1932).

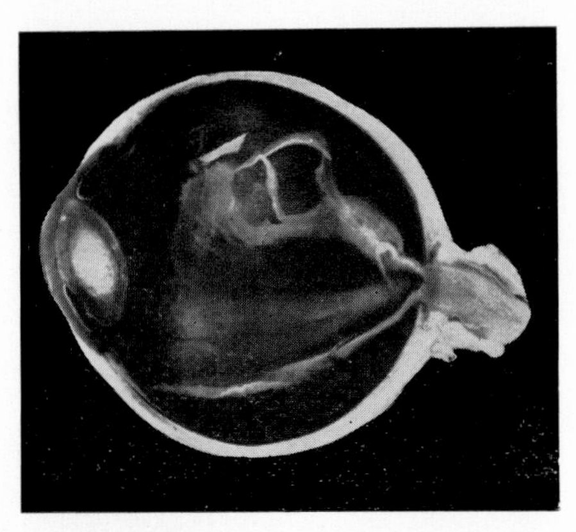

Fig. 119.—Anterior Dislocation of the Lens after a Contusion.

The lens is dislocated forwards into the anterior chamber, the iris is seen behind it above but in front of it below. There is a large retinal detachment (Museum, Inst. Ophthal.).

Figs. 120 and 121.—Posterior Dislocation of the Lens after a Contusion.

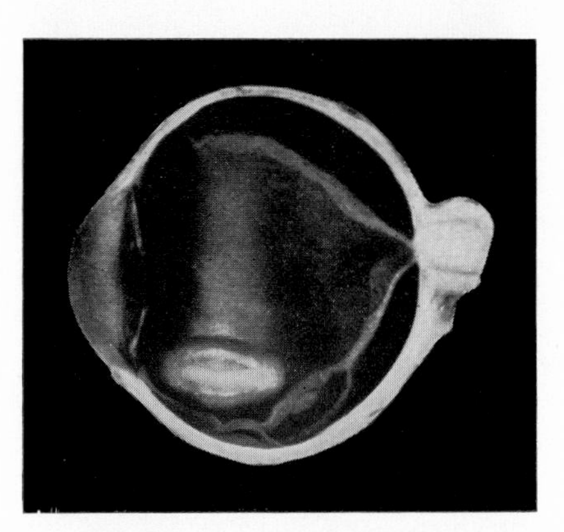

Fig. 120.—The lens lies at the bottom of the vitreous chamber; the anterior chamber is very deep (Museum, Inst. Ophthal.).

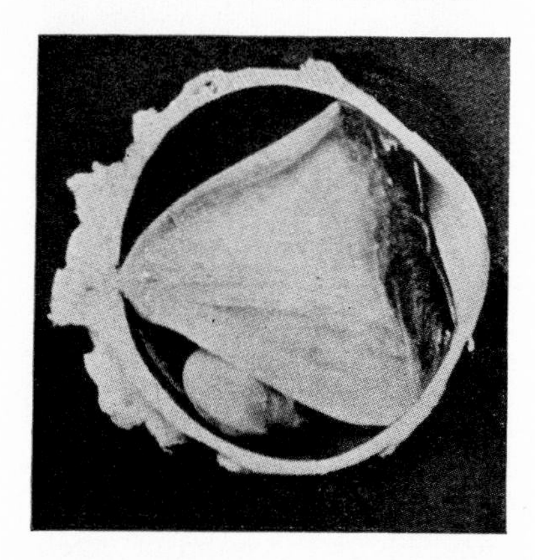

Fig. 121.—The morgagnian cataract lies beneath the retina (R. H. Elliot).

An unusual case was reported by Gutzeit (1950) in which there were two large tears in the iris at 4 and 11 o'clock; the temporal half of the lens lay in the anterior chamber blocking this segment of the angle and the nasal half lay behind the iris but pressed it against the cornea so that this portion of the angle was also occluded with a resultant acute secondary glaucoma.

Dislocation into the vitreous is twice as common as anterior dislocation and in this position the lens is more easily tolerated; it is true that the eye may remain quiet and useful for many years, but nevertheless a severe iridocyclitis may result, secondary glaucoma is by no means uncommon (90% of cases, Maggiore, 1924; Ringelhan and Elschnig, 1931; 19 of 31 cases, Kutschera and Ebner, 1964), although it may not become evident for many years (Rollet and Genet, 1913) (Fig. 118); sympathetic ophthalmitis may supervene (Dor and Paufique, 1932) and, as a delayed complication, slow degenerative changes throughout the eye usually destroy the vision (Werncke, 1903; Sievert, 1903; Elliot, 1919). At first the lens is mobile in the vitreous (*lens natans*) and may even be induced to travel from the vitreous into the anterior chamber through the dilated pupil by changing the position of the patient from the prone to the supine position (*wandering lens*) (Wolfe and Mayer, 1945; and others), a manœuvre which the patient may succeed in carrying out himself (Favory, 1952), but eventually organized membranes tend to anchor it (*lens fixata*) (Fig. 120). As a rarity the lens may slip through a retinal tear into the inter-retinal space (Ringelhan and Elschnig, 1931; Fralick, 1937) (Fig. 121); or again it may lie between the sclera and the ciliary body (*sub-scleral luxation*) (Nettleship, 1881; Lawford, 1887). Sometimes an intra-ocular hæmorrhage may preclude adequate examination; in such cases ultrasonography may help in the location of a displaced lens but the echogram may give rise to the false impression of a detachment of the retina (Goldberg and Sarin, 1967; Macoul, 1968).

The clinical signs and symptoms of posterior dislocation have already been detailed in a previous Volume.[1]

EXTRA-OCULAR DISLOCATION OF THE LENS occurs not uncommonly after contusions of sufficient severity to cause rupture of the globe, producing a clinical picture so dramatic as to have long excited interest (Dixon, 1852; and others) (Plate VIII). Once the explosive force generated inside the globe by the concussion has burst its envelope, the zonule is completely torn and the solid and relatively heavy lens is readily extruded almost invariably in its capsule (12 out of 13 cases, Mitvalsky, 1897). It may be forced into the anterior chamber, tearing the iris at its root, taking this tissue with it and then escaping into a rupture near the corneo-scleral margin (Müller 1895); here it may become incarcerated[2] or, travelling further, may lie under the conjunctiva (*lenticele, phacocele*) leaving the eye with the appearance of a wide coloboma of the iris or in a condition of aniridia and aphakia (Gangoso, 1948; and others). A lens lying subconjunctivally is usually absorbed, its site being eventually marked by calcareous deposits (Alt, 1877; d'Amico, 1925) but, particularly if the capsule is intact, it may remain practically unaltered almost indefinitely (15 years, Vieusse, 1879; 18, Collins, 1889). Such

[1] Vol. XI, p. 304.
[2] Lederle (1875), Fano (1880), Mercanti (1891), Collins (1889). Stonehill (1949).

a dislocation usually occurs in the upper quadrant somewhat to the nasal side (85% of cases, Souillard, 1910). In a further extension of the same process when the conjunctiva is also torn, the lens with a varying amount of the ocular contents is extruded altogether and is usually not seen by the surgeon; its production wrapped up in a handkerchief by the patient is an unusual event (Praun, 1899). Alternatively, the lens may be forced backwards in which case it is usually extruded through a rent in the sclera near the equator between the superior and lateral recti and comes to rest in Tenon's space.[1]

Additional cases of subconjunctival dislocation of the lens have been reported by Bhaduri (1955) in a peculiar case wherein the dislocation was caused by a leaping fish; by Chams and Sadoughi (1957), 5 cases, 1 of which presented with sympathetic ophthalmitis; by Evans (1961), a case in which two months following an injury from the handlebars of a bicycle the lens was removed via a conjunctival incision, the sclera having healed. Sédan (1961) reported having seen 9 cases in 30 years, 4 of which required immediate removal of the eye due to the gross ocular damage while the other 5 retained useful vision, although a late rise of intra-ocular pressure occurred in all of them.

Treatment of a displaced lens is a very difficult matter and, as the problems involved have been fully considered elsewhere,[2] only a short summary is required here. In general terms conservatism pays in most cases; the lens should not necessarily be removed just because it is displaced but only if complications develop. In cases of *subluxation* without complications an attempt should be made to attain reasonable vision by optical correction of the phakic or aphakic area. If the aphakic area is small the pupil can be continuously dilated by the use of weak mydriatics if the angle of the anterior chamber is open, or its area may be increased by an optical iridectomy or photocoagulation of the sphincter muscle of the iris. An alternative in young patients is a discission which may be a safe procedure up to the age of 30 (Chandler, 1964). Removal of a subluxated lens is much more difficult and should be attempted only if complications arise.

The end-results of *dislocation* into the anterior chamber are so frequently disastrous that operative removal of the lens from this site despite its technical difficulties should be attempted in all cases. Its extraction may be required although some surgeons prefer to coax the lens back into the posterior chamber followed by a peripheral iridectomy. A lens dislocated posteriorly into the vitreous is probably best left alone if complications such as secondary glaucoma do not intervene. In subconjunctival dislocations the care of the lens is usually secondary to that of the globe, a matter which will be considered in the section on ocular rupture; any attempt to remove the lens by opening the conjunctiva at an early stage is usually followed by a large loss of vitreous and atrophy of the globe. Left to itself, the lens usually slowly shrinks and its remnants may be removed if necessary after the

[1] Wadsworth (1885), Montagnon (1887), Müller (1895), Schlodtmann (1897), Ask (1911).
[2] Vol. XI, p. 307.

PLATE VIII

Rupture of the Globe and Dislocation of the Lens.

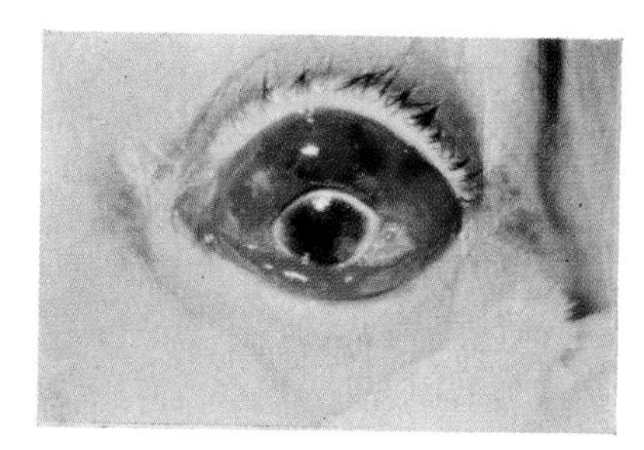

Fig. 1.—Rupture of the globe with subconjunctival dislocation of the lens, following a fall against a chair.

Figs. 2 to 5.—Rupture of the Globe and Subconjunctival Dislocation of the Lens following a Blow from a Piece of Wood.

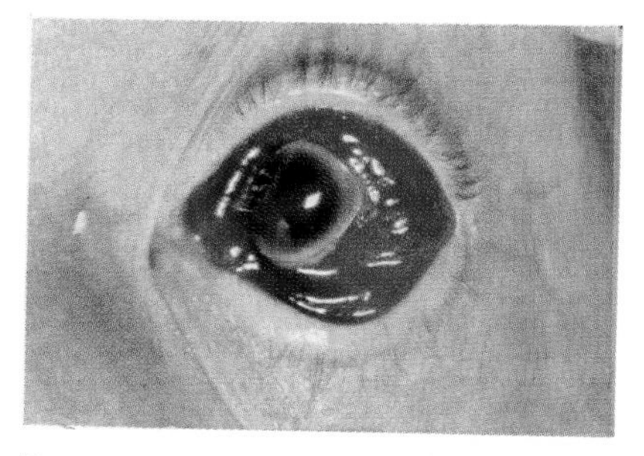

Fig. 2.—Massive subconjunctival hæmorrhage and distortion of the cornea.

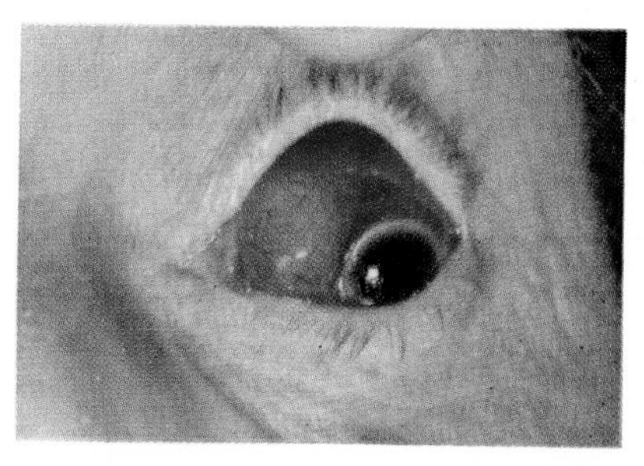

Fig. 3.—The same eye 5 days later showing a globular swelling on the nasal side.

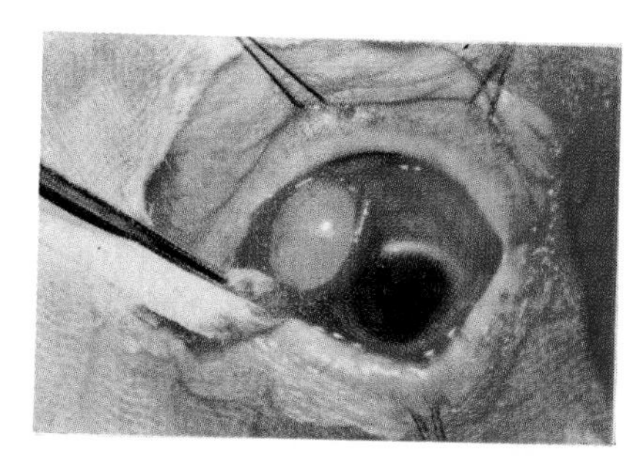

Fig. 4.—The intact lens lying outside the globe.

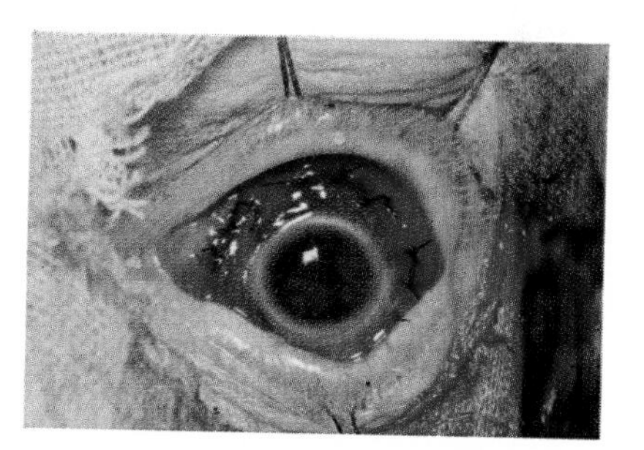

Fig. 5.—Repair of the corneo-scleral rupture extending 180° superiorly.

wound in the sclera has healed. In many of these cases, however, widespread disorganization of the globe renders enucleation necessary, but when the mutilation is less severe the eye may settle down with the retention of good vision under such conservative treatment.

Alt. *Arch. Augenheilk.*, **6**, 8, 84 (1877).
d'Amico. *Ann. Ottal.*, **53**, 665, 1190 (1925).
Ask. *Klin. Mbl. Augenheilk.*, **49** (2), 134 (1911).
Studien über path. Anat. d. erworbenen Linsensubluxationen, Wiesbaden (1913).
Augstein and Ginsberg. *Zbl. prakt. Augenheilk.*, **20**, 356 (1896).
Ayberk. *Türk. oftal. Gaz.*, **3**, 21 (1939).
Badal. *Union méd.* (Paris), **26**, 354, 365 (1878).
Beauvieux and Monod. *Arch. Ophtal.*, **41**, 266 (1924).
Bhaduri. *J. All-India ophthal. Soc.*, **3**, 17 (1955).
Burk. *v. Graefes Arch. Ophthal.*, **83**, 114 (1912).
Busacca. *Zbl. ges. Ophthal.*, **18**, 433 (1927).
Chams and Sadoughi. *Acta med. iran.*, **1**, 299 (1957).
Chandler. *Arch. Ophthal.*, **71**, 765 (1964).
Collins. *Roy. Lond. ophthal. Hosp. Rep.*, **12**, 345 (1889).
Davey. *Brit. med. J.*, **2**, 369 (1882).
Dixon. *Lancet*, **2**, 486 (1852).
Dor and Paufique. *Bull. Soc. Ophtal. Paris*, 434 (1932).
Dorsch. *Ueber angeborene u. erworbene Linsenluxation u. ihre Behandlung* (Diss.), Marburg (1900).
Elliot. *Brit. J. Ophthal.*, **3**, 49 (1919).
Evans. *Cent. Afr. J. Med.*, **7**, 164 (1961).
Fano. *Ann. Ottal.*, **9**, 364 (1880).
Favory. *Bull. Soc. Ophtal. Fr.*, 583 (1952).
Fralick. *Amer. J. Ophthal.*, **20**, 795 (1937).
Frenkel. *Ann. Oculist.* (Paris), **153**, 233 (1916); **155**, 78 (1918).
Arch. Ophtal., **48**, 205 (1931); **49**, 431 (1932).
Gangoso. *Arch. Soc. oftal. hisp.-amer.*, **8**, 402 (1948).
Goldberg and Sarin. *Ultrasonics in Ophthalmology*, Phila. (1967).
Gutzeit. *Klin. Mbl. Augenheilk.*, **116**, 213 (1950).
Habben. *Ein Beitrag z. Kenntnis d. path. Anat. d. Linsenluxationen* (Diss.), Jena (1897).
Hegner. *Beitr. Augenheilk.*, **9** (90), 707 (1915).
Heinz. *Wien. klin. Wschr.*, **59**, 819 (1947).
Jarrett. *Arch. Ophthal.*, **78**, 289 (1967).
Jess. *Klin. Mbl. Augenheilk.*, **76**, 465 (1926).
Kutschera and Ebner. *Klin. Mbl. Augenheilk.*, **144**, 277 (1964).
Lambros and Cinotti. *Amer. J. Ophthal.*, **63**, 512 (1967).
Lawford. *Roy. Lond. ophthal. Hosp. Rep.*, **11**, 327 (1887).
Lederle. *Klin. Mbl. Augenheilk.*, **13**, 30 (1875).
Macoul. *Arch. Ophthal.*, **80**, 724 (1968).
Maggiore. *Ann. Ottal.*, **52**, 817, 917 (1924).
Maxwell. *Trans. ophthal. Soc. U.K.*, **71**, 780 (1951).
Meesmann. *Arch. Augenheilk.*, **91**, 261 (1922).
Mercanti. *Ann. Ottal.*, **20**, 365 (1891).
Mitvalsky. *Arch. Ophtal.*, **17**, 337 (1897).
Montagnon. *Arch. Ophtal.*, **7**, 204 (1887).
Müller. *Über Ruptur d. Corneo-Skleralgrenze durch stumpfe Verletzung*, Leipzig (1895).
Nettleship. *Trans. ophthal. Soc. U.K.*, **1**, 24 (1881).
Pagani. *Boll. Oculist.*, **5**, 529 (1926).
Parisotti. *Bull. Acad. Med. Roma*, **18**, 602 (1891).
Peretti. *Z. Augenheilk.*, **2**, 225 (1899).
Pflüger. *Klin. Mbl. Augenheilk.*, **13**, 109 (1875).
Praun. *Die Verletzungen des Auges*, Wiesbaden (1899).
Rampoldi. *Ann. Univ. Med. Chir. Milano*, **261**, 49 (1882).
Ringelhan and Elschnig. *Arch. Augenheilk.*, **104**, 325 (1931).
Ritter. *Arch. Augenheilk.*, **37**, 348 (1898).
Rodman. *Arch. Ophthal.*, **69**, 445 (1963).
Rollet and Genet. *Rev. gén. Ophtal.*, **32**, 572 (1913).
Saunders. *Brit. med. J.*, **1**, 470 (1889).
Schlodtmann. *v. Graefes Arch. Ophthal.*, **44**, 127 (1897).
Schoeler. *Klin. Jb.*, 22 (1875). See *Jber. Ophthal.*, **6**, 481 (1875).
Sédan. *Ann. Oculist.* (Paris), **194**, 797 (1961).
Sievert. *Ueber degenerative Veränderungen d. Choroidea u. Retina bei Luxation d. Linse in dem Glaskörper* (Diss.), Freiburg (1903).
Snell. *Ophthal. Rev.*, **1**, 400 (1882).
Souillard. *Essai sur les luxations sous-conjonctivales du cristallin*, Paris (1910).
Stein. *Klin. Mbl. Augenheilk.*, **76**, 75 (1926).
Stonehill. *Amer. J. Ophthal.*, **32**, 126 (1949).
Veasey. *Ophthal. Rec.*, **10**, 8, 42 (1901).
Vieusse. *Recueil Ophtal.*, **1**, 85 (1879).
Wadsworth. *Trans. Amer. ophthal. Soc.*, **4**, 147 (1885).
Wagenhäuser. *Anatomische Untersuchungen bei acht Fällen von Linsenluxation* (Diss.), Tübingen (1912).
Walker. *Lancet*, **2**, 663 (1892).
Werncke. *Klin. Mbl. Augenheilk.*, **41**, Beil., 283 (1903).
Wolfe and Mayer. *Amer. J. Ophthal.*, **28**, 193 (1945).
Zoldan. *Ann. Ottal.*, **52**, 736 (1924).

Contusion Effects on the Choroid

As would be expected, the choroid suffers the same type of contusive and concussive effects as the more anterior portions of the uveal tract. The wave of pressure whereby the vitreous impinges upon it and forces it against the resistant sclera and the rebound of the tissues set up the same reaction with its pronounced vasomotor response—a traumatic ischæmia followed by a paretic vasodilatation with the resultant tendency to ischæmic necrosis, followed by œdema and hæmorrhage; and to this is added the purely mechanical effects of lacerations involving tearing of the blood-vessels and stroma, probably aided by sudden traction on the tissues especially round their anchorage at the optic nerve-head.

CHOROIDAL HÆMORRHAGE AND DETACHMENT

It is not surprising, therefore, that HÆMORRHAGES IN THE CHOROID are a frequent sequel of such injuries (Plate IX, Figs. 1 and 2). These may be small and intrachoroidal; blood may appear under the retina or spread between the choroid and the sclera, detaching the former from the latter (Fig. 122) while, if the retina is torn, the hæmorrhage may extend into the vitreous or, seeping through a damaged zonule, may appear in the anterior chamber (Plate IV, Fig. 4) (Zander and Geissler, 1864). If a choroidal hæmorrhage is localized and ophthalmoscopically visible, it appears as a rounded dark blotch

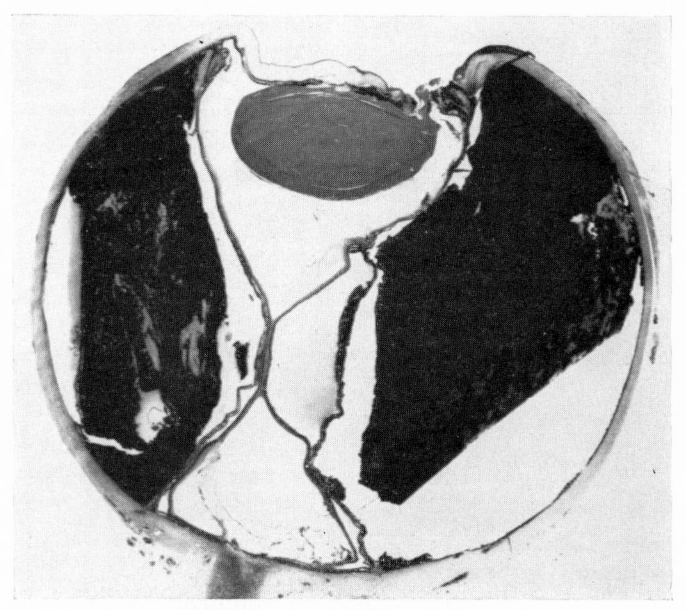

FIG. 122.—MASSIVE SUBCHOROIDAL HÆMORRHAGE.
Note that the hæmorrhage detaches the choroid and ciliary body anterior to the scleral spur (N. Ashton).

PLATE IX

CONTUSION EFFECTS ON THE CHOROID.

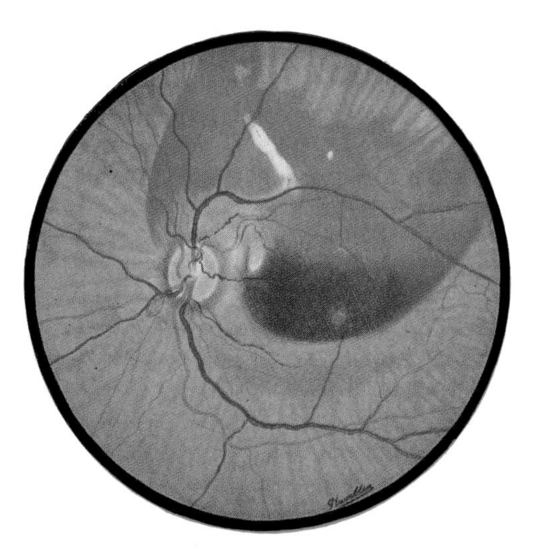

FIG. 1.—Recent choroidal rupture with a large choroidal hæmorrhage and a hole at the macula.

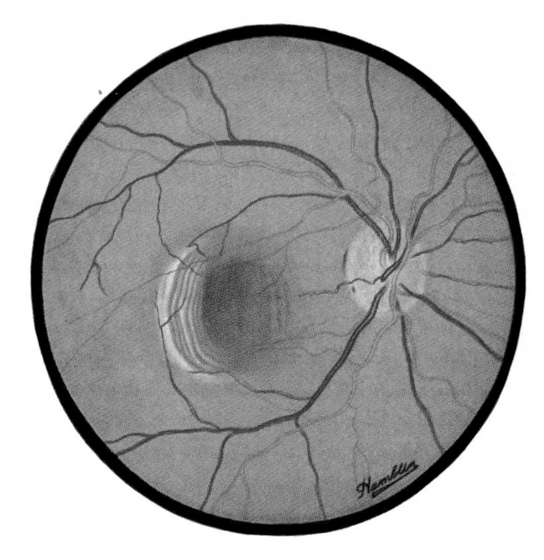

FIG. 2.—Choroidal hæmorrhage in the stage of absorption; raised 7.0 D.

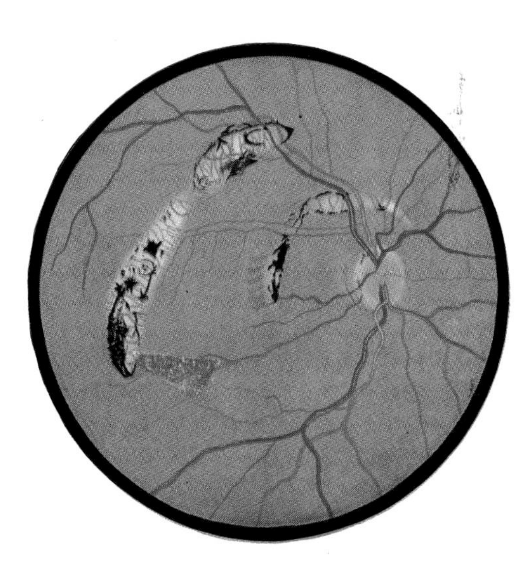

FIG. 3.—Concentric choroidal ruptures 12 years after a blow on the eye with a fist.

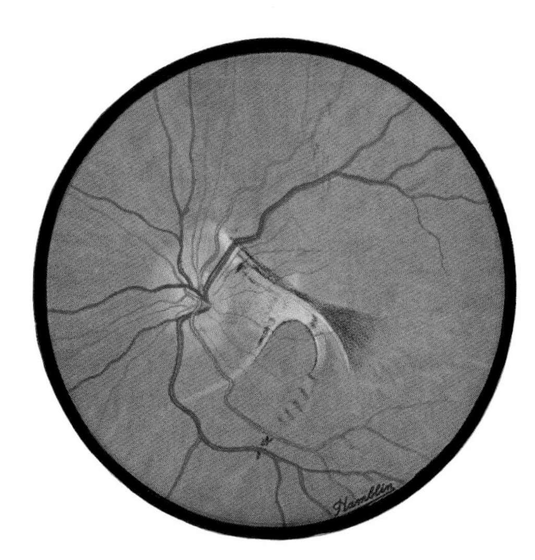

FIG. 4.—Central choroidal rupture. The eye was struck with a golf flag-stick one year previously. Central scotoma.

[*To face p.* 150.

with blurred edges over which the retinal vessels course; it slowly tends to absorb, leaving considerable pigmentation and usually some degree of atrophy which in the central area may cause substantial visual loss.[1] Treatment is expectant.

A DETACHMENT OF THE CHOROID due to bleeding from the tearing of a posterior ciliary artery occurring after a severe contusion is not unusual if the globe is ruptured, a catastrophe comparable to that occasionally complicating a cataract operation.[2] If the globe remains intact, the damage caused by the trauma and the secondary glaucoma which tends to follow the bleeding may necessitate enucleation; hypotony, however, may develop and a few cases have been reported wherein a shallow choroidal detachment has appeared and has slowly settled with retention of the eye (Michel, 1878; Sous, 1892; Mules, 1893). Occasionally the detachment is prominent and lasting (Hjort, 1882; Walter, 1883). The occurrence of such a hæmorrhage between the choroid and sclera was demonstrated experimentally in rabbits to follow a contusion of the eye by Berlin (1873), and pathological examinations have been made by Story (1881) and Collins (1916–17). The clinical picture, diagnosis and treatment of such a condition have already been detailed.[3]

In the same way, an œdematous exudation from the blood vessels dilated by the concussion may lead to a temporary serous detachment of the choroid, usually on the temporal aspect, which has the typical clinical characteristics and history[4]; such a detachment may result from an indirect trauma to the skull (Hertz, 1952).

RUPTURE OF THE CHOROID

Choroidal lesions following contusions which become evident clinically as areas of atrophy, frequently sharply defined but sometimes irregular and diffuse, have been classically described as ruptures of the choroid since their original description by von Graefe (1854). Initially a purely mechanistic hypothesis was generally accepted—that the impinging force (usually striking the globe in front) produced a direct rupture situated typically anterior to the equator, while the wave of pressure set up within the eye burst the choroid near the posterior pole by *contre-coup* injury; this tissue was said to give way more readily than the other ocular coats because of the greater toughness of the sclera and the greater elasticity of the retina (Arlt, 1875), the rupture being perhaps determined primarily by the tear in the brittle membrane of Bruch. The fact, however, that lesions similar in clinical appearance and pathology but differing in shape could be produced by the vascular disturbances caused by a contusion led later observers to suggest that the essential mechanism was not an immediate mechanical rupture but a post-traumatic necrosis (Siegrist, 1895; Østerberg, 1936; Hudelo *et al.*,

[1] Vol. IX, p. 26.
[2] Vol. IX, p. 952.
[3] Vol. IX, p. 940.
[4] Vol. IX, p. 949.

1945; Tower, 1949). It is to be remembered, however, that the clinical picture resulting from lesions caused by either of these agencies will be similar in its essentials and that the pathological changes eventually found will be much alike. It is indeed possible that both factors enter into the ætiology of most cases; but the site and shape of the typical crescentic lesion in the choroid near the posterior pole of the eye suggest a solution of the continuity of the tissues determined by mechanical forces, while the more widespread and irregular lesions seem explicable only on the basis of contusion necrosis. In the meantime, therefore, we shall discuss these under two separate headings.

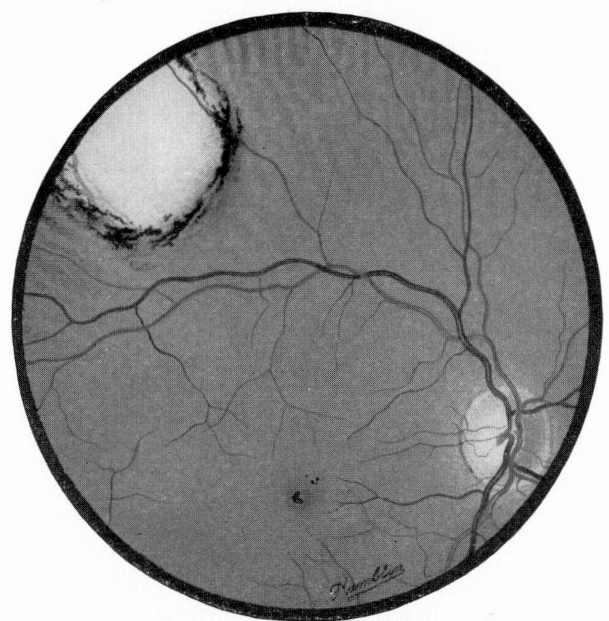

Fig. 123.—Direct Rupture of the Choroid

From a gunshot wound of the right supra-orbital region 4 years previously. A circumscribed lesion is seen in the periphery associated with a macular cyst and two pigmentary dots in the perimacular area.

DIRECT CHOROIDAL RUPTURES, presumably due to the impingement of an outside force on the globe, are relatively rarely seen in contusive injuries. A large, broad and usually irregular lesion lies near the periphery exposing the white sclera, bordered initially by hæmorrhage and eventually by heavy pigmentary changes[1] (Fig. 123). The dissolution of the choroid in such cases has been histologically verified,[2] and frequently also the overlying retina is torn. The causal injury is usually severe, and it may well be that the

[1] Schröter (1871), Genth (1871), Laqueur (1902), Nicolai (1902), Gross (1911), Oguchi (1913), Lagrange (1917), and many others.

[2] Picqué (1884), Nettleship (1904), Herrmann (1906), Kaufer and Zimmerman (1966), and others.

irregular criss-cross lesions without definite pattern seen as contusion injuries following gunshot wounds of the skull in the neighbourhood of the orbit come into this category.

INDIRECT RUPTURES OF THE CHOROID, conforming to von Graefe's (1854) description, are much more common and are a relatively frequent sequel of contusions of the globe due either to direct injury or the blast of an explosion: Hughes (1887) annotated 72 cases from the literature and Ohm (1905) 316. The initial appearance, which is usually obscured by hæmorrhage, is that of a yellowish-brown streak the edges of which are bespattered with blood and pigment covered by an œdematous retina; this gradually develops into a sharply defined white streak, usually a third or less of the diameter of the disc in width, bordered by heavily pigmented edges. Frequently, owing to the initial obscuration of the media by hæmorrhage, the lesion is first seen at this stage. As healing progresses the hæmorrhages disappear, the pigment proliferates and the surrounding region may show atrophic changes and pigmentary disturbances but in its essentials, although the width of the white floor may be observed to narrow with cicatrization,[1] the ophthalmoscopic picture remains permanently unaltered (Plate IX, Figs. 3 and 4).

Such a fissure is usually localized at or near the posterior pole and in two-thirds of all instances it is single, in a quarter of the cases double lesions appear, while multiple tears of various sizes up to six or more may be encountered (Godtfredsen, 1942). When multiple tears occur the central one is usually the largest, and the most peripheral the smallest; frequently they run concentrically or almost so but they may criss-cross one another (Hoor, 1886; Polano, 1897; and others). In such cases the more peripheral tears may be pinkish in colour, an effect said to be due to a *partial rupture* affecting the inner layers of the choroid (Figs. 124–5).

In shape the rupture is usually crescentic and runs concentrically with the margin of the optic disc, extending some two or three times the disc-diameter in length; further outwards it runs parallel with the equator, while in some 10% of cases a straight or radial rupture is seen, the latter being usually situated in the horizontal meridian. A course with the convexity towards the disc is exceptional (Ginsberg, 1893; Polano, 1897; Ohm, 1905). In the great majority of cases the fissure lies on the temporal side of the disc (82%, Hughes, 1887), in which case it may traverse the macula; a nasal crescent is more rare (14%) and a horizontal rupture exceptional (4%). The rent may extend half or three-quarters of the circumference or even encircle the optic nerve completely (Knapp, 1869; and others). As a rule it is broadest about its middle and narrows towards each end; sometimes the ends are forked; a V-shape (de Schweinitz, 1901) or Y-shape (Mills, 1903;

[1] Knapp (1869), Hersing (1872), Adamük (1878), Vossius (1883), Neubauer (1957), and many others.

FIGS. 124 and 125.—MULTIPLE RUPTURES OF THE CHOROID (H. Neame).

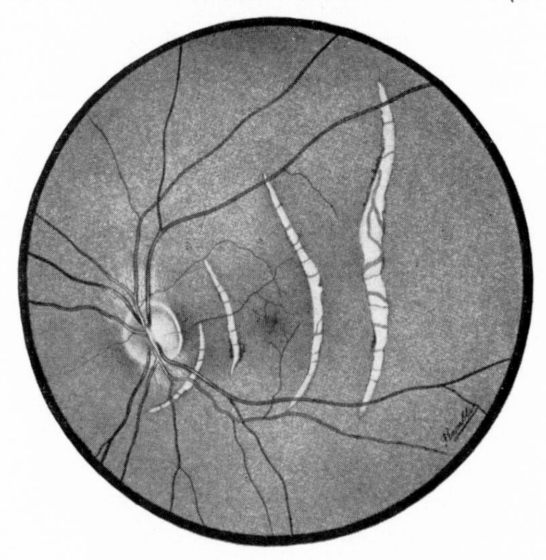

FIG. 124.—In a youth aged 19, struck in the eye with the handle of a broom, one month previously. The fovea lies between the second and third tear (vision 6/12).

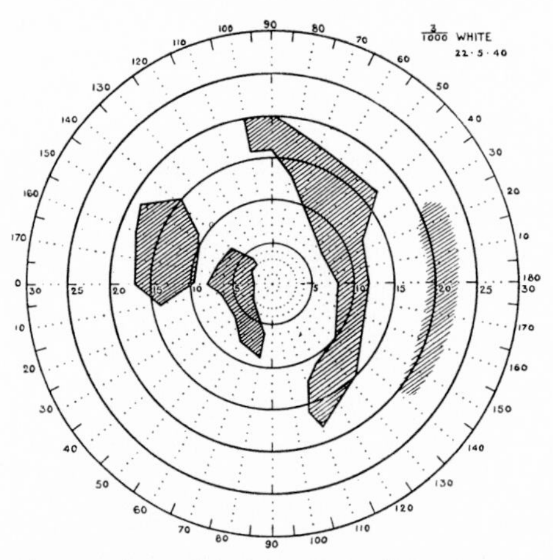

FIG. 125.—Campimetry chart of the same case; the scotoma on the left represents the blind-spot. To the right is a scotoma representing the two ruptures between the disc and the macula. The hatched area without a boundary line is an ill-defined scotoma representing the rupture furthest out on the temporal periphery (3/1,000 white).

Goar, 1938) has been recorded, or patterns so irregular as to defy description; while occasionally the tear is of immense size, so extensive as to occupy the greater part of the posterior portion of the fundus or so long that its extremities are lost to view on ordinary ophthalmoscopic examination (Mannhardt, 1875; Tower, 1949). It is interesting that an indirect rupture at the posterior pole is not uncommonly associated with a direct rupture near the periphery, the two lesions being separated by normal choroid (Aub, 1871, in a case wherein there was also a rupture of the posterior capsule of the lens).

Over the rupture the retina usually remains structurally intact and the vessels course over the rent in the choroid without any break in their continuity. Rarely, however, does the former tissue remain unscathed; initially it may show œdematous changes while at a later stage it becomes atrophic and evidences of pigmentary migration become prominent, while hæmorrhages in the neighbourhood are not infrequent. It is to be remembered, of course, that several associated injuries to the retina may occur in addition—macular lesions, tears and detachment.

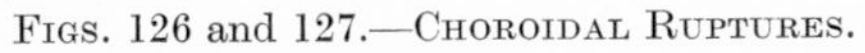

FIGS. 126 and 127.—CHOROIDAL RUPTURES.

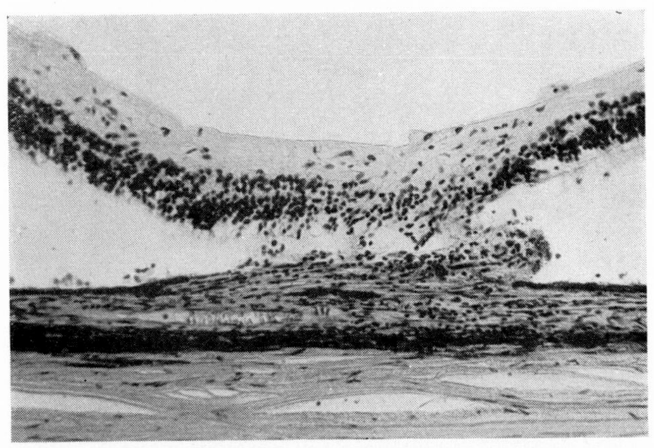

FIG. 126.—A choroidal tear; fibrous tissue from the choroid extrudes between the torn ends of the retinal pigmentary epithelium and the retina is adherent to the cicatrix in the choroid (A. Hagedoorn).

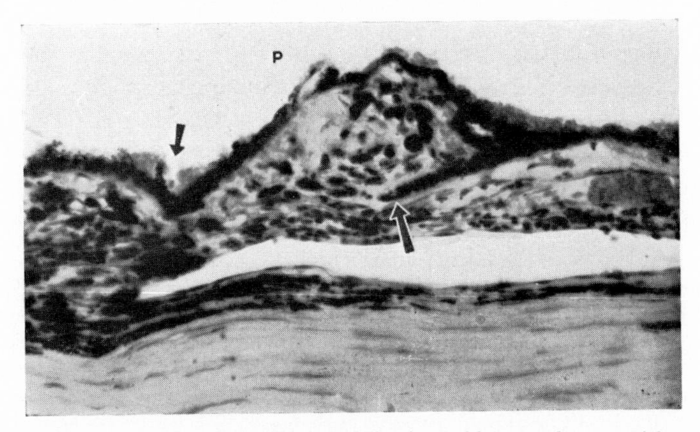

Fig. 127.—A macular choroidal tear following a blow on the eye with a piece of stone. Bruch's membrane and the pigmentary epithelium are ruptured at the sites indicated by arrows. Some choroidal tissue has extended inwards and has been covered with regenerated pigmentary epithelium (P). Six weeks after injury (H. & E.; × 250) (N. Ashton).

Pathology. The year following the original clinical description of a choroidal tear by von Graefe, the first pathological report was published by von Ammon (1855) of an indirect injury to a soldier who shot himself in the mouth with a gun loaded with water; this initial study has been followed by several others[1] (Figs. 126–7). Histologically the membrane of Bruch is torn and with it the choriocapillaris, while part or all of the vascular layer of the choroid external to this disappears; internal to the membrane the pigmentary epithelium of the retina is also lacking. In the early stages blood and exudates pour out and infiltrate between the pigmentary epithelium and the external limiting membrane of the retina, occasionally appearing on the inner aspect of the latter tissue. Even at an early stage the pigment is found

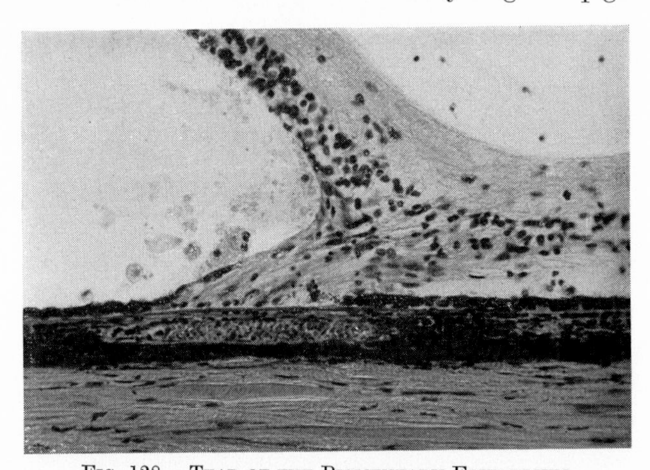

FIG. 128.—TEAR OF THE PIGMENTARY EPITHELIUM.

Showing a rupture of the pigmentary epithelium of the retina and the adherence of the retina to Bruch's membrane (A. Hagedoorn).

to be irregularly distributed and proliferated. Eventually the overlying retina becomes atrophic and degenerated showing neuroglial proliferation, wandering of pigment and the new formation of vessels. After some time it becomes adherent to and is incorporated in the fibrous tissue which fills the gap in the choroid, but in the usual lesion where this tissue is torn and the retina maintains its continuity, this fibrous tissue is always limited in amount.

A RUPTURE OF THE PIGMENTARY EPITHELIUM of the retina without other local complications was described by Tillema (1936) and Hagedoorn (1937). Clinically the lesion resembles the classical rupture of the choroid but signs of œdema and hæmorrhage are absent. Pathologically Bruch's membrane remains intact and whereas in rupture of the choroid the scar tissue is mesoblastic and formed by fibroblasts derived from the choroid, in a rupture restricted to the pigmented epithelium the scar tissue which binds the retina to Bruch's membrane is ectodermal and composed of glial tissue (Fig. 128). The underlying choroid may show some lymphocytic infiltration but is largely unaffected.

[1] Cohn (1872), Ginsberg (1897), Alt (1897), Wagenmann (1902), Nettleship (1904), Fischer (1908), Hagedoorn (1937) and many others.

FIGS. 129 to 132.—TRAUMATIC HÆMORRHAGIC DETACHMENT OF T
PIGMENTARY EPITHELIUM OF THE RETINA.

In a man aged 24 following a blow from a fist (K. A. Gitter *et al.*).

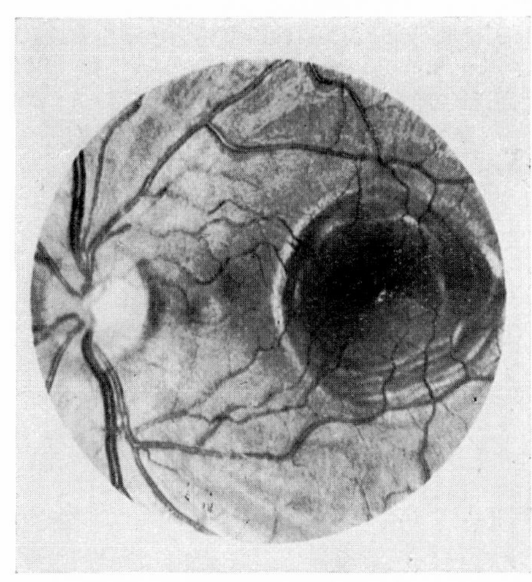

FIG. 129.—There is a dark brown mounded mass of 2 disc-diameters in the macular area elevated 2 to 3 dioptres.

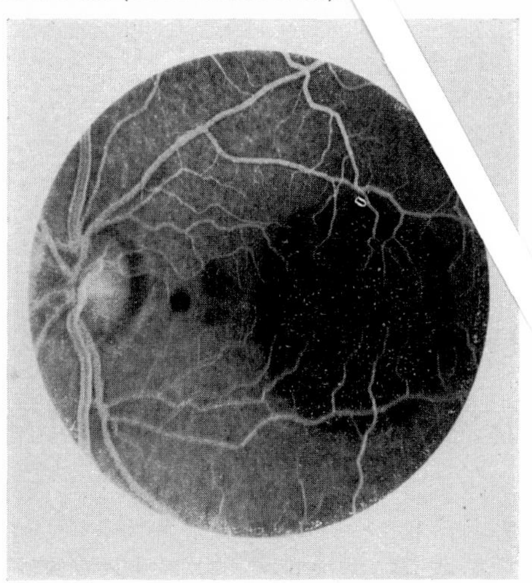

FIG. 130.—Fluorescein angiography showed a complete absence of the dye in the area occupied by the mass.

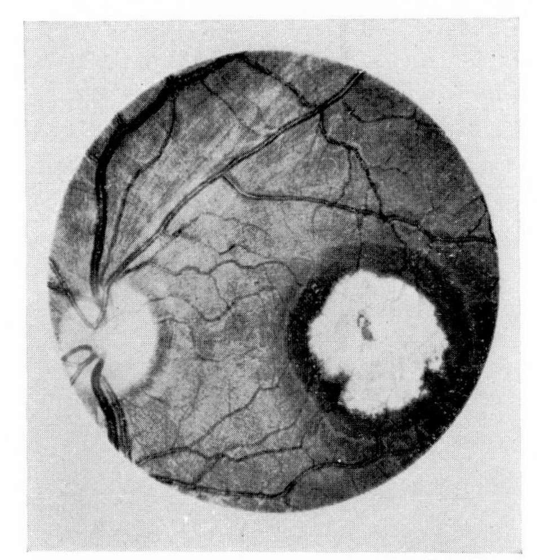

FIG. 131.—The same case 3 weeks later showing absorption of the hæmorrhage at the macula.

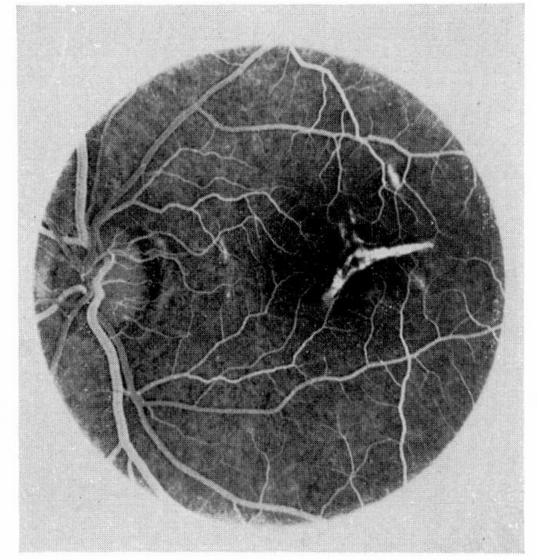

FIG. 132.—Angiographic appearance 6 months after the injury showing a leakage of the dye through a rupture of the choroid.

It was suggested by Hagedoorn (1950) that traumatic ruptures of Bruch's membrane may occur. In a case of concussive injury, after a vitreous hæmorrhage had cleared, hæmorrhagic streaks were observed in the fundus along ruptures of this membrane, an observation which indicates that some cases of angioid streaks may be of traumatic origin (Marchesani and Wirz, 1931). Maumenee (1959–66) has demonstrated that the majority of cases of hæmorrhagic detachments of the macula when studied histologically show breaks in Bruch's membrane in which vessels can be seen extending from the choroid into the subretinal mass. Focal hæmorrhagic detachments of the pigmentary epithelium occur frequently and often bilaterally as part of the clinical picture in senile choroidal macular degeneration and in other disorders of the chorio-capillaris and Bruch's membrane such as heredo-macular degeneration, myopia, Coats's disease, drusen, neoplasms, histoplasmosis, angioid streaks and other conditions wherein hæmorrhagic or serous exudation occurs beneath the pigmentary epithelium (Reese and Jones, 1961; Gass, 1967). A similar condition has been described by Gass (1967) wherein, as a result of contusion injury, blood ruptured through the overlying pigmentary epithelium. In an interesting case followed with fluorescein angiography by Gitter and his colleagues (1968) absorption of the macular hæmorrhage revealed the underlying choroidal rupture which did not progress to recurrent disciform hæmorrhagic detachment (Figs. 129–132). Reports of other cases in which fluorescein angiography has demonstrated traumatic choroidal ruptures not visible ophthalmoscopically have been made by Norton (1965–68).

DIRECT CHORIORETINAL RUPTURES

A SIMULTANEOUS RUPTURE OF BOTH THE CHOROID AND THE RETINA is rare in the usual accidents incurred in civilian life, but is frequently seen as a direct contact injury occurring as a result of a missile fracturing the orbital wall or striking a glancing blow on the globe without rupturing it; it is thus a common occurrence in war (Plate IX, Figs. 3 and 4). The impact of the missile in the peri-ocular tissues, whether passing through between the globe and the orbital wall or coming to lie close to the globe, causes a non-perforating concussive injury resulting in rupture of the choroid and retina with considerable hæmorrhage, usually exuding into and often filling the vitreous.[1] In the usual choroidal rupture and in a vitreous hæmorrhage derived from the retinal vessels the production of fibrous tissue is not great; in this lesion, however, connective-tissue proliferation is early and abundant with the formation of stout and dense fibrous tracts which run into the vitreous from the choroid resembling but more solidly formed than those characteristic of proliferating retinopathy. In the classical picture of this condition derived from a retinal hæmorrhage, the blood in the vitreous is organized by a relatively scanty amount of fibrous tissue which proliferates widely over the

[1] Several different terms have been used to describe the entity of direct choroidal and retinal injury resulting from a bullet passing adjacent to the globe but not actually penetrating it: thus *chorioretinitis plastica sclopetaria* was introduced into the German literature by Cohn (1872) and Goldzieher (1901); *chorioretinitis proliferans* (von Szily, 1917); *traumatic proliferating chorioretinitis* (Lagrange, 1917–18), a term also used by Doherty (1942) and Sommers (1949) to emphasize the proliferation of fibrous tissue from the choroid and gliosis in the damaged retina; *chorioretinitis sclopetarium* (Fuchs, 1926); *chorioretinitis sclopetaria* (Sommers, 1949; Richards *et al.*, 1968); *retinitis sclopetaria* (Nover, 1966). Despite the proliferation of terminology it is clear that all accounts are referring to the same entity of ocular damage due to the effects of missiles of high velocity passing adjacent to the globe. The derivation of the term is interesting: according to Keeney (1968) the verb " sclow " is an old English variant of " sclaw " or " claw ", meaning to scratch, pull or tear, and " sclopetaria " describes the condition of scratching or clawing against the globe. On the other hand, Shoch (1968) considered that the word has a Latin derivation, " sclopetum " being defined in the Oxford English Dictionary as a type of " culverin " which was a kind of XIVth century Italian hand-gun, although in later years this term was applied to weapons of larger bore.

fundus and frequently produces a retinal detachment by traction; after a contusion, however, the fibrous tissue is dense and localized and instead of pulling the retina from its bed on contraction, tends to anchor it more securely in place. It is probable that this massive production of fibrous tissue is due to the organization of blood-clot by the ample supply of active fibroblasts from the mesoblastic elements of the choroid, as occurs also in perforating wounds of the posterior segment of the globe. In the usual vitreous hæmorrhage derived from the retinal vessels there is a poor supply of mesoblastic elements but with the rich mesoblastic constituents of the choroid freely available, organization can proceed in the same lavish style as occurs in the other connective tissues (Parsons, 1917). Goldzieher (1901) considered that damage to the posterior ciliary vessels and nerves might be a contributory factor in the proliferation of the connective tissue and pigmentary epithelium. As a rule two areas of injury are usually present, the area directly adjacent to the path of the missile with damage from direct trauma and, in addition, indirect injury to the macula may be present (Doherty, 1942; Viallefont *et al.*, 1967; Ruedemann, 1968; Richards *et al.*, 1968), but in some cases the damage may be so severe that only one extensive lesion is seen. Although classically this injury is not perforating, the possibility that ocular penetration may have occurred should be borne in mind, since an eye damaged in this way is frequently soft, and with fragmentation of a missile within the orbit it is quite possible for penetration to have occurred.

The *causation* of choroidal ruptures has given rise to considerable speculation. Although the factors of the vascular effects of contusion and the subsequent tissue-necrosis may take part in the dissolution of the tissues, it is generally agreed that mechanical factors are important. The mechanics of the formation of a direct rupture as a contact-lesion at the site where the force impinges on the globe are relatively easy to understand, whether the force is applied directly to the wall of the globe or indirectly as a result of an associated fracture of the orbital wall. Several theories, however, have been advanced to explain the usual crescentic shape of the indirect rupture and its site at the posterior pole of the eye. In general terms this site is the region for the main *contre-coup* impact of a force impinging on the eye from in front, but the same location results as regularly from laterally directed impacts. Arlt (1875) attributed these indirect results to the deformation of the globe due to antero-posterior flattening, Becker (1878) to the effect of invagination of the optic nerve, Hughes (1887) and Parisotti (1887) to the sudden stoppage by the optic nerve of the rotation of the eye on the reception of a glancing blow, Oatman (1920) to a similar abrupt check by the oblique muscles, and Siegrist (1895) to the more unlikely effect of local anæmia caused by a rupture of the posterior ciliary arteries. It cannot be said that the matter is yet entirely satisfactorily explained.

The *symptoms* of a choroidal rupture vary with the site. The function of the overlying retina is always destroyed with the formation of corresponding scotomata in the visual field (Fig. 125). If the rupture is in the macular area the central vision is, therefore, completely and permanently lost; if the central area escapes, a defect in the peripheral field results which is usually of little consequence. If, however, the rupture is extensive, even although the macular area is undamaged, the vision is usually gravely impaired owing to the development of secondary degenerative changes in the retina and optic nerve. This, however, is not invariable for the visual acuity has remained normal or nearly so after an extensive lesion of this type (Adamük, 1878; de Schweinitz, 1901; Herrmann, 1906; Kröner, 1906–7) and good vision has been retained indefinitely after double (Talko, 1871) or quadruple ruptures even although they are near the macular area (Neame, 1940; Rosen, 1943; Kroning, 1952; Neubauer, 1957).

The *treatment* of choroidal ruptures is rest and expectancy.

TRAUMATIC CHOROIDITIS

While the crescentic rents which form the typical picture of choroidal ruptures seem determined in large part by purely mechanical factors and probably correspond to the tears in the tissue of the iris, the ciliary body or the lamina cribrosa which occur in ocular contusions, the configuration of other lesions of a similar atrophic nature following this type of injury,

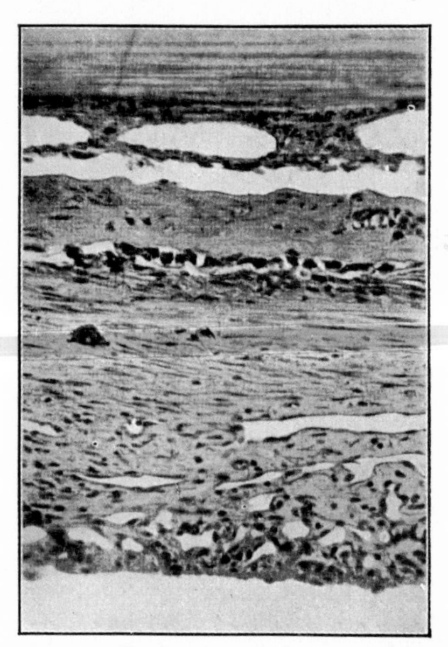

FIG. 133.—THE LATE STAGES OF TRAUMATIC CHOROIDITIS.

From a contusion 25 years previously. The choroid is atrophic but vascular and there is a thick layer of vascularized cellular tissue on its inner surface (L. Buchanan).

whether associated with direct trauma to the eye by a mechanical implement or by blast or with indirect trauma involving the orbit and the skull, suggests that the main factor in their ætiology is a tissue-necrosis usually associated with hæmorrhages of a contusional nature.[1] Such lesions may be small and discrete, round or oval and sharply defined, or they may be diffuse and widespread, assuming irregular and map-like shapes, and are always associated with a considerable degree of pigmentary proliferation and subsequent atrophy. It is probable that in these the mechanism of production is essentially the traumatic vascular reaction characteristic of a contusion followed by degeneration and necrosis in the tissue, the vitality of which has been gravely damaged by the effects of intracellular concussion (Fig. 133).

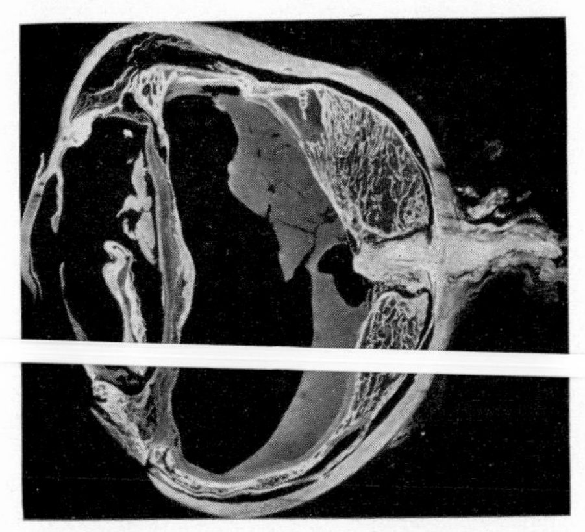

Fig. 134.—Bone Formation.

An injury sustained at the age of 7; the eye was removed at the age of 39; showing gross bone formation in the posterior segment and calcification of the shrunken lens (G. Hager and K. Ebel).

Degenerative changes of all degrees of severity may develop after a period ranging from less than one to over 70 years after the injury. The most dramatic of these are calcification and ossification which may involve large areas of the choroid, particularly near the posterior pole where the formative epithelium may proliferate, or even the entire globe including the lens[2] (Figs. 115, 134–6) (Hager and Ebel, 1964; Finkelstein and Boniuk, 1969).

BLAST INJURIES may cause a considerable disturbance of this type. As a rule they result in degeneration of the tissues of the uveal tract at the posterior pole or their actual laceration. In the first case, the common appearance is that of heavy choroidal pigmentation occurring in map-like areas irregularly over the posterior part of the fundus (Figs. 137–8); in the second, widespread necrosis of the choroid may result in the disappearance

[1] McKee (1923), Østerberg (1936), Bedell (1941), Hudelo *et al.* (1945), Tower (1949).
[2] Vol. IX, p. 740.

FIGS. 135 and 136.—POST-TRAUMATIC OSSIFICATION
(E. M. Finkelstein and M. Boniuk).

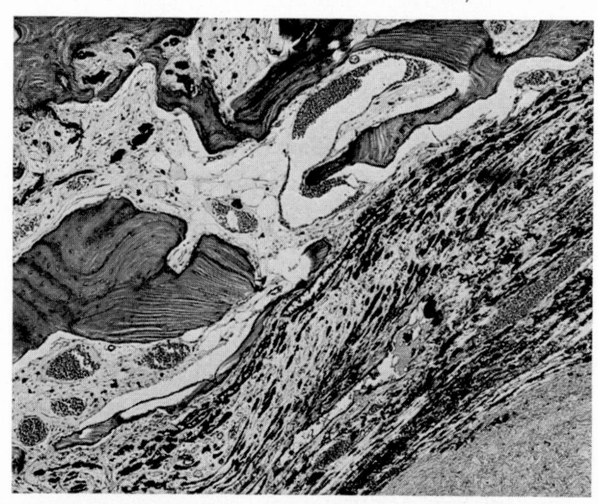

FIG. 135.—In a man aged 20 whose eye was struck by a stone 12 years previously.

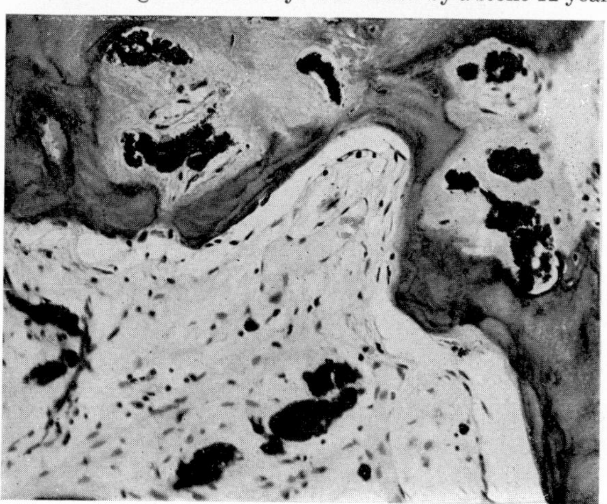

FIG. 136.—There is proliferation of the pigmentary epithelium within the areas of ossification (H. & E.).

of this tissue in irregular patches, some of which become heavily pigmented. In both cases the retina remains intact, as is shown by the normal course of its vessels (Lagrange, 1918).

A less dramatic picture has been described by Siegrist (1895), Huguenin (1916), Collins (1917) and others wherein a spherical-shaped, yellowish area with well-defined margins, which subsequently shows proliferation of the retinal pigment associated with a scotoma, develops after contusive injuries; such an area may be seen with a rupture of the choroid at a part of the fundus widely separated from the tear (Nettleship, 1904). It has been said that such a clinical appearance is due to ischæmia brought

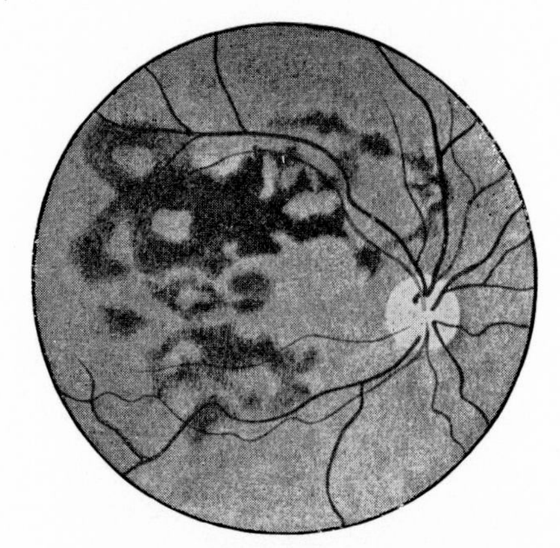

FIG. 137.—BLAST INJURY OF THE CHOROID.

Following the explosion of a torpedo. The eyes showed no external sign of injury. Around the macula and scattered over the posterior pole are localized islands of choroidal pigment. The retina is intact and its vessels normal (after F. Lagrange).

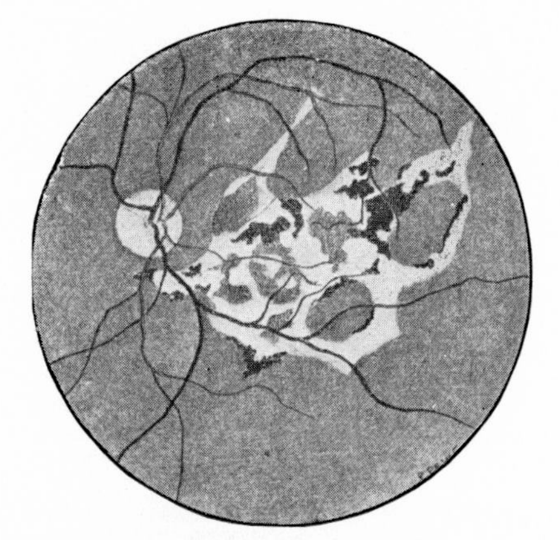

FIG. 138.—BLAST INJURY OF THE POSTERIOR POLE OF THE EYE.

Due to the explosion of a hand-grenade. In the macular region there are extensive lacerations of the choroid covered by irregularly scattered masses of pigment. The retina is intact and the retinal vessels pass over the choroidal lesion without any deviation from their normal course (after F. Lagrange).

or by a rupture of the posterior ciliary arteries (Siegrist, 1895) in view of the fact that somewhat similar appearances were produced experimentally by [illegible] by cutting these arteries in animals. From his histological studies, however, Collins (1917) concluded that a more probable cause was an obliteration of the choriocapillaris due to pressure by subchoroidal hæmorrhages.

The *symptoms* of traumatic choroiditis correspond to those of a mechanical rupture and treatment is again expectant.

Adamük. *Zbl. prakt. Augenheilk.*, **2**, 257 (1878).
Alt. *Ophthal. Rev.*, **16**, 289 (1897).
von Ammon. *v. Graefes Arch. Ophthal.*, **1** (2), 119 (1855).
Arlt. *Die Verletzungen des Auges*, Wien (1875).
Aub. *Arch. Augenheilk.*, **2**, 256 (1871).
Becker. *Klin. Mbl. Augenheilk.*, **16**, 41 (1878).
Bedell. *J. Amer. med. Ass.*, **117**, 1774 (1941).
Berlin. *Klin. Mbl. Augenheilk.*, **11**, 42 (1873).
Cohn. *Schussverletzungen des Auges*, Erlangen (1872).
Collins. *Trans. ophthal. Soc. U.K.*, **36**, 204 (1916); **37**, 112 (1917).
Doherty. *Amer. J. Ophthal.*, **25**, 135 (1942).
Finkelstein and Boniuk. *Amer. J. Ophthal.*, **68**, 683 (1969).
Fischer. *Beitrag z. Kenntnis d. Spätfolgen v. Contusio bulbi* (Diss.), Jena (1908).
Fuchs. *Lhb. d. Augenheilkunde*, Leipzig, 691 (1926).
Gass. *Amer. J. Ophthal.*, **63**, 573, 689 (1967).
Genth. *Klin. Mbl. Augenheilk.*, **9**, 143 (1871).
Ginsberg. *Vestn. oftal.*, **10**, 360 (1893).
v. Graefes Arch. Ophthal., **44** (1), 26 (1897).
Gitter, Slusher and Justice. *Arch. Ophthal.*, **79**, 729 (1968).
Goar. *Amer. J. Ophthal.*, **21**, 907 (1938).
Godtfredsen. *Acta ophthal.* (Kbh.), **20**, 337 (1942).
Goldzieher. *Z. Augenheilk.*, **6**, 277 (1901).
von Graefe. *v. Graefes Arch. Ophthal.*, **1**, 402 (1854).
Gross. *Amer. J. Ophthal.*, **28**, 97 (1911).
Hagedoorn. *Amer. J. Ophthal.*, **20**, 13 (1937).
Ophthalmologica, **119**, 245 (1950).
Hager and Ebel. *Klin. Mbl. Augenheilk.*, **144**, 513 (1964).
Herrmann. *Die Kontusionsverletzungen d. Auges in klin. u. path.-anat. Beziehung* (Diss.), Leipzig (1906).
Hersing. *Klin. Mbl. Augenheilk.*, **10**, 11 (1872).
Hertz. *Detachment of the Choroid following Contusion of the Eye*, Copenhagen (1952).
Hjort. *Nord. Med.* (Stockh.), **14**, 1 (1882).

Hoor. *Wien. med. Wschr.*, **36**, 1108 (1886).
Hudelo, Guillaumat and Maussion. *Arch. Ophtal.*, **5**, 44 (1945).
Hughes. *v. Graefes Arch. Ophthal.*, **33** (3), 21 (1887).
Huguenin. *Clin. Ophtal.*, **7**, 78 (1916).
Kaufer and Zimmerman. *Arch. Ophthal.*, **75**, 384 (1966).
Keeney. *Trans. Amer. ophthal. Soc.*, **66**, 229 (1968).
Knapp. *Arch. Augenheilk.*, **1**, 6 (1869).
Kröner. *Arch. Augenheilk.*, **55**, 308 (1906); **56**, 1 (1907).
Kroning. *Acta ophthal.* (Kbh.), **30**, 429 (1952).
Lagrange. *Les fractures de l'orbite par projectiles de guerre*, Paris (1917).
Atlas d'ophtalmoscopie de guerre, Paris (1918).
Laqueur. *Arch. Augenheilk.*, **44**, 263 (1902).
McKee. *Amer. J. Ophthal.*, **6**, 725 (1923).
Mannhardt. *Klin. Mbl. Augenheilk.*, **13**, 132 (1875).
Marchesani and Wirz. *Arch. Augenheilk.*, **104**, 522 (1931).
Maumenee. *Trans. Pac. Cst. oto-ophthal. Soc.*, **43**, 139 (1959).
Retinal Diseases (ed. Kimura and Cargill), Phila., 244 (1966).
Michel. *Klin. Mbl. Augenheilk.*, **16**, 18 (1878).
Mills. *Arch. Ophthal.*, **32**, 217 (1903).
Mules. *Trans. ophthal. Soc. U.K.*, **13**, 65 (1893).
Neame. *Brit. J. Ophthal.*, **24**, 399 (1940).
Nettleship. *Trans. ophthal. Soc. U.K.*, **24**, 241 (1904).
Neubauer. *Klin. Mbl. Augenheilk.*, **131**, 487 (1957).
Nicolai. *Arch. Augenheilk.*, **44**, 268 (1902).
Norton. *Trans. Amer. Acad. Ophthal.*, **69**, 631 (1965).
Trans. Amer. ophthal. Soc., **66**, 230 (1968).
Nover. *The Ocular Fundus* (transl. Blodi), Phila., 130 (1966).
Oatman. *Diagnosis of the Fundus Oculi*, N.Y. (1920).
Oguchi. *Beitr. Augenheilk.*, **9** (83), 75 (1913).
Ohm. *Ueber Aderhautrupturen* (Diss.), Giessen (1905).
Østerberg. *Acta ophthal.* (Kbh.), **14**, 460 (1936).
Parisotti. *Recueil Ophtal.*, **9**, 210 (1887).
Parsons. *Brit. J. Ophthal.*, **1**, 495 (1917).
Picqué. *Progr. Méd.*, **12**, 664 (1884).
Polano. *Ueber isolierte Chorioidealrupturen* (Diss.), Kiel (1897).
Reese and Jones. *Trans. Amer. ophthal. Soc.*, **59**, 43 (1961).
Richards, West and Meisels. *Amer. J. Ophthal.*, **66**, 852 (1968).
Trans. Amer. ophthal. Soc., **66**, 214 (1968).
Rosen. *Brit. J. Ophthal.*, **27**, 552 (1943).
Ruedemann. *Trans. Amer. ophthal. Soc.*, **66**, 231 (1968).
Schröter. *Klin. Mbl. Augenheilk.*, **9**, 139 (1871).
de Schweinitz. *Ophthal. Rec.*, **10**, 215 (1901).
Shoch. *Trans. Amer. ophthal. Soc.*, **66**, 231 (1968).
Siegrist. *Mitt. a.d. Klin. u. med. Inst. d. Schweiz.*, **3** (9), 554 (1895).
Sommers. *Histology and Histopathology of the Eye and its Adnexa*, N.Y., 73 (1949).
Sous. *J. Méd. Bordeaux*, **22**, 329 (1892).
Story. *Brit. med. J.*, **1**, 392 (1881).
von Szily. *Atlas d. Kriegsaugenheilkunde*, Stuttgart (1917).
Talko. *Klin. Mbl. Augenheilk.*, **9**, 48 (1871).
Tillema. *Brit. J. Ophthal.*, **20**, 193 (1936).
Tower. *Arch. Ophthal.*, **41**, 341 (1949).
Viallefont, Boudet and Philippot. *Bull. Soc. franç. Ophtal.*, **80**, 601 (1967).
Vossius. *Klin. Mbl. Augenheilk.*, **21**, 276 (1883).
Wagenmann. *v. Graefes Arch. Ophthal.*, **36** (4), 1 (1890).
Ber. dtsch. ophthal. Ges., **30**, 278 (1902).
Walter. *Ueber Ablösung d. Chorioidea v. d. Sclera* (Diss.), Würzburg (1883).
Zander and Geissler. *Die Verletzungen des Auges*, Heidelberg (1864).

Concussion Effects on the Retina

Damage to the retina after concussive injuries to the globe, affecting particularly the macula and periphery, is common. The lesions produced are of the same type as occur in other tissues and correspond precisely to those we have described in the brain—a concussion necrosis of the nerve cells, œdema and hæmorrhages causing the structural alterations characteristic of a contusion, and lacerations of the tissues themselves—but they are especially important since, although the ophthalmoscopic appearances of abnormality may be transient, their after-effects may be permanent and disastrous. Slight pigmentary changes at the macula, for example, which are seen only with difficulty and are readily overlooked—a lesion of incidental importance elsewhere—may permanently impair central vision to a degree far greater than the clinical picture would suggest. Again, degeneration in the periphery of the retina or a small tear or dialysis in this region may cause a retinal detachment with a consequent loss of vision some considerable time after the accident has been sustained. These injuries to the retina, therefore, even although slight in degree, assume an unusual medico-legal importance and careful and repeated search should be made for them after an accident.

CONCUSSION ŒDEMA OF THE RETINA

It is useful to limit the term CONCUSSION ŒDEMA (COMMOTIO RETINÆ), a condition associated with the name of Berlin, to simple concussional changes which are reversible and transient, involving œdema only; it is to be remembered, of course, that frequently their visual effects may be permanent. When the changes are so marked as to involve destruction of the tissues and are irreversible, we are using the term CONCUSSION NECROSIS.

A milky-white area of transient cloudiness with an ill-defined margin extending over the posterior region of the fundus due to the development of retinal œdema is a common sequel of concussions of the globe; sometimes it occupies a considerable area, occasionally at the site of the trauma, but more usually surrounding the optic disc and practically always involving the macula which stands out as a bright red spot in brilliant contrast to the grey background, the clinical picture resembling the typical appearance seen after an occlusion of the central artery of the retina[1] (Plate X, Figs. 1 and 2). As a general rule the cloudiness increases progressively for 24 hours after the injury, whereafter it tends slowly to fade away. Such is the typical ophthalmoscopic picture, but all variations in degree occur. In its mildest form it affects the macula alone; the retina in this area may show only minimal changes; it appears to be thicker than usual and somewhat translucent, the foveal reflex may be absent and the region may be surrounded by a circular halo-reflex or by radiating spoke-like formations indicating œdematous rucks.

No matter what the degree of œdema, while the opacity lasts the central vision is lowered considerably (Berlin, 1873), the light sense is depressed (Schmidt-Rimpler, 1884) and the peripheral field is often constricted (Makrocki, 1892). As a rule, however, with the disappearance of the œdema the vision may again become normal, but unfortunately in a large proportion of cases the lesion is followed by the appearance of pigmentary deposits, cystoid formations at the macula and even a hole, in which events central vision is either gravely impaired or permanently lost. In all cases wherein these œdematous changes are evident, therefore, the prognosis as to vision should be guarded.

The fall in vision following injury to the eye or the head was originally described as *commotio retinæ* on the analogy of *commotio cerebri*. The first careful analysis of the various causes of an impairment of function of this type was undertaken by Berlin (1873) who differentiated the effects of intracranial damage and injury to the optic

[1] Vol. X, p. 66.

nerve from those of injury to the retina. He first described œdematous retinal appearances following concussions and produced them experimentally in the eyes of rabbits by striking them with an elastic stick. Since that time the classical picture has been called BERLIN'S TRAUMATIC ŒDEMA. Clinical descriptions of the condition quickly accumulated,[1] additional experimental confirmation of its production in animals was produced by Denig (1897–99), Bäck (1899) and Lohmann (1906), while pathological verification of the mechanism involved was provided by Roscin (1931). It was also shown that the same clinical appearances may, although much more rarely, follow perforating injuries to the eye (Wagenmann, 1915) or the orbit (Dimmer, 1885).

The lesion is by no means uncommon. Thus Siegfried (1898) found that in 167 cases of concussion of the globe wherein ophthalmoscopic examination was possible, 4·7% had a macular œdema and 12·5% had a Berlin's opacity extending over a considerable area of the posterior pole; of these 12·5%, 16 cases cleared up entirely with normal vision, but in 5, pigmentary changes became evident 1, 3, 4, 8, and 19 days after the injury, and in these the best final vision was 6/60. On the other hand, Herrmann (1906) found only 17 such cases in 677 concussions; of these 10 cleared up and 7 suffered a permanent depression of vision.

The *cause* of the lesion has been disputed. Berlin (1873) attributed the disturbance to an extravasation of blood between the choroid and the sclera which brought about an ischæmia owing to pressure on the choriocapillaris and a consequent transudation of œdematous fluid into the retina, a view supported by his finding such a hæmorrhage in his experimental animals and also by the histological observations of Collins (1917). Denig (1897) assumed that the fluid was derived from the vitreous; but most authors—probably correctly—have followed the suggestion of Hirschberg (1875) that the œdema is determined by the usual vasomotor response to concussion which we have already studied—a paretic vasodilatation associated with an œdematous exudation.[2] The extreme dilatation of the small vessels of the retina and the choriocapillaris, particularly in the posterior segment of the eye, was demonstrated pathologically by Roscin (1931) in a case 48 hours after an accident which proved fatal, wherein the œdematous changes had been seen ophthalmoscipally before death. The macula is most frequently affected because of the richness of the underlying capillary network and because of the anatomical peculiarities of the structure of the retina in this region.

Treatment of such cases is purely expectant.

CONCUSSION NECROSIS OF THE RETINA

If the concussion is severe, dramatic lesions in the retina of a more destructive nature than œdema are not unusual; their rationale has already been discussed—the extreme vasodilatation with pooling of the blood and flooding of the tissues with œdema, together with the autolysis of the tissues in the condition of anoxia thus induced, combine to produce a process of necrosis and liquefaction aided, in all probability, by chromatolysis and

[1] Hirschberg (1875), Nettleship (1880), H. Knapp (1881), Schmidt-Rimpler (1885), Haab (1888), and a host of others.

[2] Ostwalt (1887), Siegfried (1898), Linde (1897), Bäck (1899), and others.

degeneration of the nerve cells induced by the impact of the force. The resulting ophthalmoscopic picture has been most clearly described by Lister (1924) in war injuries due to missiles and by Shimkin (1940) as a result of blast (Plate XI, Figs. 1 and 2; Fig. 139). Usually associated with considerable retinal hæmorrhage and sometimes with œdematous patches, large irregular but sharply demarcated areas of glistening white become evident, typically appearing adjacent to the site of impact in the periphery and, forming a separate lesion, in the macular area. After some weeks dramatic alterations are liable to occur in the ophthalmoscopic picture; the glistening areas vanish

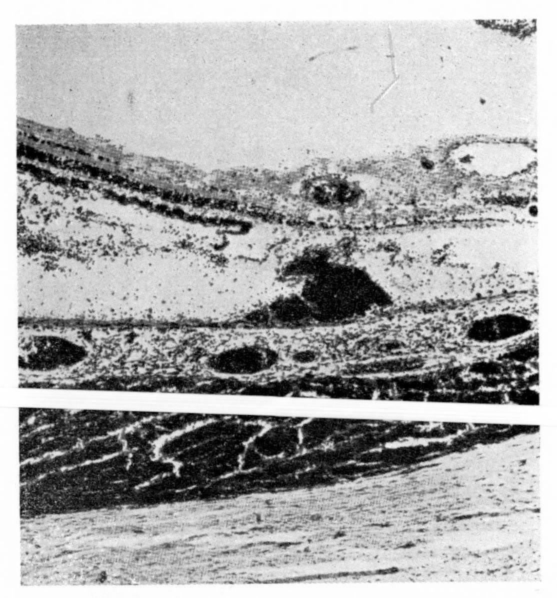

Fig. 139.—The Retina in a Concussion Injury.

A relatively slight degree of concussion injury to the retina, showing partial and patchy atrophy of the nuclei in the outer and inner plexiform layers. There are subretinal and subchoroidal hæmorrhages (W. Lister).

and are replaced by lightly coloured regions of partial atrophy, while the hæmorrhages absorb or are replaced by fine proliferating fibrous tissue.

Histologically various degrees of necrosis and atrophy are seen. The inner and outer plexiform layers of the retina are most severely affected wherein the nuclei disintegrate and disappear; the nerve-fibre, ganglion-cell and plexiform layers may become spongy, vacuolated or cystic; and in the more severely affected areas the entire retina loses its staining capacity and all traces of nuclei and cellular structure are lost (Figs. 140–1). Sometimes all the outer layers may disappear, the rods and cones being represented by degenerated structureless globules detached from their parent membrane (Tillema, 1937; Wolter, 1963). The histological appearances resemble the coagulation necrosis which occurs in the optic nerve or the central nervous system as a concussive effect after a blunt injury of considerable severity, or in the immediate vicinity of the track of a missile which has traversed these tissues. These changes, of course, are disastrous to vision in the retinal areas affected and treatment can only be expectant.

FIGS. 140 and 141.—CONTRE-COUP DAMAGE TO THE MACULAR AREA.
In a boy aged 12 who was struck in the eye with the end of a whip (the same case as Figs. 39 and 49) (J. R. Wolter).

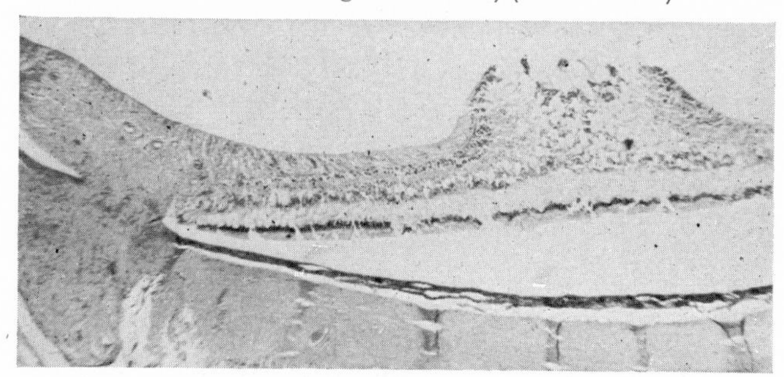

FIG. 140.—In the foveal area there is extensive cystoid degeneration with rupture of the inner limiting membrane.

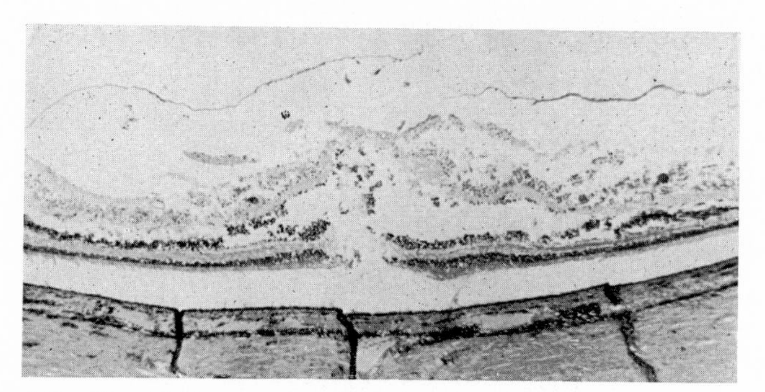

FIG. 141.—In a high-power view the ganglion cells in the affected area are seen to be absent while the rods and cones are preserved.

CONCUSSION CHANGES AT THE MACULA

MACULAR ŒDEMA

We have already seen that macular œdema is usually the most marked feature of the retinal œdema which follows a concussion of the globe. This local accentuation is probably determined by several factors. From the mechanical point of view the posterior pole is in the line of direct *contre-coup* for the force impinging on the anterior part of the eyeball, while in injuries affecting the face we have already seen that the waves of pressure throughout the soft tissues enter the orbit through the pterygo-maxillary fissure and strike preferentially the posterior part of the globe. From the anatomical

PLATES X AND XI

Concussion Effects on the Retina

PLATE X

Figs. 1 and 2.—Berlin's Œdema (W. B. Doherty).

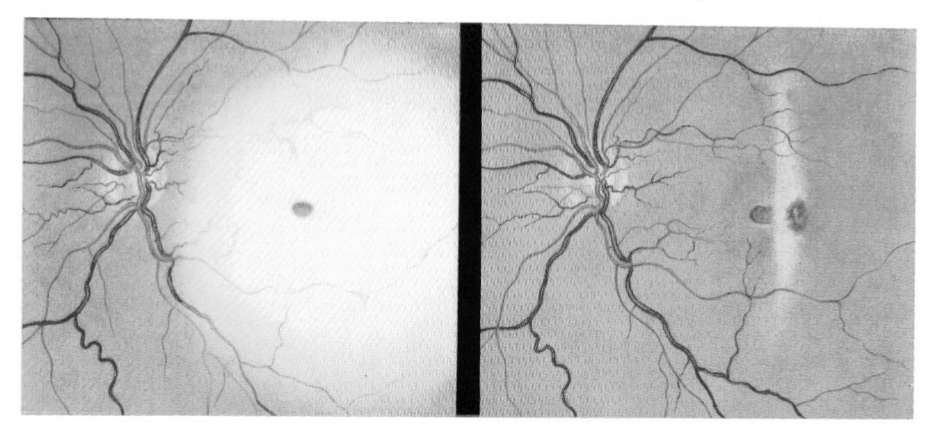

Fig. 1.—The central area of the fundus as it appeared 24 hours after the eye had been hit by a spring. There is an intense œdema with a marked cherry-red spot.

Fig. 2.—The eye as it appeared 11 days after the injury, showing that the œdema has cleared and there is now a hole in the macula towards the nasal side of a choroidal rupture. There is an absolute central scotoma.

Figs. 3 to 5.—Macular Holes following Concussion (J. Bouchat).

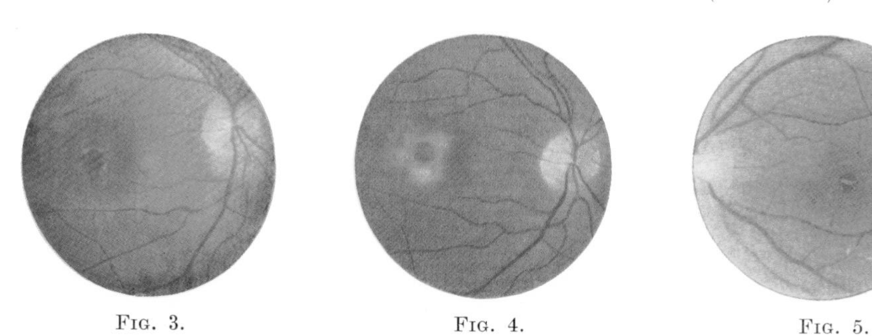

Fig. 3. Fig. 4. Fig. 5.

Figs. 3 and 4.—Caused by a metal splinter.

Fig. 3.—At an early stage, showing disturbances of the surrounding choroid. Fig. 4 after treatment by light-coagulation.

Fig. 5.—Caused by a champagne cork.

Figs. 6 to 8.—The Late Results of a Macular Concussion.

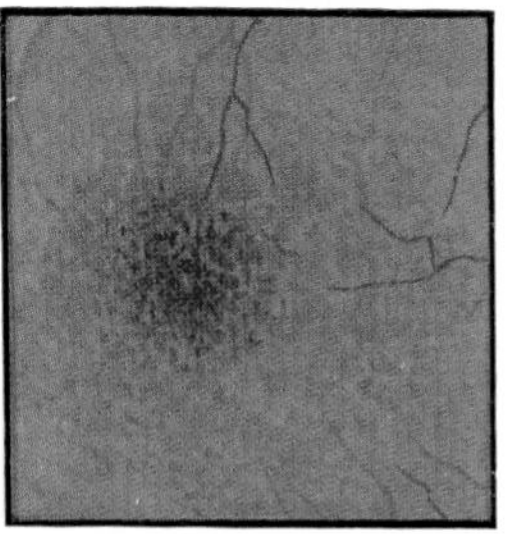

Fig. 6.

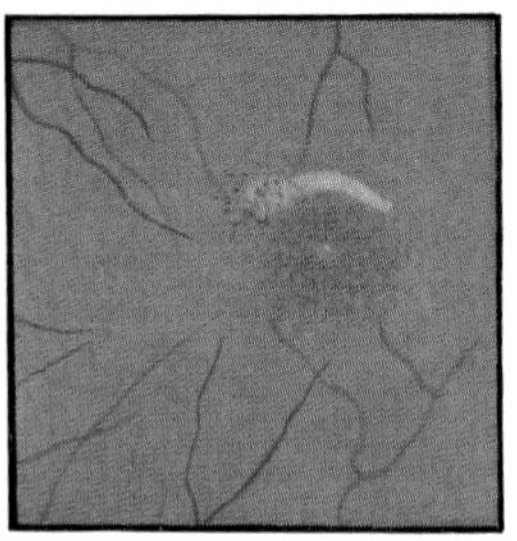

Fig. 7.

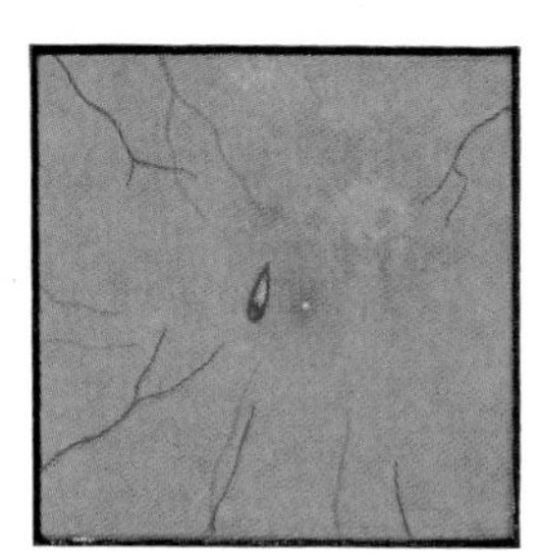

Fig. 8.

PLATE XI

Concussion Effects on the Retina.

Figs. 1 and 2.—Contusion Effects in the Retina due to the Passage of a Missile through the Orbit.

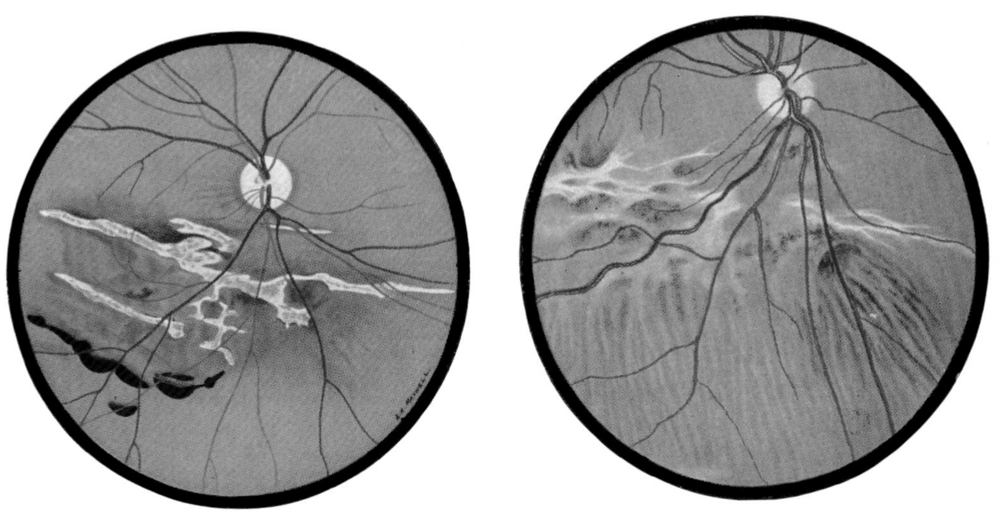

Fig. 1. Fig. 2.

Fig. 1.—The contusion seen after injury showing retinal hæmorrhages and necrotic areas. Fig. 2.—The contusion some weeks later, showing the development of [illegible] (W. Lister).

Figs. 3 and 4.—Post-concussion Retinal Changes.

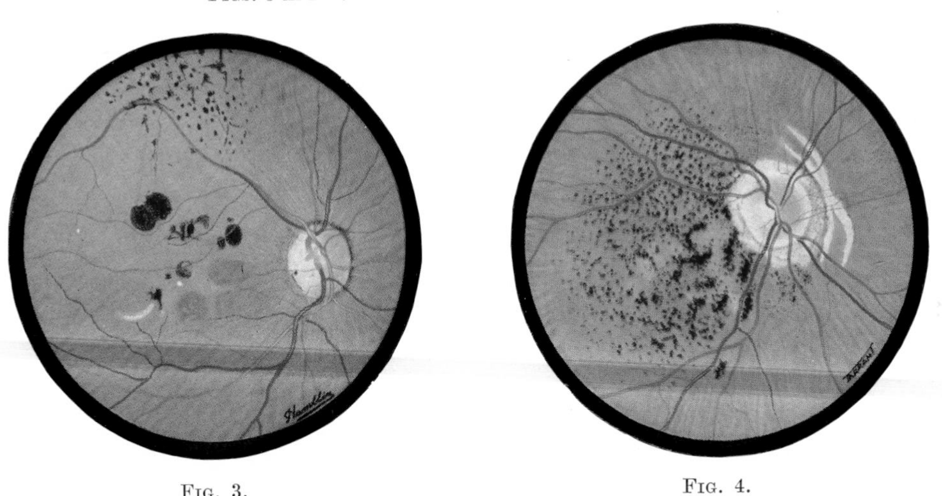

Fig. 3. Fig. 4.

Fig. 3.—Pigmentary changes eleven years after a blow with a football.

Fig. 4.—Six years after a blow with a stone. There is some optic atrophy and small choroidal ruptures on the nasal side of the disc and diffuse pigmentary changes.

point of view, also, the œdematous process tends to be particularly marked at the macula because of the richness of the choroidal capillary bed in this region so that the reactive vasodilatation is accentuated; moreover, the structure of the macular area with the thick fibre layer of Henle endows it with the ability to absorb large quantities of fluid and at the same time the avascularity of the foveal region of the retina makes resorption of the fluid more difficult. It is interesting in the last connection that the diameter of the average gross lesion here (a cyst or a hole) lies between 0·5 and 0·75 mm. which corresponds in size to the avascular area (Leber, 1916).

We have already discussed the milder degrees of macular œdema characterized by a dullness and increased translucency of the retina with œdematous rucks visible ophthalmoscopically as a halo-reflex or radial striæ, and the more severe degrees wherein the fovea stands out as a cherry-red spot in an area of milky-white retina. These changes may progress to the formation of cysts and holes, and eventually further degenerative changes with pigmentary anomalies may follow.

TRAUMATIC MACULAR CYSTS AND HOLES

The occurrence of a lesion resembling a hole at the macula has long been known. The first case probably of this type was reported by H. Knapp (1869), and sporadic unequivocal cases were recorded by Noyes (1871), Hartridge (1889) and Lawford (1893). In the year 1900, however, the accurate description of 37 examples by Kuhnt, Haab, Collins and Ogilvie firmly established the condition as a clinical entity. At first the lesion [illegible] thought to be a hole caused mechanically at the time of the accident by the rupture of the retina at its thinnest part by *contre-coup*. Two factors, however, suggested that this might not be the explanation. In the first place, the lesion has never been seen immediately after the causal accident —the earliest observation was that of Ogilvie (1900), who saw a macular " hole " after an interval of 60 hours. Moreover, in several cases an œdematous opacity in the retina without a hole had been observed soon after the trauma, and a hole was seen to develop at a later date (Reis, 1906; Twietmeyer, 1907). In the second place, an exactly similar appearance was noted in infective and degenerative conditions without any history of trauma. Fuchs (1901), from a pathological study of such a case, and Reis (1906), from the clinical appearances of a traumatic case, suggested that the lesion might result from œdema causing the formation of cysts which eventually ruptured to form a hole, a suggestion histologically proved by Coats (1907). Finally, the introduction of examination of the fundus by focal illumination showed that most of these lesions were in reality not holes but cysts (Goldmann, 1949).

The *clinical picture* presented by a macular cyst or hole is so striking and characteristic that it is always easy to recognize (Plate X). As a general rule there is a circular, dark red spot at the fovea which was aptly described by the earliest observers as if it had been made mechanically with a punch

(Noyes, 1871). At the bottom of this the dark red, finely granular surface of the choroid is visible, and frequently the phenomenon of parallax can be elicited between the floor of the circle and the surrounding retina. Its size varies from one-sixth to one-third of that of the disc, but it can be as large as this structure (Collins, 1900) or even larger (Foster Moore, 1910), and exceptionally it is situated somewhat eccentrically to one side of the fovea (Pagenstecher, 1903). While a regular circular shape is characteristic, an almond shape or pointed extremities are not unusual and, although the edges are generally clean-cut, they may have a somewhat ragged and tattered appearance; occasionally the retina is œdematous and folded in the neighbourhood and a retinal detachment, which may remain localized and shallow, may develop. In any event, once formed, the appearance is permanent, although there may be minor changes of shape in the course of years (42 years, Harman, 1901).

While the recognition of such a lesion presents no difficulty, the clinical differentiation between a cyst and a hole is often not at all easy. Occasionally the wall of a cyst may be indicated by fine structures crossing over the punched-out area or by the presence over it of ophthalmoscopic reflexes. On other occasions red-free light is of considerable value in accentuating a honeycomb appearance due to the presence of several cysts, the inner walls of which are rendered visible thereby (Vogt, 1925–34); but the surest method of differentiation is by the use of the slit-lamp adapted to fundus examination, when in the optical section the brilliant line of the surface of the retina is seen to be continuous over a cyst bulging inwards as it crosses it, while in the case of a hole this line is sharply interrupted over the foveal area[1].

The *pathology* of a traumatic lesion of this type has been investigated by Haab (1900) and Fuchs (1901) and was fully established in a classical paper by Coats (1907) whose findings have been amply confirmed (Zeeman, 1912–23; Alt, 1913; Hervouët, 1965; and others). The changes are identical with those which characterize the comparable cystic macular degeneration found in infective conditions.[2] The essential change is the presence of cystoid spaces containing œdematous fluid situated especially in the outer plexiform layer of the retina, more particularly in Henle's layer in the foveal region; there is frequently a collection of fluid, or even of blood, between the external limiting membrane and the pigment layer, producing a shallow detachment (Figs. 142 and 143). In some cases a few retinal elements remain on the inner wall of such a cyst (Collins, 1900); in others the internal limiting membrane alone may survive; while in others solution may be complete and a central gap results at which the layers of the retina end cleanly and abruptly, although cystoid spaces due to œdema may be found in the surrounding area.

In the few cases wherein there is some retinal tissue on the inner wall of a

[1] Hruby (1948), Goldmann (1949), Bonamour (1956), Hervouët (1965), Marsol and Bouchat (1967).

[2] Vol. X, p. 545.

cyst some degree of central vision may remain, but the formation of a macular hole, as would be expected, is a disability which entails a complete loss of central vision, a loss which remains as a permanent defect; some degree of useful vision, however, may return should paracentral fixation become established.

In general no treatment is of value because of the destructive nature of the retinal lesion, although differing views are held on this matter concerning the small but definite risk of subsequent retinal detachment. On the one

FIGS. 142 and 143.—THE FORMATION OF MACULAR HOLES.

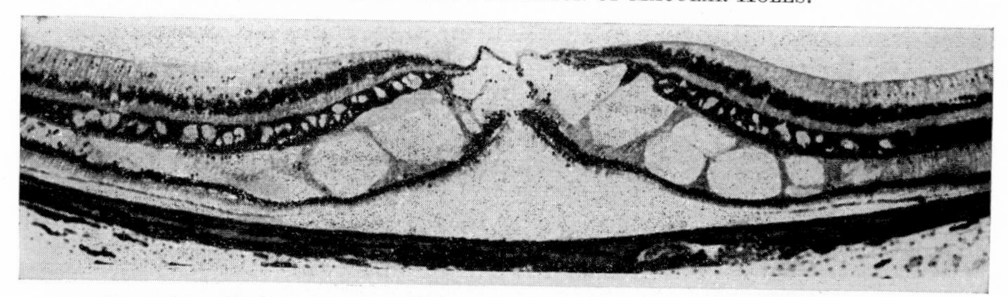

FIG. 142.—Marked post-traumatic cystoid degeneration; only the internal limiting membrane remains giving the appearance of a false hole (J. Mawas).

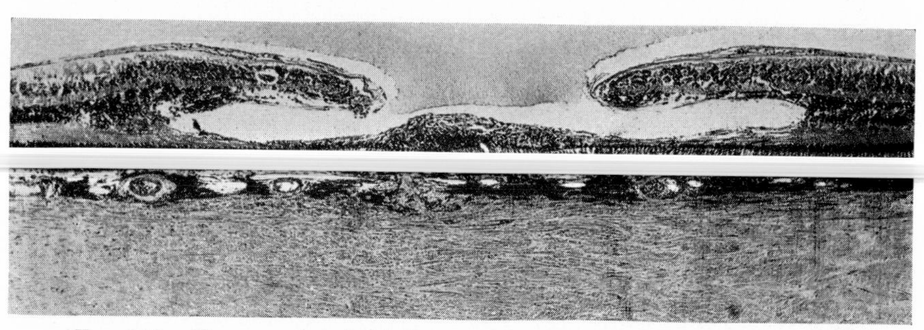

FIG. 143.—The second and third neurons in the macular area have completely disappeared and under the edges of the hole the second neuron continues to be disrupted, to be overlapped by the ganglion-cell layer. In the area of the fovea there is much gliosis but the cones and their nuclei survive. There is a considerable degree of arteriosclerosis in the choroid (F. Hervouët).

hand, an expectant attitude is adopted since a progressive retinal separation rarely follows such a lesion and any form of therapy is likely to aggravate the existing visual defect; on the other hand, prophylactic treatment by diathermy or light-coagulation around the lesion has been advocated by some authors (Marsol and Bouchat, 1967) (Plate X, Figs. 3 and 4); in the majority of cases an expectant attitude is the best policy.

It is interesting that a macular hole has been noted to form following a rapid lowering of the barometric pressure, the sudden lowering of pressure having the same mechanical effect as its increase in the usual concussion and corresponding to the vacuum element in a blast injury (Tirelli, 1948).

TRAUMATIC MACULAR ATROPHY OF HAAB

A degenerative condition of the macula characterized particularly by pigmentary changes was first described following severe concussions by Haab (1888), who found such an appearance in 24% of 192 cases of injury of this type. It is interesting that similar changes may result from an electric shock (Oliver, 1896; Haab, 1897). After a concussion such an atrophy may follow Berlin's opacity, in which case as the œdema disappears the vision does not improve as might be expected; more usually the atrophic change may not manifest itself clearly until some weeks have passed. At first the fovea and the surrounding area appear redder than normal, the reflex is absent and a fine pigmentary stippling becomes evident, occasionally accompanied by small hæmorrhages. These fine pigmentary deposits may represent the only pathological appearance but a more accentuated mottling may develop,

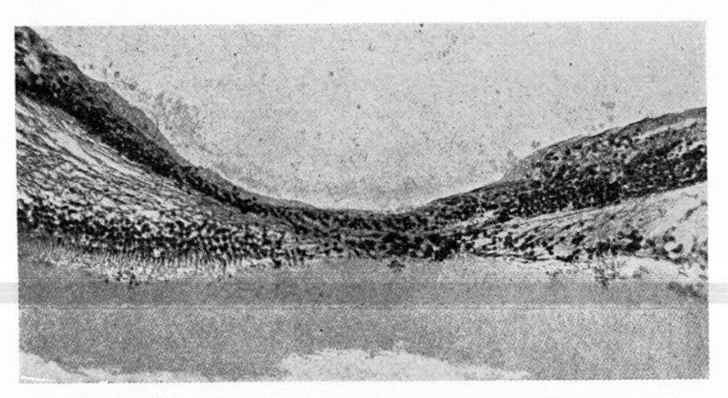

Fig. 144.—Concussion Changes at the Macula.

At the fovea the cones are missing. There is some migration of pigment, granules of which are seen in the subretinal fluid (A. Tillema).

small white atrophic patches may appear, or the migration and proliferation of pigment increase so that a dense black area may gradually form in the central area, or the region may be surrounded by a heavily pigmented ring (Plate X, Figs. 6 to 8).

The importance of such a condition depends on its serious functional effects, for as a rule central vision is slowly and permanently diminished over a period of some months, an initial relative scotoma changing in the worst cases into an absolute defect. No treatment is of value. It is of great importance, therefore, to remember that such a disability may be caused by a lesion which frequently appears to be of little moment, and may indeed be difficult to see on ophthalmoscopic examination. If complaint is made of impairment of vision after a concussion, the utmost care should therefore be taken and repeated examinations should be made for several weeks before the case is dismissed as functional or suspicions of malingering are entertained.

Finally, in more severe contusions an ACUTE CONCUSSION NECROSIS may occur at the macula, as elsewhere in the retina, wherein the neuro-epithelium disappears and is replaced by amorphous globules (Fig. 144) (Tillema, 1937).

PERIPHERAL ATROPHIC RETINAL CHANGES

CHANGES IN THE RETINAL PERIPHERY are not uncommon after ocular concussions. In this location, of course, an area of traumatic choroiditis may result in atrophy of the overlying retina, while a rupture of this tissue associated with a similar choroidal lesion may mark the site of direct injury; but in addition to such local damage the development of widespread changes in the retinal periphery of an atrophic and pigmentary nature are not uncommon, somewhat resembling the peripheral degeneration seen in high myopia or that associated with congenital or acquired syphilis. These changes readily escape notice unless specially looked for and have received little note in the literature, but Davidson (1936) found them in 58% of 34 cases of ocular concussions.

In more severe cases these atrophic changes may be generalized throughout the entire retina, particularly in the presence of a traumatic endophthalmitis, in which case the histological picture shows the usual evidence of marked degeneration—drusen on Bruch's membrane (Fig. 145), diffuse gliosis of the retina with the obliteration of its vessels (Fig. 146) and eventually complete atrophy with cystoid degeneration (Fig. 147) (Rones and Wilder, 1947).

DIFFUSE PIGMENTARY CHANGES appearing some weeks after an injury and [illegible] a large area of the retina are more unusual (Plate XXIV, Figs. 1 and 5); nevertheless their occurrence has been noted for many years since the early observations of Brailey (1876), the two Jonathan Hutchinsons (1889), Lawford (1902) and Bickerton (1904). They occur frequently as concussion effects in war injuries (McKee, 1923) and are not uncommonly caused by blast (Lagrange, 1918). The posterior region of the fundus is preferentially affected, but the migration of pigment may be widespread while localized areas may alone be affected. Sometimes the pigment is fine and dust-like, at other times it is corpuscular or arranged in clumps (Plate XI, Figs. 3 and 4), while it may carpet the whole fundus densely, being arranged without reference to blood vessels; most typically, however, it is aggregated in clumps near the vessels which occasionally may become partially obscured by the granular aggregations. Over a considerable area around the pigmentary deposits the choroidal vessels may be clearly visible, suggesting that the pigment of the hexagonal layer has been lost. If such changes are widespread, particularly if they affect the central area, they are usually associated with some degree of optic atrophy and visual failure.

The cause of these pigmentary changes probably varies in different cases. We shall see presently that an extension of the same process manifests itself in the migration of pigment granules into the vitreous, a phenomenon which

Figs. 145 to 147.—Post-concussion Atrophy of the Retina (N. Ashton).

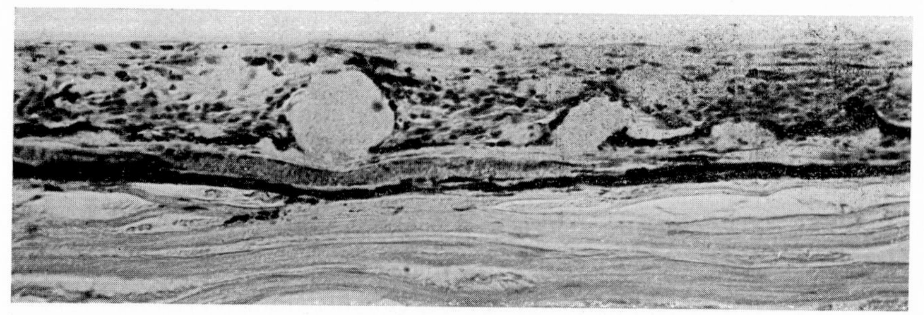

Fig. 145.—Drusen in the lamina vitrea projecting into an atrophic retina.

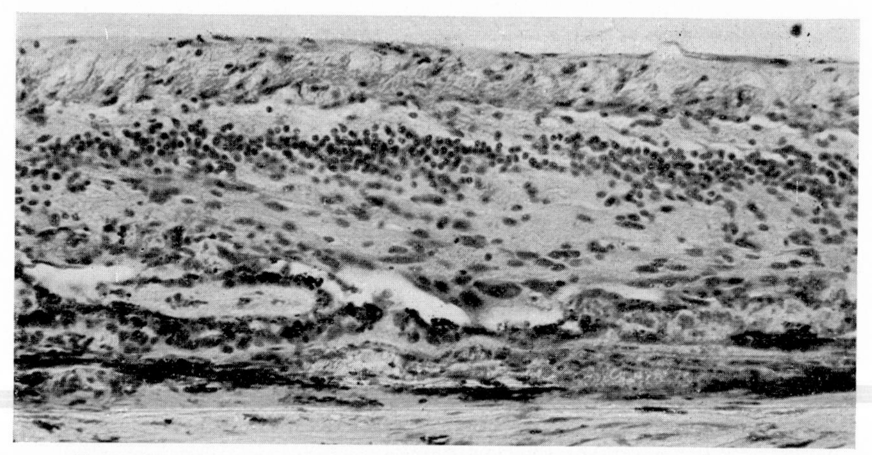

Fig. 146.—There is considerable chorioretinal atrophy and extensive gliosis.

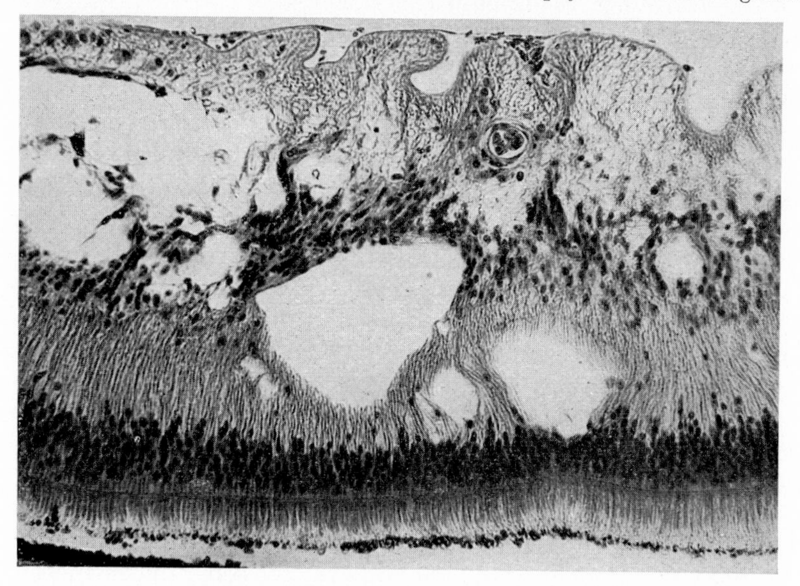

Fig. 147.—Showing marked cystoid degeneration.

is an almost constant sequel of concussions. In some cases they may result from the direct concussive effect upon the pigmentary epithelium, the cells of which may suffer necrosis and be converted into large globules or structureless masses (Fig. 148) (Tillema, 1937); in others the vascular reaction characteristic of a concussion with its subsequent necrotic changes may be the principal ætiological factor, while others may represent the effect on the retinal epithelium of choroidal or subchoroidal hæmorrhages. In any event, however they may be caused, they are permanent and are not susceptible to treatment.

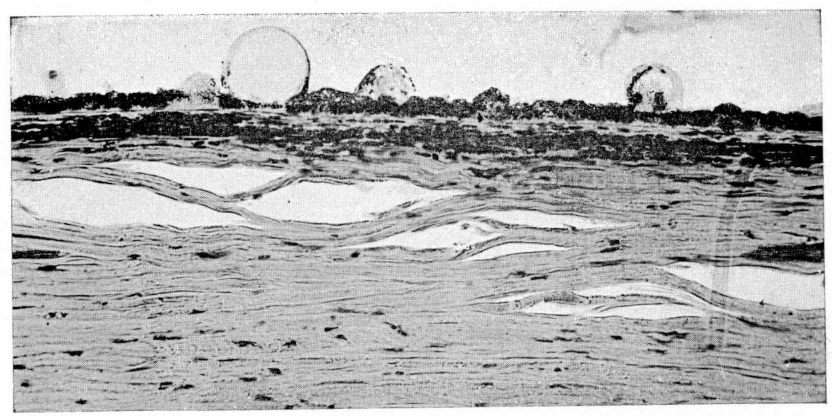

Fig. 148.—Concussion Effects on the Pigmentary Epithelium.

Showing the inflated degenerated [illegible]

VASCULAR CHANGES IN THE RETINA

We have already discussed the œdema which forms the most common vascular response in the retina to concussions even of a mild degree; a more immediate effect, however, may be a generalized and dramatic spasmodic constriction of the retinal arteries, a reaction which may disappear within a quarter of an hour (Sédan and Alliès, 1951). More gross vascular lesions characteristic of the reaction to contusion include hæmorrhages and the formation of traumatic aneurysms.

TRAUMATIC RETINAL HÆMORRHAGES

Small hæmorrhages from the retinal vessels, usually single but sometimes multiple, are common after ocular contusions; we have already seen that they are of relatively frequent occurrence as birth injuries.[1] All types of hæmorrhage may occur both after direct injuries to the globe or indirect concussions involving the head; the most common are intraretinal hæmorrhages, usually small round extravasations in the outer retinal layers or flame-shaped extravasations in the nerve-fibre layer, but preretinal

[1] p. 12.

hæmorrhages, either subhyaloid or situated between the limiting membrane and the nerve-fibre layer,[1] and extravasations into the vitreous are not unusual[2]. As a rule an intraretinal hæmorrhage clears up within a few weeks, sometimes without trace, but at other times it leaves a permanent area of atrophy with pigmentary proliferation, causing a scotoma which is disabling if in the central region; but if the bleeding is extensive, and particularly if it is associated with necrosis in the retinal tissues, much permanent damage may ensue. In these cases the blood may plough up the necrotic tissue, throwing the retina into complicated convolutions and folds and splitting its tissues so that they assume the appearance of a ghost-like tangled skein wriggling through a mass of blood clot (Lister, 1924). In such cases, and in some cases of hæmorrhage into the vitreous, absorption of the blood may be accompanied by the appearance of plaques of fine fibrous tissue which may gradually increase in density and size to simulate the picture of PROLIFERATING RETINOPATHY associated with a varying degree of pigmentary migration and proliferation (Hirschberg, 1869; Hersing, 1872; and others).[3] When retinal bleeding alone is involved, however, and the choroid does not share in the damage, such proliferation is largely glial in nature and is rarely extensive.

In cases wherein the central vessels have been ruptured, of course, bleeding is usually much more extensive and dense masses of fibrous tissue may proliferate out into the vitreous (Zimmermann, 1897). Similarly, when the membrane of Bruch has been torn and the choroid implicated, the abundant mesoblastic elements available in the latter tissue are free to take part in a luxuriant organization of the blood-clot with fibrous tissue to form the denser and more massive picture of CHORIORETINITIS PROLIFERANS.[4]

OBSTRUCTION OF THE CENTRAL RETINAL ARTERY involving a picture resembling embolism (Schapringer, 1906; Moorhouse, 1927; Arkle, 1937) and THROMBOSIS OF THE CENTRAL RETINAL VEIN (von Wiser, 1901; Hillemanns and Pfalz, 1905; Pincus, 1907; Cozzoli, 1916) have been reported after contusions as rarities.

TRAUMATIC ANEURYSMS in the retina are rare sequels of a contusion to the globe. *Miliary aneurysmal dilatations* following injury were first reported by Galezowski (1874) and Denissenko (1882), while Mannhardt (1875) noted such a development in association with a rupture of the choroid. *Traumatic arterio-venous communications* (*racemose aneurysms*) have been described by Magnus (1874) and Fuchs (1882); the degree of dilatation of the vessels is slight in such cases owing to the support afforded them by the intra-ocular pressure, but the arteries and veins are difficult to differentiate and connecting them is a pulsating anastomosis.

RETINAL TEARS

TEARING OF THE RETINA after a concussion which is frequently slight in nature has been recognized as a not uncommon occurrence since the initial observation of Lawson (1867). Such tears may occur in the young healthy

[1] Obermeier (1901), Harms (1912), Pietzker (1913), and others.
[2] Vol. X, p. 147. [3] Vol. X, p. 150. [4] p. 684.

eye after a contusion of some severity, but in the case of a retina which suffers from the degenerative changes associated with myopia, age or healed inflammatory lesions, traumata so slight as almost to pass unnoticed may act as a precipitating factor in causing this tissue to give way, particularly if vitreous adhesions exist in the area; in this event the tear is usually an irregular or angular rent. In the relatively healthy eye the sites of rupture are usually at the point of impact where the retina may be torn in association with the choroid to form a *chorioretinal rupture*, and at the anterior and

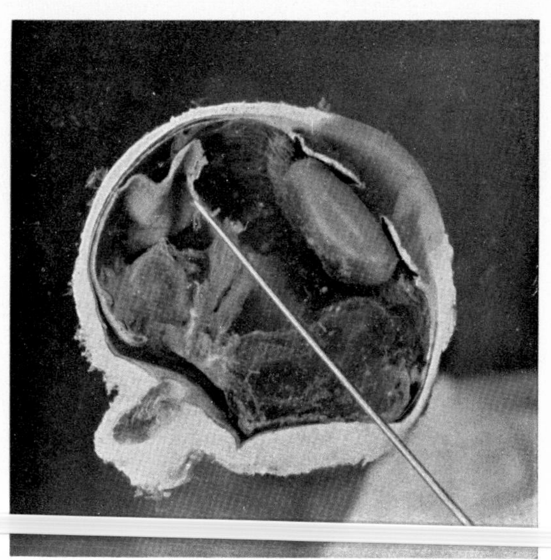

FIG. 149.—TRAUMATIC ANTERIOR RETINAL DIALYSIS.

A war injury. Section of the globe showing an anterior dialysis where the periphery of the retina is torn from the ora serrata and reflected by a probe. There is also an evulsion of the optic nerve, the sheath of which was filled by vitreous (W. Lister and M. Hine).

posterior attachments of the retina where it is firmly fixed at the ora and optic disc—usually the former.

A localized *dialysis of the ora* is relatively common, frequently situated in the infero-temporal quadrant of the globe where concussive injuries are most usually located (Figs. 149 and 150) but several authors have remarked on the high incidence of traumatic dialysis in the upper nasal quadrant of the globe.

Thus Cox and his colleagues (1966) gave the following figures for the location of the dialysis in 143 cases of traumatic retinal detachment: in the upper nasal quadrant, 37·8%; lower temporal quadrant, 27·4%; upper temporal, 22%; lower nasal, 12·8%; while Hagler and North (1968), among 131 cases with dialysis out of 1,352 cases of retinal detachment, found objective evidence of pre-existing trauma in 71% of patients with upper nasal dialysis; 50% of these cases showed an avulsed or torn strip of ciliary

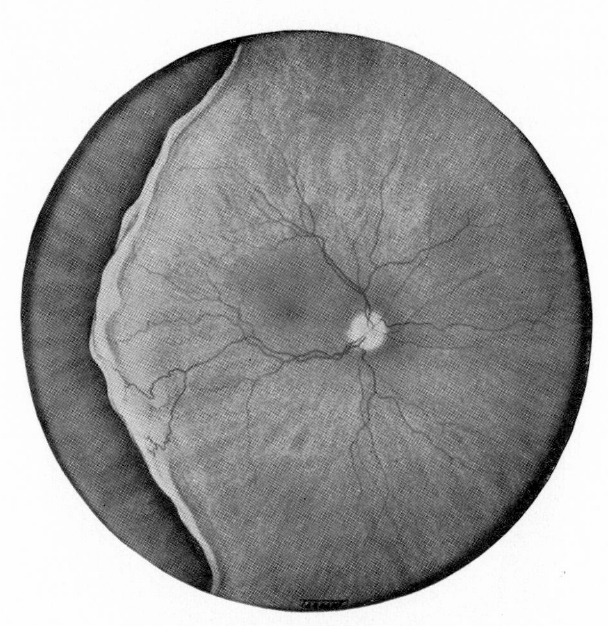

FIG. 150.—GIANT DIALYSIS.

An extensive dialysis in the temporal periphery following a contusion in a boy; the rest of the retina has remained flat (J. R. Hudson, Inst. Ophthal.).

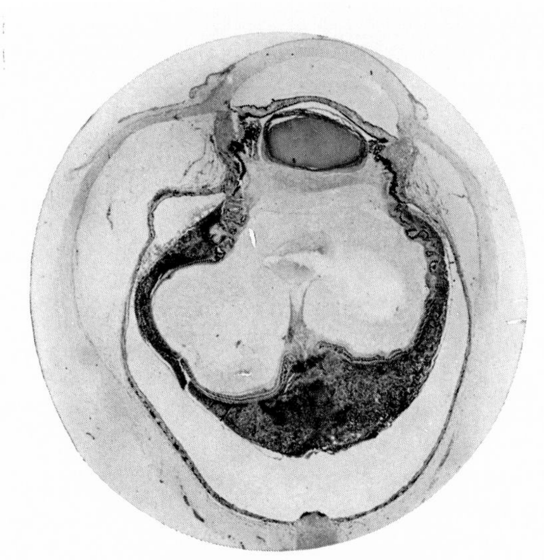

FIG. 151.—COMPLETE POSTERIOR DIALYSIS OF THE RETINA: TOTAL DETACHMENT (W. Lister).

epithelium as described by Cox and his colleagues (1966) which they regarded as pathognomonic of a contusion injury.

As a rule the tear is small, but it may extend half-way (Jeandelize *et al.*, 1931; Goldenburg, 1933; Hagler and North, 1968) or even completely round the circumference so that the retina is entirely separated from its ciliary attachment (Velhagen, 1900; Römer, 1901). A complete anterior dialysis of this type, of course, is rare, as also is a complete posterior dialysis wherein the retina is avulsed from its attachment at the optic disc (Figs. 151, 154 and 155) (Paul, 1905; Lister, 1924); but the great majority of peripheral retinal dialyses (with the exception of those resulting from the rupture of a cyst) is due to a direct contusion which is sometimes slight in degree,[1] or an indirect injury such as a fall.[2] The retina tends to give way where the mode of apposition of the two layers of the optic vesicle suddenly alters, the loose relations of the retina and the pigmentary epithelium giving place abruptly to the firm fusion between the two layers of the ciliary epithelium where the retina is thinnest, least supported by blood vessels and most prone to degeneration, and where the vitreous framework, set into violent motion by the concussion, has its fullest development and its firmest anchorage.

Apart from these relatively gross rents, the frequency of retinal tears—usually near the periphery and particularly of an angular or horse-shoe shape—in detachments following traumata indicates the clinical significance of such a lesion, their configuration suggesting that the usual causal mechanism when the force impinges on the eye is the sudden thrust and recoil of the vitreous to which the retina is often adherent, or the rapid equatorial expansion and oscillation of the ocular [illegible] following impact, while a temporal retinal dialysis is probably caused by local deformation of the sclera near the temporal limbus (Weidenthal and Schepens, 1966). This subject has already been discussed in a previous volume[3] and it will be referred to again immediately.

Alt. *Amer. J. Ophthal.*, **30,** 97 (1913).
Arkle. *Trans. ophthal. Soc. U.K.*, **57,** 353 (1937).
Bäck. *v. Graefes Arch. Ophthal.*, **47** (1), 82; **48** (2), 470 (1899).
Berlin. *Klin. Mbl. Augenheilk.*, **11,** 42 (1873).
Bickerton. *Trans. ophthal. Soc. U.K.*, **24,** 258 (1904).
Bonamour. *L'année thérap. clin. Ophtal.*, **7,** 343 (1956).
Brailey. *Roy. Lond. ophthal. Hosp. Rep.*, **8,** 534 (1876).
Coats. *Roy. Lond. ophthal. Hosp. Rep.*, **17,** 69 (1907).
Collins. *Trans. ophthal. Soc. U.K.*, **20,** 196 (1900); **37,** 112 (1917).
Cox, Schepens and Freeman. *Arch. Ophthal.*, **76,** 678 (1966).
Cozzoli. *Arch. Ottal.*, **23,** 373 (1916).
Davidson. *Amer. J. Ophthal.*, **19,** 757 (1936).
Denig. *Arch. Augenheilk.*, **34,** 52 (1897).
v. Graefes Arch. Ophthal., **47,** 678 (1899).
Denissenko. *Wien. med. Presse*, **23,** 14 (1882).
Dimmer. *Zbl. prakt. Augenheilk.*, **9,** 97 (1885).
Doherty. *Amer. J. Ophthal.*, **25,** 135 (1942).
Fuchs. *Arch. Augenheilk.*, **11,** 440 (1882).
Z. Augenheilk., **6,** 181 (1901).
Galezowski. *Recueil Ophtal.*, **1,** 368 (1874).
Goldenburg. *Arch. Ophthal.*, **9,** 256 (1933).
Goldmann. *Brit. J. Ophthal.*, **33,** 242 (1949).
Haab. *Beitr. Augenheilk.*, **22,** 8 (1888).
VII int. Cong. Ophthal., Heidelberg, 429 (1888).
Klin. Mbl. Augenheilk., **35,** 213 (1897).
Z. Augenheilk., **3,** 113 (1900).

[1] Scheffels (1891), P. Knapp (1931), Weidenthal and Schepens (1966), Cox *et al.* (1966) Hagler and North (1968).

[2] Müller (1931), Haitz (1931).

[3] Vol. X, p. 788.

Hagler and North. *Arch. Ophthal.*, **79,** 376 (1968).
Haitz. *Klin. Mbl. Augenheilk.*, **86,** 105 (1931).
Harman. *Trans. ophthal. Soc. U.K.*, **21,** 88 (1901).
Harms. *Ber. dtsch. ophthal. Ges.*, **38,** 383 (1912).
Hartridge. *Trans. ophthal. Soc. U.K.*, **9,** 144 (1889).
Herrmann. *Die Kontusionsverletzungen d. Auges in. klin. u. path.-anat. Beziehung* (Diss.), Leipzig (1906).
Hersing. *Klin. Mbl. Augenheilk.*, **10,** 171 (1872).
Hervouët. *Bull. Soc. franç. Ophtal.*, **78,** 253 (1965).
Hillemanns and Pfalz. *Klin. Mbl. Augenheilk.*, **43** (2), 373 (1905).
Hirschberg. *Klin. Mbl. Augenheilk.*, **7,** 324 (1869).
Berl. klin. Wschr., **12,** 299 (1875).
Hruby. *Ophthalmologica*, **115,** 290 (1948).
Hutchinson, J. (Sen.). *Roy. Lond. ophthal. Hosp. Rep.*, **12,** 61 (1889).
Hutchinson, J. (Jun.). *Trans. ophthal. Soc. U.K.*, **9,** 116 (1889).
Jeandelize, Baudot and Delaveuve. *Bull. Soc. Ophtal. Paris*, 202 (1931).
Knapp, H. *Arch. Augenheilk.*, **1,** 22 (1869); **10,** 337 (1881).
Knapp, P. *Klin. Mbl. Augenheilk.*, **87,** 399 (1931).
Kuhnt. *Z. Augenheilk.*, **3,** 105 (1900).
Lagrange. *Atlas d'ophtalmoscopie de guerre*, Paris (1918).
Lawford. *Trans. ophthal. Soc. U.K.*, **13,** 76 (1893); **22,** 238 (1902).
Lawson. *Injury of the Eye, Orbit and Eyelids*, London, 246 (1867).
Leber. *Graefe-Saemisch Hb. d. ges. Augenheilk.*, 2nd ed., Leipzig, **7** (2), Kap. 10A(2) (1916).
Linde. *Zbl. prakt. Augenheilk.*, **21,** 97 (1897).
Lister. *Brit. J. Ophthal.*, **8,** 305 (1924).
Lohmann. *v. Graefes Arch. Ophthal.*, **62,** 227 (1906).
Klin. Mbl. Augenheilk., **44** (2), 526 (1906).
McKee. *Amer. J. Ophthal.*, **6,** 725 (1923).
Magnus. *Virchows Arch. path. Anat.*, **60,** 38 (1874).
Makrocki. *Arch. Augenheilk.*, **24,** 244 (1892).
Mannhardt. *Klin. Mbl. Augenheilk.*, **13,** 132 (1875).
Marsol and Bouchat. *Arch. Ophtal.*, **27,** 387 (1967).
Moore, Foster. *Trans. ophthal. Soc. U.K.*, **30,** 155 (1910).
Moorhouse. *Trans. ophthal. Soc. U.K.*, **47,** 421 (1927).
Müller. *Z. Augenheilk.*, **73,** 163 (1931).
Nettleship. *Lancet*, **1,** 941 (1880).
Roy. Lond. ophthal. Hosp. Rep., **11,** 59, 60 (1886).
Noyes. *Trans. Amer. ophthal. Soc.*, **1** (6), 128 (1871).
Obermeier. *Klin. Mbl. Augenheilk.*, **39** (1), 293 (1901).
Ogilvie. *Trans. ophthal. Soc. U.K.*, **20,** 198, 202 (1900).
Oliver. *Trans. Amer. ophthal. Soc.*, **7,** 613 (1896).
Ostwalt. *Zbl. prakt. Augenheilk.*, **11,** 33, 72 (1887).
Pagenstecher. *v. Graefes Arch. Ophthal.*, **55,** 135 (1903).
Paul. *Klin. Mbl. Augenheilk.*, **43** (1), 185 (1905).
Pietzker. *Wietere klinisch-kasuistische Beitr. z. Krankheitsbilde d. sogen. präretinalen Blutung* (Diss.), Tubingen (1913).
Pincus. *Klin. Mbl. Augenheilk.*, **45** (2), 568 (1907).
Reis. *Z. Augenheilk.*, **15,** 37 (1906).
Römer. *Klin. Mbl. Augenheilk.*, **39,** 306 (1901).
Rones and Wilder. *Amer. J. Ophthal.*, **30,** 1143 (1947).
Roscin. *v. Graefes Arch. Ophthal.*, **127,** 401 (1931).
Schapringer. *Zbl. prakt. Augenheilk.*, **30,** 358 (1906).
Scheffels. *Arch. Ophthal.*, **20,** 403 (1891).
Schmidt-Rimpler. *Klin. Mbl. Augenheilk.*, **22,** 212 (1884).
Berl. klin. Wschr., **22,** 176 (1885).
Sédan and Alliès. *Rev. Oto-neuro-ophtal.*, **23,** 374 (1951).
Shimkin. *Brit. J. Ophthal.*, **24,** 265 (1940).
Siegfried. *Beitr. Augenheilk.*, **3** (22), 45 (1898).
Tillema. *Arch. Ophthal.*, **17,** 586 (1937).
Tirelli. *Rass. ital. Ottal.*, **17,** 358 (1948).
Twietmeyer. *Z. Augenheilk.*, **18,** 447 (1907).
Velhagen. *v. Graefes Arch. Ophthal.*, **49,** 599 (1900).
Vogt. *Münch. med. Wschr.*, **72,** 1101 (1925).
Klin. Mbl. Augenheilk., **84,** 305 (1930); **92,** 743 (1934).
Wagenmann. *Die Verletzungen des Auges: Graefe-Saemisch Hb. d. ges. Augenheilk.*, 3rd ed., Leipzig, 570 (1915).
Weidenthal and Schepens. *Amer. J. Ophthal.*, **62,** 465 (1966).
von Wiser. *Zbl. prakt. Augenheilk.*, **25,** 360 (1901).
Wolter. *Amer. J. Ophthal.*, **56,** 785 (1963).
Zeeman. *v. Graefes Arch. Ophthal.*, **80,** 259 (1912); **112,** 152 (1923).
Zimmermann. *Arch. Ophthal.*, **26,** 51 (1897).

TRAUMATIC RETINAL DETACHMENT

A history of trauma in the causation of a detachment of the retina[1] is an association which has been recognized ever since attention was drawn to the subject by Cooper (1859). To a large extent this was true even in the days before the mechanics of this catastrophe were fully understood; thus, Gros (1903) found that 27·7% of 170 consecutive cases of retinal detachment were due to contusions of the globe, while Casey Wood (1911) found 16·3% in 300 cases and Leber (1916), excluding perforating injuries, considered that trauma played a part in from 16 to 18% of detachments, figures which have subsequently in general been confirmed.[2] With the exception of a detachment following perforating injuries the precise relationship of trauma whether directly involving the globe or indirectly as a result of blows on the head, violent movements, shaking, straining and so on, is not simple to determine (Table XVI). A history of this nature is not necessarily reliable for it is easy

TABLE XVI

ORIGIN OF RETINAL DETACHMENT DUE TO CONTUSION
(154 cases—Cox, Schepens and Freeman, 1966)

Cause	%
Domestic Accidents	40·2%
Sporting Accidents	35·1%
Industrial Accidents	8·5%
Automobile Accidents	3·9%
Explosives	3·3%
Exact Cause Unknown	9·0%
TOTAL	100·0%

for a patient to recall some past injury and just as easy to forget it, bearing in mind that in some cases the detachment may not app[illegible] the traumatic episode. On the other hand, there may well be evidence pointing to a previous ocular contusion such as a dislocation of the lens, cataract, abnormalities of the pupil and the angle of the anterior chamber, or of pre-existing vitreo-retinal degeneration in one or both eyes (Schmöger and Hochmann, 1966; Blach and Bedford, 1966) or an inherited retinal cyst (Tulloh, 1968), observations which assume particular importance when medico-legal problems and compensation are involved (Rintelen, 1954; Nordmann, 1956; Dufour, 1961). The fact remains, however, that a traumatic retinal detachment in a healthy eye, particularly an eye unaffected by senile or myopic degeneration or old inflammatory lesions, is rare; thus Herrmann (1906) found only 16 instances in 677 cases of contusive injuries and the comparative rarity of detachments among war injuries in the young and relatively healthy army populations is striking (von Szily, 1917; Lagrange, 1918; Axenfeld, 1922; and many others). As we have seen, the choroid is

[1] See Vol. X, p. 784.

[2] Stallard (1930) found a history of trauma in 16%; Shapland (1934) in 26%; Dunnington and Macnie (1935) in 30%; Knapp (1943) and Massin (1954) in 13%; Dollfus and Clop (1956) in 10%; Thiel and Kilian (1963) in 13%; Gruber (1963) in 18%; Cox *et al.* (1966) 160 cases; Schepens and Marden (1966), in 11·5% of 2,016 unilateral cases; Tasman (1968) in 7% of 243 cases; Tulloh (1968) in 35·2% of 251 cases; Hollwich (1969) in 11·4% of 2,751 cases.

more readily ruptured than the healthy retina, and an injury may even rupture the sclera and lead to loss of vitreous while the retina remains in place.

Retinal detachment in children is uncommon and in a large proportion is due to trauma, most commonly a contusion. Thus of 59 children with retinal detachment Kadlecová (1959) found 17 of traumatic origin; Dufour (1961) 11 of 41 cases; Bernardczykowa (1966) 17 of 20 cases aged 6 to 15 years; Hudson (1965–69) 55 cases representing less than 2% of all new cases of retinal detachment seen between 1959 and 1967, of which 36 were the result of injury (24 contusions, 3 perforating and 9 indirect). The recent literature on this subject is considerable.[1]

From the pathological point of view post-traumatic detachments may be of five types:

1. Immediate detachments due to collapse of the globe through rupture, in which case the retina shares in the general disorganization.

2. Immediate detachments due to a choroidal hæmorrhage or exudation thrown out in the phase of reactive hyperæmia and increased capillary permeability following a contusion. The occurrence of this sequence has been experimentally verified in animals (Bäck, 1898); and that reposition may follow the absorption of the blood or the exudate in these cases, provided the retina is not torn, is a long-established observation.[2] Reposition, however, does not necessarily imply restoration of function since permanent atrophic changes, scarring or retinal striæ may remain in the detached area A contusion, if of sufficient severity, may well be the sole cause of a detachment in a healthy eye. Typical causes are chopping wood, blunt blows or the effects of missiles, fireworks or explosions (Thiel and Kilian, 1963) and it is a well-known hazard to boxers.[3]

3. Immediate detachments due to a gross injury which causes a tear in the retina, occasionally associated with a choroidal rupture. These tears have just been discussed, and the mechanism of the detachment in such cases is clear.

4. A remote detachment occurring secondarily to the contraction of organized tissue in the vitreous following retinal or choroidal bleeding, the cicatrization of a scleral wound or the effects of a retained intra-ocular foreign body. Such a detachment usually occurs some time after the injury (Schwarz, 1907) (Fig. 157).

5. Detachments in which the primary cause is myopia, senile or post-inflammatory degeneration and in which trauma plays a precipitating ætiological role. This is the most common type and may be immediate or remote in its incidence. The mechanism of causation has already been discussed in a previous volume[4]: the essential prelude is the existence of a localized area of inherited or acquired vitreo-retinal degeneration to which the vitreous framework has become adherent. On receipt of the trauma the sudden

[1] Tasman (1967), Hilton and Norton (1969), Gailloud *et al.* (1969), Fenton *et al.* (1969).
[2] Scheibe (1877), Schmidt-Rimpler (1883), Venneman (1898), and a host of others.
[3] p. 29.
[4] See Vol. X, p. 779.

Gonin. *Le décollement de la rétine*, Lausanne (1934).
Gros. *Bericht ü. 170 Fälle von Netzhautablösung* (Diss.), Giessen (1903).
Gruber. *Amer. J. Ophthal.*, **56**, 911 (1963).
Herrmann. *Die Kontusionsverletzungen d. Auges in klin. u. path.-anat. Beziehung* (Diss.), Leipzig (1906).
Hilton and Norton. *Mod. Probl. Ophthal.*, **8**, 325 (1969).
Hollwich. *Klin. Mbl. Augenheilk.*, **154**, 582 (1969).
Howard and Campbell. *Arch. Ophthal.*, **81**, 317 (1969).
Hudson. *Trans. ophthal. Soc. U.K.*, **85**, 79 (1965).
Mod. Probl. Ophthal., **8**, 235 (1969).
Kadlecová. *Cs. Oftal.*, **15**, 208 (1959).
Knapp, A. *Arch. Ophthal.*, **30**, 770 (1943).
Lagrange. *Atlas d'ophtalmoscopie de guerre*, Paris (1918).
Leavelle and Jungschaffer. *Amer. J. Ophthal.*, **62**, 339 (1966).
Leber. *Graefe-Saemisch Hb. d. ges. Augenheilk.*, 2nd ed., Leipzig, **7** (2), Kap. 10A (2), 1374 (1916).
McDavitt. *Sth. med. J.*, **13**, 377 (1920).
Massin. *Arch. Ophtal.*, **14**, 154 (1954).
Middleton. *Amer. J. Ophthal.*, **2**, 779 (1919).
Neblett. *Amer. J. Ophthal.*, **7**, 564 (1924).
Nordmann. *Bull. Soc. Ophtal. Fr.*, 757 (1956).
Onken. *Z. Augenheilk.*, **14**, 165 (1905).
Pfalz. *Z. Augenheilk.*, **12**, 386 (1904).
Rintelen. *Ophthalmologica*, **128**, 326 (1954).
Sachsenweger. *Klin. Mbl. Augenheilk.*, **154**, 575 (1969).
Scheibe. *Dtsch. med. Wschr.*, **3**, 113 (1877).
Schepens and Marden. *Amer. J. Ophthal.*, **61**, 213 (1966).
Schmidt-Rimpler. *Arch. Augenheilk.*, **12**, 135 (1883).
Schmöger and Hochmann. *Klin. Mbl. Augenheilk.*, **148**, 433 (1966).
Schwarz. *Z. Augenheilk.*, **17**, 54 (1907).
Shapland. *Trans. ophthal. Soc. U.K.*, **54**, 176 (1934).
Brit. J. Ophthal., **18**, 1 (1934).
Stallard. *Brit. J. Ophthal.*, **14**, 1 (1930); **30**, 419 (1946).
v. Szily. *Atlas der Kreigsaugenheilkunde*, Stuttgart, 407 (1917).
Tasman. *Trans. Amer. Acad. Ophthal.*, **71**, 455 (1967).
Brit. J. Ophthal., **52**, 181 (1968).
Thiel and Kilian. *Klin. Mbl. Augenheilk.*, **143**, 564 (1963).
Tulloh. *Brit. J. Ophthal.*, **52**, 317 (1968).
Venneman. *Ann. Oculist.* (Paris), **120**, 46 (1898).
Weidenthal and Schepens. *Amer. J. Ophthal.*, **62**, 465 (1966).
Weill. *Z. Augenheilk.*, **15**, 140 (1906).
Wood. *System of Ophthalmic Operations*, Chicago (1911).

Contusion Effects at the Optic Disc

PAPILLITIS causing considerable swelling of the disc may be associated with ocular contusions (Siegfried, 1898; Löhlein, 1908; and others), while OPTIC ATROPHY may be a sequel to widespread retinal or choroidal damage (Haab, 1902; and many others). The most typical result of a severe contusion, however, is a partial or complete rupture with partial or complete evulsion of the optic nerve.

Optic atrophy is a common sequel to indirect injuries to the skull[1]; such an atrophy may also follow slight concussive injury to the globe as in the case described by Sullivan and Helveston (1969) (Fig. 158).

In this case, concerning a 6-year-old boy, optic atrophy and total blindness in one eye followed a blow from the flat end of a long radio antenna: vision was lost completely within one hour of the accident with virtually no abnormal ocular signs other than mild bulbar hyperæmia; optic atrophy was complete within three months.

RUPTURE AND AVULSION OF THE OPTIC NERVE

The most common cause of a rupture and avulsion of the optic nerve is a penetrating injury of the orbit, a subject which will be subsequently discussed.[2] A similar lesion, however, may result from direct concussions to the globe and has been recorded as resulting from a blow on the eye with a

[1] Vol. XII, p. 273. [2] p. 440.

clothes prop (Lang, 1901), a bamboo pole (Stanton-Cook, 1953), a bat (Collins, 1914), a stone (Juler, 1916), a brick (Henderson, 1919), an accidental jab with a finger (during a polo match, Caiger, 1941). This gross injury may also follow a concussion involving the face, such as a fall (Zimmermann, 1897), a kick on the cheek from a horse (Pichler, 1910), goring by a bull (Hsu, 1952) or an automobile accident (Rones and Wilder, 1947) (Fig. 159). Since the lesion is usually associated with gross intra-ocular damage and profuse hæmorrhage it is often not immediately diagnosed and may not be discovered until a pathological examination is made (Salzmann, 1903). On the other hand, cases have been described in which, after apparently minor

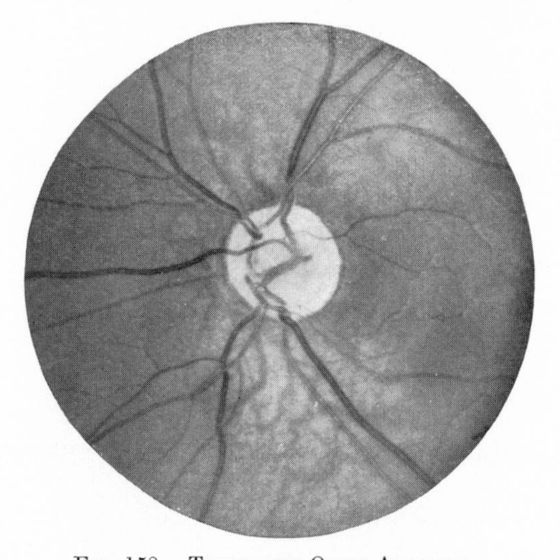

Fig. 158.—Traumatic Optic Atrophy.

Showing complete atrophy 3 months after trauma in a boy aged 6 who was struck by the tip of a radio antenna (G. Sullivan and E. M. Helveston).

trauma with little or no external evidence to show that an injury has occurred, more or less complete blindness in the affected eye has resulted from serious damage to the optic nerve.

Such an event was reported by Spizziri (1964), wherein partial avulsion of the optic nerve followed a blow from a stick; the eye showed concussive mydriasis and some intra-ocular hæmorrhage and a small fragment of wood was subsequently removed from alongside the nasal wall of the globe.

The mechanism of the injury has excited some controversy and may vary in different circumstances. It is probable that some cases are due to a direct rupture of the lamina cribrosa—the weakest portion of the ocular envelope representing one-third of the fibres of the sclera—by the explosive force generated within the eye on the impact of an outside force (Lister and Hine, 1919); in this event the optic nerve is pushed into its sheath suffering expulsion rather than avulsion. On the other hand, the blow on the eye may induce an extreme rotation of the globe which is stopped by a jerk on the nerve, thus tearing the lamina on the opposite side; in this case the nerve would be pulled out of the scleral ring (Lang, 1901; Shumway, 1917). An indirect facial injury, on the other hand, sets up concussion-waves which travel through the pterygo-maxillary fissure into the orbit and force the globe forward thus putting a sudden strain upon the nerve, a mechanism

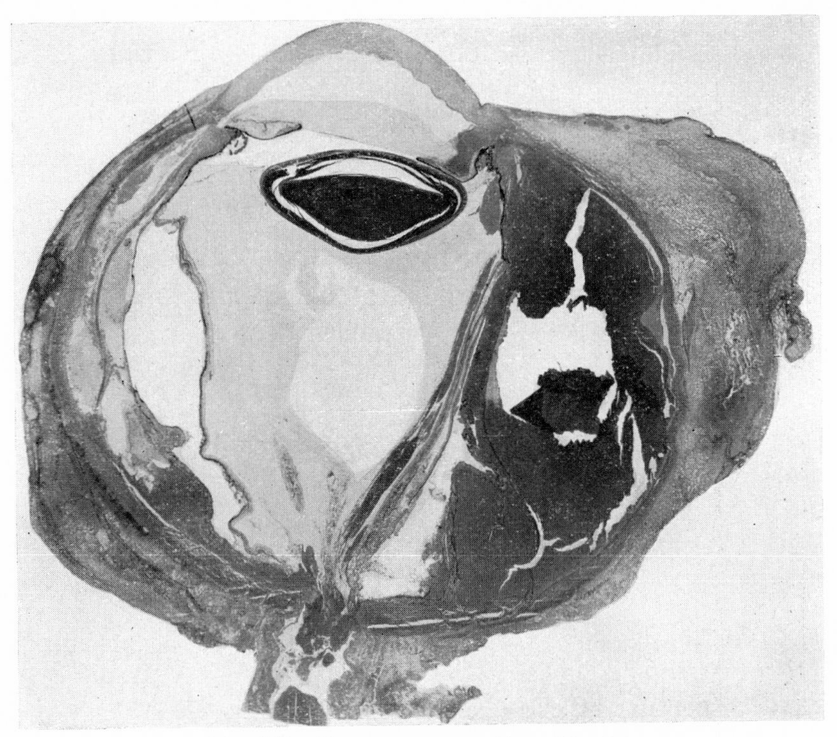

Fig. 159.—Evulsion of the Optic Nerve.

A concussion injury due to a road accident showing evulsion of the optic nerve. There is also a rupture at the filtration angle and a massive subchoroidal hæmorrhage (B. Rones and H. C. Wilder).

which has already been described (Lagrange, 1917). It is interesting that a partial cross rupture involving a portion of the nerve fibres may be caused by arterial and profuse subretinal bleeding as in a hæmorrhagic glaucoma or a post-operative expulsive hæmorrhage (Loewenstein, 1943). In all cases, whatever the mechanism, when exposed to a tensile strain the nerve fibres tend to tear at the margin of the disc, for at this point they consist merely of naked axon cylinders and, once torn, they retract for a variable distance up the sheath which, being elastic, can stretch and retain its continuity. The *clinical picture* varies with the extent of the rupture. In *marginal tears* when the configuration of the structures of the nerve-head is not grossly disturbed, the clinical evidences may be confined to the appearance of an arcuate hæmorrhage around the margin of the disc with radial extensions into the retina (Loewenstein, 1943).

It is possible that this may be the origin of the *hæmatic pigment ring at the disc* which has occasionally been described as a late result of injury (Knapp, 1868; Bunge, 1905; Lagrange, 1917; Doherty, 1942). This migration of blood pigment into Elschnig's border tissue, appearing clinically as a ring of bluish-red pigmentation at the margin of the disc, may be associated with a semi-annular paracentral scotoma and the tendency is for both the scotoma and the ring to disappear in time. These phenomena

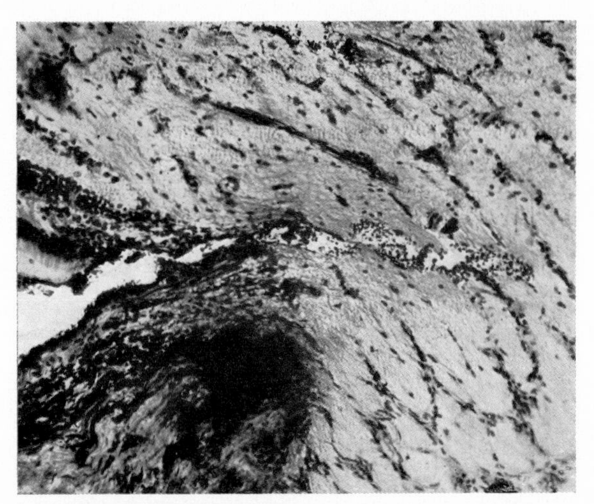

FIG. 160.—MARGINAL HÆMORRHAGE AT THE OPTIC DISC.

A man, aged 40, struck in the eye with an instrument which caused a rupture of the sclera in the lower, outer quadrant. There is a partial rupture of the tissues in a plane continuous with that of Bruch's membrane. Throughout the tear, the gap is filled with blood (A. Loewenstein).

have usually been ascribed to anterior leakage of a hæmatoma in the sheaths of the nerve, but it should be remembered that neither in subdural nor subarachnoid hæmorrhages is there continuity between the blood in the nerve sheaths and pre- or retro-retinal bleeding.[1] Lagrange (1917), on the other hand, concluded from clinical observations that the ring was probably due to the migration of blood pigment, not to the leakage of blood, from a hæmatoma of the nerve sheath of some standing; in some cases this may be an alternative explanation to that of a marginal tear.

When the injury is greater and some degree of avulsion of the nerve has occurred, the appearance of the fundus, when not entirely obscured by gross intra-ocular hæmorrhages, is characteristic (Plate XII, Figs. 1–4). In a *partial rupture with avulsion* the disc appears to be divided in two, one part (usually the lower) being depressed and dark suggesting in its appearance a

[1] Riddoch and Goulden (1925), MacDonald (1931), Ballantyne (1942), and others.

PLATE XII

EVULSION OF THE OPTIC NERVE.

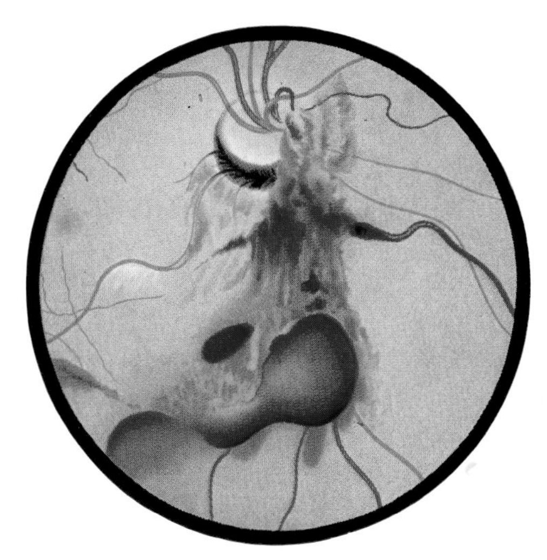

FIG. 1.

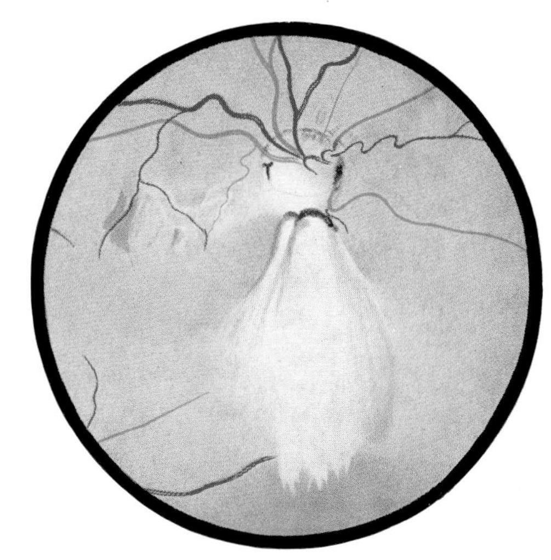

FIG. 2.

FIGS. 1 AND 2.—Partial evulsion of the optic nerve. A rupture of the lamina cribrosa after the eye had been struck with a clothes-prop. Fig. 1, the day after the injury; Fig. 2, the end-result (W. Lang).

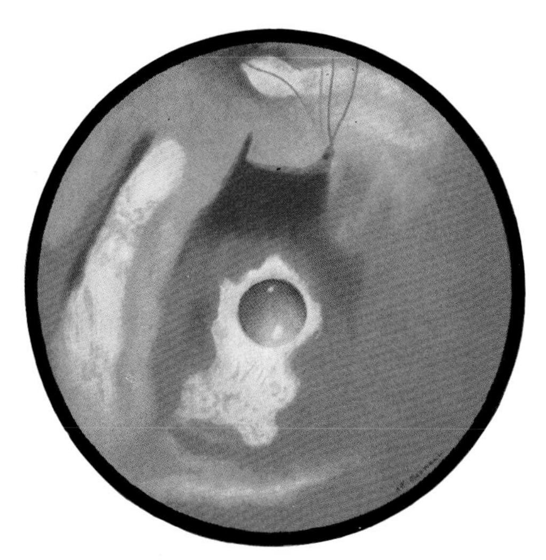

FIG. 3.—Complete evulsion of the optic nerve. The same case as Figs. 161 and 162 (W. Lister and M. Hine).

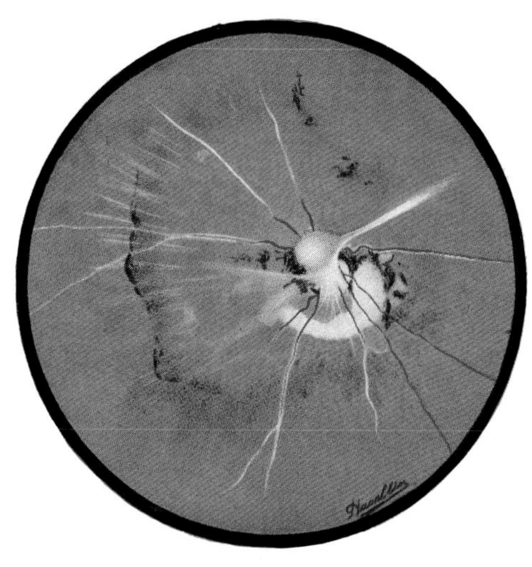

FIG. 4.—Evulsion of the optic nerve and a choroidal rupture from a fall on the handle of an umbrella 13 years previously.

Figs. 161 and 162.—Evulsion of the Optic Nerve.

A war injury wherein a fragment of shell had traversed the nose and left orbit and concussed the globe and the optic nerve. (The same case as Plate XII, Fig. 3) (W. Lister and M. Hine).

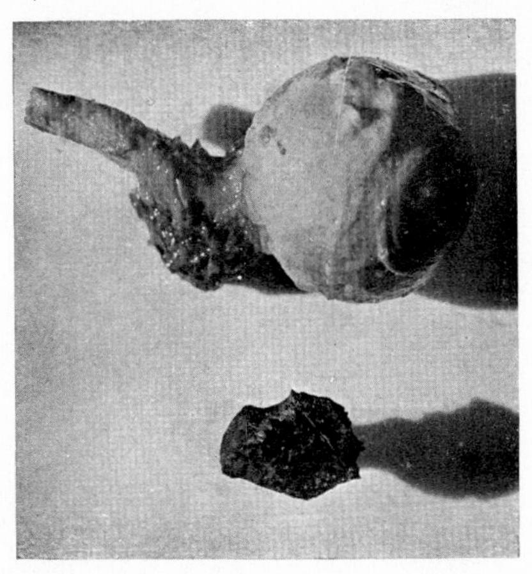

Fig. 161.—Shows the globe and the damaged nerve surrounded by a mass of inflammatory tissue. Underneath is the fragment of shrapnel which caused the injury; it was embedded at the apex of the orbit.

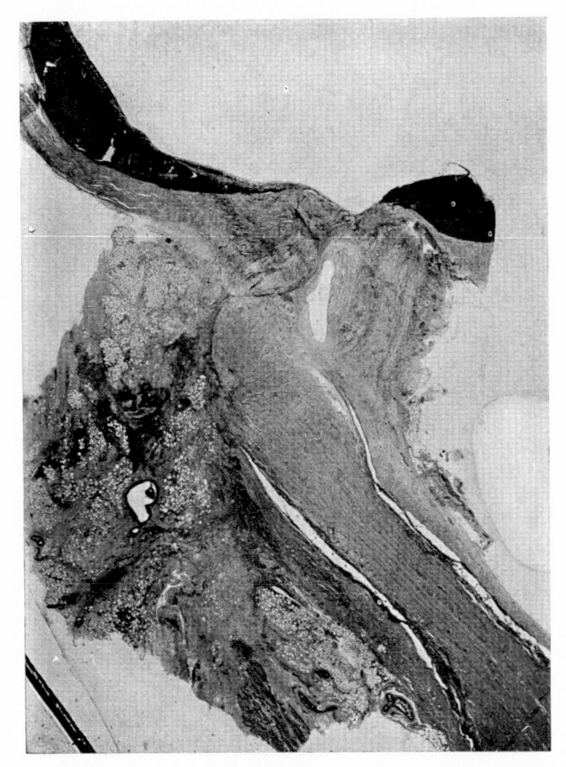

Fig. 162.—A section through the optic nerve and disc of the same eye, showing the retracted end of the nerve tucked into a gap in the nerve sheath. This tear of the sheath is surrounded by a mass of inflammatory tissue in which is embedded a fragment of bone and a small implantation cyst lined with columnar epithelium derived from the nasal mucous membrane.

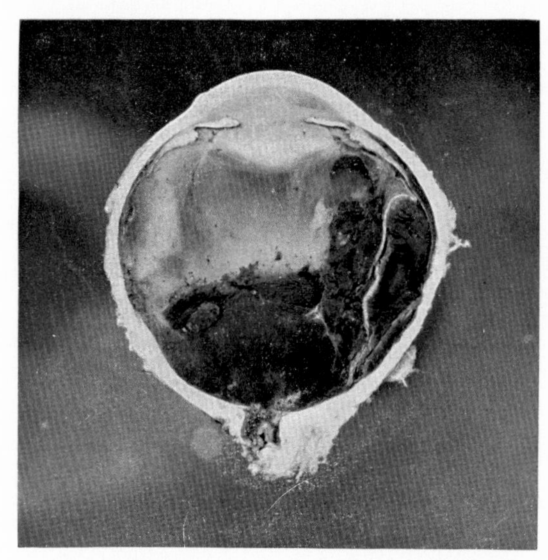

Fig. 163.—Evulsion of the Optic Nerve.

After a concussion injury. A section of the globe showing the sheath of the nerve devoid of nerve fibres and occupied by blood and coiled remnants of the retina which had been dragged back when the nerve was retracted (W. Lister and M. Hine).

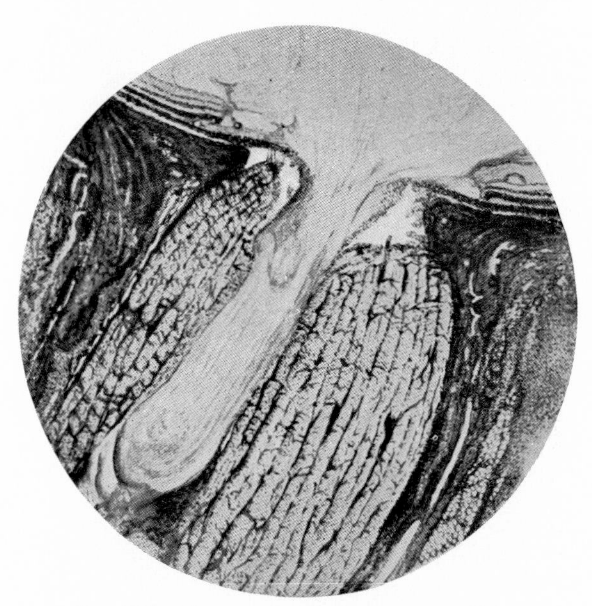

Fig. 164.—Concussion Changes at the Disc.

After a kick on the bridge of the nose. There is a vertical tear in the optic nerve-head running deeply into the nerve itself. Into the tear there is a large hernia of vitreous (V. Roscin).

deep coloboma of the nerve sheath. Elsewhere the retinal vessels course normally but in the torn area they end a little distance from the disc-margin, sometimes being curled upon themselves, sometimes dipping down into the cavern, or are buried and lost to view in hæmorrhage. Occasionally, the tear across the disc is continued beyond its margins as a rupture of the choroid (Collins, 1914). Subsequently the hæmorrhages become absorbed or organized by a massive proliferation of fibrous tissue which extends from the disc far onto the surrounding area of the retina or into the vitreous (Plate XII, Fig. 4); this newly formed tissue often has a sea-green sheen at first, probably derived from blood pigment, but it gradually becomes dull white (Stanton-Cook, 1953; and others). The retinal vessels devoid of blood ultimately appear as long, white cords.

In a *complete rupture* the ophthalmoscopic appearance in the few cases wherein it is visible corresponds to that seen in evulsion of the nerve in orbital injuries[1] (Plate XII). This is one of the most striking pictures that ophthalmoscopy reveals: the vessels are partially or completely absent from the fundus and the optic disc appears as an apparent y bottomless pit set in a background in which there are dramatic contusive changes. Eventually the cavern at the site of the disc tends to be filled up with fibrous tissue; indeed, the usual sequence—if the eye escapes excision—is that clinical examination is not possible owing to the massive hæmorrhages which fill the vitreous until the entire posterior part of the fundus is covered with a mass of fibrous tissue making it difficult to see what has happened.[2]

Pathological exam nation of cases with partial rupture of the nerve shows a fairly constant site of injury; there is an irregular transverse tear at the level of the termination of Bruch's elastic lamina; the edges are irregular as if the nerve fibres had been individually torn and the gap is filled with hæmorrhage (Fig. 160). When a complete rupture occurs the tear is situated at the same level; the fibres of the lamina cribrosa are also torn and the nerve is drawn some considerable distance up the sheath, frequently further than the length of nerve preserved in the specimen when the eye was excised so that the sheath appears as an empty sleeve. The cavity thus formed may be filled with blood clot or vitreous, or it may be partially occupied by the coiled remains of the retina which have been dragged back into it when the nerve retracted (Figs. 161–164). At a later stage, sections show a massive proliferation of newly formed, highly vascularized fibrous tissue which fills the cavity.[3]

Such an injury, of course, affects vision severely. In a partial rupture the corresponding portion of the field is permanently lost and the vision in the uninjured area is always gravely impaired; in total ruptures the sight is irretrievably destroyed. Treatment is expectant.

[1] p. 440.
[2] Compare Fig. 7, Vol. IX, p. 13.
[3] Salzmann (1903), Hesse (1907), Lister and Hine (1919), Roscin (1931), Tillema (1936), Rones and Wilder (1947), and others.

Ballantyne. *Glasg. med. J.*, **138,** 1, 52 (1942).
Bunge. *Münch. med. Wschr.*, **52,** 1266 (1905).
Caiger. *Trans. ophthal. Soc. U.K.*, **61,** 54 (1941).
Collins. *Trans. ophthal. Soc. U.K.*, **34,** 190 (1914).
Doherty. *Amer. J. Ophthal.*, **25,** 135 (1942).
Haab. *Beitr. Augenheilk.*, **5** (50), 1093 (1902).
Henderson. *Trans. ophthal. Soc. U.K.*, **39,** 205 (1919).
Hesse. *Z. Augenheilk.*, **17,** 45 (1907).
Hsu. *Chin. med. J.*, **70,** 77 (1952).
Juler. *Trans. ophthal. Soc. U.K.*, **36,** 241 (1916).
Knapp. *v. Graefes Arch. Ophthal.*, **14** (1), 252 (1868).
Lagrange. *Les fractures de l'orbite par les projectiles de guerre*, Paris (1917).
Lang. *Trans. ophthal. Soc. U.K.*, **21,** 98 (1901).
Lister and Hine. *Trans. ophthal. Soc. U.K.*, **39,** 196 (1919).
Löhlein. *Z. Augenheilk.*, **20,** 364 (1908).
Loewenstein. *Brit. J. Ophthal.*, **27,** 208 (1943).
MacDonald. *Trans. Amer. ophthal. Soc.*, **29,** 418 (1931).
Pichler. *Klin. Mbl. Augenheilk.*, **48** (2), 246 (1910).
Riddoch and Goulden. *Brit. J. Ophthal.*, **9,** 209 (1925).
Rones and Wilder. *Amer. J. Ophthal.*, **30,** 1143 (1947).
Roscin. *v. Graefes Arch. Ophthal.*, **127,** 401 (1931).
Salzmann. *Z. Augenheilk.*, **9,** 489 (1903).
Shumway. *Ophthal. Rec.*, **26,** 167 (1917).
Siegfried. *Beitr. Augenheilk.*, **3** (22), 45 (1898).
Spizziri. *Amer. J. Ophthal.*, **58,** 1056 (1964).
Stanton-Cook. *Brit. J. Ophthal.*, **37,** 188 (1953).
Sullivan and Helveston. *Arch. Ophthal.*, **81,** 159 (1969).
Tillema. *Arch. Ophthal.*, **16,** 36 (1936).
Zimmermann. *Arch. Ophthal.*, **26,** 51 (1897).

Concussion Changes in the Vitreous

Changes in the vitreous body after a concussion of any severity are invariable.[1] Corresponding to the flare in the anterior chamber there is usually, even in minor injuries, an increased relucency of the beam of the slit-lamp as it traverses the vitreous, indicating a plasmoid diffusion rich in protein resulting from the reactive vasodilatation, and this is frequently associated with disruption of the framework and liquefaction of the gel (SYNERESIS). Added to this, formed elements are usually deposited in considerable quantity on the fibrils of the vitreous framework—colourless cells frequently aggregated into clusters or star-shaped figures, erythrocytes lemon-yellow in colour and characteristically large, bright red granules of pigment derived from the pigmentary epithelium (Figs. 165 and 166). The presence of these granules in considerable numbers is a very common sequel of contusions, occurring in over 50% of cases (Kirby, 1932; 56%, Davidson, 1936). Apart from contusions, mechanical trauma as by the passage of an intra-ocular foreign body or the action of ultrasonic waves may also result in liquefaction of the vitreous (Zeiss, 1938; Kawamoto, 1947; Grün *et al.*, 1950; Lavine *et al.*, 1952).

VITREOUS HÆMORRHAGE is a common sequel to this type of injury; indeed, a tearing of the retina with or without detachment is the commonest cause of such an event. Small hæmorrhagic effusions probably derived from the ciliary region are frequently seen in the anterior vitreous and have a habit of aggregating on the posterior lens capsule either diffusely or as bright red patches (Plate IV, Fig. 4; Plate VI, Fig. 4). Occasionally such a hæmorrhage is more massive, forming a *hyphæma of the retrolental space*, the borders of which do not extend to the equator of the lens but are delimited by the arcuate line (Egger's line) where the vitreous usually comes

[1] For a résumé of the effects on the vitreous of various forms of trauma, see Vol. XI, p. 321.

into contact with the capsule.[1] Here the blood may remain fresh and red for a considerable time and may be seen to shift with movements of the head. Eventually, however, all hæmorrhagic deposits on the posterior surface of the lens change to a bronze colour and finally to a white dust, forming epicapsular deposits which may remain permanently to mark the occurrence of the injury.

In the substance of the vitreous, if the density of the hæmorrhage does not preclude slit-lamp examination, the blood cells are usually found aggregated on the framework of the gel which appears as if it were heavily dusted with lemon-coloured particles; frequently this appearance is regional when parts of the vitreous body appear dense with blood while other parts remain free (Fig. 166).

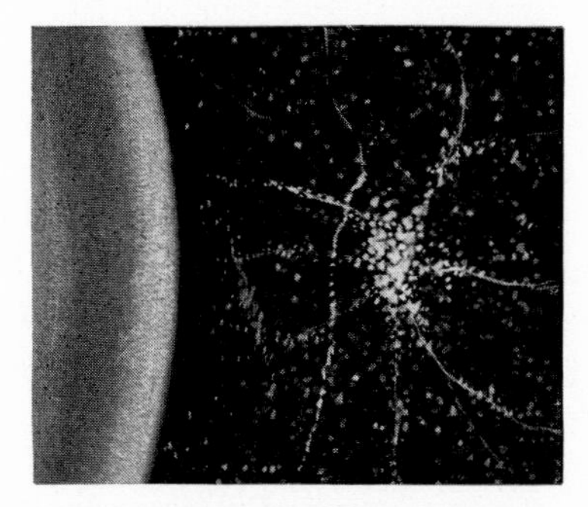

Fig. 165.—Concussion Changes in the Vitreous.

There is a deposition of white cells on the fibres of the vitreous framework with granules of pigment.

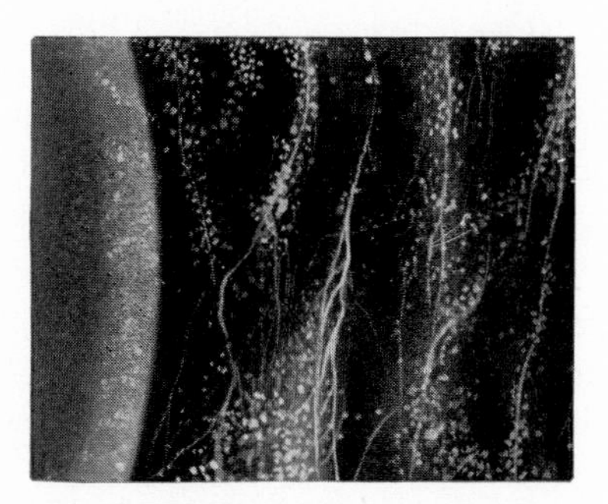

Fig. 166.—Vitreous Hæmorrhage following Concussion.

Yellowish blood cells are seen in large numbers, for the most part adherent to the vitreous framework. They are also deposited on the posterior capsule of the lens.

In one such case two months after a contusion, Hoffmann (1926) found Cloquet's canal thus filled up to the posterior pole of the lens. Eventually freely floating cholesterol crystals and fatty deposits on the retina may remain as evidence of the previous presence of blood (Rohrschneider, 1927; Gigglberger, 1937; Velhagen, 1940).

The fate of the vitreous hæmorrhages—whether they are absorbed or organized—and their treatment have already been considered.[2] In a traumatic hæmorrhage of any size absorption is usually slow, and even although it may eventually progress to the stage when vision again becomes normal, traces remain permanently in the form of cellular elements adhering to the vitreous framework. The gradual disappearance of the cellular elements and their ghosts is probably due to phagocytosis by polymorphonuclear cells from the blood and histiocytes and macrophages

[1] Mans (1922), Wirth (1922), Ascher (1923), Koby (1930), Vogt (1941).
[2] Vol. XI, p. 363.

derived from the non-pigmented ciliary epithelium and the pigmented retinal epithelium. These cells ingest the erythrocytes and transport them preferentially towards the posterior pole (Oguchi, 1913; Fuchs, 1919; Kiriyama, 1938). Organization of the blood clot by fibrous tissue to form a proliferating retinopathy is a more unfortunate occurrence which in its gross forms is typically associated with damage to the choroid and retina, while contracture of this tissue may result in a tearing and detachment of the retina. A much later complication is the reaction of *hæmosiderosis*[1] (Cibis *et al.*, 1959) associated with *hæmolytic glaucoma*, a condition due to the obstruction of the outflow channels by the debris of erythrocytes and pigmented macrophages, a complication which may in some cases be responsible for an acute glaucoma at a much earlier stage (Fenton and Zimmerman, 1963).

The *treatment* of a vitreous hæmorrhage whatever may be its cause is difficult. No matter what method is adopted, cellular elements and stromal debris, if not too abundant, eventually tend to disappear. Grosser opacities and connective tissue membranes, however, always persist and may subsequently lead to a detachment of the retina. To facilitate the disappearance of such opacities a wide variety of therapeutic measures has from time to time been advocated and their respective advantages and disadvantages have been fully considered elsewhere.[2] In recent years, however, additional techniques have been suggested to promote the disintegration of the hæmorrhage, as by the use of ultrasound (Drozdowska, 1964), or photocoagulation (Falkowska *et al.*, 1968); while the procedure of vitreous replacement[3] may be indicated in those cases in which a dense hæmorrhage shows no indication of spontaneous absorption. As a rule, particularly when the hæmorrhage is severe and in children, a period of rest in bed or at least of restricted physical activity is advisable until such time as sufficient clearing has occurred to permit inspection of the fundus for the detection of any retinal damage.

A DETACHMENT OF THE VITREOUS[4] after concussion injuries is not uncommon. Such a detachment may be localized in the posterior region only (Daily, 1970). A more gross detachment may be *infundibular* in type wherein the vitreous body assumes a tent-like shape, retaining its attachments only around its base at the ora and its apex at the optic disc; at other times the attachment at the disc gives way and a *posterior* detachment results wherein the entire gel becomes bunched up as a hemispherical mass behind the lens, leaving the posterior part of the vitreous chamber filled only with plasmoid intra-ocular fluid (Milles, 1886); while an *anterior* detachment in which the vitreous base is torn away from its attachment at the ora serrata is also a common result of a contusion or blast injury (Fig. 167).

[1] Vol. XI, p. 677.
[2] Vol. XI, p. 337.
[3] Vol. XI, p. 337.
[4] Vol. XI, p. 339.

HERNIATION OF THE VITREOUS INTO THE ANTERIOR CHAMBER, almost always a post-traumatic or post-operative condition, is common when the zonule has been injured, and in cases complicated by subluxation or dislocation of the lens or iridodialysis a prolapse of the gel is the rule (Plate IV, Fig. 4). Such a herniation may be relatively solid, forming a bead with a definitely demarcated border and a readily recognizable film-like structure which trembles jelly-like with movements of the globe and is displaced with movements of the pupil. It is always interspersed with pigment granules and frequently blood cells which remain red indefinitely; such a prolapse has been seen to diminish in size over several months (Koby, 1930).

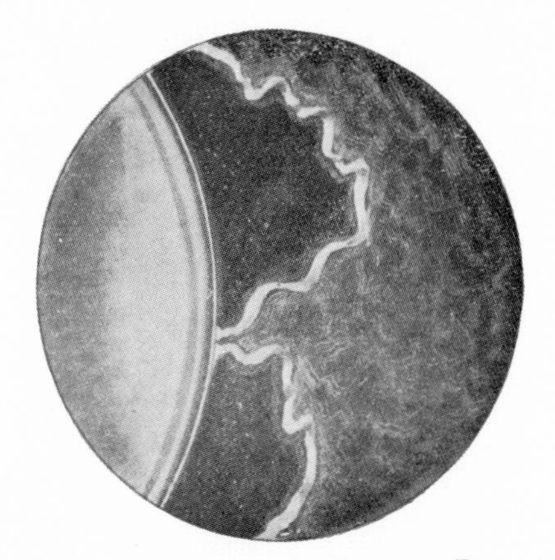

FIG. 167.—PARTIAL ANTERIOR VITREOUS DETACHMENT.
The detachment occurred after the explosion of a bomb; seen with the slit-lamp (A. S. Philps).

At other times when the gel is more fluid, its margin is ill-defined and it may fill the entire anterior chamber with a barely perceptible flocculence. In such an event, of course, the eye remains in a precarious state and is prone to suffer from secondary glaucoma, a complication giving rise to much anxiety and difficult to treat since any operative measures of relief which entail opening the globe may lead to a massive prolapse and loss of vitreous, while those designed to establish a filtering scar are liable to be nullified by blockage of the artificial drainage by vitreous humour; if a secondary glaucoma develops the best expedient—admittedly by no means always successful—is probably a cyclodialysis or a cyclodiathermy operation.[1]

Ascher. *Klin. Mbl. Augenheilk.*, **70**, 541 (1923).
Cibis, Yamashita and Rodriguez. *Arch. Ophthal.*, **62**, 180 (1959).
Daily. *Sth. med. J.*, **63**, 1197 (1970).
Davidson. *Amer. J. Ophthal.*, **19**, 757 (1936).
Drozdowska. *Klin. oczna*, **34**, 33 (1964).
Falkowska, Kecik, Malinowska and Szretter. *Brit. J. Ophthal.*, **52**, 450 (1968).
Fenton and Zimmerman. *Arch. Ophthal.*, **70**, 236 (1963).

[1] For a detailed discussion of the pathology and treatment of internal vitreous prolapse see Vol. XI, p. 368.

Fuchs. *v. Graefes Arch. Ophthal.*, **99**, 202 (1919).
Gigglberger. *Klin. Mbl. Augenheilk.*, **99**, 548 (1937).
Grün, Funder and Wyt. *Klin. Mbl. Augenheilk.*, **116**, 358 (1950).
Hoffmann. *Klin. Mbl. Augenheilk.*, **77**, 641 (1926).
Kawamoto. *Nip. Gank. Zas.*, **51**, 12 (1947).
Kirby. *Arch. Ophthal.*, **7**, 241 (1932).
Kiriyama. *Acta Soc. ophthal. jap.*, **42**, 1773 (1938).
Koby. *Slit-lamp Microscopy of the Living Eye*, London (1930).
Lagrange. *Atlas d'ophtalmoscopie de guerre*, Paris (1918).
Lavine, Langenstrass, Bowyer *et al.* *Arch. Ophthal.*, **47**, 204 (1952).
Mans. *Klin. Mbl. Augenheilk.*, **68**, 450 (1922).
Milles. *Roy. Lond. ophthal. Hosp. Rep.*, **11**, 26 (1886).
Oguchi. *v. Graefes Arch. Ophthal.*, **84**, 446 (1913).
Rohrschneider. *Z. Augenheilk.*, **61**, 296 (1927).
Velhagen. *v. Graefes Arch. Ophthal.*, **142**, 37 (1940).
Vogt. *Hb. u. Atlas d. Spaltlampenmikroskopie d. lebenden Auges*, 2nd ed., Zürich, **3** (1941).
Wirth. *Z. Augenheilk.*, **47**, 1 (1922).
Zeiss. *v. Graefes Arch. Ophthal.*, **139**, 301 (1938).

Ruptures of the Sclera

RUPTURES OF THE SCLERA may be conveniently divided into two types—*contusion ruptures* due to the direct impingement upon the globe of a slowly moving blunt force sufficiently powerful to burst it, and *ruptures caused indirectly* by the passage of a high velocity missile through the orbit sufficiently close to disintegrate the globe by concussion-waves. Since the mechanism and the results of the two accidents are very different we shall consider them separately. A rupture of the eyeball may also occur when it is actually traversed by a swiftly moving foreign body such as a bullet or a fragment of a shell; the last two types of trauma will be discussed under the heading of Gunshot Wounds.[1]

CONTUSION RUPTURES

CONTUSION RUPTURES may be divided into direct and indirect, the former, however, being much more rare than the latter.

DIRECT RUPTURES

In a DIRECT RUPTURE the ocular envelope gives way at the point of impact of an impinging force which suddenly indents it. It is obvious that such an injury will affect essentially the anterior part of the globe and this type of rupture may therefore occur in the cornea, a subject which has already been considered.[2] It will be remembered that partial ruptures of this tissue may occur involving either the superficial layers including Bowman's membrane or the deeper layers including Descemet's membrane, while a complete rupture is a rarity seen mainly in children unless the cornea is already weakened by old ulceration or other disease. Similarly if the sclera is struck it may perforate at the site of impact, an accident reported as occurring in injuries such as a fall upon a bed-post (Jessop, 1885) or the edge of a barrel (Müller, 1895) or a blow from the horn of a cow (Bertram, 1901). Such injuries are rare: thus Müller found 2 among 27 cases of scleral rupture,

[1] p. 686. [2] p. 86.

the remaining 25 being indirect in origin. They are, however, usually serious in nature for considerable damage is generally caused to the inner eye, prolapse of the uveal tissue results and the common sequel in those cases which do not require excision is atrophy of the globe; exceptionally, however, useful vision may be retained (Jessop, 1885; Simonsen, 1906).

INDIRECT RUPTURES

A COMPLETE INDIRECT SCLERAL RUPTURE is a relatively common result of severe contusions of the globe; it is a lesion usually attended by grave intra-ocular injuries and followed by prolonged and often serious complications so that, although a proportion of cases ends happily (12 out of 35, Müller, 1895), the majority requires immediate excision or the case terminates in shrinkage and atrophy of the globe.

A dramatic injury such as this would be expected to have a long history in ophthalmological literature and to have excited much attention. Early records are found in the writings of Bartisch (1583), Edmonston (1806), Beer (1813), Demours (1818), Middlemore (1835), Mackenzie (1839), and others. Sachs (1889) collected 114 cases from the literature up to his time, and in his classical paper on the subject, L. Müller (1895) described 45 cases from the Vienna clinic alone; similarly, Tempelhof (1903) reported on 20 cases from Jena. It is interesting that the accident is most common in older patients, probably because of the loss of the resilience of the sclera with increasing age. It is true that scleral ruptures may occur in the young (2 years, Nuel, 1888; 7, Tempelhof, 1903; 15, Purtscher, 1905; 17, Cooper, 1859), but in them a corneal rupture is more usual. As age advances the injury becomes more common; thus Müller (1895) found 18 cases before the age of 40 years and 26 after, and Briolat (1879) found 1 case at 17, 3 between 30 and 40, 4 between 40 and 50, 6 between 50 and 60, and 7 between 60 and 70. An interesting case was described by Bhaduri (1955) wherein a child sustained a complete indirect rupture of the sclera with a dislocation of the lens by a blow from a leaping fish.

The causal injury is always gross and is usually due to a large blunt body being driven into the orbit between the globe and the orbital wall. Ruptures are not easily caused by an impact directly on the cornea which forces the globe backwards, for in this case the blow is cushioned and its force largely lost in the soft mass of the orbital fat; the blow which bursts the eye is typically directed obliquely so that the globe is forced sideways against the unyielding orbital wall: thus in 29 cases of scleral rupture, Müller (1895) found the direction of force to be upwards (and in or out) in 22, down and in in 3, down and out in 2, and down in 2.

The type of injury varies considerably. In 97 of his cases, Sachs (1889) found 23 from cows' horns, 21 from falls against ordinary objects such as household furniture, 14 from objects such as a stick, 8 from blows with the fist, 6 from fingers thrust into the orbit, 12 from flying pieces of wood, stone, etc., 4 from animals' hoofs, 3 from whip-lashes, and so on. Other causes include a great variety of relatively slowly moving objects ranging from snowballs to soda-water and champagne corks. In the case of diseased eyes, of course, such as those with a staphyloma, high myopia, buphthalmos or absolute glaucoma, rupture is caused by less severe injury. The frequency with which an animal's horn used to figure in the ætiology is striking: one-third of Müller's (1895) cases was due to this cause; of 33 such traumata seen at Göttingen only 11 cases escaped without a rupture of the globe, 15 suffered complete and 5 partial scleral rupture, and 6 corneal rupture (Bertram, 1901). A half-century later, Moncreiff and Scheribel (1945) in America found that the most common cause was a blow from a bare fist (23 out of 52 cases) with falls ranking second; automobile accidents also figure commonly in the ætiology.

A *double rupture* of the same eye is exceptional; Shumway (1906) described a patient with one at the nasal and the other at the temporal side of the limbus, and Reïs (1926) a second case wherein two parallel ruptures occurred in the temporal quadrant, one through the sclera near the limbus and one through the cornea; both occurred after blows with the fist. Double ruptures, one in the typical position and one situated meridionally or posteriorly, have also been noted (Coroenne, 1887; Legendre, 1894; Simonsen, 1906; and others). A double rupture sustained at different times has been recorded by Praun (1899); the second followed 15 months after the first and was situated 3 mm. behind the initial scar; the eye retained useful (aphakic) vision in spite of its adventures.

Bilateral scleral ruptures occurring simultaneously have been recorded as a rarity in extensive facial injuries such as that due to the kick of a horse (Wordsworth, 1881) or cow (Lafon and Villemonte, 1906); such an accident has been recorded as inflicted by the fingers of a lunatic in an attack on a fellow patient, necessitating bilateral evisceration (Pajtas, 1951). Occurring at successive times, bilateral ruptures are more common, particularly in persons habitually exposed to the same danger.

The site of an indirect scleral rupture is remarkably constant. The TYPICAL RUPTURE runs concentrically with the limbus, starts internally from the extreme periphery of the anterior chamber and traverses the sclera obliquely to emerge upon the surface 2 to 4 mm. behind the corneo-scleral junction, and is situated in the vast majority of cases above the horizontal meridian, usually in the upper and inner quadrant of the globe (Fig. 171); the reason for this preferential incidence is the exposure of the eye to a glancing blow in the lower and outer parts of the orbit where the bony protection provided elsewhere by the prominent upper orbital rim or the nose is lacking. Although the extent of a rupture cannot be accurately assessed unless pathological examination is made, it varies as a rule between 10 and 14 mm. in length, but variations from 2 mm. (Boerner, 1902) to one-half the circumference of the limbus have been noted (20 mm., Willgeroth, 1896).

In his 114 cases, Sachs (1889) found 36 above, 20 in, 21 up and in, 11 up and out, 8 out, 2 down and in, and 2 down and out. Purtscher (1905) in 61 scleral ruptures found 24 up and in, 16 up, 7 up and out, 6 in, 1 down and out, 1 down and in, 1 down, while 1 was behind the equator.

The *mechanism of the formation of indirect ruptures* of the sclera after a contusion has excited considerable controversy, but there seems little reason to doubt the explanation offered by Arlt (1875) and substantiated by Müller (1895) who based his opinion both on clinical and experimental evidence. When the eye is struck by a slowly moving object which does not perforate it, the globe is indented in the diameter of the line of impact and if the pole opposite the point of impact is supported, the eyeball must necessarily expand in the diameter at right angles to the line of impact (Fig. 168). It is found that with a blow upon a hollow sphere the resistance of the envelope to pressure is one-third greater than its tensile strength; it therefore follows that the eyeball will not tend to burst at the point of impact where the pressure is directly applied (direct rupture) but gives way more readily at a distant point where the globe is suddenly distended to the greatest extent.

We have already seen that a blow directly from in front is largely cushioned by the orbital fat so that no rupture easily occurs; but if the blow impinges obliquely on the eye, the globe is forced against the bony orbital

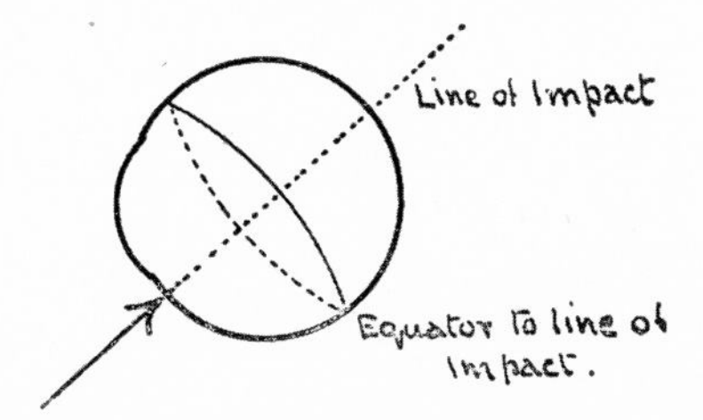

Fig. 168.—The Mechanics of Rupture of the Globe.

When the eye is compressed along the line of impact a forced expansion occurs along the equator to this line, tending to cause a rupture at the weakest point where the equator is nearest to the limbus (W. Lister).

wall and a maximum distension around the equator to the line of impact will occur. With the usual blow striking the anterior surface of the globe obliquely this meridian of expansion will generally pass as a great circle a little behind the limbus at one point and encircle the globe posteriorly at the opposite point (Fig. 168). Around this circle the sclera is supported by the extra-ocular muscles and the orbital tissues except anteriorly where the surface of the globe is exposed. Here also a weak region of the sclera exists where its continuity is broken by the canal of Schlemm and its associated perforating vessels, and the dense scleral fibres are to some extent replaced by the more open network of the trabeculæ. Moreover, in this region the peculiar arrangement of the scleral fibres, which split in a circular direction between the limbus and the insertions of the extra-ocular muscles, is probably another source of weakness tending to make the rupture run outwards and posteriorly from its starting point at the canal of Schlemm (Kokott, 1934–35). The point at which the meridian of greatest expansion approaches the corneo-scleral margin therefore tends to give way preferentially even although the sclera is thinner posteriorly; and since the usual site of impact is down and out where the least bony protection is provided by the orbital rim, the most common site of rupture is up and in about 3 mm. behind the limbus. Moreover, since the globe is burst by an explosive force from within, the rupture occurs from within outwards, the largest gap is on the internal surface, and the walls give way in the order—sclera, episclera, conjunctiva; if the rupture is partial it will affect preferentially the inner layers of the sclera. It was established by Fuchs (1905), however, that in young people the rupture, instead of being directed posteriorly to reach the surface 3 or 4 mm. behind the limbus, may run straight outwards from the

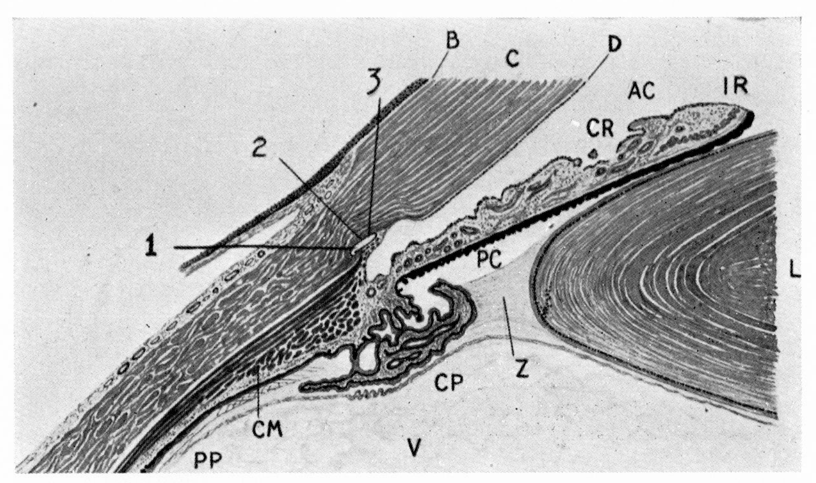

FIG. 169.—THE SITES OF INDIRECT RUPTURE OF THE SCLERA.

1. The direction of the typical rupture from the canal of Schlemm to appear on the surface of the sclera, 2 to 4 mm. behind the limbus.

2 and 3. Atypical ruptures running either directly outwards to appear near the limbus (2) or outwards and forwards to appear on the surface of the cornea itself (3, the atypical rupture of Fuchs occurring particularly in young people).

AC, anterior chamber; B, Bowman's membrane; C, corneal stroma; CM, ciliary muscle; CP, ciliary processes; CR, crypt of iris; D, Descemet's membrane; IR, iris; L, lens; PC, posterior chamber; PP, pars plana; V, vitreous; Z, zonule.

canal of Schlemm to the limbus or even somewhat forward into the cornea; such ruptures are usually small (Fig. 169).

These views have evolved after much speculation. The forcing of the globe against the orbital wall was stressed by Zander and Geissler (1864), the rupture at the unsupported part of the sclera by Manz (1865). Müller (1895) held that the weakness of the region of the corneo-scleral margin was increased owing to the abolition of the corneo-scleral groove by the sudden internal pressure, and he also attached considerable importance to the counter-pressure of the trochlea at the site of the most extreme distension of the globe in a typical rupture. Finally, the weakness caused by the presence of Schlemm's canal was particularly stressed by Fuchs (1905), to which factor Sachs (1889) added the concept of a forced rush of aqueous under great pressure through its normal channels of exit.

Experimental observations on the eyes of the human cadaver (von Seidlitz, 1873;

Berlin, 1873; Müller, 1895) have thrown little light on the subject, but they have shown that a pressure of 8–9 kg. is required to cause a rupture (25–27 kg. on the ox eye, Rouquette, 1892); similarly uninformative were investigations on the breaking strain of meridional strips of cornea and sclera which merely show that these tissues give way at their thinnest spot (Stoewer, 1892).

The *clinical picture* presented by a ruptured globe, as would be expected, is dramatic and grave. The lids are usually swollen and bruised so that even to open the eye for inspection is difficult, and the difficulties are often increased by the presence of considerable orbital hæmorrhage and proptosis. Moreover, if the conjunctiva is intact, a massive ecchymosis may obscure the rupture which may not itself be seen until the blood has absorbed, when the tear in the sclera usually appears with everted and somewhat gaping edges between which black uveal tissue bulges; alternatively, a subconjunctival dislocation of the lens may be obvious (Plate VIII). If, however, the conjunctiva has also given way, the contents of the globe may be extruded onto the cheek or lost entirely, an event usually associated with considerable hæmorrhage.

An injury so severe obviously causes much simultaneous intra-ocular damage and almost every major lesion discussed in our systematic review of contusive injuries to the globe may be found. An extensive intra-ocular hæmorrhage is the rule and the anterior chamber is usually filled with blood obscuring all view of the inner eye; to this may be added a massive vitreous hæmorrhage, and until the blood is absorbed to some extent any assessment of the damage to the eye may be impossible. In only a few cases does the lens remain in position, for it is usually dislocated into the anterior chamber or, more rarely, into the vitreous; thence it is commonly extruded from the globe, anteriorly into the subconjunctival tissues in typical ruptures or posteriorly into Tenon's capsule in atypical ruptures (Plate VIII; Figs. 170–174).[1] The iris is almost always torn and an iridodialysis is the rule at the site of the rupture, an extensive prolapse of the anterior uveal tissues into the rupture is usual, while the remainder of the iris may retain its place so that a colobomatous appearance results, pointing usefully to the site of rupture if this is obscured by subconjunctival hæmorrhage; occasionally the portion of the iris remaining in the eye suffers inversion or the whole of this tissue may be extruded (traumatic aniridia). The ciliary body may be torn or suffer dialysis, the retina and choroid usually remain intact even if all the other contents of the globe are expelled, or they may be torn or detached by massive subchoroidal hæmorrhages, while the vitreous may be lost in part or in its entirety. The cardinal sign in all cases is the softness and the collapse of the globe. In such cases, of course, the eye is immediately blinded and there is much lacrimation and pain and considerable shock.

Occasionally, however, the trauma is less gross. The lens may incarcerate itself in the rupture and prevent any extensive prolapse of the

[1] p. 206.

intra-ocular tissues. The pupil may remain round and the iris appear to be intact even if the lens has been dislocated (2 cases in 114, Sachs, 1889); sometimes, although again rarely, the lens remains in its normal position (3 cases in 114, Sachs, 1889); but the retention of the integrity of the globe to this extent, although by no means unknown, is unusual. In such cases

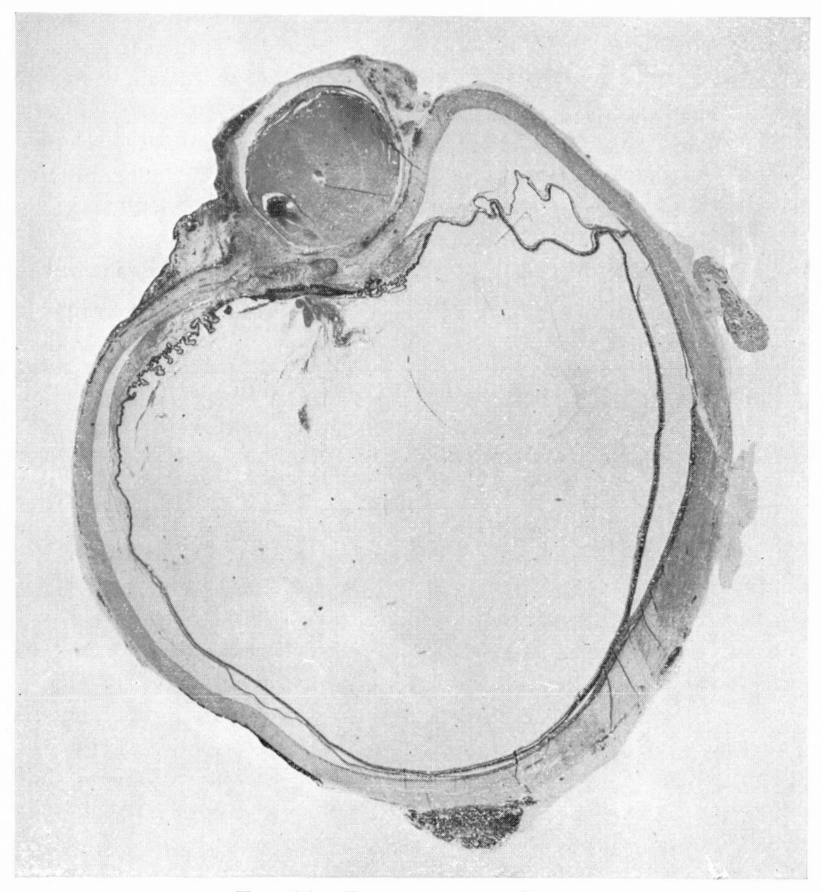

Fig. 170.—Rupture of the Globe.

Section of an eye from a man aged 34, which was struck with a heavy chain; the injury resulted in a rupture of the sclera with extrusion of the lens into the sub-conjunctival tissues (N. Ashton).

the rupture heals by the formation of fibrous tissue, the edges, initially everted, become inverted and depressed, frequently deforming the globe in their cicatrization, while some pigmentary deposition derived from the uvea may permanently mark the site.[1] Sometimes the pigmentary dispersion is very

[1] Caspar (1893), Wintersteiner (1893), Kiranow (1896), Hirsch (1897), Leonhardt (1908), Gebb (1908), Ask (1913), Kagan (1914), and many others.

FIGS. 171 to 174.—RUPTURE OF THE GLOBE (Museum, Inst. Ophthal.).

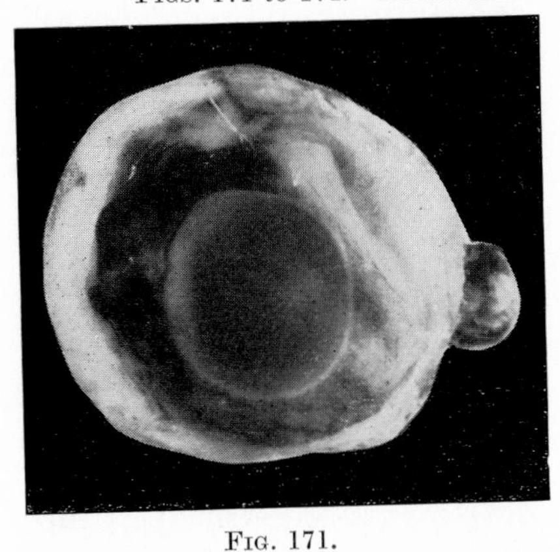

FIG. 171.

An extensive typical rupture of the globe after a contusion.

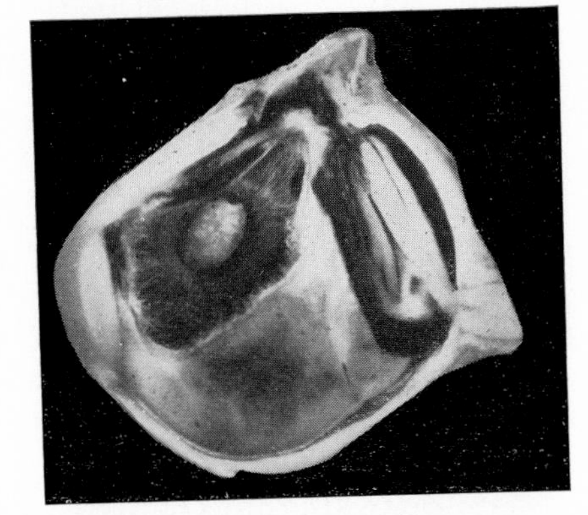

FIG. 172.—EQUATORIAL RUPTURE.

To the site of the rupture are adherent most of the intra-ocular contents, some of which are prolapsed through the wound. The iris, which has remained intact, has been dragged bodily towards it and the dislocated lens is seen in the pupil.

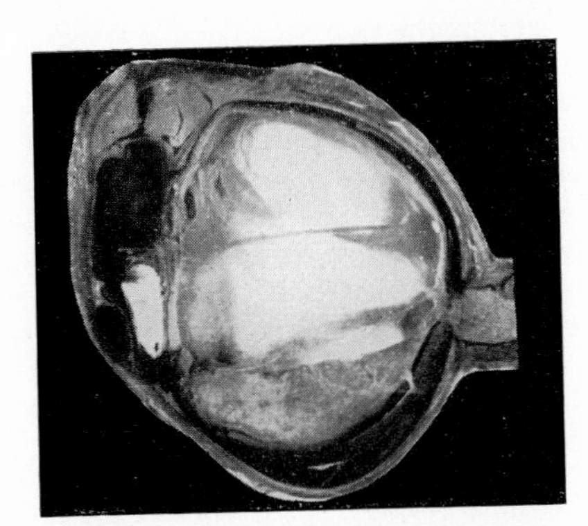

FIG. 173.—RUPTURE OF THE GLOBE ABOVE THE CORNEAL MARGIN.

In a girl of 7. The iris is largely adherent to the cornea and the lens has been almost entirely absorbed. Above the cornea there is a gap in the sclera through which the uvea protrudes. Above this, there is a large cyst lined by conjunctival epithelium which covers the uvea at its inner side and insinuates itself between the cornea and the iris, breaking through the rupture in the sclera.

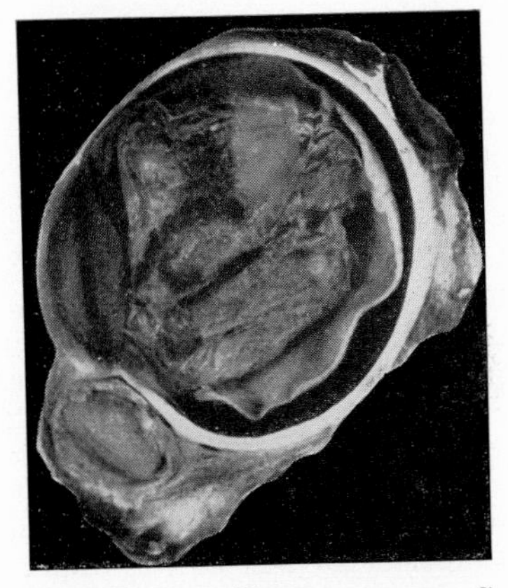

FIG. 174.—TYPICAL RUPTURE OF THE GLOBE WITH SUBCONJUNCTIVAL DISLOCATION OF THE LENS.

After an injury by an iron hook. There is a rupture of the sclera below the limbus and an extensive rupture of the choroid. The iris is torn at its root and is rolled up in the anterior chamber. The suprachoroidal space is filled with hæmorrhage raising up the retina by blood clot.

extensive and it has been observed to affect large areas of the palpebral conjunctiva and even the skin of the lids up to the orbital margin (Cashell, 1948). Occasionally the wound may become staphylomatous (Landesberg, 1887; and others), a sequel which has had the unusual effect of producing a high degree of myopia in an atypical posterior rupture reported by Schrag (1870).

The *pathological anatomy* of scleral ruptures has attracted much attention (Figs. 171–174). The typical rupture starts internally in the extreme periphery of the anterior chamber, traverses the trabeculæ and the canal of Schlemm and runs through the sclera posteriorly and obliquely to reach the surface 3 or 4 mm. behind the cornea. The inner aspect of the wound is always larger than the outer, and in it is usually incarcerated a variable amount of intra-ocular tissue.[1]

ATYPICAL RUPTURES at the corneo-scleral margin, occurring particularly in young people, were described by Fuchs (1905), wherein the tear starts internally in the usual way in the region of the canal of Schlemm and, instead of running through the sclera backwards to reach the scleral surface 2 to 4 mm. behind the limbus, runs in an obliquely forward direction to appear externally at the limbus or in the cornea itself (Fig. 169). Such ruptures are usually small, some 2 to 4 mm. in length, and have a relatively good prognosis partly because of their small size and partly because the associated prolapse if present is usually confined to the iris.

Although ruptures of the choroid are common in the posterior part of the globe, *atypical contusion ruptures* running meridionally at or behind the equator involving the sclera are less frequent (Nuel, 1888; Purtscher, 1905; and others); 41 such cases were collected by Riffenburgh (1963). They are caused by such injuries as the thrusting into the orbit of a finger (Oeller, 1880; Axenfeld, 1899) or the horn of an ox (Pagenstecher, 1879; Schlodtmann, 1897; B. Schäfer, 1926) and automobile accidents (Riffenburgh, 1963). Such a lesion may be determined by local weakness due to a posterior staphyloma in a highly myopic eye (Wintersteiner, 1903; Casanovas, 1933) or buphthalmos (Casanovas, 1933). An atypical posterior rupture of this type may escape discovery until the eye is enucleated (Cooper, 1859; Legendre, 1894) or a pathological examination is made (Weeks, 1886; Ask, 1913; and others); such a lesion has, however, been diagnosed by ultrasound (Oksala and Lehtinen, 1958). The rupture is frequently found to be complicated by a dislocation of the lens into Tenon's capsule (Wadsworth, 1885; Montagnon, 1887; Ask, 1913). To this category ruptures of the lamina cribrosa[2] properly belong. It is interesting that Mules (1887) reported a case due to an injury with a brick wherein the optic disc was dislocated backwards with a surrounding frill of sclera.

Pathological examinations of atypical ruptures at and behind the equator were recorded by Weeks (1886), Schlodtmann (1897), Wintersteiner (1903), Ask (1913), B. Schäfer (1926), Riffenburgh (1963), and others.

The general *prognosis* of a ruptured globe is poor; if the eye does not require immediate excision the usual ultimate result is phthisis and atrophy or, more rarely, infection and panophthalmitis. If the globe remains intact

[1] Schiess-Gemuseus (1868), Alt (1877), Mitvalsky (1897), Fehr (1898), Henderson (1904), Gross (1907), Fuchs (1911), and many others.

[2] p. 187.

the dangers of a subluxated or luxated lens have to be overcome and secondary glaucoma may follow, while vision may be grossly impaired by permanent vitreous opacities and the proliferation of fibrous tissue in the posterior segment of the globe. A traumatic uveitis is an invariable complication, and sympathetic ophthalmitis has been recorded in a significant number of cases.[1] Schirmer (1900) collected 27 cases in the literature up to his time. This tragedy may occur even if the conjunctiva remains intact: among 17 ruptured globes thus affected Müller (1895) found 9 with the conjunctiva torn and 8 with this membrane undamaged. The onset of tetanus is an exceptional additional tragedy (Müller, 1895).

Not every case, however, follows this somewhat gloomy history and the number of cases which are reported with a healed scleral rupture is testimony to the recuperative powers of the eye although gravely damaged. As a rule such cases have had a subconjunctival dislocation of the lens and retain aphakic vision. It may be said that about one-quarter or one-third of ruptured eyes retain some vision, although this is usually poor (12 out of 35, Müller, 1895; 10 in 35, Eversheim, 1906; 12 in 52, Moncreiff and Scheribel 1945); only occasionally does normal (but usually aphakic) vision result,[2] and may exceptionally follow an injury so severe as to cause aniridia, or aniridia and aphakia (Simkova and Zahn, 1951). The best prognosis attaches to the small limbal ruptures, in which the ciliary body is not involved in the prolapse. Nevertheless, even after a prolapse of the iris and ciliary body normal vision has been attained (El-Naggar, 1961).

Thus in a bilateral rupture caused by the kick of a horse, a patient observed by Wordsworth (1881) eventually obtained bilateral normal aphakic vision; Fuchs (1889) recorded a similar case in a farmer who had his eyes ruptured on successive occasions by a cow's horn; each eye was healed and aphakic but had retained good vision, two excellent intracapsular extractions having been performed by the animal. As we have noted, an eye has survived a double rupture with the retention of useful vision (Praun, 1899). Würdemann (1932) also reported an interesting case of a man with cataract in one eye who was struck with a cow's horn in the other; he "felt the water of the eye run out" and put on a home-made bandage without consulting a doctor. Some time later, when the vision returned, he obtained spectacles from an optician and with these he saw sufficiently well to continue his activities happily.

The only *treatment* possible in too many cases of a rupture of the eyeball is immediate excision; but if the globe is not disorganized an attempt may be made to retain the eye. In this event rest with bandaging is probably the best course to adopt for 24 hours, antibiotics being administered locally and systemically to avoid the development of infection, and tetanus toxoid, particularly if the injury has been received in rural surroundings. If the wound does not gape widely, prolapse of uveal tissue has not occurred

[1] Bartisch (1583), Lawson (1865), Gunn (1886), Sachs (1889), Müller (1895), and many others.

[2] Jeaffreson (1871), Eales and White (1899), Rowan (1900), Schreiber (1904), de Schweinitz (1905), Cashell (1948), and others.

and the conjunctiva is intact, the eye may be left alone even although a luxated lens lies under the conjunctiva. If, however, the uvea herniates through or is prolapsed, operative measures are necessary. A conjunctival flap is prepared, scleral sutures inserted, any prolapsed tissue excised or healthy herniating uveal tissue reposed, and the scleral wound closed and covered by a conjunctival flap.

INCOMPLETE CONCUSSION RUPTURES

Since, as we have seen, a rupture of the sclera starts internally and bursts outwards, a partial rupture will affect the inner layers only. Such an occurrence is obviously difficult to prove clinically; for a certain diagnosis an anatomical examination is essential.

A DIRECT INCOMPLETE RUPTURE is said to occur at the region of the canal of Schlemm often as a result of relatively minor traumata at the limbus from light bodies such as a pencil, or flying objects with a small velocity such as a piece of metal or spent shot. Such a lesion was produced experimentally by Berlin (1873) and the early literature was collected by Czermak (1889). Mechanically the lesion forms the first stage of the process of the classical typical rupture of the globe. The clinical picture ascribed to this accident is the sudden accumulation of a large hyphæma which is followed by the appearance of red lines of hæmorrhage running into the posterior layers of the cornea from the limbus, associated with œdematous corneal opacities and folds in Descemet's membrane. Initially there is slight pain and obscuration of vision due to the hyphæma which is rapidly resolved, but normal vision does not return until the corneal opacity eventually disappears. The prognosis is good with expectant treatment. That such an injury may occur is undoubted, but that all the cases described as such in the literature (before the days of gonioscopy), some of them associated with visible intra-ocular lesions such as iridodialysis, are in fact due to such a rupture is problematical.

INDIRECT TYPICAL INCOMPLETE RUPTURES are also rare and, since most of the cases reported as such depend on the clinical appearance only, the true diagnosis must be open to doubt; in this case the trauma involved is usually considerable. The usual criterion has been that after an injury a bluish-black line has appeared in the sclera in the typical position concentric with the limbus, and this has usually developed into a staphylomatous condition at a later date.[1] Anatomical studies demonstrating the occurrence of such a lesion, however, have been published by several observers[2]; a rupture has been demonstrated running from the periphery of the anterior chamber through the trabeculæ (Fig. 70) or traversing the canal of Schlemm and running some distance into the sclera. Burk (1912) described the pathology of a small partial rupture at the limbus itself, corresponding to the first stage of the atypical ruptures in this locality described by Fuchs (1905).

INDIRECT ATYPICAL INCOMPLETE RUPTURES are very rare indeed; Garnier (1891) described a case which may have been of this nature, wherein a localized staphyloma

[1] Arlt (1875), Müller (1895), Bertram (1901), Fuchs (1905), Purtscher (1905).

[2] H. Schäfer (1883), Buchanan (1907), Fuchs (1911), von Szily (1918), Tillema (1936), and Rones and Wilder (1947).

was found in the upper and inner quadrant when an eye was excised two weeks after a blow. Axenfeld (1899) described a tearing of the inner layers of the sclera at the equator in the eye of a lunatic who had gouged it out with his finger; this may have been a direct injury. Tillema (1936) described two cases in eyes removed for painful traumatic glaucoma; one had knocked his eye against a wooden box on falling, and the other was hit in the eye with a piece of wood; in both, pathological examination revealed a partial rupture of the inner layers of the sclera in the upper and inner quadrant running towards the equator, a lesion complicated in the first case by a typical partial rupture running backwards and outwards from Schlemm's canal along the line of the perforating vessels.

Alt. *Arch. Augenheilk.*, **6**, 8, 84 (1877).
Arlt. *Ueber d. Verletzungen d. Auges*, Wien (1875).
Ask. *Klin. Mbl. Augenheilk.*, **51** (2), 331 (1913).
Axenfeld. *Z. Augenheilk.*, **1**, 128 (1899).
Bartisch. Οφθαλμοδουλεια, *Das ist Augendienst*, Dresden, 204 (1583).
Beer. *Lehre v. d. Augenkrankheiten*, Wien, **1**, 176 (1813).
Berlin. *Klin. Mbl. Augenheilk.*, **11**, 42 (1873).
Bertram. *Ueber Kuhhornverletzungen d. Auges* (Diss.), Göttingen (1901).
Bhaduri. *J. All-India ophthal. Soc.*, **3**, 17 (1955).
Boerner. *Ueber Kuhhornverletzungen d. Auges* (Diss.), Halle (1902).
Briolat. *Étude sur la luxation sous-conjonctivale du cristallin* (Thèse), Paris (1879).
Buchanan. *Trans. ophthal. Soc. U.K.*, **27**, 103 (1907).
Burk. *v. Graefes Arch. Ophthal.*, **83**, 114, 131 (1912).
Casanovas. *Z. Augenheilk.*, **80**, 35 (1933).
Cashell. *Trans. ophthal. Soc. U.K.*, **68**, 241 (1948).
Caspar. *Klin. Mbl. Augenheilk.*, **31**, 395 (1893).
Cooper. *On Wounds and Injuries of the Eye*, London (1859).
Coroenne. *Bull. Clin. Ophtal. Hosp. Quinze-Vingts*, **5**, 97 (1887).
Czermak. *Klin. Mbl. Augenheilk.*, **27**, 132 (1889).
Demours. *Traité des maladies des yeux*, Paris (1818).
Eales and White. *Lancet*, **2**, 412 (1899).
Edmonston. *Treatise on Varieties and Consequences of the Ophthalmy*, Edinburgh (1806).
El-Naggar. *Bull. ophthal. Soc. Egypt*, **54**, 226 (1961).
Eversheim. *Ueber Kuhhornstossverletzungen d. Auges* (Diss.), Bonn (1906).
Fehr. *Zbl. prakt. Augenheilk.*, **22**, 375 (1898).
Fuchs. *Lhb. d. Augenheilkunde*, Wien, 247 (1889).
Wien. klin. Wschr., **18**, 985 (1905).
v. Graefes Arch. Ophthal., **79**, 53 (1911).
Garnier. *Wratsch.*, **12**, 636 (1891).
Gebb. *Arch. Augenheilk.*, **59**, 223 (1908).
Gross. *Arch. Augenheilk.*, **57**, 9 (1907).
Gunn. *Roy. Lond. ophthal. Hosp. Rep.*, **11**, 78 (1886).
Henderson. *Trans. ophthal. Soc. U.K.*, **24**, 80 (1904).
Hirsch. *Beitr. Augenheilk.*, **3** (26), 477 (1897).
Jeaffreson. *Roy. Lond. ophthal. Hosp. Rep.*, **7**, 191 (1871).
Jessop. *Trans. ophthal. Soc. U.K.*, **5**, 199 (1885).
Kagan. *Pathologisch-anatomische Untersuchung eines Falles v. indirekter subconjunctivaler Skleralruptur* (Diss.), Heidelberg (1914).
Kiranow. *Beitr. Augenheilk.*, **3** (24), 348 (1896).
Kokott. *Klin. Mbl. Augenheilk.*, **92**, 177 (1934); **95**, 33 (1935).
Lafon and Villemonte. *J. Méd. Bordeaux*, **36**, 934 (1906).
Landesberg. *Arch. Augenheilk.*, **17**, 202 (1887).
Lawson. *Med. Times Gaz.*, **1**, 570, 596 (1865).
Legendre. *Contribution à l'étude des ruptures de la sclérotique* (Thèse), Bordeaux (1894).
Leonhardt. *v. Graefes Arch. Ophthal.*, **68**, 484 (1908).
Lister. *Brit. J. Ophthal.*, **8**, 305 (1924).
Mackenzie. *Practical Treatise on the Diseases of the Eye*, London (1839).
Manz. *Klin. Mbl. Augenheilk.*, **3**, 170 (1865).
Middlemore. *Treatise on Diseases of the Eye*, Birmingham, **2**, 44 (1835).
Mitvalsky. *Arch. Ophtal.*, **17**, 337 (1897).
Moncreiff and Scheribel. *Amer. J. Ophthal.*, **28**, 1212 (1945).
Montagnon. *Arch. Ophtal.*, **7**, 204 (1887).
Mules. *Trans. ophthal. Soc. U.K.*, **7**, 298 (1887).
Müller. *Ueber Ruptur des Corneo-Skleralgrenze durch stumpfe Verletzung*, Leipzig (1895).
Nuel. *Ann. Oculist.* (Paris), **99**, 264 (1888).
Oeller. *Zbl. prakt. Augenheilk.*, **4**, 255 (1880).
Oksala and Lehtinen. *Acta ophthal.* (Kbh.), **36**, 37 (1958).
Pagenstecher. *Arch. Augenheilk.*, **8**, 65 (1879).
Pajtas. *Cs. oftal.*, **7**, 137 (1951).
Praun. *Die Verletzungen des Auges*, Wiesbaden (1899).
Purtscher. *Beitr. Augenheilk., Fest. J. Hirschberg*, 227 (1905).
Reïs. *Arch. Ophtal.*, **43**, 544 (1926).

Riffenburgh. *Arch. Ophthal.*, **69**, 722 (1963).
Rones and Wilder. *Amer. J. Ophthal.*, **30**, 1143 (1947).
Rouquette. *Contribution à l'étude clinique des blessures de l'oeil pars corps étrangers* (Thèse), Lyons (1892).
Rowan. *Ophthal. Rev.*, **19**, 121 (1900).
Sachs. *Arch. Augenheilk.*, **20**, 367 (1889).
Schäfer, B. *v. Graefes Arch. Ophthal.*, **117**, 693 (1926).
Schäfer, H. *v. Graefes Arch. Ophthal.*, **29** (1), 13 (1883).
Schiess-Gemuseus. *v. Graefes Arch. Ophthal.*, **14** (1), 91 (1868).
Schirmer. *Graefe-Saemisch Hb. d. ges. Augenheilk.*, 2nd ed., Leipzig, **6** (2) Kap. VIII (1900).
Schlodtmann. *v. Graefes Arch. Ophthal.*, **44** (1), 127 (1897).
Schrag. *Einige Fälle von Rupturen d. Sklera u. d. Choroidea* (Diss.), Leipzig (1870).
Schreiber. *Münch. med. Wschr.*, **51**, 1177 (1904).
de Schweinitz. *Ophthal. Rec.*, **14**, 195 (1905).
von Seidlitz. *Experimentaluntersuchungen ü. Zerreissung d. Choroidea* (Diss.), Kiel (1873).
Shumway. *Ophthal. Rec.*, **15**, 534, 611 (1906).
Simkova and Zahn. *Cs. oftal.*, **7**, 109 (1951).
Simonsen. *Zur Prognose u. Therapie d. Bulbusrupturen* (Diss.), Giessen (1906).
Stoewer. *Arch. Augenheilk.*, **24**, 255 (1892).
von Szily. *Atlas d. Kriegsaugenheilkunde*, Stuttgart (1918).
Tempelhof. *Weiterer Beitrag z. Kenntnis d. subkonjunktivalen Bulbusrupturen* (Diss.), Jena (1903).
Tillema. *Brit. J. Ophthal.*, **20**, 193 (1936).
Wadsworth. *Amer. J. Ophthal.*, **2**, 144 (1885).
Weeks. *Arch. Augenheilk.*, **16**, 125 (1886).
Willgeroth. *Beitrag z. Kenntnis d. subkonjunktivalen Bulbusrupturen* (Diss.), Jena (1896).
Wintersteiner. *Wien. klin. Wschr.*, **6**, 101 (1893).
v. Graefes Arch. Ophthal., **40** (2), 1 (1894).
Klin. Mbl. Augenheilk., **41** (1), 499 (1903).
Wordsworth. *Roy. Lond. ophthal. Hosp. Rep.*, **10**, 204 (1881).
Würdemann. *Injuries of the Eye*, London (1932).
Zander and Geissler. *Die Verletzungen des Auges*, Heidelberg (1864).

Concussion Effects on the Refraction

Post-traumatic changes in refraction are well-known, occasionally involving a hypermetropia, but more commonly myopia.

TRAUMATIC HYPERMETROPIA is usually associated with paralysis of accommodation and, as we have seen, may be either temporary or permanent, due usually to an injury of the ciliary nerves or, in more severe cases, to organic lesions in the ciliary muscle itself. In such cases if the disability is prolonged and accommodation is lost, it may be advisable to prescribe bifocal lenses to assist with near work. Very occasionally a traumatic hypermetropia is due to a raising of the retina with organized material after a rupture of the choroid (Grimsdale, 1912), and other cases occur wherein an explanation of the refractive change, which may measure 2 or 3 D, is not obvious (Huber, 1929–32). A posterior dislocation of the lens with an increased depth of the anterior chamber will, of course, alter the refraction in the direction of hypermetropia. The effect of an ocular contusion on accommodation was studied by Jorgensen and Tönjum (1967); the amplitude of accommodation in 39 eyes showing some recession of the angle of the anterior chamber as the result of a contusion was compared with the normal fellow eye, and a difference of −0·7 dioptre was found.

TRAUMATIC MYOPIA is the commonest refractive change following a concussion to the globe. As a rule it involves an increase in myopic refraction of from 1 D to 6 D and disappears within a week or two, so that in the great majority of cases the refraction again becomes normal within a space of a month; only very occasionally does the condition persist for one year (Fromaget, 1911; Fox, 1942) or two years (Sourdille, 1908; Fox, 1942), or apparently permanently (Bourgeois, 1904; Janson, 1935). This occurrence has excited a great deal of interest since its original observation by Kugel (1870), and a considerable literature has accumulated which has been correlated by Frenkel (1905) (41 cases) and Fox (1942) (60 cases), in which much ingenuity has been expended on devising ætiological theories; but it is certain that all the cases are not due to the same cause. The more important factors may be briefly classified as follows.

Ciliary spasm undoubtedly accounts for the majority of cases, due most probably to irritation of the muscle fibres themselves or the IIIrd nerve, and perhaps sometimes to paresis of the cervical sympathetic. In this event the spasm of accommodation is associated with the spastic miosis which so commonly follows trauma of this nature. Such a spasm would account for a myopia varying from 1 D to 4 D associated with a loss of accommodative amplitude; it disappears under atropine and in the vast majority of cases is temporary, although there is evidence that it may be prolonged for periods up to a year by the superimposition of functional factors (Tange, 1913–14; Morgan, 1940).

Damage to the suspensory apparatus of the lens involving an increase of the lenticular curvature explains the occurrence of myopia in a number of cases wherein the refractive change persists and shows no diminution with atropine.[1] If the zonule is actually ruptured and the lens remains in place, the myopia may amount to 5 D or 6 D and be permanent (Møller, 1926–27; Cosserat, 1938), while a higher degree may be caused by an anterior dislocation of the lens (Manfredi, 1871; Bourgeois, 1904; Janson, 1935).

Traumatic concussion opacities in the lens possibly account for a few cases of the development of myopia (Morgan, 1940).

Ruptures of Descemet's membrane leading to an increase in the corneal curvature may have the same effect (Bailey, 1921).

A *loss or diminution of the anterior chamber* associated with hypotony will also cause a myopia so long as this condition lasts (Knapp, 1883; Fromaget, 1911; Brøns, 1931).[2]

Aub. *Arch. Augenheilk.*, **2**, 252 (1871).
Bailey. *Amer. J. Ophthal.*, **4**, 363 (1921).
Bourgeois. *Ann. Oculist.* (Paris), **132**, 267 (1904).
Brøns. *Zbl. ges. Ophthal.*, **25**, 534 (1931).
Cosserat. *Bull. Soc. Méd. milit. franç.*, **32**, 526 (1938).
Damel. *Arch. Oftal. B. Aires*, **8**, 497 (1933).
Darier. *Clin. Ophtal.*, **5**, 85 (1899).
Fox. *Arch. Ophthal.*, **28**, 218 (1942).
Frenkel. *Ann. Oculist.* (Paris), **134**, 1 (1905).
Fromaget. *Bull. Soc. franç. Ophtal.*, **28**, 346 (1911).
Grimsdale. *Trans. ophthal. Soc. U.K.*, **32**, 187 (1912).
Guende. *Marseille-Méd.*, **37**, 449 (1900).
Huber. *Klin. Mbl. Augenheilk.*, **83**, 523 (1929); **88**, 230 (1932).
Janson. *Klin. Mbl. Augenheilk.*, **94**, 517 (1935).
Jorgensen and Tönjum. *Acta ophthal.* (Kbh.), **45**, 159 (1967).
Knapp. *Arch. Augenheilk.*, **12**, 85 (1883).
Kugel. *v. Graefes Arch. Ophthal.*, **16**, 323 (1870).

[1] Aub (1871), Schiess-Gemuseus (1881), Darier (1899), Guende (1900), Damel (1933).
[2] For the triad of myopia, hypotension and mydriasis, see Vol. XI, p. 735.

Manfredi. *Ann. Ottal.*, **1**, 189 (1871).
Møller. *Acta ophthal.* (Kbh.), **4**, 60 (1926); **5**, 258 (1927).
Morgan. *Brit. J. Ophthal.*, **24**, 403 (1940).
Schiess-Gemuseus. *Klin. Mbl. Augenheilk.*, **19**, 384 (1881).
Sourdille. *Gaz. Méd. Nantes*, **26**, 945 (1908).
Tange. *Ned. T. Geneesk.*, **1**, 1305 (1913). *Arch. Ophtal.*, **34**, 463 (1914).

The Effects of Concussion on the Ocular Tension

The effects of concussion on the ocular tension may be dramatic and, indeed, may be the dominant factor in determining the fate of the eye. A disturbance of the normal equilibrium is usual and may occur in the absence of any observable intra-ocular lesion; as a rule after such an injury the tension is unstable, sometimes being raised, sometimes lowered, and occasionally alternating between the two extremes. This instability may be shared to some extent by the other (uninjured) eye, both varying within considerable limits for a number of days, periods of mild and transient hypertony alternating with periods of hypotony until stability is again attained. Usually the instability passes away without serious effects, but not infrequently a traumatic glaucoma may develop either so severe and intractable as to involve rapid loss of sight and even necessitating excision of the eye owing to pain or, as we have already seen, a delayed and insidious rise of the intra-ocular pressure may result from damage to the structures of the angle of the anterior chamber and other lesions of traumatic origin. On the other hand, a persistent hypotony may as surely lead to changes which eventually render the eye useless.

As this subject has already been dealt with at length in the volume on Glaucoma[1] wherein full bibliographies will also be found, no further discussion is required here.

CONCUSSIONS AND CONTUSIONS OF THE OCULAR ADNEXA

Injuries to the ocular adnexa by blunt force follow a multitude of accidents, great and small—the impact of a ball, a blow from a fist or a kick, a fall upon the edge of a table or a projecting piece of furniture, a collision with a door in the dark or with another person in sport, a crash in a road or air accident, and innumerable other events associated with everyday activities. Their effects are most conveniently discussed under five headings—injuries to the soft tissues of the lids, fractures of the orbital bones, orbital hæmorrhages and emphysema, and secondary injuries caused to the orbital contents and lacrimal passages.

Contusions of the Lids

ŒDEMA AND HÆMORRHAGE OF THE LIDS

After a contusion the laxity of the structures of the lids and their paucity of subcutaneous tissue permit an almost instantaneous swelling due to

[1] Vol. XI, p. 705, for traumatic glaucoma including that due to concussions, perforating wounds and retained foreign bodies; p. 659 for glaucoma associated with traumatic displacements of the lens; p. 733 for traumatic ocular hypotension.

œdema and hæmorrhage, frequently so marked in degree as to close the eye with such tautness that to open the lids for purposes of examination is usually difficult and sometimes impossible. When blood extravasates into the subcutaneous tissue in any quantity the everyday picture of a " black eye " is produced, and occasionally if a vessel of some size is torn a hæmatoma is formed which generates enough pressure to give rise to pain (Plate III, Fig. 1; Fig. 175). Although diffusion of fluid through the loose subcutaneous cellular tissue of both lids occurs with great ease, the blood is held up by the anchorage of the fascia at the eyebrows, preventing its spread onto the forehead, and at the naso-jugal and the malar folds, preventing expansion to the cheek and upper lip unless these tissues are also injured; the only point of

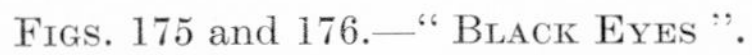

FIGS. 175 and 176.—" BLACK EYES ".

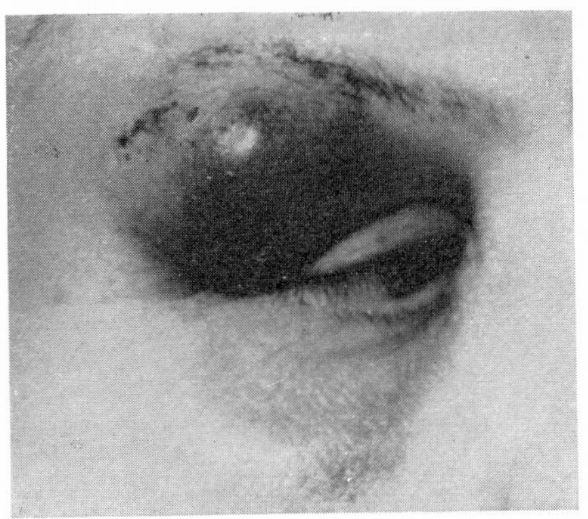

FIG. 175.—Encysted hæmatoma of the eyebrow following a blow from a stick.

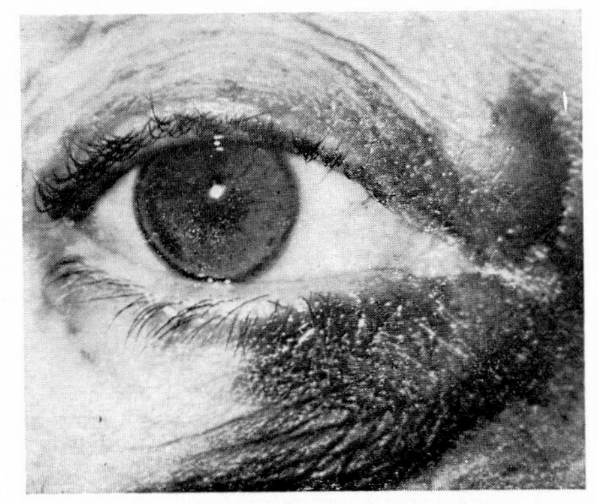

FIG. 176.—The seepage of blood across the nose from an injury of the other eye by a blow from a fist, causing hæmorrhage in the lids of the undamaged eye.

egress from this somewhat constricted territory is across the bridge of the nose into the tissue of the lids of the other eye (Fig. 176). Since the skin over the bridge of the nose is thick and firmly bound down, this region does not undergo swelling and the subcutaneous blood is not visible so that the continuity of the seepage from one eye to the other is not apparent and a second and independent hæmorrhage on this side is simulated. Initially the suffusion is purple in colour, but within a few days the degradation products of hæmoglobin give it a greenish-brown and eventually a yellowish appearance before it finally disappears in some two or three weeks. Only occasionally are isolated spots of pigment left as a permanent legacy.

As a general rule the hæmorrhage absorbs without complications but if the surface of the skin is broken infection may develop. Pain, tenderness, fluctuation and fever indicate the development of a cellulitis or an abscess which may on occasion progress to gangrene; such a complication is, however, fortunately rare. Other complications include the subsequent formation of fibrous tissue, which may lead to cicatrization or exuberant keloid overgrowth, and (exceptionally) a fusion of the upper border of the tarsus with the orbital margin (Cramer, 1931). Damage to the levator palpebræ muscle involving a certain amount of traumatic ptosis is a relatively common sequel.

A supra-orbital *subperiosteal bleeding* leading to the development of a hæmatoma which may form a widespread fluctuating swelling deeply in the forehead may result from a contusion in this region.

A *subconjunctival ecchymosis* may accompany the suffusion into the tissues of the lids. This is usually fleeting and generally disappears without trace, although permanent pigmentation leading to pseudo-melanosis has been observed (Sous, 1897).

The *diagnosis* of a hæmorrhage into the lids after an injury presents no difficulty, but the differential diagnosis as to the source of the blood may cause some anxiety. A similar extravasation into the palpebral tissues may arise from an orbital hæmorrhage or an extravasation of blood reaching the orbit from a fracture of the base of the skull. This matter will be discussed more fully subsequently,[1] but in general terms a hæmorrhage into the lids due to local damage appears immediately after the injury, while blood tracking through the tarso-orbital fascia from the deeper tissues becomes evident in the lids only after a day or two, is more diffuse in distribution and is associated with less œdematous swelling.

The *treatment* of a traumatic hæmorrhage into the lids is expectant; the suffusion is self-limiting and is best left alone to absorb. Cold compresses initially, followed in 24 hours by warm applications and massage, are usually recommended; these may not be of much value but they are as effectual as more impressive applications such as the old expedients of lotions of lead and opium and hamamelis or alcohol. Attempts at evacuation of the blood by incision or aspiration are best discouraged, since they are usually of little value and may allow the entry of infection. The rather unsightly appearance can usually be disguised by dark glasses and to some extent by grease-paint or other cosmetic applications, while painting the skin with guaiacol may help to obscure the discoloration by its blanching effect.

CRUSH WOUNDS

A blunt force striking the orbital margins may compress the tissues between the impinging object and the bone, the soft tissues being ruptured or stretched so that they are torn; the most typical result is the formation of a sharply defined wound running along the rim of the orbit at the outer part of the brow; a contusion of the forehead may cause a similar wound usually running vertically through the aponeurosis down to the frontal bone. The appearance of such wounds frequently suggests that they have been inflicted by a sharp instrument and it may be difficult to appreciate that they have

[1] p. 268.

been due to a fall or a blunt force—a matter of considerable medico-legal importance. The differential diagnosis between a lacerated wound of this type and an incised wound inflicted by a sharp instrument depends upon four features: a lacerated wound always runs down to the bone, it is more extensive at its deepest part next to the bone than superficially, it does not gape as does a cut, and it is frequently bridged across by attenuated strands of tissue which are absent in an incised wound; moreover, if a lacerated wound due to a crush-injury is at the orbital margin it is always associated with an intense œdema and usually with ecchymosis of the lids so severe as to close the eye completely (Fig. 177).

More severe damage may be done if sufficient force is involved. A common and disfiguring occurrence is a *dislocation of one or other of the canthi*. This is due to an injury involving the palpebral ligaments and occurs not infrequently in major accidents complicated by fractures of the orbital rim or comminution of the nasal bones, and is occasionally seen in extreme degrees of trauma associated with avulsion of the eyelids. The deformity produced is considerable, for the palpebral fissure is shortened and the affected canthus usually pulled downwards by cicatrization; not uncommonly the eye is also damaged and frequently requires excision, in which case the difficulties of a contracted socket eventually arise (Figs. 178–9). If the inner canthus is involved there is an asymmetrical widening of the intercanthal distance (*traumatic telecanthus*), and damage of this nature to the medial palpebral ligament is usually associated with tearing of the lacrimal passages.

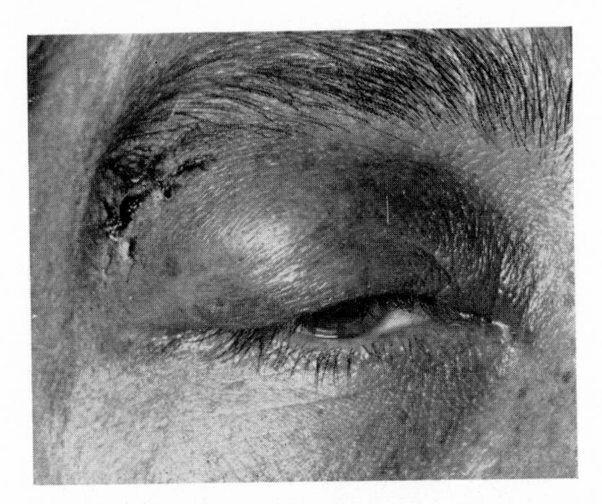

Fig. 177.—Lacerated Wound of the Eyebrow.
Following a collision with the head of a companion in the gymnasium.

A common result of such contusive lacerations is a rupture of the posterior portion of the internal canthal ligament from its insertion into the posterior lacrimal crest; a similar accident may follow a pull on the lid as by a button-hook or a meat-hook, or may be caused by a simple penetrating wound or a fracture involving the lacrimal crest. The importance of the deformity which results from such an injury is that the lower lid loses its apposition to the globe so that epiphora results; it will be remembered that in lacrimal surgery the anterior portion of this ligament can be cut with impunity but if the posterior portion is also severed this annoying deformity results. The condition is best left alone until the tissues have healed whereafter the lower lid should be carried upwards, backwards and inwards and reattached to a convenient part of the periosteum behind the lacrimal crest (Kirby, 1940).

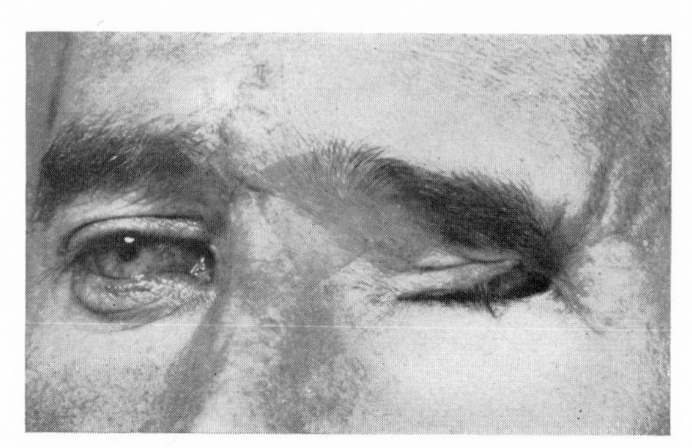

Fig. 178.

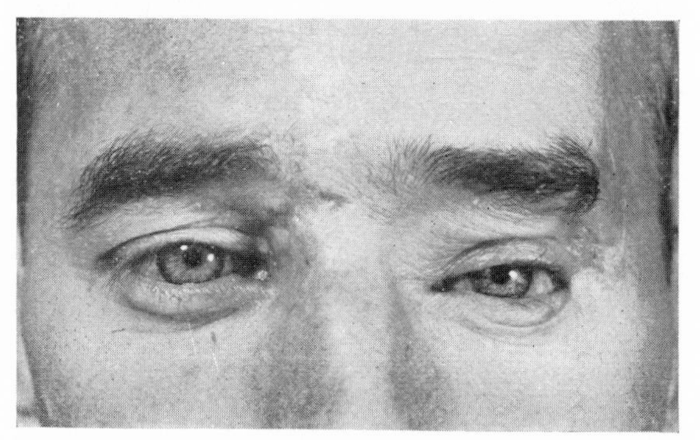

Fig. 179.

Figs. 178 and 179.—Severance of the Canthal Ligaments.

Resulting from an explosion in which the left eye was lost. The right medial and left lateral palpebral ligaments were severed and the right upper lid fixed in a scar (Fig. 178).

Fig. 179.—Shows the post-operative appearance with the improvement of both canthi. A plastic eye has been inserted on the left side (A. Callahan).

A less frequent injury is a *vertical splitting of the upper tarsus*; this has followed a blow from a curtain-rail or knuckle-duster (Cauer, 1907), a wooden stick or a crotchet-hook (Collier, 1965), and is a not infrequent accident in war when it may be due to the blast of a nearby explosion. Sometimes the lid is split throughout its entire thickness vertically at the junction of its medial and middle thirds, the tarsal plate being rent from its upper to its lower margin; the tarsus may be similarly split subcutaneously leaving the skin and orbicularis muscle unharmed (Pannarale, 1951, from the horn of a bull). More rarely the tear runs horizontally concentric with the orbital margin above the tarsal plate and involves the skin and the orbicularis muscle down to the orbital septum.

A *traumatic ptosis* is a frequent sequel of a concussive injury of the orbital rim and may be due to damage to the levator tendon or injury to the palpebral branch of the oculomotor nerve (Fig. 180).

On recovery from traumatic ptosis, Halpern (1934) noted the interesting phenomenon of a *paradoxical elevation of the upper lid.* Such a phenomenon occasionally follows a traumatic IIIrd-nerve palsy, and in the recovery stage both a pseudo-Graefe and a Marcus Gunn phenomenon have been observed; these will be noted when we are discussing injuries to the IIIrd nerve.[1]

Complications occasionally met with in injuries of this type are the occurrence of a fracture of the orbital rim, the onset of sepsis which is

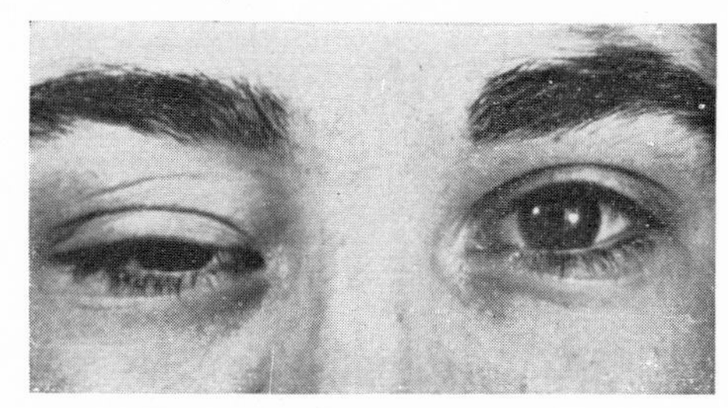

FIG. 180.—TRAUMATIC PTOSIS.

From a laceration of the upper lid, severing the levator palpebræ, due to a kick by a horse 7 months previously (A. McIndoe).

facilitated by the fact that the edges of the wound are contused, the development of periostitis which may be followed by caries and necrosis of the bone and, when the injury is of the nature of a severe crush and infection is absent, the development of necrosis or dry gangrene. Sepsis, if it does develop, may lead to cellulitis, abscess formation and even gangrene of the soft tissues, which on occasion has resulted in a fatal septicæmia (Valude, 1890). A relatively rare sequel in modern times is the development of tetanus, of which there are many cases in the early literature; these have been summarized by von Wahl (1882) and Fromaget (1894). Finally, it is undoubtedly the case that in susceptible subjects an injury of this type may lead to an activation of a tuberculous or syphilitic periostitis.

Treatment. The treatment of such injuries is with the usual techniques applied in traumatic surgery. If the skin surface is broken, anti-tetanic prophylaxis should be immediately undertaken by the toxoid if the patient is non-immune or by a boosting dose of toxoid if he has been previously

[1] p. 299.

immunized, and the wound treated as indicated in a later section.[1] It is to be noted that if there is extensive contusive damage the edges of the wound may be freshened, but any excision of tissues should be most conservative for their viability in this region is surprisingly great owing to their rich blood supply, and unnecessary removal leads to cicatrization and the need for subsequent plastic procedures, sometimes on a large scale.

Although it is by no means always possible, an immediate attempt should be made to reduce any bony deformity[2] and to reconstitute the lacrimal passages if these are involved.[3] These procedures will be dealt with more fully at a later stage.

When injury to the palpebral ligaments has occurred, involving dislocation of the canthi, immediate repair of the deformity is advisable. If the ligament is severed it should be reunited and if, as frequently happens, it is torn from the periosteum it should be reunited to this membrane by sutures. If, however, the deformity is of some standing and much cicatricial tissue has developed, it is probable that stitches to the periosteum will not hold; in this event, or if the periosteum is torn, bone should be used for anchorage and the ligaments secured by wire or nylon sutures inserted through holes bored through the bone by a dental drill. On the medial side these holes will be located in the region of the anterior or posterior lacrimal crest, whichever is indicated, and neither they nor the wire should perforate the nasal mucosa; but if the nasal wall is extensively damaged or absent, steel sutures can be passed through the nasal septum and anchored temporarily in the opposite nasal bone. A tarsal plate dislocated from its attachment to the palpebral ligament may be anchored in the same way. If much cicatricial deformity also exists canthoplasty may be necessary in addition[4] (Figs. 178 and 179). Where there is gross loss of tissue plastic reconstruction of the lids may be required after an interval, the problems of which will be discussed elsewhere.[5]

In many cases, of course, the eye is damaged and will require treatment on the lines indicated earlier in this section, or its excision may be advisable; in the latter case plastic repair may be necessary to reconstitute a useful socket. In all cases cerebral damage should be excluded and general treatment instituted as indicated by the condition of the patient.

SUPRA-ORBITAL AMAUROSIS AND AMBLYOPIA. There is an old and delightfully ingenuous theory, the literature regarding which goes back to the Hippocratic writings,[6] that a blow in the supraciliary region produces amblyopia or blindness by reflex irritation of the supra-orbital nerve. Among early writers the theory excited much clinical speculation and experimental work (see Beer, 1813; Platner, 1841; Praun, 1899). It is true that a contusion of the forehead frequently does entail grave visual consequences but it is probable that this is usually due to such lesions as a commotio

[1] p. 408. [2] p. 272. [3] p. 435.
[4] Blair *et al.* (1932), Hildreth (1935), Wheeler (1939), Converse (1944), Callahan (1946–50), Converse and Smith (1963), Mustardé (1966).
[5] p. 431. [6] *De morbis vulgaribus.*

retinæ or damage to the optic nerve by concussion changes, tearing of its blood vessels and occasionally a fracture of the orbital roof in the region of the apex of the orbit; it should also be remembered that in some such cases a considerable functional element may be superimposed.

Beer. *Lehre v. d. Augenkrankheiten*, Wien, **1** (1813).
Blair, Brown and Hamm. *Amer. J. Ophthal.*, **15**, 498 (1932).
Callahan. *Sth. med. J.*, **39**, 681 (1946).
Trans. Amer. Acad. Ophthal., **53**, 486 (1948).
Plast. reconstr. Surg., **3**, 456 (1948).
Surgery of the Eye, Injuries, Springfield (1950).
Cauer. *Klin. Mbl. Augenheilk.*, **45** (2), 80 (1907).
Collier. *Bull. Soc. franç. Ophtal.*, **78**, 497 (1965).
Converse. *Arch. Ophthal.*, **31**, 323 (1944).
Converse and Smith. *Trans. Amer. Acad. Ophthal.*, **67**, 622 (1963).
Cramer. *Kurzes Hb. d. Ophthal.*, Berlin, **4**, 440 (1931).
Fromaget. *Arch. Ophtal.*, **14**, 657 (1894).
Halpern. *Harefuah*, **8**, 111 (1934).
Hildreth. *Amer. J. Ophthal.*, **18**, 437 (1935).
Kirby. *Surg. Clin. N. Amer.*, **20**, 573 (1940).
Mustardé. *Repair and Reconstruction in the Orbital Region*, Edinburgh (1966).
Pannarale. *Boll. Oculist.*, **33**, 751 (1951).
Platner. *De vulneribus superciliis*, Lipsiae, 184 (1841).
Praun. *Die Verletzungen des Auges*, Wiesbaden (1899).
Sous. *Ann. Oculist.* (Paris), **117**, 137 (1897).
Valude. *Ann. Oculist.* (Paris), **103**, 204 (1890).
von Wahl. *St. Petersburg med. Wschr.*, **7**, 333 (1882).
Wheeler. *Collected Papers*, N.Y., 425 (1939).

Fractures of the Orbit

Most of the serious injuries to the ocular adnexa involve fractures in the region of the orbit and in our knowledge of these, two famous names stand out which are worthy of mention, one a French surgeon of the past generation who delineated the lines of weakness along which gross fractures in the facial or orbital skeleton occur, and the other an American surgeon of our own time who first stressed the importance of those fractures of the delicate walls of the orbit itself that follow less severe trauma.

RENÉ LE FORT [1869–1951] (Fig. 181) was one of the greatest surgeons France has produced. Born in Lille to a medical family, he graduated in the university of that city, receiving his doctorate in 1890 for a remarkable thesis on cranio-cerebral topography and its surgical applications; incidentally, at the age of 21 he was the youngest doctor in France at that time. He first served in the Army and in 1899 returned to Lille where he acted as a surgeon in several hospitals, but in 1912 he resumed military service and served in the Balkan war; thereafter he indulged in a world tour, studying leprosy in China and visiting Japan and North and South America. Once more at Lille he occupied surgical posts including those in infantile and orthopædic clinics until the first World War broke out in 1914 when he became chief of the Ambulance Division of the 1st Corps of the French Army and distinguished himself in overcoming enormous difficulties in evacuating all the wounded from Lille during the retreat to the Marne. After the war he occupied the Chair of Clinical Surgery at the Charité in Paris until he reached retiring age in 1937. The commencement of the second World War found him on a voyage to Tierra del Fuego; he immediately returned to France to replace his more junior colleagues in their civilian surgical work. Le Fort's contributions to surgery were manifold, particularly in its orthopædic and plastic aspects, his enthusiasm for his work, for travelling and for the whole of life was unbounded, and his kindliness and geniality endeared him to everyone who knew him.

JOHN MARQUIS CONVERSE [1909—] (Fig. 182), like Le Fort, underwent his apprenticeship to traumatic surgery in war. He was born in San Francisco but from the age of 9 to 24 he lived in France where his father was head of the American Hospital in Paris. In this city he studied medicine and received his early training in surgery under Thiery

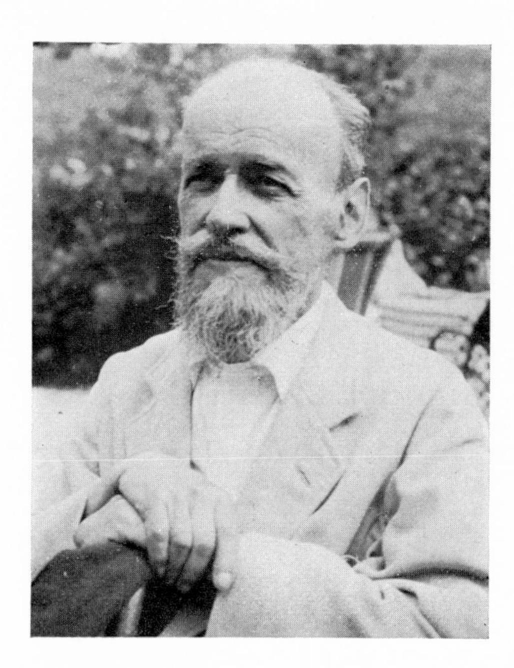

FIG. 181.—RENÉ LÉON LE FORT [1869–1951].
(From a photograph in the possession of his son, Jacques Le Fort.)

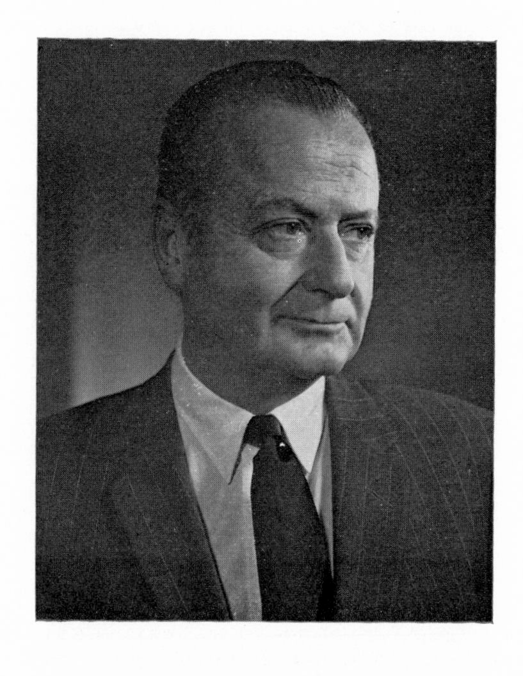

FIG. 182.—JOHN MARQUIS CONVERSE [1909—].

de Martel. Returning to America in 1935 he became a house officer at the Massachusetts General Hospital and the Eye and Ear Infirmary. In Boston he studied plastic surgery and in the second World War he joined the American Hospital in Britain in 1940 where he worked in Basingstoke with Sir Harold Gillies and at East Grinstead with Sir Archibald McIndoe. In 1942 the American unit established the Churchill Hospital at Oxford and at the end of that year he returned to America. He was then sent to Algiers in 1943 to start a unit in plastic surgery for the French Army. On his return to the United States he joined the American Army and returned to France in 1944 where he established a unit in the Hôpital Foch. Returning finally to the United States he became Professor of Plastic Surgery at New York University Medical Center and Director of the Institute of Reconstructive Plastic Surgery there and at the Manhattan Eye, Ear and Throat Hospital. His industry has been immense and, in addition to publishing some 200 papers up to the present date, he was co-author with Dr. V. H. Kazanjian of a classical text-book *The Surgical Treatment of Facial Injuries*, the first edition of which appeared in 1949, as well as editing the five-volumed text-book, *Reconstructive Plastic Surgery*.

FRACTURES OF THE ORBIT and in the surrounding region of the skull are common. In addition to the ordinary risks of industry or sport the classical causes have usually been falls from a height or a crushing blow from the fist or the boot or the implements of war, but in an age of impatiently accelerating travel, high-speed crashes and collisions account for an ever-increasing number of such incidents. Today a head-on crash in an automobile accident is the most common cause; indeed, some 50% of orbital fractures may arise in this way (Converse *et al.*, 1967; Rowe and Killey, 1968). As would be expected in such injuries the damage to bone may be extensive, but trauma elsewhere may be so severe that the local condition may have of necessity to be neglected temporarily in order to take urgent measures to save the patient's life. A fatal outcome is nowadays an uncommon result of fractures of the facial skeleton; if death does occur it is usually due to intracranial hæmorrhage. As a general rule, therefore, in the absence of respiratory obstruction, surgical interference with the fracture in an unconscious patient is best deferred until his general and cerebral condition has improved. Immediate responsibility for the patient may lie primarily with a general or orthopædic surgeon and the extent of the damage frequently necessitates cooperation with the neurosurgeon, the thoracic surgeon, the rhinologist and the maxillo-facial surgeon.

The high incidence of multiple and serious associated injuries in patients with head and facial trauma sustained in road accidents has been noted by Kulowski (1956), Lundquist (1960), Buzzard and his colleagues (1964), Plewes (1967) and Sevitt (1968). Dawson (1962) emphasized that, in addition to facial injuries, such cases may have "stove-in chests" from impaction against the steering wheel, fractured spines from acute flexion, buckled legs due to floorboards coming up and the engine being forced back, and ruptured internal organs caused by the engine and dashboard coming backwards, together with trauma from behind resulting from forward movement of the rear occupants. In a study of fatal accidents on a motorway, Gissane and Bull (1964) also pointed out the importance of looking for other injuries, especially to the thorax and abdomen; in 73 necropsies of such cases injuries to the skull and face were present in

86·3% and about one-third also showed evidence of damage to the lungs, great vessels and major viscera, with each fatality receiving an average of 5·6 injuries. In a post-mortem study of 250 road accidents, Sevitt (1968) found that the most frequent causes of death were a contusion of vital centres in the midbrain or third ventricular region, and tentorial herniation; the first is not and the second ought to be amenable to treatment.

Although the problems involved may therefore be complicated it should always be remembered that early and efficient treatment of the local fracture, if it is at all possible, is of the utmost urgency in order to prevent gross disabilities of the eyes, nose and mouth, for if this is delayed until a later date these may be of such magnitude that reconstructive surgical procedures on a major scale may be necessary for their repair; and sometimes if these measures are deferred for long, even the most heroic efforts at reconstruction may in the end be unsatisfactory. Throughout this section we shall repeatedly emphasize the importance of early diagnosis and treatment of injury to the eye associated with facial fractures: a blind eye is a heavy price to pay for a straight face.

The clinical evaluation of these injuries at the time of the accident frequently presents a problem of great difficulty; the patient may be concussed, mentally confused or unconscious and, owing to the enormous swelling and suffusion of the surrounding area, clinical examination may not provide exact information; moreover, radiographic evidence is difficult to interpret and the necropsy material from other apparently similar cases which might serve as a guide has seldom been fully investigated. In general, however, the type and extent of the fracture vary with the force, its velocity, duration, and the extent of its surface contact. A sudden trauma over a limited area tends to produce a local fracture with much comminution of the bone; in this way the margin of the orbit may be splintered and pieces of bone driven into the orbital cavity. The less the velocity of the force and the more extensive its impact, the more widespread the fracture tends to be and, indeed, a crushing force spread over a wide area on the forehead (for example) may fissure the orbital roof, leaving the part of the bone which was struck and the orbital rim intact. The effect of the trauma also varies with the resistance of the bone upon which the force falls, its mode of fixation, the difficulty of its displacement and, in general, on the arrangement and construction of the bony structures with which it is connected, which may serve as buttresses to distribute and dissipate local stresses.

From the ophthalmological point of view such injuries may be divided into two types, direct and indirect, the former being due to blunt violence falling directly upon the orbit, the latter resulting from an involvement of the orbital bones in a radiating fracture of the vault of the skull or the bones of the face. Since, however, the two frequently involve the same type of fracture so far as the orbit is concerned, in this discussion we shall divide fractures of the orbital bones into four types:

1. Fractures involving the upper third of the skull due to direct injury in the frontal region.
2. Fractures involving the middle third of the skull due to direct injury in the facial region either medially or laterally.
3. Internal orbital fractures due to direct injury to the orbit.
4. Indirect orbital fractures associated with head injury.

A considerable volume of literature has now accumulated concerning the incidence and classification of facial fractures and their associated injuries. Among many such reports the following may be of interest to the ophthalmic surgeon: Kazanjian and Converse (1949–70), Dawson and Fordyce (1953), Kulowski (1956), Herman *et al.* (1960), McCoy *et al.* (1962), P. François (1965), Schuchardt *et al.* (1966), Rowe and Killey (1968), Fanjul (1968), Reny and Stricker (1969).

FRONTAL FRACTURES INVOLVING THE ORBITAL ROOF

An understanding of the functional architecture of the skull is of great importance in appreciating the effects of an impinging force, for the distribution of the areas of density in the bone and its arrangement in curves and buttresses disperse the strains and stresses set up by the blow in well-defined directions so that the effects are felt not only in the immediate area but may travel far afield; indeed, the distant effects may be more important than the local damage. A blow upon the frontal region or the upper orbital rim may cause a local fracture, frequently involving the frontal sinus (Schultze, 1970). If the inner table of the bone is also fractured the fragments are usually depressed, the dura of the anterior cranial fossa may be penetrated and the brain injured. It is important to remember that the structure of the skull is such that the inner table is frequently more widely damaged than the outer, so that care must be taken lest a fracture which seems to have few implications superficially may have profound intracranial significance. Occasionally the levator muscle or its nerve supply may be damaged resulting in a traumatic ptosis.

Apart, however, from this local damage, the studies of Lagrange (1917) showed that a force impinging in this area is distributed by way of the internal and external processes of the frontal bone to dissipate itself in the facial mass. The globe, the orbital contents and the brain thus largely escape direct concussive injury, but the thin orbital roof gives way, particularly in its posterior part in the region of the superior orbital fissure and the optic foramen; further radiation may take place along the base of the skull. A fracture of this type, therefore, tends to injure the optic, motor and sensory nerves entering the orbit in this region, a circumstance first stressed by Berlin (1879–81) and giving rise to what is now known as *the syndrome of the orbital apex*. Such a fracture is usually confined to the same side but may be bilateral: thus bilateral visual damage occurred in 7·5% of 225 traumatic lesions of the optic nerve of this type studied by Cantonnet and Coutella (1906), and in 12% of 42 cases reported by Davidson (1938).

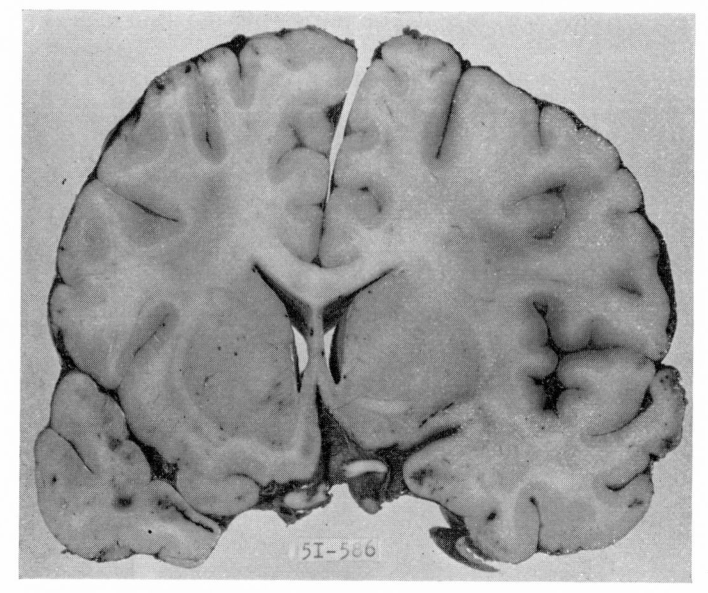

FIG. 183.—RUPTURE OF THE CHIASMA.

There was an extensive fracture of the base of the skull (F. B. Walsh and J. D. Gass).

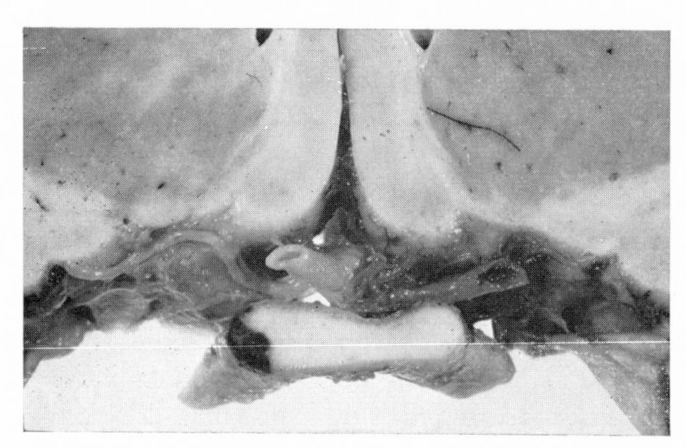

FIG. 184.—CONTUSION OF THE CHIASMA WITH HÆMORRHAGE.

In a man aged 66 after a fall. There was a fracture of the skull through the right orbital roof (F. B. Walsh and J. D. Gass).

It is important to remember that such a fissured fracture, involving the orbital roof and the anterior fossa as a result of the impact of blunt violence on the forehead so that the skull is flattened in an antero-posterior direction, may occur without a local fracture of the superciliary arch; and although the causal injury is usually severe, leading to a loss of consciousness, it may on occasion be trivial so that the patient is only momentarily dazed and no external marks of violence are seen (Thoral, 1924; Davidson, 1938; Turner,

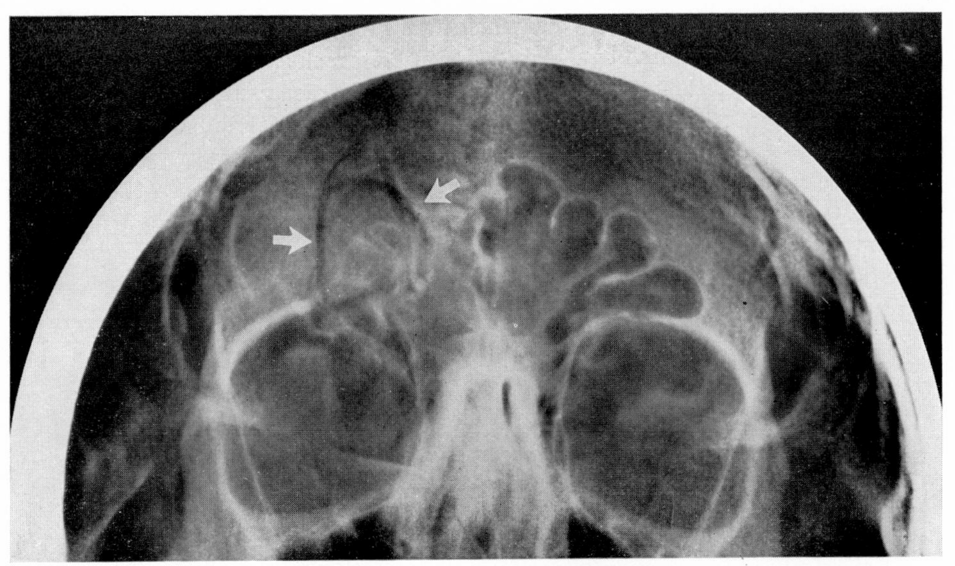

Fig. 185.

Figs. 185 and 186.—Fracture of the Frontal Bone.

Involving the superior rim and roof of the orbit and the anterior aspect of the anterior cranial fossa. An adult struck his forehead on the dashboard in an automobile accident and sustained the fracture shown by arrows. In this type of fracture it is essential to consider the possibility of subdural hæmatoma or other intracranial injury (S. L. Trokel).

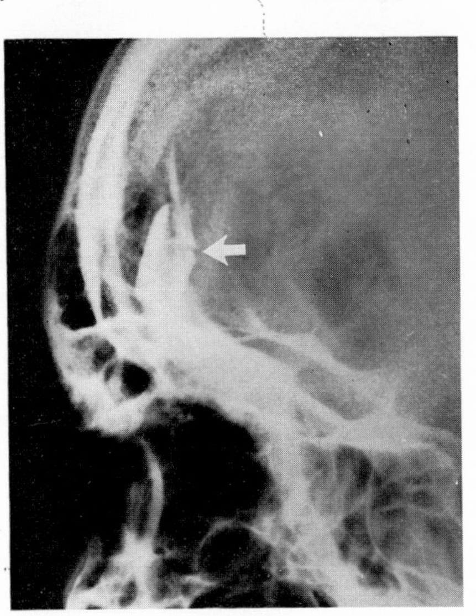

Fig. 186.

1943). Reports of such injuries have been few: Cantonnet and Coutella (1906) collected 8 cases from the literature, Bollack (1920) 17, and Traquair and his colleagues (1935) 27, with 3 of their own; the largest series (of 7 cases) was seen by Hughes (1962). On the other hand, if the injury is more severe, as results from a crash in a high-speed collision or a fall from a great height, the line of the fracture may extend beyond the orbit into the chiasmal region, a rare and frequently fatal event which was first reported by Nieden (1883) and anatomically verified by Körber (1889), Liebrecht (1906) and Walsh and Gass (1960) (Figs. 183–4). Such an injury, however, may be survived and a frontal fracture may cause a displacement of the sella, resulting in a compression atrophy of the optic nerve (Streiff and Buffat, 1951) or longitudinal fractures throughout the sella with resultant chiasmal defects in the visual fields, typically bitemporal hemianopia.[1] It is interesting that a similar injury on the forehead may involve a comparable type of distant fracture of the floor of the orbit, also without implicating its upper rim, a matter which will be dealt with later[2] (DeVoe, 1947).

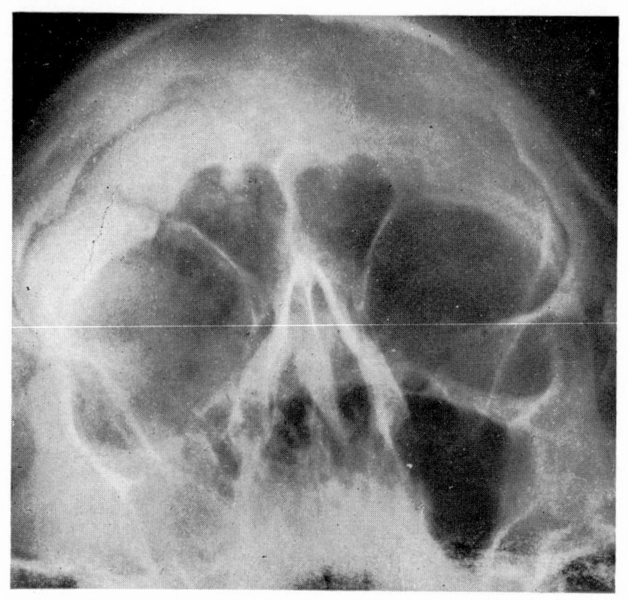

FIG. 187.—MULTIPLE ORBITAL FRACTURES.

Depressed rotated fracture of the zygoma with an opaque antrum, fractures of the frontal bone and supra-orbital margin communicating with the frontal sinus resulting in surgical emphysema (R. L. G. Dawson).

In severe cases the clinical condition is usually dominated initially by shock and the results of cranial injury by concussion, while the bony damage, although sometimes obvious and palpable, is frequently obscured by the swelling of the tissue; the frontal fracture, however, is usually demonstrated by local tenderness, discontinuity of the contour and the elicitation of crepitation on manipulation. Epistaxis is an indication of a tear in the mucosa of the nose or its associated sinuses, while cerebro-spinal rhinorrhœa carries the more serious implication of a fracture of the anterior fossa with its

[1] Apollonio (1951), Anderson and Lloyd (1964), Walsh (1966), Logan and Gordon (1967), J. François and Verriest (1969).

[2] p. 243.

accompanying danger of meningeal infection (Schjelderup, 1950). If consciousness is maintained, visual damage may be the most alarming symptom; the cause and pathology of injury to the optic nerve in these circumstances will be discussed subsequently.[1] On the other hand, in the less severe type of injury no symptoms may be evident even although the orbital roof, floor or apex has been fractured; indeed, the whole occurrence may have seemed to be so trivial that it may be difficult to associate the subsequent discovery of visual failure with the causal accident.

Radiological diagnosis of fractures of this type is easy when they affect the frontal region (Figs. 185–7), but the interpretation of radiographs of the orbital roof and apex

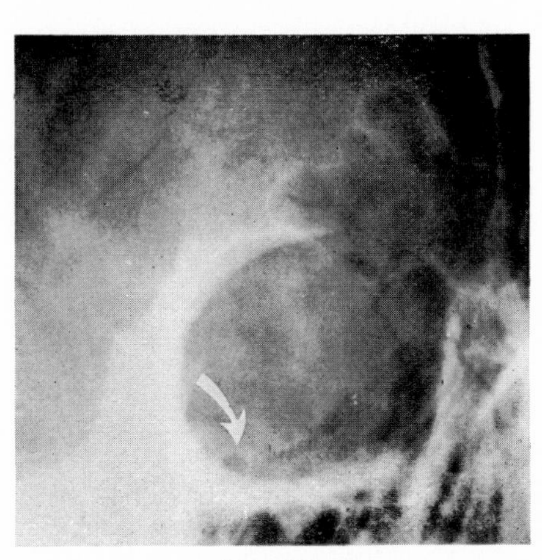

Fig. 188.

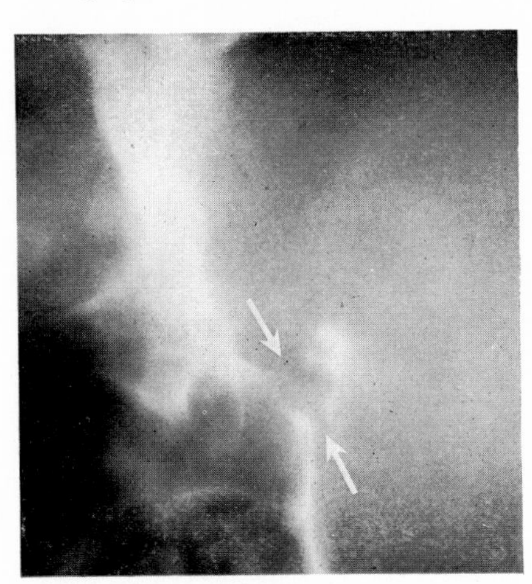

Fig. 189.

Figs. 188 and 189.—Fracture of the Optic Canal.

Trauma to the skull which involved total loss of vision of the right eye. Fig. 188 is a plain x-ray of the optic canal (curved arrow); it is partly obscured by the zygomatic arch. Fig. 189 is a tomographic section and shows the fracture in the canal at its junction medially with the body of the sphenoid bone. It is seen that hypocycloid blurring is necessary for adequate tomographic demonstration of the optic canal (S. L. Trokel).

is usually difficult owing to the complicated architecture of the bones and their obscuration by denser surroundings. With the special techniques which have been evolved for the radiography of the optic foramen, however, the presence of a fracture in this region can be demonstrated in a considerable number of cases (Rodger, 1943; Trokel and Potter, 1969) (Figs. 188–9), and even although it has escaped detection at the time of the injury, its presence has on occasion been proved at a later date by deformations of the bone due to the formation of callus (Lillie and Adson, 1934). At the same time it seems certain that many cases of damage to the optic nerve and the chiasma following this type of injury are unassociated with fracture of the bone; the mechanism of this damage is considered elsewhere.[2]

Complications. Overshadowing local events in the orbit, the most urgent complication is *cerebral damage*, both local and general. It is to be re-

[1] p. 437. [2] Vol. XV

membered that focal damage may not be confined to the frontal area only but, particularly as a result of a diffused force, may involve the occipital lobes, thus resulting in the appearance of homonymous scotomata. These may be transient and may not become manifest until a few weeks after the injury; their probable mechanism is injury by *contre-coup* and sudden rotation of the skull in the horizontal plane (Holbourn, 1943).

Of the events which may occur in the orbit itself, much the most dramatic and important is *injury to the optic nerve.* This may be evident as soon as clinical examination is possible when, in the worst cases, unilateral blindness is discovered; the pupil is inactive to direct light and although the disc looks normal at the time, optic atrophy eventually makes its appearance, sometimes after a few days but usually not until towards the end of the 3rd week. As a rule, however, the injury is less severe and the vision gradually recovers, sometimes rapidly, sometimes slowly over a period of some four weeks; in other cases irregular permanent defects remain in the visual field. This subject is considered more fully elsewhere.[1]

Further immediate orbital complications include orbital hæmorrhage, emphysema from involvement of the frontal sinus (Middeldorpf, 1886), ptosis, which may be due to damage either to the levator muscle or its nerve supply (Reber, 1899; and others), and derangement of the mobility of the globe with diplopia due sometimes to a paresis of the superior rectus (Lyle, 1941; Neely, 1947), sometimes to a displacement of the trochlea of the superior oblique muscle, at other times to an injury to the motor nerves as they traverse the superior orbital fissure and not infrequently to a depressed fracture of the orbital floor (Figs. 259–61). Of considerable importance from the practical point of view, however, is the development of infection which if not introduced at the time of the injury may be derived from the frontal sinus; in the days before the introduction of antibiotics a fatal meningitis was a frequent result of severe fractures of this type and even today with all the improvements in our therapeutics this termination is by no means unknown.

Injury to the nerves traversing the sphenoidal fissure can give rise to *the sphenoidal fissure syndrome* in which damage to any one or all of the IIIrd, IVth, or VIth cranial nerves or of the ophthalmic division of the Vth nerve may result in muscular palsies or sensory impairment without loss of vision; while in the fully developed *orbital apex syndrome* in addition to these effects blindness may result from damage to the optic nerve or the ophthalmic artery (Badal, 1894; Fromaget, 1894). Trauma as a cause of the orbital-apex syndrome, although uncommon, has been described on a number of occasions.[2] The probable mechanism of blindness in these cases is that rupture of an intra-orbital vessel causes severe hæmorrhage into the muscle-cone, the ensuing severe progressive and irreducible proptosis

[1] Vol. XII, p. 273.

[2] Hirschberg (1880), Lagrange (1917), Kjoer (1945), Wüst (1949), Gordon and Macrae (1950), Jefferson and Schorstein (1955), Mortada (1961), Lakke (1962), Banks (1967), Watson and Holt-Wilson (1968).

stretches the optic nerve and induces spasm or compression of the central retinal artery leading to acute retinal ischæmia. Inevitably there follow a loss of vision, abolition of the pupillary reflexes and cycloplegia. Left to itself the arterial occlusion will in time relax but only after permanent damage has been caused so that urgent measures are required if blindness is to be prevented. Retrobulbar injections of anti-spasmodics or vasodilators are clearly inappropriate; on the other hand, anti-spasmodic drugs delivered directly to the artery may be beneficial; this can be achieved by the intra-arterial infusion of papavarine via the supra-orbital artery as advocated by Watson and Holt-Wilson (1968), while in those cases wherein proptosis has resulted from severe intra-orbital hæmorrhage decompression of the orbit should be undertaken without delay, preferably via the trans-antral route so that the blood clot may be evacuated, and at the same time any fracture of the orbital floor can be dealt with.

The technique of continuous intra-arterial infusion of papavarine with heparin combined with trans-antral decompression has been described by Watson and Holt-Wilson (1968) who successfully treated two cases with visual failure following severe orbital trauma. In both cases the visual acuity and the visual field returned to normal. The whole question of serious ocular damage resulting from fractures in and around the orbit will be considered later in this section.

A serious complication of a fracture of sufficient severity to shatter the floor of the anterior fossa is a prolapse of brain-substance into the orbit to form a *traumatic encephalocele*. In such cases the brain pushes aside the bony fragments and displaces the orbital contents forwards and downwards so that proptosis and limitation of ocular movements result, signs, however, which may not be immediately apparent but may develop gradually some months after the injury. A typical case of this nature was reported by King (1951) following an automobile accident wherein such an encephalocele invaded the orbit and the ethmoid sinuses so that brain tissue could be seen protruding into the posterior nares (Figs. 190 and 191). In such cases, of course, infection of the protruding brain and meninges becomes a major hazard demanding the prophylactic use of antibiotics. Treatment of such a complication consists of removal of the prolapsed portion of the brain and extensive repair of the dura and of the orbital roof.[1]

Delayed complications of such frontal fractures are less common. *Chronic infection* may establish itself, resulting in a low-grade arachnoiditis which may bring about a slowly progressive deterioration of vision due to atrophy of the optic nerves caused by the compressing embrace of inflammatory adhesions.[2] Indeed, chronic infection arising from a fracture of the frontal sinus may lead to arachnoid adhesions so massive and widespread over the chiasmal region that damage initially uniocular has become binocular

[1] p. 275.

[2] Holmes (1929), Malbran and Balado (1933), Malbran (1935–37), Belloni and Fasiani (1940), and others.

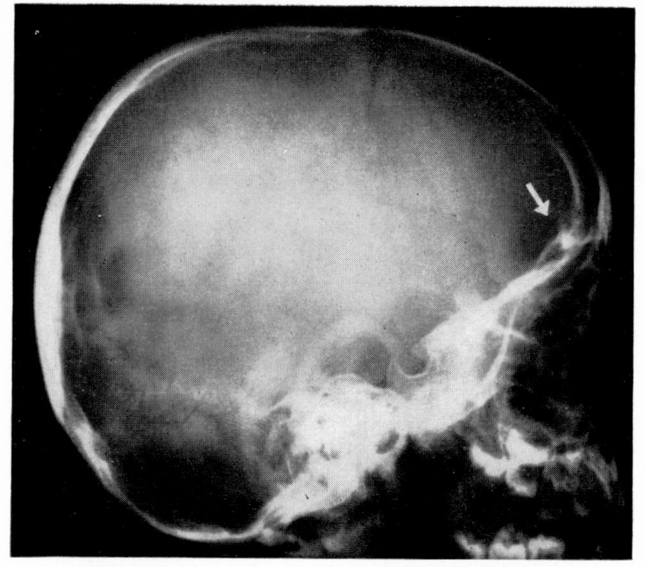

Fig. 190.

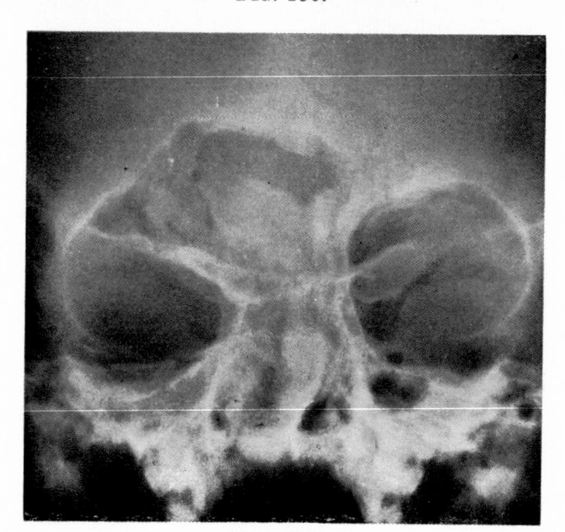

Fig. 191.

Figs. 190 and 191.—Traumatic Encephalocele of the Orbit.

Radiographs showing the destruction of the floor of the anterior fossa, the supra-orbital ridge and the base of the nose on the right side. The depression and tilting of the roof of the orbit on this side are very obvious (see Fig. 245) (A. B. King).

(Hughes, 1943). The formation of callus may cause damage by compressing important structures; we have already seen that this may involve a gradual deterioration of vision owing to compression of the optic nerve in the optic canal, a disability which has been relieved by operative removal of the newly formed bone through a transfrontal approach (Lillie and Adson, 1934).

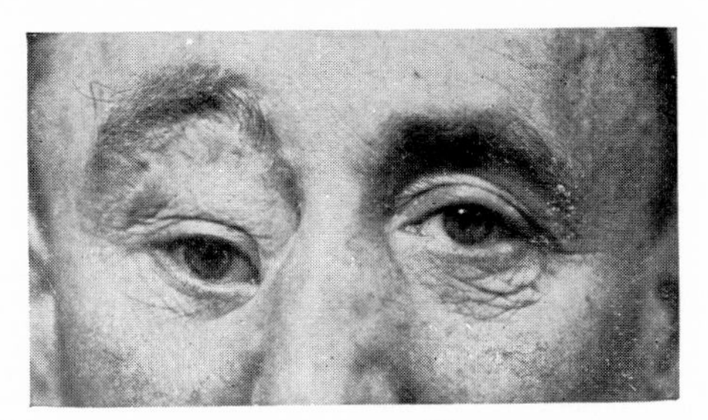

FIG. 192.—FRONTAL MUCOCELE.

Associated with a trauma involving a fracture of the floor of the orbit (W. H. Summerskill).

Stenosis of the supra-orbital foramen by the formation of callus after a fracture of the supra-orbital margin may similarly cause a supra-orbital neuralgia, a condition which may be cured by chiselling the foramen into a widely open notch (Dowling, 1910). Finally, injury to a sinus may result in the slow development of a mucocele which occasionally may attain enormous dimensions (Fig. 192); an intra-orbital hæmorrhage may result in the formation of a hæmorrhagic cyst which may appear clinically as an orbital tumour or the accumulated products of trauma may excite granulomatous proliferation resulting in a traumatic granuloma.

The general treatment of these fractures will be discussed subsequently.[1]

Anderson and Lloyd. *Canad. med. Ass. J.*, **90,** 110 (1964).
Apollonio. *Riv. Oto-neuro-oftal.*, **26,** 404 (1951).
Badal. *Gaz. Sci. méd. Bordeaux*, **15,** 283 (1894).
Banks. *Oral Surg.*, **24,** 455 (1967).
Belloni and Fasiani. *Riv. Oto-neuro-oftal.*, **17,** 491 (1940).
Berlin. *Ber. dtsch. ophthal. Ges.*, **12,** 9 (1879); **13,** 81, 87 (1881).
Graefe-Saemisch Hb. d. ges. Augenheilk., 1st ed., Leipzig, **6,** 586 (1880).
Bollack. *Ann. Oculist.* (Paris), **157,** 27 (1920).
Buzzard, Crampton-Smith, Hayton-Williams *et al. Brit. dent. J.*, **116,** 63 (1964).
Cantonnet and Coutella. *Arch. gén. Méd.*, **2,** 2177 (1906).
Converse, Smith, Obear and Wood-Smith. *Plast. reconstr. Surg.*, **39,** 20 (1967).
Davidson. *Amer. J. Ophthal.*, **21,** 7 (1938).
Dawson. *Brit. dent. J.*, **113,** 345 (1962).
Dawson and Fordyce. *Brit. J. Surg.*, **41,** 254 (1953).
DeVoe. *Trans. Amer. ophthal. Soc.*, **45,** 502 (1947).
Dowling. *Ophthalmology*, **6,** 633 (1910).
Fanjul. *Arch. Oftal. B. Aires*, **43,** 39 (1968).
François, J. and Verriest. *Proc. III Cong. Europ. Soc. Ophthal.*, Amsterdam, 332 (1969).
François, P. *Bull. Soc. Ophtal. Fr.*, **65,** 707 (1965).
Fromaget. *Gaz. Sci. Méd. Bordeaux*, **15,** 352 (1894).
Gissane and Bull. *Brit. med. J.*, **1,** 75 (1964).
Gordon and Macrae. *Plast. reconstr. Surg.*, **6,** 228 (1950).
Herman, Grasser and Beissiegel. *Dtsch. Zahnärztl.*, **15,** 657 (1960).
Hirschberg. *Berl. klin. Wschr.*, **17,** 169 (1880).
Holbourn. *Lancet*, **2,** 438 (1943).
Holmes. *XIII int. Cong. Ophthal.*, Amsterdam, **3** (3), 65 (1929).
Hughes, B. *Bull. Johns Hopk. Hosp.*, **111,** 98 (1962).
Hughes, E. B. C. *Brit. J. Ophthal.*, **27,** 367 (1943).
Jefferson and Schorstein. *Brit. J. Surg.*, **42,** 561 (1955).
Kazanjian and Converse. *The Surgical Treatment of Facial Injuries*, Baltimore (1949; 1970).
King. *Arch. Ophthal.*, **46,** 49 (1951).
Kjoer. *Acta ophthal.* (Kbh.), **23,** 357 (1945).
Körber. *Dtsch. Z. Chir.*, **29,** 545 (1889).
Kulowski. *J. Amer. dent. Ass.*, **53,** 32 (1956).
Lagrange. *Les fractures de l'orbite par les projectiles de guerre*, Paris (1917).
Lakke. *Arch. Neurol.*, **7,** 289 (1962).
Liebrecht. *Arch. Augenheilk.*, **55,** 36 (1906).

[1] p. 272.

Lillie and Adson. *Arch. Ophthal.*, **12,** 500 (1934).
Logan and Gordon. *Brit. J. Ophthal.*, **51,** 258 (1967).
Lundquist. *Int. dent. J.*, **10,** 476 (1960).
Lyle. *Trans. ophthal. Soc. U.K.*, **61,** 189 (1941).
McCoy, Chandler and Magnan. *Plast. reconstr. Surg.*, **29,** 381 (1962).
Malbran. *Arch. Oftal. B. Aires*, **10,** 632 (1935); **12,** 150 (1937).
Malbran and Balado. *Arch. Oftal. B. Aires*, **8,** 199 (1933).
Middeldorpf. *Breslauer aerztl. Z.*, No. 22 (1886). See *Jber. Ophthal.*, **17,** 563 (1886).
Mortada. *Brit. J. Ophthal.*, **45,** 662 (1961).
Neely. *Brit. J. Ophthal.*, **31,** 581 (1947).
Nieden. *Arch. Augenheilk.*, **12,** 30 (1883).
Plewes. *Proc. roy. Soc. Med.*, **60,** 945 (1967).
Reber. *Ophthal. Rec.*, **8,** 545 (1899).
Reny and Stricker. *Fractures de l'orbite*, Paris (1969).
Rodger. *Brit. J. Ophthal.*, **27,** 23 (1943).
Rowe and Killey. *Fractures of the Facial Skeleton*, 2nd ed., Edinburgh (1968).
Schjelderup. *Acta chir. scand.*, **99,** 445 (1950).
Schuchardt, Schwenzer, Rottke and Lentrodt. *Fortschr. Kiefer- u. Gesichtschir.*, **11,** 1 (1966).
Schultze. *Plast. reconstr. Surg.*, **45,** 227 (1970)
Sevitt. *Brit. J. Surg.*, **55,** 481 (1968).
Streiff and Buffat. *Rev. méd. Suisse rom.*, **71,** 531 (1951).
Thoral. *Clin. Ophtal.*, **13,** 192 (1924).
Traquair, Dott and Russell. *Brain*, **52,** 398 (1935).
Trokel and Potter. *Arch. Ophthal.*, **81,** 797 (1969).
Amer. J. Roentgenol., **106,** 530 (1969).
Turner. *Brain*, **66,** 140 (1943).
Walsh. *Invest. Ophthal.*, **5,** 433 (1966).
Walsh and Gass. *Amer. J. Ophthal.*, **50,** 1031 (1960).
Watson and Holt-Wilson. *Trans. ophthal. Soc. U.K.*, **88,** 361 (1968).
Wüst. *Klin. Mbl. Augenheilk.*, **114,** 140 (1949).

MIDDLE FACIAL FRACTURES

The general structure of the bones of the face is important in determining the lines of fracture caused by an impinging force. For our present purpose the face may be considered as being composed of an outer framework of hard bony elements surrounding a complicated arrangement of fragile central bones which enclose the nasal cavities and sinuses and partly surround the orbits, the whole complex being lightly attached to the skull in such a way as to receive and absorb blows without excessive jarring of the cranial base. It is probable that this arrangement is biologically determined to protect the cranium and the enclosed brain from constant trauma from the activities of the jaws; the upper jaw is designed to transmit over a wide area of the skull, through bony columns of which the zygomatic bones are the keystones, the mechanical stresses sustained in the act of biting—an activity which in civilized man rarely involves the violence necessary for the biological survival of his progenitors. Below, the upper jaw, braced transversely by the palatal arch, is specially toughened to carry the teeth. Above, two heavily built bones join with the frontals to constitute the solid lower orbital rim, the two sides being linked together by the less compact but still stout arch formed by the nasal processes of the maxillæ and the nasal bones.

Between these two, a fragile framework of thin plates of bone forms the walls of the maxillary antra, the nasal cavity and the ethmoid recesses. These delicate structures are not accessible to direct violence and since they are clothed by soft adherent tissues which greatly augment their strength, the elasticity of the whole is enhanced and impinging forces are distributed over a wide area. Indeed, the extreme tenuity of these bony elements increases the resistance of the whole structure. The arrangement is therefore one of functional strength rather than weakness, for even although the facial structure is smashed, the cushioning effect of the easily telescoped central area allows severe blows to be absorbed without irreparable damage to important organs such as the brain and the eyes, to protect which the bony framework is specially thickened. Thus a blow on the alveolus will result in this structure being sheared away from, or impacted into the crushable central mass; a blow on the bridge of the nose similarly thrusts the nasal arch into the nasal cavity and ultimately may cause a separation of the entire face from the cranium; while a similar blow on the lateral bastion of the malar is widely distributed throughout the cranial vault through the orbital processes of the frontal bone or, alternatively, the malar bone is driven into the antrum and the force dissipated in the crushing of non-vital structures. It therefore follows that few fractures of the face and only those associated with violent force, are continued into the skull, and frequently when both the cranium and the face are fractured, two separate fractures occur simultaneously.

It might be thought that fractures of this complicated structure would elude classification; but this is not so. The subject was first scientifically analysed by René Le Fort[1] (1900–1) who, conducting an elaborate series of 40 experiments on the cadaver skull whereby different parts of the face were subjected to blows of differing violence and direction, found on subsequent dissection that three lines of weakness exist, the presence of which allow such injuries to be grouped into a relatively small number of characteristic types. His " lines of weakness " thus determined are seen in Figs. 193 and 194.

Le Fort I. The Low Transverse Fracture. This line of weakness determines the commonest facial fracture (*Guérin's fracture*) and is present in most extensive lesions involving the face below the malar bones. Starting from the lower part of the nasal cavity, the line crosses the canine fossa and runs upwards and backwards to the pterygo-maxillary fissure. The fragment involved comprises the alveolar border, the vault of the palate and the pterygoid processes. This fracture, however, is without ophthalmological interest.

Le Fort II. The pyramidal fracture (also called a *floater*) separates the whole of the lower block of the middle third of the face from its supports. The line of weakness runs across the midline of the face, leaving the zygomatic arch uninjured. It involves or runs below the inferior part of the nasal bones, crosses the frontal process of the maxilla and the lacrimal bone usually above the naso-lacrimal canal, traverses a variable and sometimes extensive area of the floor of the orbit which shatters without offering much resistance, crosses the lower orbital margin in the region of the maxillo-zygomatic suture (leaving the latter bone unbroken), traverses the infra-orbital foramen, and fractures the pyramidal process of the maxilla and the pterygoid process, to end in the pterygo-maxillary fissure. In a complete fracture, the fragment thus involves part of the nasal bones, the lower part of the frontal process of the maxilla and part of the lacrimal bone. This type of fracture is of considerable importance to the ophthalmic surgeon since the injury may damage the medial orbital margin, the area of the lacrimal sac and the medial canthal ligament, resulting in lacrimal obstruction and displacement of the eyelids.

[1] p. 219.

FIGS. 193 and 194.—LE FORT'S LINES OF WEAKNESS.

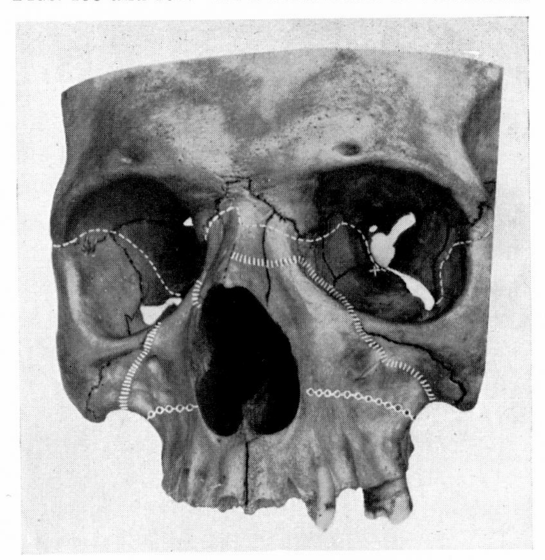

FIG. 193.—Antero-posterior view.

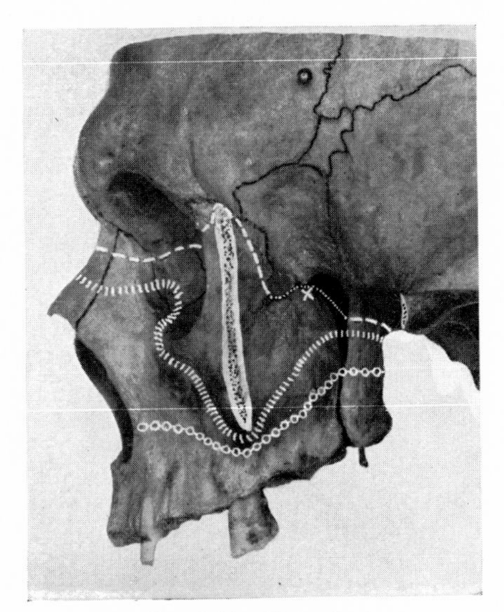

FIG. 194.—Lateral view.

Le Fort I, circles. Le Fort II, hatching. Le Fort III, broken line.

Le Fort III. The High Transverse Fracture. In its essentials this line of weakness allows a separation of the face from the cranium above the zygomatic arch, a condition known as *cranio-facial dysjunction.* The line starts through the upper part of the nasal bones; the upper cranial extremities of these bones are very resistant indeed, and if these give way the line of fracture traverses the cribriform plate and the floor of the anterior fossa. From the nasal bones the line runs through the medial wall of the orbit

FIGS. 195 to 198.—FACIAL FRACTURES.

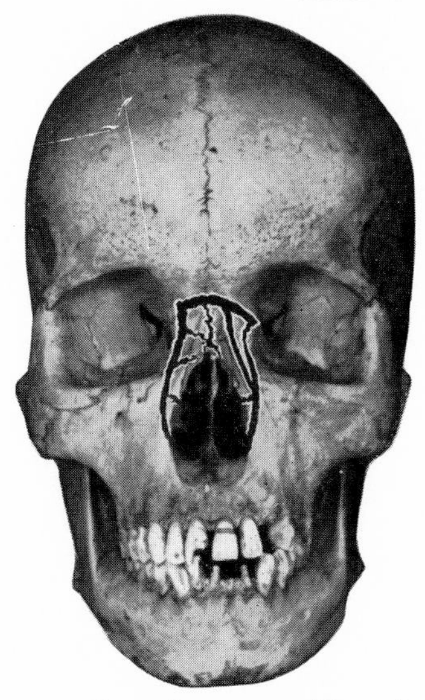

FIG. 195.—Central naso-maxillary fracture, first degree.

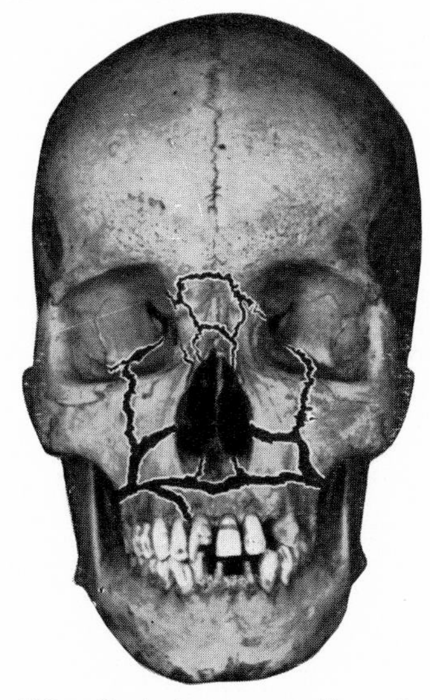

FIG. 196.—Central naso-maxillary fracture, second degree.

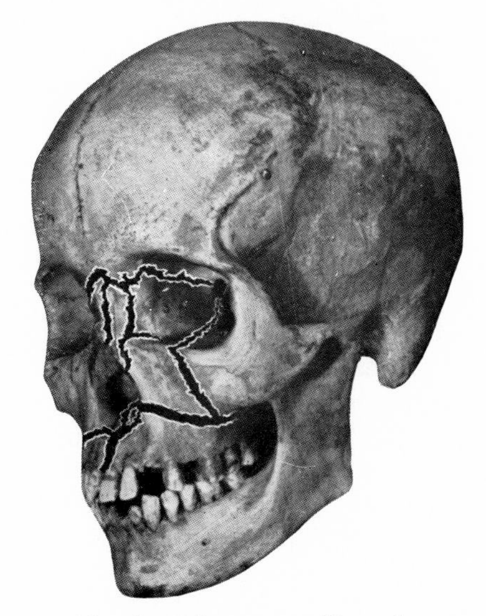

FIG. 197.—Central naso-maxillary fracture, third degree.

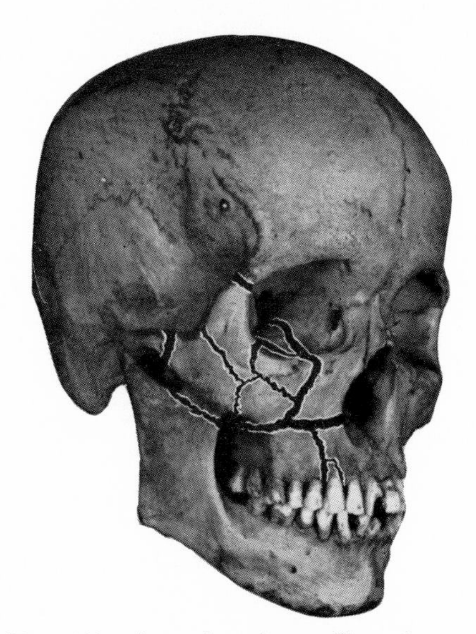

FIG. 198.—Lateral malo-maxillary fracture (after A. McIndoe).

in the neighbourhood of, or below the fronto-maxillary suture, the upper part of the lacrimal bone, across the ethmoid which is extensively fissured so that the ethmoid cells are exposed, and then descends below the optic canal (which escapes) to the infra-orbital fissure where the line of weakness bifurcates, one arm running upwards and forwards, separating the roof of the orbit from its lateral wall to terminate just below the fronto-malar suture at the external angular process, the other running downwards and backwards from the pterygo-maxillary fissure to divide the pterygoid processes near their bases. The bulk of this fragment therefore consists of the mass of the zygomatic arch.

These conclusions of Le Fort have been studied and amplified by many authors.[1] While these lines of weakness exist in the bony framework of the face and determine the general lines of structural weakness, they do not represent the actual form assumed in clinical practice by fractures, the type of which is determined in each individual accident by the incidence and nature of the impinging force and to a considerable extent by the degree of crushing injury entailed. Minor localized blows, which are of relatively common occurrence, produce localized fractures at the site of impact, often with a considerable degree of comminution. Major injuries, particularly of the crushing type so common in traffic accidents, produce effects which vary with the direction of the force and, so far as the orbital region is concerned, are usefully divided into two types depending on whether the violence is frontal or lateral.[2]

NASO-MAXILLARY FRACTURES—*due to frontal violence*

Frontal violence such as is sustained in a head-on crash causes bony damage varying in degree from a localized nasal fracture to a severe injury involving the anterior fossa of the skull; in either case the medial wall and floor of the orbit are frequently implicated. These fractures can usefully be classified into three groups according to the degree of force involved (Figs. 195–198) (McIndoe, 1941). This classification, however, does not help from the radiological point of view which is concerned more with the pattern of the fracture and the degree and direction of the displacement of the fragments involved (Campbell, 1964).

First degree. Moderate violence falling on the front or side of the nose produces a localized fracture which tends to involve a circle including the lower part of the nasal arch and the naso-maxillary processes which may be collapsed into the nasal cavity. Such a fracture may result in nasal obstruction and frequently in damage to the lacrimal sac and the naso-lacrimal canal (Fig. 195) or unsightly derangements at the inner canthus such as a traumatic telecanthus or epicanthus (Converse and Smith, 1966) (Fig. 199).

Second degree. If the violence is not absorbed by the collapse of the nasal arch into the nasal cavity, the narrow circle of the fracture is widened to the next line of weakness and runs backwards from the nasal bone, across the frontal process of the maxilla, and perhaps the upper part of the lacrimal bone; it crumbles the lamina papyracea of the ethmoid to reach the sphe-

[1] Wassmund (1927), Zarenko (1928), Wuhrmann (1932), Sonntag (1936), Link (1937), Kjoerholm (1938), James and Fickling (1941), and others.

[2] For a comprehensive description of the pathology, diagnosis and treatment of these injuries together with an extensive bibliography see *Fractures of the Facial Skeleton*, Ed. Rowe and Killey, 2nd ed., Edin. (1968) and *Orbital Fractures*, Hötte, Assen (1970).

noidal fissure from which it traverses the orbital floor to emerge at the malo-maxillary junction; thence it extends vertically downwards usually through the infra-orbital canal, and then across the anterior antral wall to the floor of the nasal cavity (Fig. 196). The line of such a fracture may be extended by running posteriorly along Le Fort's line beneath the malo-maxillary junction to the pterygo-maxillary fissure, or a complete Guérin's fracture may result (Fig. 197). Not infrequently the lateral malo-maxillary complexes are sprung open at the moment of impact so that the central portion

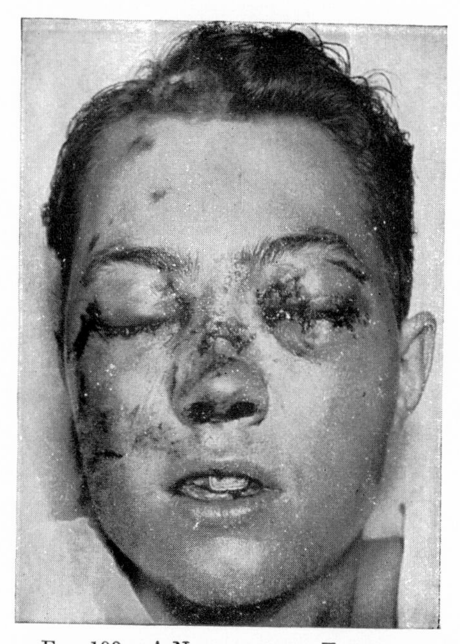

FIG. 199.—A NASO-ETHMOID FRACTURE.

Causing an increased intercanthal distance (traumatic telecanthus) (N. Rowe and H. Killey, *Fractures of the Facial Skeleton*, Livingstone).

of the face is driven between the two lateral portions and is there trapped by their recoil (Figs. 200–204).

Third degree. If the violence is more severe than can be absorbed by the underlying bony sinuses it will be transmitted to the cranial base so that the cribriform plate and the anterior fossa are involved.

The *clinical deformity* produced by such a fracture is essentially determined by the depression of the bridge of the nose and the widening of the intercanthal distance to produce the characteristic appearance traditionally known as " dish-face " (Figs. 205–207). Bleeding from the nose is common and, as a rarity, bleeding into the conjunctival sac from the puncta may occur (Urbantschitsch, 1946).

FIGS. 200 and 201.—SEVERE INJURY TO THE FACIAL SKELETON
(N. Rowe and H. Killey, *Fractures of the Facial Skeleton*, Livingstone).

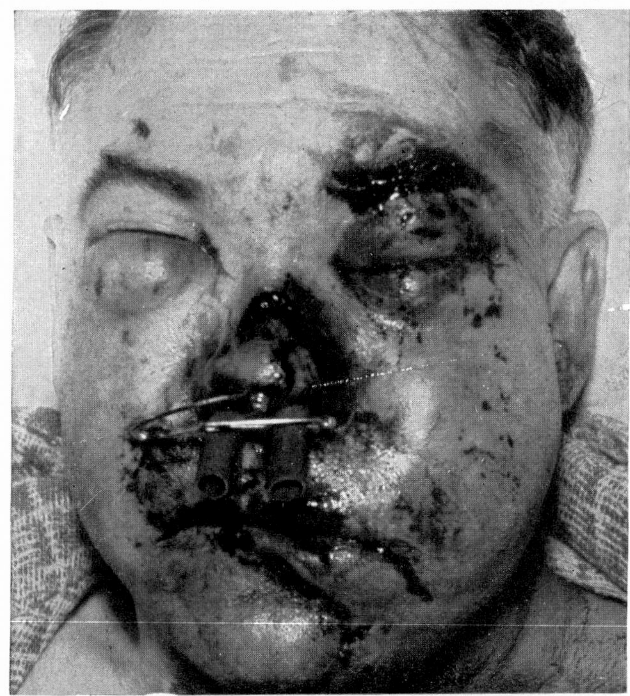

FIG. 200.—Four hours after the accident. There is œdema of the eyelids and middle third of the face with circumorbital ecchymosis. The left inner canthus is displaced downwards and outwards. Cyanosis resulting from obstruction to the airway by displacement of the palate and swelling of the tongue was relieved by two naso-pharyngeal tubes. The skeletal injuries include Le Fort fractures I, II and III, fractures of the cribriform plates of the ethmoid bone, the nasal bones, the body of the left mandible and posterior displacement of the left zygoma.

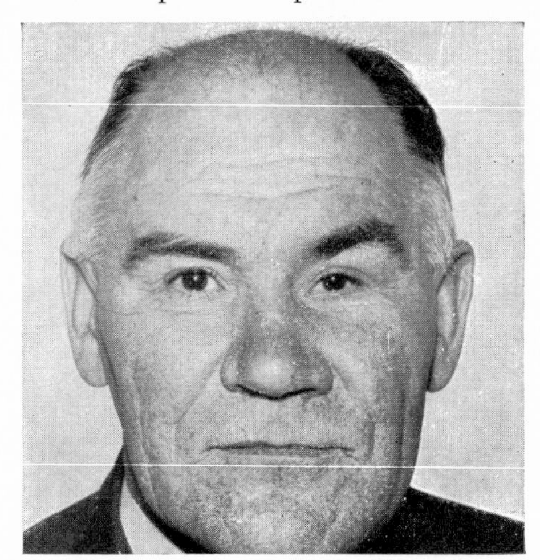

FIG. 201.—The same patient, showing full recovery.

Figs. 202 to 204.—Multiple Facial Fractures (W. Campbell).

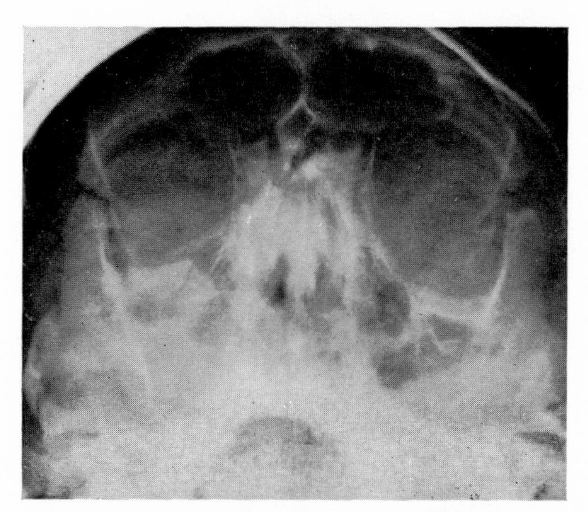

Fig. 202.

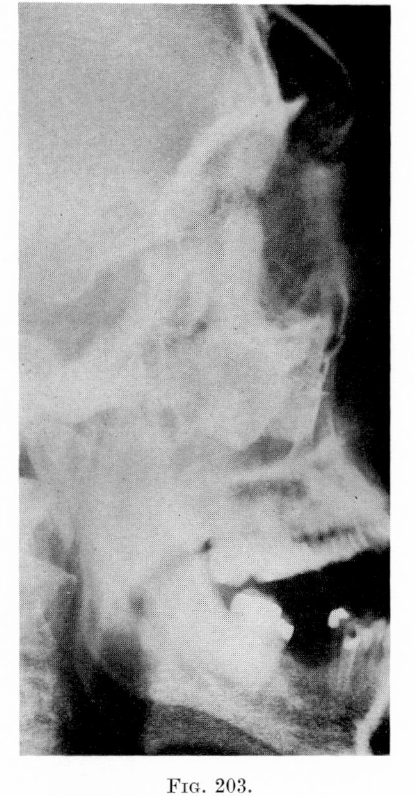

Fig. 203.

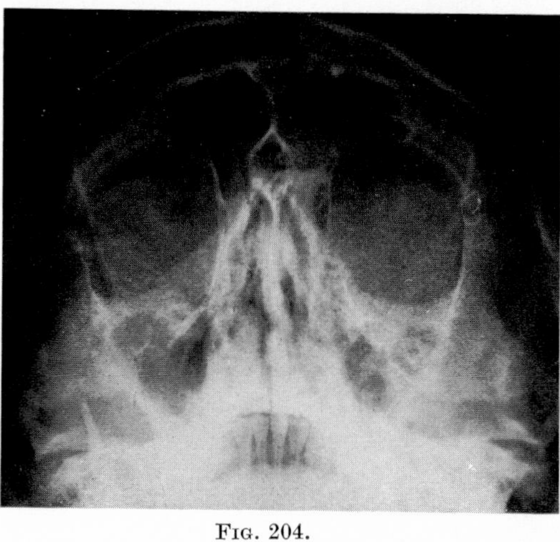

Fig. 204.

Figs. 202 and 203.—Severe facial injury showing a high transverse fracture of the face separating the whole bony structure from the floor of the frontal fossa. There is also a pyramidal fracture of the central middle third of the face and a low transverse fracture separating the alveolar processes of the maxillæ. The middle third of the face has been displaced backwards and downwards.

Fig. 204.—The same case one year later, showing almost complete restoration of the bony contour.

FIGS. 205 to 207.—MIDDLE FACIAL FRACTURES.

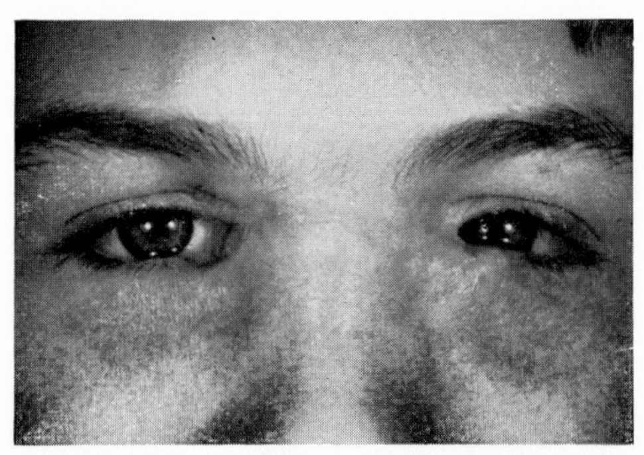

FIG. 205.—The appearance of " dish-face " resulting from a middle third facial fracture sustained in a motor accident one year previously. There is mal-alignment of the inner canthi which are displaced laterally (A. McIndoe).

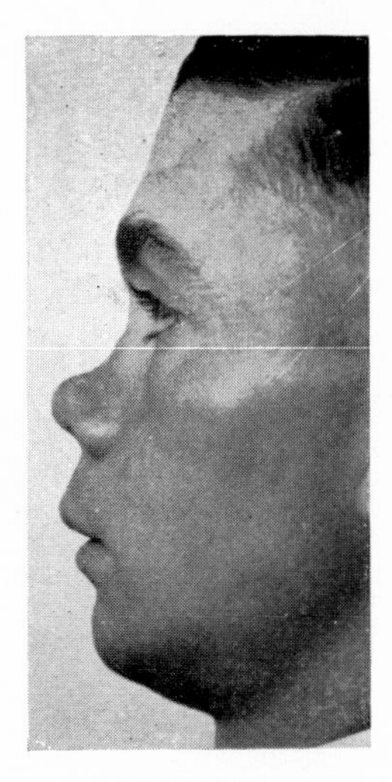

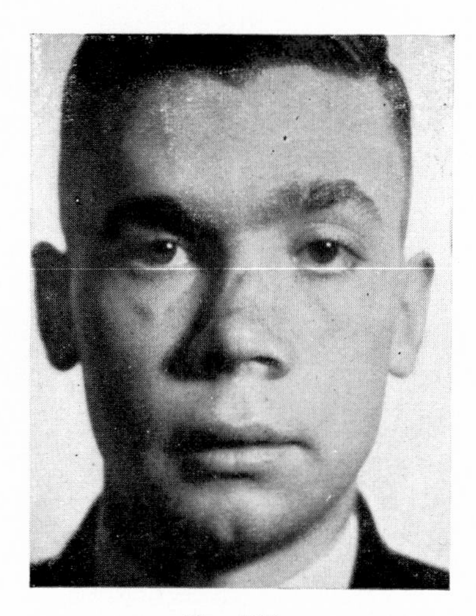

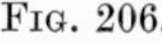

FIG. 206. FIG. 207.

FIGS. 206 and 207.—The typical " dish-face " deformity following naso-maxillary fracture of the third degree.

MALAR FRACTURES—*due to lateral violence*

In lateral violence the blow falls upon the malar bone which forms the prominence of the cheek. Fractures in this region have long been known and were first mentioned by Duverney (1751); before the advent of the automobile they were rare and were usually due to such an injury as a kick from a horse, but today they have become very common indeed. The usual line of fracture involves the malar processes of the frontal and maxillary bones; from the external angular process it runs backwards along the outer wall of the orbit, sometimes encroaching on the sphenoidal and frontal bones, to reach the infra-orbital fissure; thence it runs forwards along the orbital floor to reach the malo-maxillary attachment at the orbital rim whence it is directed obliquely downwards and outwards, usually traversing the infra-orbital canal through the malar process of the maxilla. If the force is moderate the malar bone is left intact, but in a more severe injury this bone is comminuted and is frequently impacted into the maxillary antrum and sometimes into the infra-temporal fossa (Fig. 234). If this occurs there is always a comminution of the orbital floor with a prolapse of the orbital contents into the antrum; further violence may involve in addition a fracture of the alveolus, while extreme degrees of crushing may determine an associated fracture of the skull involving one or more of the frontal and parietal bones and the great wing of the sphenoid (Fig. 198).

The deformity thus produced is frequently overlooked at the time of the accident owing to the swelling of the tissue of the cheek and lower lid. When

Figs. 208 and 209.—The Deformity produced by a Malar Fracture (modified from J. M. Converse and B. Smith).

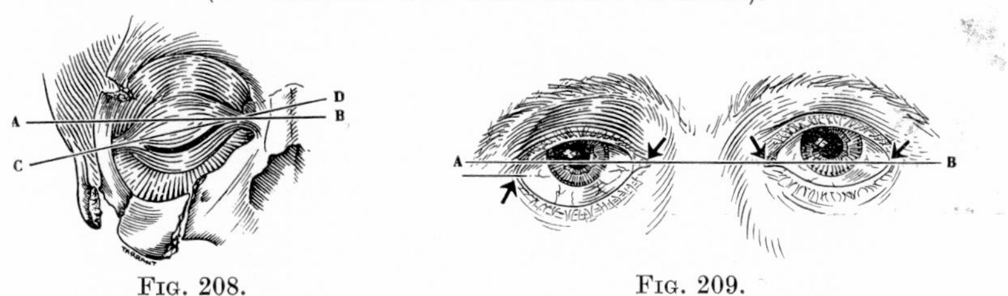

Fig. 208. Fig. 209.

Fig. 208.—Showing the disposition of the parts after fracture, particularly the downward displacement of the outer canthus. AB indicates the normal canthal level; CD the obliquity of the displacement.

Fig. 209.—Showing the external appearance in a malar fracture on the right side. The arrows indicate the position of the canthi. AB is the normal canthal level.

this swelling subsides, however, it is found that the malar prominence is flattened, the external canthus is displaced downwards, the eye has sunk backwards and downwards often with diplopia, the lower lid is retracted downwards and the superior palpebral sulcus is deeply hollowed (Figs. 208–212); the backward displacement of the globe may entail a mechanical ptosis wherein the upper lid, deprived of its normal support, falls downwards (Fig. 211). The antrum itself is filled with blood and opaque to trans-illumination, sometimes obscuring the fracture in the x-ray picture; there is bleeding from the nose, while the depression of the zygoma sometimes interferes with the movement of the coronoid process of the mandible so that the mouth can be opened or closed only with difficulty. Occasionally considerable deformities may persist such as the conversion of the usual downward displacement of the outer canthus into a condition of permanent avulsion (Fig. 212). In addition to the cosmetic deformity of flattening of the cheek and displacement of the globe, the signs and symptoms of such a fracture are therefore occasional diplopia, disturbance of the mobility of the jaw and sometimes anæsthesia throughout the area of distribution of the infra-orbital nerve when the fracture has involved the infra-orbital canal. Generally speaking, the eye itself escapes serious ill-effects unless the original injury directly involves the globe in a concussion or penetrating wound, but in a

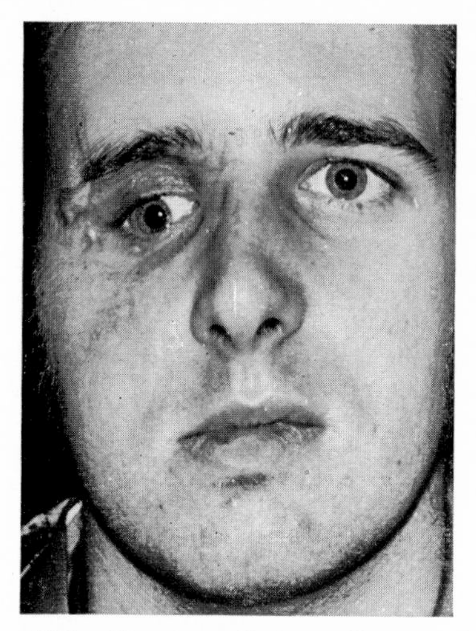

FIG. 210.—MULTIPLE ORBITAL FRACTURES.

In a road accident; there resulted fractures of the frontal bone, zygoma and floor of the orbit causing downward displacement of the globe (Inst. Ophthal.).

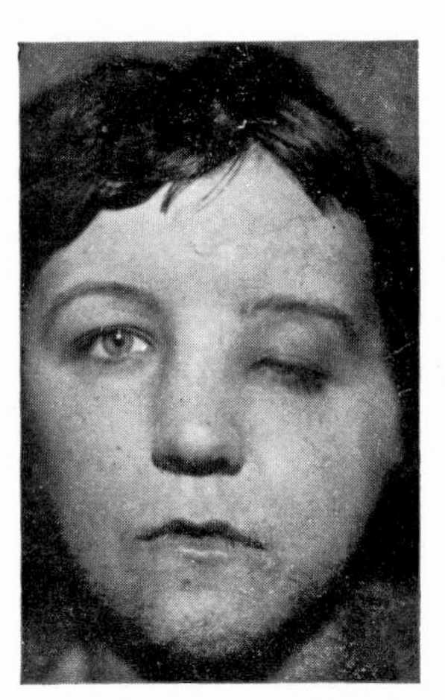

FIG. 211.—MALAR FRACTURE.

Long-term result showing depression of the cheek, downward and inward displacement of the globe and a mechanical pseudo-ptosis on the left side (T. Pomfret Kilner).

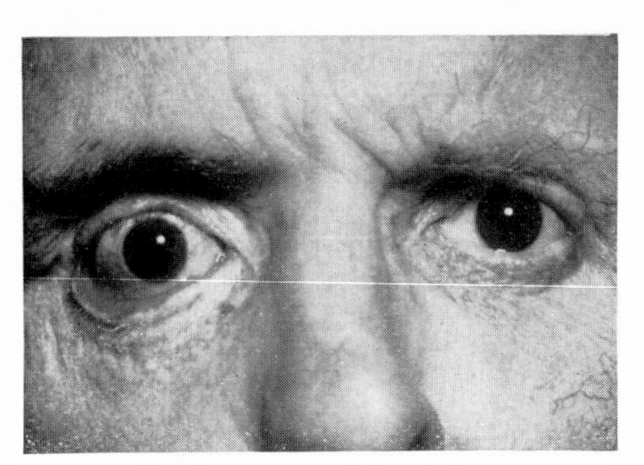

FIG. 212.—AVULSION OF THE OUTER CANTHUS.

The deformity produced by a facial injury received 10 years previously. There is a right malar fracture with depression of the eye, right-sided facial palsy and evulsion of the right outer canthus (A. McIndoe).

case reported by Gordon and MacRae (1950) uniocular blindness followed the surgical reduction of a fractured zygoma, probably due to obstruction of the central retinal artery. This problem will be discussed more fully in a subsequent section.[1]

[1] p. 277.

It is interesting that the malar bone which is developed from cartilage and contains red marrow may give rise to considerable callus formation on healing after a fracture. A hyperplasic growth of this type may fill the temporal fossa and encroach upon the orbit, producing proptosis and requiring operative removal (Eagleton, 1935). Exostoses and hyperostoses may also follow such a trauma (Baltin, 1935); while the development of the syndrome of the sphenoidal fissure (ocular motor pareses, trigeminal anæsthesias and neuralgia and occasionally disturbances of the optic nerve), due presumably to a periostitis of the orbital apex, has been noted to occur at a later date.

An unusual and exceptional complication of an orbital fracture is the development of a mucocele or pyocele arising from the displacement into the orbit of a portion of the mucoperiosteum of a sinus and the subsequent formation of a cyst. Such a sequence was reported by Shuttleworth and King (1951) wherein a mucocele, symptom-free for seven years but displacing the globe, was formed from the detached antral mucoperiosteum.

Treatment is by operative removal.

Baltin. *Auerbach Jub. Vol.*, 53 (1935). See *Zbl. ges. Ophthal.*, **36,** 440 (1936).
Campbell. *Recent Advances in Radiology* (ed. Lodge), London, 239 (1964).
Converse and Smith. *Plast. reconstr. Surg.*, **38,** 147 (1966).
Duverney. *Traité des maladies des yeux*, Paris, **1,** 182 (1751).
Eagleton. *Arch. Ophthal.*, **14,** 1 (1935).
Gordon and MacRae. *Plast. reconstr. Surg.*, **6,** 228 (1950).
James and Fickling. *Proc. roy. Soc. Med.*, **34,** 205 (1941).
Kjoerholm. *Ugeskr. Laeg.*, **100,** 659 (1938).
Le Fort. *Echo méd. Nord*, **4,** 470 (1900).
XIII Cong. int. Méd., Paris (1900), *Sect. Chir. gén.*, 275 (1901).
Le Fort. *Rev. Chir.*, **23,** 208, 360, 479 (1901).
Link. *Zbl. Chir.*, **64,** 467 (1937).
McIndoe. *Brit. dent. J.*, **71,** 235 (1941).
Rowe and Killey. *Fractures of the Facial Skeleton*, 2nd ed., Edinburgh (1968).
Shuttleworth and King. *Brit. J. Ophthal.*, **35,** 427 (1951).
Sonntag. *Mschr. Unfallheilk.*, **43,** 369 (1936).
Urbantschitsch. *Wien. klin. Wschr.*, **58,** 488 (1946).
Wassmund. *Frakturen u. Luxationen des Gesichtsschädels*, Berlin (1927).
Wuhrmann. *Schweiz. med. Wschr.*, **62,** 767 (1932).
Zarenko. *Arch. klin. Chir.*, **153,** 161 (1928).

INTERNAL ORBITAL FRACTURES

Neither the internal wall nor the floor of the orbit both of which are of paper-thinness can be considered as a barrier to impinging violence. A fracture of these orbital walls occurring without involving the stout orbital rim or other bones of the face is thus a relatively common event, probably much more common than is supposed (Pfeiffer, 1943; E. F. King, 1944; DeVoe, 1947). We have already seen that frontal injury may determine a fracture of the orbital roof and this may be further complicated by a splintering of the floor leaving the orbital margin both above and below unaffected, while Pfeiffer (1943) found that among 120 fractures of the orbit the floor alone was implicated in 24 cases. Similarly, the medial wall may be fractured alone or in association with an injury involving the orbital floor or the nasal bones (Cramer *et al.*, 1965; Dodick *et al.*, 1969).

In recent years as a result of the work of J. M. Converse and Byron Smith in the United States a new term has been added to the nomenclature of orbital fractures. In a series of publications dating from 1957 they introduced the concept of a *blow-out fracture* of the floor of the orbit resulting from blunt trauma producing a fracture of the orbital process of the maxilla (Converse and Smith, 1957; Smith and Converse, 1957). As we have already seen, fractures of the orbital floor are common in association with other fractures of bones of the middle third of the face and they have been classified in many ways, such terms as pure and impure, simple and complicated, internal and external, primary and secondary, being generally used. The term "blow-out" fracture of the orbit, however, refers to a specific syndrome in which a *fracture of the orbital floor occurs on its own without a fracture of the orbital rim*, usually as a result of a blow from in front impinging on the soft tissues of the orbit. This condition is to be distinguished from an injury to the orbital floor associated with fractures of the zygoma, maxilla or nasal bones (impure, rim and wall fractures). Whereas the orbital floor is most commonly involved in a blow-out fracture, a similar injury may involve the medial orbital wall either in continuity or alone.[1]

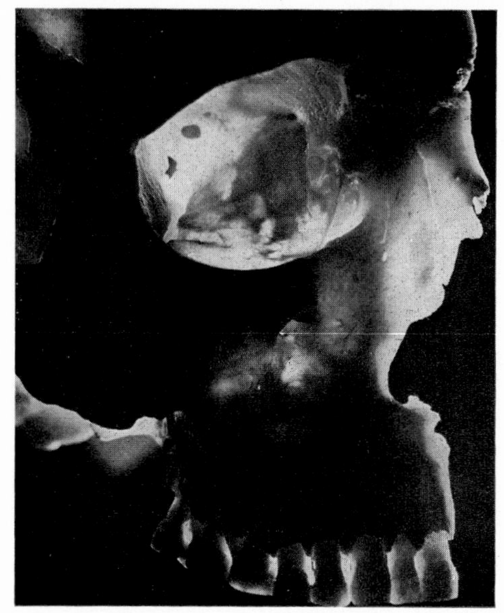

FIG. 213.—THE APPEARANCE ON TRANSILLUMINATION OF THE SKULL.
Demonstrating the thinness of the walls of the orbit and the thickness of its margins (E. W. Walls).

Historically the complications resulting from blow-out fractures were described long before the fracture or its exact causation was understood; Lang (1889) held that every case of traumatic enophthalmos with limitation of ocular movement was due to a fracture of the orbital floor. Pfeiffer (1941–43) found among 120 cases of facial fracture involving the orbit, 53 with enophthalmos in 24 of which only the orbital floor was fractured, the rim remaining intact; he also observed the increase in radio-density of the ipsilateral maxillary antrum in cases of enophthalmos and suggested that the thin posterior orbital floor could be broken by the sudden impact on it of the eyeball.

[1] The literature dealing with blow-out fractures of the orbit is now very extensive. A detailed account of the problems involved in the diagnosis and treatment of these cases, particularly those with late complications, together with a comprehensive bibliography up to 1967, can be found in an important review by Converse and his colleagues (1967) and Fanjul (1968), and the management of these injuries has also been described in detail by Mustardé (1966), Rowe and Killey (1968), Milauskas (1969), Reny and Stricker (1969) and Lerman (1970).

It is, however, to the clinical and experimental work of Smith and Converse and their colleagues that we owe much of our present understanding of the mechanism of the fracture and its complications, on which the principles of management are now based.

At this point it is convenient to recapitulate certain points concerning the anatomy of the bony orbit[1] which are relevant to an understanding of the mechanism of blow-out and other types of orbital fracture. In antero-posterior section the orbit is cone-shaped. The orbital contents are protected anteriorly by a strong rounded rim of bone, the superior orbital rim of the frontal bone above, the zygoma laterally, the frontal process of the maxilla medially, and inferiorly the relatively thick rim of the orbital floor formed medially by the maxilla and laterally by the zygoma. Situated between the two strong bony abutments, the zygoma and frontal process of the maxilla, the inferior orbital rim is supported from below by relatively thin bone which constitutes the anterior wall of the maxillary sinus. The floor of the orbit extends backwards and upwards on an inclined plane, the posterior portion of which is an area of thin bone situated immediately anterior to the inferior orbital fissure. This area which is the thinnest part of the bony orbit is continued medially by the lamina papyracea of the ethmoid, a portion of the medial wall which, as its name implies, is of paper-like thinness. These differences in structural thickness are well demonstrated in Fig. 213. The medial half of the orbital floor is further weakened by the canal or groove for the passage of the infra-orbital nerve; the bone overlying the infra-orbital canal is reduced to a thickness of only 0·5 mm. (Bowers, 1964). This nerve is in a precarious position; it enters the orbit through the inferior orbital fissure, continues forward in the infra-orbital groove and canal and pierces the maxilla at the infra-orbital foramen. In addition to the posterior orbital floor inferiorly and the lamina papyraces and orbital plate of the ethmoid medially, there is a third weak area laterally in the thin bone adjacent to the temporal fossa.

BLOW-OUT FRACTURES result from a sudden increase of intra-orbital pressure secondary to a blow to the eye and soft tissues of the orbit, from a non-penetrating convex object such as a tennis ball, a fist or other bodies of greater diameter than the orbital margin. Smaller objects such as a golf-ball are more likely to produce a severe contusion or rupture of the globe. The tissues of the orbit are suddenly compressed and the increased pressure is transmitted to the walls, of which the more delicate portions are fractured and blown outwards. As a rule the floor is the usual site of fracture, possibly because the weak area is convex in shape and bulges slightly upwards behind the eyeball (Figs. 214–217). Bony fragments and orbital soft tissues may be displaced downwards into the underlying maxillary antrum, usually giving rise to a hæmorrhage. Sometimes the blow-out fracture involves the medial orbital wall in the area of the lamina papyracea and the orbital plate of the ethmoid, resulting in the medial displacement of the bony fragments and the orbital soft tissues with local hæmorrhage and œdema in the plane of the ethmoid air-cells.

The basic mechanism responsible for this type of orbital floor injury was first suggested by Pfeiffer (1943) from a study of the radiological appearances in a series of cases of traumatic enophthalmos associated with vertical diplopia and infra-orbital paræsthesia; in the same year Linhart (1943) put

[1] Vol. II, p. 389.

Figs. 214 to 216.—Blow-out Fractures of the Orbital Floor.

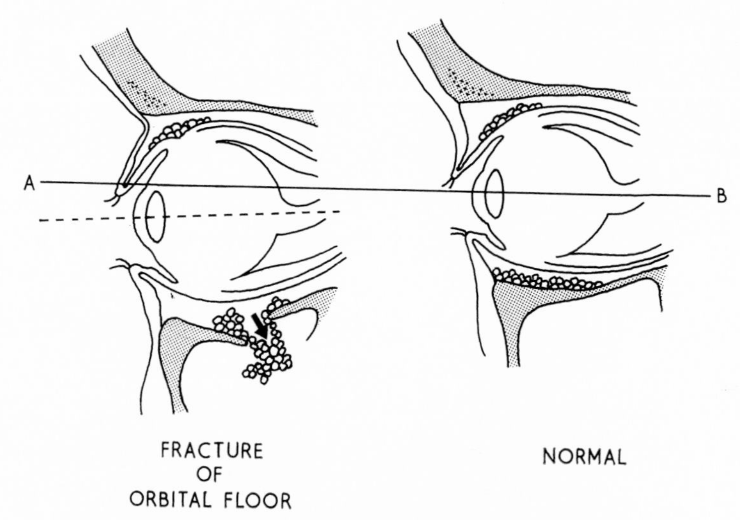

Fig. 214.—The figure illustrates the displacement of the eyeball and the visual axis. The line AB represents the visual axis in the normal position (right) and the dotted line that in the displaced position (left) (T. K. Lyle).

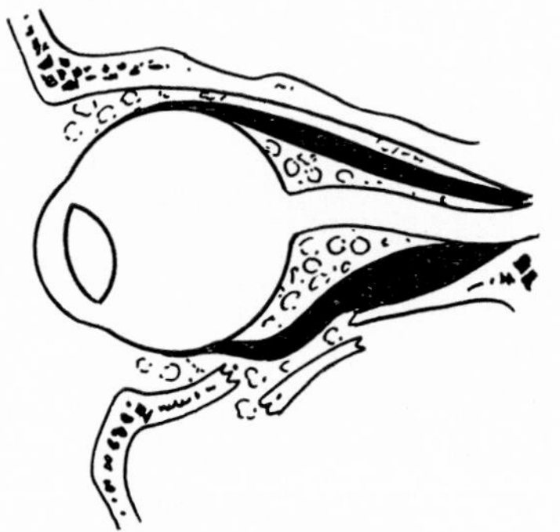

Fig. 215.—A fractured bone of the orbital floor has projected downwards into the maxillary antrum as though it had been punched out (D. K. Whyte).

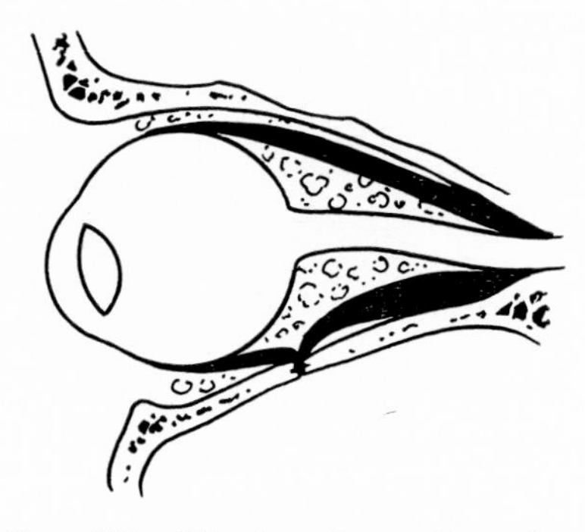

Fig. 216.—The trap-door effect showing that the inferior rectus is nipped as the fractured floor springs back into its original position (D. K. Whyte).

forward a similar explanation to account for fractures of the medial wall. Evidence in support of the theory that a blow-out fracture is the result of increased intra-orbital pressure and not due to direct bony transmission was first produced by Smith and Regan (1957) in experiments on a cadaver. They showed that a *sudden* increase of pressure within the orbit was necessary, and that the striking body must occlude the anterior orbital aperture; moreover, repetition after removal of the eyeball did not rupture the orbital floor until sufficient force had been applied to fracture the orbital rim as well. The degree of force required to cause a blow-out fracture was also investigated by Bessière and his colleagues (1964), and D. Jones and Evans (1967) produced blow-out fractures in the orbits of cadavers by means of a firm blow from a hammer to an applicator placed in position over the closed eyes in order to determine the commonest site of fracture. In 79% of cases the main site of fracture was situated in the posterior part of the orbital floor medial to the infra-orbital groove and canal. According to Jones and Evans (1967) and Whyte (1968) the reason for the high incidence of fractures at this site is a combination of the extreme thinness of the bone at this point, the close proximity of the upwardly inclined bone of the posterior orbital floor to the globe and the fact that the site of the fracture lies directly beneath the

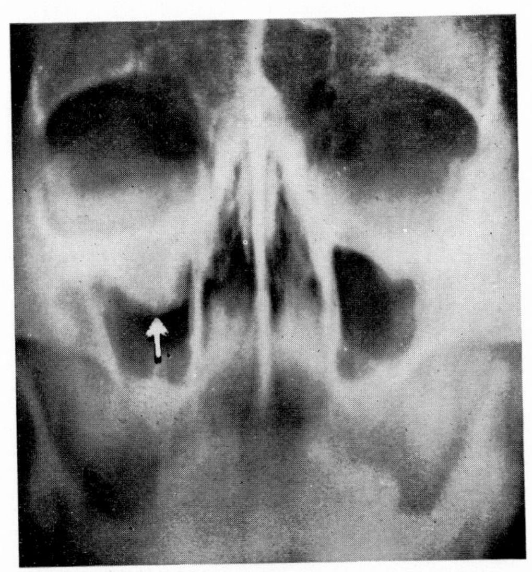

Fig. 217.—Blow-out Fracture of the Orbital Floor.

Tomogram showing the orbital contents herniated into the maxillary antrum comprising the characteristic " hanging drop " opacity (arrowed) (J. M. Converse and B. Smith).

geometrical orbital axis along which it is presumed the eyeball is pushed as a result of a direct frontal blow. It is interesting that a blow-out fracture of the ethmoid occurred in 6 of the 33 orbits studied by Jones and Evans (1967), similar to the case described by Smith and Regan (1957), in 11 out of 24 cases studied radiologically by Pfeiffer (1943), and in 8 of 14 cases examined with the technique of hypocycloid tomography by Dodick and his colleagues (1969).

In the typical case of internal orbital fracture the causal injury is comparatively slight, a blow by a ball in games or by a fist or elbow which has perhaps left few external marks of injury and excited little attention at the time. On the other hand, the injury may be severe, particularly in children (Wolter and Chamichian, 1970). Increasingly, however, this fracture is a result of a road traffic accident; thus, in 100 cases such a cause was responsible in 49 (Converse *et al.*, 1967). A detailed analysis of large numbers of such cases was given by Rowe and Killey (1968).

On very rare occasions the causal injury does not fit into any of the above categories—as in the case reported by Consul and his colleagues (1968) wherein a fracture of the floor of the orbit resulted from the bite of a camel—the damage was successfully repaired with a graft of autogenous bone from the iliac crest.

Fracture of the medial orbital wall is a common result of naso-orbital injuries (Converse and Smith, 1963) and should be suspected if there is bleeding from the nose with or without surgical emphysema, and as we have already seen the ethmoid may be involved in a blow-out fracture of the orbital floor (Cramer *et al.*, 1965; Dodick *et al.*, 1969). Cases have occurred, however, in which the medial wall alone has been the site of such a fracture with the characteristic sign of limitation of movement due to the incarceration in it of the medial rectus muscle (Figs. 218–219).

In a case reported by Miller and Glaser (1966) incarceration of Tenon's capsule and the medial rectus muscle was associated with retraction of the globe and narrowing of the palpebral fissure on attempted abduction, amounting to a traumatic retraction syndrome, a lesion accompanied by a fracture of the orbital floor entrapping the inferior rectus and the inferior oblique muscles; freeing the medial rectus and reconstitution of the orbital floor by a methyl methacrylate implant restored normal motility. In another case described by Edwards and Ridley (1968) following blunt trauma to the orbit from a bottle, diplopia associated with limitation of adduction and of abduction was found on exploration to be due to imprisonment of the medial rectus muscle and its sheath within the line of a fracture in the ethmoid bone; removal of a small piece of the ethmoid plate allowed the muscle to be set free whereupon the forced duction test became normal. A similar situation occurred in a case reported by Fischbein and Lesko (1969) wherein the forced duction test suggested incarceration of the medial rectus, although there was, in fact, also a fracture of the orbital floor. At a second exploration a fracture in the lamina papyracea of the ethmoid was found with a spicule of bone interfering with the action of the muscle; release of this obstruction restored normal ocular rotation. A further case of the retraction syndrome with gross limitation of adduction due to entrapment of the medial rectus, in which the exact location of the fracture in the lamina papyracea was demonstrated by hypocycloid tomography, was reported by Trokel and Potter (1969) (Figs. 218–9). These cases emphasize the importance of incarceration of the medial rectus as shown by limitation of voluntary movement or of forced duction as evidence of a fracture of the medial orbital wall even when radiological confirmation is absent; it should be regarded as an indication for surgical exploration.

In this connection it should be remembered that the floor of the anterior cranial fossa consists of relatively thin bone which can readily be fractured; this applies particularly to children in whom the superciliary arch is not fully developed. Even penetrating wounds of the lids may thus be complicated by intracranial damage.[1]

BLOW-IN FRACTURE OF THE ORBIT. Dingman and Natvig (1964) drew attention to a very unusual type of injury of the orbital floor, similar in ætiology and clinical

[1] p. 443.

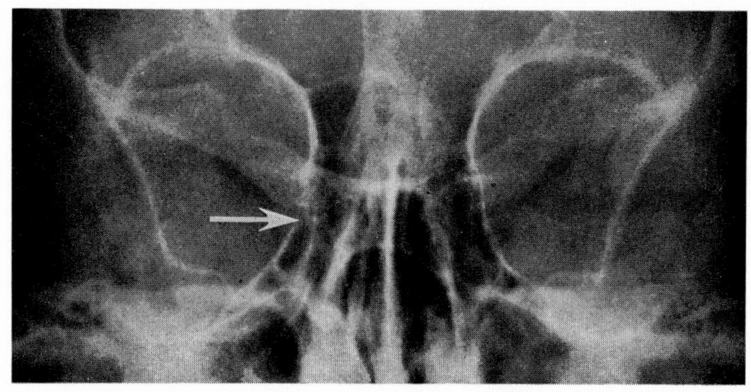

Fig. 218.

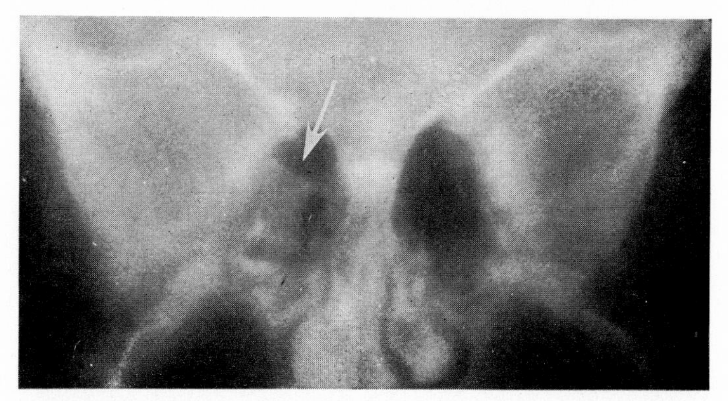

Fig. 219.

Figs. 218 and 219.—Fracture of the Medial Wall of the Orbit.

A youth aged 17 jammed his knee into his right orbit while doing acrobatics. The eye and visual acuity were normal but there was a gross limitation of adduction. The plain radiograph (Fig. 218) revealed only a slight clouding of the right ethmoid sinus (arrowed); but the tomogram (Fig. 219) showed a discontinuity of the medial wall of the orbit through which there was a prolapse of the orbital contents with incarceration of the medial rectus through the lamina papyracea of the ethmoid bone (S. L. Trokel and G. B. Potter).

appearance to the more usual depressed blow-out fracture, but where the orbital floor is elevated. Treatment is by surgical exposure and instrumental depression of the fragment to its normal level.

Clinical Picture

The clinical picture of fractures of the middle third of the face is usually so dominated by multiple injuries, the enormous swelling and suffusion of the soft tissues and by the general condition of shock and concussion that the fracture itself, particularly if it involves the orbital floor and the malar region, may be overlooked. The presence of a fracture is indicated by local tenderness and the demonstration of the loss of continuity or the deformity around the orbital margin in comparison with its fellow while the elicitation of crepitation indicates its site with certainty. *Hæmorrhage* into the lids appearing some hours after an injury suggests underlying damage to the bone (Fig. 220); a profuse hæmorrhage, particularly into the orbit involving proptosis, is of considerable diagnostic significance, while *surgical emphysema* indicates a fracture involving one or other of the nasal sinuses usually in a fracture of the medial orbital wall (Figs. 221, 257).

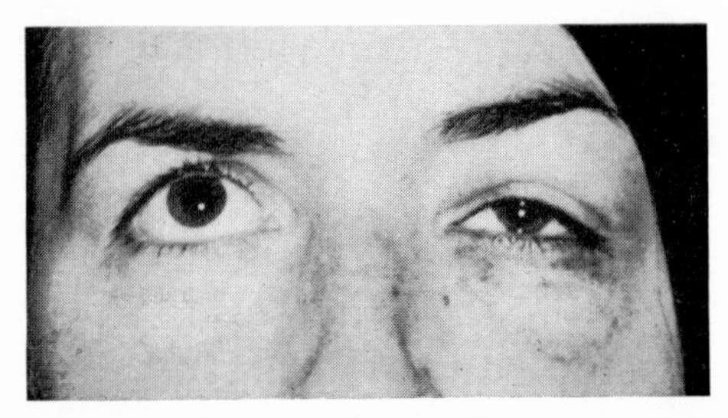

Fig. 220.—Fracture of the Orbital Floor of the Left Eye.
There is a hæmorrhage into the lids in the malar region.

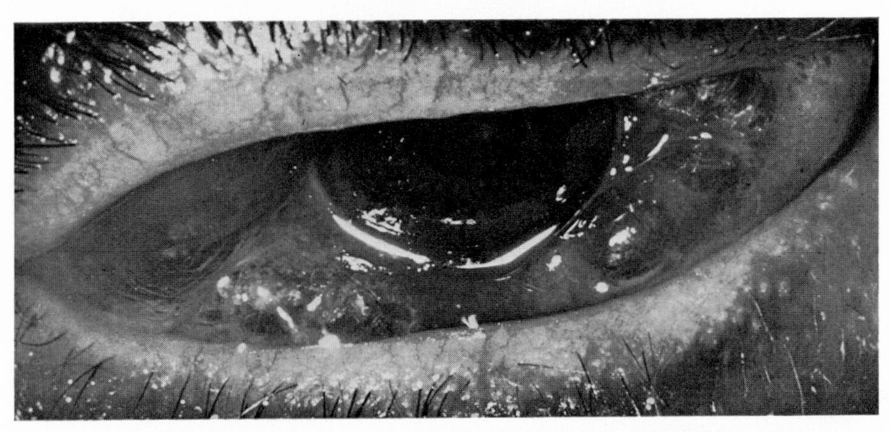

Fig. 221.—Subconjunctival Emphysema (Inst. Ophthal.).

Displacement of the globe is a frequent occurrence: either proptosis due to intra-orbital hæmorrhage or a staving-in of the orbital walls; enophthalmos due to comminution of the floor with herniation of the orbital contents into the maxillary antrum or the nasal cavity; a vertical displacement which may be upwards caused by the presence of bony fragments in the orbit or, more usually, downwards due to the loss of the supporting action of the ligament of Lockwood which stretches like a hammock from the medial to the lateral bony margins of the orbit (Mustardé, 1966). Of these, enophthalmos is the usual type of displacement following an orbital fracture although it may not become obvious until the hæmorrhage and swelling of the soft tissues have subsided. A number of factors may contribute to this occurrence; thus an escape of fat from the orbital cavity through a rupture of the periorbita into the maxillary sinus, or an enlargement of the orbital cavity as may occur in any type of orbital fracture results in a redistribution of the orbital soft tissues so that they no longer effectively maintain the normal position of the globe. Necrosis of the orbital fat may result from a low-grade inflammation or be caused by the pressure from an orbital hæmatoma. Finally, the globe may

FIGS. 222 and 223.—AN ORBITAL FRACTURE BELOW THE LIGAMENT OF LOCKWOOD (J. C. Mustardé).

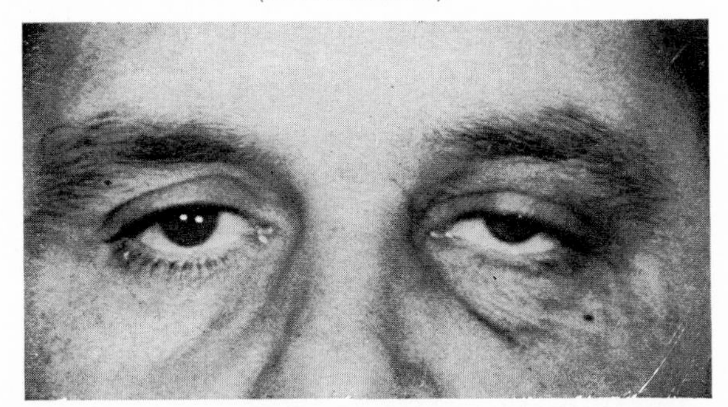

FIG. 222.—The eyes are level in the primary position.

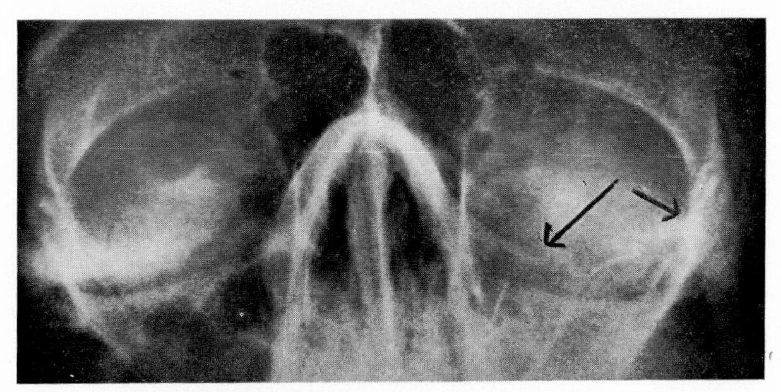

FIG. 223.—Radiograph demonstrating the fracture.

be held in a backward position by incarceration of one or more of the extra-ocular muscles in a fracture-line; the affected muscle tends to become fibrotic and shortened while similar changes may eventually affect the other extra-ocular muscles. When enophthalmos is gross, as may occur with massive downward displacement of the orbital contents, a pseudo-ptosis of the upper lid may result giving rise to a deepening of the supratarsal fold and a shortening of the horizontal dimension of the palpebral fissure, while in the presence of a naso-orbital fracture and damage to adjacent bones the deformity may be even more complicated.

The important role of the suspensory ligament of Lockwood in maintaining the normal position of the eye has been stressed by Mustardé (1968); if this structure and its attachments to the orbital walls are intact, the level of the eye within the orbital cavity is unlikely to be affected (Figs. 222 and 223). If the fracture occurs above the line of attachment of Lockwood's ligament, a downward displacement of the globe will certainly follow (Figs. 224 and 225). Such a displacement may be considerable but is unlikely to be as severe as occurred in an extraordinary case cited by Converse and his colleagues (1967): a fireman turned on his hose while inspecting the nozzle and received the full power of the water-jet in his face, the resulting blow-out fracture was

Figs. 224 and 225.—An Orbital Fracture Above the Ligament of Lockwood on the Left Side (J. C. Mustardé).

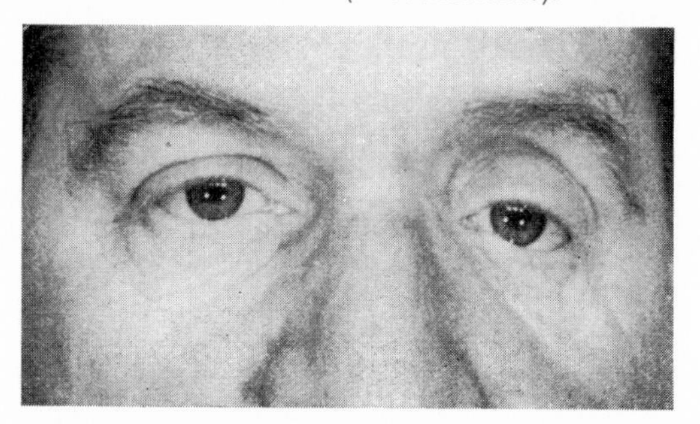

Fig. 224.—The eye is displaced downwards.

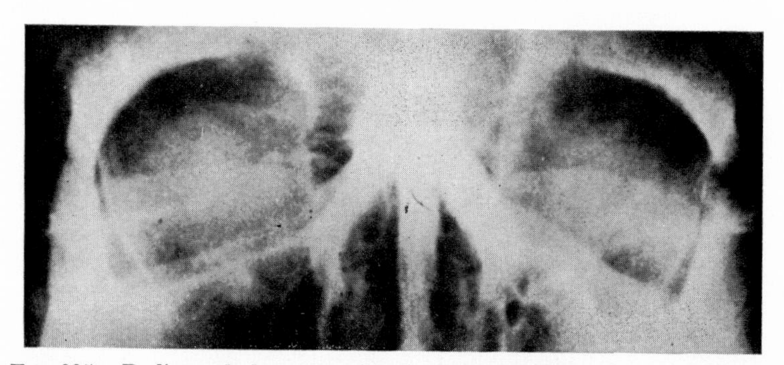

Fig. 225.—Radiograph demonstrating the fracture involving a displacement of the ligament of Lockwood.

so severe that the whole eyeball disappeared from the orbital cavity and was at first thought to have been enucleated by the blast of water; exploration, however, revealed the globe within the maxillary antrum, intact apart from several choroidal tears; the eye was restored to its natural position and the orbital floor repaired; virtually normal vision was regained.

Diplopia is a common and important ocular symptom of orbital injury, usually due to restriction of vertical movements (Figs. 226–230); in some cases it may become the dominant permanent disability, the management of which will be discussed subsequently.[1] At this point, however, it is convenient to

[1] p. 302.

FIGS. 226 to 228.—BLOW-OUT FRACTURE OF THE ORBITAL FLOOR.
Following a blow with a fist (M. A. Bedford).

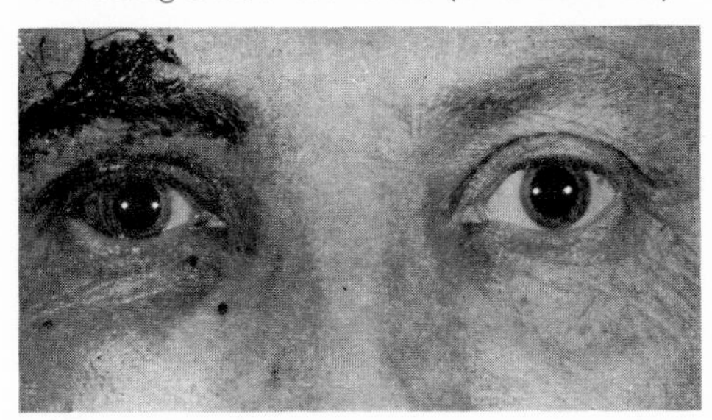

FIG. 226.—Subconjunctival and palpebral hæmorrhages with laceration of the eyebrow.

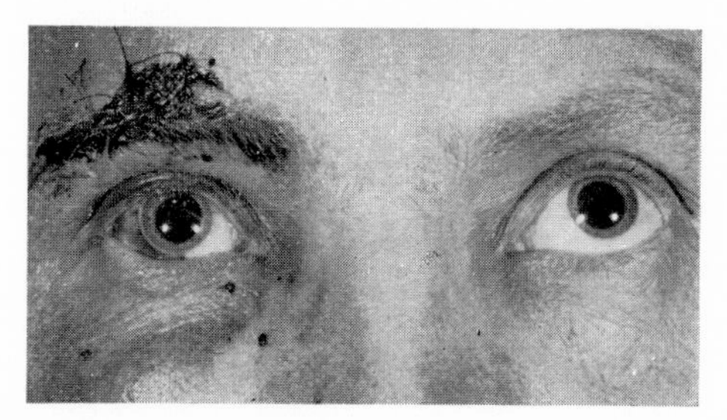

FIG. 227.—Defective elevation of the eye on the injured side due to incarceration of the inferior rectus in the fracture.

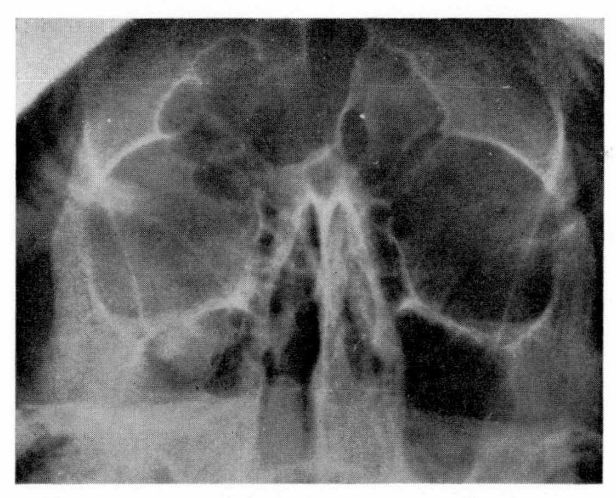

FIG. 228.—Characteristic radiological appearance showing an opacity due to orbital tissue in the right antrum.

summarize the main factors responsible for this distressing complication. (1) Incarceration within the fracture-line of the extra-ocular soft tissues particularly the inferior rectus and oblique muscles, displacement of the suspensory ligament of Lockwood, the periorbita, the muscle sheaths and their connections, which in the case of a fracture of the orbital floor results in a failure of upward rotation of the affected eye, while in a fracture of the medial wall the medial rectus muscle and its sheath may be similarly involved resulting in limitation of horizontal movement of the globe. (2) Direct injury to the muscles through laceration by bony fragments, hæmorrhage into their substance or severance of their attachments; paresis of the superior oblique muscle may result from damage to or displacement of the trochlea in a medial wall or a frontal fracture. (3) Damage to the nerve supply to the muscles, either as they enter the muscle or at the orbital apex, may result in a paralytic squint. (4) Diplopia may also be aggravated by the secondary deviation due to overaction of the conjugate muscles of the opposite eye. (5) Apart from the types of squint due to mechanical interference with the action of the muscles and damage to their nerve supply, any injury to the head or orbit may cause decompensation of an existing latent

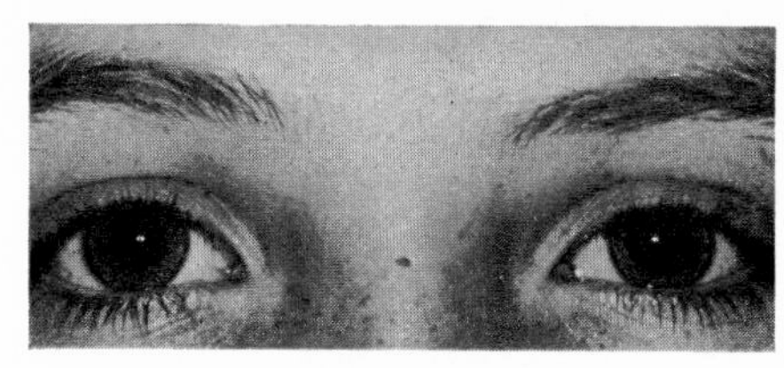

Fig. 229.

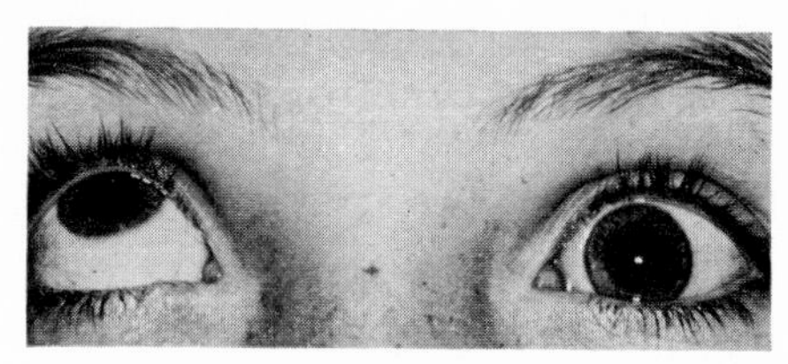

Fig. 230.

Figs. 229 and 230.—Late Result of a Blow-out Fracture of the Orbital Floor

In the primary position the eyes are normal (Fig. 229), but there is a complete failure of elevation of the left eye (Fig. 230) (Inst. Ophthal.).

squint, particularly if temporary immobilization or occlusion of the affected eye as by bandaging or swelling of the soft tissues has removed the stimulus for fusion. (6) Displacement of the globe is unlikely of itself to result in double vision if the visual axes remain parallel; if, however, there is also limitation of the action of the extrinsic muscles double vision will result. The appreciation of diplopia is of course dependent on the previous presence of binocular vision; its absence may therefore occasionally be due to severe damage to the eye itself and in such cases cannot be regarded as indicative of intact muscular function. It should also be remembered that a type of *uniocular diplopia* may be caused by subluxation or opacification of the lens or macular œdema.

The *muscle traction test* is useful in the detection of the incarceration of a muscle as distinct from the limitation of movement due to swelling of the soft tissues or hæmorrhage. It is performed as follows: a drop of local anæsthetic is placed in the conjunctival sac or if under general anæsthesia the test should be done before exploration is started; with toothed-forceps the tendon of the muscle is grasped and an attempt is made to move the globe; incarceration is suggested if there is marked limitation of movement as compared with the uninjured eye. The *forward traction test* may be helpful in assessing the possibility of the surgical correction of cases of enophthalmos seen at a late stage after injury: the medial and lateral rectus muscles are grasped simultaneously and resistance to forward traction suggests that there is fibrosis and shortening of the muscles with a correspondingly poor outlook for surgical correction. In a blow-out fracture of the orbital floor restriction of vertical movement leading to limitation of upward gaze is common. The inferior rectus is most usually involved due to its mid-line position over the infra-orbital canal where such fractures most frequently occur (Fig. 216), but as there is usually some fibrous connection between the inferior rectus and the inferior oblique muscles where they cross each other, limitation of both muscles usually results so that limitation of downward gaze may also be apparent.[1] Diplopia on attempted depression may also result from entrapment of the inferior rectus when it occurs with the eye in a position of elevation (Feore, 1965).

Electromyography may be useful in the investigation of an ocular palsy following an orbital fracture: a normal record suggests the incarceration of a muscle and is an indication for surgical exploration, while an abnormal tracing may suggest a neurological cause (Reny and Stricker, 1969).

Sensory loss. An important sign of a maxillary fracture is anæsthesia over the region of skin and oral mucosa supplied by the infra-orbital nerve although this may be difficult to elicit satisfactorily owing to the effects of swelling of the soft tissue following contusion of the cheek. Infra-orbital anæsthesia usually suggests a fracture in the central part of the floor of the orbit; the absence of such sensory loss in the presence of other signs of a fracture of the orbital floor indicates that the injury may be either medial or lateral to the infra-orbital canal. In the case of a fracture of the lateral orbital floor sensory loss in the distribution of the zygomatic nerve may be found.

Two further clinical manifestations of fractures of the facial skeleton remain to be considered—*epistaxis* and *cerebro-spinal rhinorrhœa.*

Bleeding from the nose is a frequent occurrence in fractures of the facial skeleton, a naso-maxillary injury or a fracture of the medial orbital wall. In a fracture of the zygomatico-maxillary complex, unilateral epistaxis is usually due to the escape of blood from the maxillary antrum arising from a laceration of its mucosal lining; in severe gunshot wounds of the maxilla hæmorrhage may be sufficiently severe to require blood transfusion, and particularly in this type of injury the risk of secondary hæmorrhage from infection is considerable. Persistent hæmorrhage most probably indicates a fracture of the nasal skeleton itself perhaps involving the palatine or septal vessels, and in a fracture of the ethmoid bone serious epistaxis may result from a laceration of the anterior ethmoidal arteries or from a fracture involving the sphenoid sinus. In the majority of cases nasal hæmorrhage ceases spontaneously although occasionally packing of the nasal cavity with layers of ribbon gauze soaked in 1 : 1,000 adrenaline introduced through the nostril will be required; in some cases the introduction of a post-nasal pack may also be indicated. In view of the possibility of infection no pack should

[1] Converse and Smith (1960), Cole and Smith (1963), Morton and Turnbull (1964), D. Jones (1966), Lerman (1970).

be left *in situ* for more than 24 hours. Exceptionally, hæmorrhage may be so severe that blood transfusion will be required pending preparation for surgical control of the bleeding either by deeply placed sutures including the vessels and periosteum in a single bite or in exceptional cases by proximal ligation on the arterial side as of the maxillary artery.

The triad of unilateral blindness, orbital fracture and massive epistaxis has been described by Maurer and his colleagues (1961) and Voris and Basile (1961); Hitchcock (1965) reported two such cases with a fracture involving the sphenoid sinus and pointed out that, although the hæmorrhage may, indeed, be alarming, it usually settles without

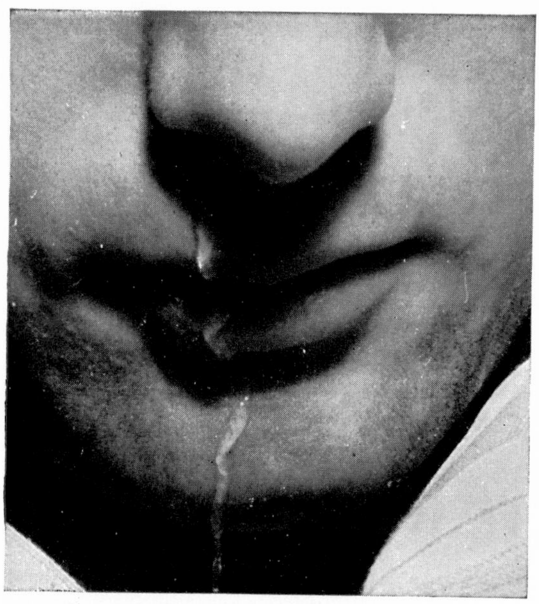

Fig. 231.—Cerebro-spinal rhinorrhœa associated with a fracture of the cribriform plate of the ethmoid bone in a patient who sustained a fracture of the fronto-naso-ethmoid region (N. Rowe and H. Killey, *Fractures of the Facial Skeleton*, Livingstone).

operative interference, whereas in an exsanguinated patient carotid ligation carries a serious risk of producing hemiplegia. Delayed epistaxis occurring some days or weeks after such an injury may be due to damage to the carotid artery resulting in a traumatic aneurysm which subsequently gives way; the mortality in these cases is high (10 of 21 cases, Weaver *et al.*, 1961) and the treatment involves either a clamping procedure on the affected artery or proximal carotid ligation (Petty, 1969).

Cerebro-spinal rhinorrhœa. A fracture frequently passes through one or other of the air-sinuses, be it the frontal, sphenoid or ethmoid, and since the dura is firmly attached to the base of the skull a tear of the meninges is a common result. The development of a clear watery discharge from the nose (or ear) following an injury to the head indicates that a communication exists between the subarachnoid space and the exterior. The recognition of CSF rhinorrhœa may at times be difficult: while nasal bleeding usually occurs on its own, it may be associated with the simultaneous escape of cerebro-spinal fluid, although recognition of the nature of the fluid may be rendered difficult by the presence of blood clot, and at a later stage serous or purulent nasal discharge may further complicate matters (Figs. 231–2).[1] Moreover the CSF may pass backwards down into the throat and not be detected until a clear watery fluid is seen to drip from the nostril when the patient sits up. When there is radiological evidence of a fracture involving the base of the skull those concerned should be on the look out for this complication. Approximately 25%

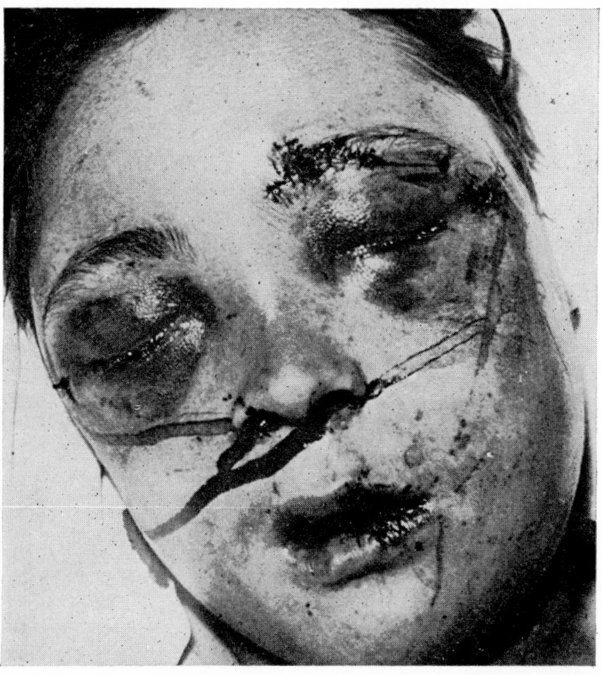

FIG. 232.—Fracture of the middle third of the face, showing gross œdema, cerebrospinal and hæmorrhagic rhinorrhœa and circumorbital hæmatomata (R. O. Walker).

of cases sustaining a facial injury involving the paranasal air-sinuses can be expected at some time to develop such a rhinorrhœa; in the majority this will be obvious within 48 hours, in others its appearance may be delayed for some days or even weeks until absorption of blood clot has taken place. In general the flow ceases spontaneously within about 7 to 10 days, although in cases in which extensive damage has occurred to the cribriform plate of the ethmoid it may persist for much longer. Two relatively rare complications

[1] Chemical tests with Benedict's solution for the presence of reducing substances may be helpful; there is a level of 50–70 mg. glucose per 100 ml. in the CSF and little or no glucose in mucus (Schurr, 1963). Alternatively, chemical test-papers as for urine analysis may be used; another test using radio-active sodium has been described (Crow *et al.*, 1956).

of this condition can be noted: an effusion of CSF into the orbit through a fracture of the ethmoid can give rise to a fluctuant swelling above and medial to the globe, and an intracranial aerocele may develop indicating a large fistula.

The management of this complication is a neurosurgical matter and in all such cases the advice of a neurosurgeon should be sought at an early stage, but certain principles may be stated here. In many instances the flow of

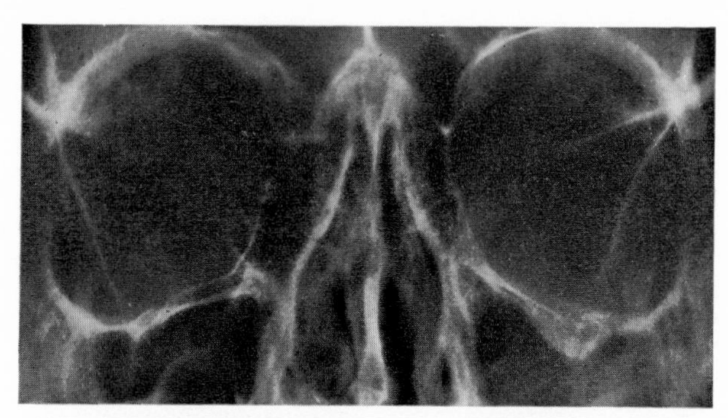

Fig. 233.—Fracture of the Floor of the Left Orbit (G. Lloyd).

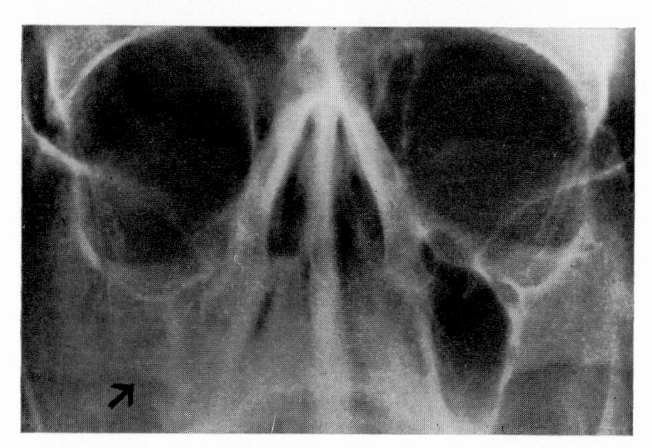

Fig. 234.—Impacted Malar Fracture (arrowed) (G. Lloyd).

cerebro-spinal fluid is transient and ceases spontaneously and in other cases repositioning and fixation of the fractured bones may be all that is required to arrest the flow. When the leak persists for longer than two weeks exploration and closure of the fistula are probably required either by direct suture or, when a large defect of the dura exists, by the application of a graft of fascia lata or other material. The question of the timing of surgical interference, whether for treatment of the fracture or of the tear in the dura, is difficult and requires the opinion of a neurosurgeon at an early stage. In all cases, however, measures to prevent infection with the consequent risk of meningitis are vital. Nursing of the patient in isolation is probably desirable and the prophylactic administration of antibiotics and sulphonamides is mandatory.[1]

The RADIOLOGICAL DIAGNOSIS of orbital fractures is a matter of considerable importance and in recent years following the elucidation of the mechanism of blow-out fractures considerable attention has been directed to this subject (Figs. 233–239).[2] To be of value the radiological technique must be above the average standard; moreover, if it is to be conclusive the examination must be comprehensive. The bony walls in this region are thin and are often obscured by thicker bones while the fracture lines, which are readily confused with the many suture lines and bony septa in this area, may at one time appear as rarefactions in the film and at another as lines of increased density where the fragments overlap; occasionally pre-existing sinus disease may further complicate the picture: moreover, the bony surfaces are not only thin and broad but are joined in a multi-angular relationship which renders their demonstration on a single radiograph almost impossible. In the majority of cases, therefore, ordinary direct postero-anterior and lateral views of the skull are insufficient and stereoscopic and other special views are required to demonstrate the profile of the orbital floor, supplemented on occasion by the techniques of tomography, while in other cases when the details of the bony structure are obscured by hæmorrhagic effusion into the paranasal sinuses or into the soft tissues of the face the exact nature of the injury may be most clearly demonstrated by positive contrast orbitography. If the clinical signs and preliminary routine films indicate that gross bony displacement is not present, it is probably better to delay more detailed radiological examination for a few days until at least some of the swelling of the soft tissues has subsided, bearing in mind that in cases in which incarceration of the extra-ocular muscles has occurred early surgical intervention may be indicated.

For the detailed radiological techniques the reader is referred to standard works on the subject[3]; the most useful techniques and some of their advantages and limitations are as follows:

1. *Caldwell's nose-forehead position* (Fig. 235), a postero-anterior view with the head positioned so that the forehead and nose touch the plate and with the incident ray angled 10° downwards, superimposes the petrous portions of the temporal bones

[1] Calvert (1942), Dandy (1944), Dawson and Fordyce (1953), W. Lewin (1954), Schurr (1963), O'Connell (1968), Ray and Bergland (1969), MacGee *et al.* (1970).

[2] Important contributions dealing with the radiological aspects of orbital fractures are those of Hoffmann and Loepp (1935), Baltin and Sviadocz (1940–41), Culler (1940), Pfeiffer (1941–43), Linhart (1943), Samuel (1944), McGrigor and Samuel (1945), Murray (1949), Hartmann and Gilles (1959), J. R. Lewin *et al.* (1960), Zizmor *et al.* (1962), I. Jones (1963), Lerman and Cramer (1964), Campbell (1964), Brown *et al.* (1965), Feore (1965), Lloyd (1966–70), Vigario (1966), Vinik and Gargano (1966), Fueger *et al.* (1966), Milauskas *et al.* (1966), Gould and Titus (1966), Freimanis (1966), Converse *et al.* (1967), Lombardi (1967), Meulemans (1967), Rowe and Killey (1968), Dodick *et al.* (1969), Reny and Stricker (1969), Milauskas (1969), Trokel and Potter (1969), and others.

[3] Merrill: *Atlas of Roentgenographic Positions*, St. Louis, 405 (1959). Clark: *Positioning in Radiography*, London (1964).

FIGS. 235 and 236.—FRACTURE SUSTAINED BY A FALL FROM A HORSE (S. L. Trokel).

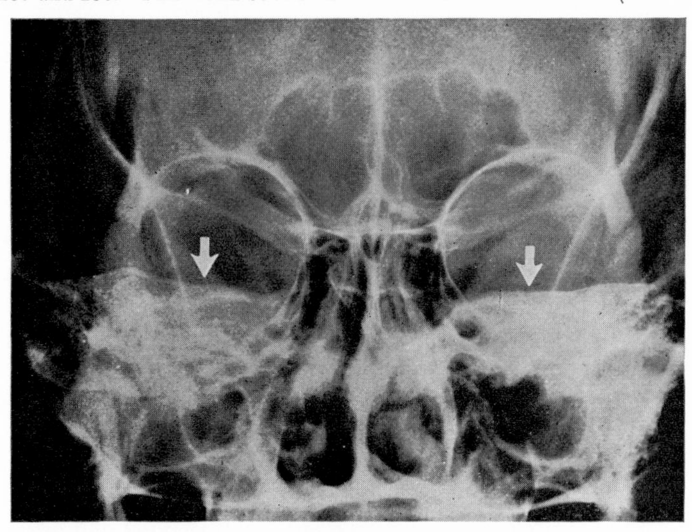

FIG. 235.—In Caldwell's view the dense petrous pyramids (arrowed) project through the orbits and obscure all detail of their lower third.

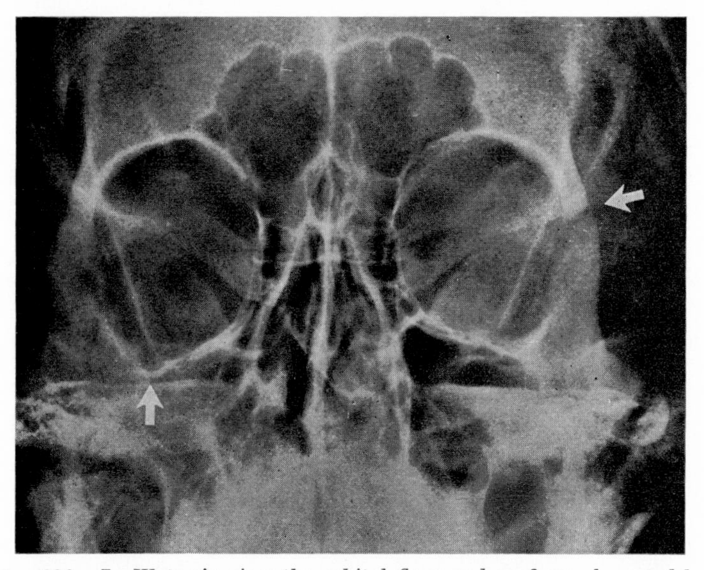

FIG. 236.—In Waters's view the orbital floor and roof are elongated but the petrous pyramids are projected below the maxillary sinuses making the orbital floors clearly visible where the fracture of the right orbital floor as well as of the left outer wall are clearly seen.

upon the maxillæ and gives an undistorted view of the orbital margins; the superior orbital fissures, the sphenoidal ridges and the lines of the temporal fossæ are well seen, while a clear view is given of the frontal and ethmoid sinuses and the nasal fossæ. With this view, however, the orbital floor is not well demonstrated because of the superimposition of the petrous temporal bone on the superior maxilla, while the presence of blood in the maxillary antrum or extensive periorbital œdema and bruising may further obscure the picture (J. R. Lewin *et al.*, 1960; Vigario, 1966).

2. *Waters's nose-chin position* (Fig. 236) allows a good view of the entire maxillary bone without superimposition of the petrous bones; the antra are clearly defined and although the orbits are distorted their floors and boundaries and particularly the zygomatic bones and temporal arches are clearly delineated. This view will show a fracture of the orbital floor and a prolapse of soft tissue into the antrum, especially if tomograms are done in this position (Brown *et al.*, 1965; Freimanis, 1966; and others).

3. *Occipito-mental views* are the most generally valuable. Two angles of incidence may be taken.

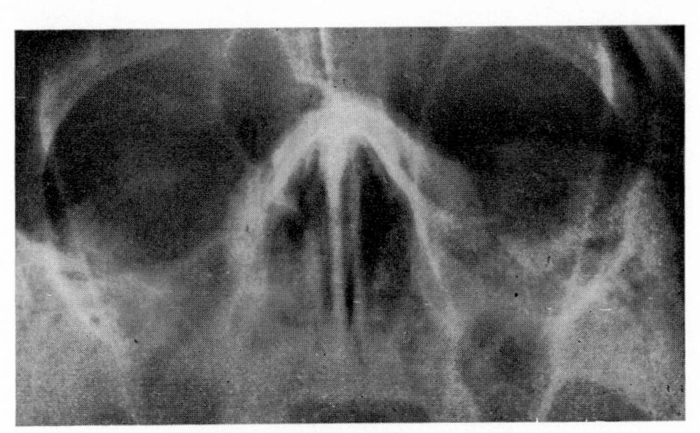

FIG. 237.—MALAR FRACTURE.

Over-tilted occipito-mental radiograph showing a comminuted fracture of the malar bone and inferior orbital margin (G. Lloyd).

(*a*) In the standard 10° occipito-mental view the head is positioned so that the radiological base-line (the line joining the external canthus to the external auditory meatus) is at an angle of 45° to the horizontal. If the incident beam is horizontal and is first centred at the occipital protruberance and then at a point 3 centimetres on either side of the mid-line, a film taken in each position results in a stereoscopic pair allowing good demonstration of the orbital rim and roof.

(*b*) In the 30° occipito-mental view with the head positioned in a similar way and the incident beam inclined from the horizontal at an angle of 30° and centred in the mid-plane of the orbit, a distorted view of the orbital margin but an excellent demonstration of the orbital floor is obtained through the maxillary antrum (Fig. 237).

The floor of the orbit is not a simple plane but consists of two separate regions, the antero-lateral plane portion and a posterior portion that inclines upward; these two regions are not clearly distinguishable from each other on either Caldwell's or Waters's views. Based on this anatomical observation two special views to demonstrate the profile of the orbital floor, particularly when a blow-out fracture is suspected, have been described by Fueger and his colleagues (1966) using a postero-anterior projection which permits evaluation of the separate parts of the orbital floor: the patient's head is placed in the nose-brow position and the central ray is angulated 30° caudally so that it emerges about 1 in. below the nasion; a 20° oblique view is also obtained with the injured orbit placed directly on the cassette with the central ray angled 35° caudally through it, thereby demonstrating the lateral half of the orbital floor and the underlying facial bones.

4. A *lateral view* with the head placed with its sagittal plane parallel to the film and the affected orbit next to it and with the incident rays directed horizontally centres the latter through the mid-point of the affected orbit. The amount of distortion, however, is considerable and the value of such a picture is frequently disappointing when

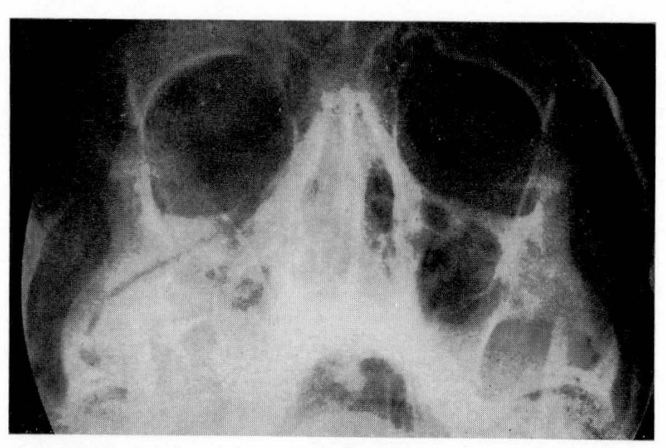

Fig. 238.

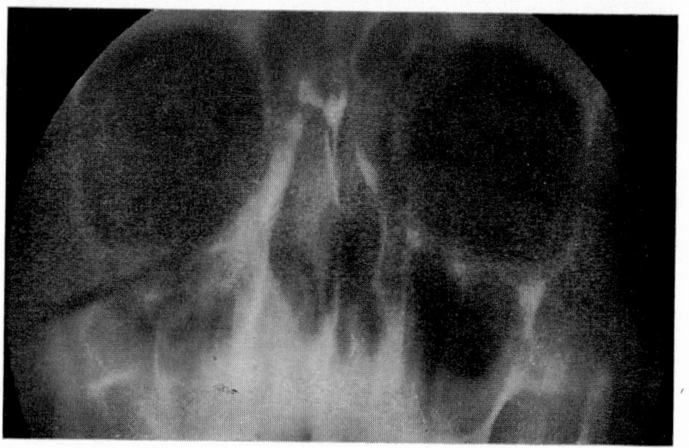

Fig. 239.

Figs. 238 and 239.—A Fracture of the Orbital Floor on the Right Side associated with Diplopia.

Seen by plain x-ray (Fig. 238) and tomography (Fig. 239) (W. Campbell).

orbital fractures are concerned, but it may be of use in the interpretation of a series of pictures and should certainly be included with the other views. A soft-tissue lateral projection taken from a distance of 6 ft. is ideal for demonstrating a fracture of the nasal bones and in a low transverse or Guérin type of fracture at the anterior nasal aperture it may show up road-grit embedded in the soft tissues of the face.

5. *Dental films* may be used with advantage in studying fractures of the nasal bones, hard palate and zygoma.

6. *Tomography* (*laminography*). The principle of this method is that the x-ray

tube and film are moved around a fulcrum so that only those structures in the plane of the fulcrum are clearly delineated in the resulting radiograph (Figs. 238–9). By this means it is possible to obtain a section of the body at varying depths with blurring of all the overlying and underlying structures except those in the plane desired. This technique is of some value in studying fractures of the orbital floor in the postero-anterior or lateral plane and may provide information which is difficult to obtain otherwise, particularly when several fractures are present at different levels.[1] Although tomography picked up only 11 of 18 cases in one series (Fueger *et al.*, 1966), in another group of 21 cases a positive result was obtained in 95% (Gould and Titus, 1966). The recent development of hypocycloid tomography has proved useful in the demonstration of ethmoid fractures (Trokel and Potter, 1969) and fractures of the orbital floor (Dodick *et al.*, 1968–69). With this radiographic technique the x-rays arise from an infinite number of points thereby striking the object from an infinite number of directions, whereas in the case of linear tomography the movement of the x-ray tube is linear resulting in the characteristic streaking seen in linear tomograms. Since the thickness of the layer varies directly with the arc through which the x-ray tube travels, a thinner section results from the use of multi-directional hypocycloid tomography producing films of high diagnostic quality.

7. *The Radiography of Emphysema.* The accumulation of air in the tissues of the lids or the orbit (surgical emphysema) indicates a communication between them and one or other of the nasal sinuses, a circumstance which is usually the result of trauma. The deliberate production of surgical emphysema by asking the patient to exhale forcibly while his nose is held closed may be the only way of demonstrating a small fracture of the medial wall of the orbit. The collection of air within the orbit shows up clearly on the film (Murray, 1949). This is an important diagnostic sign in cases of fracture of the paranasal sinuses and orbital injury and is commonly found in blow-out fractures (Lange, 1965; 50% of cases, Lloyd, 1966), and when the air is situated in the deeper orbital tissues it may be most clearly demonstrated by taking a radiograph with the patient in the erect position. The presence of air in the cranial cavity indicates a fracture involving one of the paranasal sinuses and the possibility of cerebro-spinal rhinorrhœa.

8. *Orbitography.* The situation may arise when opacification of the paranasal sinuses due to hæmorrhage prevents demonstration of the detailed bony structure and may delay the exact anatomical diagnosis of an orbital fracture even when this is clearly present on the basis of the clinical signs and perhaps some surgical emphysema visible on routine radiographs. In these cases positive contrast orbitography may be of considerable help and, indeed, this technique is regarded by some workers as the most generally reliable means of demonstrating orbital blow-out fractures (Fueger and his colleagues, 1966; Milauskas and his co-workers, 1966; Milauskas, 1969; and others). With this method a small quantity of contrast medium (about 4 to 5 ml.) is injected along the orbital floor after local anæsthesia to the skin and orbital rim. A convenient mixture consists of 3·5 ml. of 50% diatrizoate (hypaque), 3·0 ml. of 2% lignocaine, and 0·5 ml. of diluent, containing 150 units of hyaluronidase. The needle is placed so that it is outside the muscle-cone, the syringe containing local anæsthetic is replaced with another containing the contrast medium which is then injected slowly along the orbital floor, first posteriorly, then laterally after withdrawing about one-half inch and then medially. At the same time palpation with the needle may locate an actual break in the bones. After completion of the injection, routine and specially angled radiographs are taken to demonstrate whether the dye has leaked into the maxillary antrum. Of 51 cases of surgically proved blow-out fractures Milauskas and his colleagues (1966) found that orbitography revealed the fracture in 94% compared with an accuracy of

[1] Culler (1940), Samuel (1944), Lloyd (1966), Gould and Titus (1966).

only 28% with radiographs and 55% when tomographs were carried out as well. The advantages claimed for this radiological technique are that it demonstrates a high percentage of blow-out fractures, it provides the opportunity to determine the integrity of the orbital floor at the time of injection, there is a good delineation of any prolapse of the soft tissues, and radiographs are provided which are easier to interpret than those obtained by tomography. On the other hand, if the needle is placed within the muscle-cone the dye may not reach the site of the fracture and the incarceration of soft tissues within the fracture may prevent the passage of the dye into the maxillary antrum. As with any orbital injection, serious complications such as perforation of the globe, retrobulbar hæmorrhage and spasm of the retinal artery are theoretically possible but have not been seen by these workers and, although no case of idiosyncrasy to the contrast medium occurred in a total of 90 orbitographies, they recommended that a skin-test should be performed before the orbital injection is made. A further rare complication is the entrance of the contrast medium into the subdural space (Kaufer and Augustin, 1966; Lombardi, 1967; Reed *et al.*, 1969); and finally the development of a lipid granuloma (Eifrig, 1968) emphasizes the importance of using only water-soluble contrast media.

Although it is undoubtedly true that a significant proportion of these fractures can be diagnosed accurately with plain radiographs or tomograms using special views, nevertheless there are cases clinically or radiologically negative or equivocal in which the information derived from positive contrast orbitography may be of considerable value and, indeed, occasionally lead to a diagnosis when the simpler methods have failed. There is thus available a variety of radiological procedures which may aid in the evaluation of a patient with a known or suspected orbital fracture. As a routine at Moorfields Eye Hospital the following views are taken: (1) occipito-oral, (2) under-tilted occipito-mental (to demonstrate blow-out fractures), (3) over-tilted occipito-mental (to demonstrate malar fractures), and (4) a lateral view. For special cases more refined techniques are required.

Radiological diagnosis of a fracture of the orbit depends on the observation of any displacement and the interruption or fragmentation of bone in *one or more* of the orbital walls. Additional evidence of a fracture is represented by any or all of the following signs: orbital emphysema, clouding of the paranasal sinuses due to hæmorrhage, and localized displacement of the soft tissues into the roof of the maxillary antrum or the ethmoid sinuses. According to Vigario (1966) obliteration of the infra-orbital foramen on the injured side invariably means disruption of the orbital floor, while the presence of globules of fat in the antral cavity has the same significance. The special 30° postero-anterior view described by Fueger and his colleagues (1966) may in the presence of a blow-out fracture show the following signs: an absence of the anterior orbital line with a pseudo-polyp (" hanging drop ") in the antral roof due to herniation of orbital tissue, a divergence of the two lines representing the orbital floor, a defect in the posterior bulge of the floor and the depression of this bulge; a fragment of bone may be seen within the maxillary antrum below the lines of the orbital floor and there may be diffuse widening and opacification of the contours of the orbital floor, while there may also be asymmetry of the ethmo-maxillary septum and opacification of the infero-medial ethmoid air-cells; the medial orbital wall may be fragmented with or without opacification of the ethmoid sinuses while emphysema of the orbit is commonly seen.

Not all blow-out fractures, however, are radiologically evident. This is particularly true of the " trap-door " variety in which there is a minimal bony displacement and no deficiency in the orbital floor (Soll and Poley, 1965). In this type of case the rise in the intra-orbital pressure results in a linear fracture of the floor with herniation of the orbital contents and, in particular, of the inferior rectus muscle; when the force is discontinued the displaced bone springs back and traps the herniating tissues, leaving the floor apparently intact (Whyte, 1968) (Fig. 216).

INDIRECT ORBITAL FRACTURES ASSOCIATED WITH HEAD INJURY

Associated with a head injury such as results from a heavy blow, a fall or a traffic collision, two types of orbital fracture may result without direct violence to the region of the orbit itself. In the first place, an extensive

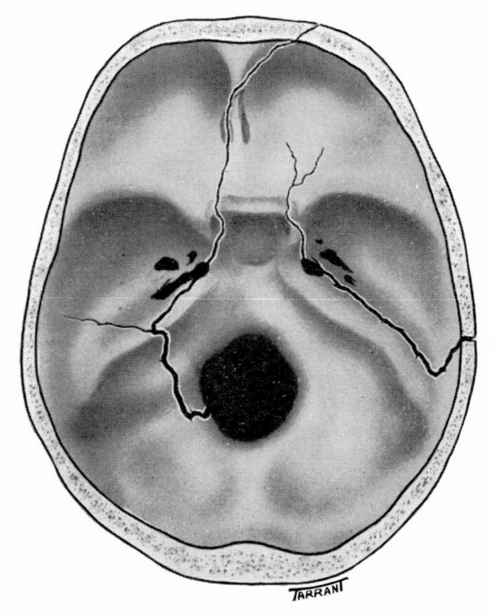

Fig. 240.—Typical fracture lines in the base of the skull showing the implication of the orbital roof.

fracture of the base of the skull commonly radiates to involve the floor of the anterior fossa and the roof of one or both orbits (Fig. 240). The fracture line usually runs irregularly but adopts a general postero-anterior direction bearing one of three relationships to the orbit; it runs either on the medial aspect along the cribriform plate, in an intermediate position between the inner and middle thirds of the orbital roof, or more temporally in the orbital roof involving the lesser wing of the sphenoid. Greder (1885) found that in about three-quarters of these cases the optic canal was involved, but his observations have not been confirmed; thus Rawling (1904) found that basal fractures extending to this region habitually tended to run on either side of the optic canal, medially along the cribriform plate or laterally through the sphenoidal fissure, throwing only occasional and minor fissures into the canal itself.

In the second place, and more rarely, an isolated indirect fracture of the orbital roof may occur, usually but not invariably associated with a separate fracture of the base or the occipital region, in which case the factor of *contre-coup* is involved, the vault giving way preferentially in this area where the bones comprising the orbital roof are very thin.[1] In such an accident both roofs may be simultaneously involved[2]. Such fractures are not uncommon. The frequency of orbital extensions of basal fractures was first noted by Prescott Hewett (1858) who confirmed their presence in 33% of 68 cases of fracture of the base of the skull, an incidence considerably increased in the observations of subsequent writers (90% of 88 cases, Berlin, 1880; 69% of 13 cases, Körber, 1889; and others).

Isolated indirect fractures are much more rare. Berlin (1880) collected 14 cases from the literature, Ipsen (1898) 25 cases of which 10 were due to blunt force and 15 to gunshot wounds, and Tilman (1902) 49 cases of which 29 were due to gunshot injury, 11 to falls on the occiput or vertex, 2 followed a blow on the head, one (Friedberg, 1864) was a birth injury, while in 6 the fracture of the orbital roof was not indubitably proved to be continuous with a radiating fracture of the base. Axenfeld's case (1902) was interesting since it involved an orbito-cerebral hernia.

In these cases, of course, the fracture of the orbit is merely an incident in a clinical picture dominated by events characteristic of a severe head injury with its associated signs of cerebral concussion and contusion. It is true that in some cases the accident appears trivial and the patient resumes his activities apparently unscathed; but even in these as well as in the obviously serious cases, over him hangs the shadow of the cumulative effects of cerebral hæmorrhage with evidences of increasing intracranial pressure on the timely relief of which by operative interference his survival may depend. From the purely ophthalmological point of view one incident may occur of sufficient drama to compel attention even at a time when life and death may be balanced—injury to the optic nerve which may result in partial or complete blindness, a complication which is by no means exceptional (30 cases in 750 basal fractures (4%), Birch-Hirschfeld, 1930). The implications of this, whether occurring as a temporary or a permanent disability, has been discussed elsewhere,[3] as also has the other ophthalmological signs of head injury

[1] von Bergmann (1880), Stierlin (1900), Tilman (1902), Doepfner (1912), and others.
[2] Morian (1883), Ipsen (1898), Axenfeld (1902), von Szily (1918) in war injuries.
[3] Vol. XII, p. 273.

FIGS. 241 and 242.—SUBCONJUNCTIVAL HÆMORRHAGES IN CRANIAL FRACTURES (D. B. Archer).

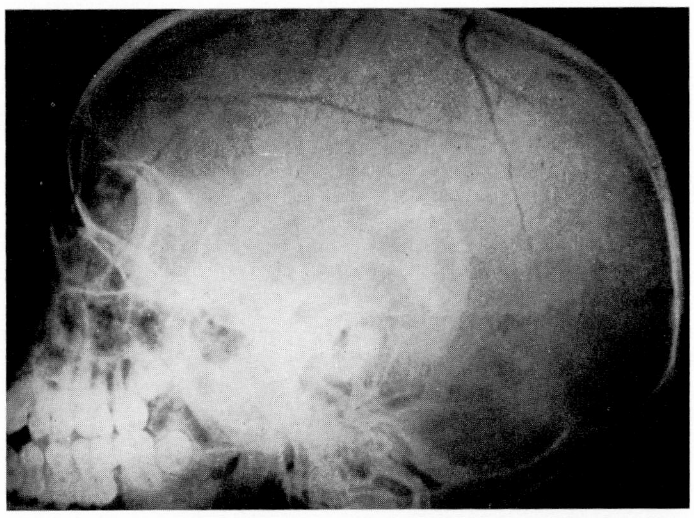

FIG 241.—Multiple fractures of the skull including the orbit.

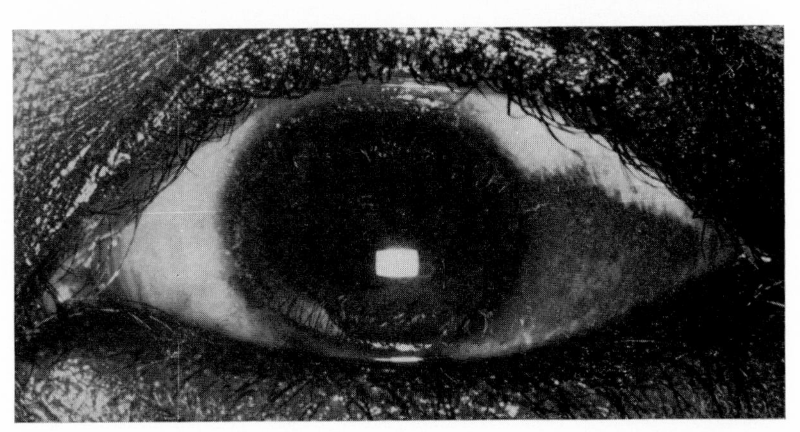

FIG. 242.—The resulting subconjunctival hæmorrhage in the same case.

affecting particularly the pupils and the ocular motor system, some of which are of considerable significance in the assessment of diagnosis and prognosis, while others, such as the development of an arterio-venous aneurysm, may have long-term and far-reaching consequences. It is important to remember, however, that from the local point of view, in addition to the cerebro-spinal rhinorrhœa which indicates an open communication between the anterior fossa and the nose, a fracture of the orbital roof, although usually symptomless, may be suggested by the occurrence of an intra-orbital hæmorrhage which, although it may remain subperiosteal and appear clinically as an orbital tumour (Postempski, 1889), may become apparent subconjunctivally as it seeps from the roof along the levator muscle or from the orbital apex along the lateral rectus muscle some 24 to 48 hours after the accident (Morison, 1894; Kehl, 1921; and others) (Figs. 241–2). On the other hand, a hæmorrhage due to a distant fracture of the base of the skull is usually first seen at the medial border of the lower lid whence it gradually diffuses (A. B. King and Walsh, 1949).

The *diagnosis* of the seepage of blood from a fracture of the base of the skull in contradistinction to that due to the local effects of an orbital contusion (that is, a " black eye ") is important. The main points of differentiation are that blood from a fractured base:

(1) usually appears first at the medial border of the lower lid,

(2) is limited sharply by the palpebral fascia to the orbital margins so that the suffused area is circular in outline (in local injury there is no such limitation),

(3) is related to the amount of palpebral œdema (in local injury œdema is usually more marked and unrelated to the bleeding),

(4) is subconjunctival in site (not intra-conjunctival moving with this membrane),

(5) is purple in colour from its first appearance (not bright, beefy red as in a " black eye "),

(6) has no posterior visible limit, being least extensive towards the cornea, and

(7) usually appears after an interval.

According to Rowbotham (1964) subconjunctival hæmorrhages are of diagnostic significance only (1) when they cause œdema of the conjunctiva, (2) when they are so extensive that it is impossible to see beyond their posterior limits in any position of the eye, and (3) when they are so large that they cause displacement of the globe or limitation of its movement. Furthermore, a fracture of the base of the skull may not lead to an intra-orbital hæmorrhage but frequently is associated with a "black eye ". It is to be remembered also that subgaleal bleeding due to fracture of the vault or to scalp trauma may cause the delayed appearance of hæmorrhage in the eyelids.

OCULAR INJURY IN ORBITAL FRACTURES

Usually in most cases of orbital fracture the eye escapes serious injury. We have already referred to the *extra-ocular* problems associated with orbital and mid-facial fractures which can be summarized as follows—œdema and hæmorrhage into the periorbital soft tissues, surgical emphysema, sub-conjunctival hæmorrhage, enophthalmos, ptosis, diplopia due to paresis of the ocular muscles and mechanical limitation of ocular rotation, laceration of the eyelids and detachment or severance of the medial palpebral ligament with or without damage to the lacrimal passages. Under this heading should also be noted damage to the blood vessels at the orbital apex and to the optic nerve, either from bony fragments, hæmorrhage or concussion-necrosis which may result in partial or complete loss of vision in the affected eye.

It is important to remember, however, that occasionally *intra-ocular damage* may be caused by the injury responsible for the facial fracture, as for instance with a gunshot wound of the orbit causing either a penetrating wound of the globe or severe concussion of the choroid and retina with intra-ocular hæmorrhage, while in a blow-out fracture of the orbital floor ocular contusion may result from a protruding object or if the missile happens to strike the relatively exposed temporal side of the globe. As the clinical picture is so often dominated by the facial fracture and by injuries elsewhere in the body, significant damage to the eye itself may be missed unless it is specifically sought. It is, therefore, imperative that in every case of a " black eye " a careful ophthalmic examination should be made as soon as possible, preferably before surgical management of the associated fractures and before the increasing swelling of the soft tissues in the lids and conjunctiva

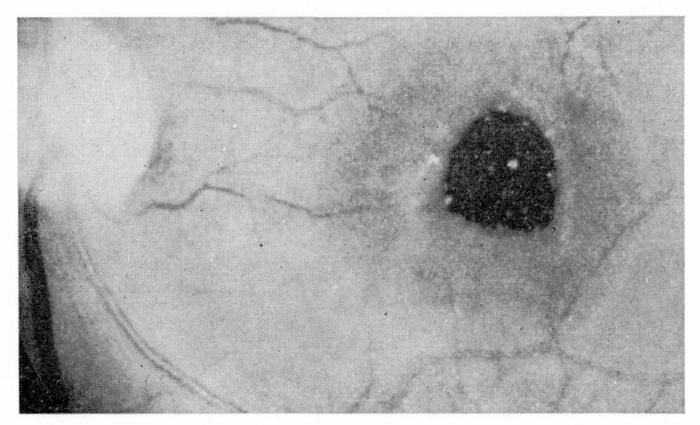

Fig. 243.—Retinal Complications of Orbital Fractures.

Fundus photograph showing a large hole at the macula and a surrounding ring of shallow retinal detachment associated with a blow-out fracture of the left orbital floor (G. R. Miller and R. R. Tenzel).

makes it impossible to separate the lids for inspection of the globe. The general condition of the patient may preclude a detailed examination but it is essential to exclude a perforating wound and to make at least some assessment of the visual function bearing in mind the possibility of subsequent medico-legal and compensatory problems. Impairment of vision may result from any of the numerous lesions which can be caused by an ocular contusion and which have already been dealt with at length; among these may be noted damage to the optic nerve or vessels of the orbital apex as a result of fracture, hæmorrhage or concussion-necrosis, retinal damage by direct ocular contusion (Fig. 243), hæmorrhage or a retinal tear, displacement of the lens and rupture of the globe. If it is impracticable to test the visual acuity in the usual way, simple tests such as the ability to read a newspaper and the confrontation test for the visual field in the four diagonal quadrants and examination of the pupillary responses to light may give valuable information concerning the integrity of the optic nerve although a traumatic mydriasis may make evaluation of the last sign difficult

(Miller and Tenzel, 1967). In the presence of a head injury and particularly when consciousness is impaired, mydriatics should not be used to facilitate examination of the fundus because of subsequent interference with the interpretation of pupillary changes indicating cerebral compression.

Reports in the literature concerning the incidence of serious intra-ocular complications associated with facial trauma are few. In a series of 337 mid-facial fractures McCoy and his colleagues (1962) found only 3 cases of blindness and 1 of cycloplegia, giving an incidence of approximately 1%. It seems likely, however, that this is an underestimate; thus loss of the eye occurred in 4 out of 145 cases of blow-out fracture reviewed by Converse and his colleagues (1967). The importance of an early diagnosis of intra-ocular complications is borne out by several recent reports.[1] Jones and Evans (1967) noted injury to the globe in 10% of their cases and considered that the relatively low incidence of ocular injury in blow-out fractures was probably due to the fact that the eyeball does not usually directly strike the orbital wall. Finally, the possibility should be mentioned that the visual loss may result from the treatment of a fracture in this region; uniocular blindness complicating the reduction of a fractured zygoma was noted by Gordon and MacRae (1950) and other similar reports have appeared[2]; the possibility of damage to the optic nerve as a result of over-enthusiastic packing of the maxillary antrum has been reported (Romanes, 1968). Severe bleeding from orbital blood vessels after the blood in the antrum from the original injury has clotted or where the healing of fracture-lines has created a fibrous seal may result in considerable proptosis and perhaps a rise in the intra-orbital pressure necessitating urgent decompression of the orbit. In order to achieve this Fry (1967) recommended a curved incision through the lateral third of the eyebrow made sufficiently deep to cut through the periorbita into the orbital cavity which can thus be drained for three days.

Aiello and Myers. *Arch. Otolaryng.*, **82**, 638 (1965).
Aubry. *Arch. Ophthal.*, **25**, 79 (1968).
Axenfeld. *Ber. dtsch. ophthal. Ges.*, **30**, 276 (1902).
Baltin and Sviadocz. *Vestn. oftal.*, **16**, 39 (1940); **18**, 306 (1941).
Barclay. *Brit. J. plast. Surg.*, **11**, 147 (1958).
von Bergmann. *Die Lehre v. d. Kopfverletzungen*, Stuttgart (1880).
Berlin. *Graefe-Saemisch Hb. d. ges. Augenheilk.*, 1st ed., Leipzig, **6**, 586 (1880).
Bessière, Depaulis, Vérin and Lauzeral. *J. Méd. Bordeaux*, **141**, 227 (1964).
Birch-Hirschfeld. *Kurzes Hb. d. Ophthal.*, Berlin, **3**, 107 (1930).
Bowers. *Surv. Ophthal.*, **9**, 237 (1964).
Brown, Longman, De Stefano *et al.* *Radiology*, **85**, 908 (1965).
Calvert. *Proc. roy. Soc. Med.*, **35**, 805 (1942).
Campbell. *Recent Advances in Radiology* (ed. Lodge), London, 239 (1964).
Cole and Smith. *Amer. J. Ophthal.*, **55**, 930 (1963).
Consul, Sharma, D. and R. *J. All-India ophthal., Soc.*, **16**, 245 (1968).
Converse and Smith. *Brit. J. plast. Surg.*, **9**, 265 (1957).
Trans. Amer. Acad. Ophthal., **64**, 676 (1960); **67**, 622 (1963).
Plast. reconstr. Surg., **38**, 147 (1966).
Converse, Smith, Obear and Wood-Smith. *Plast. reconstr. Surg.*, **39**, 20 (1967).
Cramer, Tooze and Lerman. *Brit. J. plast. Surg.*, **18**, 171 (1965).
Crow, Keogh and Northfield. *Lancet*, **2**, 325 (1956).
Culler. *Trans. Amer. ophthal. Soc.*, **38**, 348 (1940).
Dandy. *Arch. Surg.*, **49**, 75 (1944).
Dawson and Fordyce. *Brit. J. Surg.*, **41**, 254 (1953).
DeVoe. *Trans. Amer. ophthal. Soc.*, **45**, 502 (1947).
Dingman and Natvig. *Surgery of Facial Fractures*, Phila. (1964).
Dodick, Berrett and Galin. *Surg. Forum*, **19**, 484 (1968).

[1] Six cases of orbital fracture with severe ocular injury (Erdbrink *et al.*, 1963); Aiello and Myers (1965); in 84 cases of blow-out fracture reported by Milauskas and Fueger (1966) 14% sustained severe ocular injury including rupture of the globe, intra-ocular hæmorrhage and displacement of the lens; 5 cases out of 30 consecutive mid-facial fractures (Miller and Tenzel, 1967); of 69 cases treated by Jackson (1968), 5 lost the sight of one eye; in 10 cases Whyte (1968) observed severe contusive injuries in 4.

[2] Penn and Epstein (1953), Gordon (1957), Barclay (1958), Stockdale (1959), Nysingh (1960), Magoon (1963), Fry (1967), Watson and Holt-Wilson (1968).

Dodick, Galin and Berrett. *Canad. J. Ophthal.*, **4,** 370 (1969).

Dodick, Galin and Kwitko. *Canad. J. Ophthal.*, **4,** 377 (1969).

Doepfner. *Dtsch. Z. Chir.*, **116,** 44 (1912).

Edwards and Ridley. *Amer. J. Ophthal.*, **65,** 248 (1968).

Eifrig. *Arch. Ophthal.*, **79,** 163 (1968).

Erdbrink, Smith, Walker and Gossett. *Amer. J. Ophthal.*, **56,** 982 (1963).

Fanjul. *Arch. Oftal. B. Aires*, **43,** 39 (1968).

Feore. *Clin. Radiol.*, **16,** 347 (1965).

Fischbein and Lesko. *Arch. Ophthal.*, **81,** 162 (1969).

Freimanis. *Radiol. Clin. N. Amer.*, **4,** 341 (1966).

Friedberg. *Virchows Arch. path. Anat.*, **31,** 344, 357 (1864).

Fry. *Med. J. Aust.*, **1,** 264 (1967).

Fueger, Milauskas and Britton. *Amer. J. Roentgenol.*, **97,** 614 (1966).

Gordon. *Plast. reconstr. Surg.*, **20,** 65 (1957).

Gordon and MacRae. *Plast. reconstr. Surg.*, **6,** 228 (1950).

Gould and Titus. *Amer. J. Roentgenol.*, **97,** 618 (1966).

Greder. *Dtsch. Z. Chir.*, **21,** 491 (1885).

Hartmann and Gilles. *Roentgenologic Diagnosis in Ophthalmology*, Phila. (1959).

Hewett. *Med. Times Gaz.*, **16,** 311 (1858).

Hitchcock. *Brit. J. Surg.*, **52,** 197 (1965).

Hoffmann and Loepp. *v. Graefes Arch. Ophthal.*, **134,** 82 (1935).

Ipsen. *Die indireckten Orbitaldach Frakturen*, Greifswald (1898).

Jackson. *Proc. roy. Soc. Med.*, **61,** 497 (1968).

Jones, D. *Trans. ophthal. Soc. U.K.*, **86,** 271 (1966).

Jones, D., and Evans. *J. Laryng.*, **81,** 1109 (1967).

Jones, I. *Trans. Amer. Acad. Ophthal.*, **67,** 635 (1963).

Kaufer and Augustin. *Amer. J. Ophthal.*, **61,** 795 (1966).

Kehl. *Beitr. klin. Chir.*, **123,** 203 (1921).

King, A. B., and Walsh. *Amer. J. Ophthal.*, **32,** 191, 379 (1949).

King, E. F. *Trans. ophthal. Soc. U.K.*, **64,** 134 (1944).

Körber. *Dtsch. Z. Chir.*, **29,** 545 (1889).

Lang. *Trans. ophthal. Soc. U.K.*, **9,** 41 (1889).

Lange. *Plast. reconstr. Surg.*, **35,** 26 (1965).

Lerman. *Brit. J. Ophthal.*, **54,** 90 (1970).

Lerman and Cramer. *Amer. J. Ophthal.*, **57,** 264 (1964).

Lewin, J. R., Rhodes and Pavsek. *Amer. J. Roentgenol.*, **83,** 628 (1960).

Lewin, W. *Brit. J. Surg.*, **42,** 1 (1954).

Linhart. *J. Amer. med. Ass.*, **123,** 89 (1943).

Lloyd. *Brit. J. Radiol.*, **39,** 933 (1966); **43,** 1 (1970).

A Textbook of Radiology (ed. Sutton), Edinburgh (1968).

Lombardi. *Radiology in Neuro-ophthalmology*, Baltimore, 95 (1967).

McCoy, Chandler and Magnan. *Plast. reconstr. Surg.*, **29,** 381 (1962).

MacGee, Cauthen and Brackell. *J. Neurosurg.*, **33,** 312 (1970).

McGrigor and Samuel. *Brit. J. Radiol.*, **18,** 65, 284 (1945).

Magoon. *Amer. J. Ophthal.*, **55,** 370 (1963).

Maurer, Mills and German. *J. Neurosurg.*, **18,** 837 (1961).

Meulemans. *Ophthalmologica*, **154,** 461 (1967).

Milauskas. *Diagnosis and Management of Blowout Fractures of the Orbit*, Springfield (1969).

Milauskas and Fueger. *Amer. J. Ophthal.*, **62,** 670 (1966).

Milauskas, Fueger and Schulze. *Trans. Amer. Acad. Ophthal.*, **70,** 25 (1966).

Miller and Glaser. *Arch. Ophthal.*, **76,** 662 (1966).

Miller and Tenzel. *Plast. reconstr. Surg.*, **39,** 37 (1967).

Morian. *Dtsch. Z. Chir.*, **18,** 803 (1883).

Morison. *Lancet*, **1,** 16 (1894).

Morton and Turnbull. *Canad. med. Ass. J.*, **90,** 58 (1964).

Murray. *J. Fac. Radiol.*, **1,** 121 (1949).

Mustardé. *Repair and Reconstruction in the Orbital Region*, Edinburgh (1966).

Brit. J. plast. Surg., **21,** 73 (1968).

Nysingh. *Zygomatico-maxillaire Fracturen*, Utrecht (1960).

O'Connell. *Fractures of the Facial Skeleton* (ed. Rowe and Killey), Edinburgh, 634 (1968).

Penn and Epstein. *Brit. J. plast. Surg.*, **6,** 65 (1953).

Petty. *J. Neurosurg.*, **30,** 741 (1969).

Pfeiffer. *Trans. Amer. ophthal. Soc.*, **39,** 492 (1941).

Arch. Ophthal., **30,** 718 (1943).

Postempski. *Riforme Med.*, **5,** 585 (1889).

Rawling. *Lancet*, **1,** 1097 (1904).

Ray and Bergland. *J. Neurosurg.*, **30,** 399 (1969).

Reed, MacMillan and Lazenby. *Arch. Ophthal.*, **81,** 508 (1969).

Reny and Stricker. *Arch. Ophtal.*, **28,** 477 (1968).

Fractures de l'orbite, Paris (1969).

Romanes. *Fractures of the Facial Skeleton* (ed. Rowe and Killey), Edinburgh, 676 (1968).

Rowbotham. *Acute Injuries of the Head*, Baltimore (1964).

Rowe and Killey. *Fractures of the Facial Skeleton*, 2nd ed., Edinburgh (1968).

Samuel. *Trans. ophthal. Soc. U.K.*, **64,** 140 (1944).

Schurr. *Recent Advances in Surgery of Trauma* (ed. Matthews), London, 376 (1963).

Smith, B., and Converse. *Trans. Amer. Acad. Ophthal.*, **61,** 602 (1957).

Smith, B., and Regan. *Amer. J. Ophthal.*, **44,** 733 (1957).

Soll and Poley. *Amer. J. Ophthal.*, **60,** 269 (1965).

Stierlin. *Dtsch. Z. Chir.*, **55,** 198 (1900).
Stockdale. *Brit. J. plast. Surg.*, **12,** 78 (1959).
von Szily. *Atlas der Kriegsaugenheilkunde*, Stuttgart (1918).
Tilman. *Arch. klin. Chir.*, **66,** 750 (1902).
Trokel and Potter. *Amer. J. Ophthal.*, **67,** 772 (1969).
Arch. Ophthal., **81,** 797 (1969).
Vigario. *Brit. J. Radiol.*, **39,** 939 (1966).
Vinik and Gargano. *Amer. J. Roentgenol.*, **97,** 607 (1966).
Voris and Basile. *J. Neurosurg.*, **18,** 841 (1961).
Watson and Holt-Wilson. *Trans. ophthal. Soc. U.K.*, **88,** 361 (1968).
Weaver, Gates and Nielsen. *Trans. Amer. Acad. Ophthal.*, **65,** 759 (1961).
Whyte. *Brit. J. Ophthal.*, **52,** 721 (1968).
Wolter and Chamichian. *J. pediat. Ophthal.*, **7,** 37 (1970).
Zizmor, Smith, Fasano and Converse. *Trans. Amer. Acad. Ophthal.*, **64,** 802 (1962).
Amer. J. Roentgenol., **87,** 1009 (1962).

The Treatment of Orbital Fractures

If we can forget the horror, the devastation and the prolonged wretchedness which it causes, war frequently does some good in stimulating men to purposeful inventiveness in devising new techniques to aid them to survival or victory or to alleviate the distress. We have already seen that the first modern surgeon to awake this subject out of its mediæval sleep, Ambroise Paré (Fig. 30), was a creation of war; the Crimean war created nursing; in the first World War the intensive shelling of millions of men in crowded trenches over a period of four years produced such a holocaust of injuries that it was natural that traumatic surgery received a dramatic fillip.

In this SIR HAROLD GILLIES [1882–1960] (Fig. 244) was a pioneer. Born of an old Scottish family from the Isle of Bute, his grandfather migrated to New Zealand; Gillies returned to Britain for his medical education at Cambridge University and St. Bartholomew's Hospital in London where he became interested in the newly created Department of Otolaryngology, to the staff of which he was appointed. It was natural that during the first World War this introduction to surgery led him to specialize in the treatment of facial wounds and he established a unit of maxillo-facial surgery in which ideally a surgeon of his specialty combines forces with a neurosurgeon, an ophthalmologist and a dental surgeon. After the war Gillies specialized in plastic surgery; he would not have had to if he had lived so see the present era of traffic accidents. Gillies was extraordinarily richly endowed with many gifts. His ingenuity was unusual, his painstaking efforts and sympathy for his patients great, while his surgical craftsmanship was superb. With the effortlessness of an apparently inherent expertise rather than as the result of laboriously acquired skill, he was strangely proficient at cricket, golf, billiards, wood-carving and fishing, as well as painting in both water-colours and oils. No one could call him handsome but he was a gay spirit and a good companion who thoroughly enjoyed his life.

In most of these injuries particularly when severe the general condition of the patient absorbs the attention of everyone concerned, so much so, indeed, that there is a tendency to leave the orbital fracture untreated until a later date, even although considerable deformity is apparent. Cases do occur when such conservatism is necessary if life is to be saved, but such cases are rare and are confined to those in which a cerebro-spinal rhinorrhœa indicates that the anterior fossa is freely opened. It is true that an indirect fracture of the orbital roof associated with radiating fractures of the base of the skull is an incident in a clinical picture completely dominated by more important events. In direct fractures, however, particularly when bones are displaced, the case is often different. It is to be remembered that the healing of the orbital and facial bones is rapid so that if repositioning is not done at

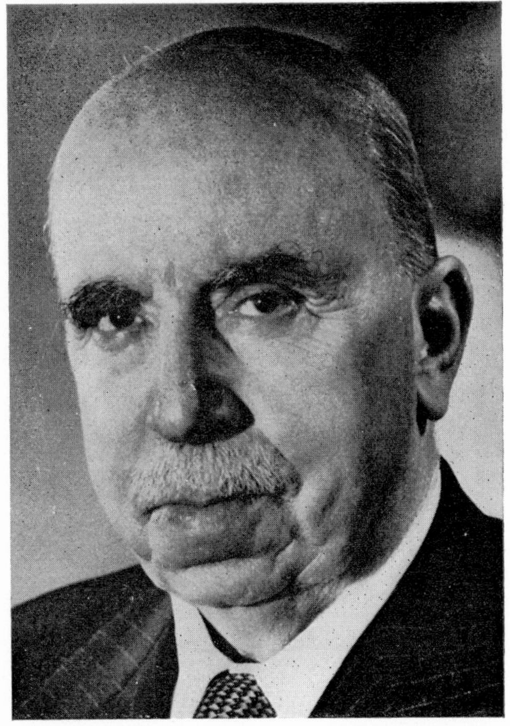

Fig. 244.—Sir Harold Gillies [1882–1960].

an early stage and the fragments are allowed to consolidate in their abnormal position considerable force may be required to refracture and replace them, or alternatively, major surgical procedures may be necessary to get rid of the deformity. If definite treatment is long delayed such procedures may be impossible and all that can be done thereafter is to attempt to camouflage the deformity so far as plastic surgery will allow. It is curious that it is sometimes considered that in a patient with a head injury, fractures of the limbs can reasonably be set while fractures of the facial bones cannot. It should be emphasized that repositioning should be undertaken as soon as the period of shock has passed provided the general condition of the patient allows and before the local swelling of the lids and face has subsided.

In the treatment of all types of facial injury three fundamental principles apply—the preservation of life, the maintenance of function and the restoration of the appearance. The detailed treatment of specific types of fracture is now such a complex matter involving specialized techniques in several inter-related fields, usually within special accident-units or centres devoted to the care of maxillo-facial injuries, that it is impossible here to deal with all aspects of this problem. In this section we shall outline the essential principles of the treatment of these cases which should be generally understood; for the detailed management of individual types of fracture the reader is referred to more specialized works.[1] The ophthalmic surgeon has an important role in the management of these cases; while it is true that measures for the preservation of life take precedence over all other considerations, the early surgical treatment of an injury to the eye, particularly where perforation of the globe has occurred, is essential and, indeed, may be most conveniently undertaken at the same time as the initial treatment of the facial injury. At a later stage he will be concerned with the problems presented by obstruction to the lacrimal passages, the restoration of the bony walls of the orbit and the surgical relief of diplopia. In all cases the maintenance of the air-way is essential, whether by posture, the removal of clot and debris from the mouth and larynx, suction, intubation and in certain cases tracheotomy. Measures for the control of hæmorrhage are important, particularly in a fracture of the nasal bones and medial orbital wall wherein it may be a serious problem; as a rule, nasal hæmorrhage usually ceases spontaneously but in some cases packing with ribbon-gauze soaked in 1:1,000 adrenaline may be required, while in severe cases direct occlusion of the responsible vessels by suture or proximal ligation may be necessary.

Infection. In all cases wherein a surface wound exists the immediate treatment should include attention to prophylaxis against tetanus,[2] the systemic administration of antibiotics to combat infection and the cleansing of superficial wounds with warm saline or cetrimide with as little debridement as possible, followed by their careful suturing in layers as will be indicated in the treatment of injuries to the eyelids. Despite the wide variety of antibiotics currently available penicillin is still the most generally useful prophylactic and should be given in appropriate dosage pending the result of sensitivity tests unless a previous history of hypersensitivity to this drug is known. Penicillin, however, has the serious drawback that it does not usually reach a satisfactory level in the cerebro-spinal fluid. In those cases of facial or cranial fractures in which cerebro-spinal rhinorrhœa is present or if a communication is suspected between the cranial cavity and the naso-pharynx, air-sinuses or middle ear, prophylactic treatment with sulphonamides is indicated[3]; indeed, it is probably wise to use both penicillin and the sulphonamides routinely in all cases of fracture involving the facial bones.

Fractures of the different parts of the orbit or the associated bones require specific techniques in their treatment.

Fractures of the orbital roof and superior orbital rim

Fractures in this region are usually the result of severe local violence and the associated injuries therefrom may require the services of a neurosurgeon

[1] See particularly Dawson (1963), Stallard (1965), Mustardé (1966), Rowe and Killey (1968), Reny and Stricker (1969). [2] p. 408.

[3] As sulphadiazine 2 g. initially, followed by 1 g. six-hourly taken with mist. pot. cit. 15 ml. and as liberal a fluid intake as the condition of the patient will allow.

or an otorhinologist. If the outer table of the frontal bone is fractured it may be elevated and the wound closed in layers after the establishment of drainage, if this is indicated. If the inner table is involved it may also be elevated but in such a case damage to the dura is almost certainly present and the treatment of this should be left to the neurosurgeon. If the upper rim of the orbit is broken and displaced inwards without losing its periosteal connections it may be replaced and held in position by periosteal sutures (Schultze, 1970); particular care should be taken if the region of the trochlea is involved, for unless it is accurately replaced to its original position the consequent impairment of the action of the superior oblique

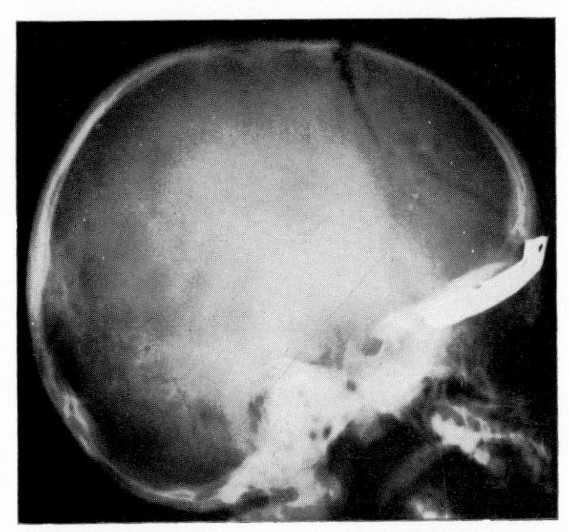

Fig. 245.—The Use of a Tantalum Plate in Repair.

The tantalum plate has been used to repair the gross defect in the floor of the anterior fossa and roof of the orbit and forms a new supra-orbital ridge. In the case of traumatic encephalocele of the orbit seen in Figs. 190 and 191 (A. B. King).

muscle will cause a disturbing diplopia. Completely detached fragments of bone which have been stripped of their periosteal covering are generally removed but with great care lest in the process the dura should be damaged. The resulting bony defect in the supra-orbital ridge or orbital roof will require replacement with a bony or alloplastic implant at a later date (Fig. 245). Alternatively, instead of debridement of damaged bony fragments, some neurosurgeons advocate their primary replacement and frequently cases treated in this way do well.[1] If the frontal sinus is involved in the fracture the possibility of infection is great; infection at the site of injury and the more serious spread of infection into the intracranial cavity may result if

[1] A full discussion of the principles of reconstruction of the frontal bone using bony or alloplastic implants is given by Dickinson and Cipcic (1966), and Dickinson *et al.* (1969).

FIGS. 246 and 247.—THE TREATMENT OF FRACTURES
(N. Rowe and H. Killey, *Fractures of the Facial Skeleton*, Livingstone).

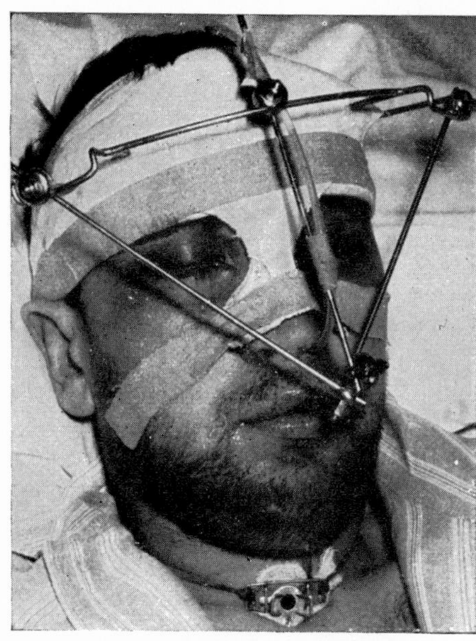

FIG. 246.—Multiple facial injuries including Le Fort II and III fractures, bilateral mandibular and nasal fractures. Fixation by triple anterior rod. A tracheotomy has been performed.

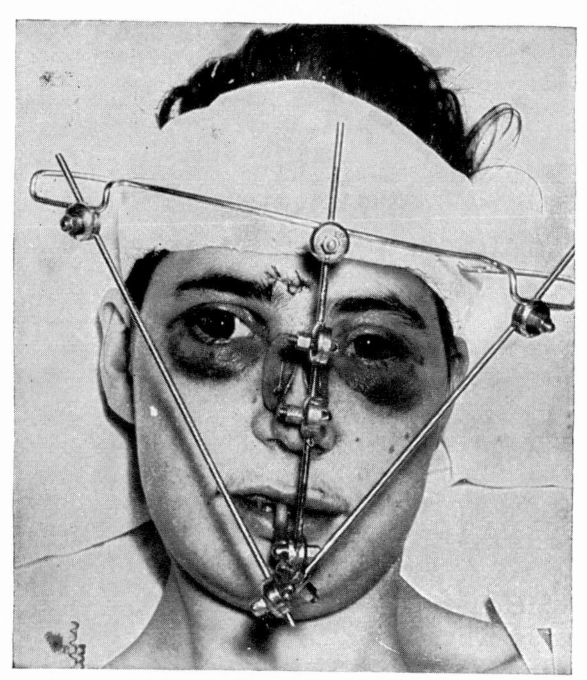

FIG. 247.—Similar injuries to those seen in Fig. 246 but with depression of the naso-ethmoidal complex, showing medial compression using lead plates with stainless steel wire fixation to prevent traumatic telecanthus. The wires are secured to the vertical rod connecting the maxillary splint to the plaster-of-Paris headcap.

there should be a tear in the dura. In all these cases, as we have already emphasized, treatment with penicillin and sulphonamides is essential.

Naso-maxillary fractures should if possible be replaced at the earliest possible moment. The particular method by which such fractures are dealt with depends on the time at which treatment is undertaken. Within the period up to the first 14 days or so after the injury, primary treatment is likely to be successful. The principles of treatment in these cases involve disimpaction of the fracture and replacement of the bones in their normal anatomical position, followed by immobilization of the fragments until a satisfactory degree of bony union has occurred. If only one maxilla is fractured and the contralateral maxilla remains firmly attached to the base

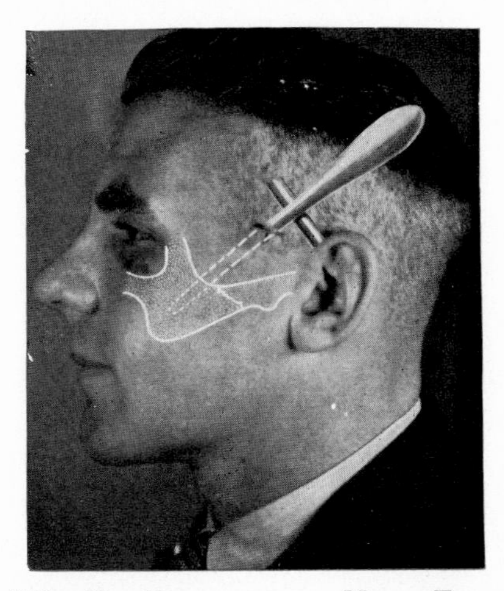

FIG. 248.—THE ELEVATION OF A MALAR FRACTURE.

The bony fragment is repositioned by a lever introduced through a temporal approach and passed down behind the temporal fascia (R. Watson Jones, *Fractures and Joint Injuries*, Livingstone, Edinburgh).

of the skull, immobilization of the fracture can be achieved by splinting it to the normal side by means of a connecting bar. With a bilateral fracture, however, and when both maxillæ are separated from the skull more complex methods are required; in these cases immobilization may be achieved by external skeletal fixation using a system of metal rods and universal joints connecting a splint applied to the teeth, maxilla or mandible with a framework embedded within a plaster-of-Paris headcap, or internal skeletal suspension, transfixion of the fragments or trans-osseous wiring (Rowe and Killey, 1968) (Figs. 246–7).

Zygomatic Fractures. Early treatment in this type of fracture is desirable for in most cases the depressed bone can be replaced with relative ease if it has insufficient time to become consolidated in its displaced position. The most generally satisfactory method of treatment is by open reduction through a temporal approach; the bony fragment may be replaced by means of an elevator inserted through an incision in the temporal area and passed down behind the temporal fascia till it lies beneath the zygoma (Fig. 248). If treatment has been delayed for more than 2 or 3 weeks such a manœuvre may be difficult or even impossible; in such a situation and in those cases wherein the bone is comminuted, or if a previously successful reduction becomes unstable, open reduction and fixation of the fragments to the lateral orbital margin by wire may be required together with packing of the maxillary antrum. It is to be remembered that in all procedures involving the insertion of a pack into the maxillary antrum great care should be taken lest damage to the optic nerve should occur; blindness has been reported following such a manœuvre, probably due to injury to the optic nerve or its blood vessels (Gordon and MacRae, 1950; McCoy *et al.*, 1962).

Medial Orbital Wall Fracture (*Naso-orbital Fracture*). Occasionally in a fracture through the infero-medial angle of the orbit involving the medial part of the maxillary component of the inferior orbital margin, sometimes associated with a fracture of the nose, reduction is best achieved by the use of forceps through the nasal cavity. More serious, however, is the fracture of the medial orbital wall as a result of direct violence to the nose or associated with a blow-out fracture of the orbital floor; in these cases the whole naso-ethmoid region may be involved, usually on both sides. There may be comminution of the naso-lacrimal bones, lateral displacement of the medial canthus and damage to the lacrimal passages. Immediate treatment should include exploration of the lacrimal sac and fossa and replacement of any displaced bony fragments which should be immobilized by trans-osseous wiring through the nasal septum (Converse and Smith, 1966; Dingman *et al.*, 1969; Stranc, 1970).

Orbital Floor Fracture

(1) When the inferior orbital margin and adjacent bones are fractured the bones should be realigned; in such lesions a portion of the rim is usually depressed and after reduction of the deformity inter-osseous wiring may be required.

(2) Blow-out fracture. Cases of blow-out fracture of the orbital floor seen *recently* after injury can be divided into two groups (Jones, 1966; and others). (*a*) Those cases in which there are no or only minimal signs of restriction of ocular movements and the diagnosis depends essentially on radiological findings. In this group surgical treatment is not usually required but they should be kept under observation lest further signs develop; Bowers (1964) followed up 13 untreated blow-out fractures of this type and showed that they remained symptom-free. The incidence of pathological sequelæ to untreated fractures that were initially asymptomatic, however, has not yet been established (Goldberg, 1969). (*b*) A second group includes those cases which have significant enophthalmos or marked restriction of

movement, confirmed by the duction test, particularly of elevation, or radiological evidence of the incarceration of orbital tissues. In this group early surgery (within 14–21 days) is advisable to free the trapped inferior ocular muscles and to repair the defect in the orbital floor.[1]

The orbital floor may be explored in two ways—either through an incision in the lower eyelid or through the maxillary antrum by the Caldwell-Luc technique. The *antral approach* through the canine fossa and the maxillary antrum enables the surgeon to liberate the prolapsed orbital contents from below and to elevate the downwardly displaced orbital floor; following reduction and removal of any blood and clot from the antral cavity, the orbital floor may be held in its correct position by means of gauze packing or an

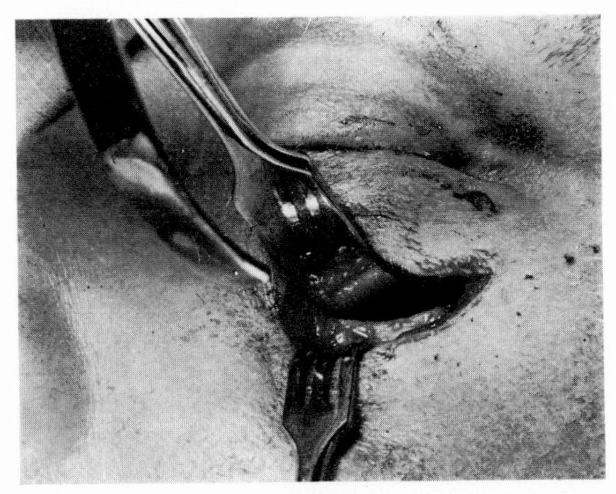

FIG. 249.—BLOW-OUT FRACTURE OF THE ORBITAL FLOOR.

When a muscle is incarcerated in the fracture it should be immediately liberated to prevent its atrophy and avoid the development of scar-tissue. A spatula is introduced between the periorbital fascia and the floor and as soon as it touches the hernia a second spatula is introduced and the incarcerated muscle is detached from the fracture by delicate " hand-over-hand " manipulation (G. M. Bleeker).

inflatable balloon (Fisher, 1957; Cunningham and Marden, 1962; Converse *et al.*, 1967). The prevention of post-operative antral infection is important; no loose fragments should be left behind and an intra-nasal antrostomy is advisable supplemented by systemic antibiotics and the instillation of 1% ephedrine as nasal drops. The antral approach, however, is not entirely satisfactory for the release of trapped orbital soft tissues or for the insertion of an orbital floor implant, and is probably best combined with an approach through the eyelid. In the *eyelid approach* the incision is made following the natural fold of the lower lid, leaving intact a wide strip of skin between it and the lid-margin to preserve the lymphatic and venous drainage (Fig. 249). The orbicularis oculi muscle is split along the line of its fibres, the

[1] E. F. King (1944), Smith and Regan (1957), Converse and Smith (1960–61), Jones (1966), Converse *et al.* (1967), Whyte (1968), Reny and Stricker (1969), Goldberg (1969), Lerman (1970).

septum orbitale is exposed and followed downward to its point of attachment to the inferior orbital rim. If the orbital septum is inadvertently penetrated, the defect should be repaired so as to prevent herniation of the orbital fat into the eyelid. The periosteum is incised and raised backwards over the floor of the orbit until the area of the blow-out fracture is demonstrated. The incarcerated tissues are liberated from the site of the fracture and, if necessary, the defect in the orbital floor is repaired using either a bone-graft or an alloplastic implant. It is essential to verify (as by the muscle traction test) that the orbital contents have been freed and that normal ocular movements have been restored.

More difficult problems occur in those cases which present for treatment at a *late stage* after injury or after inadequate or unsuccessful primary treatment (Obear, 1967; and others). Malunion of the fracture, fibrosis of the soft tissues, enophthalmos and persistent diplopia, together with palpebral and lacrimal complications may all have to be dealt with. In these cases definitive surgical management is best postponed until all traces of œdema and inflammatory reaction in the tissues have subsided. In general the same techniques are to be used as in the case of recent fractures and the majority will most probably require a combined antral and eyelid approach. The aim of treatment in these late cases includes restoration of the continuity of the orbital floor and the reduction in the size of the orbital cavity thereby correcting enophthalmos, while operations on the extra-ocular muscles will probably be required to correct residual diplopia. Reduction of the fracture and replacement of the bony fragments to their normal position will relieve most cases of post-traumatic diplopia. When double vision persists despite adequate reduction and replacement of the orbital floor, further surgical procedures on the extra-ocular muscles will be required, a subject which is considered fully in a subsequent section.[1]

THE REPAIR OF BONY DEFECTS. Numerous materials are now available for the reconstruction of defects of the orbital walls or margin or of the associated facial bones, but whatever material is chosen satisfactory results demand a very high standard in the techniques of plastic surgery. Autografts of bone or cartilage from the patient's own body are certainly the most suitable but satisfactory results are frequently obtained by the use of various alloplastic implants.

(1) *Bone grafts* were first employed for the reconstitution of the zygoma by the American surgeon, John B. Murphy, in 1915 who used a tibial-osteo-periosteal graft. The most suitable form is cancellous bone taken from the smooth inner aspect of the iliac crest which is easy to mould into shape; eventually a certain amount of absorption and remodelling of the graft may be expected so that a piece larger than the existing defect must be inserted. Nevertheless it is the method of choice when extensive damage has to be repaired. For smaller defects bone removed from the anterior

[1] p. 302.

wall of the maxillary sinus in the canine fossa and the perpendicular plate of the ethmoid may also be used. Whether fresh or preserved bone is used it serves merely as a framework and is, in time, entirely replaced by vascularized living bone from the host[1] (Fig. 250).

(2) *Cartilage grafts* were used in the first World War to a considerable extent for the reconstruction of the orbital rim, particularly the zygomatic arch and occasionally for the reconstitution of the orbital floor (Morestin, 1916; Lagrange, 1917; Gillies, 1920), and since that time a great deal of experience has been gained in the method.[2] Cartilage is more flexible than bone, it can be easily carved into thin slices for small defects and is the material of choice in children; their iliac crest is still cartilaginous in nature but it is an active centre of growth and it should, if possible, be left undisturbed (Rowe and Killey, 1968). If cartilage is required it should be obtained from the tips of the ribs, a suitable site being the point where the 8th and 9th or 9th and 10th costal cartilages fuse together. If necessary human bone or cartilage taken post-mortem and preserved by freezing may be used, as also may preserved bovine cartilage.

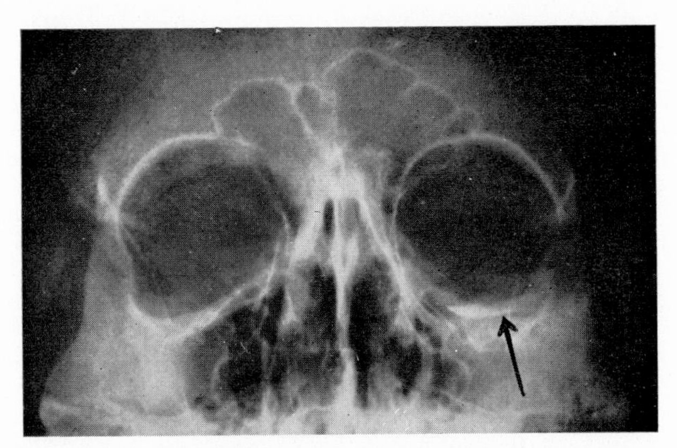

FIG. 250.—FRACTURE OF THE ORBITAL FLOOR.
An implant from the mastoid bone shaped to fit the orbital floor has been inserted (G. M. Bleeker).

(3) *Alloplastic implants.* A considerable variety of foreign materials has from time to time been employed in the reconstruction of defects in the orbital region, although in the case of some of these substances histological and clinical proof of the absence of adverse tissue reactions has been lacking.

(*a*) *Metals.* Implants constructed from tantalum, stainless steel and vitallium have all had their advocates. Tantalum which is strong, resistant to corrosion and chemical attack, of high malleability and ductility, is an eminently suitable material. Its use in this way was initially explored by Burke (1940), and it was extensively applied in orbital repair by Callahan (1950) and A. B. King (1951). It is used in sheets 0·015 in. thick, made into the correct shape from a model of the patient's defect, superimposed on that of the normal orbit. Such a sheet perforated for purposes of fixation can be used for reconstituting the anterior table of the frontal bone and the orbital margin and it may be extended inwards to replace much of the orbital roof; in the form of a gauze mesh it has also been recommended for the immediate reconstruction of the orbital floor and is also suitable for the restoration of the medial orbital wall (Prowler,

[1] Gillies (1920), Mowlem (1941–44), Converse (1944), Neely (1947), Converse and Smith (1950), Mustardé (1966), Converse *et al.* (1967), Bleeker (1968).

[2] McIndoe (1937), Mowlem (1941), DeVoe (1947), Callahan (1950), Rowe and Killey (1968).

1965). Regeneration of bone around the tantalum may occur but, although this metal is non-toxic, it may not be tolerated in the presence of infection. In such circumstances an infected granuloma may develop after a period varying from 1 week to 3 months after its insertion, a complication which may necessitate its subsequent removal (Meirowsky *et al.*, 1950). Its insertion and, indeed, the use of any alloplastic material should therefore be delayed until the presence of infection is excluded.

(*b*) *Terylene wool* has also been used for the building up of orbital defects; it has the disadvantage, however, of inducing a severe fibrotic reaction in the presence of sepsis and may thus increase any existing adhesions in the region of the orbital floor. It is therefore not recommended.

(*c*) A *fibre-glass* material was used by Walser (1960–62); extrusion occurred in 4 out of 37 patients treated in this way.

(*d*) *Methylmethacrylate*, a plastic resin, was first used at the beginning of the second World War for elevation of the orbital floor. A plate of the plastic material is cut to the required size and inserted subperiosteally and held in place initially by sutures, perforations being made through the plate to allow for the subsequent ingrowth of fibrous tissue. This has been used with success in the treatment of enophthalmos (Callahan, 1950; and others) but it is not always tolerated and cases have occurred wherein the graft has been expelled. A form of rapidly polymerizing methylmethacrylate was used by Ballen (1964); in this procedure powdered acrylic is mixed with a liquid catalyst, the resulting material is moulded *in situ* and hardened by a process of polymerization but in so doing gives off heat.

(*e*) Considerable success has been reported with implants constructed from *Teflon* (a polytetrafluorethylene resin) and *silicone rubber* (dimethylpolysiloxane). Several histological studies[1] and clinical reports[2] have confirmed the satisfactory nature of these substances. Teflon and silicone are available in thin sheets which may be easily carved or moulded to fit a specific defect and are, in addition, virtually inert in the tissues.

Finally, the old method of attempted reconstruction by the injection of paraffin wax is quite useless (Sallmann, 1928) if not dangerous, while the employment of grafts of fat for reconstituting the orbital floor (Pichler, 1920) is usually unsatisfactory although in certain cases they may be of value when padding out of the area round the orbit is all that is required (Mustardé, 1966).

Whatever material is used for reconstruction of bony defects resulting from injury certain precautions must be observed. It is essential to ensure that no part of the actual graft is left exposed, either within the antrum, the nose or the conjunctival fornices: exposure in this way is likely to result in its extrusion and in more serious cases to infection. Where the defect is extensive as may occur with a blow-out fracture, the implant may slide forwards on rotation of the globe; to prevent this complication the implant should be secured to the orbital rim. Similarly, the implant should be so placed that it bridges over the defect and rests on the stable adjacent portions of the orbital floor. Finally, care should be taken to avoid a dead space between the implant and the orbital wall since such a cavity may provide a space in which infection can occur.

These operations can produce remarkable results from a cosmetic point of view and are eminently satisfactory when the eye has been excised and

[1] Brown *et al.* (1960), Calnan (1963), Rees *et al.* (1965), among others.

[2] Freeman (1962), Browning and Walker (1965), Cramer *et al.* (1965), Mustardé (1966), Converse *et al.* (1967), Lerman (1970).

the only necessity is to have a prosthesis with an adequate appearance. Although reconstruction of the orbital floor may not completely overcome diplopia, satisfactory functional results have been obtained.[1] It is true that the power of fusion may be sufficient to overcome a considerable residual displacement but in the majority of cases diplopia, although considerably lessened, is not completely abolished. Before resort is made to occlusion of the eye, which in the end may be necessary, orthoptic exercises may be tried, for these occasionally stimulate the capacity for fusion sufficiently to produce a functional cure (E. F. King, 1944). Little relief is usually obtained from prisms since their effects rarely extend far outside the primary position; most frequently the residual defect must be corrected by muscle surgery which in the majority of cases gives satisfactory results.

For completeness, the treatment of a number of additional complications associated with fractures of the orbit and adjacent bones should be mentioned here, although the details of their management will be found in subsequent sections of this volume.

(1) PTOSIS. A pseudo-ptosis occurs when the globe is displaced downwards and backwards, but is corrected by its replacement. True ptosis is usually due to paresis of the levator palpebræ superioris from damage to its nerve supply or to a rupture of the tendon of the muscle from a severe contusion of the upper lid. The defect may require either resection of the levator, repair of the tendon or, if no function remains in this muscle, some procedure based on the suspension of the upper lid from the frontalis muscle. In general, any existing extra-ocular muscular imbalance should be dealt with before the ptosis is corrected.

(2) EPIPHORA. Persistent and troublesome watering may result from obstruction to the lacrimal apparatus at any site from the puncta to the opening of the naso-lacrimal duct into the nose. Such may result from lacerations in the region of the inner margins of the eyelids and the inner canthal tissues, or from fractures in the naso-orbital area and of the maxilla. Simple obstruction of the naso-lacrimal duct below the sac is best treated by dacryocystorhinostomy; canalicular obstructions resulting from scarring and fibrosis are more complex problems, for which various types of intubation or operations designed to by-pass the block may be required.

[1] Illustrative reports of cases treated in this way include Reeh and Tsujimura (1966) using a Supramid plate; Lerman and Cramer (1964), 10 cases successfully treated with a subperiosteal silastic implant; Pinkerton *et al.* (1967), 39 cases; Stranc (1968), 33 cases with a subperiosteal polythene plate inserted via an eyelid incision; Harrison (1968), bone grafting in 8 cases, only 1 relieved of diplopia; Jackson (1968), polythene plates inserted in 31 cases, resulting in a useful field of single vision in them all, but in 13 persistent diplopia necessitated extra-ocular muscle surgery; Whyte (1968), 10 cases with a silicone rubber plate; Lerman (1970) obtained excellent results in 50 cases with no evidence of infection or extrusion of the implant up to three years after its insertion.

(3) MEDIAL AND LATERAL CANTHAL DEFORMITIES occur most commonly as a result of multiple facial fractures, particularly when the root of the nose is involved. Fracture-dislocation of the zygoma may dislocate the attachment of the lateral palpebral raphe producing an anti-mongoloid slant of the eyelids, while the complete detachment of this structure results in a rounded lateral canthus and a decreased intercanthal distance. The medial palpebral ligament is inserted in front onto the anterior lacrimal crest and behind onto the posterior lacrimal crest: naso-orbital fractures, fractures of the frontal process of the maxilla, lacrimal or nasal bones may disrupt the stability of the medial insertion of the eyelids so that the medial canthus is pulled laterally and occasionally downward, producing the condition of traumatic telecanthus. The lacrimal sac is frequently involved in this type of injury. Treatment will require careful dissection of the tissues at the medial canthus, removal of free bony fragments, refixation of the medial palpebral ligament to the nasal bone and appropriate surgery on the lacrimal apparatus.

(4) RETRACTION OF THE LOWER EYELID. A vertical shortening of the lower eyelid with exposure of sclera below the limbus in the primary position may result from scar formation, from downward and backward displacement of the fractured inferior orbital rim or from inadvertent inclusion of the periorbita in the septum orbitale after the insertion of an orbital floor implant. Release of the scar-tissue and replacement of the orbital rim in the correct position will restore the lower lid to its natural position; if there is bony malunion, release of the attachment of the septum orbitale to the orbital rim followed by reconstruction of the orbital margin by a bone graft will result in elevation of the lid margin, while in some cases a tarso-conjunctival graft from the same or opposite upper eyelid may be required to produce the same result.

(5) INFRA-ORBITAL NERVE ANÆSTHESIA. Persistent sensory loss extending from the lower eyelid over the cheek and the lateral side of the nostril to the upper lip may be a distressing symptom; in such cases exploration of the orbital floor and decompression of the infra-orbital nerve may be required, although it should be remembered that sensation may return spontaneously up to 12 months after injury (Converse and Smith, 1966; Mustardé, 1966; Converse *et al.*, 1967).

Ballen. *Plast. reconstr. Surg.*, **34**, 624 (1964).
Bleeker. *1st. int. Cong. Orthoptists* (1967), London, 207 (1968).
Bowers. *Surv. Ophthal.*, **9**, 237 (1964).
Brown, Fryer and Ohlwiler. *Plast. reconstr. Surg.*, **26**, 264 (1960).
Browning and Walker. *Amer. J. Ophthal.*, **60**, 684 (1965).
Burke. *Canad. med. Ass. J.*, **43**, 125 (1940).
Callahan. *Surgery of the Eye: Injuries*, Springfield (1950).
Calnan. *Brit. J. plast. Surg.*, **16**, 1 (1963).
Converse. *Arch. Ophthal.*, **31**, 323 (1944).
Converse and Smith. *Arch. Ophthal.*, **44**, 1 (1950).
Trans. Amer. Acad. Ophthal., **64**, 676 (1960).
J. Florida med. Ass., **47**, 1337 (1961).
Plast. reconstr. Surg., **38**, 147 (1966).
Converse, Smith, Obear and Wood-Smith. *Plast. reconstr. Surg.*, **39**, 20 (1967).

Cramer, Tooze and Lerman. *Brit. J. plast. Surg.*, **18,** 171 (1965).
Cunningham and Marden. *Arch. Ophthal.*, **68,** 492 (1962).
Dawson. *Recent Advances in the Surgery of Trauma* (ed. Matthews), London, 217 (1963).
DeVoe. *Trans. Amer. ophthal. Soc.*, **45,** 502 (1947).
Dickinson and Cipcic. *Trans. Amer. Acad. Ophthal.*, **70,** 495 (1966).
Dickinson, Cipcic and Kimber. *Laryngoscope*, **79,** 1019 (1969).
Dingman, Crabb and Oneal. *Arch. Surg.*, **98,** 566 (1969).
Fisher. *Trans. Amer. Acad. Ophthal.*, **61,** 607 (1957).
Freeman. *Plast. reconstr. Surg.*, **29,** 587 (1962).
Gillies. *Plastic Surgery of the Face*, London (1920).
Goldberg. *Diagnosis and Management of Blowout Fractures of the Orbit* (ed. Milauskas), Springfield, 121 (1969).
Gordon and MacRae. *Plast. reconstr. Surg.*, **6,** 228 (1950).
Harrison. *Proc. roy. Soc. Med.*, **61,** 493 (1968).
Jackson. *Proc. roy. Soc. Med.*, **61,** 497 (1968).
Jones, D. *Trans. ophthal. Soc. U.K.*, **86,** 271 (1966).
King, A. B. *Arch. Ophthal.*, **46,** 49 (1951).
King, E. F. *Trans. ophthal. Soc. U.K.*, **64,** 134 (1944).
Lagrange. *Les fractures de l'orbite par les projectiles de guerre*, Paris (1917).
Lerman. *Brit. J. Ophthal.*, **54,** 90 (1970).
Lerman and Cramer. *Amer. J. Ophthal.*, **57,** 264 (1964).
McCoy, Chandler and Magnan. *Plast. reconstr. Surg.*, **29,** 381 (1962).
McIndoe. *Surg. Gyn. Obstet.*, **64,** 376 (1937).
Meirowsky, Hazouri and Greiner. *J. Neurosurg.*, **7,** 485 (1950).
Morestin. *Bull. Soc. Chir. Paris*, **42,** 1700 (1916).
Mowlem. *Brit. J. Surg.*, **29,** 182 (1941).
Lancet, **2,** 746 (1944).
Murphy. *Clinics of J. B. Murphy*, Chicago, **4,** 125 (1915).
Mustardé. *Repair and Reconstruction of the Orbital Region*, Edinburgh (1966).
Neely. *Brit. J. Ophthal.*, **31,** 581 (1947).
Obear. *Plastic and Reconstructive Surgery of the Eye and Adnexa* (ed. Smith and Converse), St. Louis, 237 (1967).
Pichler. *Klin. Mbl. Augenheilk.*, **65,** 891 (1920).
Pinkerton, Rosen, de Margerie *et al. Canad. J. Ophthal.*, **2,** 103 (1967).
Prowler. *J. oral Surg.*, **23,** 5 (1965).
Reeh and Tsujimura. *Amer. J. Ophthal.*, **62,** 79 (1966).
Rees, Platt and Ballantyne. *Plast. reconstr. Surg.*, **35,** 131 (1965).
Reny and Stricker. *Fractures de l'orbite*, Paris (1969).
Rowe and Killey. *Fractures of the Facial Skeleton*, 2nd ed., Edinburgh (1968).
Sallmann. *Z. Augenheilk.*, **65,** 298 (1928).
Schultze. *Plast. reconstr. Surg.*, **45,** 227 (1970).
Smith and Regan. *Amer. J. Ophthal.*, **44,** 733 (1957).
Stallard. *Eye Surgery*, 4th ed., Bristol, 859 (1965).
Stranc. *Proc. roy. Soc. Med.*, **61,** 494 (1968).
Brit. J. plast. Surg., **23,** 8, 339 (1970).
Walser. *Klin. Mbl. Augenheilk.*, **136,** 89 (1960); **141,** 252 (1962).
Whyte. *Brit. J. Ophthal.*, **52,** 721 (1968).

ORBITAL HÆMORRHAGE

A hæmorrhage into the orbit is a common sequel of a contusion in the immediate neighbourhood and may produce a dramatic clinical picture (Figs. 251–2). The bleeding may be subperiosteal or into the orbital tissues; in the first case it is usually, and in the second frequently associated with a bony fracture which may entail considerable laceration of the tissues if the fragments are displaced, but this is by no means an invariable antecedent as was long ago demonstrated experimentally in rabbits and on post-mortem examination in man by Berlin (1880) and Morian (1883). It may be taken as a general rule, however, that a severe orbital hæmorrhage is usually associated with a fracture, but it is to be remembered that arterial branches in the orbit may be torn by *contre-coup* (Rollet, 1909), while the possibility of a rupture of the ciliary vessels just before they enter the eye must also be kept in mind (Busacca, 1947).

If the hæmorrhage is small, signs and symptoms may be few or absent, but if the bleeding is of any size it is characterized by some proptosis which

FIGS. 251 and 252.—ORBITAL HÆMORRHAGES.

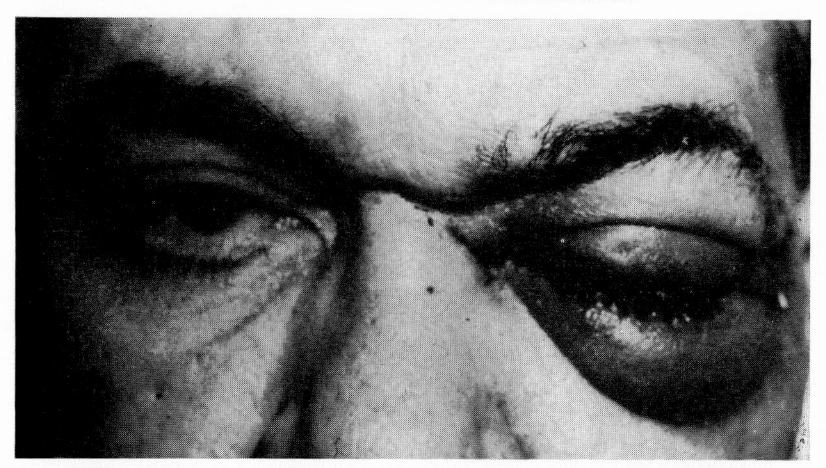

FIG. 251.—In the early stages, showing gross swelling of the eyelids after a blow.

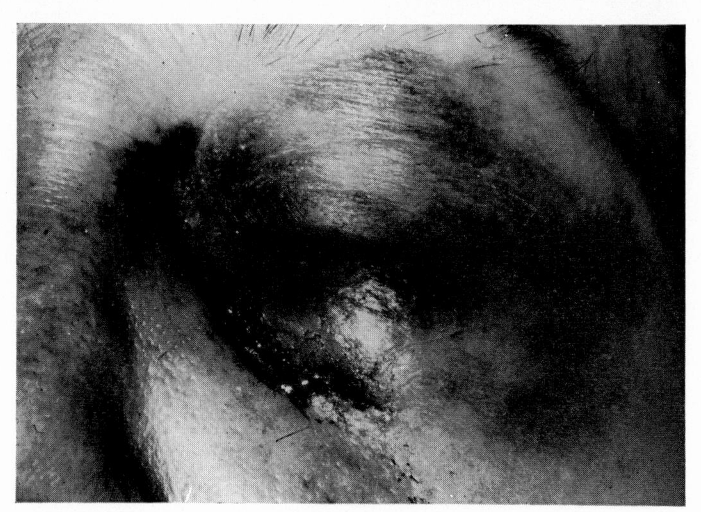

FIG. 252.—In the early stages, showing gross orbital hæmorrhages and laceration of the lid after a blow.

may be moderate or severe, an extravasation of blood under the conjunctiva which may be sufficient to raise up this membrane with the formation of a hæmatoma, a seepage through the tarso-orbital fascia to produce an ecchymosis of the lids which usually appears some hours (12 to 24) after the injury, a loss of movement of the globe with resulting diplopia, and occasionally a loss of vision owing to pressure on the optic nerve or damage to its supplying blood vessels associated perhaps with bleeding into its sheath. The proptosis, which is of sudden onset and irreducible, is usually eccentric, particularly if the bleeding is subperiosteal, but if the hæmorrhage is extensive and the orbital tissues themselves are infiltrated, axial protrusion of the globe will result. The plugging action of the eyeball usually generates sufficient pressure to control the bleeding before it has progressed to an alarming extent but occasionally the proptosis increases until the cornea is endangered through exposure; indeed, the globe has even been dislocated outside the lids. An extreme proptosis of this type may occur in hæmophiliacs (Priestley Smith, 1888).

Damage to the eyeball itself is comparatively rare. The pressure generated in the orbit may give rise to a traumatic mydriasis and the abolition of the pupillary reflexes (Rochon-Duvigneaud and Veil, 1923); papillœdema and occasionally hæmorrhages in the retina may occur; while a case has been reported wherein pressure upon the globe produced indentation of the sclera resulting in a detachment of the retina and a deformation leading to the development of 6 D of myopia (Ulrich, 1882).

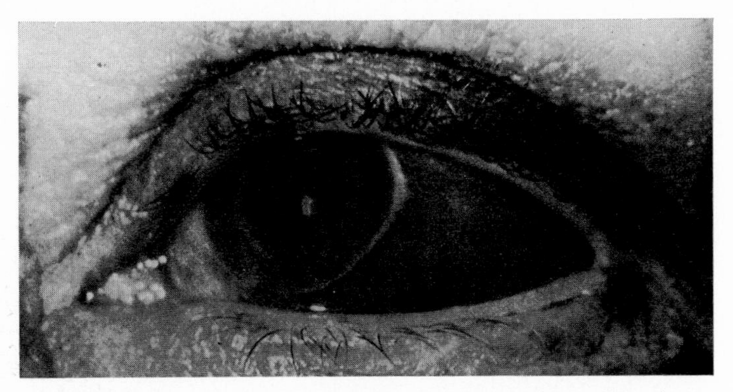

Fig. 253.—Subconjunctival hæmorrhage and a black eye following a concussion injury.

Corneal damage may occur due to exposure accentuated perhaps by the neurotropic effects of compression-paresis of the ophthalmic branch of the trigeminal nerve.

The *differential diagnosis* of an orbital hæmorrhage is usually easy but the determination of the origin of the bleeding may present difficulties. We have already seen that local contusion of the lids produces an immediate swelling of the tissues; an orbital hæmorrhage does not reach the superficial tissues until after the lapse of some hours. Hæmorrhage derived from an orbital fracture, which usually appears some 12 to 24 hours after the accident, may have some localizing significance: from a fracture of the roof it tends to track along the levator muscle and the upper lid; of the apex, along the lateral rectus; from the orbital surface of the sphenoid, along the temporal aspect of the orbit (Fig. 253); from the floor, into the lower lid (Kehl, 1921–23).

Hæmorrhage derived from a fracture of the base of the skull may present a somewhat similar picture, but in this case the extravasated blood, which seeps along the floor of the orbit and appears typically towards the nasal side in the subconjunctival tissues and in the lower lid, does not usually become evident until the lapse of a day or two after the injury. Such an event is relatively common; in 100 basal fractures, Liebrecht (1906) found that 34% had bleeding into the lids (22 unilateral and 12 bilateral), 10% had subconjunctival hæmorrhages in addition, and 4% subconjunctival ecchymosis alone. *Such an extravasation appearing at an interval greater than 24 hours after a head injury with or without unconsciousness is pathognomonic of a fracture of the base of the skull.* It is to be remembered that a hæmorrhage into the optic nerve-sheath between the dura and arachnoid derived from a similarly situated intracranial hæmorrhage with or without a fracture of the skull, may lead to compression of the central vein of the retina and papillœdema (Priestley Smith, 1884; Silcock, 1884). It is seldom difficult to differentiate the origin of a subconjunctival hæmorrhage due to local injury; in this case the blood is densest at one part, usually anteriorly, and it fades posteriorly towards the equator of the globe, whereas if the bleeding is of retrobulbar or basal origin the subconjunctival hæmorrhage is more widespread and denser posteriorly and sometimes may not even reach the limbus.

The *symptoms* of a severe orbital hæmorrhage include some pain, which occasionally is acute and radiating; in the worst cases, when considerable pressure is generated, vomiting and slowing of the heart may occur owing to implementation of the oculo-gastric and oculo-cardiac reflexes through the trigeminal and vagus (Rollet and Paufique, 1929). Loss of vision, as we have seen, may occur, which is usually transient and rarely permanent. The absorption of blood from this region is generally slow compared with other parts of the body, partly because of the poverty of blood vessels and phagocytic reticulo-endothelial elements in the orbital fat, and partly owing to the obliteration of the available circulation because of the increased pressure generated in a closed space, an effect accentuated by a rapidly spreading œdema. In the average case, however, absorption is complete in 3 or 4 weeks, the proptosis becoming less and the mobility of the eye and the vision slowly returning; occasionally the proptosis may not resolve for some months (7 months, Spicer, 1892).

Permanent loss of vision is rare: thus in a series of 2,750 retrobulbar injections of local anæsthetics, Klecker (1956) found only two instances of optic atrophy resulting from retrobulbar hæmorrhage. In hæmophiliacs, however, the risk of permanent visual loss following a severe orbital hæmorrhage is considerable; thus optic atrophy due to intra-orbital hæmorrhage and occlusion of the central retinal artery have followed a head injury (Bonnet, 1957). A similar sequence of events occurred in a 14-year-old hæmophiliac boy who struck his right eye on a door-knob; the rapid onset of proptosis was followed within three weeks by optic atrophy due to hæmorrhage into the nerve-sheath and obliteration of the central retinal artery from the pressure of the intra-orbital hæmatoma (Zimmerman and Merigan, 1960). In other types of blood dyscrasia characterized by defective coagulation, orbital hæmorrhage may be very severe; treatment by replacement therapy may be effective and prevent the loss of vision.

Complications, however, may occur. Infection, usually derived from the nasal sinuses, is indicated by the onset of pain, tenderness and fever, and may progress to the development of cellulitis or an abscess (Aydin, 1952; and others). Absorption of the hæmorrhage has been said to be followed by enophthalmos due perhaps to stretching of one or more of the check

Figs. 254 to 256.—Post-traumatic Granuloma.

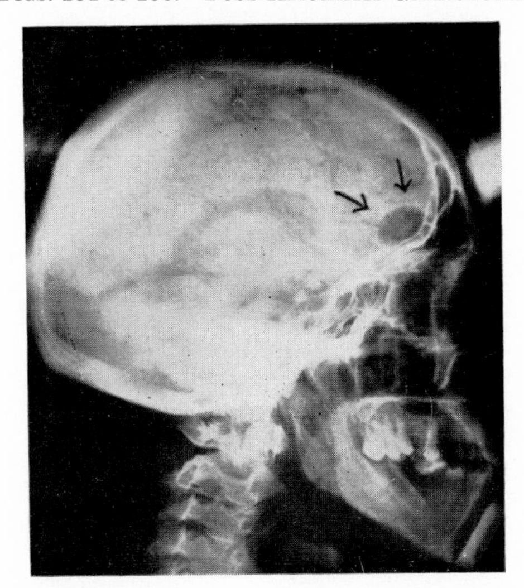

Fig. 254.

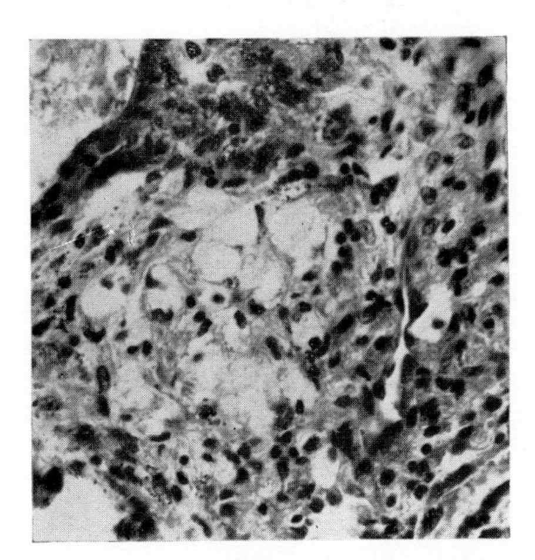

Fig. 255.

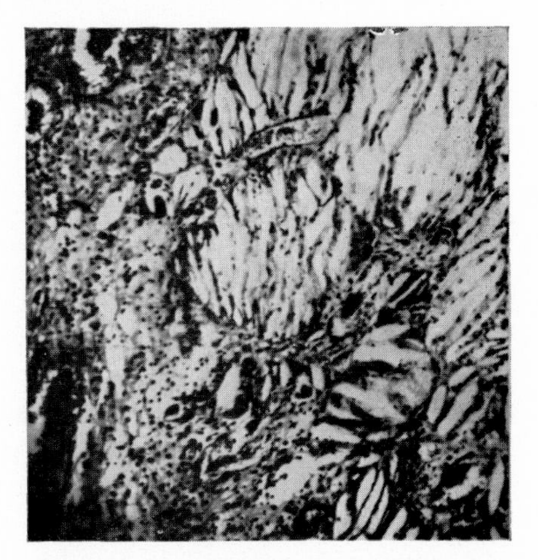

Fig. 256.

Fig. 254.—X-ray showing an expanding rarefying lesion of the left frontal bone. The patient had a baseball injury 35 years previously and was hit over the orbital margin with a knuckle-duster 13 years previously. Clinically there was a palpable swelling in the upper and outer corner of the orbit displacing the eye downwards and forwards.

Fig. 255.—Section of the lesion in Fig. 254, showing chronic granulomatous tissue with many foam cells.

Fig. 256.—Section of a granuloma somewhat similar to that illustrated in Figs. 254 and 255, following a fracture of the upper orbital margin in an automobile accident. The tumour contains chronic granulation tissue with innumerable acicular clefts (cholesterol crystals) and many foreign-body giant cells (Stuart Ramsey and others).

ligaments, absorption of the retrobulbar fat by pressure-atrophy or to the formation of cicatricial fibrous tissue. Occasionally a granuloma or an encapsulated cyst remains as a permanent legacy simulating an orbital tumour (Wolter *et al.*, 1966) and a rare sequel is the development of an intermittent proptosis, presumably due to varicose stasis in periods of venous congestion encouraged by laxity of the atrophic retrobulbar tissues (Caesar, 1929).

AN ORBITAL GRANULOMA of a non-specific nature (the so-called *inflammatory pseudo-tumour*) may result from an orbital hæmorrhage, particularly if chronic infection is derived from the neighbouring nasal sinuses. This chronic hyperplasic reaction is particularly associated with depositions of crystals of cholesterol and other irritative decomposition products of blood (Lafon, 1908), and the reaction may occur not only in the orbital tissues but also intra-ocularly in the uveal tract, simulating a true neoplasm therein (Williamson-Noble, 1926). In the presence of a fracture of the orbital wall an extensive osteolytic reaction may occur wherein fragments of dead bone may increase the irritative response to form an orbital tumour of sufficient size to necessitate surgical removal; such a mass consists of fibrous tissue heavily infiltrated with cells, including multinucleated giant cells and foam cells surrounding particles of dead bone, cholesterol crystals and blood pigment (Ramsey *et al.*, 1948) (Figs. 254–256).

BLOOD CYSTS are occasional sequels of orbital hæmorrhages resulting from the breakdown of a hæmatoma[1]; occasionally they arise from an injury which appears slight, such as a small fracture of the ethmoid sustained with a perforating injury of the cornea (Svoboda, 1948). They may be situated subperiosteally, particularly in the roof of the orbit, or in the orbital tissue-spaces. As a rule they are surrounded by a dense coat of fibrous tissue, on the inner aspect of which is a layer of richly vascularized granulation tissue containing foam cells loaded with lipids or cholesterol crystals, while the cyst contains a yellowish-green fluid with degenerated blood-cells. From the clinical point of view such a cyst may appear suddenly but more usually grows slowly, behaving as an orbital tumour; aspiration may supply a clue to the diagnosis.

Treatment. As a rule an orbital hæmorrhage requires only expectant treatment; iced compresses in the initial stages are usually recommended, but it is questionable if their value is great. If, however, the proptosis becomes dangerous, operative measures may be desirable, but they should not be undertaken lightly in view of the possibility of introducing sepsis. Aspiration may be practised but is only occasionally of value, as in a case reported by Causé (1905), wherein 10 mm. of proptosis developed in a child after being struck by a stone and rapid resolution followed the aspiration of 15 ml. of partially clotted blood. Incisions designed to evacuate the blood frequently lead to disappointing results so that in cases wherein proptosis is extreme and the vision is endangered, decompression of the orbit may be indicated, either laterally into the temporal fossa (Wüst, 1949; List, 1951) or downwards into the maxillary antrum (Watson and Holt-Wilson, 1968), while an incision in the outer third of the eyebrow is also practicable (Fry, 1967). Augstein (1917) claimed rapid absorption of a hæmatoma with

[1] Berlin (1880), Ulrich (1882), Denig (1902), Golowin (1928), Awerbach (1933), Wolter *et al.* (1966), Mortada (1969), and others.

x-ray therapy. A post-traumatic granuloma or cyst usually requires surgical excision.

Augstein. *Klin. Mbl. Augenheilk.*, **59,** 593 (1917).
Awerbach. *Ann. Oculist.* (Paris), **170,** 863 (1933).
Aydin. *Göz. Klin.*, **10,** 113 (1952).
Berlin. *Graefe-Saemisch Hb. d. ges. Augenheilk.*, 1st ed., Leipzig, **6,** 558 (1880).
Bonnet. *Bull. Soc. Ophtal. Fr.*, 492 (1957).
Busacca. *Atti Soc. Oftal. Lomb.*, **2,** 336 (1947).
Caesar. *Cas. Lék. ces.*, **2,** 1211 (1929).
Causé. *Arch. Augenheilk.*, **52,** 313 (1905).
Denig. *Ophthal. Rec.*, **11,** 187 (1902).
Fry. *Med. J. Aust.*, **1,** 264 (1967).
Golowin. *Klin. Mbl. Augenheilk.*, **81,** 1 (1928).
Kehl. *Beitr. klin. Chir.*, **123,** 203 (1921).
Virchows Arch. path. Anat., **246,** 194 (1923).
Klecker. *Klin. Mbl. Augenheilk.*, **129,** 393 (1956).
Lafon. *Bull. Soc. franç. Ophtal.*, **25,** 502 (1908).
Liebrecht. *Arch. Augenheilk.*, **55,** 36 (1906).
List. *J. Neurosurg.*, **8,** 340 (1951).
Morian. *Dtsch. Z. Chir.*, **18,** 803 (1883).
Morison. *Lancet*, **1,** 16 (1894).
Mortada. *Brit. J. Ophthal.*, **53,** 398 (1969).
Ramsey, Laws, Pritchard and Elliott. *Canad. med. Ass. J.*, **59,** 206 (1948).
Rochon-Duvigneaud and Veil. *Ann. Oculist.* (Paris), **160,** 658 (1923).
Rollet. *Encyl. franç. Ophtal.*, Paris, **8,** 434 (1909).
Rollet and Paufique. *Ann. Oculist.* (Paris), **166,** 745 (1929).
Silcock. *Trans. ophthal. Soc. U.K.*, **4,** 274 (1884).
Smith, Priestley. *Trans. ophthal. Soc. U.K.*, **4,** 271 (1884).
Roy. Lond. ophthal. Hosp. Rep., **12,** 70 (1888).
Spicer. *Trans. ophthal. Soc. U.K.*, **12,** 33 (1892).
Svoboda. *Cs. Oftal.*, **4,** 291 (1948).
Ulrich. *Klin. Mbl. Augenheilk.*, **20,** 242 (1882).
Watson and Holt-Wilson. *Trans. ophthal. Soc. U.K.*, **88,** 361 (1968).
Williamson-Noble. *Brit. J. Ophthal.*, **10,** 65 (1926).
Wolter, Fralick and Tanton. *Amer. J. Ophthal.*, **62,** 528 (1966).
Wüst. *Klin. Mbl. Augenheilk.*, **114,** 112 (1949).
Zimmerman and Merigan. *Arch. Ophthal.*, **64,** 949 (1960).

ORBITAL EMPHYSEMA

The *accumulation of air in the tissues of the lids or the orbit* indicates a communication between them and one or other of the nasal sinuses, a circumstance which can only be achieved by a solution of the continuity of the bony walls and a laceration of the mucosa. The entrance of air does not occur spontaneously with the fracture but intermittently when the pressure in the upper respiratory passages is increased, typically on blowing the nose or sneezing. Such an event is not rare, but relatively few cases have been reported in the literature; most of them have been due to the effect of trauma, occasionally operative trauma, but a few have been " spontaneous " in the sense that an action which would usually not be considered traumatic, as a violent sneeze, has been sufficient to fracture an unusually thin wall of a sinus. Indeed, blowing the nose has had this result in an apparently normal individual (Cawthorne, 1938) and a sneeze has produced a spontaneous emphysema of such violence as to cause a dislocation of the globe (Desmarres, 1845; Dépoutot, 1885; Schanz, 1899; Cotlier, 1940). Bony caries due to infection has resulted in recurring leakages of air in this way, and even in traumatic cases the occurrence of a fracture and therefore of emphysema is assisted by disease of the nose such as an atrophic rhinitis (Rampoldi, 1884).

The injury causing emphysema is frequently slight. As a rule it is a direct injury such as a blow by a fist (Baudry, 1882; Reber, 1899; 7 cases incurred in boxing,

Linhart, 1943), a piece of wood or iron (von Graefe, 1854; Hirschberg, 1884; Jocqs, 1901; Salus, 1908), a stone (Löwenstein, 1916), or a ball (Humphrey, 1884; Salus, 1908); a more severe injury, as from a revolver shot, has been recorded (Berlin, 1880; Marcus, 1886), as also has an indirect injury such as a fall on the back of the head on a stone pavement (Hilbert, 1884). Lloyd (1966) found that 7 out of 20 cases were due to a blow-out fracture of the orbital floor and 9 of the lamina papyracea.

Emphysema in the region of the eye may be divided into three types (Heerfordt, 1904):

1. EMPHYSEMA OF THE LIDS. This is very rare and results from a fracture of the lacrimal bone in front of the tarso-orbital fascia, causing a rupture of the lacrimal sac; the air finds its way from the nose up the lacrimal canal and into the tissues of the lids.

2. ORBITAL EMPHYSEMA. An orbital emphysema is due to a fracture of the bony orbital walls behind the tarso-orbital fascia which itself remains

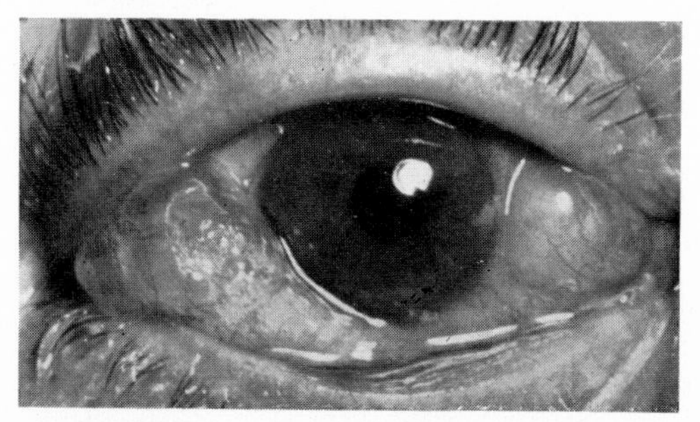

FIG. 257.—SUBCONJUNCTIVAL EMPHYSEMA.

Resulting from fracture of the orbital margin which was dislocated into the antrum (F. G. Badger, Birmingham Accident Hospital).

intact. In the majority of cases the fracture occurs in the floor or inner wall and involves the tenuous lamina papyracea, thus bringing the orbital tissues into communication with the ethmoid cells; occasionally the sphenoid sinus is involved. Much more rarely a fracture of the orbital roof communicates with the frontal sinus (Middeldorpf, 1886; Jocqs, 1901). In either event the air collects in the fatty tissues of the orbit and within the muscle cone, increasing the intra-orbital tension with a consequent proptosis and causing a widening of the palpebral aperture so that the lids become tense, the part of the upper lid between the orbital margin and the upper edge of the tarsus being characteristically stretched. In such cases the immobility of the globe may give rise to diplopia. The proptosis may to some extent be diminished by pressure through the lids on the globe, and when this is done there is a characteristic feeling of crepitation and a faint sound as of crunching snow.

3. ORBITO-PALPEBRAL EMPHYSEMA. In this type the air from the orbit traverses the tarso-orbital fascia and causes a variable degree of swelling of the tissues of the lids and conjunctiva. In these cases the orbital tension is

usually less, there is little or no proptosis, despite the swelling the lids can be opened, and palpation does not betray the same degree of tenseness but the tissues feel soft and crepitate and crackle under the fingers when they are manipulated (Fig. 257).

Heerfordt (1904) pointed out that to enter the orbit the air must be under a pressure higher than that of the orbital tissues, a circumstance which accounts for its intermittent accumulation. The air, however, is never under very great pressure since this is limited by the pressure which can be generated in the respiratory system. The highest air pressure which he measured in the orbit was 80 mm. Hg. For this reason

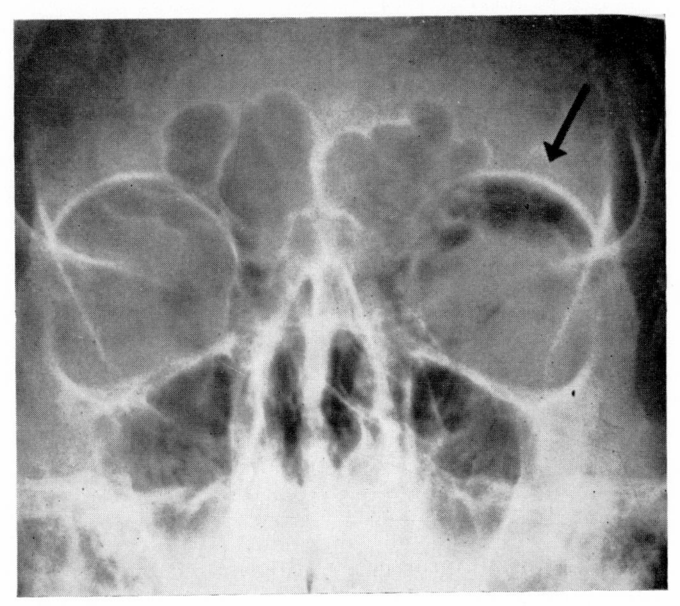

FIG. 258.—ORBITAL EMPHYSEMA.

Emphysema following a fracture of the ethmoid. The collection of air in the upper part of the orbit is indicated by an arrow (R. S. Murray).

the condition is harmless. If, however, air is introduced into the orbit under greater pressure in experimental conditions, considerable harm may result such as tearing of the ophthalmic veins, on one occasion with fatal effects (Marcus, 1886).

The *diagnosis* of the condition is usually easy, although when it suddenly appears it may at first seem sufficiently serious to cause anxiety. This, however, is not always so, for the local effects of the contusion combined with considerable proptosis may so simulate a cellulitis that the orbit has been opened to allow only the escape of gas (O'Malley, 1943). The essential diagnostic point is the presence of a proptosis which can, to some extent at any rate, be reduced by pressure on the lids, is lessened by free breathing and is increased by forced expiration, blowing the nose or sneezing. The crepitant feeling in the tissues of the lids or conveyed to the fingers on pressing the globe deeply into the orbit is also pathognomonic. The diagnosis is confirmed by radiography which clearly demonstrates the air pockets (Fig. 258). It is to be remembered that a severe degree of emphysema may be caused by an injury so trivial that it has escaped notice so that the history of trauma may be difficult to obtain, but the radiographic demonstration of air in the orbit constitutes a proof of the solution of the continuity of its bony walls at one point, usually on the medial side (Murray, 1949; King and Walsh, 1949; Heslop, 1955; Lloyd, 1966–68).

No *treatment* is required apart from the application of a pressure bandage and the avoidance of forcible and particularly spasmodic expiration. The air is rapidly absorbed and the swelling disappears, usually in a few days; only very rarely does it persist for periods up to one month (Baudry, 1882; Hirschberg, 1884).

Baudry. *Note sur un cas d'emphysème de l'orbite et des paupières*, Lille (1882).
Berlin. *Graefe-Saemisch Hb. d. ges. Augenheilk.*, 1st ed., Leipzig, **6** (1880).
Cawthorne. *Trans. ophthal. Soc. U.K.*, **58**, 19 (1938).
Cotlier. *Arch. argent. Oftal.*, **1**, 5 (1940).
Dépoutot. *J. Méd. Chir. prat.*, **56**, 114 (1885).
Desmarres. *Ann. Oculist.* (Paris), **14**, 97 (1845).
von Graefe. *v. Graefes Arch. Ophthal.*, **1** (1), 288 (1854).
Heerfordt. *v. Graefes Arch. Ophthal.*, **58**, 123 (1904).
Heslop. *Brit. J. plast. Surg.*, **8**, 243 (1955).
Hilbert. *Zbl. prakt. Augenheilk.*, **8**, 242 (1884).
Hirschberg. *Zbl. prakt. Augenheilk.*, **8**, 243 (1884).
Humphrey. *Brit. med. J.*, **2**, 1190 (1884).
Jocqs. *Clin. Ophtal.*, **7**, 231 (1901).
King and Walsh. *Amer. J. Ophthal.*, **32**, 191, 379 (1949).
Linhart. *J. Amer. med. Ass.*, **123**, 89 (1943).
Lloyd. *Brit. J. Radiol.*, **39**, 933 (1966).
Textbook of Radiology (ed. Sutton), Edinburgh (1968).
Löwenstein. *Klin. Mbl. Augenheilk.*, **57**, 77 (1916).
Marcus. *Dtsch. Z. Chir.*, **23**, 169 (1886).
Middeldorpf. *Breslauer aerztl. Z.*, No. 22 (1886). See *Jber. Ophthal.*, **17**, 563 (1886).
Murray. *J. Fac. Radiol.*, **1**, 121 (1949).
O'Malley. *Brit. J. Ophthal.*, **27**, 222 (1943).
Rampoldi. *Ann. Ottal.*, **13**, 344 (1884).
Reber. *Ophthal. Rec.*, **8**, 545 (1899).
Salus. *Z. Augenheilk.*, **20**, 342 (1908).
Schanz. *Beitr. Augenheilk.*, **4** (34), 335 (1899).

Contusion Injuries to the Orbital Contents

Injuries to the orbital contents from a contusion are relatively rare because of the protection offered by the surrounding bone; gross damage is therefore confined to cases wherein the orbital rim is fractured and driven inwards. Apart from injuries to the eyeball itself, which we have already considered, several sequelæ may follow injuries of this type affecting the position of the eye, involving occasionally proptosis and even luxation, but more frequently enophthalmos; affecting the optic nerve, resulting in visual damage; the extra-ocular muscles, resulting in diplopia and sometimes ptosis; the lacrimal gland, resulting occasionally in inflammation or in luxation, as well as the lacrimal passages, which are not infrequently torn.

CHANGES IN POSITION OF THE EYEBALL

PROPTOSIS, as we have seen, may follow a contusion in the region of the eye with the occurrence of an orbital hæmorrhage, emphysema or, at a later date, the development of infection with a resulting cellulitis or abscess, or the development of a granulomatous " pseudo-tumour ".

LUXATION OF THE GLOBE from an injury of this type is rare. We have already seen that it occurs uncommonly as a birth injury, usually as a result of the application of forceps to the side of the head. Occasionally such an accident follows what appears to be a relatively slight injury, such as the case reported by Zorab and Burns (1940), wherein the lids closed spasmodically behind the luxated globe after a light fall on a box. Several such cases have appeared in the literature involving little or no external injury (Rothenpieler, 1899, references dating from the 16th century; Baldwin, 1903; Lawford, 1903; and others). As a general rule, however, luxation is due to a severe accident wherein a violent blow causes an extensive fracture of the orbital rim. Such an accident has been reported as resulting from the kick of a horse in the malar region (Würdemann, 1932) or at the upper border of the orbital margin, which resulted in its fracture and an avulsion of the medial rectus muscle from the sclera (von Hippel, 1907); in an elevator crash when both globes protruded and one was luxated (Würdemann, 1932), or in a traffic accident (Cramer, 1931).

A curious incident was reported by de Beck (1900): a stream of water from a fire hose hit a fireman in the face and knocked him unconscious 20 feet away; no trace of his eyeball was found, but he recovered. In another incident (Greene, 1948) a man left a dance-hall and, hitting a peg in a dark cloakroom, evulsed his eye; he was transported to hospital with his eye in a parcel. For a similar case, see White Cooper's story.[1] Further examples of evulsion of the eyeball have occurred as self-inflicted injuries in psychotic patients[2] or as the result of an assault (Vinger and Seelenfreund, 1969).

In less severe injuries the luxation of the globe may do little harm. Occasionally, during the period of luxation, the fundus is pale in colour, but on reposition of the globe it is not uncommon for function to be rapidly resumed.[3] Sometimes it is easy with traction on the lids and the application of gentle pressure to induce reposition of the globe which springs back into the socket with a click, although the manipulation may be more readily accomplished after inducing akinesia of the lids by blocking the facial nerve. Such a happy termination, however, may well be out of the question if the associated trauma to the bony or soft tissues of the orbit is severe.

TRAUMATIC ENOPHTHALMOS

A common result of contusive injuries is a downward and inward displacement of the globe, the ætiology of which has given rise to a great deal of speculation in the earlier literature. There seems to be little doubt that the condition is almost invariably, or perhaps invariably, due to fracture of the orbital floor with a *prolapse of some of the orbital contents into the maxillary antrum*, followed subsequently by a drawing downwards of the comminuted fragments and the periorbita by cicatricial contraction of the mucous mem-

[1] p. 311.
[2] p. 58.
[3] See the case cited by Converse *et al.* (1967) described on p. 252.

brane of the antrum in the process of its healing (Figs. 214–216). Many of the older discussions on the cause of the deformity were speculative, but it is to be remembered that they were carried out before radiographic examination was known or was developed to the high degree of usefulness to which we are accustomed today.

Since the original report of Nieden (1881) the early literature which accumulated on this subject is considerable: Lederer (1902) analysed 52 reported cases, Birch-Hirschfeld (1907) 71, Lukens (1907) 78, and Grönholm (1910) 96, a number to which

FIGS. 259 to 261.—FRACTURE OF THE FLOOR OF THE ORBIT.

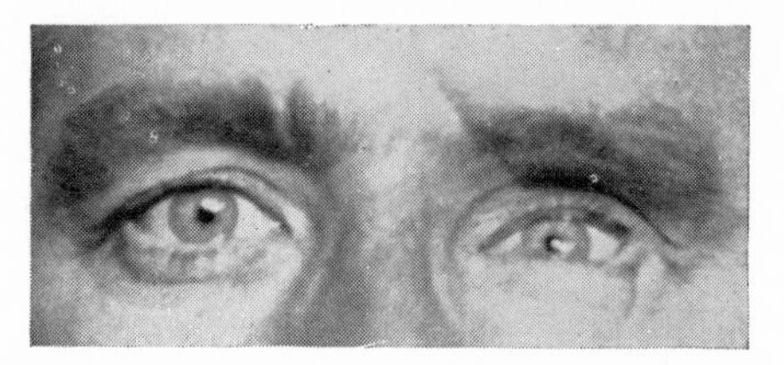

FIG. 259.

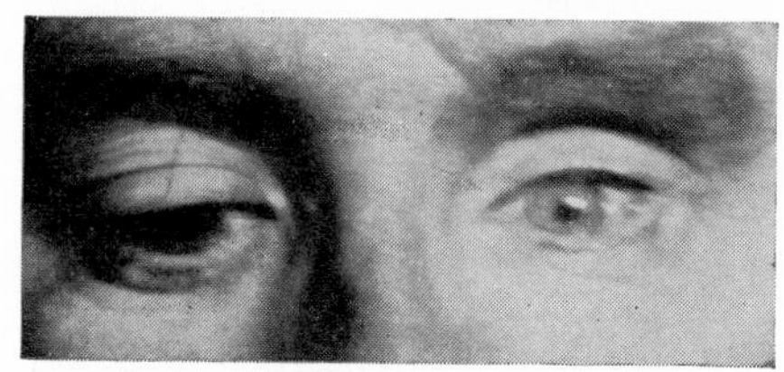

FIG. 260.

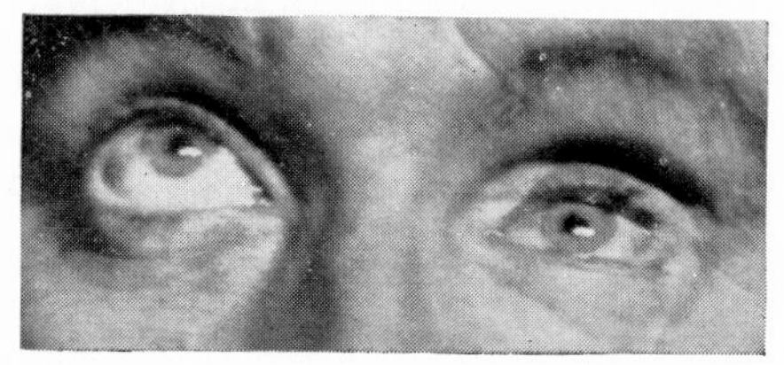

FIG. 261.

FIG. 259.—The fracture caused a gross deformity of the floor of the left orbit so that the eyeball was displaced downwards and backwards, tilting the visual axis upwards, producing a left hyperphoria of 45Δ.

FIG. 260.—To show the absence of depression of the left eye on looking downwards.

FIG. 261.—To show the deviation with the patient looking upwards; curiously, this was the only position of the eyes in which single binocular vision could be obtained (T. Keith Lyle).

Wagenmann (1915) added 13 others. Throughout the old literature the enophthalmos has been variously ascribed to such factors as palsy of the sympathetic, pressure-atrophy of the orbital tissues, the contraction of cicatricial tissue or damage to the fascial ligament of Tenon's capsule. In more recent years the refinements of radiographical techniques have made it apparent that the deformity is practically invariably due to a blow-out fracture of the floor of the orbit frequently associated with injury to the ligament of Lockwood (Pfeiffer, 1943; King, 1944; DeVoe, 1947; Callahan, 1950; Mustardé, 1966).

The appearance of this deformity with the sunken, depressed eye is characteristic (Figs. 259–262). It is interesting that the cicatricial depression of the periorbita of the orbital floor frequently drags upon the orbital septum which in turn retracts the lower lid, thus increasing the deformity. A further

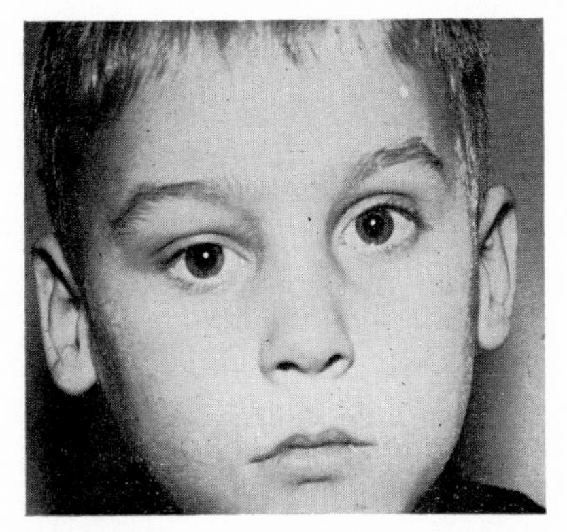

FIG. 262.—FRACTURE OF THE ORBITAL FLOOR.
The late appearance of the deformity.

consequence is a hollowing of the upper tarsal sulcus, the upper lid falling backwards owing to lack of its normal support with displacement of the eyeball, thus producing an appearance somewhat reminiscent of that usually associated with a prosthesis. The symptoms associated with this deformity, the diplopia which it causes and its treatment by reconstruction of the orbital floor, and if necessary orthoptic treatment or surgical rectification of the extra-ocular muscles to compensate for any residual misalignment of the globe, have already been discussed[1] and will again be noted.[2]

Baldwin. *Trans. ophthal. Soc. U.K.*, **23,** 281 (1903).
de Beck. *Cincinn. Lancet-Clin.*, **44,** 377 (1900).
Birch-Hirschfeld. *Graefe-Saemisch Hb. d. ges. Augenheilk.*, 2nd ed., Leipzig, **9** (2), 149 (1907).
Callahan. *Surgery of the Eye: Injuries*, Springfield (1950).
Converse, Smith, Obear and Wood-Smith. *Plast. reconstr. Surg.*, **39,** 20 (1967).
Cramer. *Kurzes Hb. d. Ophthal.*, Berlin, **4,** 444 (1931).
DeVoe. *Trans. Amer. ophthal. Soc.*, **45,** 502 (1947).
Greene. *Trans. ophthal. Soc. U.K.*, **68,** 352 (1948).
Grönholm. *Z. Augenheilk.*, **24,** 479 (1910).
von Hippel. *Dtsch. med. Wschr.*, **33,** 1922 (1907).
King. *Trans. ophthal. Soc. U.K.*, **64,** 134 (1944).
Lawford. *Trans. ophthal. Soc. U.K.*, **23,** 319 (1903).
Lederer. *Arch. Augenheilk.*, **53,** 241 (1902).
Lukens. *Ophthalmology*, **3,** 30 (1907).
Mustardé. *Repair and Reconstruction in the Orbital Region*, Edinburgh (1966).
Nieden. *Klin. Mbl. Augenheilk.*, **19,** 72 (1881).
Pfeiffer. *Arch. Ophthal.*, **30,** 718 (1943).
Rothenpieler. *Beitr. Augenheilk.*, **4** (31), 1 (1899).
Vinger and Seelenfreund. *Amer. J. Ophthal.*, **68,** 630 (1969).
Wagenmann. *Graefe-Saemisch Hb. d. ges. Augenheilk.*, 3rd ed., Leipzig, **1,** 685 (1915).
Würdemann. *Injuries of the Eye*, London (1932).
Zorab and Burns. *Brit. J. Ophthal.*, **24,** 286 (1940).

INJURIES TO THE OPTIC NERVE

Concussion injuries at the optic disc have already been discussed[3]; those to the nerve itself and the visual pathways have been fully described in the Volume on Neuro-ophthalmology.

[1] pp. 250, 278. [2] p. 300. [3] p. 187.

CONCUSSION INJURIES TO THE ORBITAL MUSCLES AND NERVES

Involvement of the extra-ocular muscles is common after concussion injuries to the orbit; similar palsies, of course, are also caused by injury within the skull, an event which will be discussed subsequently.[1] So far as orbital events are concerned, the ocular motility may be affected in four ways. (1) Direct damage to a muscle or its nerve is rare, apart from those cases in which as we have already seen there is incarceration of the muscle within a fracture line. (2) Post-traumatic cicatricial contraction of the orbital tissues involving the muscles is similarly rare, while (3) an orbital fracture, frequently not suspected, resulting in the displacement either of the origin or potential origin of a muscle or of the globe so that a group of muscles acts at a mechanical disadvantage, is much more common. It follows that the usual disability is due to paresis rather than paralysis of a muscle or muscle group. It is always to be remembered, however, that the resulting disability is not confined to the disturbance of the action of the muscle concerned but also, and to a greater degree, (4) to the secondary changes which occur in the other muscles—overaction of the contralateral synergist, contraction of the ipsilateral (direct) and inhibitional palsy of the contralateral antagonist.[2]

INJURY TO THE NERVES may be due to a fracture involving the bones at the apex of the orbit or occasionally to direct injury when the orbital walls are driven in, as may occur when the malar bone is forced inwards and damages the nerve to the lateral rectus or when a fracture of the roof injures the nerve to the levator muscle with a resulting traumatic ptosis. The nerves most commonly affected in this way are the abducens (Battle, 1890; Franke, 1898; Krauss, 1909) and the oculomotor (van Nes, 1898). The nature of the lesion of the nerve must frequently remain a matter for conjecture; undoubtedly in some cases a solution of its continuity occurs but the fact that many such cases recover in time to a greater or less degree suggests that the more common lesions are concussion changes or hæmorrhages into or stretching of the nerve fibres. An alternative cause of palsy suggested by several authors is compression of a nerve by external hæmorrhage, an ætiology often lightly assumed when the impairment of mobility is partial and transient; it would seem unlikely, however, that hæmorrhage alone would produce a lesion of this type (Cairns, 1938). In these traumatic palsies the recovery rate is good; thus Falbe-Hansen and Gregersen (1959) found that 14 out of 18 IIIrd nerve palsies resolved, and 5 out of 10 with multiple pareses.

The *diagnosis* of the site of such injuries is frequently difficult but paresis of a single muscle associated with a fracture of the orbital wall is suggestive of a local injury, while a composite disability, such as a combination of paralysis of nerves III, IV and VI, points to a bony accident in the superior orbital fissure (Silex, 1888; and many others). The occurrence of the full

[1] p. 709. [2] Vol. VI.

syndrome of the orbital apex involving one or more of the IIIrd, IVth and VIth cranial nerves as well as the first division of the Vth and occasionally the optic nerve localizes the lesion with certainty to the region of the sphenoidal fissure and the optic foramen.

PARADOXICAL MOVEMENTS of the eye occasionally arise in the healing stage of traumatic ocular motor palsies caused both by intra-orbital and intracranial lesions; the most common explanation is an aberrant regeneration of nerve fibres whereby those destined for one nerve go astray and grow into the sheath of another.[1] One of the most common nerves thus affected is the branch of the IIIrd nerve to the levator palpebræ, so that an upper lid which had suffered from a paralytic ptosis exhibits a paradoxical spasmodic elevation in association with another movement of the eye (*Fuchs's phenomenon*, 1895). This has been observed in the healing stage of a traumatic IIIrd nerve palsy when the eyes are moved to either side in cases wherein, presumably, regenerating nerve fibres which should have reached the medial or lateral rectus muscle find themselves diverted to the levator (Cords, 1930); but the usual manifestation occurs on looking downwards when the upper lid flips suddenly upwards (*the pseudo-Graefe phenomenon*, Fuchs, 1895). Post-traumatic cases of this type following intracranial or intra-orbital injury to the IIIrd nerve have been reported by several authors[2]; Hinkel (1902) recorded its occurrence after a birth injury.

An interesting case wherein the trauma appeared to affect the levator alone, causing ptosis, was described by Halpern (1934): as the ptosis disappeared it was replaced by a paradoxical elevation of the lid.

Such a paradoxical reaction appears to be most common after a traumatic ocular motor palsy but may occur when this condition follows a ruptured intracranial aneurysm; it occurs rarely in syphilis and with neoplasms and apparently not at all in diabetic ophthalmoplegia (Forster *et al.*, 1969). The signs of aberrant regeneration of the IIIrd nerve may include any of the following:

(1) Dyskinesis of the lid in horizontal gaze: elevation of the involved lid on adduction of the globe.

(2) The pseudo-Graefe sign: retraction and elevation of the lid on downward gaze.

(3) Limitation of upward and downward gaze with attempted retraction of the globe on vertical movement.

(4) Adduction of the involved eye on attempted depression or elevation.

(5) A pseudo-Argyll Robertson pupil wherein the dilated pupil will not react to light but will contract on convergence and also on adduction in conjugate gaze.

(6) A uniocular vertical optokinetic response wherein the normal eye responds as usual but the involved eye shows suppressed vertical responses.

The Marcus Gunn phenomenon (the jaw-winking phenomenon) wherein an elevation of the upper lid is associated with movements of the jaw[3]—a condition usually congenital—may occasionally develop after trauma (Lagrange and Pesme, 1924). It has also been reported as a birth injury (Gasteiger, 1950).

INJURIES TO THE MUSCLES themselves may follow contusion or crushing against the orbital wall or laceration by fractured fragments of bone. Occasionally the muscle is completely ruptured and torn from its insertion into the sclera (Panas, 1902); more commonly it is crushed and an effusion

[1] An alternative explanation is a mass response through a glial scar (See Vol. VI).

[2] Sattler (1906), Feingold (1926), Bielschowsky (1935), Spaeth (1947), Filho (1947), Nutt (1958), and others.

[3] Vol. III, p. 900.

into the sheath or intramuscular hæmorrhages with subsequent cicatrization lead to an impairment of function. Such an injury may occur to the lateral rectus in a malar fracture, but the most commonly affected muscles are the levator palpebræ or the superior rectus or both together in fractures of the orbital roof, and the inferior rectus and inferior oblique in fractures of the floor.[1] The levator may be bruised or even torn in a direct contusion affecting the upper lid, a palsy which is usually temporary[2]; and, as we have already seen, the medial rectus may also be damaged in a fracture of the medial orbital wall.

THE ORIGIN OR POTENTIAL ORIGIN OF A MUSCLE MAY BE DISPLACED by a fracture, an accident particularly liable to happen in the case of the inferior oblique in the relatively common depressed or blow-out fracture of the orbital floor, or the superior oblique the motility of which is impaired by a displaced fracture of the superior orbital rim involving the attachment of the trochlea which may either diminish or enhance the action of the muscle[3] (Figs. 263–264). The disability thus entailed usually disappears within a few weeks, but if it is permanent the trochlea should be refixed in its proper position by suturing to the periosteum.

INCARCERATION OF THE MUSCLE IN THE LINE OF A FRACTURE may occur, thus the inferior rectus and inferior oblique may become trapped in a fracture of the orbital floor, while the medial rectus may be similarly involved in a fracture of the medial wall of the orbit, giving rise to a form of traumatic retraction syndrome.[4]

A DISPLACEMENT OF THE GLOBE may result in an impairment of ocular motility even although the neuro-muscular system is structurally undamaged, since a group of muscles may thus be placed at a mechanical disadvantage. This applies particularly to traumatic enophthalmos wherein the depression of the eye may gravely impair its movements, particularly elevation, the defect in mobility appearing clinically to resemble a paresis of the inferior oblique and the superior rectus (Figs. 259–261).

Finally, as a delayed result it is possible that CICATRICIAL CONTRACTION after an orbital hæmorrhage, inflammatory sequelæ or laceration of the tissues may involve muscles in scar-tissue to such an extent that their motility is impaired.

In concussion injuries the muscles which are most affected are those underlying the roof of the orbit, while a common combination involves the elevators of the affected eye. Cross (1945) gave the following incidence in 71 cases: paresis of superior rectus 21, inferior oblique 8, superior oblique 7, lateral, medial and inferior rectus each 2, inferior division of nerve III 3, total nerve III 2, total nerves III and IV 2, various combinations of muscles without nervous relationship 22. Neely (1947) in 49 cases

[1] Terson (1901), Alexander (1904–11), Rollet and Grandclément (1909), Fage (1912), Müller (1912), Lagrange (1917), and many others.

[2] Kempner (1897), Alexander (1901), Purtscher (1905), Roche (1905), and others.

[3] Panas (1902), Garipuy (1905), Kimura (1911), Müller (1912), Neely (1947), and many others.

[4] p. 248.

Figs. 263 and 264.—Injury to the Right Trochlea (T. Keith Lyle).

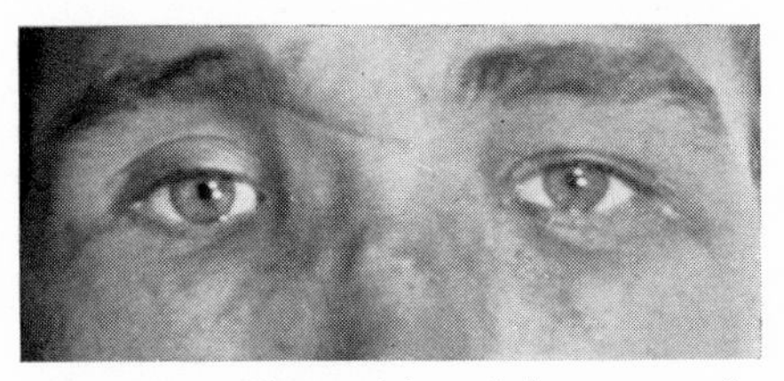

Fig. 263.—The position of the eyes on forward regard. There were 5△ of right hyperphoria but no diplopia.

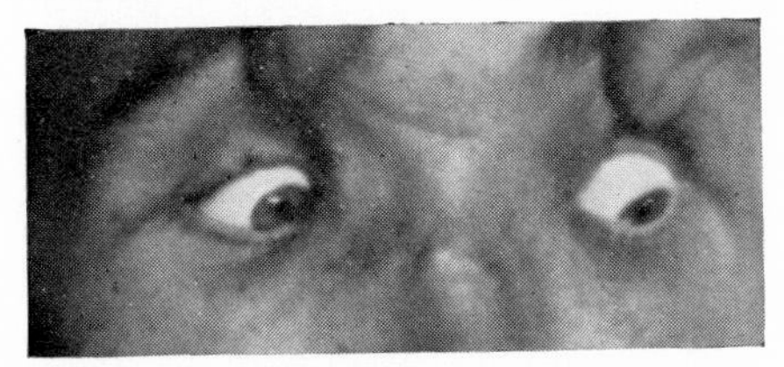

Fig. 264.—The position of the eyes in lævo-depression. The movement is so defective on the right side that a vertical diplopia resulted. This was cured by a graded tenotomy of the left inferior rectus.

Figs. 265 to 268.—Traumatic Palsy of the IVth Nerve (J. C. Neely).

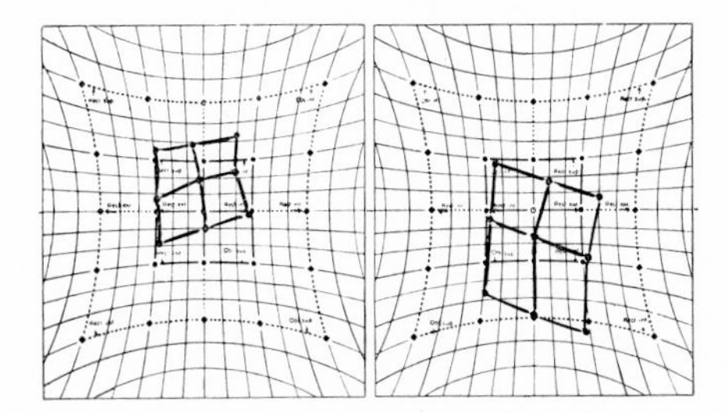

Fig. 265.

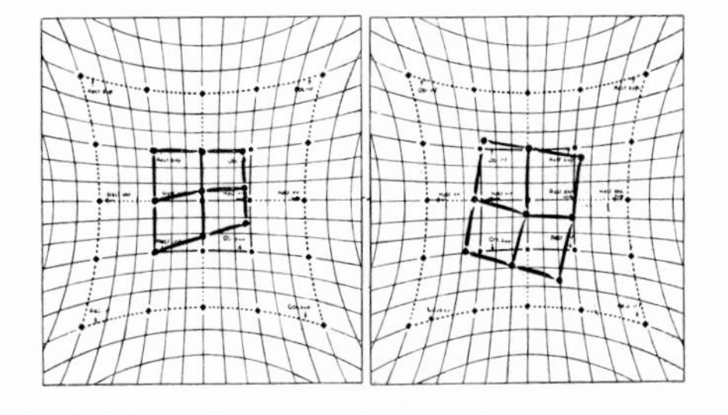

Fig. 266.

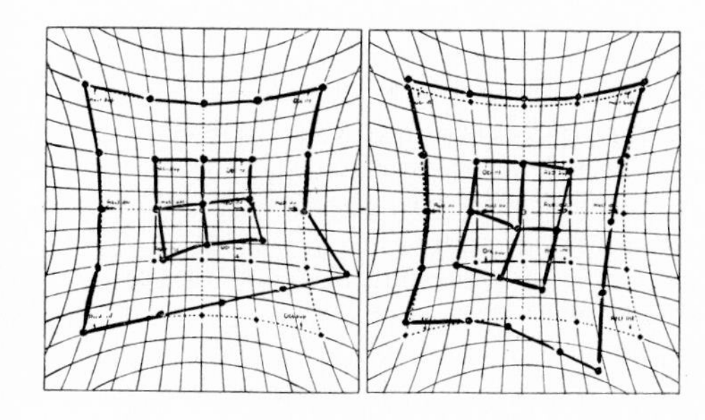

Fig. 267.

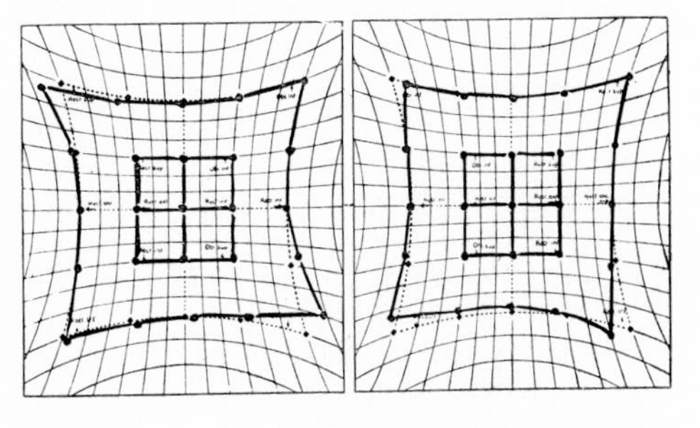

Fig. 268.

Fig. 265.—Hess chart before first operation showing primary paresis of left superior oblique and secondary palsy of right superior rectus.

Fig. 266.—After recession of right inferior rectus.

Fig. 267.—After myectomy of left inferior oblique.

Fig. 268.—After further recession of right inferior rectus; patient asymptomatic.

found paresis of the superior oblique in 17, superior rectus 14, inferior and lateral rectus each 2, both elevators 8, both depressors 2, both medial recti 2, both lateral recti 2.

The essential symptom of all such cases, of course, is the *diplopia* which usually results, a condition which causes much misery and incapacity, particularly when the dissociation has a cyclotropic element. In the majority of cases it is transient and the disability improves, even if it does not disappear within 3 or 4 months; its persistence beyond this period suggests an orbital fracture, a solution in the continuity of a nerve or a central origin. Apart from obvious measures such as the replacement of the trochlea by reconstitution of the orbital rim (when this is possible) and periosteal suturing with the most scrupulous accuracy (Rosengren, 1933), or restoring the orbital floor to its normal position, it is usually wise to defer treatment until this period has elapsed; thereafter the disability must be accepted as permanent unless binocular function can be restored by operative measures. It is usually not advisable to delay operative interference beyond 4–6 months for if left too long the palsy becomes complicated by the consolidation of a marked secondary contraction of the ipsilateral antagonist, and this in turn produces a relative paresis of its contralateral synergist with consequent disorientation of the harmonious working of the entire team of muscles (Figs. 265–8).

The clinical pictures presented by the various disorders of ocular mobility and the methods of analysing the various types of paresis which occur are described in detail elsewhere in this *System*[1] but it is appropriate here to emphasize the importance of careful and repeated orthoptic examinations in the assessment of these conditions and in the selection of the appropriate surgical treatment which may well have to be carried out in several stages. Regular charting of the ocular deviation by the Hess screen is invaluable, since it not only demonstrates the muscle or muscles primarily affected but also indicates the sequelæ of the initial palsy affecting other muscles. It provides a diagrammatic record of the condition of the extra-ocular muscles at any one period so that progression or retrogression of the deviation and the results of surgical treatment can be clearly estimated. In patients seen early after injury or in those cases wherein the presence of a complicated fracture requires the use of cranio-maxillary fixation, the recording by the Hess chart may be impossible; in such a situation the cover-test, recording a description of the ocular movements and noting the presence or absence of diplopia, may be all that can be done. Examination of ambulant patients by means of the synoptophore is of considerable value. The most important information obtained in this way relates to the state of binocular vision, to the presence of suppression and to the fusional duction power; the angle of deviation can be measured not only in the primary position but also in the other positions of conjugate gaze. Finally, considerable valuable information in assessing the results of or need for surgical treatment can be obtained from the field of binocular single vision. In some cases the forced duction test and electromyography of the extra-ocular muscles may help to distinguish between muscle or nerve damage and mechanical limitation of movement due to tethering or incarceration of soft tissue.

In many cases, and particularly in those wherein misalignment of the globe is the cause of the disability and the neuro-muscular system is un-

[1] Vol. VI.

FIGS. 269 and 270.—DISPLACEMENT OF THE GLOBE AFTER A LACERATING INJURY.

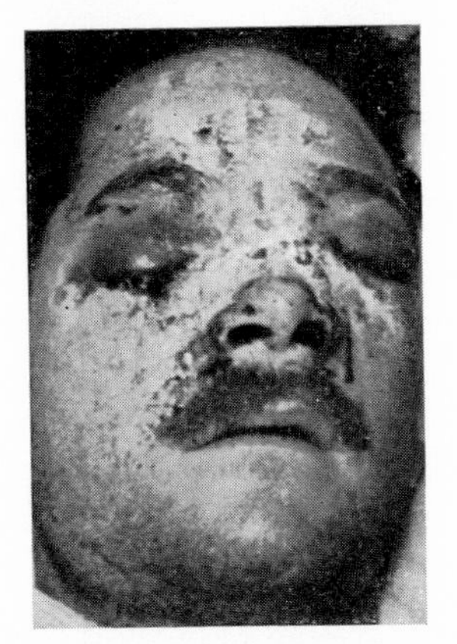

FIG. 269.

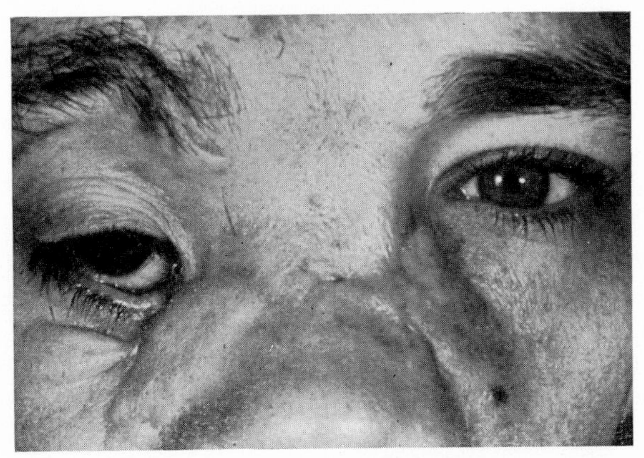

FIG. 270.

The face was severely lacerated by the propellor of an aircraft (Fig. 269), resulting in a fracture and displacement of the lacrimal and nasal bones. Despite the gross displacement of the right eye, there was full stereoscopic vision and full movement in all directions, with only an insignificant degree of diplopia on extreme excursions of the eye (Fig. 270).

The lacrimal sac and the upper punctum remained intact despite the fracture-dislocation of the surrounding bone, and syringed through easily; the lower punctum, however, was destroyed (A. McIndoe).

damaged, diplopia may be overcome on occasion to a surprising extent by the adaptability of a well-developed capacity for fusion (Lancaster, 1941; Alabaster *et al.*, 1942; DeVoe, 1947) (Figs. 269 and 270), but it is always to be remembered that, although fusion may be maintained in the primary position, perhaps with some discomfort or fatigue, it may well happen that it becomes strained beyond the breaking point when the eyes are moved in the direction of action of the paretic muscle, while from time to time diplopia may appear even in the primary position in conditions of stress. In this type of case the ability to fuse may be consolidated or a functional cure may be attained (although rarely) by orthoptic exercises (King, 1944; Neely, 1947); these, it will be remembered, may increase the fusional amplitude but do nothing to strengthen a weakened muscle. Prisms may afford some relief but, unless the deviation is small, their effect is usually limited to a restricted area of the field around the primary position and they cannot eliminate the element of torsion so frequently the cause of the greatest distress.

If the correction of gross deformities such as reposition of the trochlea or reconstruction of the orbital floor by bony or cartilaginous grafts or the insertion of an alloplastic implant has not already been attempted, these should be undertaken at this stage; they may relieve the diplopia in some cases but normal function is very difficult to attain when a considerable time has elapsed since the injury.

The most hopeful method of treatment for most cases, when paralysis is not complete and the disalignment is relatively small or has been reduced to manageable proportions by plastic surgery, is by muscle surgery; this is usually required to supplement plastic surgery when the deformity is large. Operations on the extrinsic muscles in cases of orbital injury are based on the same principles as if the lesion had been primarily nervous in origin. In the case of a nerve lesion overaction of the contralateral synergist is usually obvious, but this is not always the case with an orbital injury; in these cases it is unlikely that a satisfactory result will be obtained merely by weakening the contralateral synergist and, in general, it is necessary to operate upon more than one muscle, usually including a shortening or strengthening operation on the affected muscle.[1] In order to overcome diplopia completely it is essential to aim at securing a state of equilibrium of the extrinsic ocular muscles so that the two eyes move symmetrically, equally and comfortably in all directions of the gaze. It matters little if movement is slightly limited in one or other direction provided that the movement of each eye is similarly limited. The second aim of treatment is to secure as large a field of binocular single vision as possible, particularly including the lower half of the visual field. Operation should be undertaken when sufficient time has been allowed to elapse to ensure that spontaneous improvement due to the resolution of hæmorrhage and bruising of muscles is no longer possible; this usually means a minimum interval of 3 or 4 months after injury. The surgical techniques are discussed in another Volume[2] but it is important to remember that several operations may be necessary and it is wise to carry these out in stages although the entire course of treatment may last a year or more. It frequently happens that if the deviation can be reduced to manageable proportions by surgery, the binocular reflexes, strengthened by orthoptic

[1] For detailed discussion of the principles of the treatment of traumatic diplopia see the following: Lyle (1941–63), Neely (1945–47), Cross (1945–48), Lyle and Cross (1951), Lyle and Wybar (1967).

[2] Vol. VI.

training, will enable fusion to be maintained within a sufficiently wide range of movements to ensure reasonable comfort. It should also be remembered that the possible range of movement of the eyeballs is greatly in excess of that normally required in ordinary everyday life so that the production of a slight artificial defect in extreme movements is of little importance.

Cases of orbital injury causing positional diplopia and relative ocular palsy may be classified as follows (Lyle, 1963; Lyle and Wybar, 1967): (1) unilateral fracture of zygoma and maxilla. The affected eye is hypotropic—*i.e.*, there is downward displacement of the eyeball and downward deviation of the visual axis, resulting in the elevator muscles, particularly the superior rectus, being placed at a mechanical disadvantage with consequent defective elevation. As a rule the operation of choice is one designed to strengthen the affected muscle—resection of the superior rectus—because there is usually no gross overaction of the contralateral synergist. It may, however, be necessary in addition or alternatively to weaken the direct antagonist by a small recession of the inferior rectus, the aim being to secure symmetrical and equal ocular movements in all directions; (2) unilateral fracture of zygoma, maxilla and frontal bone—the affected eye is hypotropic with defective depression and markedly defective elevation frequently with abnormal horizontal movement also; (3) unilateral fracture of zygoma and maxilla with defective depression, the affected eye being hypotropic; (4) central naso-maxillary fracture leading to a dish-faced depression of the root of the nose with increase of the interpupillary distance and exotropia or exophoria; (5) temporary hypotropia due to orbital hæmorrhage; (6) blow-out fracture of the orbital floor with restriction of elevation and depression due to tethering of the soft tissues to the floor of the orbit; early operation to separate the adhesions is essential.

INJURY TO THE SENSORY NERVES within the orbit is rare. The first division of the Vth nerve may be injured by a fracture at the apex of the orbit in association with one or more of the motor nerves, sometimes with the optic nerve and occasionally with the olfactory nerves when the fissure extends into the floor of the anterior fossa (Hirschberg, 1880; and others). The frequent damage to the infra-orbital branch of the second division of the Vth, involving anæsthesia of the lower lid and upper part of the cheek, in fractures of the malar bone has already been mentioned, as also has a similar involvement of the supra-orbital branch of the first division, the compression of which by callus may give rise to neuralgia in fractures of the upper orbital rim. Infra-orbital neuralgia is often associated with a retained foreign body; this condition will be discussed subsequently.[1]

INJURY TO THE CILIARY GANGLION may give rise to an Argyll Robertson pupil exhibiting isolated light-rigidity.[2]

A TRAUMATIC ANEURYSM OF THE OPHTHALMIC ARTERY producing a pulsating exophthalmos due to a fall causing a fracture of the orbital bones is a rarity. Such a case was reported by de Vincentiis (1894). This rare lesion is more typically caused by a direct injury to the vessels following a penetrating wound.

A SEROUS TENONITIS, usually of a transient nature, has been noted to follow a contusion injury to the orbit.[3]

[1] p. 664. [2] Vol. XII, p. 662. [3] Vol. XIII.

Finally, a note on the OCULO-CARDIAC REFLEX is of some importance. It will be remembered that firm pressure on the globe may stimulate the vagus to produce an inhibitory action on the heart, the vasomotor tone and the gut. An ocular contusion or the pressure generated by an orbital hæmatoma may similarly induce a bradycardia, and if this is associated with an enlarged pupil caused by the trauma, some confusion in diagnosis between the possible systemic effects of head injury involving increased intracranial pressure may thus arise (King and Walsh, 1949; Kacetl, 1968).

Alabaster, Rudd and Tree. *Brit. J. Ophthal.*, **26,** 304 (1942).
Alexander. *Münch. med. Wschr.*, **48,** 729, 819 (1901); **51,** 1579 (1904).
Dtsch. med. Wschr., **37,** 238 (1911).
Battle. *Lancet*, **2,** 1, 57, 107 (1890).
Bielschowsky. *Arch. Ophthal.*, **13,** 33 (1935).
Cairns. *Trans. ophthal. Soc. U.K.*, **58,** 464 (1938).
Cords. *Kurzes Hb. d. Ophthal.*, Berlin, **3,** 626 (1930).
Cross. *Trans. ophthal. Soc. U.K.*, **65,** 20 (1945).
Ann. roy. Coll. Surg., **2,** 233 (1948).
DeVoe. *Trans. Amer. ophthal. Soc.*, **45,** 502 (1947).
Fage. *Arch. Ophtal.*, **32,** 282 (1912).
Falbe-Hansen and Gregersen. *Acta ophthal.* (Kbh.), **37,** 359 (1959).
Feingold. *Contrib. to Ophthal. Science* (Jackson Birthday Vol.), Wisconsin, 1 (1926).
Filho. *Arch. Ophthal.*, **38,** 308 (1947).
Forster, Schatz and Smith. *Amer. J. Ophthal.*, **67,** 696 (1969).
Franke. *Klin. Mbl. Augenheilk.*, **36,** 265 (1898).
Fuchs. *Beitr. Augenheilk.*, **2** (11), 12 (1895).
Garipuy. *Recueil Ophtal.*, **27,** 705 (1905).
Gasteiger. *Dtsch. Gesundh-Wes.*, **5,** 616 (1950).
Halpern. *Harefuah*, **8,** 111 (1934).
Hinkel. *Ueber d. Pseudo-Graefe'sche Symptom im Anschluss an Lähmungen d. Augenmuskeln* (Diss.), Jena (1902).
Hirschberg. *Berl. klin. Wschr.*, **17,** 169 (1880).
Kacetl. *Wien. klin. Wschr.*, **80,** 821 (1968).
Kempner. *Klin. Mbl. Augenheilk.*, **35,** 10 (1897).
Kimura. *Klin. Mbl. Augenheilk.*, **50** (1), 266 (1911).
King, A. B. and Walsh. *Amer. J. Ophthal.*, **32,** 379 (1949).
King, E. F. *Trans. ophthal. Soc. U.K.*, **64,** 134 (1944).
Krauss. *Zur Kasuistik d. traumatischen Augenmuskellähmungen nach Schädelverletzungen* (Diss.), Tübingen (1909).
Lagrange. *Les fractures de l'orbite par les projectiles de guerre*, Paris (1917).
Lagrange and Pesme. *Arch. Ophtal.*, **41,** 673 (1924).
Lancaster. *Amer. J. Ophthal.*, **24,** 485 (1941).
Lyle. *Trans. ophthal. Soc. U.K.*, **61,** 189 (1941).
Brit. J. Ophthal., **45,** 341 (1961).
Brit. J. plast. Surg., **16,** 221 (1963).
Lyle and Cross. *Brit. J. Ophthal.*, **35,** 511 (1951).
Lyle and Wybar. *Practical Orthoptics in the Treatment of Squint*, 5th ed., London (1967).
Müller. *Arch. Augenheilk.*, **69,** 178 (1911); **70,** 54 (1912).
Neely. *Trans. ophthal. Soc. U.K.*, **65,** 47 (1945).
Brit. J. Ophthal., **31,** 581 (1947).
van Nes. *Dtsch. Z. Chir.*, **44,** 593 (1898).
Nutt. *Brit. orthopt. J.*, **15,** 61 (1958).
Panas. *Arch. Ophtal.*, **22,** 229 (1902).
Purtscher. *Beitr. Augenheilk., Festschr. J. Hirschberg*, Leipzig (1905).
Roche. *Recueil Ophtal.*, **27,** 73 (1905).
Rollet and Grandclément. *Rev. gén. Ophtal.*, **28,** 413 (1909).
Rosengren. *Acta ophthal.* (Kbh.), **11,** 161 (1933).
Sattler. *Rosenthalsche Festschr.*, Leipzig, **2,** 223 (1906).
Silex. *Klin. Mbl. Augenheilk.*, **26,** 429 (1888).
Spaeth. *Amer. J. Ophthal.*, **30,** 143 (1947).
Terson. *Arch. Ophtal.*, **21,** 514 (1901).
de Vincentiis. *Zbl. prakt. Augenheilk.*, **18,** 208 (1894).

Concussion Injuries to the Lacrimal Apparatus

THE LACRIMAL GLAND

Damage to the lacrimal gland in concussion injuries involving the orbit is rare. A DACRYOADENITIS may result which is difficult to diagnose; direct injury to the gland in a fracture of the orbital rim in its neighbourhood may result in the formation of a traumatic fistula,[1] while the development after many years of a traumatic cyst has been reported (McMullen, 1920); but the most common lesion is a dislocation and prolapse of the gland itself.

LUXATION OF THE LACRIMAL GLAND occurs generally after a blow, a fall or especially a collision between children in whom the upper and outer orbital rim is slightly developed (10 out of 13 cases, Jackson, 1904); this applies particularly to the age group between 10 and 14 years in whom boisterousness in sport is usually most marked but after this age the protection offered by the bones is usually a sufficient prevention. In adults, luxation of the gland is usually the result of perforating injuries under the brow or occurs when the fascial anchorage of the gland is lax, in which case a minor injury may precipitate an event which can more correctly be described as a spontaneous luxation (as in blepharochalasis).[2] It is not surprising that the accident has been recorded as a birth injury when the orbit has been severely compressed (Würdemann, 1932).

The luxated gland prolapses into the tissues of the upper lid where it is felt as a mobile tumour in the lacrimal region, freely movable upwards and laterally but not downwards. It is usually replaceable by steady pressure, but on release of the pressure it usually prolapses again. Constant pressure for a period of some two weeks may result in its permanent reposition, as in the case reported by Crowder (1906) wherein a prolapse occurred in a young girl who collided with another in a game of basket-ball; but usually the most effective treatment is surgical removal of the gland.

The literature on traumatic luxation of the lacrimal gland, an event first noted by von Graefe (1866), is meagre—Rampoldi (1884), Haltenhoff (1895), Bistis (1895), Ahlström (1898), Hilbert (1900), Villard (1903), Coppez (1903), Jackson (1904), Santucci (1904), Crowder (1906), and others.

THE LACRIMAL PASSAGES

A disturbance of the lacrimal passages is common in concussion injuries. Sometimes the lower punctum is displaced with consequent epiphora as a result of a deformation of the inner canthus such as occurs most typically in an avulsion of the internal palpebral ligament; occasionally the canaliculi may be torn when the lower lid is avulsed; but much more commonly the passages are torn across in the typical naso-maxillary fracture resulting from frontal injury for, as we have seen, the common fracture line runs across the lacrimal bone. It occasionally happens that the tear in the lacrimal sac is small and confined to its posterior wall so that the passages retain their patency; in this case radio-opaque media when injected for diagnostic purposes may extravasate widely into the tissues of the lower lid and orbit and at the same time may reach the inferior meatus of the nose. In the absence

[1] Vol. XIII. [2] Vol. XIII.

of infection and functional disability this may be left without treatment. More usually, however, the tear is more extensive and the continuity of the passages is completely disrupted. In this event, as soon as the effects of the trauma have subsided, epiphora becomes obvious; this is permanent, and frequently to this inconvenience is added the development of a mucocele or a suppurative dacryocystitis which may progress to the formation of a lacrimal fistula (Figs. 271–4). This sequence has long been recognized (Dürr, 1879; and others) and traumatic epiphora of this type is common, particularly after traffic accidents (13 cases in 65 naso-maxillary fractures or 20%, Rycroft, 1949; epiphora in 12 out of 100 cases of middle facial fracture, Campbell, 1964; Converse and Smith, 1966).

Treatment for the relief of epiphora in such cases can only be by surgical reconstruction of the lacrimal channels or, if this is not attempted or fails, by

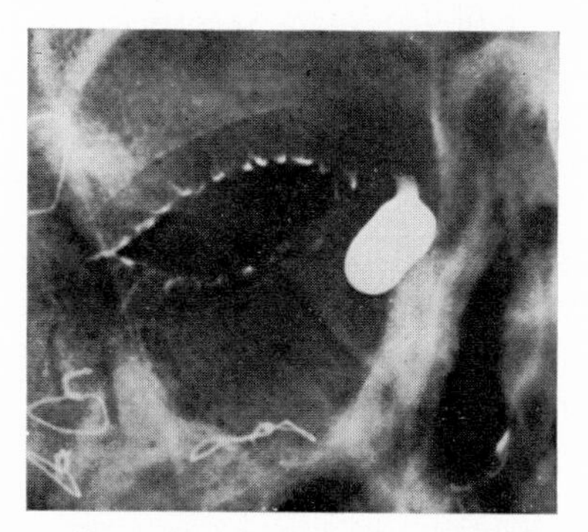

Fig. 271.—Traumatic Mucocele of the Lacrimal Sac.

Dacryocystogram showing a displaced and grossly dilated right lacrimal sac resulting from rupture of the naso-lacrimal duct associated with severe injuries to the middle third of the face; the wiring of the fractures can also be seen (W. Campbell).

excision of the lacrimal gland or occlusion of its efferent ducts. Probing the lacrimal passages in this type of case is valueless. The various techniques which have been employed for this purpose are discussed in another Volume[1] and need not be repeated in detail here.

Briefly, if the canaliculi are torn, their immediate and accurate repair may be possible by direct suture with the aid of a retained silk seton or a polythene tube; alternatively, a conjunctivo-dacryocystostomy may be attempted. If the canaliculus and the sac are intact while the duct is damaged, a dacryocystorhinostomy usually gives good results; if the canaliculus is intact while the sac and duct are damaged, a canaliculo-rhinostomy may be attempted or, as well as in cases wherein the canaliculus is also destroyed, completely new drainage channels may be reconstituted by a conjunctivo-rhinostomy or by the use of plastic or other tubing leading from the lacus lacrimalis to the nasal cavity.[2]

[1] Vol. XIII.

[2] Worst (1962), Jones (1965), Beard (1965–67), Converse and Smith (1966), Smith and Dodick (1968), Stranc (1970), and others.

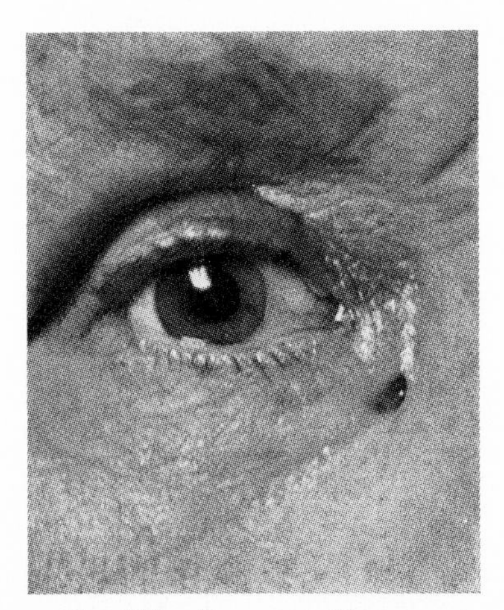

Fig. 272.—Lacrimal Fistula.

In a man aged 63 who sustained a naso-maxillary fracture of the skull on falling from scaffolding. A purulent dacryocystitis followed with the formation of a fistula lying in the retracted scar. Excision of the mucous membrane of the fistula and of the lacrimal sac resulted in recovery (C. Wesley).

Figs. 273 and 274.—Traumatic Lacrimal Fistulæ (W. Campbell).

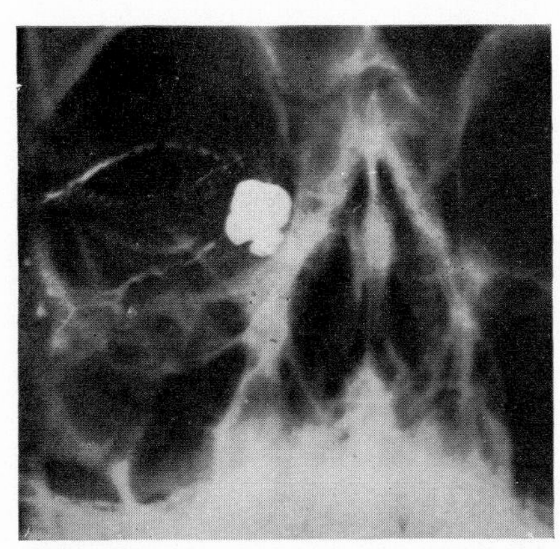

Fig. 273.—A fracture of the face was followed by a persistent watery discharge from an opening on the cheek for one year. The dacryocystogram shows a distended and distorted lacrimal sac communicating by way of a long track over the malar bone. The symptoms were entirely relieved by dacryocysto-rhinostomy.

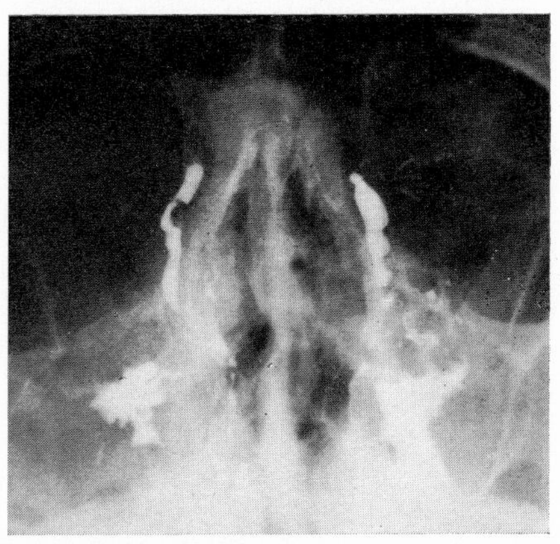

Fig. 274.—There are communications between the lacrimal passages and the antra on both sides after a fracture of the middle third of the face sustained in a road accident.

Ahlström. *Zbl. prakt. Augenheilk.*, **22,** 300 (1898).
Beard. *Trans. Amer. Acad. Ophthal.*, **69,** 970 (1965).
Plastic and Reconstructive Surgery of the Eye and Adnexa, (ed. Smith and Converse), St. Louis, 171 (1967).
Bistis. *Ann. Oculist.* (Paris), **114,** 457 (1895).
Campbell. *Brit. J. Radiol.*, **37,** 1 (1964).
Converse and Smith. *Plast. reconstr. Surg.*, **38,** 147 (1966).
Coppez. *Arch. Ophtal.*, **23,** 348 (1903).
Crowder. *Ophthal. Rec.*, **15,** 422 (1906).
Dürr. *Kln. Mbl. Augenheilk.*, **17,** 367 (1879).
von Graefe. *v. Graefes Arch. Ophthal.*, **12** (2), 224 (1866).
Haltenhoff. *Ann. Oculist.* (Paris), **113,** 319 (1895).
Hilbert. *Klin. Mbl. Augenheilk.*, **38,** 478 (1900).
Jackson. *Ophthal. Rec.*, **13,** 345 (1904).
Jones. *Amer. J. Ophthal.*, **59,** 773 (1965).
McMullen. *Proc. roy. Soc. Med.*, **13,** Sect. Ophthal., 64 (1920).
Rampoldi. *Ann. Ottal.*, **13,** 68 (1884).
Rycroft. *Trans. ophthal. Soc. U.K.*, **69,** 507 (1949).
Santucci. *Zbl. prakt. Augenheilk.*, **28,** 137 (1904).
Smith and Dodick. *Canad. J. Ophthal.*, **3,** 263 (1968).
Stranc. *Brit. J. plast. Surg.*, **23,** 339 (1970).
Villard. *Rev. gén. Ophtal.*, **22,** 193 (1903).
Worst. *Amer. J. Ophthal.*, **53,** 520 (1962).
Würdemann. *Injuries of the Eye,* London (1932).

CHAPTER III

INCISED WOUNDS

WE ARE introducing this chapter with the portrait of WILLIAM WHITE COOPER [1816–1886] (Fig. 275), who founded the ophthalmological department of St. Mary's Hospital, London, because he wrote the first book on ocular injuries—*Wounds and Injuries of the Eye* (London, 1859). And a delightful book it is. Although now more than a century old, it is still a mine of information; beautifully illustrated with woodcuts and full of shrewd observations, it maintains the interest of the reader with its succession of anecdotes each of which is a concise clinical study—now of the Peninsular War and Waterloo, now of the Crimean War, now of the intoxicated traveller in Ostend who, falling on the key of his bedroom door, enucleated his eye, went to bed and slept profoundly and at peace until his eye was found on the floor in the morning (both the eye and the key are illustrated, the latter slightly bent!), or again of the "fearful injuries" sustained by a "very pleasing young lady" who left her home and went to Paris where her pursuing "unreasonably jealous husband" threw sulphuric acid in her face on one of the bridges of that city. Our predecessors of a hundred years ago were sound clinicians and certainly had opportunities to practise their art; and not the least of the distinguished company in London at about that time—Bowman, Tyrrell, Lawrence, Dalrymple, Critchett, Lawson, Jonathan Hutchinson and others—was White Cooper who, in the woodcut overleaf, at the age of 37, looks for all the world as if he had walked out of Dickens's contemporaneously published "Tale of Two Cities".

For descriptive purposes wounds of the eye and its adnexa may be divided into two main classes, superficial and deep. The first class comprises abrasions and cuts of the cornea, conjunctiva and sclera which do not perforate the eyeball, or similar injuries to the skin and subcutaneous tissues which do not enter the orbit; deep wounds involve such a perforation. The latter may be of the nature of a sharply defined cut caused by a sharp body, a minute perforation caused by a small body travelling with a high velocity, a contused and lacerated wound whereby the globe is impaled by a blunt object driven in with immense force, or the shattering wound caused by a relatively large high-velocity projectile. We have already considered the fracture of the cornea or the rupture of the globe caused by a contusion or blast injury. In this section we shall not consider the effects of gunshot injuries or the complications introduced by the retention of a foreign body on or in the eye or in the orbit; the discussion of these events which are associated with problems of their own will be reserved for later sections.

The pathology of the processes involved in the healing and regeneration of wounds of the ocular coats is described in detail elsewhere in this *System*, so that no further discussion is required here.[1]

[1] See Vol. VIII, p. 5, for conjunctival wounds, p. 604 for corneal and p. 996 for scleral wounds; Vol. IX, p. 5, for wounds of the uvea; Vol. X, p. 40, for wounds of the retina.

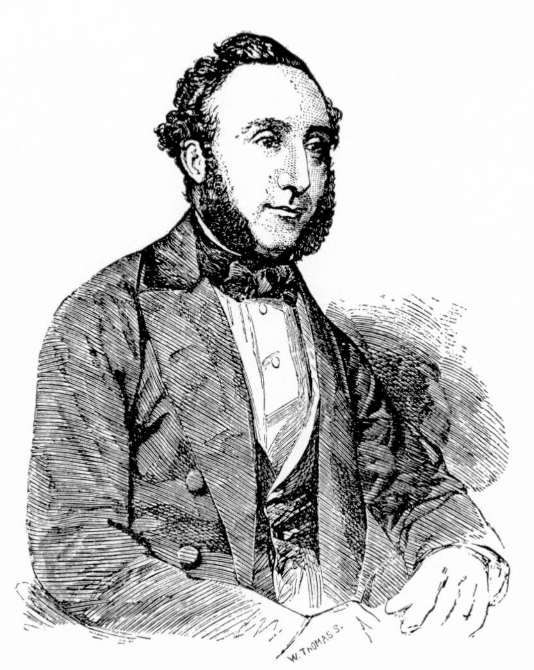

FIG. 275.—WILLIAM WHITE COOPER
[1816–1886]
(From a daguerreotype by Mayall.)

NON-PERFORATING WOUNDS OF THE EYE

Non-perforating Wounds of the Cornea

NON-PERFORATING WOUNDS OF THE CORNEA can be divided into two classes—superficial abrasions in which the epithelium is denuded from Bowman's membrane, and wounds penetrating into the substance of the cornea which leave Descemet's membrane intact.

CORNEAL ABRASIONS

A CORNEAL ABRASION—a stripping of the epithelium from Bowman's membrane, leaving this structure intact (Fig. 276)—is a common result of the thousand and one minor traumata that occur in everyday experience: the grazing of the corneal surface by such objects as a foreign body retained under the upper lid, a finger nail, the edge of a piece of paper, the bristles of a brush,

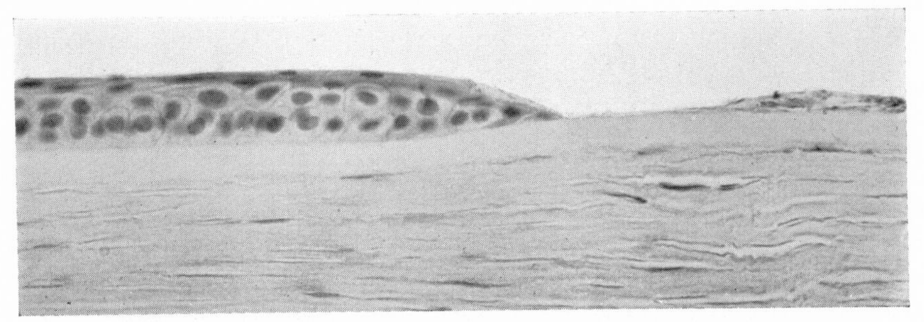

FIG. 276.—CORNEAL ABRASION.

A recent corneal abrasion received just before enucleation. There is a smooth epithelial margin and an extension of the basal cells into the defect (Armed Forces Inst. of Path., Washington).

a piece of clothing or such small objects as are in continuous use in domestic life, twigs or straws in rural life, or small objects such as abound in industrial surroundings, to which may be added the increasingly common corneal abrasions due to the injudicious manipulation of contact lenses. The condition is in a sense parallel with the exfoliation which follows injuries due to chemicals and radiant energy.

An important cause which should always be preventable is the occurrence of an abrasion during an operation on the eye (frequently for squint) when the speculum exposes for some time an anæsthetized cornea which is allowed to become dry; the entire epithelium may be exfoliated in this way. The " anæsthetic eye " produced by sticking an inquisitive finger into the eye of a patient under general anæsthesia to test the corneal reflex is similarly deplorable; a severe abrasion can be caused in this way, particularly if the cornea is exposed to a high concentration of anæsthetic vapour.

That such an incident should easily occur is understandable, for so readily does the epithelium slip over Bowman's membrane that epithelial folds caused by blinking movements of the lids can be observed entoptically or recorded photographically by the distortion of the corneal reflex (Fischer, 1928). The cohesive forces binding the two tissues together are not yet fully elucidated, but it would seem that they are not due to passive adhesion by an intercellular cement but depend rather on the presence of protein-lipid multilayers, the maintenance of which is probably related to intrinsic proteolytic activity (Herrmann and Hickman, 1948; Buschke, 1950). This metabolic requirement may account for the frequent development of recurrent erosions if the vitality of the epithelial cells is impaired. The speed and security of healing would also seem to depend largely on whether the basement membrane has survived intact so that it can be utilized by the new epithelium (Khodadoust *et al.*, 1968).

The *clinical picture* presented by a corneal abrasion is much more alarming than the simple pathology of the condition would seem to warrant, owing to the free exposure of the sensory nerve endings and their constant mechanical stimulation by the rubbing of the eyelid over them. There are acute pain, photophobia and blepharospasm immediately on the receipt of the injury, accompanied by profuse lacrimation, in which the other eye tearfully participates; associated with this is a reflex miosis and usually a circumcorneal ciliary congestion.

The history is usually so typical as to suggest the diagnosis, but a small or even a large abrasion may be difficult to see unless it is delineated by vital staining. The most useful dye for this purpose is a 2% watery solution of *fluorescein* in 2% sodium bicarbonate, a procedure introduced by Pflüger (1882) and applied clinically by Straub (1888)[1]; the dye leaves the normal corneal surface unaltered but stains a brilliant green any area in which the superficial layer of epithelial cells is absent or devitalized; this effect is considerably enhanced if the examination is made with blue or violet light (Anderson, 1949). Other dyes have been employed (æscorcin, Fröhlich, 1892; pyoktanin, Faure, 1895; methylene blue, eosin, toluidine blue, and others) but they show no advantages for this purpose over fluorescein. In the absence of such a dye, keratoscopy may reveal a distortion of the reflex of a Placido disc or, if instrumental aids are unavailable, careful inspection may betray irregularities in the corneal image of a window.

The prognosis in general is good, for the vast majority of corneal abrasions heals rapidly; the pain and photophobia gradually subside, for a small abrasion will heal within 12 hours, and even if the epithelium is completely denuded re-epithelialization may be sufficiently advanced in 48 hours to allow clinical comfort. Certain complications, however, may occur, the most common of which is infection. This may not necessarily be introduced by the traumatic agent but may be already present in the conjunctival sac, particularly in cases of dacryocystitis, and is often introduced subsequently by the patient's attempts to comfort himself by rubbing

[1] Vol. VII, p. 243.

the eye with dirty fingers or a soiled handkerchief. This is particularly prone to occur in certain trades, such as miners and quarrymen (" miners' ulcer ") (Paterson, 1931; Cameron, 1949; Scott, 1954), in agriculturists (" reapers' ulcer ") (Perez Toril, 1949) and is also frequently encountered in the debilitated, the alcoholic, the aged, or in sufferers from such diseases as diabetes. Such a development is ushered in by the appearance of a grey sloughing area at the margin of the erosion and may progress to the formation of a deep ulcer, a severe iridocyclitis with hypopyon, and even loss of the eye. These infections are usually bacterial, but in rural injuries the possibility of infection by such organisms as the *Aspergillus fumigatus* or *Actinomyces* should be remembered.

Apart from infection, slowly progressive degenerative changes may occur, resulting in chronic ulceration and sometimes superficial calcareous degeneration, but the most common complications of a corneal abrasion are its periodic breakdown subsequently as a recurrent corneal erosion, the development of filamentary degeneration, epithelial streaks, and a painful scar.

Occasionally blepharospasm is severe at the time of the injury and persists long after the causal lesion has organically healed; the muscular spasm, indeed, may be continued indefinitely as a hysterical manifestation. Such a spasm has been observed after a trauma without apparent injury (Crookes, 1946); the milder cases are usually readily relieved after akinesia has been induced by injection of the facial nerve.

RECURRENT CORNEAL EROSION

The condition of RECURRENT CORNEAL EROSION, which may follow not only trauma but many inflammatory, degenerative and œdematous conditions of the cornea and may occasionally be hereditary (Franceschetti, 1928), has already been described.[1] It was originally called *intermittent keratitis vesiculosa neuralgica* by Hansen (1872), who found that it followed a scratch by a baby's finger-nail so frequently that he suggested the colloquial description " *nail keratitis*". The exciting injury may be so small that it had attracted little or no attention at the time; the abrasion appeared to have healed well and quite suddenly some weeks or months afterwards, almost invariably in the morning when the patient wakes, he is acutely uncomfortable with pain, lacrimation and photophobia—with all the symptoms, in fact, of a typical abrasion. The symptoms last from 1 to 36 hours and then gradually disappear and the eye quietens—until the next attack. This occurs apparently quite spontaneously and without reason, and the incident repeats itself in this way every few days, weeks or months for an indefinite period up to 20 years or more; but the attacks generally tend to decrease in frequency and intensity and eventually fade away. Sometimes the abraded area is large, in which case the attacks tend to recur at long intervals and to

[1] Vol. VIII, p. 694.

be severe; more commonly, however, the affected area is minute and the recurrences more frequent but milder in nature.

Histologically the condition is marked by vesiculation of the epithelium followed by exfoliation, leaving an eroded area which stains with fluorescein; frequently the vesicles have burst and are not seen when the eye is inspected, but a looseness of the surrounding area of epithelium is constantly found, and sometimes epithelial filaments. The cells are swollen and necrotic, showing some nuclear fragmentation with œdematous vacuoles between them.[1] This sudden epitheliolysis need not necessarily be confined to the area originally traumatized, for successive recurrences may appear on different parts of the cornea, a circumstance which suggests that the epithelial weakness may be due to irregular and unsatisfactory restitution of the terminal nerve filaments as if the lesion had a neurotropic basis (von Szily, 1913; Salus, 1922; Gifford, 1925; and others). It seems reasonably certain, also, that its typical occurrence on waking in the morning is due to the mechanical stripping of the unstable epithelium by the first movements of the upper lid.

The same symptoms may arise without a gross exfoliation of the epithelium that is clinically demonstrable, a condition termed *traumatic keratalgia* (or *cicatrix dolorosa*) by Grandclément (1888). Slit-lamp examination, however, has shown in most cases that there are minute punctate or linear dehiscences in the superficial layers of the epithelium which take on a fluorescein stain (*epithelial streaks*: von Szily, 1913–18), dehiscences which have been demonstrated histologically (Schulte, 1929). Similar symptoms may also be associated with the appearance of *epithelial filaments* which tend to change their site and orientation from day to day (Czermak, 1891; Hess, 1892; Wagenmann, 1892; and others).

The *treatment* of uncomplicated corneal erosions is usually a simple matter: the instillation of antibiotics to prevent infection, the instillation of homatropine to overcome the miotic spasm if there is ciliary injection and neuralgia—the prolonged cycloplegia of atropine is rarely necessary—and, most important of all, sufficiently firm bandaging (which should not be disturbed for 24 hours) to immobilize the lids and prevent their movements from mechanically tearing away the regenerating epithelium. We have already seen that the inhibitory effect of anæsthetics on epithelial regeneration should discourage their use; for the same reason the instillation of antiseptics is unwise; indeed, it has been amply shown that treatment should be as simple as possible. With this simple regime most abrasions heal well and rapidly, and of the three measures detailed above, immobilization of the lids is the most important. Indeed, if the abrasion is extensive, occupying one-third or more of the cornea—particularly if it is in the pupillary area—binocular bandaging with rest in bed is the most satisfactory procedure.

In the presence of infection an antibiotic ointment (penicillin, the tetracyclines, etc.) gives a more prolonged effect, and the bandages may be

[1] von Szily (1900), Peters (1904), Franke (1906), von Szily, jun. (1913).

removed to repeat the instillation periodically; and if a grey sloughing area has already appeared, cauterization (as with carbolic acid) will leave a less conspicuous scar than will an ulcer. When doubt exists this should be done early. The lacrimal sac should also be investigated for the presence of infection.

Many remedies have been proposed for the treatment of recurrent erosions or the less obvious recurrent degenerations, varying from the instillation of quinine (Hirsch, 1898) to the use of the galvanocautery (Nettleship, 1889). In view of the fact that epithelial œdema may precede the breakdown of the smaller type of lesion, Chandler (1945) suggested the nightly application of a 10% boric ointment. The most effective treatment, however, particularly for an extensive lesion, is chemical cauterization, using an agent such as carbolic acid, trichloracetic acid (10%) or an alcoholic solution of iodine, which should be used freely over the eroded area and its surrounds, so that all the unstable epithelium is destroyed down to Bowman's membrane and an entirely new epithelium is allowed to regenerate. If it is found that after anæsthetization a relatively small area of epithelium can be easily rubbed away by a cotton applicator, leaving a clear-cut circumscribed margin, the prognosis after such chemical destruction is usually good. The procedure is not without subsequent pain but, even although the whole of the corneal epithelium is denuded in this way, re-epithelialization will occur within four days. An alternative and less drastic method which may be successful in preventing or postponing recurrences is the application of small doses of X-rays (Greeves, 1930; Lederman, 1951; Rougier, 1953). In resistant cases wherein all other methods fail, recourse may be had to a lamellar corneal graft (François and Neetens, 1953; Leigh, 1959).

Anderson. *Ophthalmologica*, **118**, 444 (1949).
Buschke. *Acta XVI int. Cong. Ophthal.*, London, **2**, 1363 (1950).
Cameron. *Brit. J. Ophthal.*, **33**, 368 (1949).
Chandler. *Amer. J. Ophthal.*, **28**, 355 (1945).
Crookes. *Brit. med. J.*, **1**, 486 (1946).
Czermak. *Klin. Mbl. Augenheilk.*, **29**, 229 (1891).
Faure. *Indépendance Méd.*, 10 (1895).
Fischer. *Arch. Augenheilk.*, **98**, 41 (1928).
Franceschetti. *Z. Augenheilk.*, **66**, 309 (1928).
François and Neetens. *Bull. Soc. belge Ophtal.*, No. 104, 271 (1953).
Franke. *Klin. Mbl. Augenheilk.*, **44** (1), 508 (1906).
Fröhlich. *Arch. Augenheilk.*, **24**, 318 (1892).
Gifford. *Arch. Ophthal.*, **54**, 217 (1925).
Grandclément. *Bull. Soc. franç. Ophtal.*, **6**, 145 (1888).
Greeves. *Trans. ophthal. Soc. U.K.*, **50**, 111 (1930).
Hansen. *Hospitalstidende*, **15**, 201 (1872).
Herrmann and Hickman. *Bull. Johns Hopk. Hosp.*, **82**, 182 (1948).
Hess. *Ber. dtsch. ophthal. Ges.*, **22**, 34 (1892).
Hirsch. *Wschr. Therap. Hyg. Auges*, **1**, 169 (1898).
Khodadoust, Silverstein, Kenyon and Dowling. *Amer. J. Ophthal.*, **65**, 339 (1968).
Lederman. *J. belge Radiol.*, **34**, 450 (1951).
Leigh. *Trans. ophthal. Soc. U.K.*, **79**, 439 (1959).
Nettleship. *Ophthal. Rev.*, **8**, 221 (1889).
Paterson. *Trans. ophthal. Soc. U.K.*, **51**, 341 (1931).
Perez Toril. *Arch. Soc. oftal. hisp.-amer.*, **9**, 534 (1949).
Peters. *v. Graefes Arch. Ophthal.*, **57**, 93 (1904).
Pflüger. *Klin. Mbl. Augenheilk.*, **20**, 69 (1882).
Rougier. *Bull. Soc. Ophtal. Fr.*, 635 (1953).
Salus. *Klin. Mbl. Augenheilk.*, **68**, 673 (1922).
Schulte. *Klin. Mbl. Augenheilk.*, **82**, 49 (1929).
Scott. *Trans. ophthal. Soc. U.K.*, **74**, 105 (1954).
Straub. *Zbl. prakt. Augenheilk.*, **12**, 75 (1888).
von Szily (Sen.). *v. Graefes Arch. Ophthal.*, **51**, 486 (1900).
von Szily (Jun.). *Ber. dtsch. ophthal. Ges.*, **39**, 56 (1913); **41**, 394 (1918).
Wagenmann. *Ber. dtsch. ophthal. Ges.*, **22**, 43 (1892).

DEEP NON-PERFORATING CORNEAL WOUNDS

Deep non-perforating corneal wounds which traverse the substance of the cornea sometimes as far as to Descemet's membrane but do not perforate the globe are relatively rare. They may be *incised or puncture wounds* inflicted accidentally by sharp instruments (knives, needles, pins, etc.) or caused by flying particles of metal or glass (as from spectacles or in a motor accident), *flap wounds* splitting the cornea into two layers, caused by a sharp object such as a knife striking the cornea tangentially or a finger-nail or an animal's claw, or *excised wounds* as occur when an object, grazing the cornea tangentially, shaves off a portion of the tissues. It is noteworthy that a child's finger-nail may tear away a flap extending from the limbus to the centre of the cornea and involving a quarter or a third of the corneal thickness. The first two types of wound may be complicated by the presence of a retained foreign body, a problem which will be discussed subsequently, while a more rare occurrence is the imprisonment of air bubbles in a tangential wound causing a localized CORNEAL EMPHYSEMA (Gallenga, 1911; Wagenmann, 1911); the bubbles of air can be seen by the corneal microscope and disappear by absorption in a few hours. Clean cuts running directly into the corneal surface give rise to the least symptoms; there is little pain, lacrimation or redness, particularly if the wound is in a part of the cornea not covered by the lids, and the patient may not seek advice until the lapse of some days, when infection may have established itself. In lacerated or flap wounds the symptoms are more severe, sometimes resembling those of a corneal erosion; but even if a portion of the cornea has been excised the subjective effects are usually less than those characteristic of an epithelial lesion which exposes the rich interepithelial nerve plexus.

The *clinical course* of such an injury is usually characteristic. Initially the margins of the wound become cloudy and swollen owing to the imbibition of fluid so that the edges tend to pout open, but as the epithelium covers the defect, the haziness disappears and repair is speedy. In an incised wound the lips may thus become gummed together in a few hours and the œdematous opacity may disappear within a day or so. Lacerated or flap wounds may entail more extensive distortion and widespread œdema and opacity, and may result in some permanent bulging of the cornea with considerable astigmatism (Lans, 1898), but even when a large portion of the surface of the cornea has been lost, epithelialization is usual before the end of a week. In these cases, it is true, the new epithelium may break down, either in the centre or the periphery of the wound, but in a few weeks, in the absence of complications, it becomes consolidated. When epithelialization has occurred and the œdema and swelling have disappeared, there is always some permanent scarring and, even in the most favourable cases, examination with the slit-lamp will disclose a fine tracery in the corneal stroma resembling floss silk, due to the invasion of the cornea by cellular elements; but in uncomplicated wounds, particularly in young people, this tends to diminish or disappear after some 4 to 5 weeks. Even an extensive flap wound, splitting the substantia propria into two layers, may heal in position and become almost transparent, allowing useful vision (Ulbrich, 1904); but when the loss of tissue is considerable, complete reparation is slow and the irregularity of the new-formed elements involves a permanent defect in transparency. When the damage is gross, however, and particularly in the presence of complicating infection, vascularization of the cornea occurs and subsequent healing leaves a scar varying in density from a diffuse nebula to a dense leucoma but always involving some degree of optical defect. When loss of tissue has occurred some opacification of the cornea invariably results which, however, may eventually be small; and if a considerable amount of tissue has been lost a keratectasia may develop at a later date.

Complications, however, are always to be feared—*the retention of a foreign body*, particularly a piece of glass or wood, *misalignment of the edges*, especially in the case of large flap wounds, resulting in deformity with much optical disability, and above all, *infection*, the virulence of which varies not with the degree of trauma but with the type of organisms already present in the conjunctival sac or introduced at the time of the accident. If this infection runs a violent and stormy course, it may result in extensive ulceration, intra-ocular inflammation with hypopyon and even loss of the eye, and if it materializes more leisurely it may result in the development of a traumatic keratitis, the torpid chronic disciform keratitis of Fuchs (1901) which, after a smouldering inflammation lasting many months, may leave a permanent and disabling opacity. A severely infected ulcer with a hypopyon is a common result of an injury of this type; the very violently destructive condition of ring abscess of the cornea, which leads to rapid and massive necrosis of the cornea, is a more rare sequel of a superficial injury. The occasional occurrence of a fungal infection, particularly aspergillosis, in injuries received in rural surroundings, with the development of *mycotic keratitis*, should not be forgotten (Fig. 277). This type of infection should always be remembered when a traumatic corneal ulcer maintains a torpid course in spite of treatment with antibiotics and particularly when topical corticosteroid drops have been used (Jones *et al.*, 1969). Until the possibility of infection is eliminated the prognosis should always be guarded, a reservation which applies particularly to flap wounds which have fallen back into place, for the edges may become gummed together, enclosing within them an infective nidus.

The *treatment* of such wounds should entail a thorough exploration of their extent, aided if necessary by the instillation of fluorescein and the elimination of any foreign material. The first step should be the adoption of prophylactic measures against infection by the instillation of antibiotic drops. Thereafter, in small uncomplicated wounds, immobilization of the lids by bandaging usually allows rapid repair. In extensively lacerated wounds or flap wounds, since the degree of scarring is inversely proportional to the accuracy of coaptation, it may be advisable to unite the edges by sutures; if sharp atraumatic corneal needles are used, the resultant damage is negligible, and this procedure is generally wiser than the employment of a conjunctival flap since it ensures more accurate apposition while the adhesion of the subconjunctival tissue to the edges of the wound may interfere with rapid re-epithelialization. In extensive flap wounds, particularly if the flap hangs downwards and has undergone opacification, it may be preferable to excise the loose portion rather than to attempt its reposition. If infection has developed, treatment should be instigated as for an infected corneal ulcer; but it is always to be remembered that if the infection is

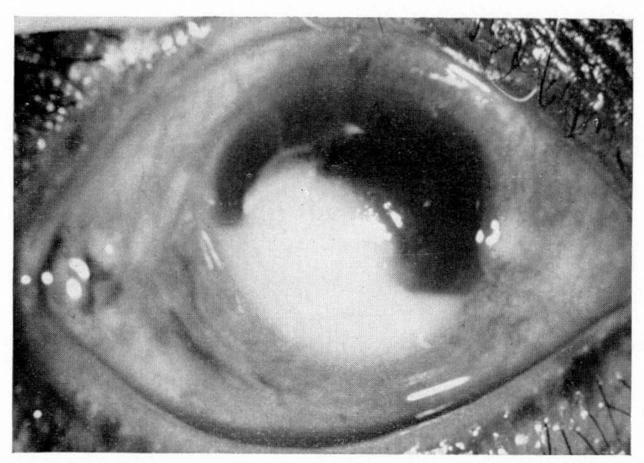

Fig. 277.—Infection by *Cephalosporium* following Corneal Injury.

In a man aged 59 whose cornea was injured with a corn stalk. There is a large hypopyon ulcer (J. L. Byers).

violent even the most efficient treatment by chemotherapy and antibiotics may not suffice to retain useful vision although the eye itself may be saved (Alvarez, 1950, in a case of ring abscess of the cornea developing after a superficial trauma from the branch of a tree).

The treatment of the scar which is invariably left by such a wound depends upon its position in the cornea and the vision of the other eye. Medicaments (dionine, yellow oxide of mercury, quinine bisulphate, etc.) are useless, as also are physical methods (iontophoresis with iodine, ultra-violet light, x-rays, etc.) which from time to time have been advocated for this purpose. Three methods of approach are possible—an optical iridectomy, the results of which are rarely spectacular owing to the inefficiency of peripheral refraction; tattooing with platinum, which may diminish the annoying dispersive properties of a nebula and may be a welcome cosmetic disguise for a leucoma; or an excision of the superficial lamellæ of the cornea containing the scar and their replacement by a lamellar graft. The last expedient is the most practical and efficient if any therapeutic measures are considered desirable.

Wounds of the Conjunctiva

As a general rule wounds of the conjunctiva are in themselves trivial, usually exciting few symptoms and healing rapidly without reaction or complications; the amenability of this membrane to surgical insult—cutting, stretching, transplantation and so on—is a matter of everyday experience. They are most commonly caused by sharp objects which strike the globe a glancing blow, and on occasion a jagged flap of considerable size may be torn off. *Abrasions* are rare since, unlike the corneal epithelium, the loose conjunctiva slides along before a gentle impact; cuts and piercing wounds rapidly close, so rapidly indeed that restitution of the conjunctiva may mask the entrance of a foreign body into the eye within a day; even wounds which penetrate into Tenon's capsule quickly epithelialize. A conjunctival flap-wound will become adherent in about an hour, and smooth, almost unrecognizable healing occurs within a few days, so that in the ordinary course of events the scars are scarcely visible, being perhaps recognizable by their ivory-like appearance. Ragged and irregular wounds, however, should receive prompt attention, for if they are neglected adhesions and exposure of the sclera, except for a thin layer of epithelialized cicatricial tissue, tend to result. Any of these wounds may be associated with a considerable amount of sub- or intra-conjunctival ecchymosis which, indeed, may be the only clinical indication of its presence.

Complications, although rare, sometimes arise. *Hæmorrhage*, which sometimes may be widespread, although it looks alarming to the uninitiated, is of no importance. Occasionally, particularly in puncture wounds, the reparative process is exuberant and polypoid nodules of *granulation tissue* appear, or enfolding and burying of the epithelium may result in the formation of a *traumatic implantation cyst* which may require subsequent excision, sometimes after several years.

Such an event is not uncommon[1]; a cyst may develop in this way after a simple conjunctival wound (Collins, 1896; Lange, 1903) but this development is more usually seen if a foreign body is retained and is particularly prone to occur in the rare event of an eyelash being buried in the wound. An insect-bite is an exceptional cause (Uhthoff, 1879) and such cystic formation is not very unusual after operations involving a conjunctival incision, as for strabismus, and has been encountered after enucleation of the globe (Aosima, 1937). A type of retention cyst of imprisoned glandular debris has been reported after a wound which led to cicatrization between the bulbar and palpebral conjunctiva in the lower fornix (Xilo, 1920). In the usual case the epithelium, buried in the submucous tissue, grows and proliferates into a mass which eventually

[1] Rombolotti (1895), Collins (1896), Ballaban (1901), Lange (1903), Langhorst (1904), Alt (1909), Carlini (1910), Lindahl (1910), Rolandi (1912), Shoda (1924), Grom (1949), Werner (1950), and many others.

degenerates in the centre, leaving a cyst containing clear fluid surrounded by laminated epithelium adherent to the conjunctiva and usually also to the sclera by inflammatory reaction (Wolff, 1928), and occasionally extends deeply into the sclera and even the cornea (Grom, 1949).

Infection, however, is the main complication of a conjunctival wound and, although it is usually a transient affair readily controlled without specific therapeutic measures by the highly vascular tissues, cases have been reported wherein a *subconjunctival abscess* has formed (scratch by the paw of a dog, Langhorst, 1904), or an *orbital abscess* with gangrene of the lids (scratch from a finger-nail, Vossius, 1902); the spread of such an infection to form a *suppurative tenonitis* has occasionally occurred (Gallemaerts, 1899; Capolongo, 1899; Puech, 1902; and others).

Infections by specific organisms have occasionally occurred. A very rare event is the infection of a conjunctival wound with tubercle bacilli so that a primary *tuberculous ulcer* results.[1] Conjunctival *glanders* may develop when an abrasion is infected by the *Pf. mallei* (Neisser, 1892; Gourfein *et al.*, 1897–1902), or a primary chancre of *syphilis* may be thus acquired (Denti, 1883; Campart, 1885; Morel-Lavallée, 1886). *Tetanus* has been reported as arising in this way (Samelsohn, 1879).

The *treatment* of conjunctival wounds is a straightforward matter. In all cases infection or potential infection should be combated by a preliminary irrigation with saline followed by the instillation of antibiotics. Small wounds may be left to epithelialize themselves assisted by immobilization of the lids by bandaging; after irregular tags have been trimmed away, the edges of more extensive wounds should be apposed by silk sutures to prevent adhesion to the underlying sclera; and in order to secure good coaptation in widespread defects, no hesitation need be felt in wide undermining or in the mobilization of flaps so that bared areas are covered without tension. Granulomata or traumatic cysts can be treated only by excision; in the latter case removal must be complete if recurrences are to be avoided.

Non-perforating Wounds of the Sclera

Non-perforating wounds of the sclera are also of minor importance and usually take the form of scratches from pins or pencils or the claws or teeth of animals. They are, of course, associated with conjunctival wounds and add little to their clinical symptoms. The dark uveal pigment may be apparent in the depth of a wound which almost penetrates the globe, but so long as this does not actually occur scleral wounds heal rapidly and without mishap, leaving little scar formation. Complications occasionally occur if a virulent infection is present, such as the development of a necrotic scleritis following a wound incurred while chopping wood by a patient with dacryocystitis (Levy, 1900) or in the presence of a fungal infection (*Aspergillus fumigatus*) (Köllner, 1906); but with the simple routine treatment adopted

[1] Walb (1877), Pergel (1893), Stutzer (1898), Jessop (1900), Lagrange and Cabannes (1900), Greeff (1902), Hancock (1906), and others.

for conjunctival injuries—the maintenance of asepsis and conjunctival suturing if necessary—the prognosis is generally good.

Alt. *Ophthal. Rec.*, **18,** 141 (1909).
Alvarez. *Ophthalmologica*, **120,** 206 (1950).
Aosima. *Acta Soc. ophthal. jap.*, **41,** Suppl., 374 (1937).
Ballaban. *Arch. Augenheilk.*, **43,** 167 (1901).
Campart. *Bull. Clin. Ophtal. Hôp. Quinze-Vingts*, 48 (1885).
Capolongo. *Arch. Ottal.*, **6,** 410 (1899).
Carlini. *v. Graefes Arch. Ophthal.*, **73,** 288 (1910).
Collins. *Researches*, London (1896).
Denti. *Ann. Ottal.*, **12,** 567 (1883).
Fuchs. *Klin. Mbl. Augenheilk.*, **39** (2), 513 (1901).
Gallemaerts. *Ann. Oculist.* (Paris), **121,** 57 (1899).
Gallenga. *Klin. Mbl. Augenheilk.*, **49** (1), 150 (1911).
Gourfein, Marignac and Valette. *Rev. med. Suisse rom.*, **17,** 737 (1897); **22,** 447 (1902). *Ann. Oculist.* (Paris), **119,** 157 (1898).
Greeff. Orth's *Lhb. d. spez. path. Anat.*, Berlin, Erg. **1,** 198 (1902).
Grom. *Ann. Oculist.* (Paris), **182,** 52 (1949).
Hancock. *Trans. ophthal. Soc. U.K.*, **26,** 33 (1906).
Jessop. *Trans. ophthal. Soc. U.K.*, **20,** 51 (1900).
Jones, Richards and Morgan. *Trans. ophthal. Soc. U.K.*, **89,** 727 (1969).
Köllner. *Z. Augenheilk.*, **16,** 441 (1906).
Lagrange and Cabannes. *Arch. Ophtal.*, **20,** 353 (1900).
Lange. *Klin. Mbl. Augenheilk.*, **41** (2), 199 (1903).
Langhorst. *Zur Kasuistik d. Lidverletzungen* (Diss.), Jena (1904).
Lans. *v. Graefes Arch. Ophthal.*, **45,** 117 (1898).
Levy. *Klin. Mbl. Augenheilk.*, **38,** 840 (1900).
Lindahl. *Mitt. a. d. Augenklin. d. Carol. Inst.*, Stockholm, **11,** 69 (1910).
Morel-Lavallée. *Ann. Derm. Syph.*, **7,** 85 (1886).
Neisser. *Berl. klin. Wschr.*, **29,** 321 (1892).
Pergel. *Wien. med. Wschr.*, **43,** 475 (1893).
Puech. *Bull. Soc. franç. Ophtal.*, **19,** 117 (1902).
Rolandi. *Ann. Ottal.*, **41,** 741 (1912).
Rombolotti. *Arch. Augenheilk.*, **31,** 9 (1895).
Samelsohn. *Zbl. prakt. Augenheilk.*, **3,** 325 (1879).
Shoda. *Klin. Mbl. Augenheilk.*, **73,** 223 (1924).
Stutzer. *Beitr. Augenheilk.*, **3** (30), 884 (1898).
Uhthoff. *Berl. klin. Wschr.*, **16,** 729 (1879).
Ulbrich. *Klin. Mbl. Augenheilk.*, **42** (1), 256 (1904).
Vossius. *Ber. dtsch. ophthal. Ges.*, **30,** 210 (1902).
Wagenmann. *Klin. Mbl. Augenheilk.*, **49** (1), 368 (1911).
Walb. *Klin. Mbl. Augenheilk.*, **15,** 285 (1877).
Werner. *Acta ophthal.* (Kbh.), **28,** 203 (1950).
Wolff. *Proc. roy. Soc. Med.*, **22,** 22 (1928).
Xilo. *Boll. Sci. med. Bologna*, **8,** 496 (1920).

PERFORATING WOUNDS OF THE EYE

Perforating wounds of the eye are common, whether they be small punctures or extensive lacerations; they occur particularly among children at play or adults engaged in industry, but accidents incurred while travelling or injuries sustained in war contribute largely to the total. The causes are innumerable and often bizarre: knives and forks, needles and pins, sharp toys and glass among children; a multitude of sharp instruments and flying bodies in adults, even a whip-lash or a cat's claw or the teeth of a dog (Schmidt-Rimpler, 1875). The types of such wounds encountered in day-to-day practice are therefore very varied. Incised and punctured wounds form the majority, such as are inflicted by knives, pieces of glass, the points of scissors or other sharp instruments, and they vary in size from gaping or flap-like lacerating gashes or the virtual bisection of the globe by a rotary saw (Petersen and Raagaard, 1951) to punctures so small as to be discerned only with difficulty. No matter how small, however, such injuries are never to be considered trivial but are always to be treated as surgical emergencies. Too often the globe is disorganized at the time of the accident; if it is not, the introduction of infection with subsequent loss of vision is common. The clinical picture is frequently complicated by a prolapse of some of the intra-ocular contents, an event which, although it may aid at the time in the immediate closure of the wound and the avoidance of infection, is a suicidal method of repair in its consequences (Plate XIII). Even although the structural damage does not appear to be catastrophic at the time, the subsequent development of a traumatic endophthalmitis may slowly and remorselessly lead to a painful, atrophic and useless organ; while in many instances the possibility of the development of sympathetic ophthalmitis, with its potentialities of bilateral blindness, adds to the anxieties of both the patient and the surgeon. If to these problems are added the complications of a retained foreign body the difficulties are further increased; the consideration of this matter, however, will be left to a subsequent section.

Injuries of the human eye resulting from the pecking of birds are rare, and are mostly caused by owls and roosters; the mother owl is particularly dangerous when defending her young (Rodewald, 1896; Janiszewska-Zygier, 1966). Long-legged shore-birds such as storks and cranes have been said to defend themselves against children by pecking exactly in the centre of the cornea, resulting in a triangular injury with prolapse of the uveal tissue. On the other hand, injuries from domestic fowls are much less frequently seen (Paul, 1964; Kuhl, 1970); the case of pecking injury of the cornea by a cock described by Samuels (1954) was complicated by a septic abscess of the lens and that reported by Seefried (1951) by a tear of the retina with a detachment. These are, of course, unusual injuries but their treatment should follow general principles. It is advisable, however, to determine whether or not the responsible species of bird is subject to viral disease or is a carrier, for instance, of Newcastle disease or psittacosis.

Perforating Wounds of the Ocular Coats

UNCOMPLICATED CORNEAL WOUNDS

The UNCOMPLICATED HEALING OF A PERFORATING CORNEAL WOUND is a simple and straightforward matter provided the edges are in apposition (Fig. 278). The most interesting work on this subject has been done on keratome and cataract sections.[1] Immediately the wound is made the imbibition of fluid by the corneal lamellæ makes the edges swell and turn opaque; this, together with the outpouring of exudative material, tends to bring the edges into apposition with the result that, particularly if the wound is oblique and valvular, coaptation is rapid and in favourable circumstances cohesion may be sufficient to withstand the intra-ocular pressure within half an hour (Clarke, 1898). When the edges of the wound are in apposition, coaptation occurs first in the central area, while anteriorly and posteriorly the peripheral parts, retracted by the elasticity of the

[1] Weinstein (1903) on dogs, Henderson (1907) on man, Tooke (1914) and Collins (1914) on rabbits, Maggiore (1940–41) and Purtscher (1942) on man, Dunnington (1951) and Dunnington and Regan (1952) on monkeys, and Ashton and Cook (1951) on rabbits. See Vol. VIII, p. 604.

PLATE XIII

Perforating Injuries.

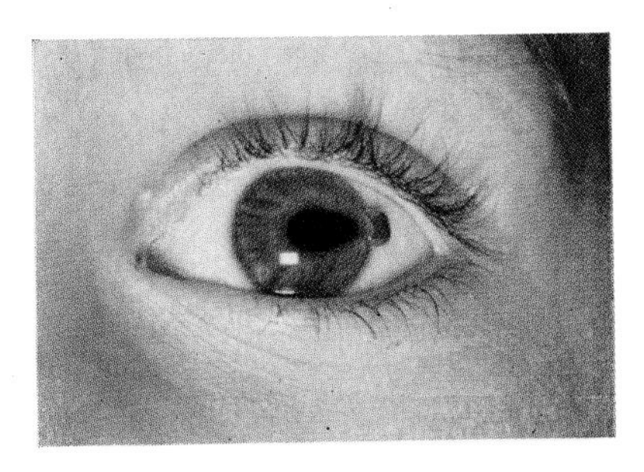

Fig. 1.—Prolapse of the iris after a perforating injury with scissors

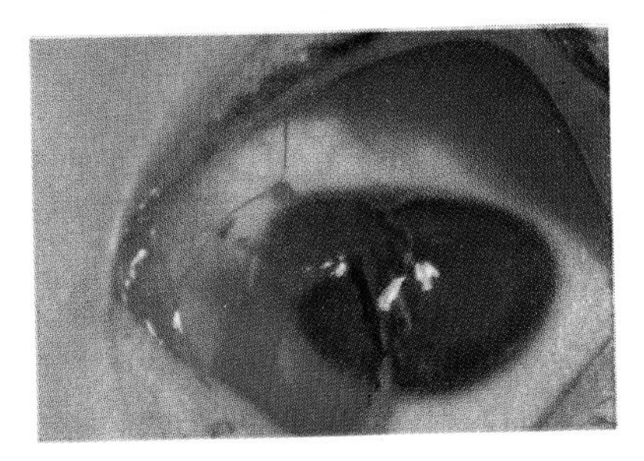

Fig. 2.—Collapse of the globe with loss of intra-ocular contents due to penetration by an arrow.

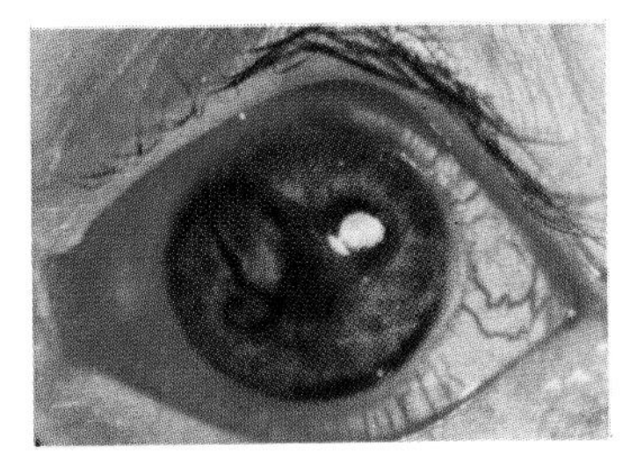

Fig. 3.—Laceration of the cornea, iris and lens caused by scissors.

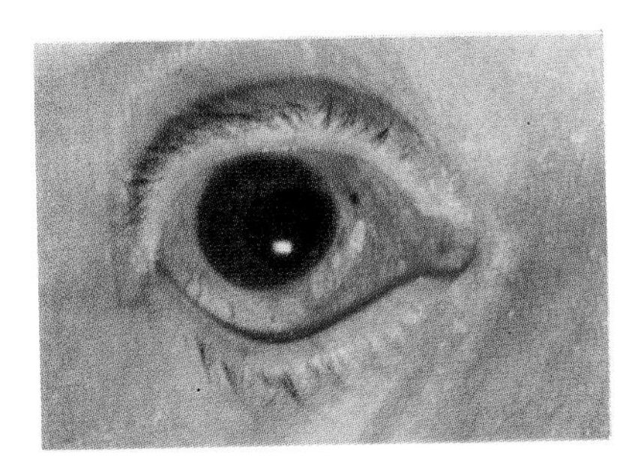

Fig. 4.—Delayed dehiscence due to secondary glaucoma of a repaired corneo-scleral perforating wound.

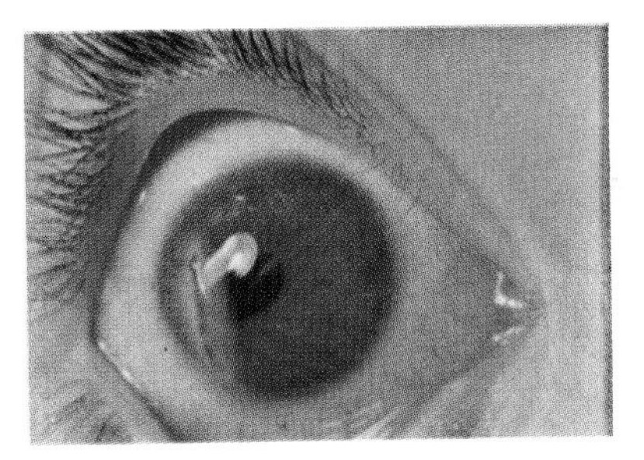

Fig. 5.—Healed corneal laceration with incarceration of the iris.

[*To face p.* 324.

tissue, tend to gape, leaving an anterior and posterior triangle where the lips of the wound pout open. The anterior triangle is rapidly filled by epithelium, partly by mechanical sliding and partly by mitotic multiplication of cells, a process which is usually consolidated at the end of two days (Fig. 279). At the same time the posterior triangle, sometimes filled with a fibrinous clot derived possibly in part from fluid from the corneal stroma and in part from the newly formed plasmoid aqueous, is bridged over by endothelial growth (Henderson, 1907; Collins, 1914; and others); at other times the triangular gap remains open without the formation of a fibrinous plug and becomes lined by endothelium more slowly (Dunnington, 1951); but in either case a new Descemet's membrane is simultaneously secreted, a process which takes some 3 months to become complete. In the meantime, the approximated edges of the substantia propria, now sealed together with a

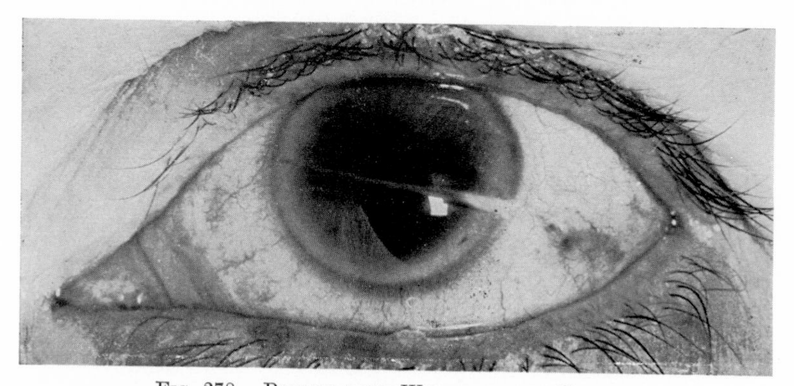

Fig. 278.—Perforating Wound of the Cornea.

Caused by the windscreen in a car accident. The injury was bilateral (see Fig. 14) (Inst. Ophthal.).

fibrinous matrix, become infiltrated with leucocytes and macrophages which appear in great numbers on the 5th or 6th day, and new fibrous lamellæ are slowly laid down (Fig. 280). In general terms there is thus rapid epithelial closure of the anterior part of the wound before the deeper structures participate in reparative activity. As time goes on the new connective tissue derived from the stroma pushes the epithelial plug towards the surface and simultaneously fills out the posterior triangle so that the cornea gradually returns to its normal layering, but it is at least a month before this new connective tissue has fully consolidated (Maggiore, 1941; Purtscher, 1942). The eventual contraction of this tissue which binds the two lips of the wound together makes the scar dwindle in extent and may even make the edges of Bowman's membrane, originally retracted, over-ride each other and become convoluted (Fig. 280). Ultimately the bundles of fibres, at first disposed somewhat irregularly, tend to assume a more even pattern in conformity with the system of corneal lamellæ, but a residual irregularity always leaves a perman-

Figs. 279 and 280.—Perforating Corneal Wounds (N. Ashton).

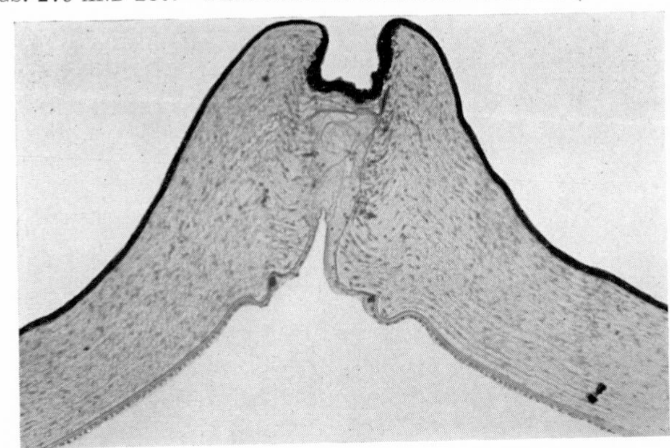

Fig. 279.—The appearance on the second day after corneal section in the rabbit. Epithelial regeneration had progressed to form a continuous surface. The wound is filled with a fibrinous coagulum. Descemet's membrane has retracted and curls forward accompanied by its endothelium.

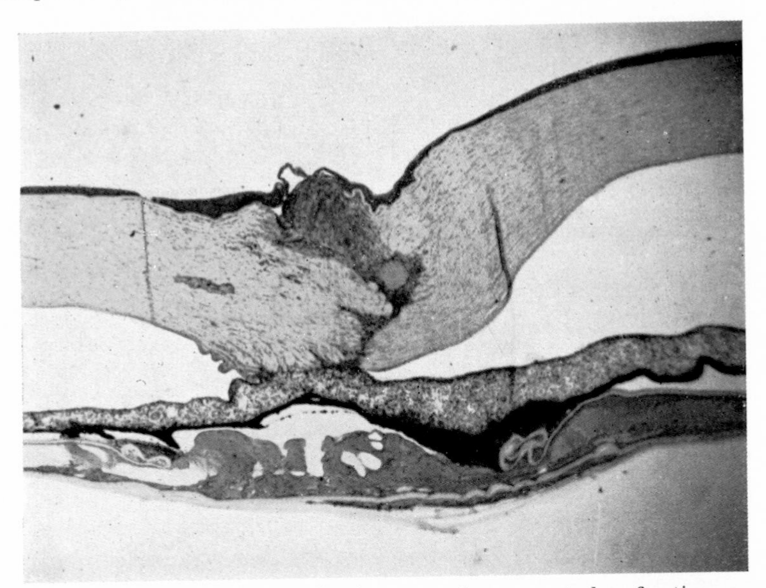

Fig. 280.—The human cornea showing a scar of a paracentral perforating wound. Scar-tissue binds both sides of the wound together sending out conical processes between the lamellæ. Bowman's membrane is seen to be curled up on the right side immediately underneath the epithelium. To the internal surface is adherent the œdematous and chronically infiltrated iris. The lens shows a traumatic cataract.

ent opacity which, however, in the most favourable circumstances may be very tenuous.

Post-traumatic astigmatism, as would be expected, is a usual and almost constant result of a perforating corneal wound. If the wound is near the periphery, as is seen typically after an operative incision, the astigmatism is usually regular, a fact first noted by Donders (1864) and measured ophthalmometrically by Reuss and Woinow (1869). The meridian at right angles to the wound is usually flattened and, while the astigmatism may initially be as much as 4 or 6 dioptres, it usually diminishes to 1 or 2 D within 4 to 6 months.[1] In central wounds, however, and in complicated cases particularly when a prolapse of the iris has occurred, the astigmatism is always irregular and may be of high degree (10 D, Laqueur, 1884; 14 D, Seidel, 1913; 32 D, Aschheim, 1897).

COMPLICATED CORNEAL WOUNDS

Such is the method of healing of a typical corneal wound; but when *the edges of the wound are in faulty apposition* events do not take this ideal course and a number of misadventures may follow. Imperfect apposition occurs when the edges overlap or when they gape widely apart. If this takes place anteriorly while the posterior parts of the wound are in apposition, the defect tends to be rapidly filled by epithelium; in the opposite case, healing is slower and the gap is only gradually made good by new stromal tissue. If, however, apposition of the lips is grossly defective, the tendency for a profuse *ingrowth of epithelium* is great; while, if the posterior hiatus is extensive, a similar *exuberance of growth may affect the regenerative elements of the substantia propria.* An almost constant further complication of a gaping wound is the *incarceration within it of one or more of the intra-ocular tissues*, particularly the iris, a complication which, if extensive, may lead to the development of an *ectatic cicatrix* or an *anterior staphyloma* or, in the presence of ingrowing or incarcerated tissue, a *cystoid cicatrix* or a *fistula.*

EPITHELIAL INGROWTHS

In view of the virility of the regeneration of the corneal epithelium, it is not surprising that if the edges of the wound are not rapidly apposed, these cells do not confine themselves to covering the outer aspects of the wound but swarm inwards to clothe the lips of the wound entirely (Fig. 281); indeed, they may do this to such purpose that they may proliferate along the inner aspect of the cornea, fill up (and block) the angle of the anterior chamber and creep along the anterior surface of the iris whereon they grow most rapidly and luxuriantly (Fig. 282); or, particularly if the iris is adherent to the cornea, they may cover the posterior surface of the former tissue and spread over the ciliary body and lens (Fig. 285). In this way a veritable " epithelial cyst " of the anterior or posterior chamber may be formed (Fig. 376). In such a case, in the remarkable enthusiasm of its growth the epithelium tends to invade every nook and cranny available to it and swarms over exudative deposits. The wall of the cyst thus formed may remain continuous with the surface epithelium along the track of the wound (Stölting, 1885; Kümmell, 1907), it may communicate with a cyst-like formation in the substance of the cornea, or the cavity of the cyst may

[1] Treutler (1900), van Lint (1914), Alexiadès (1920), Andreae (1923), Tron (1925), and others.

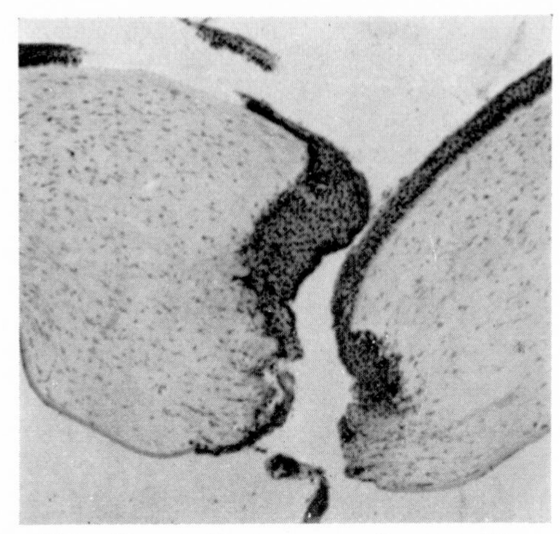

Fig. 281.—Recent Perforating Corneal Wound.

Showing proliferation and ingrowth of the epithelium into the anterior half of the wound. A small length of epithelium on the left has become artificially detached (H. & E.) (N. Ashton).

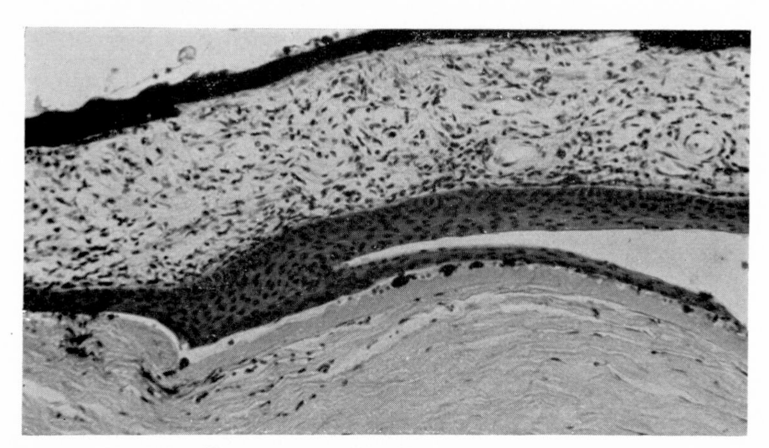

Fig. 282.—Epithelialization of the Anterior Chamber.

Squamous epithelium can be seen growing along the corneal endothelium blocking the filtration angle and growing over the anterior surface of the iris (H. & E.; ×170) (N. Ashton).

protrude under the conjunctiva resulting in a bi-locular formation (Parsons, 1904) (Fig. 283); the proliferating epithelium may invade the lens if the capsule is torn (Wintersteiner, 1900) and in exceptional circumstances it may eventually line the entire cavity of a shrunken eye (Collins, 1891).

If the lips of the wound gape widely the epithelium may grow inward in great sheets varying in thickness from one to six or more layers deep in stratified formation, occasionally showing goblet cells indicating a conjunctival origin (Terry *et al.*, 1939) (Figs. 282, 284–5); if the dehiscences in the wound are small, irregular and tortuous, columns of cells may traverse the cornea giving the impression of the formation of epithelial tubes or localized cysts unless the true condition is revealed by serial sections. Sometimes the process of ingrowth is extraordinarily rapid; thus Meller (1901) found both lips of a wound completely clothed by epithelium in four days. At other times it takes several years before the anterior chamber becomes lined with cells (Fuchs, 1902; Terry *et al.*, 1939). On the other hand, if the even spread of the epithelial growth is obstructed by mechanical barriers such as lens capsule, vitreous or organized exudate, the logical consequence is the formation of a localized epithelial cyst which eventually becomes enlarged by the accumulation within it of exfoliated, degenerated cells associated

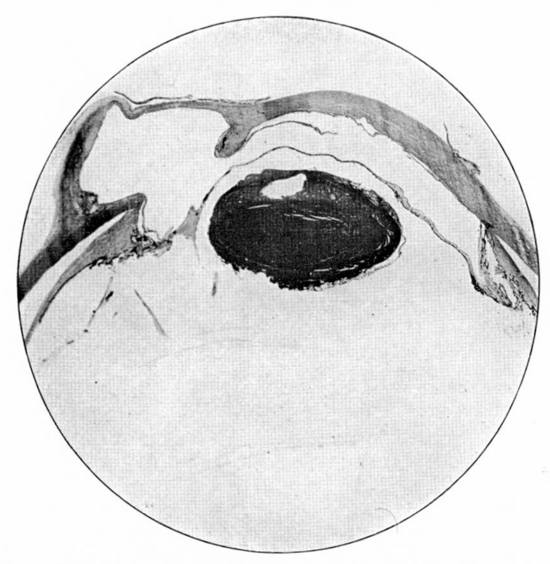

FIG. 283.—EPITHELIAL CYST OF THE ANTERIOR CHAMBER.

Two and a half years after a corneal wound with prolapse of the iris. The cyst lined with multi-layered epithelium occupies the entire anterior chamber, being continuous over the iris, and protrudes under the conjunctiva (×5) (J. H. Parsons).

sometimes with phagocytic and pigmented cells and cholesteatomatous material. Several cysts of this type may occur together in the same eye, some purely corneal, some iridic and some bounded by various portions of the anterior chamber (Clausnizer, 1911).

Fortunately such epithelial ingrowths are not common. Terry and his colleagues (1939) found only 28 cases of epithelialization of the anterior or posterior chamber in 45,500 consecutive cases of perforating wounds of the eye, traumatic and surgical (0·06%). The condition was first noted by Collins (1891–92), who considered it to be an implantation phenomenon, and Guaita (1893) who mistook the epithelium for endothelium; Meller (1901) was the first to appreciate its full significance and the pathological features of the condition are now fully established.[1] Until the advent of

[1] Elschnig (1903), Morax and Duverger (1909), Nagano (1910), Collins (1914) and Speciale-Cirincione (1924).

Figs. 284 and 285.—Epithelialization of the Anterior Chamber after Cataract Extraction (N. Ashton).

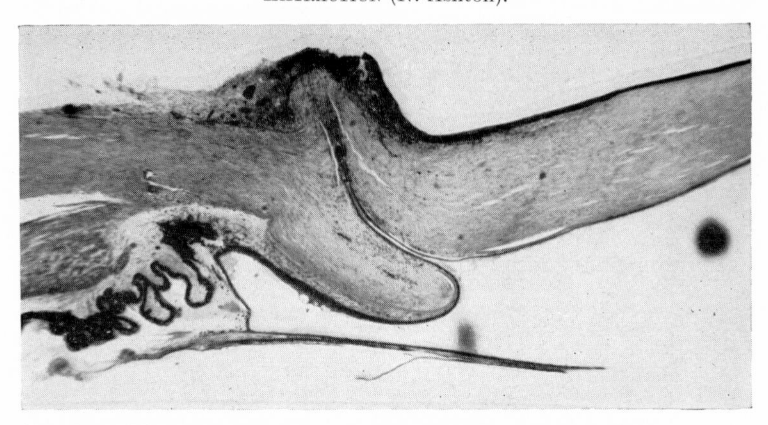

Fig. 284.—The corneal section has healed only superficially and the deeper portion of the wound, the corneal endothelium and the posterior surface of the iris stump are completely lined with squamous epithelium (H. & E.; ×30).

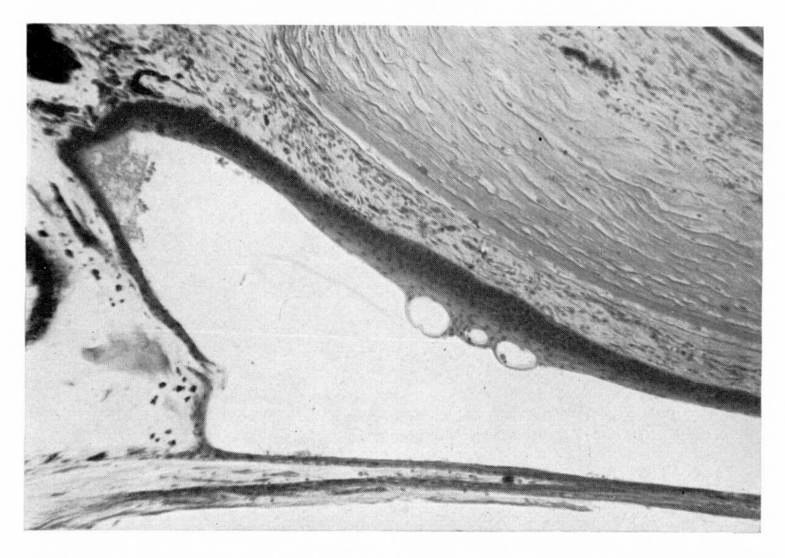

Fig. 285.—High-power view showing the squamous epithelium on the posterior aspect of the iris which is adherent to the cornea. The epithelium can be traced round the surface of the ciliary body and over a fine cyclitic membrane. Bullous formation is present in the epithelium (H. & E.; ×135).

the slit-lamp such ingrowths were difficult to diagnose clinically so that most cases were recognized and studied only in the histological stage after the eye had been excised for secondary glaucoma; with the aid of the slit-lamp, however, the thin, veil-like appearance of the epithelium can be seen growing from the wound along the posterior surface of the cornea and over the iris as a fine film-like tissue frequently spotted with pigment granules or minute, pearl-like globules representing goblet cells or bullous degeneration.[1] Confirmation of the diagnosis may be made by immediate histological examination of a biopsy of the membrane obtained through a small keratotomy (Calhoun, 1966); while Maumenee (1964) drew attention to the diagnostic value of the reaction of an epithelial membrane on the surface of the iris to light-coagulation which causes it to fluff up in a characteristic manner. Epithelialization of the anterior chamber following intra-ocular surgery is rare (probably under 1%); it is most common after a cataract extraction, but cases have been observed after iridencleisis, iridectomy and penetrating keratoplasty (Leibowitz *et al.*, 1967).

The essential precursor of such an ingrowth is delayed closure of the wound usually associated with hypotony of the globe, due sometimes to mal-apposition of the lips of the wound and frequently to the incarceration of tissues within them; the accident therefore tends to occur particularly in severely lacerating injuries although linear wounds such as a cataract section are by no means exempt. Thus if a tag of conjunctiva intrudes into the wound it usually either becomes expelled or completely absorbed without exerting a pronounced influence upon healing; but on the other hand, if it is of sufficient bulk to prevent approximation or if it seriously delays the healing process, epithelial ingrowth may well develop, a circumstance demonstrated experimentally by Suzuki (1934) in rabbits and verified clinically by several observers (Perera, 1937; Theobald and Haas, 1948; Calhoun, 1949; and others). In the same way, a similar result follows the incarceration into the deeper part of the wound of iris tissue, vitreous and particularly lens capsule which is inert and therefore excites little tissue-reaction[2] (Fig. 293). The implantation of a cilium (Collins and Cross, 1892) (Plate XXII, Fig. 2) or a celluloid plaque into the wound has had a like effect (Corrado, 1931) and there is little doubt that the increased use of sutures in the closure of corneal wounds, providing a portal of entry for the epithelial ingrowth if they are deep, has made the condition more common in recent years (Fig. 286) (Dunnington, 1951; Berliner, 1951; Gördüren and Tosunoglu, 1951; and others). Finally, the formation of a fistula is a direct encouragement to epithelial proliferation of this type (Dunnington and Regan, 1950–52).

Whatever the cause, the results are almost invariably disastrous. If the extent of the ingrowth is wide, union is prevented by the epithelialization and a fistula tends to develop; while as soon as the epithelium begins to grow over the endothelium, a dystrophic keratitis tends to develop in association with an irritative iritis, which may rapidly and inexorably destroy the usefulness of the cornea. Once the anterior chamber becomes lined with cells the iritis becomes progressively destructive, and ultimately the onset of a secondary glaucoma which is generally unresponsive to treatment necessitates excision of the eye.

[1] Salus (1927), Papolczy (1930), Custodis (1932), Fazakas (1932), Michaïl (1932), Vail (1936) and others.

[2] Tooke (1914), Collins (1914), Corrado (1931), Terry *et al.* (1939), and others.

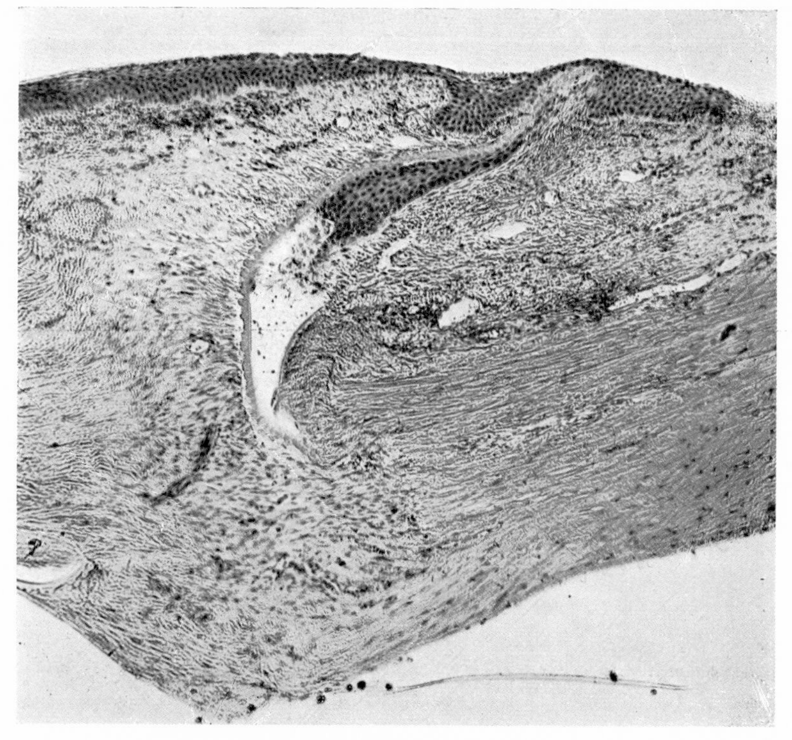

Fig. 286.—Corneal Sutures.

The eye of a monkey two days after a corneal wound as for cataract extraction, showing the corneal epithelium growing along the track of a suture (J. Dunnington and E. Regan).

STROMAL OVERGROWTH

An exuberant overgrowth of the stromal tissues of the cornea is not an uncommon event if the lips of a perforating wound are badly apposed particularly in their posterior parts; although it has been remarked after a cataract extraction (Wood, 1932), it is a phenomenon which largely escaped attention until Levkoieva (1947) and Tichomirov (1948) drew attention to its frequency (occurring to some extent in 25% of all eyes enucleated for perforating wounds) and to the damage it may cause. We have discussed elsewhere the processes of regeneration in the substantia propria,[1] and it is not unnatural when the posterior part of a wound gapes, and particularly when the raw surfaces face the anterior chamber over a wide area, that these regenerative activities should run astray. The newly formed cells and fibrils grow into the anterior chamber; the cells become narrow, arrow-like elements, and the fibrils at first argyrophil eventually become collagenous in nature, the new tissue resembling in every way the reparative elements which normally

[1] Vol. VIII, p. 615.

FIGS. 287 AND 288.—PERFORATING COR[illegible] WOUNDS (N. Ashton).

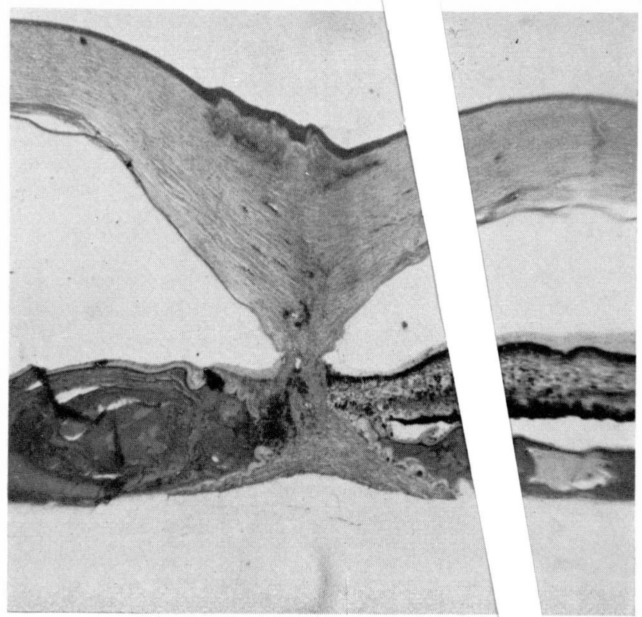

FIG. 287.—Perforating wound passing through the centr[illegible] the cornea and the lens. A corneal proliferation traversing the anterior chamber [illegible]grown through and is extending to both sides of the remnants of the cataractous [illegible]. On one side the pupillary margin of the iris is adherent to the corneal prolifer[illegible] (H. & E.; ×27).

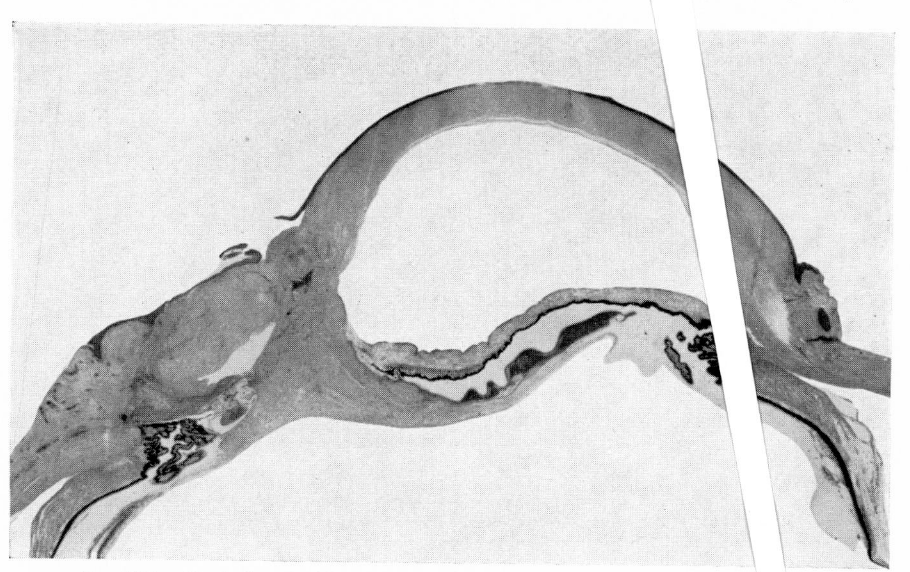

FIG. 288.—Both the nasal limbus and the adjacent peripheral cornea show[illegible]e scars of perforating wounds. The nasal part of the iris is missing and is replaced [illegible] a mass of fibro-vascular tissue derived from the corneal stroma which, extending b[illegible]wards from the wound, passes through the pupil and partially encloses the remnan[illegible] of the lens.

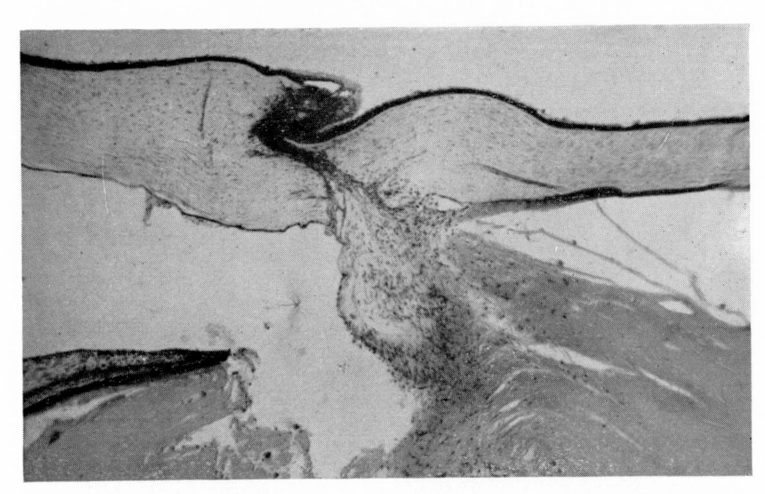

FIG. 289.—PERFORATION OF THE CORNEA WITH SCISSORS.

The healing wound is mal-apposed and there is a corneal proliferation traversing the anterior chamber and growing into the shrunken lacerated cataractous lens (H. & E.; ×43) (N. Ashton).

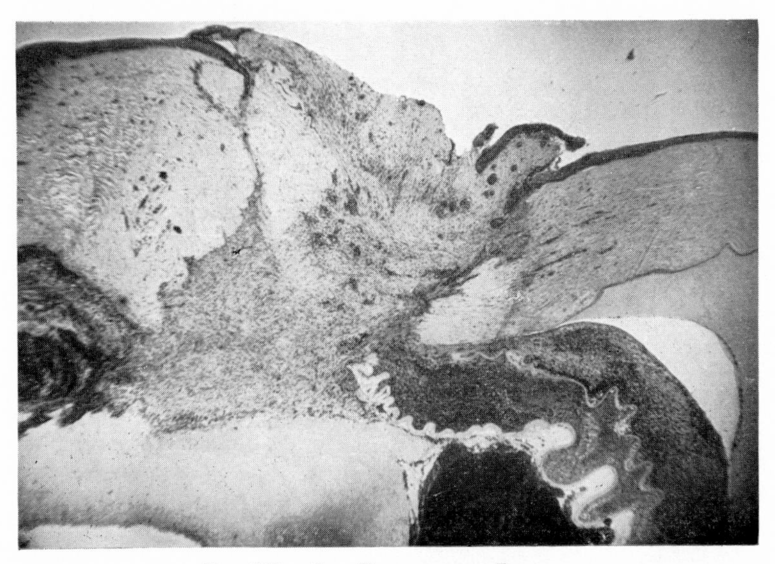

FIG. 290.—OLD PERFORATING INJURY.

The section shows a mal-apposed corneal wound covered by a conjunctival flap from which there is fibrous-tissue proliferation extending into the anterior chamber, where it joins with a dense cyclitic membrane in which remnants of the cataractous lens and its capsule are embedded (H. & E.; ×28) (N. Ashton).

replace damaged corneal stroma and heal a wound therein. The process closely resembles growth in a tissue-culture, and on occasion so virile and tempestuous is the proliferation of this tissue in the favourable milieu provided within the eye that immense damage occurs which may eventually result in the destruction of the globe. Quite commonly this exuberant growth spans the anterior chamber and spreads itself over the iris; it may clothe the posterior surface of the cornea and block the angle of the anterior chamber (Fig. 288); if the lens is wounded it may traverse the substance and at the same time cover the anterior and posterior surfaces of this issue (Figs. 287–290); and it may occasionally penetrate to the posterior parts of the eye.

In the meantime, violent inflammatory and exudative changes are usually absent from the uveal tissues, for the iris and ciliary body, encased in the mass of regenerative tissue, remain relatively passive and suffer slow atrophy; but chronic irritative changes eventually ensue, the contraction of the newly formed tissue pulls upon the corneal scar, flattening and depressing it and deforming the globe until it becomes atrophic or is removed in fear of the development of sympathetic ophthalmitis or because of the onset of a recalcitrant secondary glaucoma due to the embarrassment of its drainage channels.

THE INCARCERATION OF INTRA-OCULAR TISSUES IN THE WOUND

As would be expected, a perforating wound of the cornea is very frequently complicated by the incarceration of one or more of the intra-ocular tissues which are swept between its lips with the rush of escaping aqueous humour. If left to its own devices this incarcerated tissue consolidates with the fibrous tissue formed in the regeneration of the cornea to form a dense opaque mass (an ADHERENT LEUCOMA) which, although it aids in the mechanical closure of the wound initially, may lead eventually to chronic irritative changes which may well endanger the safety of the eye (Plate XIII, Fig. 5).

INCARCERATION OF THE IRIS is the most common event. This tissue is either caught in the posterior part of the wound to form an ANTERIOR SYNECHIA (Figs. 280 and 291) or is carried outwards to protrude from the wound as a PROLAPSE OF THE IRIS (Plate XIII, Fig. 1); such a prolapse may involve a portion of the body of the iris which then protrudes as a knuckle, or the free margin of the iris in which case a tag hangs freely over the cornea. A small marginal wound may thus involve the incarceration of a localized portion of the iris to form a *partial synechia* or prolapse which, when the anterior chamber re-forms, puts the iris under considerable tension creating a pear-shaped pupil, incidentally thereby acting as a constant source of irritation; alternatively, in a large or central wound the entire pupillary margin may be involved so that a *total synechia* results, the pupil becomes completely occluded and the whole or the greater part of the iris is incorporated in the corneal scar, with grave consequences to the future of the eye and to vision (Figs. 296–7).

If the iris remains in contact with the wound it is at first glued down with a greyish-yellow, exudative coagulum which renders the wound water-tight so that the anterior chamber re-forms. Eventually it becomes firmly fixed with newly formed granulation and then fibrous tissue, the corneal epithelium rapidly grows over the surface and a PSEUDO-CORNEA eventually results in which iridic elements become blended with corneal to form a uniform mass in which only the pigmentary layer of the posterior

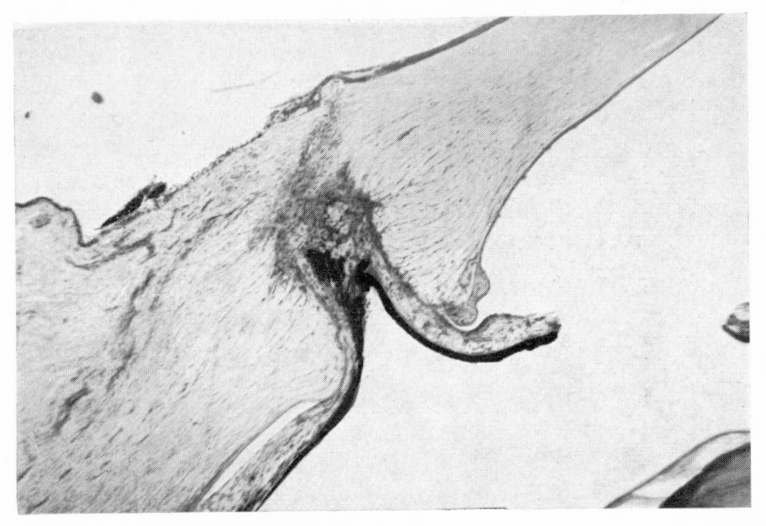

FIG. 291.—PERFORATING WOUND OF THE CORNEA.

The middle third of the iris is deeply incarcerated between the lips of the corneal wound (H. & E.; ×53) (N. Ashton).

surface of the iris retains its individuality. Meantime at the margins of the wound the endothelium proliferates as spindle-shaped cells with rod-shaped nuclei which are reflected over the surface of the iris, secreting a cuticular membrane simultaneously with their growth, so that at the margin of the synechia Descemet's membrane may eventually appear to pass over onto the surface of the iris or to split at the edge of the adhesion to form more than one layer.

A loss of the iris constituting a type of traumatic aniridia is a great rarity after a perforating wound. An interesting case was reported by Wagenaar (1952) wherein an assailant's finger nail perforated the eyeball, hitched onto the iris and subsequently drew it out; it was found prolapsed into the subconjunctival tissue. In the globe, no trace of iris tissue remained and after the total hyphæma had absorbed the vision returned to normal (Fig. 292). Additional cases of traumatic aniridia have been described by Hermann (1954), Kelly (1955) and Papapanos (1958) (Fig. 67).

INCARCERATION OF THE LENS AND ITS CAPSULE in the wound is less common, and is practically always associated with a prolapse of the iris. In the most favourable cases when the wound is small and the capsule itself is uninjured, the opening may be occluded by a prolapse of the lens which becomes gummed to the back of the cornea by a coagulum. Here it may remain and a *subcapsular cataract* may develop at the site of the adhesion, and on occasion the corneal endothelium has grown over the surface of the lens secreting a cuticular layer corresponding to Descemet's membrane so that the lens becomes clothed with two membranes, this newly formed structure of endothelial origin and the other, the true capsule, lined by cubical epithelium. Alternatively, as the anterior chamber is re-formed, the exudate which binds it to the cornea may be stretched so that separation of the two tissues ensues, an *anterior polar cataract* marking the original site

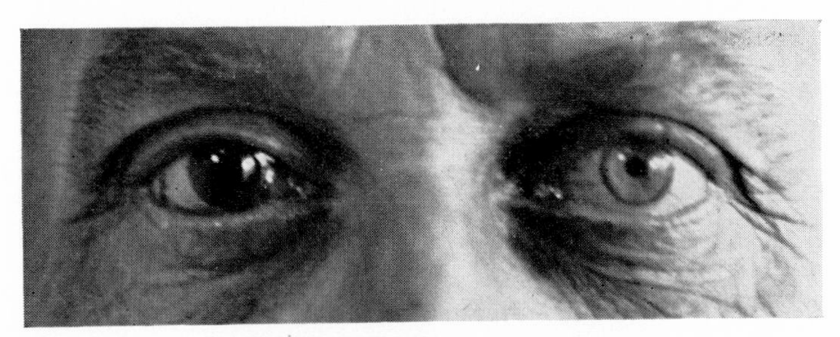

FIG. 292.—TRAUMATIC ANIRIDIA.

After rupture of the right eye by a blow from a hand in which a finger nail perforated the globe. Apart from the loss of the iris the eye was not irretrievably damaged. Corrected vision finally was 5/5 (J. W. Wagenaar).

of apposition opposite the corneal scar; in the worst cases, of course, the entire lens may be extruded and lost.

More usually, however, in perforating injuries the lens capsule is torn, in which case it may prolapse into the wound. There it may remain inert for some time and the most serious immediate effect is the obstruction thus caused to the normal healing of the wound and the stimulus given to epithelial ingrowth[1] (Fig. 293). Eventually, however, the retention of capsule within the wound tends to result in a persistent and intractable iridocyclitis. If the lens substance is also wounded the incarceration of cortical matter excites a much more violent reaction, acting as a potent stimulus to the exuberant proliferation of regenerative fibrous tissue from the corneal stroma (Fig. 290); a firm scar may then rapidly consolidate, but frequently the reparative elements proliferate exuberantly into the substance of the lens, this tissue swells and undergoes partial absorption, and the whole mass eventually becomes bound to the wound with a thick zone of granulation

[1] Tooke (1914), Collins (1914), Corrado (1931), Terry *et al.* (1939).

FIGS. 293 AND 294.—WOUNDS OF THE CORNEA AND LENS (N. Ashton).

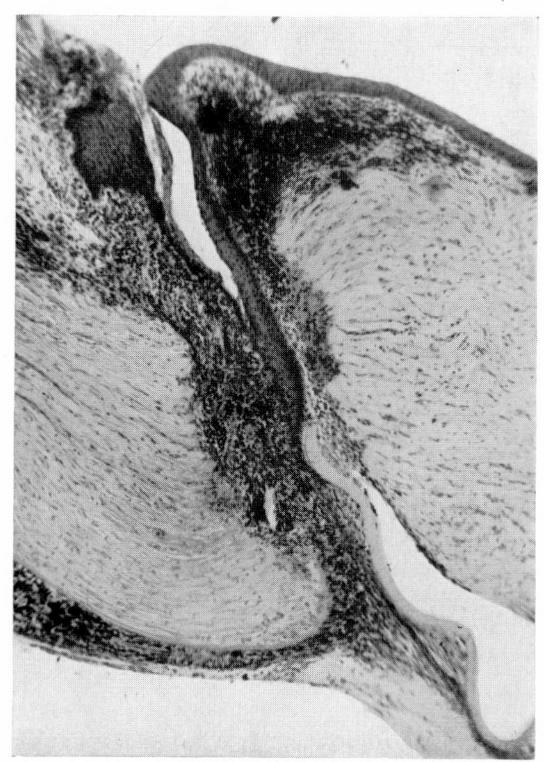

FIG. 293.—Situated in the region of the corneo-scleral junction there is an old gaping operation wound into which the lens capsule has prolapsed. The surrounding tissue is densely infiltrated with plasma cells and lymphocytes; the corneal epithelium has grown into the outer two-thirds of the wound (H. & E.).

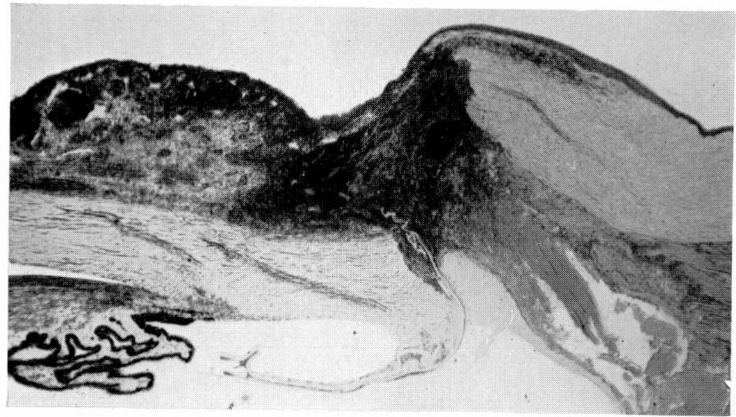

FIG. 294.—Non-united perforating wound of the cornea. The gap is filled with granulation tissue and remnants of the damaged lens have been drawn into the wound (H. & E.).

and fibrous tissue containing multi-nucleated giant cells in which the convoluted capsule is usually discernible (Figs. 293–4).

INCARCERATION OF THE VITREOUS INTO THE WOUND occurs when the zonule is ruptured or the lens is absent. It has a variable effect, but always delays healing. If the vitreous is fluid, this effect is slight when the edges of the wound are in apposition, but if the gel is intact, the reaction is considerable and resembles that caused by lens substance. The adherent vitreous stimulates fibroblastic formation from the cornea and is freely invaded by these cells so that a dense scar may result sometimes extending backwards by bands of fibrous tissue radiating from the wound; such a new formation tends to perpetuate an irritative iridocyclitis and frequently results in a localized area of corneal œdema which persists with the recurrent formation of large epithelial bullæ which repeatedly break down (DELAYED TRAUMATIC BULLOUS KERATOPATHY) (Fig. 295).

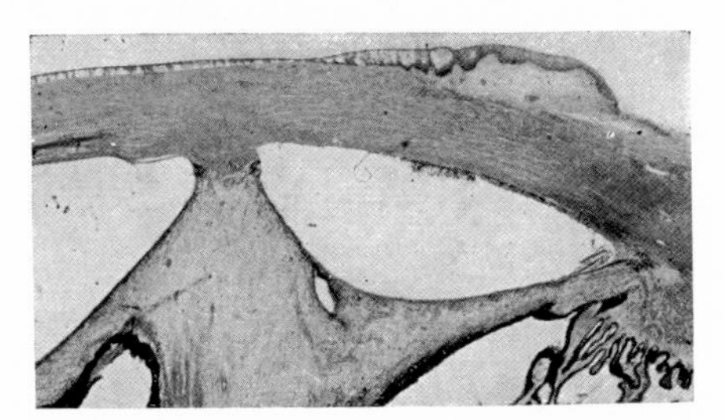

FIG. 295.—GROSS CORNEAL ŒDEMA.

In an old perforating wound complicated by synechiae of the iris and vitreous. The whole epithelium is grossly œdematous and desquamating ($\times$ 10·5) (J. H. Parsons).

In more extensive lesions the CILIARY BODY, the CHOROID and the RETINA may become widely detached after expulsion of the lens and incarcerated in the wound or even prolapsed out of the globe (Figs. 296–301); in such cases, of course, the damage to the eye is irreparable. Such an accident is greatly facilitated if there has been a considerable hæmorrhage within the eye, and if this has been so extensive as to assume the proportions of an *expulsive hœmorrhage* much of the intra-ocular structures may be extruded through the wound with the blood (Fig. 302).

ECTASIAS AND STAPHYLOMATA

In an extensive corneal wound when the edges have not remained in apposition, considerable stretching may occur before the scar-tissue finally consolidates. If the resultant scar is formed of corneal tissue alone, it is termed an ECTASIA; if, as usually happens, the wound is complicated by the incarceration of uveal tissue, the ectatic cicatrix thus formed is termed a STAPHYLOMA (σταφυλή, a bunch of grapes), so called from the tendency of the dark uveal tissue to shine through and the frequent occurrence of lobulation owing to the uneven contraction of fibrous bands. More rarely

FIGS. 296 to 299.—PERFORATING OCULAR WOUNDS.
(Museum, Inst. Ophthal.)

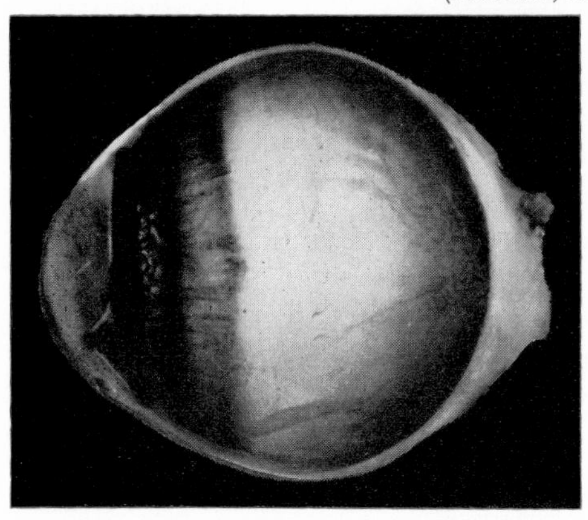

FIG. 296.

There is a tent-like anterior synechia at the site of perforation, causing occlusion of the angle which resulted in secondary glaucoma. The lens has been entirely absorbed.

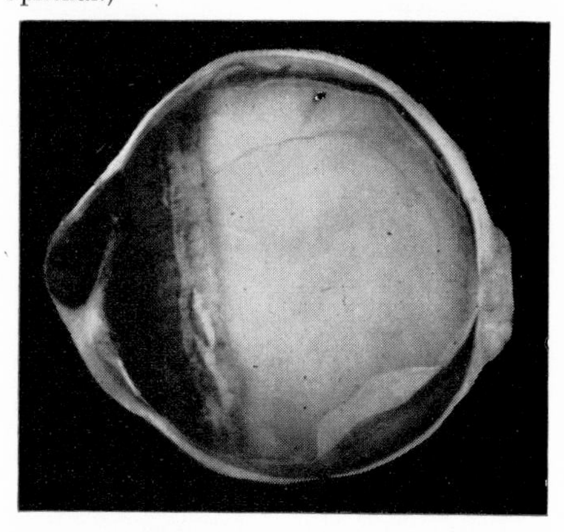

FIG. 297.

Resulting in a dense central corneal scar, adherent to which are the remains of the lens. The cornea is completely lined by iris tissue and is distended above the wound to form a corneal staphyloma. The obliteration of the anterior chamber resulted in a secondary glaucoma.

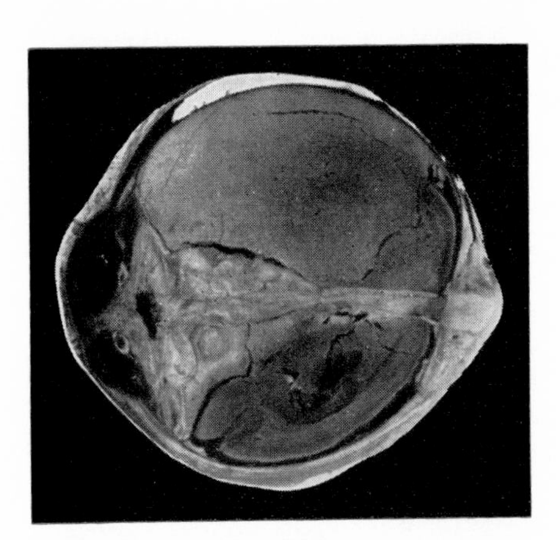

FIG. 298.

To the wound is adherent a mass of fibrous tissue in which are embedded the remains of the iris and the lens. The anterior chamber is obliterated by total adhesion of the iris to the cornea. There is a total retinal detachment and the posterior part of the globe is filled with blood clot.

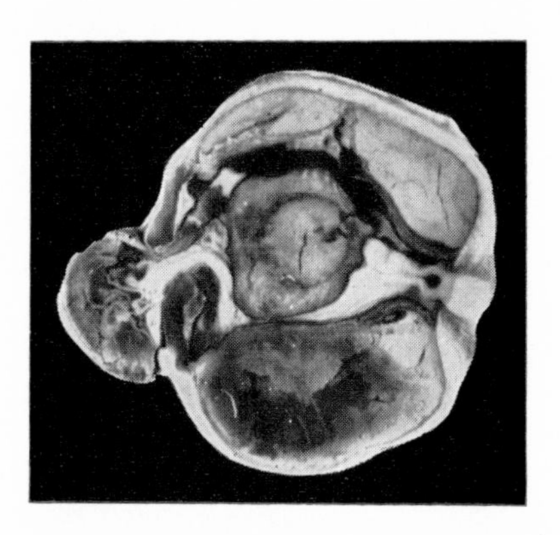

FIG. 299.

In a child of 9, from a penknife. The globe is disorganized and through the wound protrudes a mass of uveal and retinal tissue, the folds of which can be readily seen embedded in blood clot. The whole of the inner eye is occupied by hæmorrhagic clots.

FIGS. 300 AND 301.—PERFORATING WOUNDS OF THE CORNEA AND LENS (N. Ashton).

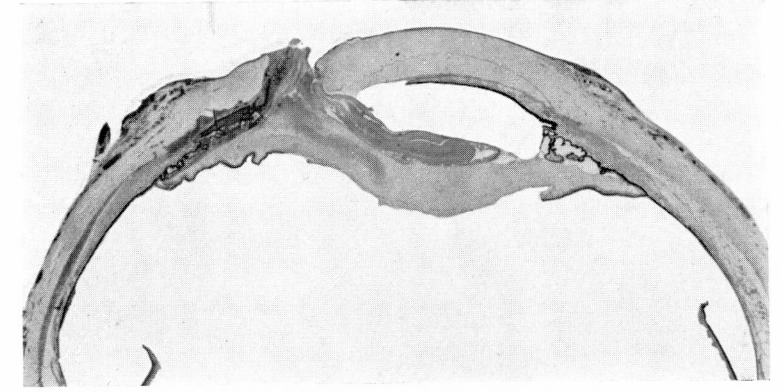

FIG. 300.—There is a widely gaping wound of the peripheral cornea through which a mass of uveal tissue, soft lens material and vitreous is protruding (H. & E.).

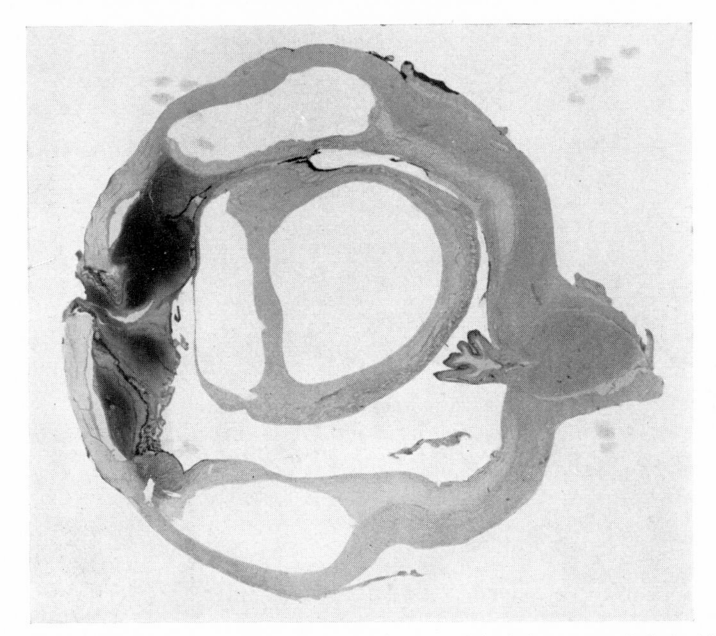

FIG. 301.—There is a prolapse of uveal tissue and incipient panophthalmitis.

cicatrization is so rapid and dense that it can withstand the intra-ocular pressure and the cornea becomes flattened or even indented by the contraction of fibrous bands (APPLANATIO CORNEÆ), or rapidly degenerative changes take place so that the whole tissue shrinks into a small contracted and shrunken scar (PHTHISIS CORNEÆ).

A CORNEAL ECTASIA, while relatively common as a result of the softening of the tissues which follows ulceration or degenerative processes, is rare after trauma, in which case it usually follows a small perforating or punctured wound. Such a result, for example, following a perforation by a hat-pin whereafter a conical deformity developed, was described by Würdemann (1894).

CORNEAL STAPHYLOMATA, on the other hand, are common and may involve a portion or the whole of the cornea (Figs. 297, 303 and 304). Their pathological development has been most comprehensively studied by Fuchs (1918). In the earliest stages the staphyloma is composed merely of prolapsed iris directly covered with epithelium. Eventually the proliferating epithelium fills all the crevices available to it and usually becomes much

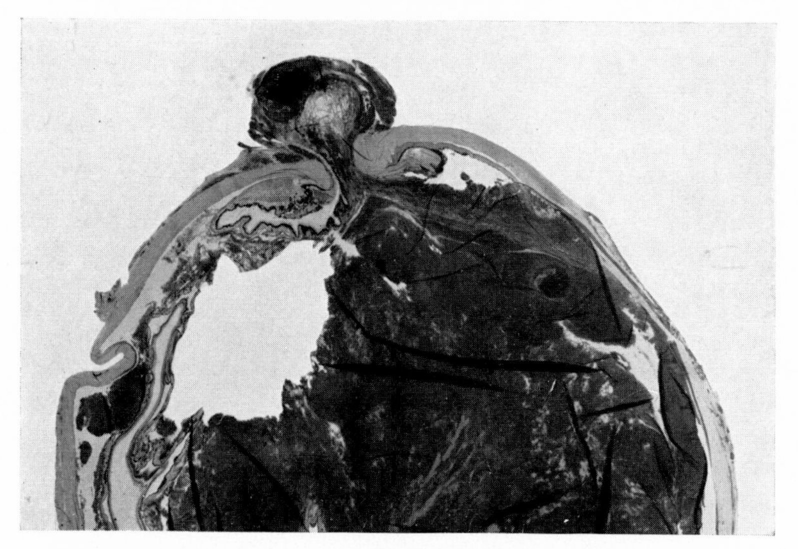

FIG. 302.—EXPULSIVE HÆMORRHAGE.

There is a gaping perforating wound in the region of the limbus. Within the eye there has been an expulsive hæmorrhage; the blood fills up the vitreous cavity and has poured through the wound from which a mass of uveal tissue protrudes. The lens has been extruded from the eye. The dark folds in the mass of blood-clot are artefacts (H. & E.) (N. Ashton).

thickened, sending numerous downgrowths into the tissue underneath. Meantime an intense inflammation of the iris sets in, its tissues become packed with leucocytes, granulation tissue forms sometimes in large masses on its surface, and this gradually develops into scar-tissue merging with similar tissue derived from the cornea, binding the whole mass with any remnants of the lens or its capsule which may be incarcerated into a fibrous PSEUDO-CORNEA. As time goes on the iris stroma gradually atrophies and is replaced by fibrous tissue, while the pigmentary epithelium breaks down and pigment granules are taken up by leucocytes and travel into the epithelium or become embedded in the scar-tissue where they remain sometimes for years, sometimes permanently. The thickness of the staphyloma varies

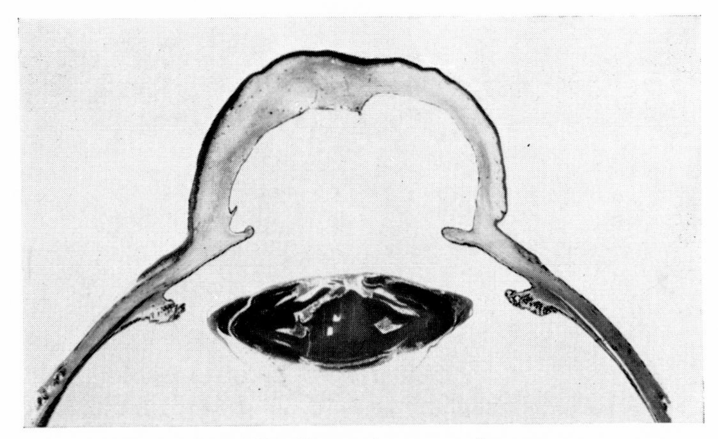

Fig. 303.—Total Anterior Staphyloma.

In an agricultural worker, following an infected wound with chaff while threshing (N. Ashton).

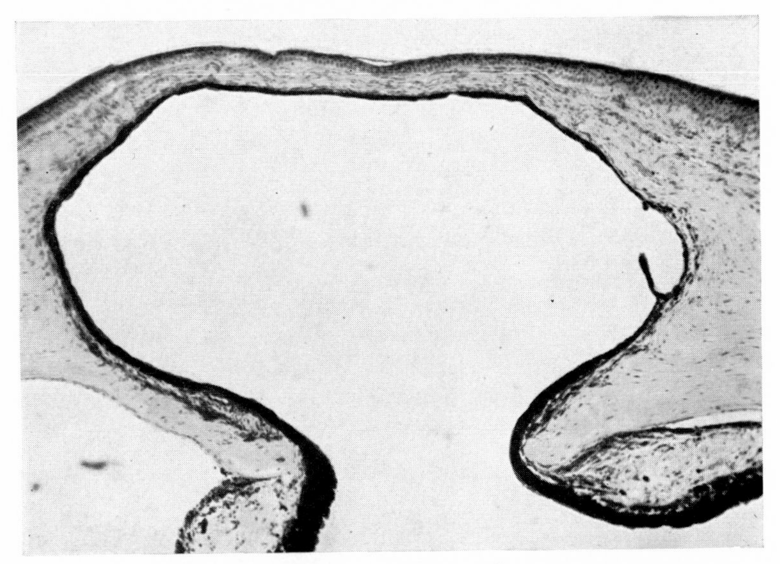

Fig. 304.—Localized Anterior Staphyloma.

Localized anterior staphyloma following injury. The staphyloma communicates with the anterior chamber through a narrow neck (below); it is lined with degenerate iris tissue from which the thin anterior wall is formed (H. & E.) (N. Ashton).

with the amount of scar-tissue thus formed; the pseudo-cornea may be immensely thick or thin as paper where the epithelium grows directly over the prolapsed iris with the interposition of a minimal amount of granulation tissue. In this event the scar-tissue may not be strong enough to withstand the intra-ocular pressure, so that the bulging increases. When it is thin the uveal pigment becomes more obvious so that, depending on the thickness, the

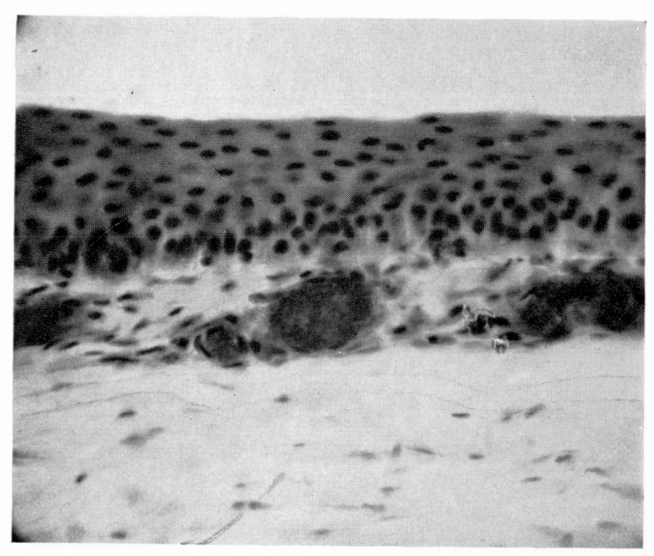

Fig. 305.—Traumatic Degenerative Pannus.

Pannus degenerativus in a case of perforating corneal injury. A mass of vascularized new-formed connective tissue is seen lying upon Bowman's membrane under a thickened epithelium (H. & E.; ×333) (N. Ashton).

colour may vary from slate-grey to a deep blue-black, and since great differences may occur in the same staphyloma, bulging dark areas may be separated by retracted fibrous bands giving a picture justifying the name of a " bunch of grapes ".

Degenerative changes are prone to occur in the course of time in such staphylomatous corneæ—vascularization to form a degenerative pannus (Fig. 305), a thickening and cornification of the epithelium which may show papillary downgrowths so that it assumes an epidermoid appearance (Fig. 306), and changes such as hyaline or calcareous degeneration in the sub-

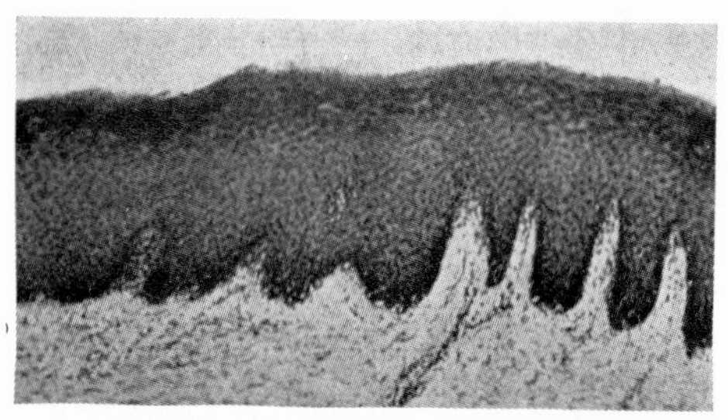

Fig. 306.—Cornification of the Epithelium in an Anterior Staphyloma.

The eye was injured 12 years previously and a dense anterior staphyloma formed. The corneal epithelium is typically epidermoid with well-marked true papillæ. The superficial cells are corneous and devoid of nuclei; the layer below this contains granules of kerato-hyalin. Note the large blood vessels in the connective tissue of the pseudo-cornea (×55) (J. H. Parsons).

stance of the pseudo-cornea. Such an eye rarely remains quiet indefinitely; there is a tendency for the formation of torpid atheromatous ulcers, frequently associated with recurrent attacks of inflammation which may eventually involve considerable necrosis and sloughing, a progressive process which may ultimately terminate in panophthalmitis (Fuchs, 1902).

CYSTOID CICATRIX: CORNEAL FISTULA

Occasionally in the healing of a corneal wound which is complicated by the incarceration of uveal tissue, when the scar-tissue is minimal or remains loosely arranged, spaces are left, the anterior walls of which are frequently formed by epithelium and the posterior by the pigment layer of the iris. Such an area may not be strong enough to withstand the intra-ocular pressure, in which event the cicatrix becomes progressively more thin and ectatic in this region and the uveal pigment almost invariably shines through. In this event the aqueous may percolate the iridic tissue, fill up the cystoid spaces in the scar and persistently leak under the epithelium making it œdematous and sometimes forming bullæ underneath it (a CYSTOID CICATRIX). At other times as the aqueous seeps through the loose scar-tissue of the cicatrix, it eventually bursts through the epithelium to form a CORNEAL FISTULA, the opening of which may be so small that it readily escapes detection; the anterior chamber is lost and, as the intra-ocular pressure falls profoundly, the fistula closes again; as the pressure rises, a bleb is again formed showing up as a small dark point in the white scar-tissue and again bursts; and so the cycle is repeated until it is ended by the development of an intra-ocular infection or a hæmorrhage. An adherent iris is the almost invariable accompaniment of such a fistula (Czermak, 1890–91; Oguchi, 1909)—perhaps the pull of the iris sometimes prevents consolidation. In such a fistula a downgrowth of epithelium is facilitated, in which case the track becomes permanent and complete cicatrization is prevented unless the epithelium is destroyed; at the same time the epithelium may invade the globe and line the iris resulting in the development of a recalcitrant secondary glaucoma.[1]

PERFORATING CORNEO-SCLERAL WOUNDS

Wounds near the limbus show the same processes of healing as are found in the cornea and the sclera with the exception that the epithelial plug which fills the open anterior triangle in a corneal wound is partially replaced by a mass of highly vascularized granulation tissue derived from the episclera; the same process occurs when the healing of a corneal wound occurs underneath a conjunctival flap. The size of such a plug depends upon the degree of apposition of the lips of the wound, and if this is poor the granulation and fibrous tissues thus formed may not only fill the hiatus but may grow exuberantly and extend through the wound into the anterior

[1] Vol. XI, p. 719.

chamber where they blend with incarcerated uveal or lenticular tissue (Fig. 307). Such wounds are liable to be complicated with a massive prolapse of important ocular tissues, the ciliary body, vitreous, and even the retina being not infrequently drawn into the scar or suffering prolapse—a circumstance, of course, which frequently jeopardizes the fate of the eye. Apart from the immediate traumatic disorganization thus produced, such a wound, if its edges are badly apposed, tends to develop into an intercalary staphylomatous scar or a cystoid cicatrix through which the aqueous oozes out

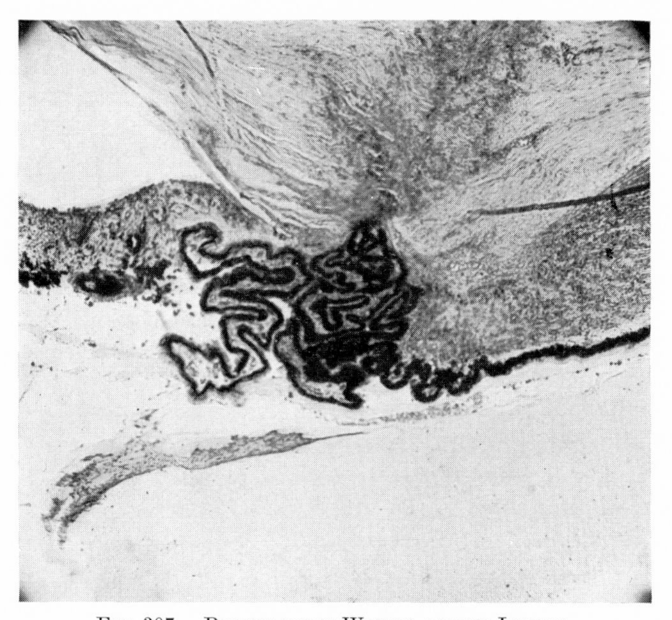

Fig. 307.—Perforating Wound at the Limbus.

There is a scar of a perforating wound of the sclera in the region of the limbus, infiltrated by chronic inflammatory cells. Some of the ciliary processes are incarcerated in the posterior lips of the wound (H. & E.; ×48) (N. Ashton).

under the conjunctiva, raising it up in an œdematous bleb; a recalcitrant post-traumatic iridocyclitis is not unusual, and when the injury involves the ciliary region a sympathetic ophthalmitis is prone to result.

PERFORATING SCLERAL WOUNDS

We have already seen[1] that if a scleral wound is uncomplicated and its edges remain apposed, infection is rare, healing is rapid, the resultant scar is inconspicuous and function is unimpaired. If, however, the wound gapes and if uveal or retinal tissue is incarcerated, as is almost invariably the case, complications arise. Initially the uveal tissues become heavily infiltrated with leucocytes and other inflammatory cells, and shortly there-

[1] Vol. VIII, p. 996.

FIGS. 308 to 310.—PERFORATING WOUNDS OF THE SCLERA.

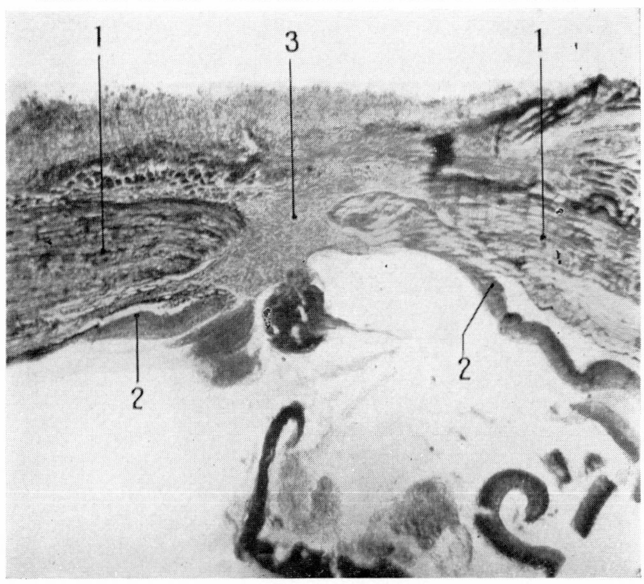

FIG. 308.—Showing excessive fibrous proliferation at an early stage. Eight days after an injury to a young rabbit. The cut ends of the sclera are sharply defined (1,1) and the gap is filled by a proliferation of fibrous tissue from the episclera and subconjunctiva (3). From this tissue fibroblasts are beginning to spread into the cavity of the eye in a process of excessive regeneration. In the eye there are traces of hæmorrhage and in the region of the wound the retina is swollen and œdematous (2) (G. Renard *et al.*).

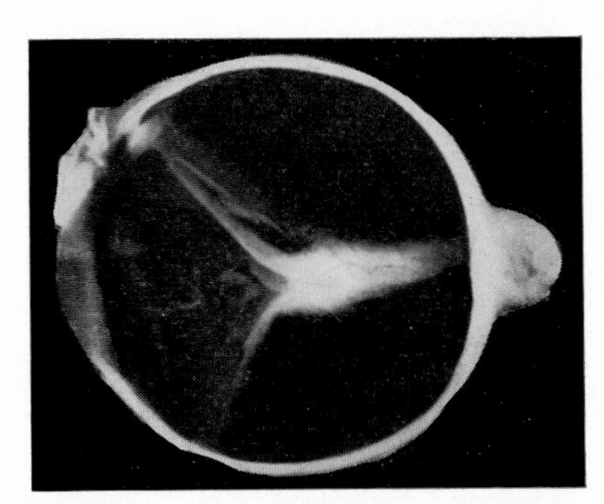

FIG. 309.—After perforation with a piece of iron there was a prolapse of iris and ciliary body which was excised and covered with a conjunctival flap. Five months later the eye was excised. Uveal tissue is incarcerated in the wound, the lens is absorbed and there is a complete cicatricial detachment of the retina (Museum, Inst. Ophthal.).

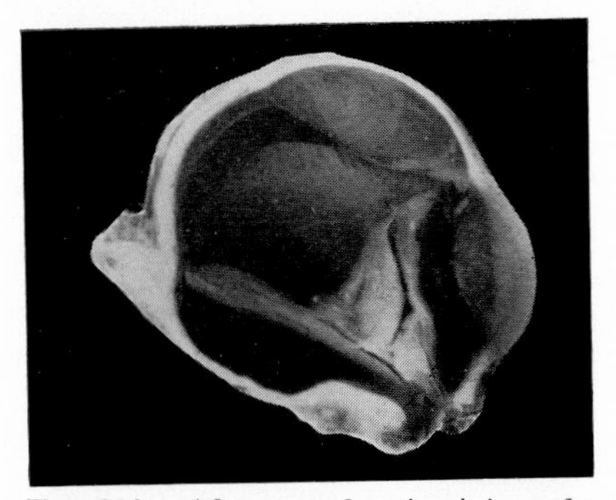

FIG. 310.—After a perforating injury there have developed a complete retinal detachment, which has become incarcerated in the wound, and an extensive detachment of the choroid (Museum, Inst. Ophthal.).

after the vascular elements of the ciliary body or the choroid throw out fibroblasts which permeate the blood clot filling the wound, mingling with the reparative elements supplied by the episcleral and scleral tissues and thus increasing the amount of organizing tissue so that the uvea is incorporated into the mass of granulations forming the scar; the process thus resembles an anterior staphyloma (Fig. 308). If the edges of the wound are nearly apposed, this activity may be localized; but the pigmented cells of the uvea usually proliferate, the pigment granules being profusely scattered

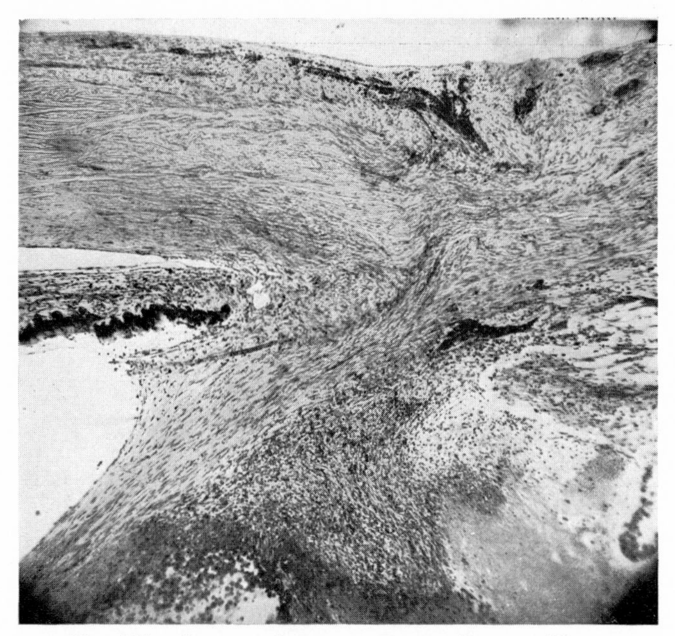

Fig. 311.—Stromal Overgrowth in a Scleral Wound.

Immediately in front of the ora serrata there is the healed scar of a perforating wound of the sclera and ciliary body from which a fibrous proliferation extends into the vitreous space (H. & E.; ×48) (N. Ashton).

throughout the scar, some of them intracellular but most of them lying free in the meshes of the scar-tissue or engulfed in phagocytic cells. Meantime the retina is essentially inert but becomes fused in the scar-tissue, and the end-result after 3 or 4 weeks is the formation of a fibrous scar in which the conjunctiva, sclera, uvea and retina are fused together; this, when the new-formed vessels are obliterated, eventually consists merely of layers of imbricated spindle cells closely packed together interspersed with particles of pigment. Subsequent contraction, of course, may lead to a retinal detachment, a complication more prone to occur if the injury has entailed a loss of vitreous (Figs. 309 and 310).

At other times, however, particularly if mal-apposition of the edges of the wound has occurred, this reparative process runs amok. Just as may happen in the cornea, the new-formed fibrous tissue, here reinforced profusely by fibroblastic elements from the episclera and uvea, may grow exuberantly from the wound over the inner surface of the retina and extend far into the vitreous, sending out long proliferative processes forwards to the ciliary body and backwards towards the optic disc, a process which may lead to a chronic uveitis, massive detachment of the retina and eventually to shrinkage and atrophy of the globe (Michel, 1890; Levkoieva, 1947; Renard *et al.*, 1952) (Figs. 308 and 311).

Alexiadès. *Arch. Ophtal.*, **37,** 554 (1920).
Andreae. *Der postoperative Astigmatismus nach Staroperationen* (Diss.), Marburg (1923).
Aschheim. *Klin. Mbl. Augenheilk.*, **35,** 108 (1897).
Ashton and Cook. *Brit. J. Ophthal.*, **35,** 708 (1951).
Berliner. *Amer. J. Ophthal.*, **34,** 899 (1951).
Calhoun. *Trans. Amer. Acad. Ophthal.*, **54,** 498 (1949).
Amer. J. Ophthal., **61,** 1055 (1966).
Clarke. *Trans. ophthal. Soc. U.K.*, **18,** 307 (1898).
Clausnizer. *Klin. Mbl. Augenheilk.*, **49** (2), 434 (1911).
Collins. *Trans. ophthal. Soc. U.K.*, **11,** 133 (1891); **12,** 64 (1892); **34,** 21 (1914).
Collins and Cross. *Trans. ophthal. Soc. U.K.*, **12,** 175 (1892).
Corrado. *Ann. Ottal.*, **59,** 706 (1931).
Custodis. *Klin. Mbl. Augenheilk.*, **89,** 612 (1932).
Czermak. *v. Graefes Arch. Ophthal.*, **36** (2), 163 (1890); **37** (2), 58 (1891).
Donders. *On the Anomalies of Accommodation and Refraction of the Eye*, London (1864).
Dunnington. *Amer. J. Ophthal.*, **34,** 36 (1951).
Dunnington and Regan. *Arch. Ophthal.*, **43,** 407 (1950).
Amer. J. Ophthal., **35,** 167 (1952).
Elschnig. *Klin. Mbl. Augenheilk.*, **41** (1), 247 (1903).
Fazakas. *Orvosi Hetil.*, **76,** 776 (1932).
Z. Augenheilk., **88,** 315 (1936).
Fuchs. *Trans. ophthal. Soc. U.K.*, **22,** 15 (1902).
v. Graefes Arch. Ophthal., **53,** 61 (1902); **95,** 215 (1918).
Gördüren and Tosunoglu. *Göz. Klin.*, **9,** 27 (1951).
Guaita. *Arch. Ophtal.*, **13,** 507 (1893).
Henderson. *Ophthal. Rev.*, **26,** 127 (1907).
Hermann. *Bull. Soc. Ophtal. Fr.*, 474 (1954).
Janiszewska-Zygier. *Klin. oczna*, **36,** 613 (1966).
Kelly. *Trans. Canad. ophthal. Soc.*, **7,** 335 (1955).
Kümmell. *Klin. Mbl. Augenheilk.*, **45,** 421 (1907).
Kuhl. *Klin. Mbl. Augenheilk.*, **157,** 810 (1970).
Laqueur. *v. Graefes Arch. Ophthal.*, **30** (1), 99 (1884).
Leibowitz, Elliott and Boruchoff. *Arch. Ophthal.*, **78,** 613 (1967).
Levkoieva. *Brit. J. Ophthal.*, **31,** 336 (1947).
van Lint. *Bull. Soc. franç. Ophtal.*, **31,** 448 (1914).
Maggiore. *Ann. Ottal.*, **68,** 481, 561, 641, 721, 881 (1940); **69,** 1, 65 (1941).
Maumenee. *Trans. Amer. ophthal. Soc.*, **62,** 153 (1964).
Meller. *v. Graefes Arch. Ophthal.*, **52,** 436 (1901).
Michaïl. *Ann. Ottal.*, **60,** 553 (1932).
Michel. *Lhb. d. Augenheilkunde*, Wiesbaden, 695 (1890).
Morax and Duverger. *Ann. Oculist.* (Paris), **141,** 1 (1909).
Nagano. *Arch. Augenheilk.*, **65,** 116 (1910).
Oguchi. *v. Graefes Arch. Ophthal.*, **70,** 88 (1909).
Papapanos. *Klin. Mbl. Augenheilk.*, **132.** 256 (1958).
Papolczy. *Klin. Mbl. Augenheilk.*, **84,** 266 (1930).
Parsons. *Pathology of the Eye*, London, **1,** 151 (1904).
Paul. *Klin. Mbl. Augenheilk.*, **144,** 723 (1964).
Perera. *Trans. Amer. Acad. Ophthal.*, **42,** 142 (1937).
Petersen and Raagaard. *Ugeskr. f. Laeger*, **113,** 753 (1951).
Purtscher. *v. Graefes Arch. Ophthal.*, **144,** 669 (1942).
Renard, Lelièvre and Naneix. *Arch. Ophtal.*, **12,** 5 (1952).
Reuss and Woinow. *Ophthalmometrische Studien*, Wien (1869).
Rodewald. *Drei Fälle v. Bissverletzungen d. Auges* (Diss.), Kiel (1896).
Salus. *Klin. Mbl. Augenheilk.*, **78,** 368 (1927).
Samuels. *Acta. XVII int. Cong. Ophthal.*, Montreal, **3,** 1481 (1954).
Schmidt-Rimpler. *Klin. Mbl. Augenheilk.*, **13,** 315 (1875).
Seefried. *Wien. klin. Wschr.*, **63,** 210 (1951).
Seidel. *v. Graefes Arch. Ophthal.*, **84,** 312 (1913).
Speciale-Cirincione. *Atti Cong. Soc. ital. oftal.*, 180 (1924).
Stölting. *v. Graefes Arch. Ophthal.*, **31** (3), 99 (1885).

Suzuki. *Acta Soc. ophthal. jap.*, **38**, 553 (1934).
Terry, Chisholm and Schonberg. *Amer. J. Ophthal.*, **22**, 1083 (1939).
Theobald and Haas. *Trans. Amer. Acad. Ophthal.*, **53**, 470 (1948).
Tichomirov. *Vestn. oftal.*, **27** (1), 22 (1948).
Tooke. *Trans. Amer. ophthal. Soc.*, **13**, 742 (1914).
Treutler. *Z. Augenheilk.*, **3**, 484 (1900).
Tron. *Klin. Mbl. Augenheilk.*, **75**, 333 (1925).
Vail. *Arch. Ophthal.*, **15**, 270 (1936).
Wagenaar. *Ophthalmologica*, **124**, 193 (1952).
Weinstein. *Arch. Augenheilk.*, **48**, 1 (1903).
Wintersteiner. *Ber. dtsch. ophthal. Ges.*, **28**, 4 (1900).
Wood. *Brit. J. Ophthal.*, **16**, 546 (1932).
Würdemann. *Ann. Ophthal. Otol.*, **3**, 372 (1894).

Wounds of the Intra-ocular Tissues

From the pathological point of view perforating injuries, whether caused by the entrance into the globe of a sharp instrument or a body travelling at a velocity sufficiently high to penetrate the ocular coats, may wound any of the ocular tissues each of which reacts with individual peculiarities.

WOUNDS OF THE IRIS are unique in the paucity of the reaction which they excite, a characteristic well seen in the complete lack of change throughout the remainder of life in the wound of an iridectomy or in the indefinite persistence of a punctate hole which marks the track of a foreign body which has traversed this tissue. We have already seen that the iris is eminently capable of forming granulation and scar-tissue in profusion, a phenomenon frequently encountered as a sequel to iritis and constantly evident in the formation of an anterior staphyloma; it may be that its passivity after an aseptic wound is due to the absence of such irritative factors as might excite a reaction while it remains bathed in the aqueous humour to which it is normally freely permeable; alternatively, inhibitory substances may be present in the anterior chamber (Snell, 1955–56). Whatever the cause, hæmorrhage is usually absent or slight owing to the active retraction of the severed blood vessels, and any small amount of blood-clot formed is rapidly absorbed. Thereafter the edges of the wound may become somewhat thickened and retracted owing to the contraction of the posterior layers, but in general the edges remain free, neither the endothelium on the anterior surface nor the epithelium on the posterior makes any attempt to cover the raw area, and there is no evidence of the new formation of fibrous tissue or other sign of reparative activity (Fuchs, 1896; Parsons, 1904; Henderson, 1907; McBurney, 1914; and others).

This passivity occurs either when the wound is small (as in a small perforation which leaves the lens intact, Schoute, 1899) or when extensive damage is caused, such as, for example, when the iris is torn away in whole or in part. A rarer injury is a tearing apart of the posterior pigmentary layer from the mesodermal stroma as is more usually seen after a contusion (Gelpke, 1887; Boerma, 1893; Hack, 1909; and others).

WOUNDS OF THE CILIARY BODY AND CHOROID, on the other hand, display an immediate reaction and considerable reparative activity. This we have already discussed in dealing with perforating scleral wounds so that a full description is not necessary here. The usual reaction of a highly vascularized tissue to the insult of trauma becomes evident. Initially, hæmorrhage is usually considerable, an intense leucocytic infiltration appears at the edges of the wound, new vessels and fibroblasts throw out granulation tissue into the blood-clot and healing ultimately takes place by the consolidation of fibrous tissue in which pigment granules from the proliferated pigmentary epithelium are buried in considerable quantities in a scar in which retina, choroid and sclera are usually fused into a uniform mass. If, however, the wound is extensive, particularly if it involves the ciliary body, progressive cicatrization frequently leads to an irritative uveitis which may be followed by shrinkage of the globe or, on the other hand, excessive proliferation of scar-tissue may lead to equally disastrous results.

WOUNDS OF THE RETINA are dominated by the reparative processes in the choroid usually with the participation of the episclera as well. In the immediate neighbourhood of the wound the nervous elements of the retina show degenerative changes only, the ganglion cells peripheral to the injury undergo degeneration as also do the affected nerve fibres (Tepljaschin, 1894; Parsons, 1903; Collins, 1928) and, as is seen clinically after the formation of a retinal tear, active healing is absent. A secondary gliosis may occasionally occur (Krückmann, 1905; von Hippel, 1918) but any such abortive attempts at proliferation are without essential significance in the reparative process. Mesoblastic retinal elements, however, may participate in the profuse fibrosis derived from the uvea and episclera, and when such newly formed tissue is abundant and spreads widely over and pulls upon the retina, this structure may suffer considerable atrophy and frequently becomes detached.

WOUNDS OF THE LENS: PERFORATING TRAUMATIC CATARACT

Owing to the exposed position of the lens, wounds of this tissue are common in injuries which penetrate the globe and the damage thus caused may vary from a localized or transient opacity caused by a puncture to a complete break-up of the lens substance following a lacerating injury; such damage to the lens is of considerable importance as it exerts a profound influence on the prognosis of the case.

It is not surprising that after a penetrating injury of the globe, typical CONCUSSION CHANGES such as we have already described[1] are frequently seen in the lens, for an injury of this type must almost invariably have a considerable concussive effect. Indeed, in perforating injuries whether caused by cuts or the entry of foreign bodies, Davidson (1940) found that the majority showed lenticular lesions characteristic of the morphology of concussive injuries; in only 7 out of 29 penetrating injuries and 6 out of 33 perforations by intra-ocular foreign bodies where the lens showed traumatic changes was this tissue actually wounded. As a rule the concussion is probably indirect, but occasionally a direct injury may in fact occur in this way as when a penetrating foreign body strikes the capsule of the lens tangentially without perforating it (Michaïl,

[1] p. 121.

1931). It is also to be remembered that when the lens itself is perforated, considerable concussion is involved at the same time, the effects of which are added to those of the actual perforation. Finally, the frequent occurrence of capsular rents in the former type of injury makes the end-results of both often indistinguishable.

LOCALIZED STATIONARY CATARACT

LOCALIZED NON-PROGRESSIVE CHANGES (CATARACTA TRAUMATICA CONSCRIPTIVA) are not uncommon after small puncture injuries such as are inflicted by a perforating needle or thorn, a small foreign body traversing the lens, or in the operation for discission; they are much more common in many lower vertebrates, such as the rabbit, than in man, perhaps because, owing to their lower accommodative power, the capsule is less taut and thus tends to gape less when pierced. Such changes are, however, frequently evident after perforating accidents to the human eye and assume two typical forms—scars in the capsule and opacities in the lens along the track of the wound, and disturbances farther afield, either amorphous or stellate in design, usually in the region of the posterior pole.

CAPSULAR DAMAGE is, of course, invariable in such injuries, but in the stationary type of cataract the hiatus in this membrane seals up before permanent and widespread damage is done, a circumstance which seems to occur with the greatest ease when the puncture wound has traversed the iris so that exudate from this tissue may aid the occlusive process. The mechanism of this healing activity and its histology have already been described in the section on concussion cataract.[1] From the clinical point of view the tear in the capsule at first tends to gape and its edges to roll outwards, while between them the lens fibres sometimes protrude mushroom-like into the anterior chamber (Pagenstecher, 1865; Wagenmann, 1905). If the changes are not progressive, these bulging fibres take on a granular form while the higher magnifications of the slit-lamp may show the presence of a greying halo around the area indicating the deposition of a fibrinous exudate. If healing proceeds, a small cicatrix forms wherein the anterior line of disjunction is lost and around which the capsule may show multiple traction folds (Fig. 312) (Rosen, 1945; and others), while in the neighbourhood radiating lines may accentuate the design of the lens fibres. A wound of the posterior capsule is less dense; from it lens fibres may protrude into the vitreous and on healing it may show a backward concave bulge resembling a posterior lenticonus, sometimes heavily encrusted with opacity (Rosen, 1945).

At a later date degenerative changes may occur in a scar of the anterior capsule, the most typical of which are small blister-like spherules which protrude outwards (Vogt, 1931) (Fig. 313). Such changes indicate an area of weakness and Vogt (1931) recorded the spontaneous rupture of such a scar two years after the original perforating injury with the protrusion of lens masses into the anterior chamber and the rapid development of cataract.

[1] p. 123.

FIGS. 312 AND 313.—THE END-RESULTS OF CAPSULAR WOUNDS.

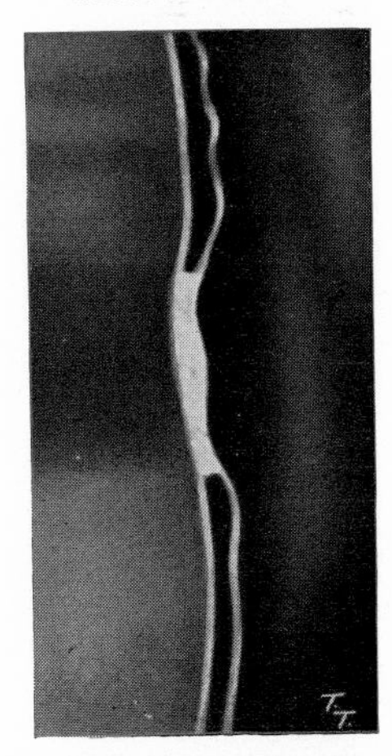

FIG. 312.—Post-traumatic changes, showing a dense capsular scar indenting the lens. There are folds in the capsule around the scar and the anterior line of disjunction disappears at the site of the scar.

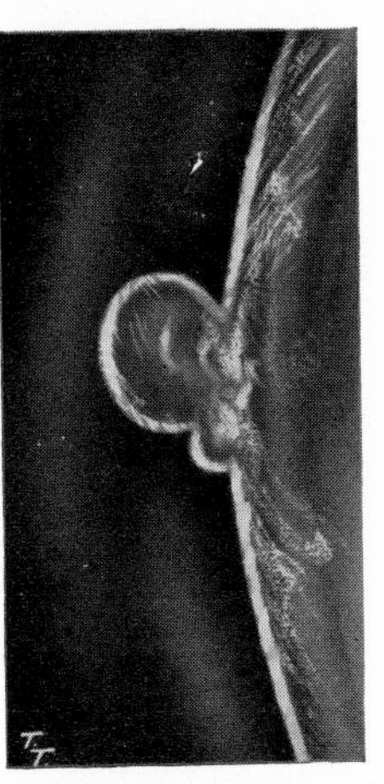

FIG. 313.—Blister-like spherule on the anterior lens capsule, seen in optical section with the slit-lamp.

FIGS. 314 to 316.—PARTIAL STATIONARY TRAUMATIC CATARACTS.

Examples of stationary lenticular opacities following perforating wounds of the lens (after M. Davidson).

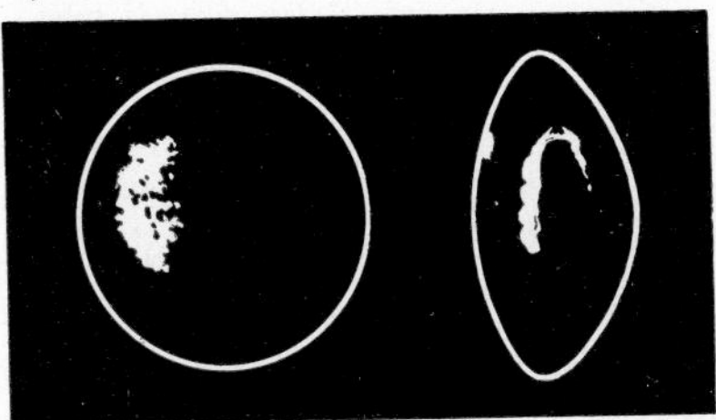

FIG. 314.—A perforating injury of 25 years' standing seen in diffuse illumination and optical section.

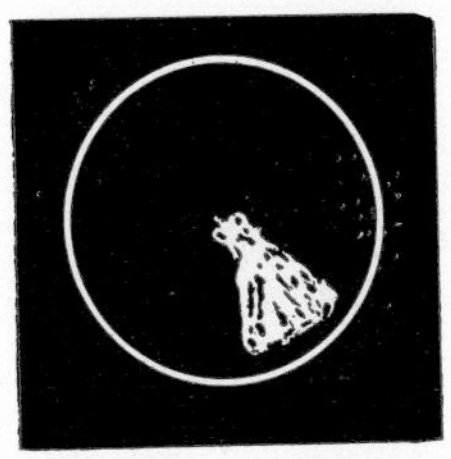

FIG. 315.—A sector-like anterior subcapsular opacity, 1 year after a perforating injury.

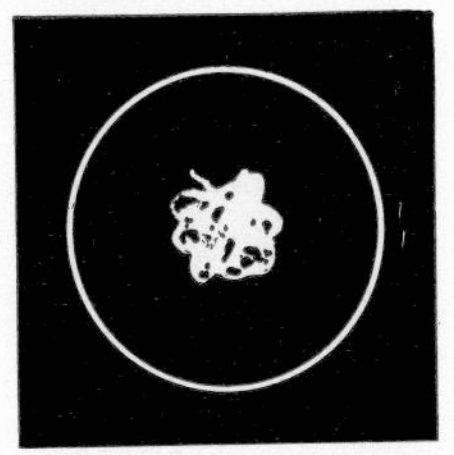

FIG. 316.—Anterior axial rosette-shaped opacity, 2 years after a perforating injury.

LOCALIZED CHANGES IN THE LENS SUBSTANCE along the track of the wound take on many morphological forms, varying from small dots or linear opacities to cloud-like masses of considerable size (Figs. 314–316; Plate XIV). Sometimes the opacities, retaining their sectoral distribution, pass round the equator to the posterior cortex. The track of a perforating injury may be marked out by a localized linear opacity, sometimes the lesion takes on a somewhat characteristic spear-shape, and at other times it is surrounded by a cloud-like haze without sharp delineation which shows no tendency to progress. As a rule such opacities show no pattern of the fibres, vacuoles or fluid-clefts.

At other times more diffuse changes develop in the cortex, usually in the posterior but sometimes in the anterior region, which may disappear after some time leaving the vision and even the accommodation unimpaired. This is an old observation which has been repeatedly verified[1]; in such cases the imbibition of fluid has not led to irreversible changes. The most typical appearance, however, follows the tracery of the lens fibres to form a star-shaped rosette somewhat resembling the rosette cataract seen after a concussion.

ROSETTE (STAR-SHAPED) CATARACT

A frequent sequel of a perforating wound of the lens is a ROSETTE-SHAPED OPACITY occurring in the subcapsular region, sometimes at the anterior but more commonly and typically at the posterior pole, even although the wound is localized anteriorly. This is best seen after a small puncture wound, such as is inflicted by a small foreign body or a needle, wherein the opening through the capsule has become rapidly closed so that diffuse opacification of the lens does not occur, but it is probable that such changes may accompany a generalized opacification of the lens and remain clinically invisible. The rosette is situated axially and, lying in one circumscribed plane, outlines with great clarity the architectural design of the fibres (Fig. 108). The sutures appear dark, and from them radiate grey feathery lines which glitter in focal illumination, forming " petals " of the rosette, and intermingled with them in the figure may be found large areas of vacuole formation, also regularly arranged in a pattern, the whole giving the impression of subcapsular accumulations of fluid between the fibres (Plate XIV; Fig. 317). The rosette appears rapidly after the injury, sometimes within a few hours and always within the first few days, starting in the axial region of the lens and radiating rapidly outwards to the periphery. Thereafter its clinical evolution varies; sometimes it shrinks in size so considerably that eventually it can hardly be distinguished (Vogt, 1931) or even disappears entirely (Fuchs, 1888; Schmidt-Rimpler, 1898; zur Nedden,

[1] Krückow (1878), Bresgen (1881), Franke (1884), Landesberg (1886), Fuchs (1888), von Pflugk (1902), Strickler (1911), Black (1911), Cusner (1912), Bergmeister (1914), Sédan and Farnarier (1947), and many others.

PLATE XIV

CATARACT FROM PERFORATING INJURIES.

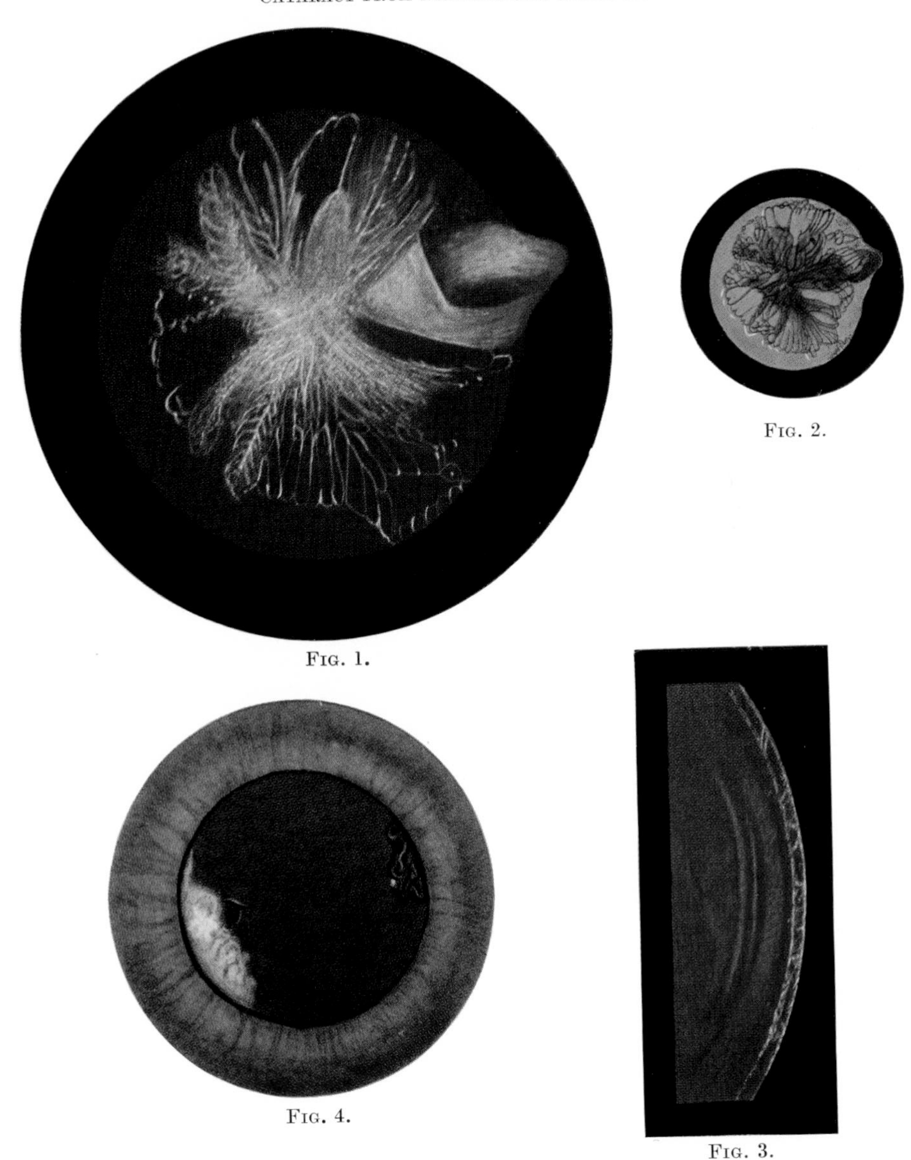

FIG. 1.

FIG. 2.

FIG. 4.

FIG. 3.

FIGS. 1 TO 3.—PERFORATION ROSETTE CATARACT.

Resulting from a fragment of stone which penetrated the temporal portion of the lens of the left eye 8 days previously (H. Sautter).

FIG. 1.—The general appearance of the lens by focal illumination.
FIG. 2.—Shows the ophthalmoscopic picture by transmitted light.
FIG. 3.—The optical section as seen by the slit-lamp.

FIG. 4.—LOCALIZED TRAUMATIC CATARACT.

A perforating injury by a broken spectacle lens in a man aged 32. The cut on the cornea is faintly seen in the region of the localized opacity in the lens at the point of injury; the rest of the lens remained transparent with 6/6 vision but diminished accommodation.

[*To face p.* 354.

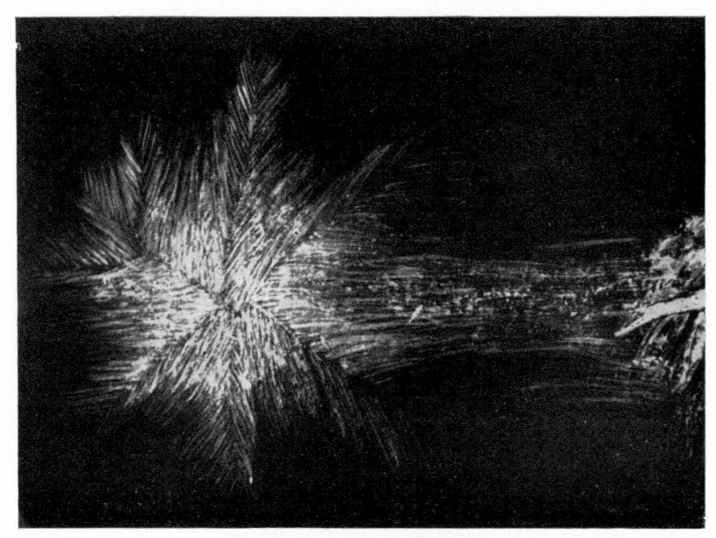

FIG. 317.—PERFORATION ROSETTE CATARACT.

In the posterior pole of the lens which had been transfixed by a needle piercing the cornea near the temporal limbus and penetrating into the vitreous. The drawing was made 5 days after the injury (after A. Vogt).

1904–5; Avizonis, 1923); at other times it remains permanently to become buried in the substance of the lens as new layers are laid down more superficially. In time, however, it changes its form, the stellate arrangement being slowly replaced by a lacework of vacuoles arranged generally in palisade-formation with their axes in conformity with those of the lens fibres, gradually becoming more discrete and smaller until all that finally remains is a collection of fine granules in which, however, some suggestion of the antecedent stellate figure may be retained (Hudson, 1910).

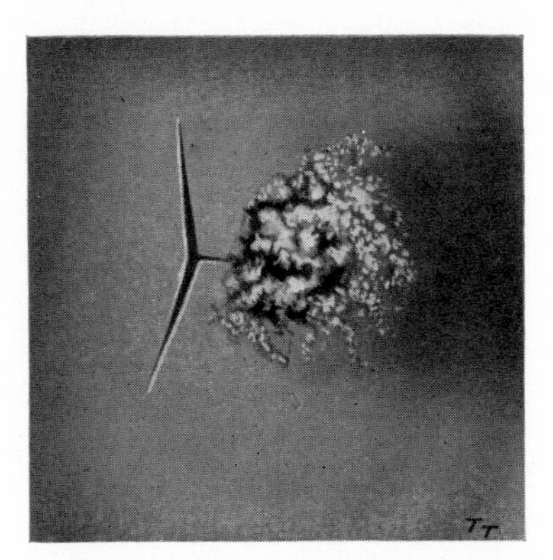

FIG. 318.—POSTERIOR CORTICAL OPACITIES AFTER A PERFORATING INJURY.

Seen by retro-illumination.

Amorphous opacities of an irregular crumb-like morphology are occasionally seen at the posterior pole after perforating injuries of the lens resembling a complicated cataract (Fig. 318).

TOTAL TRAUMATIC CATARACT

INTUMESCENT CATARACT. Sometimes, apparently for no reason, a relatively small puncture of the capsule will become sealed and, as we have seen, result in the formation of a localized opacity; at other times equally for no apparent reason, the process of imbibition proceeds apace and the

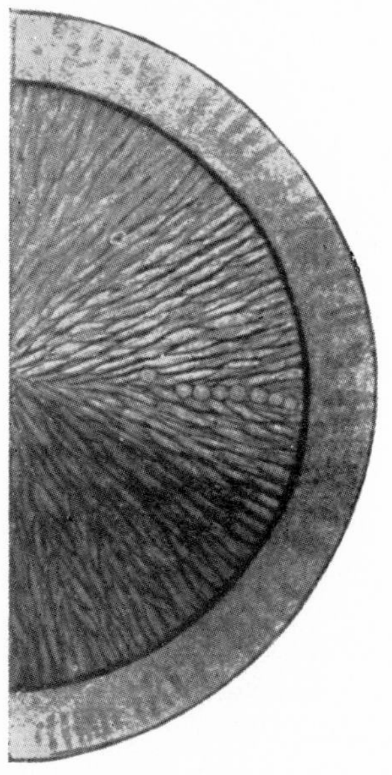

FIG. 319.—INTUMESCENT TRAUMATIC CATARACT.

A drawing of the lens as seen with oblique illumination 14 days after it had been perforated by a piece of steel. The whole of the anterior surface of the lens is divided into small areas, elongated in the direction of the course of the lens fibres (A. C. Hudson).

whole lens gradually swells up and becomes milky and opaque. Throughout the lens the bundles of fibres become separated by clefts of fluid as if the process of imbibition had forcibly torn the fibres apart, while large vacuoles may form underneath the anterior capsule. Occasionally, in the earlier stages the cortex of the lens may be seen to be divided into innumerable small areas elongated in the direction of the course of the lens fibres (Fig. 319); but eventually the entire cortex tends to become a uniform milky white. In young people absorption gradually occurs and the whole tissue may eventually disappear leaving a condition of aphakia, a happy result which may sometimes occur in mid-adult life (36 years, Klein, 1910); but after the third decade the persistence of much of the cortex and the whole of the nucleus may provide complicating problems such as the development of a

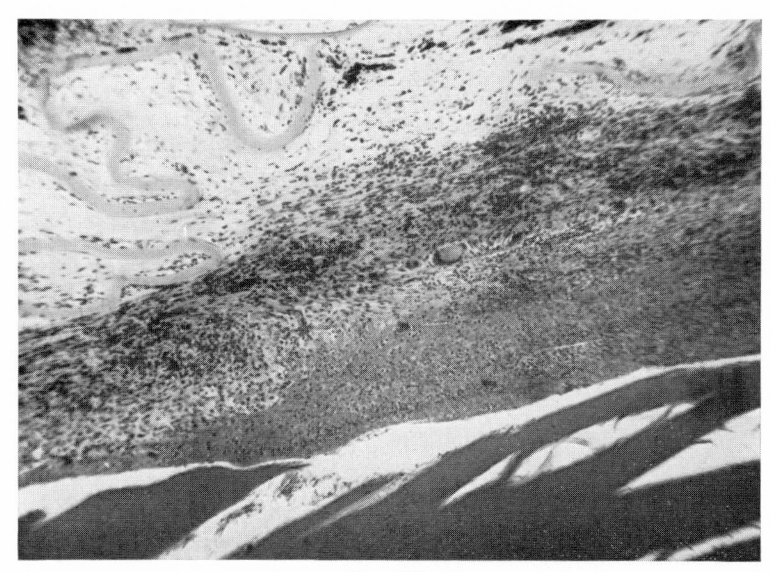

FIG. 320.

Perforating injury of the eye resulting in rupture of the lens capsule which can be seen folded in the picture. There is a thick zone of granulation tissue underneath the lens capsule in which a few multi-nucleated giant cells may be seen. The lens substance is swollen and undergoing absorption (H. & E.) (N. Ashton).

secondary glaucoma or a recalcitrant iridocyclitis so that the operative removal of the lens may become imperative.

LACERATED CATARACT. When the injury is more severe, so that the capsule is widely torn and the lens substance ploughed up, disintegration and opacification of the lens are inevitable. In these circumstances the cortical material usually herniates into the anterior chamber, sometimes in considerable quantity. In many such cases the lens matter becomes incarcerated in the corneal wound together with the iris, and excites a marked reaction in the surrounding tissues (Figs. 289–90 and 320). In such circumstances,

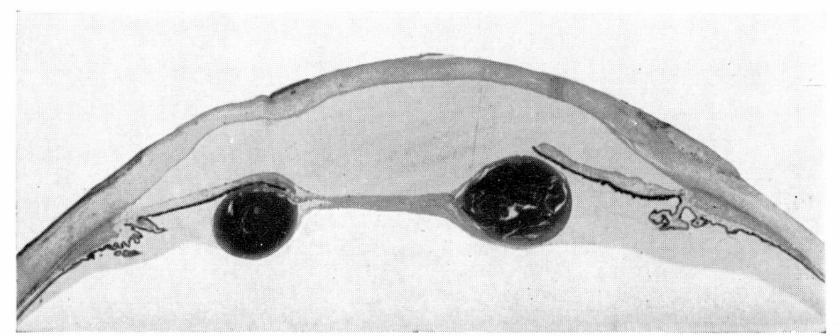

FIG. 321.—SOEMMERRING'S RING.

Following a perforating injury with a steel foreign body (N. Ashton).

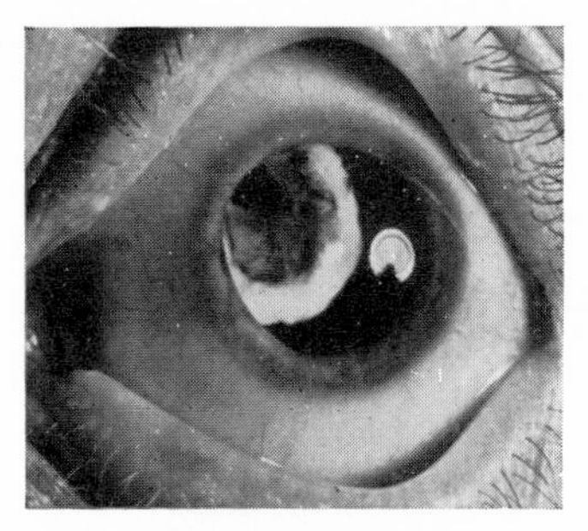

FIG. 322.—DISLOCATION OF SOEMMERRING'S RING.

After a blow on the head. The pupil is widely dilated. The light reflex of the camera is towards the right (Inst. Ophthal.).

especially in older patients, the formation of granulation tissue is abundant, a violent iridocyclitis is the rule, a secondary glaucoma common and the prognosis for resolution of the injury is usually serious, particularly if it is complicated by the introduction of infection which thrives in the culture medium provided by the lens substance.

If the eye survives the injury, a variable amount of "after-cataract" may remain behind. In young people this may consist of little more than the capsule; at other times this structure may be agglutinated in a mass of organizing tissue derived from cyclitic exudates and post-traumatic hæmorrhage so that a dense scar is formed; and occasionally when the wound has been central the main mass of the lens is absorbed but a considerable amount of its substance remains imprisoned around the periphery between the anterior and posterior capsule to form a RING OF SOEMMERRING (1828)[1] lying behind the iris (Fig. 321). As a rarity, even although the eye remains quiet in these circumstances, the anterior dislocation of a ring of Soemmerring at a later date may lead to a sharp inflammatory reaction with raised tension[2] (Fig 322).

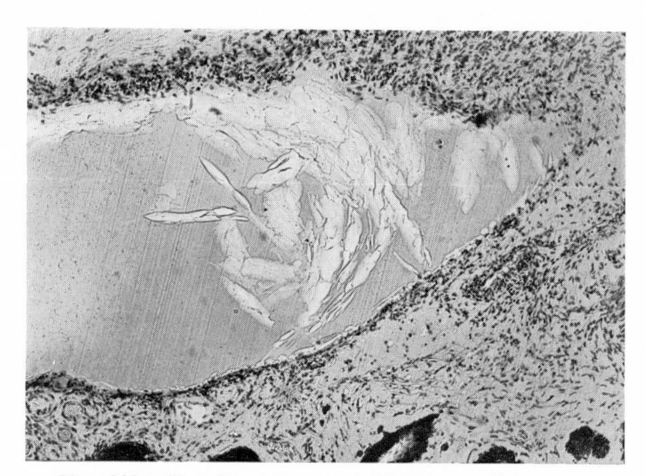

FIG. 323.—THE END-RESULT OF TRAUMATIC CATARACT.

In a man of 70 years whose eye had been perforated 40 years previously by a piece of steel which had been removed. The vision was nil and the eye was enucleated for endophthalmitis. In the anterior chamber were many proliferated and degenerated lens-epithelium cells (Elschnig's pearls) as well as chains and clumps of partially collapsed cystic bodies. These degenerated cells have lost their nuclei and consist only of an attenuated wall (Bertha Klien).

[1] Vol. XI, p. 238.
[2] Jess (1931), Poos (1931), Tooke (1933), Jacoby and Wolpaw (1935), and others.

In all these cases degenerative changes tend to occur in any lens substance which remains, the most common of which are liquefaction and the appearance of cholesterol crystals or of calcareous masses (von Reuss, 1907); while occasionally, proliferative changes in the capsular epithelium may form the large bladder-like CELLS OF ELSCHNIG (1911)[1] (Fig. 323).

The sum of damage thus inflicted on the ocular tissues by a perforating wound may be very considerable. The iris may be torn, a part of its tissue may be avulsed and carried into the vitreous body (Chisholm, 1886), an iridodialysis may occur (Haase, 1900) or the entire tissue is not uncommonly torn away from the ciliary body, leaving a condition of traumatic aniridia.[2] The lens may be dislocated into the anterior chamber or the vitreous cavity or even extruded from the eye; the vitreous may fill the anterior chamber (Waldhauer, 1885) or be lost through the wound; while the ciliary body may be avulsed (Salzmann, 1907; Markbreiter, 1908) and the choroid or the retina torn, widely detached or even extruded from the eye. A complete tearing of the retina from the ora to form a total anterior dialysis is a rare event (Velhagen, 1900; Römer, 1901; Vossius, 1901; Wintersteiner, 1901), as also is a semi-complete dialysis so that the upper half of the retina is retroflexed and lies upon the lower half (Larmande *et al.*, 1952). Even the optic disc may suffer direct injury. It is to be remembered that a retinal detachment may follow such a wound as a late sequel (Zarkin, 1905, 2 years; Schwarz, 1907, 8 years).

Avizonis. *Z. Augenheilk.*, **50,** 113 (1923).
Bergmeister. *Klin. Mbl. Augenheilk.*, **52,** 535 (1914).
Black. *Ophthal. Rec.*, **20,** 257 (1911).
Boerma. *Klin. Mbl. Augenheilk.*, **31,** 381 (1893).
Bresgen. *Arch. Augenheilk.*, **10,** 265 (1881).
Chisholm. *Amer. J. med. Sci.*, **64,** 125 (1872). *Med. Rec.*, **29,** 90 (1886).
Collins. *Trans. ophthal. Soc. U.K.*, **48,** 107 (1928).
Cusner. *Bull. Soc. belge Ophtal.*, No. 33, 31 (1912).
Davidson. *Amer. J. Ophthal.*, **23,** 1358 (1940).
Elschnig. *Klin. Mbl. Augenheilk.*, **49** (1), 444 (1911).
Folker. *Brit. med. J.*, **2,** 372 (1872).
Franke. *Berl. klin. Wschr.*, **21,** 71 (1884).
Frost. *Ophthal. Rec.*, **20,** 276 (1911).
Fuchs. *Wien. klin. Wschr.*, **1,** 53. 86 (1888). *Ber. dtsch. ophthal. Ges.*, **25,** 179 (1896).
Gelpke. *v. Graefes Arch. Ophthal.*, **33** (3), 159 (1887).
Green. *Ophthal. Rec.*, **20,** 219 (1911).
Guilford. *Ophthal. Rec.*, **18,** 579 (1909).
Haase. *Ein Fall von Spontanheilung einer Iridodialyse* (Diss.), Kiel (1900).
Hack. *Arch. Augenheilk.*, **68,** 343 (1909).
Henderson. *Ophthal. Rev.*, **26,** 191 (1907).
von Hippel. *v. Graefes Arch. Ophthal.*, **95,** 173 (1918).
Hudson. *Roy. Lond. ophthal. Hosp. Rep.*, **18,** 112 (1910).
Jacoby and Wolpaw. *Arch. Ophthal.*, **13,** 634 (1935).
Jess. *Klin. Mbl. Augenheilk.*, **86,** 98 (1931).
Klein. *Zbl. prakt. Augenheilk.*, **34,** 65 (1910).
Kretschmer. *Zbl. prakt. Augenheilk.*, **26,** 268 (1902).
Krückmann. *v. Graefes Arch. Ophthal.*, **60,** 350, 452 (1905).
Krückow. *Zbl. prakt. Augenheilk.*, **2,** 66 (1878).
Landesberg. *Klin. Mbl. Augenheilk.*, **24,** 318 (1886).
Lange. *Petersburger med. Wschr.*, **4,** 389 (1879).
Larmande, Toulant and Timsit. *Arch. Ophtal.*, **12,** 692 (1952).
McBurney. *Arch. Ophthal.*, **43,** 12 (1914).
Markbreiter. *Klin. Mbl. Augenheilk.*, **46** (1), 637 (1908).
Michaïl. *Klin. Mbl. Augenheilk.*, **86,** 606 (1931).

[1] Vol. XI, p. 235.

[2] Chisholm (1872), Folker (1872), Lange (1879), Kretschmer (1902), Guilford (1909), Frost (1911), Green (1911), Wagenaar (1952, with a finger-nail), and others.

zur Nedden. *Z. Augenheilk.*, **11**, 389 (1904).
Ber. dtsch. ophthal. Ges., **32**, 320 (1905).
Pagenstecher. *Klin. Mbl. Augenheilk.*, **3**, 1, 71 (1865).
Parsons. *Roy. Lond. ophthal. Hosp. Rep.*, **15** (3), 215 (1903).
Pathology of the Eye, London, **1**, 286 (1904).
von Pflugk. *Münch. med. Wschr.*, **49**, 854 (1902).
Poos. *Klin. Mbl. Augenheilk.*, **86**, 449 (1931).
von Reuss. *Klin. Mbl. Augenheilk.*, **45** (2), 272 (1907).
Römer. *Klin. Mbl. Augenheilk.*, **39** (1), 306 (1901).
Rosen. *Brit. J. Ophthal.*, **29**, 370, 373 (1945).
Salzmann. *Klin. Mbl. Augenheilk.*, **45** (2), 602 (1907).
Schmidt-Rimpler. *Berl. klin. Wschr.*, **35**, 965 (1898).
Schoute. *Z. Augenheilk.*, **1**, 374 (1899).
Schwarz. *Z. Augenheilk.*, **17**, 54 (1907).
Sédan and Farnarier. *Bull. Soc. franç. Ophtal.*, **60**, 140 (1947).
Snell. *Trans. Amer. ophthal. Soc.*, **53**, 489 (1955).
Amer. J. Ophthal., **41**, 499 (1956).
Soemmerring. *Beobachtungen ü. d. organischen Veränderungen im Auge nach Staaroperationen*, Frankfurt (1828).
Strickler. *Ophthal. Rec.*, **20**, 33 (1911).
Tepljaschin. *Arch. Augenheilk.*, **28**, 353 (1894).
Tooke. *Brit. J. Ophthal.*, **17**, 466 (1933).
Velhagen. *v. Graefes Arch. Ophthal.*, **49**, 599 (1900).
Vogt. *Lhb. u. Atlas d. Spaltlampenmikroskopie d. lebenden Auges*, 2nd ed., Berlin, **2** (1931).
Vossius. *Beitr. Augenheilk.*, **5** (47), 850 (1901).
Wagenaar. *Ophthalmologica*, **124**, 193 (1952).
Wagenmann. *Ber. dtsch. ophthal. Ges.*, **32**, 320 (1905).
Waldhauer. *Zbl. prakt. Augenheilk.*, **9**, 141 (1885).
Wintersteiner. *Ber. dtsch. ophthal. Ges.*, **29**, 260 (1901).
Zarkin. *Vestn. oftal.*, **22**, 27 (1905).

Clinical Picture of Perforating Wounds

A composite clinical picture of perforating wounds of the eye is impossible to draw, for they may vary from a fine puncture without clinical symptoms or detectable signs to an extensive lacerating wound which may disorganize the entire globe. Indeed, a minute puncture by a fine needle or a small foreign body may never be remarked by the patient; it may never excite symptoms and its occurrence may be shown only by the presence of a hole in the iris, sectoral damage to the lens or a retinal lesion, or may be inferred at the time by the occurrence of intra-ocular bleeding or, at a later date, by the subsequent appearance of changes such as the gradual evolution of lens opacities, the development of an organized lesion in the fundus or a detachment of the retina. Even although minute, a perforating corneal wound always leaves some trace of scarring which can be detected on sufficiently close scrutiny; but a similar anterior scleral wound may be quite invisible, particularly if obscured by subconjunctival hæmorrhage or œdema, and a posterior scleral perforation can be inferred only from subsequent events such as a vitreous hæmorrhage, retinal changes or persistent hypotony. It is to be remembered, however, that most of these changes including the fall in tension may follow a contusion; on the other hand, while hypotony persists as long as a wound leaks, a minute puncture may allow no escape of fluid and the tension may remain normal.

If the wound is of considerable extent, however, the condition is obvious. In the cornea the appearance of the wound, the fall in the ocular tension, the usual disappearance of the anterior chamber (in recent cases) and the frequent incarceration of uveal tissue make a classical clinical picture with which are generally associated palpebral œdema, conjunctival chemosis and ciliary injection accompanied by pain which may be severe, profuse lacrimation, some photophobia and frequently loss of vision. At first the cut edges of the cornea are clear and sharply defined, but within a few hours they become cloudy, swollen and macerated, while from them may protrude the darkly pigmented uveal tissue; a smaller incarceration may be betrayed by a deformation of the pupil which becomes drawn up into an elongated pear shape. Vitreous appearing in the wound is at first bright and glistening, but it gradually clouds over when it hangs out of the eye, looking for some days or weeks like a shred of mucus adhering to the wound before it is eventually cast off.

A few hours after the injury grey lines deep in the corneal stroma may be seen to radiate from the wound, or a diffuse cloudiness may become evident in the substantia propria. This appearance of STRIATE KERATOPATHY[1] is due to a separation of the corneal lamellæ by œdematous fluid; sometimes the lines are parallel and radiate star-like from the wound, at other times they branch or cross each other in an irregular pattern cut across by dark bands produced as optical reflexes by folds and rucks in Descemet's membrane.[2] Only occasionally after perforating wounds does the cornea become discoloured with blood (de Schweinitz, 1896; Wadsworth, 1905; Barlay, 1907).

Small wounds of the anterior part of the sclera are frequently obscured by chemosis or hæmorrhage, but if they gape, dark uveal tissue from the iris or ciliary body usually herniates outwards from their depths, while the anterior chamber is lost; if the wound is situated wholly behind the ciliary body the anterior chamber increases in depth, the iris may even become partially retroflexed (van der Hoeve, 1902) and the choroid and frequently the vitreous protrude, the first initially as a shiny black membrane, the second as a clear bead, both eventually becoming grey and cloudy. Larger wounds usually gape widely and the herniation of the tissues is greater so that the lens and much of the vitreous may be extruded, a process which may be progressive with each movement of the lids or on the application of external pressure.

The state of the inner eye varies within equally wide limits, but frequently the damage to its tissues is obscured by the presence of intra-ocular bleeding; a hyphæma may be present, the entire anterior chamber may be filled with blood or the fundus reflex obscured by a vitreous hæmorrhage. A rare occurrence is the temporary appearance in the upper part of the anterior chamber of air bubbles introduced at the time of perforation (Viefhaus, 1894; Dimitriou, 1950). If the intra-ocular structures can be seen, damage to the lens may be discernible and injury to the iris obvious, but in the most severe cases wherein prolapse of the ocular tissues has occurred the precise topographical details of the injury are usually difficult to differentiate clinically although the gravity of the damage is clear (Plate

[1] Vol. VIII, p. 705.

[2] Becker (1875), Nuel (1892), Hess (1892–96), Schirmer (1896), Fuchs (1902), and others.

XIII, Figs. 2 and 3). In all cases, of course, a post-traumatic uveitis is invariable, the course of which should be closely followed for the first few months lest the danger of sympathetic inflammation arise. Persistent and increasing signs of irritation are always to be viewed with anxiety, as also is the appearance of keratic precipitates, even in a relatively quiet eye; in this connection, however, in the presence of a traumatic cataract, care must be taken to differentiate these harbingers of danger from the innocuous deposition of small particles of lens cortex on the corneal endothelium.

The Treatment of Perforating Wounds

While a careful survey of a wounded eye is a necessary preliminary to a decision on the lines of treatment, it is to be remembered that the application of pressure on the lids by the surgeon or the patient's natural reflex of protective blepharospasm may cause considerable damage: uveal tissue may become incarcerated in the wound, a portion of iris may be prolapsed or herniating vitreous may be profusely extruded. It is obvious, therefore, that the examination of the globe should be conducted with the utmost care and gentleness, the lids being drawn apart and raised from the globe by retractors, preferably after local analgesia and akinesia by blocking the facial nerve, or under general anæsthesia prior to surgery.

The first question that arises, the answer to which is often difficult and fraught with anxiety, is whether conservative treatment is justified or immediate excision should be performed. If the globe is disorganized, uveal tissue freely prolapsed, the lens gravely injured or extruded, or approximately one-fifth of the vitreous lost so that it is obvious that the eye can retain no useful vision, excision is the wisest course as soon as the condition of the patient warrants such a procedure. Again, if despite immediate surgical repair the tension remains low, the eye remains filled with blood and projection of light fails, denoting a loss of retinal function, retention of the globe is of no practical value. But if the damage is less severe and the orientation of incident light proves the survival of retinal function, the advantages of excision with subsequent rapid healing and lack of danger to the other eye, although associated with the psychological and cosmetic effects of mutilation, must be carefully weighed against the disadvantages of a long and stormy convalescence, perhaps eventually resulting in insignificant functional advantage, to which may be added the anxiety of the possible loss of the vision of both eyes through sympathetic ophthalmitis. It is true that recent methods of therapeusis appear to have made sympathetic disease a less dreadful event than formerly, but even with treatment by corticosteroids it is a complication which none can afford to view lightly, a much greater evil than an unnecessary primary excision of an eye that might perhaps have been retained. It is also true that the shortest recorded interval between the infliction of an ocular wound and the development of sympathetic inflammation is five days (Joy, 1935–37; Thies, 1947), so that in doubtful cases a period of a week may be allowed to pass without danger, during which the healing powers of the eye may be given a chance. Since many eyes, even although severely traumatized, heal with remarkable rapidity and unexpected ease, this course may be safely adopted when the fellow eye is a useful organ; when it has no useful vision or is absent, every endeavour should be made to retain the injured eye so long as any hope remains of the survival of any degree of vision. In civilian practice immediate enucleation is thus rarely justified.

The Immediate Treatment of a Perforated Eye

THE IMMEDIATE TREATMENT OF A PERFORATED EYE is all-important, for the possibility of the retention of visual function and, indeed, of the eye itself, depends primarily on early and efficient toilet of the wound and the prevention of infection. Thus in an extensive statistical study of perforating injuries of all kinds, Alsen (1913) found that of eyes treated on the day of injury, 39·3% retained a visual acuity of 1/3 and 17·4% required enucleation, while if treatment were delayed for five days or more 11·9% retained 1/3 visual acuity and 30·9% were enucleated.

Such treatment should be directed towards five ends: the washing away of any obvious dirt or contaminating material by gentle irrigation with warm saline, the freeing of incarcerated tissues from the wound and the reposition of the intra-ocular contents so far as possible to their normal anatomical position, the adequate closure of the wound, the instillation of atropine and corticosteroids (if indicated) to control post-traumatic inflammation, and the prevention of exogenous infection so far as possible by the use of systemic and subconjunctival antibiotics.

Whatever the nature of the wound *adequate exposure* is essential, both to demonstrate the full extent of the injury which particularly in the case of limbal wounds may not be immediately apparent, and to facilitate accurate closure. Exposure of scleral wounds requires a generous conjunctival incision and possibly the detachment of extra-ocular muscles, while a lateral canthotomy is frequently of value not only for the exposure of more posteriorly situated wounds but also to relieve pressure on the globe from the eyelids.

In every case of perforating wound the possibility exists of the retention of an intra-ocular foreign body; every effort therefore should be made to exclude or confirm this complication at the earliest possible moment by careful consideration of the history of the exact causation of the injury (use of a hammer or chisel, drills), and by radiological examination.

Finally, in the initial assessment of a perforating wound and, indeed, of every case of ocular injury the extreme importance of the determination and recording of the vision of the damaged and the normal eye should be emphasized. Apart from the diagnostic information derived in this way, a change in vision is of prognostic significance and may herald the onset of delayed complications, and it is important to establish whether or not the injured eye possessed normal vision before the injury; in all these cases medico-legal considerations including compensation render the measurement of the visual acuity absolutely essential *before* any therapeutic measures are undertaken.

THE ADEQUATE CLOSURE OF A CORNEAL OR SCLERAL WOUND is a matter of extreme importance in the attainment of rapid and uncomplicated healing of a perforating wound of the globe. If firm coaptation is secured and maintained from the outset, healing of the corneo-scleral envelope is usually uncomplicated; most of the unfortunate sequels of such injuries are direct results of mal-apposition, over-riding or gaping of the lips of the wound—failure of the re-formation of the anterior chamber and the subsequent incarceration of tissue occurring as a delayed event, the ingrowth of epithelium, overgrowth of regenerating connective tissue within the globe, the formation of gross residual scarring and astigmatism, and often the development of infection and sometimes of sympathetic inflammation. Unless the wound is small and its edges are in good coaptation and seem likely to remain so, the immediate and future safety provided by artificial closure should thus be secured. Wounds near the posterior pole are, of course, not accessible to such treatment; but anterior to the equator two methods of wound closure are available—direct suturing and the use of conjunctival flaps.

CORNEAL OR SCLERAL SUTURES have long been applied in the reparative traumatic surgery of perforating wounds. Virgin silk is the most generally useful material in that it excites less reaction than catgut, and it should always be used attached to fine atraumatic needles; these, used with a sharp scleral hook or bi-pronged scleral forceps between which the needle is passed in order to provide counter-pressure when the tough envelope is pierced, are an absolute necessity and impart little trauma when used with reasonable manipulative delicacy: coarse needles used crudely with pressure upon the open globe are liable to do more damage than good. Moreover, adequately introduced sutures leave scars so minute as to be distinguished only with difficulty after a few weeks and cause much less functional disability than a broad scar or a staphylomatous wound.

The sutures should penetrate only the outer half of the tissues. In the cornea this is especially important, since epithelialization may occur along their tracks (Fig. 286); and it is noteworthy that in the sclera a perforating stitch (in an operation for strabismus) has led to the formation of retinal tears or detatchment (McLean *et al.*, 1960; Gottlieb and Castro, 1970) or an intra-ocular epithelial implantation cyst with ultimate loss of the eye (Brownlie and Neame, 1923). To forestall such epithelial downgrowth all stitches should be removed about the 7th day. Moreover, if a deeply placed suture which has been tightly tied is allowed to remain in place too long, necrosis of the surrounding tissues results and the associated increase in round-celled infiltration and decrease in fibroblastic repair produce a weakened area resulting in sloughing and, if sufficiently deep, in fistulization (Dunnington and Regan, 1952). Interrupted sutures suffice for the sclera, but in an extensive wound in the cornea a continuous suture eliminates the irritation of knots and allows the anterior chamber to be rapidly refilled, usually immediately the operation is completed, thus offering an opportunity of making sure that the wound is free from adherent iris tissue or for introducing antibiotics into the eye if infection is suspected. To accomplish this accurately the operating microscope is very useful.

THE USE OF CONJUNCTIVAL FLAPS as an alternative to suturing was introduced at an early date (Schöler, 1877; Snellen, 1894; and others) and was eventually elaborated and largely popularized by Kuhnt (1898–1906). Any flap should be designed to suit the particular wound in question, but certain general principles should be observed. In scleral wounds SLIDING FLAPS should be used, cut in such a manner that their edges are clear of the wound and the conjunctival sutures are not directly over it (Figs. 339 and 340).

Corneal wounds may be covered by one of four types of conjunctival flap. A HOOD FLAP is applicable to peripheral corneal wounds: the conjunctiva is incised round the nearest portion of the limbus, undermined, drawn well over the wounded area and stitched into place as shown in Figs. 324 and 325 (H. Knapp, 1868). Such a flap, frequently termed a *van Lint flap* (1912) since it was popularized by this surgeon to secure a cataract section, usually recedes so that the conjunctiva regains its normal position within seven days.

PEDICLE and BRIDGE FLAPS are applicable to central corneal wounds; in the first case, a pedicle is formed, turned over the corneal wound and secured by mattress stitches at the opposite point in the limbus; in the second (which, used alone, provides little support), a bridge of conjunctiva surrounding one half of the cornea is dissected up, placed across the cornea and secured in the correct position by stitches at its extremities (Figs. 326 and 327). A pedicle flap may be reinforced by passing it beneath bridges of conjunctiva on either side of the cornea and suturing it in place (Figs. 328 and 329); the tension exerted may be increased by the use of two conjunctival tongue-flaps cut one from each side of the cornea of such lengths that when they are sutured over it the suture line does not correspond to the wound (Figs. 330 and 331); and if the wound is extensive and particularly if there is a considerable defect of corneal tissue which will take time to regenerate, any of these flaps may be strengthened by the incorporation of Tenon's capsule with the conjunctiva. In more extensive wounds the entire cornea may be covered by freeing and undermining the conjunctiva extensively all round the limbus and securing it by a central purse-string (tobacco-pouch) suture as a TOTAL FLAP (de Wecker, 1879).

Other expedients for reinforcing a wound have been suggested from time to time—the passage of a long-distance, double-armed suture fixed on either side of the globe near the equator so that it crosses over the wound (Nuel, 1888), the use of fascia lata or the saphenous vein as flap material (Krückmann, 1911; Kuhnt, 1919), or of the skin of a boiled egg (Oxilia and Carlevaro, 1950); none of these, however, has the general efficiency of the first two methods. An alternative method of splinting which may be very effective even in severe cases involving considerable loss of vitreous is an extensive medial tarsorrhaphy which may be allowed to remain for 7 to 8 days; it has the advantage that it allows a limited inspection of the globe as well as the instillation of drugs.

A further method of reinforcing the adhesive power of a corneal wound, particularly if a conjunctival flap is used, is the application of *thrombin* (500 units per ml. in normal saline) to its lips so that, uniting with the autogenous plasma or the fibrinogen in the plasmoid aqueous, a coagulum of fibrin is formed which acts as if it were a physiological glue. Originally used in the suture of nerves (J. Z. Young and Medawar, 1940) and in skin grafting (Sano, 1943; and others), the method was applied experimentally to the closure of corneal wounds by Brown and Nantz (1944–46). Byrnes (1948) employed it in corneal lacerations and leaking wounds, and it has been used to assist the closure of cataract incisions (Tassman, 1950; Town and Naidoff, 1950; and others) or to improve the adherence of corneal grafts (Tassman, 1949). Its tensile strength is, however, very limited, and its slight advantage may be more than counterbalanced by the experimental finding of Dunnington and Regan (1952) (in monkeys)

Figs. 324 to 331.—Conjunctival Flaps for Corneal Wounds.

Figs. 324 and 325.—The Hood Flap.

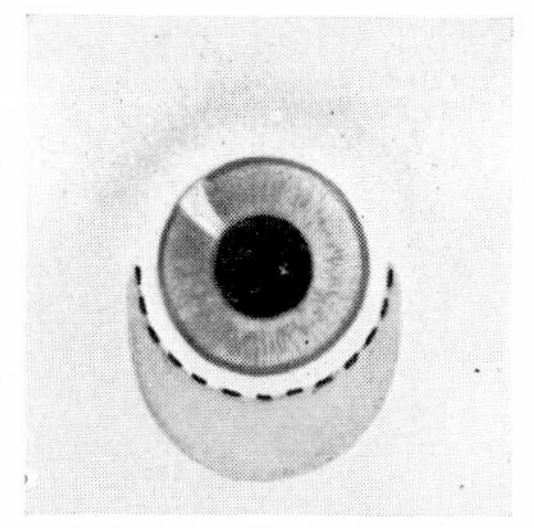

Fig. 324.—The dotted line represents the incision in the flap; the shadowed area the undermined portion of conjunctiva.

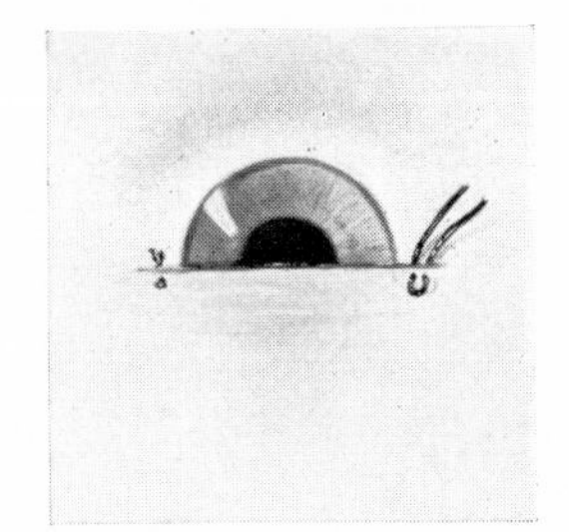

Fig. 325.—The flap in place.

Figs. 326 and 327.—The Bridge Flap.

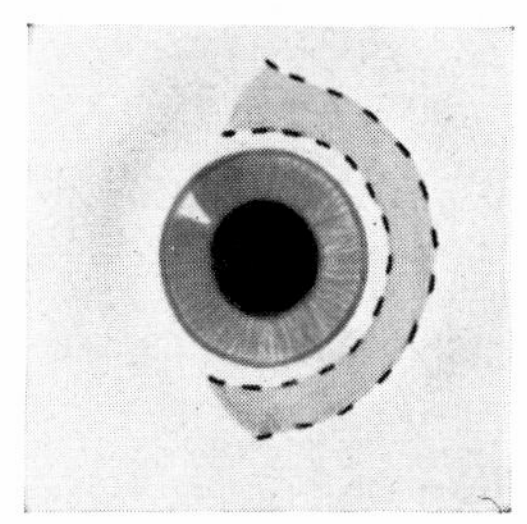

Fig. 326—The outline of the flap prepared from conjunctiva around the limbus.

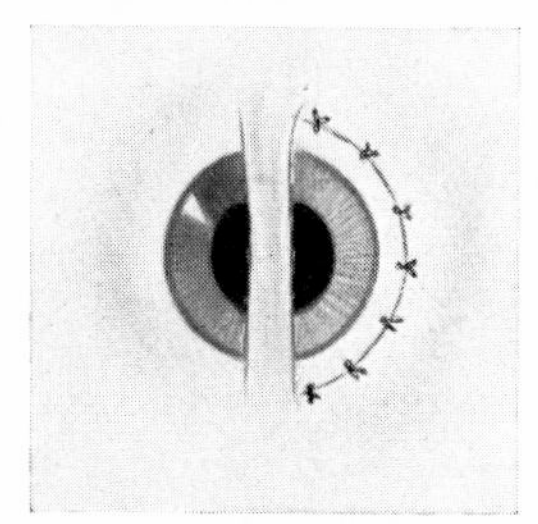

Fig. 327.—The flap crossing the cornea; the conjunctiva is sutured over the bare area of sclera.

Figs. 328 and 329.—Bridge Pedicle Flap.

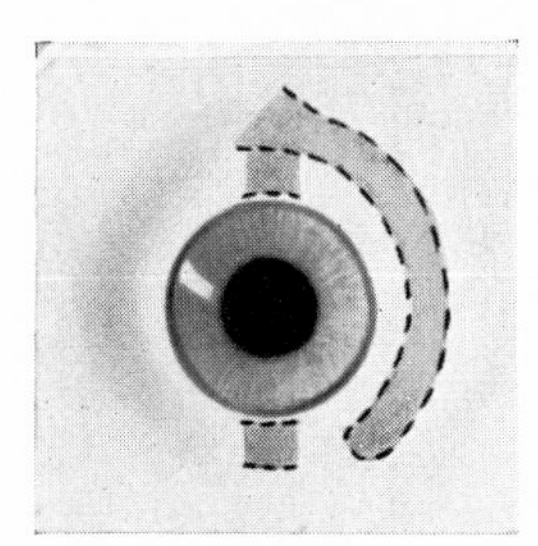

Fig. 328.

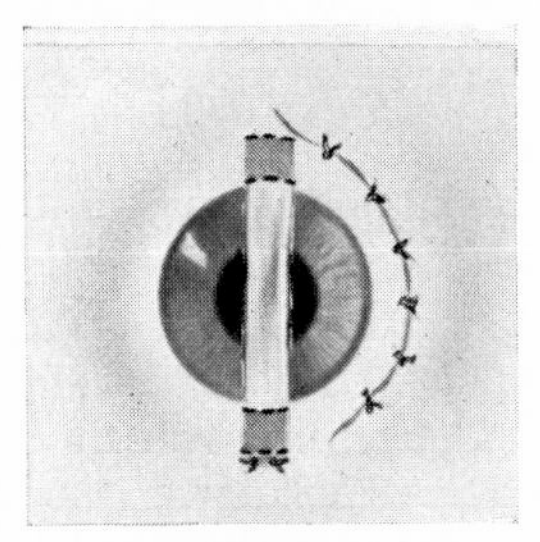

Fig. 329.

Figs. 328 and 329.—The two shadowed areas at either pole of the cornea are undermined bridges of conjunctiva. The outline of the pedicle flap half surrounding the limbus is shown in Fig. 328. The pedicle flap is threaded through the upper bridge, traverses the cornea and is tucked underneath the lower bridge where it is stitched in place (Fig. 329).

Figs. 330 and 331.—Reinforced Pedicle Flaps.

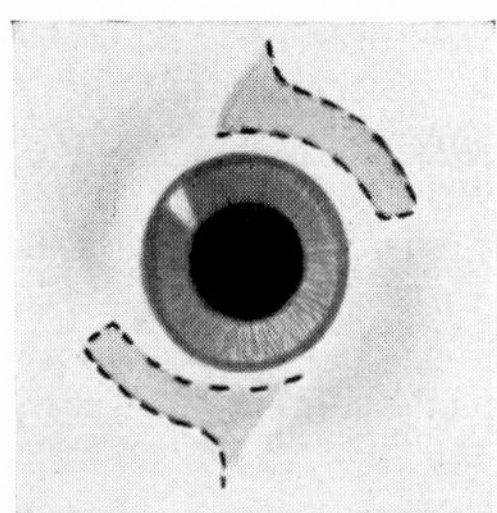

Fig. 330.—Two pedicle flaps are cut from the conjunctiva on each side as indicated.

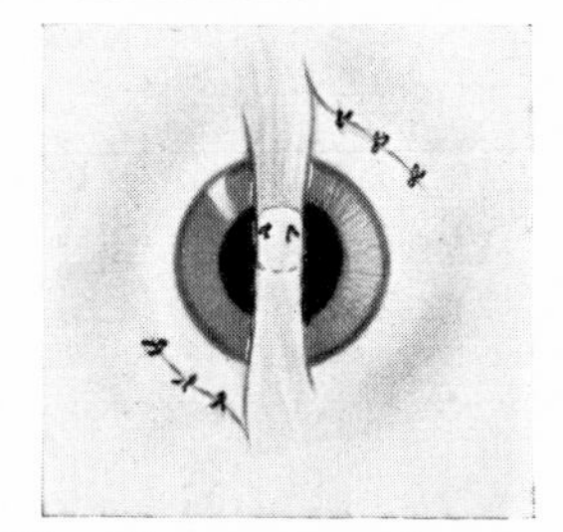

Fig. 331.—The flaps are placed across the cornea and sutured one on top of the other in order to gain tension.

that the coagulum tended to prevent apposition of the surfaces of the wound (Fig. 332). If it is used, it may be employed to reinforce sutures, not to replace them.

Recent work by Dohlman and his colleagues[1] has resulted in the development of an adhesive substance which can be used instead of sutures in the repair of corneal wounds or for the sealing of small corneal perforations. Earlier work by Straatsma (1963) resulted in the use of a cyanoacrylate monomer as an adhesive in tarsorrhaphies, but the toxicity of the substance precluded its use on the globe. Dohlman utilized n-heptylcyanoacrylate, a higher monomer, which polymerizes more rapidly and is much less toxic to the surrounding tissues. Experimental work on rabbits showed that corneal

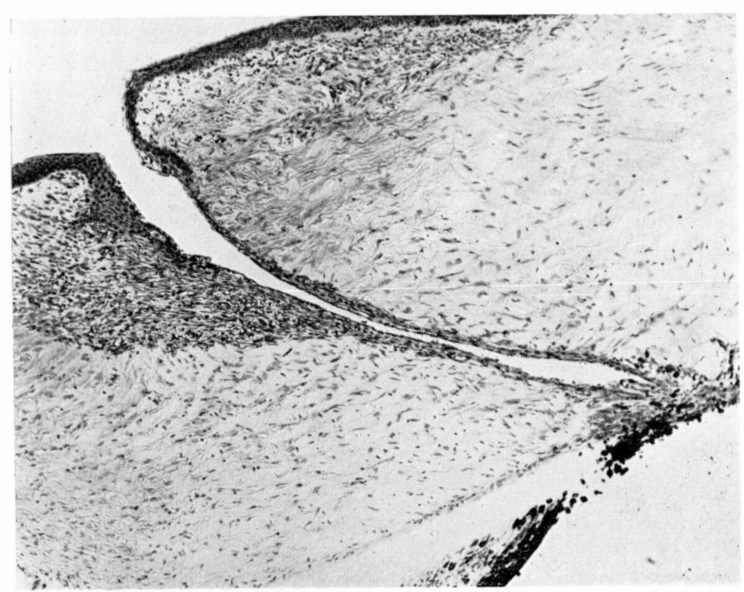

FIG. 332.—THE EFFECT OF FIBRIN IN THE HEALING OF A CORNEAL WOUND.

An occasional effect of fibrin is to form a large subepithelial plug which may cause separation of the edges of the wound. The illustration shows the eye of a monkey 7 days after a corneal wound as for a cataract extraction to which fibrin was applied. The separation of the edges and the gross subepithelial fibroblastic proliferation, seen particularly on the left, resulted in an epithelial downgrowth (J. Dunnington and E. Regan).

trephine wounds 2·5 mm. in diameter may be bridged with this substance resulting in immediate sealing of the wound and rapid restoration of the anterior chamber. Tissue from the rabbit's own cornea rapidly bridges the gap and healing takes place; no toxic effects were noted after the adhesive had been placed within the anterior chamber for a period of twelve months. Dohlman's technique has been used to restore corneal integrity and the anterior chamber in patients with perforations or small lacerations; treatment is carried out with the patient seated at the slit-lamp microscope or reclining in a chair, while seriously ill patients have been treated in their hospital beds. The area of the corneal ulcer or laceration is carefully debrided of any necrotic or loose material and the surface is then thoroughly dried. An applicator stick and disc bearing

[1] See Webster *et al.* (1968), Refojo *et al.* (1968), Price and Wadsworth (1969), Refojo and Dohlman (1969); *Highlights Ophthal.*, **11,** 252 (1968) See p. 1049.

the fluid glue is then applied against the base of the wound overlying the perforation and held in place for about 15 seconds. As soon as the glue has solidified and bonded itself onto the cornea the applicator is withdrawn. If a drop of fluorescein solution reveals a residual leak this can be sealed by a further application of the adhesive. The glue remains adherent for several weeks and if spontaneous loosening of the glue has not occurred after about one month it can easily be removed with forceps. At the present time this new method of dealing with corneal perforations is still under investigation.

In the choice of the method of closure to be adopted, each case should be considered on its own merits. A small wound, the edges of which are in good coaptation, uncomplicated by uveal incarceration, should be left alone; a flap support may well be the only practical method of dealing with a wound which has jagged, irregular and contused edges, which involves a considerable loss of tissue, or which takes the form of a puncture from which it is desirable to stop a leakage of aqueous; for the rest, suturing is generally the method of choice, but it should never be attempted in the absence of suitable atraumatic needles. A flap rarely secures perfect coaptation; it may increase any existing tendency for the lips of the wound to over-ride and it encourages the proliferation of granulation tissue in the gap if the wound gapes beneath it (Fig. 290). Suturing, on the other hand, provided the technique employed is sufficiently delicate, secures better apposition and quicker healing, is a more effective insurance against the subsequent prolapse of tissue or the entrance of infection, inhibits the intra-ocular growth of fibrous tissue and, by making the anterior chamber immediately water-tight, permits its rapid re-formation so that the anatomical position of the intra-ocular contents is immediately restored and allows the anterior chamber to be reconstituted with air or saline to prevent the formation of synechiæ (Rouher, 1949).

THE FREEING OF INCARCERATED TISSUE FROM THE WOUND is of primary importance, for the presence of prolapsed or adherent tissue prevents rapid healing, facilitates the entrance of infection, leads to chronic or recurrent inflammatory episodes which may ultimately destroy the function of the eye, and undoubtedly encourages the development of sympathetic ophthalmitis, which may eventually, even after some years, destroy the function of both eyes.

As a general rule if a wound in the cornea or near the limbus is of some size, preparations to close it should be completed—sutures inserted but not tied or a flap prepared—before the prolapsed tissue is dealt with so that the wound can thereafter be rapidly closed. Because of the risk of introducing infection into the eye, prolapsed tissue should usually be excised; after its surface has been swabbed to clear it of mucus or exudate, it should be gently pulled forward, first away from one side of the wound and then from the other, to free it, a process which may require the additional help of an iris repositor in neglected cases when adhesions have formed; thereupon it should be cut cleanly with scissors tangentially to the surface of the wound, all the time being held on the stretch so that the cut ends tend to spring back freely into the eye. If this does not occur satisfactorily, the pillars of the coloboma thus formed should be stroked back with an iris repositor; thereafter the sutures (if these are employed) should be tightened and tied and the area, if necessary, consolidated with a

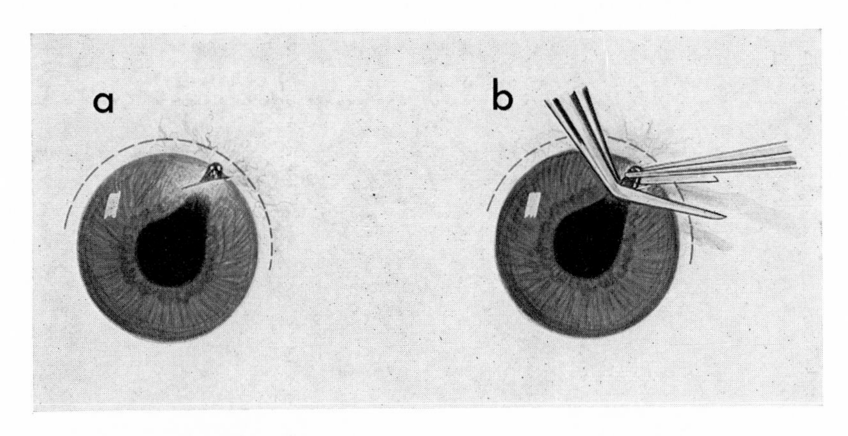

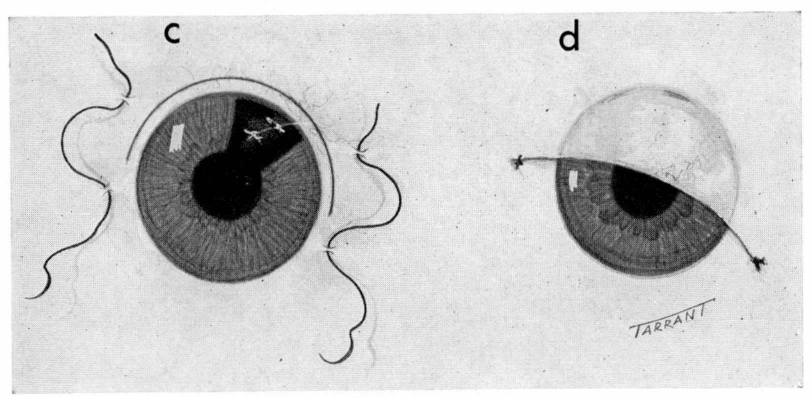

Fig. 333.—Perforating Injury with Prolapse of the Iris and its Surgical Treatment.

(a) Linear wound with iris prolapse. (b) Incision for a conjunctival flap indicated by a dotted line. Abscission of the prolapse. (c) Coloboma after abscission of prolapse and closure of corneo-scleral wound with interrupted sutures. (d) Conjunctival flap secured in position.

conjunctival flap (Fig. 333). On the other hand, cases seen within a few hours after a perforating wound may occasionally permit replacement of the iris into the anterior chamber with the aid of a strong miotic and the passage of a repositor through a separate keratotomy provided that the wound is not grossly contaminated by foreign material, blood or damaged tissue, and that the iris is not actually protruding but merely plugging the base of the wound (Fig. 334).

If these manipulations are not possible, as may occur when the iris is adherent to the inner surface of a shelving wound or when a synechia leads to a punctured wound, the adherent iris may be freed by means of a repositor passed through a small valvular incision made by a keratome or corneal needle through the cornea near the limbus some distance away from the

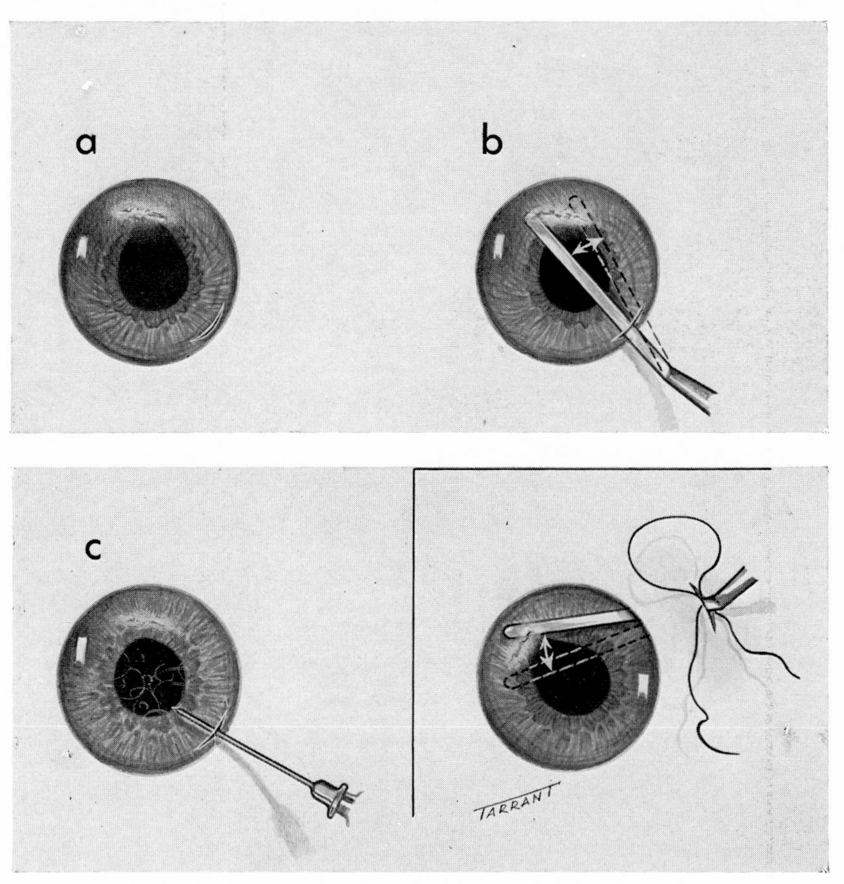

FIG. 334.—THE MANAGEMENT OF INCARCERATION OF THE IRIS.

(a) Corneal wound with incarceration of the iris. (b) Iris repositor inserted through a peripheral keratotomy incision showing the movement required to free the iris from the wound. (c) Re-formation of anterior chamber with air. (Inset) An alternative method using a cyclodialysis approach.

injured area—an easy matter if the anterior chamber is retained or is rapidly re-formed after suturing; an alternative is a cyclodialysis approach (Fig. 334). In all cases when sutures are used and the anterior chamber does not rapidly re-form, advantage may be taken of such a secondary incision to fill the anterior chamber with air and force the iris and lens back so that the dangers of the formation of further synechiæ are minimized.

FIGS. 335 to 337.—CLOSURE OF A CORNEO-SCLERAL WOUND.

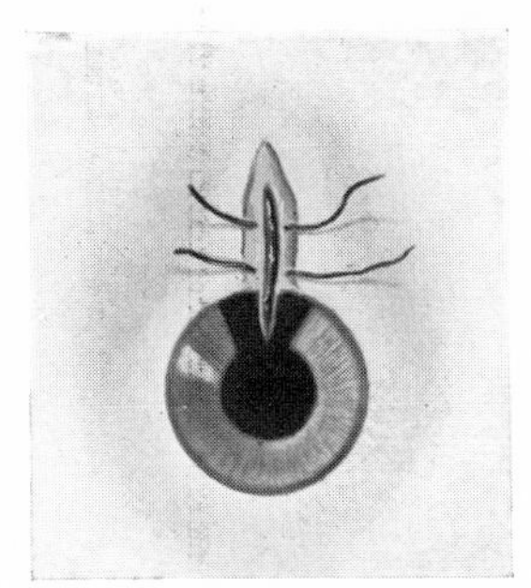

FIG. 335.

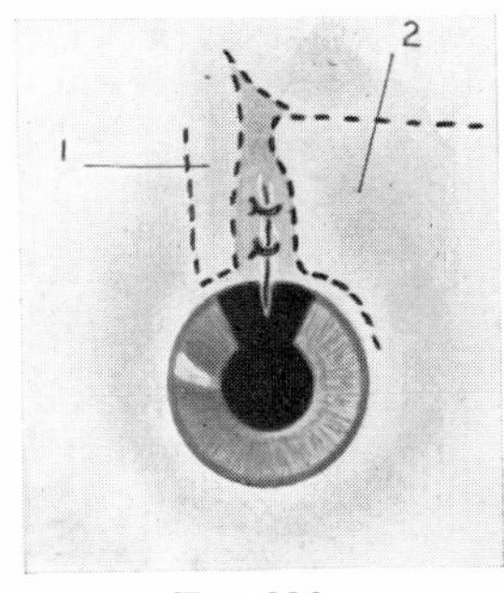

FIG. 336.

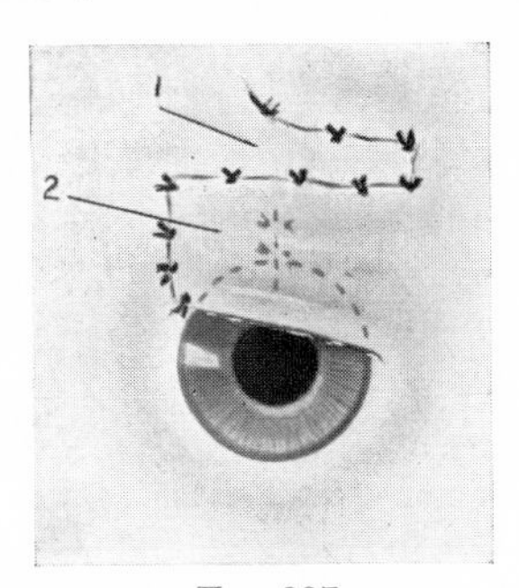

FIG. 337.

FIG. 335.—The corneo-scleral wound is shown at 12 o'clock. There has been a prolapse of the iris which has been excised. The scleral sutures traversing half the thickness of the sclera are seen in place. The conjunctiva is slightly retracted.

FIG. 336.—The two scleral sutures are tied and two conjunctival flaps are cut, (1) a vertical flap on one side of the scleral wound, and (2) a large horizontal flap the lower margin of which skirts the limbus to the horizontal meridian.

FIG. 337.—Flap (2) is pulled tightly across the upper part of the cornea covering the corneo-scleral wound and sutured into place. Flap (1) is swivelled around to the horizontal position to cover the area of sclera denuded by the stretching of flap (2).

FIGS. 338 to 340.—CLOSURE OF A SCLERAL WOUND.

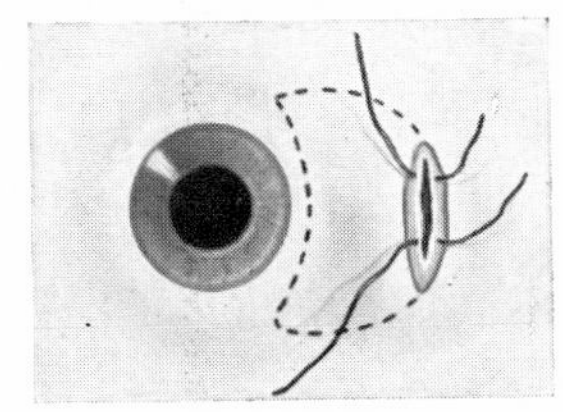

FIG. 338.

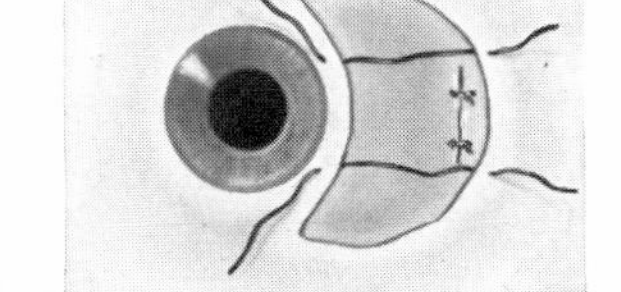

FIG. 339.

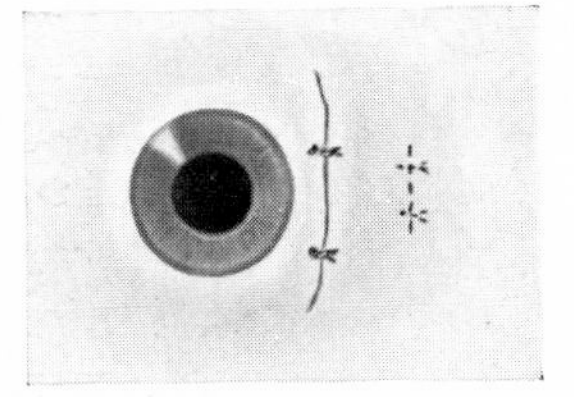

FIG. 340.

FIG. 338.—Shows the scleral wound with sutures traversing half the thickness of the sclera in place. The area of conjunctiva to be excised is outlined.

FIG. 339.—The scleral wound is closed and the conjunctival sutures are in place.

FIG. 340.—The posterior lip of the conjunctival wound is drawn forward and tied with sutures so that it lies between the scleral wound and the limbus.

Scleral wounds should be treated similarly, and it is to be remembered that, unless surgically closed, every such wound over 3 mm. in length tends to gape, favouring such complications as the immediate entrance of infection, secondary re-opening during healing and the subsequent development of chronic post-traumatic uveitis, retinal detachment or the formation of a staphylomatous scar. Interrupted sutures are inserted into the superficial half of the sclera with the aid of counter-pressure with a scleral hook or scleral forceps, any loose or torn tags of uveal tissue or prolapsed vitreous abscised, and as the sutures are tightened bulging uveal tissue is eased back into the eye with the aid of a repositor; it is important that the lips of the wound should be closely apposed without the intervention of blood clot, uveal tissue, vitreous or lens capsule. It is often a wise precaution to ring round the area with a circle of diathermic or cryotherapeutic applications as a prophylactic measure against the occurrence of a later retinal detachment. Thereafter a conjunctival flap is made and secured by appropriate sutures, reinforcing the closure in such a way that the two suture lines, scleral and conjunctival, do not coincide (Figs. 335–340).

When panophthalmitis has developed and attempts to preserve the eye have been abandoned, its removal must be contemplated. In cases wherein suppuration is violent with much orbital reaction, such an operation is not always easy and frequently involves bursting the globe: the orbit will therefore almost certainly become flooded with the infected ocular contents which may lead to the spread of infection up the sheaths of the optic nerve to the meninges, a sequence which has had fatal results. In these cases it is better to eviscerate the eye in the usual way, scooping out its contents, and thereafter to remove most of the sclera without opening the sheath of the optic nerve (Lister's *frill operation*). In this procedure, when the contents of the eye have been scooped out and the inner surface of the sclera cleaned, the cavity of the globe is packed with ribbon gauze and the conjunctiva and muscles removed from the outer aspect. The packing is then removed and the sclera cut away just anterior to the optic nerve, leaving a small frill around it so that the nerve sheath is not opened. If the sclera is not removed in this way it will gradually slough and the wound will persistently discharge. After such an operation packing should never be inserted into the orbit.

MEASURES TO PREVENT THE DEVELOPMENT OF INFECTION of a perforating wound have become much more effective since the introduction of antibiotic drugs; these have rendered obsolete the older methods of repeated irrigation with antiseptics, the instillation of silver preparations, painting the lips of the wound with carbolic acid or iodine, the use of the cautery, the intra-ocular injection of iodoform or the subconjunctival injection of substances such as mercuric cyanide, used with the hope of inducing an intra-ocular vasodilatation.[1]

A culture of the conjunctival sac should be taken when possible and the instillation of antibiotic drops should be a routine in every case; ointments are best avoided initially lest they should penetrate into the anterior chamber through a corneal wound and interfere with inspection of the interior of the globe, although they may well be used after the wound has been repaired. A subconjunctival injection of an antibiotic with a wide range of activity (such as framycetin or neomycin) should be given whenever intra-ocular infection seems likely and, indeed, is probably a wise precaution in all cases wherein ocular penetration has occurred. Although the subconjunctival injection of antibiotics is generally sufficient, systemic antibiotic therapy may be indicated as, for instance, in grossly contaminated wounds or those sustained in agricultural and similar occupations, or when repair of the ocular injury has to be delayed by necessary travel or pending the assessment of other injuries. In such a situation penicillin (or one of its newer derivatives) or a tetracycline may be given but chloramphenicol is the drug of choice for

[1] Ostwalt (1897) Haab (1899) van Millingen (1899), Krauss (1904), and many others.

ease of penetration into the eye (Ellis, 1968). It is to be remembered, however, that severe toxic effects may occur when this drug is used in high dosage for a considerable period (for instance optic neuritis, hepatic damage, blood dyscrasias); an alternative choice lies with one or other of the sulphonamides. Tetanus immunization should be carried out whenever the opportunity for contamination by this organism seems likely.[1]

It must be remembered, however, that it is by no means possible to forestall the development of infection in every case, even with the most efficient antibiotic and chemotherapy, and that once infection has become established, even if it is subsequently overcome, the eye may be so severely damaged as to be virtually useless; it follows that if it is to be of any use antibacterial therapy must be instituted early as a prophylactic measure. The principles of the management of an established intra-ocular infection will be subsequently discussed.

THE IMMEDIATE TREATMENT OF INTRA-OCULAR DAMAGE usually resolves itself into relatively simple measures apart from the abscission of prolapsed tissue and the reposition of incarcerated uveal tissue as far as is possible to its normal anatomical arrangement; as we have already seen, gross intra-ocular damage demands removal of the eye. If a hyphæma is total or nearly so, it may be advisable to wash the blood from the anterior chamber through a corneal wound if it already exists, and it is useful after suturing to refill the chamber, partially at any rate, with air; but the only intra-ocular tissue which may require additional immediate attention is a damaged lens. Injury to this tissue is always to be considered a serious menace to the eye, but as a general rule a traumatic cataract is usually best left alone until the eye has become quiet, if such a course is possible. If, however, the injury has involved a laceration of the lens and its substance is extruding into the anterior chamber or has become incarcerated in the wound, and if in these circumstances an effort is to be made to save the eye, as much as possible of the lens matter should be removed by irrigation, aided perhaps by corneal massage or aspiration before the wound is closed. In such cases extreme care should be taken lest pieces of lens capsule or tags of vitreous, both of which are usually invisible, remain in the wound. If the wound requires no closure and the lens has not become intumescent, it is often wise to leave the eye for 2 or 3 days until a linear extraction becomes more feasible, *provided infection can be prevented by adequate antibiotic therapy.* After this lapse of time the prolapsed iris can be abscised and the lens matter more easily removed, while the unpleasant necessity of opening the eye after some days to remove the irritating lens matter is avoided.

The Delayed Treatment of a Perforated Eye

THE DELAYED TREATMENT OF PERFORATING WOUNDS with badly apposed edges, which have not received adequate emergency care initially,

[1] p. 408.

resolves itself into the treatment of the complications of wound healing—epithelial ingrowth, fibrous-tissue overgrowth, corneal scars, adherent leucoma, ectatic cicatrix or staphyloma, and cystoid cicatrix or fistula.

Epithelial Ingrowths. The treatment of this condition whether following surgery or perforating injury is extremely difficult.[1] The following procedures, however, have been recommended: surgical removal of the epithelium from the inner surface of the cornea (Long and Tyner, 1957); destruction of the membrane by alcohol and curetting (Maumenee, 1957; Sullivan, 1967) or, more effectively, by cryosurgery which may also be used for the destruction of a localized cyst (Ferry and Naghdi, 1967); photocoagulation of an epithelial membrane on the anterior surface of the iris has also been successful (Maumenee, 1964); irradiation of the anterior segment either by x-rays or beta rays has long been recommended in an attempt to control the epithelial proliferation (Custodis, 1932; Suzuki, 1934; Gördüren and Tosunoglu, 1951; Anton, 1967; and others) and may well be undertaken as a drastic measure in a desperate clinical situation, although the results of this form of therapy are uncertain. If x-ray treatment is used it is important that this should be applied in fractionated doses over a period of several weeks so that radiational side-effects may be minimized and so as to destroy the newly formed epithelial cells in the stage of mitosis. Beta radiation with its limited depth of penetration is unlikely to be successful in destroying an epithelial membrane on the surface of the iris. In all cases when these forms of treatment are adopted it is, of course, essential to eliminate a fistulous wound. When glaucoma supervenes little can be done other than a cyclodiathermy; in a high proportion of these cases enucleation of the affected eye is eventually required (Blodi, 1954; Paufique and Hervouët, 1964; and others).

Treatment for fibrous-tissue overgrowth extending into the eye either from a corneal or scleral wound is most unsatisfactory; prophylaxis by adequate and early apposition is the only satisfactory method of tackling this problem, although the early exhibition of topical corticosteroids may diminish the tendency for proliferation. We have already seen that this condition leads to continued irritation and frequently to eventual shrinkage of the globe. When the ingrowth is confined to the region of the wound it is best to excise or cauterize its edges and to close it securely with corneal sutures, reinforced, if necessary, by a conjunctival flap. In the posterior part of the eye such bands may easily cause a widespread retinal detachment quite unresponsive to the usual methods of operative reposition. In cases (as of an only eye) wherein it seems necessary to make a heroic attempt to retain some vision, an encircling procedure offers the best prospect of success, in order to minimize the effect of traction by the fibrous bands through decreasing the size of the globe.

[1] Vol. XI, p. 283 and p. 719.

Treatment of corneal scars, whether diffuse and nebulous or dense and leucomatous, is frequently indicated for optical or cosmetic reasons; it is to be remembered that a diffuse nebula may be more incapacitating than a dense circumscribed leucoma owing to the visual distortion caused by irregular refraction and the dispersion of light. Left to themselves such scars may clear up to a considerable extent during the first few months after the accident, but usually this occurs to a small degree only and, as we have seen, some sequelæ always remain.

Medicaments and physical methods of treatment being on the whole useless, considerable improvement may be obtained from *operative measures*. Three procedures are available. In the first place, if the scar is central and localized, an *optical iridectomy* may be of value, although the peripheral refraction which must be utilized to a large extent lowers the practical efficiency of what should theoretically give a good result.

In the second place, *tattooing* may disguise an unsightly leucoma and at the same time, by converting a diffuse nebula into a sharply defined opaque plaque, it may improve the visual efficiency. For this purpose two techniques are available whereby a chemical reaction involving the precipitation of a pigment is brought about in the corneal tissues or a colouring pigment is directly introduced into the corneal tissues; these have been discussed.[1]

The final and best procedure is *excision of the scar.* A superficial scar may be dealt with by a simple keratectomy, the defect being allowed to epithelialize, but the best results are obtained by *corneal grafting*, using lamellar or full-thickness grafts as may be indicated; in perforating wounds the latter are usually required, and although grafting of the entire cornea is surgically practicable, severe immunological reactions follow this procedure with such frequency as to make its final outcome somewhat unsatisfactory at present. The general principles and historical development of this technique have already been discussed.[2]

The treatment of an adherent leucoma in which the synechiæ have been allowed to remain and consolidate until the wound has healed introduces problems which require considerable judgment. In general, if a prolapse of uveal tissue lies outside the wound it should be destroyed, and if an anterior synechia is found to exist some days after the accident it should be divided, if possible, as soon as consolidation of the wound has reached a stage which permits the necessary manipulations without re-opening it. If this is not done the eye may sometimes remain quiet indefinitely but too frequently the constant traction of the iris tends to keep up irritation and predisposes to sympathetic inflammation, while a broad synechia provides an avenue for the entrance of infection and predisposes to the development of secondary glaucoma. If the centre of the cornea is extensively involved in an adherent leucoma a satisfactory result may be obtained by excision of the scar and the

[1] Vol. VIII, p. 645. [2] Vol. VIII, p. 648.

iris tissue adherent to it followed by the insertion of a penetrating corneal graft.

An old prolapse extending out of the wound may have become so consolidated that it is impossible to free it and abscise it adequately without excessive trauma. If the prolapse is small and localized it may be completely abscised in an elliptical excision embracing the entire wound with the prolapse, combined with an iridectomy performed as the ellipse of tissue containing the prolapse is removed. The operative wound is closed by sutures previously inserted after half the thickness of the cornea or sclera has been cut through, reinforced, if necessary, by a prepared conjunctival flap.

If, however, the prolapse was extensive, its destruction used to be advised. Cauterization with the galvano-cautery at a dull red heat was the classical method to employ in such cases, a prepared conjunctival flap being available to cover the wound immediately thereafter and thus consolidate healing. Such a technique, however, is traumatizing and has led to the development of sympathetic inflammation (Trousseau, 1897; and others); the alternative of cauterization by trichloracetic acid suggested by Gifford (1910) and popularized by Bettman and Barkan (1937) is probably a safer substitute which excites much less reaction.

By this method a few hygroscopic crystals of the acid are dissolved in a drop of saline to form a saturated solution, and the prolapsed tissue, previously dried by swabbing, is touched over the whole of its extent by a wooden applicator soaked in the solution. The prolapsed tissue thus treated immediately turns a milky-white colour, and if the process is repeated daily for a week or more, it diminishes in size, flattens and becomes covered with a white, firm, non-irritating eschar sufficiently solid to prevent the entrance of bacteria. Synechiæ adherent to the posterior lips of the wounds can be dealt with subsequently.

If a synechia incarcerated in the inner surface of the wound is small and delicate, it may be cut as closely as possible to the posterior surface of the cornea by a small knife passed through this tissue some distance from the limbus at a site convenient for the manipulations so that the point of entrance serves as a fulcrum from which the knife cuts. The point of election for the introduction of the knife is usually about the junction of the middle and peripheral thirds of the cornea, since if it pierces the cornea nearer the limbus a further synechia readily forms.

Lang's twin knives are useful and safe for this purpose; the corneal incision is made with a sharp-pointed knife which is then withdrawn without the loss of the anterior chamber, and the synechia cut with a second blunt-pointed knife of identical size introduced into the valvular opening made by its twin. Ziegler's knife-needle is an alternative; but if the adhesion is broad, Wheeler's knife-needle or a thin Graefe knife may be necessary.

If the synechia is extensive and dense, particularly if it is situated near the limbus, the most effective method of cutting it is to pass a thin cataract knife through the anterior chamber with puncture and counter-puncture at either limbus suitably placed with respect to the adhesion and with the cutting edge towards it; with the sawing movements appropriate for a cataract section the knife is then carried through the adherent iris and preferably withdrawn before the section is completed, if that is possible. If such a method is inapplicable owing to the extent of the synechia, a wide iridectomy may be attempted or the incarcerated segment of the iris may be isolated from the remainder of the tissue by an iridectomy on either side (Denig, 1944). If, unfortunately, the anterior chamber is lost in any of these manipulations, it may be wise to reconstitute it immediately with air in order to forestall the formation of further adhesions. The same method may be employed to free an attenuated adhesion of vitreous to the posterior aspect of the wound, for if sufficient air is injected, the strand may be ruptured and the vitreous held in position for a sufficient length of time to allow consolidation to take place (Dunphy, 1949; Briggs, 1952).

The treatment of an ectasia or a staphyloma of the cornea is frequently difficult and, if it is to be effective, calls for somewhat heroic measures. In its initial stages its progress may be checked to some extent by repeated paracenteses and pressure bandaging (see Terry and Chisholm, 1940, as applied to keratoconus); a rise of intra-ocular pressure may occasionally be prevented by a wide iridectomy, a procedure which, unfortunately, is not by any means always possible. In favourable circumstances, however, while the scar-tissue is still young and capable of contraction, this operation may check its progress and even induce some shrinkage (Kuhnt, 1898), while in some cases excision of the staphyloma and its replacement by a corneal graft may be possible (Raïs, 1955). Other operations for the relief of pressure, such as trephining, are rarely of value. Once a staphyloma has become fully established, its gradual increase and the occurrence of repeated attacks of irritation may call for surgical intervention by partial or total excision. Most of these procedures, however, must be heroic in nature and are generally of doubtful value. Thereby a protuberant staphyloma may, indeed, be replaced by a flat scar, but in the first place this also is unsightly, and frequently the resulting globe is small and shrunken requiring to be covered by a prosthesis. Further, if the conditions determining a raised intra-ocular pressure persist, the scar will again stretch, while if they do not, a lowered tension may well be maintained at the price of a plastic endophthalmitis or progressive atrophy of the globe, conditions about which little easiness can be felt. In most cases the eye has eventually to be enucleated; and in a few sympathetic ophthalmitis has developed. If surgical treatment is necessary the wisest course, therefore, is enucleation or one of the operations which may be substituted for it.

Scleral ectasias and staphylomata present an equally difficult problem in surgical therapeusis, and again in these cases serious consideration should be given to the relative values of heroic surgical measures followed by a long and anxious convalescence with little prospect of useful vision on the one hand, and simple excision of the eye on the other. If, however, the ectatic area is small and the eye otherwise good, a sclerectomy of the staphyloma is a possibility (Vail, 1946); if sufficiently small it may be buckled inwards (C. A. Young, 1955); alternatively, it may be excised and replaced by a scleral graft (Payrau and Remky, 1961).

The treatment of a cystoid cicatrix or a fistula follows much the same lines. Repeated paracenteses may be tried to control the tension and encourage healing, together with the superimposition of a conjunctival flap; but as a rule the condition is recalcitrant to curative efforts, persisting until it is destroyed either by cauterization with the actual cautery, by diathermy or chemicals (as trichloracetic acid, Bothman, 1937, or 10% silver nitrate, Wiener and Alvis, 1939) or by paring its edges with the knife. Such a cauterization or excision followed by suturing (Gradle, 1921; Dunnington and Regan, 1950) or the protection of a conjunctival flap usually succeeds in closure unless in the meantime the eye has become infected.

The delayed treatment of intra-ocular damage caused by a perforating wound devolves into the therapeutic measures which may be undertaken for traumatic cataract, iridodialysis, retinal detachment and glaucoma. The treatment of traumatic *cataract* caused by an aseptic perforating injury should in general be conservative until the eye is quiet, a procedure always indicated if the cataract is partial and stationary, in which case, of course, treatment is frequently unnecessary. Such a routine is by no means invariably possible, particularly in older people since the presence of lens material in the eye frequently gives rise to a severe uveitis[1] or a secondary glaucoma; the latter complication may also be associated with an intumescent cataract when a rupture in the capsule is small or absent and in these circumstances early measures of relief by aspiration will be necessary. The early removal of extruded lens material not only reduces the chances of complications in the anterior segment but also permits early observation of the fundus and in some cases the earlier restoration of useful vision with a contact lens (Gass, 1969), but it should be noted that removal of a cataractous lens in an acutely injured eye is a difficult and hazardous procedure which should be done only when it is necessitated by a serious complication such as acute glaucoma (Havener and Gloeckner, 1969). On the whole, however, more satisfactory ultimate results are obtained if surgical intervention is delayed until the post-traumatic inflammatory phase has passed, although a careful watch for the development of complications is necessary, and delay is more desirable if hypotony persists as this is frequently associated with a latent uveitis. The use of steroids either by subconjunctival injection or the instillation of drops may be of considerable value in hastening the disappearance of the clinical evidences of irritation.

[1] Vol. IX, p. 501.

In young people total absorption of the lens matter from the pupillary area frequently occurs without surgical intervention but in older patients a linear extraction with a keratome section followed by curette evacuation and irrigation or aspiration of free lens substance from the anterior chamber is usually indicated. If the tension is high, repeated paracenteses with the expression of as much cortical matter as possible are a safe procedure. In older people, although an intracapsular extraction may be the method of choice when the capsule is not torn and in cases with luxated or subluxated lenses,[1] the classical extracapsular extraction is occasionally necessary, the capsule being freely opened to allow the escape of the large nucleus. In all these cases extreme care should be taken to avoid entanglement of the lens capsule or the vitreous in the wound for such a synechia may jeopardize the result of the operation. Such a complication arises easily when considerable intra-ocular disorganization has followed the perforation of the globe and for this reason King (1943) advocated that the keratome incision should be located in the upper nasal quadrant some distance from the limbus to allow easy access if a second intervention is necessary to cut any adhesions which may form subsequently. It is also advisable if an extracapsular method of extraction is performed to make discission of the posterior capsule a final stage in the operative treatment after all loose cortex has been absorbed since such a procedure undertaken at a later date when thickening of the capsule has occurred is frequently difficult and may involve much trauma.

An alternative method of evacuation is by *aspiration*, a procedure practised by the Arabs in the second century and advocated in the nineteenth century by a number of French surgeons (Coppez, 1885; Motais, 1886; and others), and recently revived for the treatment of cataract in young people by several American surgeons (Scheie, 1960; Troutman, 1961; Hogan, 1967; and many others). To avoid the complication of synechiæ Leonardi (1948) entered the anterior chamber by the operative technique of cyclodialysis 5 mm. behind the limbus in the lower temporal quadrant and, introducing a cannula attached to a syringe into the anterior chamber, through this approach sucked out the soft lens matter. The main factor determining the practicability of aspiration of the lens is the absence of nuclear sclerosis; it can thus be used in most cases at least up to the age of thirty years and it is, therefore, a particularly suitable technique for the treatment of traumatic cataract (including that which follows therapeutic irradiation) in children and young adults.

The following procedure as advocated by Rice (1967) may be used (Fig. 341); under general anæsthesia and with the pupil dilated as widely as possible, retraction sutures are placed in the eyelids and bridle sutures through the superior and inferior rectus muscles; thereafter all manipulations are carried out with the aid of the operating microscope. A corneal puncture is made with a goniotomy knife just in front of the limbus in the 3 or 9 o'clock meridian. The knife is directed downwards as far inferiorly

[1] Vol. XI, p. 307.

as the size of the pupil allows and the anterior capsule of the lens is incised vertically. If the upward sweep of the knife does not create a sufficiently large incision in the lens capsule it may be enlarged by re-engaging the knife at 12 o'clock and cutting downwards, following which the knife is withdrawn. A blunt-ended cannula mounted on a syringe loaded with 1 ml. of Ringer's solution is then passed through the same limbal puncture, the tip is directed into the substance of the lens and aspiration commences, using gentle suction and taking great care not to perforate the posterior capsule. Repeated injection and withdrawal of Ringer's solution may be necessary before the lens matter is sufficiently broken up to permit aspiration. As the lens matter is removed the anterior chamber collapses and the cannula is withdrawn; another cannula is inserted and the anterior chamber re-formed with Ringer's solution followed by a further aspiration of lens matter, which should be continued until the pupillary

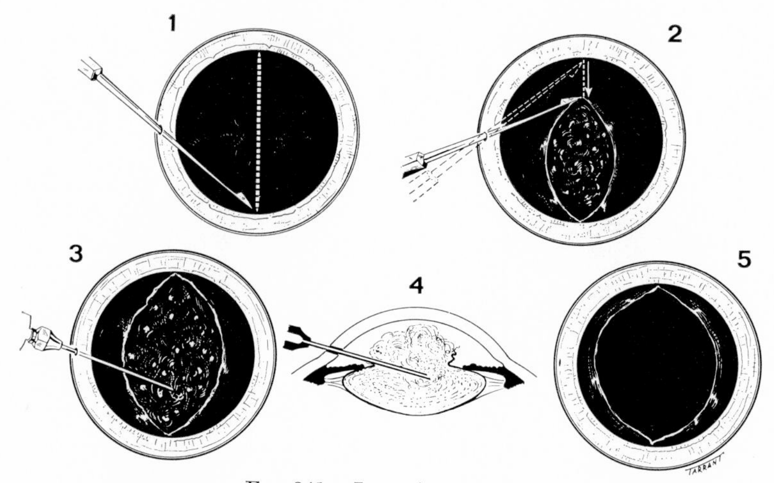

Fig. 341.—Lens Aspiration.

(1) A vertical capsulotomy with a goniotomy knife. (2) Completion of the capsulotomy. (3) and (4) Aspiration of the lens matter through a No. 17 cannula. (5) The black pupil on the completion of the aspiration (N. S. C. Rice).

area is completely clear. At the completion of the operation the anterior chamber is left filled with Ringer's solution and a mydriatic and antibiotic are instilled into the conjunctival sac. No suture is required for the corneal puncture. The advantages of this relatively simple and atraumatic procedure are that a wide opening of the globe is eliminated thereby simplifying the post-operative management, the ease with which all the lens matter can be removed thereby reducing the risk of post-operative uveitis and development of synechiæ which might lead to secondary glaucoma, and the usual absence of a dense after-cataract. An iridectomy is not generally necessary but if full mydriasis cannot be achieved pre-operatively, a sector iridectomy should be performed prior to the aspiration.

The main operative hazard of aspiration of the lens is accidental rupture of the posterior capsule and the anterior hyaloid face of the vitreous; to avoid this complication the tip of the cannula should be blunt (Rice, 1967) or the side-opening needles of Gass (1969) and Hart (1970) may be employed; the use of the operating microscope is generally desirable (Harms and Mackensen, 1967; Rice, 1967).

The complications which may arise through *dislocation of a ring of Soemmerring* have already been mentioned.[1] Laibson and McDonald (1965) removed such a ring by first transfixing it with a needle passed through the pars plana with the patient in the prone position, thereafter removing it through an anterior incision with an iris hook. Persistent capsulo-lenticular remnants may present considerable problems in the management of a retinal detachment by preventing an adequate view of the fundus; removal of a Soemmerring's ring followed by re-formation of the anterior chamber with air, the use of mannitol to produce ocular hypotension, Flieringa's ring, alpha-chymotrypsin and the division of vitreo-retinal bands under the operating microscope was successfully carried out in a small number of cases by Henderson and his colleagues (1969).

The problems involved in the rehabilitation of the patient with uniocular aphakia following removal of a traumatic cataract, including the question of contact lenses and intra-ocular implants, are fully considered in the Volume on Optics.[2]

Apart from incarceration of tissue in the wound the only injury to the uveal tract which is amenable to delayed surgical treatment is an extensive iridodialysis; the operative techniques for dealing with this injury have already been described.[3]

Retinal detachments following perforating injuries are sometimes amenable to treatment. If the tear in the retina is small the usual methods of reposition should be tried (diathermy, cryosurgery, light-coagulation). If the detachment is gross with extensive or invisible tears and particularly if it is caused by the proliferation of bands in the vitreous cavity, scleral infolding or an encircling procedure may be the most hopeful technique in those cases wherein it is felt that every effort should be made to retain some vision. Persistent vitreous opacities due to unabsorbed hæmorrhage may demand treatment in bilaterally injured or uniocular cases; if the opacities persist in spite of expectant treatment resort may be had to the somewhat hazardous and unreliable technique of vitreous replacement.[4]

The management of *traumatic glaucoma* is described in Volume XI of this *System*.

Alsen. *Klinische Erfahrungen ü. Augenverletzungen a. d. Zeit v. 1909 bis 1912* (Diss.), Kiel (1913).
Anton. *Klin. Mbl. Augenheilk.*, **150**, 675 (1967).
Barlay. *Z. Augenheilk.*, **18**, 90 (1907).
Becker. *Atlas d. path. Topog. d. Auges*, Wien (1875).
Bettman and Barkan. *Amer. J. Ophthal.*, **20**, 131 (1937).
Blodi. *J. Iowa St. med. Soc.*, **44**, 514 (1954).
Bothman. *Arch. Ophthal.*, **18**, 65 (1937).
Briggs. *Amer. J. Ophthal.*, **35**, 411 (1952).
Brown and Nantz. *Amer. J. Ophthal.*, **27**, 1220 (1944).
Trans. Amer. ophthal. Soc., **44**, 85 (1946).
Brownlie and Neame. *Brit. J. Ophthal.*, **7**, 497 (1923).
Byrnes. *Amer. J. Ophthal.*, **31**, 1261 (1948).
Calhoun. *Amer. J. Ophthal.*, **61**, 1055 (1966).
Coppez. *Arch. Ophtal.*, **5**, 174 (1885).
Custodis. *Klin. Mbl. Augenheilk.*, **89**, 612 (1932).
Denig. *Arch. Ophthal.*, **31**, 232 (1944).
Dimitriou. *Bull. Greek ophthal. Soc.*, **18**, 82 (1950).
Dunnington and Regan. *Arch. Ophthal.*, **43**, 407 (1950).
Amer. J. Ophthal., **35**, 167 (1952).

[1] Vol. XI, p. 239.
[2] Vol. V, pp. 377, 530.
[3] p. 198.
[4] Vol. XI, p. 337.

Dunphy. *Amer. J. Ophthal.*, **32**, 940 (1949).
Ellis. *Surv. Ophthal.*, **13**, 157 (1968).
Ferry and Naghdi. *Arch. Ophthal.*, **77**, 86 (1967).
Fuchs. *Beitr. Augenheilk.*, **1** (3), 201 (1891).
Trans. ophthal. Soc. U.K., **22**, 15 (1902).
Gass. *Arch. Ophthal.*, **82**, 87 (1969).
Gifford. *J. Amer. med. Ass.*, **55**, 368 (1910).
Gördüren and Tosunoglu. *Göz. Klin.*, **9**, 27 (1951).
Gottlieb and Castro. *Arch. Ophthal.*, **84**, 151 (1970).
Gradle. *Arch. Ophthal.*, **50**, 154 (1921).
Haab. *IX int. Cong. Ophthal.*, Utrecht, 425 (1899).
Harms and Mackensen. *Ocular Surgery under the Microscope*, Chicago (1967).
Hart. *Brit. J. Ophthal.*, **54**, 212 (1970).
Hartmann. *Klin. Mbl. Augenheilk.*, **118**, 530 (1951).
Havener and Gloeckner. *Atlas of Diagnostic Techniques and Treatment of Intraocular Foreign Bodies*, St. Louis (1969).
Henderson, Crock and Galbraith. *Brit. J. Ophthal.*, **53**, 296 (1969).
Hess. *v. Graefes Arch. Ophthal.*, **38** (4), 1 (1892).
Arch. Augenheilk., **33**, 204 (1896).
Hogan. *Amer. J. Ophthal.*, **63**, 821 (1967).
van der Hoeve. *Festschrift f. Rosenstein*, Leiden, 167 (1902).
Joy. *Arch. Ophthal.*, **14**, 733 (1935); **17**, 677 (1937).
King. *Trans. ophthal. Soc. U.K.*, **63**, 76 (1943).
Knapp. *v. Graefes Arch. Ophthal.*, **14** (1), 273 (1868).
Krauss. *Z. Augenheilk.*, **12**, 97 (1904).
Krückmann. *Ber. dtsch. ophthal. Ges.*, **37**, 366 (1911).
Kuhnt. *Ueber d. Verwertbarkeit d. Bindehaut ü. d. prakt. u. operativen Augenheilkunde*, Wiesbaden (1898).
Z. Augenheilk., **15**, 312 (1906); **24**, 516 (1910); **41**, 148 (1919).
Laibson and McDonald. *Arch. Ophthal.*, **73**, 643 (1965).
Leonardi. *Chirurgia dell'apparato oculare*, Rome, **1**, 515 (1948).
van Lint. *Ophthalmoscope*, **10**, 563 (1912).
Long and Tyner. *Arch. Ophthal.*, **58**, 396 (1957).
McLean, Galin and Baras. *Amer. J. Ophthal.*, **50**, 1167 (1960).
Maumenee. *Trans. Amer. Acad. Ophthal.*, **61**, 51 (1957).
Trans. Amer. ophthal. Soc., **62**, 153 (1964).
van Millingen. *Zbl. prakt. Augenheilk.*, **23**, 161 (1899).
Motais. *Gaz. méd. Paris*, No. 35, 412 (1886).
Nuel. *Ann. Oculist.* (Paris), **99**, 264 (1888).
Bull. Soc. franç. Ophtal., **10**, 37 (1892).
Ostwalt. *Arch. Augenheilk.*, **35**, 308 (1897).
Oxilia and Carlevaro. *Ann. Ottal.*, **76**, 29 (1950).
Paufique and Hervouët. *Ann. Oculist.* (Paris), **197**, 1, 105 (1964).
Payrau and Remky. *Klin. Mbl. Augenheilk.*, **138**, 797 (1961).
Price and Wadsworth. *Amer. J. Ophthal.*, **68**, 663 (1969).
Raïs. *Bull. Soc. franç. Ophtal.*, **68**, 410 (1955).
Refojo and Dohlman. *Amer. J. Ophthal.*, **68**, 248 (1969).
Refojo, Dohlman, Ahmad *et al. Arch. Ophthal.*, **80**, 645 (1968).
Rice. *Trans. ophthal. Soc. U.K.*, **87**, 491 (1967).
Rouher. *Bull. Soc. franç. Ophtal.*, **62**, 179 (1949).
Sano. *Amer. J. Surg.*, **61**, 105 (1943); **64**, 359 (1944).
Scheie. *Amer. J. Ophthal.*, **50**, 1048 (1960).
Schirmer. *v. Graefes Arch. Ophthal.*, **42** (1), 131 (1896).
Schöler. *Jb. ü. d. Augenklin. zu Berlin* (1876), 15 (1877).
de Schweinitz. *Amer. J. Ophthal.*, **13**, 41 (1896).
Snellen. *VIII int. Cong. Ophthal.*, Edinburgh, 9 (1894).
Straatsma. *Trans. Amer. Acad. Ophthal.*, **67**, 320 (1963).
Sullivan. *Trans. ophthal. Soc. U.K.*, **87**, 835 (1967).
Suzuki. *Acta Soc. ophthal. jap.*, **38**, 553 (1934).
Tassman. *Trans. Amer. Acad. Ophthal.*, **54**, 134 (1949).
Amer. J. Ophthal., **33**, 870 (1950).
Terry and Chisholm. *Amer. J. Ophthal.*, **23**, 1089 (1940).
Thies. *Klin. Mbl. Augenheilk.*, **112**, 185 (1947).
Thomas, Cordier and Michel. *Bull. Soc. franç. Ophtal.*, **60**, 173 (1947).
Town and Naidoff. *Amer. J. Ophthal.*, **33**, 879 (1950).
Trousseau. *Recueil Ophtal.*, **19**, 249 (1897).
Troutman. *Highlights Ophthal.*, **4**, 293 (1961).
Vail. *Amer. J. Ophthal.*, **29**, 785 (1946).
Viefhaus. *Ueber Lufteintritt bei Bulbusverletzungen* (Diss.), Kiel (1894).
Wadsworth. *Ophthal. Rec.*, **14**, 368 (1905).
Webster, Slansky, Refojo *et al. Arch. Ophthal.*, **80**, 705 (1968).
de Wecker. *Arch. Augenheilk.*, **2** (2), 84 (1870).
Chirurgie oculaire, Paris, 189 (1879).
Wiener and Alvis. *Surgery of the Eye*, Phila. (1939).
Young, C. A. *Amer. J. Ophthal.*, **40**, 12 (1955).
Young, J. Z. and Medawar. *Lancet*, **2**, 126 (1940).

The Post-traumatic Complications of Perforating Wounds

In addition to the misadventures which we have already discussed arising from the healing of a corneal or scleral wound when the edges are badly apposed, the incorporation in it of intra-ocular tissues or direct damage to the ocular contents by the injury, a number of further complications may arise subsequently and disturb the convalescence of the patient. The most important of these are the secondary rupture of the original wound, the development of post-traumatic uveitis or of chronic hæmophthalmitis, the introduction of infection, the development of sympathetic ophthalmitis and the formation of intra-ocular cysts.

SECONDARY RUPTURE OF THE WOUND is not an uncommon event, the cicatrix giving way on a slight trauma or the application of pressure to the lids, or sometimes apparently stretching or gaping spontaneously when the normal intra-ocular pressure re-establishes itself. Even after the lapse of some weeks a relatively slight trauma may be sufficient to re-open the original scar (4 weeks, Praun, 1899). Such an accident is always unpleasant and usually results in an extensive prolapse of the iris or even of the vitreous; moreover, healing activity having passed its height, reparation is frequently torpid and a cystoid cicatrix tends to result. In these circumstances a fistula may form, so tiny, perhaps, as to evade recognition, a complication which favours epithelial ingrowth with all the dangers that this entails (Gradle and Sugar, 1941; Theobald and Haas, 1948; and others).

A unique case was reported by Sattler (1921) wherein, 28 years after a perforating injury, the wound was re-opened and a corneal fistula formed apparently by internal trauma from the sharp edge of a calcified lens.

In view of the probable consequences of such an accident—the establishment of a fistulous or staphylomatous scar, the development of an irritative uveitis, the entrance of infection or the possible onset of sympathetic inflammation—surgical methods of treatment are usually indicated. These follow the lines already indicated: the abscission of prolapsed and the reposition of incarcerated tissue, and the adequate closure of the wound after any necessary trimming of its edges by pre-placed corneal or scleral sutures reinforced by a pre-prepared conjunctival flap, the manipulations being carried out preferably with a microscope under anæsthesia.

POST-TRAUMATIC NON-INFECTIVE UVEITIS

While some uveal irritation and vasodilatation making themselves clinically evident by ciliary injection and an aqueous flare are invariable results of every penetrating wound, a frank post-traumatic uveitis may develop and assume proportions which dominate the clinical picture and may endanger the functional survival of the eye and even occasionally implicate its fellow. Apart from the retention of foreign bodies, a subject which will be considered subsequently,[1] the most potent ætiological factors determining the onset of such a condition are the incarceration of uveal tissue in the wound, the irritation caused by free lens matter or persistent hæmorrhage, and the proliferation into the globe of exuberant connective tissue from the corneal stroma or the sclera of the wounded area. The first two of these may be surgically remediable but the presence of any of them may well result in the development of a progressive iridocyclitis at first congestive and exudative in nature and eventually plastic, leading sometimes to secondary glaucoma but more usually to hypotension and atrophy of the globe and often amenable to no treatment other than excision of the eye.

From the clinical point of view, post-traumatic uveitis may develop continuously from the immediate traumatic reaction, in which case the generalized vasodilatation characteristic of this initial phase gradually gives place to a fully developed exudative iridocyclitis. This sequence is seen most dramatically in cases wherein the penetrating injury has not been a clean cut with a sharp instrument but has been *associated with a considerable amount of contusion*: in this event the clinical picture is often complicated by a persistent and unresolved hyphæma, and the pathological changes include extensive areas of tissue-necrosis such as we have seen to be characteristic of post-concussive inflammation. The prognosis in such cases is not good, and the usual clinical course is a progressive increase of the inflammation until the eye is excised (Figs. 346–347).

More usually, however, the eye whitens after the first few days following the injury and subsequently relapses to become heavily injected, keratic precipitates sometimes appear and a uveitis develops which may be most recalcitrant to treatment—the *post-traumatic serous iritis* of Fuchs (1913). This chronic uveitis unaccompanied by concussive necrosis usually runs a less stormy course but too frequently the end-result is the same. In uncomplicated cases the inflammation may slowly resolve and the eye gradually whiten; in others the onset of a secondary glaucoma presents considerable anxiety; but the more usual sequence is the progressive development of a plastic iridocyclitis which gradually occludes the pupil and leads too frequently to a chronically irritable globe which shrinks and eventually loses the power of light perception. Even if the eye appears likely to do well at first, too often it remains constantly weak, watery and irritable, and acute exacerbations occur with the most annoying persistence, the symptoms clearing up only to relapse again, each recurrence being accompanied by the same acute pain and irritation until eventually the eye is removed, a decision frequently hastened by the fear of sympathetic inflammation.

The pathological changes in such eyes have been fully studied.[2] The

[1] p. 477.

[2] Collins (1891), E. Fuchs (1910–13), A. Fuchs (1924), Samuels (1936), Klien (1945), and many others.

FIGS. 342 and 343.—POST-TRAUMATIC UVEITIS.

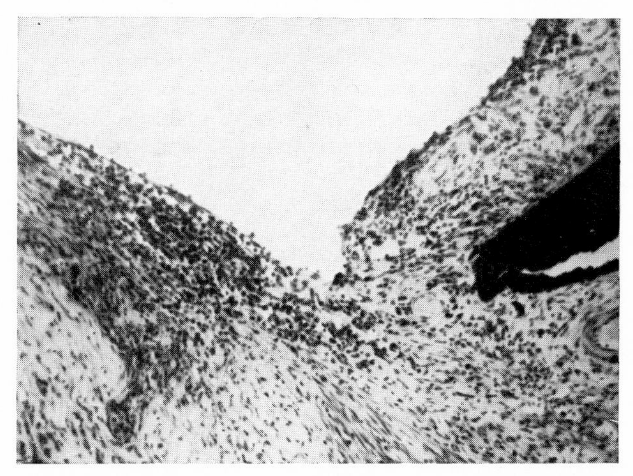

FIG. 342.

Chronic inflammatory infiltration in the root of the iris and in the uveo-scleral meshwork in a case of chronic iridocyclitis following an old perforating injury (H. and E.; × 120) (N. Ashton).

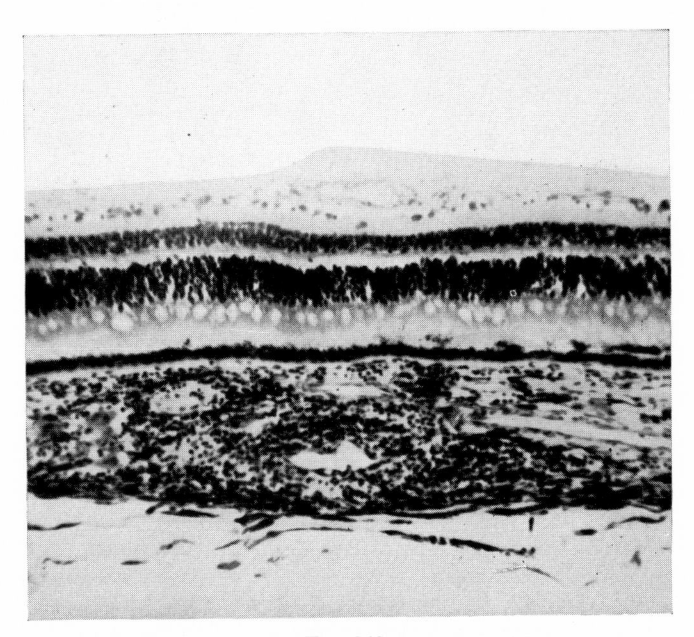

FIG. 343.

The choroid is infiltrated with chronic inflammatory cells (H. and E.; × 160) (N. Ashton).

FIGS. 344 and 345.—RETINAL INFILTRATION AFTER PERFORATING INJURIES (N. Ashton).

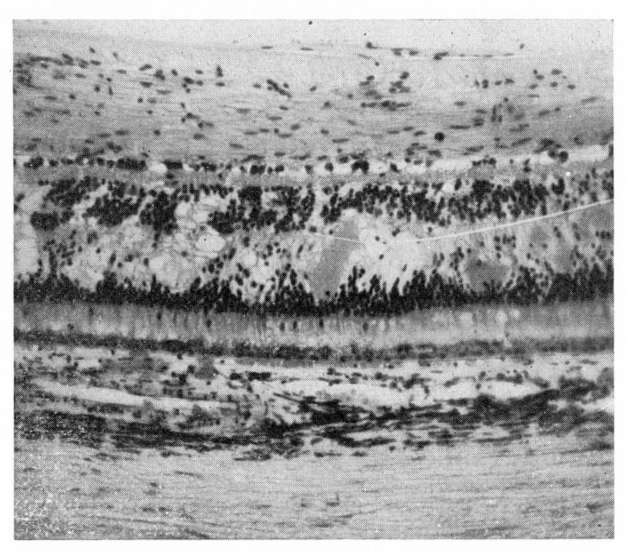

FIG. 344.—Retinal œdema associated with a perforating wound of the cornea (H. & E.; × 140).

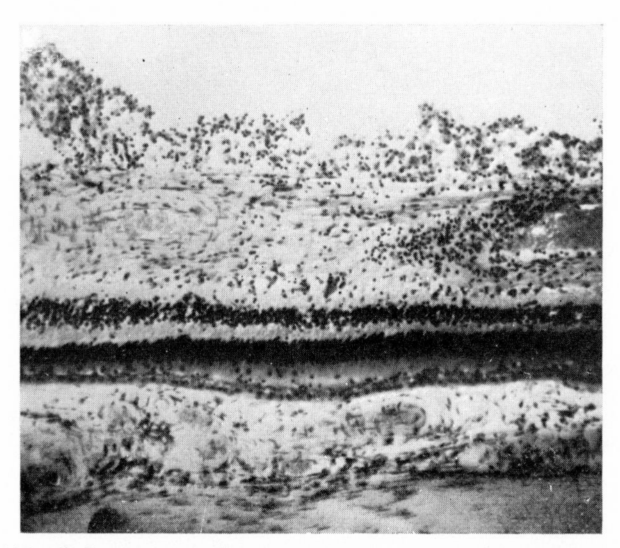

FIG. 345.—Inflammatory cells upon the surface and within the substance of the retina; these changes were associated with a perforating wound of the limbus (H. & E.; ×120).

outstanding characteristic is the round-celled infiltration with lymphocytes and plasma cells which pack the iris; here they are frequently aggregated into nodules, but are usually less conspicuous in the ciliary body and choroid (Figs. 342 and 343). A similar infiltration may also be prominent in the retina, the nerve-fibre layer and the ganglion-cell layer being peculiarly affected and the vessels being surrounded with cuffs of densely packed cells determining a picture of perivasculitis (Fig. 345). This intense retinal involvement

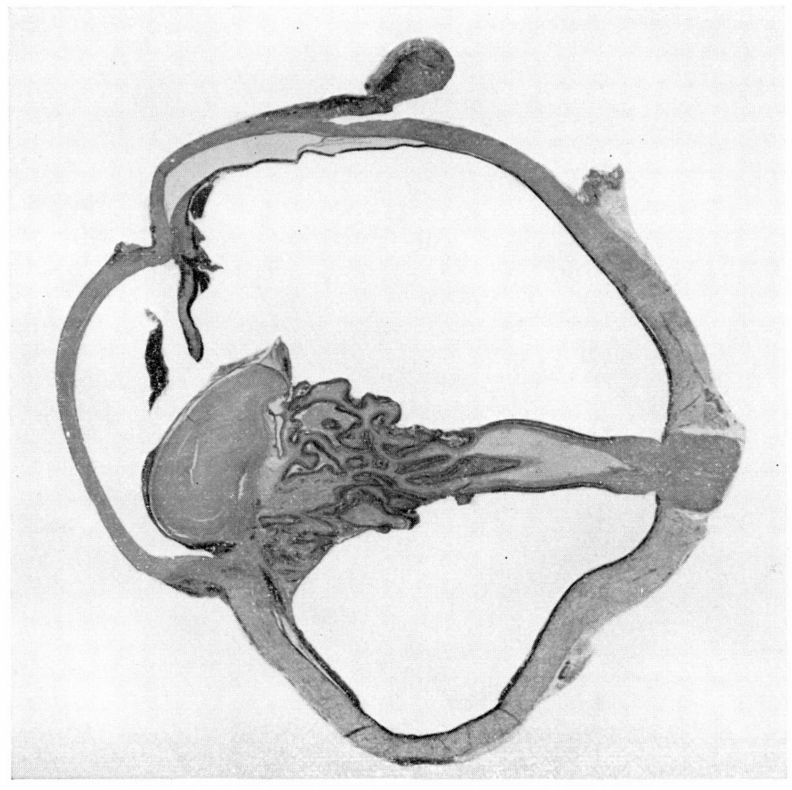

Fig. 346.—Perforating Wound of the Sclera and Ciliary Body.

From the back of the wound a dense mass of fibrous tissue projects into the vitreous space and is adherent anteriorly to the dislocated and cataractous lens and posteriorly merges into a cyclitic membrane. The totally detached retina is degenerate and is adherent anteriorly to the newly formed fibro-vascular tissue (N. Ashton).

which was particularly stressed by Samuels (1936) (*retinitis serosa*) is unusual and is often accompanied by considerable general œdema of this tissue which may become separated from the pigmentary epithelium by an albuminous exudate, a complication seen characteristically at the macula. On the surface of the retina exudates are sometimes deposited, often aggregated into spherical or mushroom-shaped clumps (Elliot, 1917; Lister, 1921)[1] while

[1] Vol. X, p. 213.

the vitreous is usually densely powdered with cells (Fig. 344 and 345). The optic nerve-head is almost constantly involved in the inflammatory reaction, the papillitis taking on the aspect of an œdematous swelling or a frankly exudative infiltration. This implication of the optic nerve-head which occurs even in injuries affecting only the anterior segment of the globe is an old observation and has been variously ascribed to toxic absorption or œdema induced

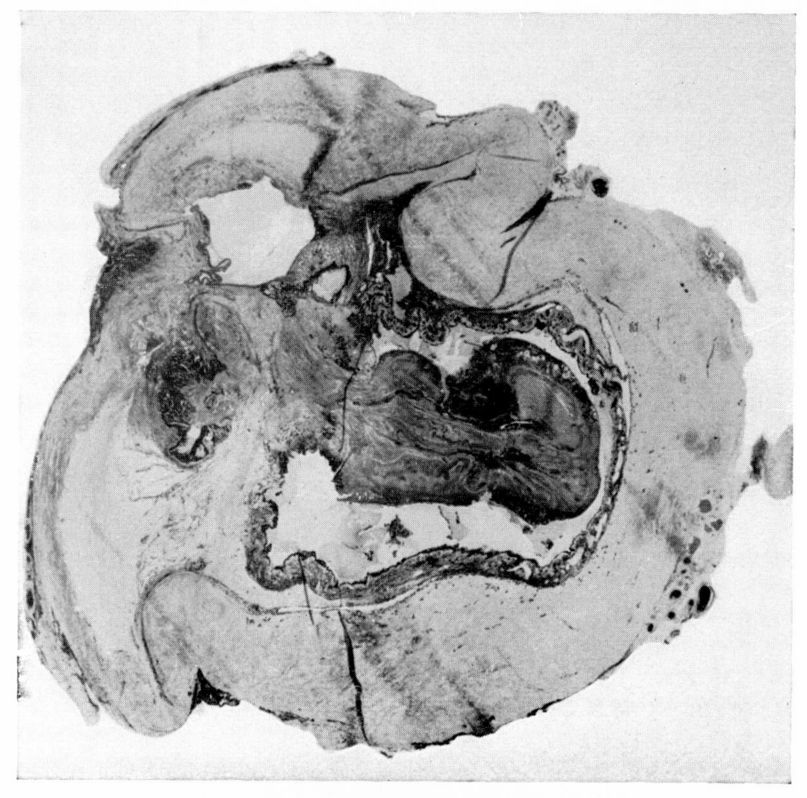

Fig. 347.—Atrophia Bulbi.

Following an old perforating wound of the globe. The intra-ocular contents are disorganized and distorted. In the anterior segment remnants of the cornea have become partially invaginated to form a cystic space lined by corneal epithelium. The anterior chamber is completely obliterated and the totally detached retina and uvea show advanced degenerative changes. There is hæmorrhagic exudate in the suprachoroidal and subretinal spaces (N. Ashton).

statically owing to the sudden lowering of the intra-ocular pressure.[1] These marked and progressive changes in the retina and optic nerve probably account for the unusually rapid deterioration of vision in this type of uveitis and the end-result is frequently widespread degeneration of all the tissues (Figs. 346 and 347).

[1] van der Borg (1908), Happe (1908), Gilbert (1910), Natanson (1910), Behr (1912), Leber (1914), and others.

The mechanism of these changes is not thoroughly understood for the fairly characteristic picture suggests some specific cause. That tissue-reaction alone in the absence of infective micro-organisms may cause a plastic uveitis of this type is well established; thus Manna and Capolongo (1951) cultured 14 such eyes after enucleation and found them sterile. In a great many cases the lens has suffered injury, and it is possible that in

FIGS. 348 and 349.—PHACO-ANAPHYLACTIC ENDOPHTHALMITIS (P. Henkind and B. Jay).

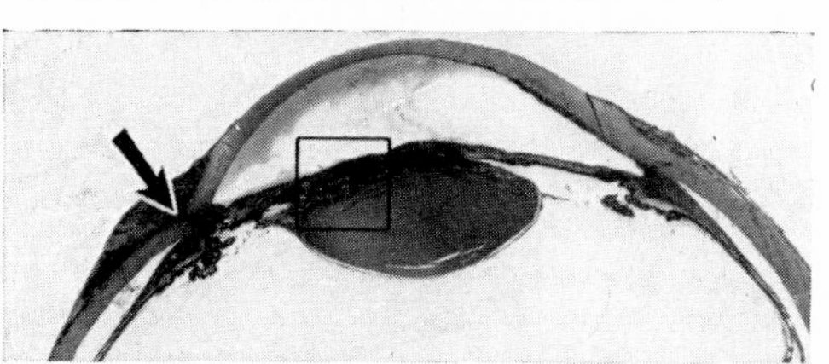

FIG. 348.—The anterior segment of the globe, showing a perforating wound (arrowed), exudate in the anterior chamber and an inflammatory reaction involving the lens and the iris (H. & E.).

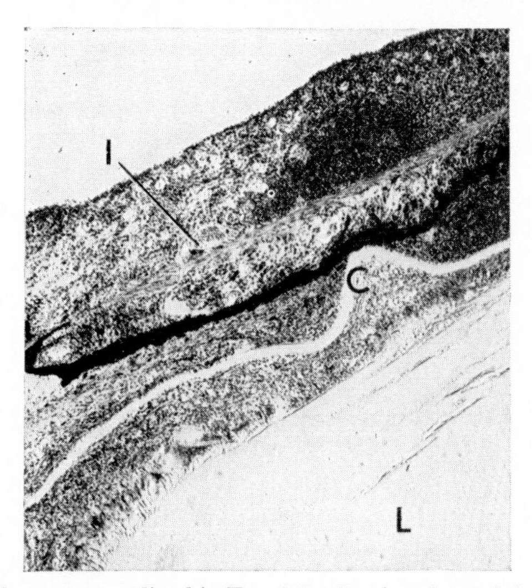

FIG. 349.—The square outlined in FIG. 348, showing the periphery of the lens (L) invaded by polymorphonuclear leucocytes, the distorted capsule of the lens (C) and the granulomatous reaction surrounding the lens and involving the adjacent iris (I).

these the reaction represents the response of the tissues to irritation by lens protein (*endophthalmitis phacoanaphylactica*)[1] (Figs. 348 and 349); the possibility of a similar reaction to uveal pigment must also be remembered. When the lens is grossly damaged the tissue-response may be violent, and the absorbing lens substance is often rapidly engulfed by a mass of granulation and fibrous tissue containing an abundance of multi-nucleated giant cells (Fig. 290).

[1] Vol. IX, p. 501.

On the other hand, other cases are associated with an uncontrolled proliferation of connective tissue which spreads profusely from the area of the wound into the interior of the eye as if in a tissue-culture[1]; irritation may therefore enter into the ætiology (Fig. 346). A further complication is the presence of blood derived from the original traumatic hæmorrhage or recurrences of bleeding; this, however, tends to produce a pathological picture with characteristics of its own (hæmophthalmitis) which will be described immediately.

An interesting but very rare complication of traumatic iridocyclitis following an ocular perforation is *alopœcia* involving loss of the hair, eyebrows and lashes. Such a sequence has been known for some time to be an unusual complication of head injuries not involving the eye (Wechselmann, 1908; Steindorf, 1914), but after ocular injuries it is still more rare. A temporary alopœcia occurring three weeks after a perforating wound of the eye was reported by Khavin (1940) and a second more dramatic case by McGrath (1951). In the latter case, six weeks after a foreign body had been removed and the eye had become quiet, an almost complete alopœcia occurred dramatically, the scanty remnants of hair, lashes and brows being thin and colourless, while scattered over the trunk were several depigmented macules. The cause of such a widespread change following an ocular injury is unknown, but such cases obviously have a parallel with the alopœcia which has long been recognized to occur in the Vogt-Koyanagi syndrome, sympathetic ophthalmitis and other types of chronic uveitis.

Four conditions simulating post-traumatic uveitis must always be remembered in the differential diagnosis—the reaction caused by the presence of a foreign body, a chronic infective endophthalmitis due to the lodgment of infection which does not run a frankly purulent course, the development in tissues damaged by trauma of an infective uveitis from an extra-ocular source, and sympathetic ophthalmitis. A clinical differentiation may be extremely difficult and is often impossible. In the first case, keratic precipitates are less common, in the last, the fellow eye is involved; but in all cases anxiety lest a bilateral affection develop usually leads to excision of the injured eye if it shows signs of persistent inflammation—and the wisdom of such a course cannot be gainsaid.

CHRONIC HÆMOPHTHALMITIS

In the presence of a profuse intra-ocular hæmorrhage or of recurrent bleedings, post-traumatic irritation tends to be prolonged and, although the eye may become quiescent, it is not uncommon for relapses of the inflammation to occur during the following years. A characteristic feature in such a sequence is the presence of conglomerate granulomatous masses on the iris or around the periphery of the anterior chamber, while small refractile bodies resembling cholesterol crystals may sometimes be seen suspended in the aqueous (Eyb, 1949; and others). Each recurrent attack of pain, photophobia and redness may be relatively easily controlled by treatment with rest, heat and atropine, but the incapacity caused by their repetition, the anxiety associated with the persistence of irritation, and the fact that the retinal function gradually but surely disappears usually lead sooner or later to the excision of the globe.

Pathological examinations of such cases show that the cause of the condition is the presence of the degenerated products of blood and the

[1] p. 332.

FIGS. 350 and 351.—POST-TRAUMATIC CHRONIC HÆMOPHTHALMITIS.

In a boy of 13 whose eye was perforated by a piece of glass from an exploding bottle. There was a profuse intra-ocular hæmorrhage; recurrent attacks of inflammation occurred during the following 4 years (Bertha Klien).

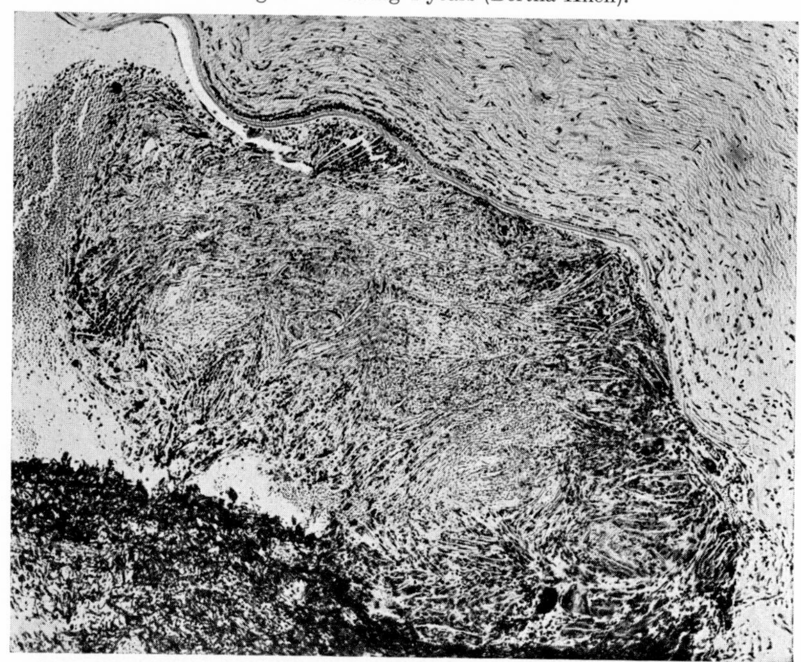

FIG. 350.—Shows a cholesterol tumour in the anterior chamber with several necrotic areas (the cornea is above and to the right, the iris below and to the left). It appeared clinically as a conglomerate mass of yellowish refractile bodies and particles resembling cholesterol crystals were suspended in the aqueous. The tumour itself consists of clumps of foreign-body giant cells, monocytes and round cells surrounding the empty slit-like spaces which always indicate cholesterol crystals *in vivo*.

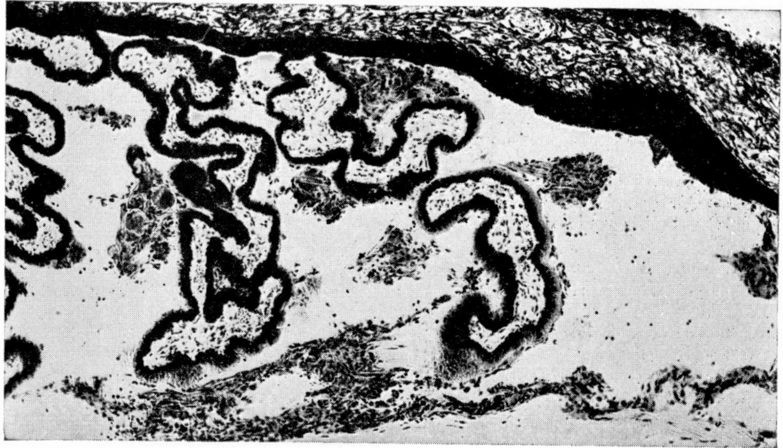

FIG. 351.—Shows similar but smaller cholesterol tumours associated with the ciliary processes.

chronic granulomatous inflammation to which they give rise. Tumour-like masses of granulation tissue may be seen particularly in the anterior chamber, the iris and ciliary body, wherein monocytes, round cells and fibroblasts, usually with a plentiful sprinkling of clumps of large foreign-body giant cells, are massed around the empty slit-like spaces which are characteristic of the presence of cholesterol crystals: in such tumours necrotic areas are common and with them round-celled or polymorphonuclear infiltration is abundant (Klien, 1945) (Figs. 350 and 351).

Such changes are similar to the post-traumatic granulomata sometimes seen to develop from a hæmorrhage into the orbit.

The *treatment of post-traumatic non-infective uveitis* can rarely be dramatic. The standard methods—mydriasis, heat, rest and sedatives—should always be fully exploited but too often they are only of temporary benefit. A more effective blocking of the inflammation and exudative phases of the post-traumatic reaction may result from the systemic use of corticosteroids or ACTH or, more easily and economically, by the topical use of the former either as drops or more effectively by subconjunctival injections; both of these agents may act dramatically if given at an early stage, or in established cases may occasionally give a sufficient fillip to the healing process so that an uneventful recovery ensues, but more usually, once organized changes have become established within the eye, their effect is only temporary and relapses follow their cessation.[1] If permanent control of the inflammation cannot be secured, the remorseless progress of the disease and its tendency to recurrent exacerbations, as well as the anxiety felt for the fate of the other eye, usually indicate enucleation as the treatment of expediency.

Behr. *Klin. Mbl. Augenheilk.*, **50** (1), 56 (1912).
van der Borg. *Klin. Mbl. Augenheilk.*, **46** (1), 359 (1908).
Collins. *Roy. Lond. ophthal. Hosp. Rep.*, **13**, 166 (1891).
Duke-Elder. *Brit. J. Ophthal.*, **35**, 637 (1951).
Elliot. *Lancet*, **1**, 325, 361 (1917).
Eyb. *Wien. klin. Wschr.*, **61**, 606 (1949).
Fuchs, A. *Atlas of Histopathology*, Vienna (1924).
Fuchs, E. *v. Graefes Arch. Ophthal.*, **77**, 304 (1910); **84**, 201 (1913).
Gilbert. *v. Graefes Arch. Ophthal.*, **77**, 199 (1910).
Gradle and Sugar. *Trans. Amer. ophthal. Soc.*, **39**, 94 (1941).
Happe. *Ber. dtsch. ophthal. Ges.*, **35**, 141 (1908).
Klin. Mbl. Augenheilk., **47**, Festschr., 140 (1909).
Khavin. *Vestn. oftal.*, **17**, 140 (1940).
Klien. *Amer. J. Ophthal.*, **28**, 1193 (1945).
Leber. *Graefe-Saemisch Hb. d. ges. Augenheilk.*, 2nd ed., Leipzig, **7** (10), 582 (1914).
Lister. *Trans. ophthal. Soc. U.K.*, **41**, 275 (1921).
McGrath. *Arch. Ophthal.*, **46**, 319 (1951).
Manna and Capolongo. *Arch. Ottal.*, **55**, 59 (1951).
Natanson. *Klin. Mbl. Augenheilk.*, **48** (1), 512 (1910).
Praun. *Die Verletzungen d. Auges*, Wiesbaden, 178 (1899).
Samuels. *Amer. J. Ophthal.*, **19**, 493 (1936).
Sattler. *v. Graefes Arch. Ophthal.*, **105**, 502 (1921).
Steffensen, Wishbow, Nagle *et al.* *Amer. J. Ophthal.*, **34**, 345 (1951).
Steindorf. *Klin. Mbl. Augenheilk.*, **53**, 188 (1914).
Theobald and Haas. *Trans. Amer. Acad. Ophthal.*, **53**, 470 (1948).
Wechselmann. *Dtsch. med. Wschr.*, **34**, 1982 (1908).
Woods. *Amer. J. Ophthal.*, **33**, 1325 (1950).

[1] Woods (1950), Steffensen *et al.* (1951), Duke-Elder (1951).

INFECTED PERFORATING WOUNDS

The infection of an eye which has suffered a perforating injury is a common and always a serious complication. It may occur in three ways: a *primary infection* may become established at the time of the injury, a *secondary infection* may be incurred before the wound has healed, and a *late infection* may affect a badly consolidated scar, an unfortunate event seen most commonly in the presence of a fistula or an attenuated staphyloma.

Of these a primary infection is the most common. Apart from small metallic fragments travelling at a high velocity, few of the objects which cause such a wound are sterile and the conjunctival sac of most people contains organisms which, although frequently innocuous and saprophytic in their usual environment, rapidly become pathogenic in the interior of the eye; for these reasons every penetrating wound should be initially treated as potentially infected. In addition, in many cases touching or rubbing the eye with soiled fingers or surgically unclean handkerchiefs introduces a secondary infection before the patient comes under informed control, and the possibility of contamination of the wound is considerably increased if it gapes or if uveal tissue is prolapsed. The virulence of the ocular reaction is, of course, augmented if gross intra-ocular damage has occurred, particularly if the lens has been injured, for free lens matter not only causes considerable intra-ocular irritation on its own account but forms an excellent culture medium; moreover, the absence of the normal immunological defences in the vitreous body allows organisms introduced into the posterior segment of the eye to flourish with little inhibition or control. Finally, in addition to the introduction of exogenous infection, it must be remembered that an injured eye becomes a *locus minoris resistentiæ*, and it is not uncommon for an infective endogenous iridocyclitis to be activated by trauma (Axenfeld, 1894; Panas, 1897; and others).

From the ætiological point of view infections introduced at the time of injury may be discussed under two headings—those due to pyogenic organisms, and those due to specific organisms, such as gas-gangrene and tetanus.

PYOGENIC INFECTIONS OF THE WOUND

Depending on the virulence of the invading organisms the clinical picture varies considerably and can conveniently be divided into three types—acute, subacute and chronic. In the most acute and fulminating cases, such as are typically caused by the streptococcus, the pneumococcus or the *Ps. pyocyanea*, a dramatic and rapidly destructive inflammation of the wound may cause a ring abscess of the cornea or a necrotic scleritis, while infection of the inner eye may result in an uncontrollable panophthalmitis. In the less acute cases the infective process may assume a fibrinoplastic character and be limited to a segment of the eye; and in more attenuated infections a chronic septic endophthalmitis may result, but even this condition too frequently results in a functionally useless organ.

RING ABSCESS (PERIPHERAL ANNULAR INFILTRATION) of the cornea[1] is a rare but distressing complication of perforating injuries, particularly relatively small corneal wounds. It is an acutely destructive condition wherein the greater part of the cornea necroses rapidly and in mass, the necrotic centre being surrounded by an annular girdle of purulent infiltration; the usual termination is panophthalmitis. As a rule it follows rapidly on the injury, sometimes within 12 hours, the interval varying from 1 to 11 days; in a case recorded by Fuchs (1903) it appeared as a late infection three years after a perforating injury which involved incarceration of the iris in the sclera.

Various organisms have been implicated—the *Bacillus subtilis* most commonly (Happe, 1907; Kodama, 1910; Flieringa, 1922; Gifford and Hunt, 1929; Hoffmann, 1933), the *Ps. pyocyanea* (Happe, 1907; R. Schneider, 1926; Safar, 1927), and a member of the proteus group (Hanke, 1903). The introduction into the inner eye of the rabbit of these organisms has led to the development of the typical condition.[2]

The clinical picture is dramatic; with great rapidity the cornea becomes hazy, the conjunctiva chemotic and the eye fixed, and soon there appears a yellow ring of infiltration, usually from 1 to 2 mm. wide, separated from the limbus by about 1 mm. of clear cornea. No matter what the position of the wound, the ring is always peripheral; the clear zone of cornea round it always remains, and the edges of the wound are usually little infiltrated. Meantime the corneal epithelium disappears en bloc, panophthalmitis sets in, the cornea assumes the consistency of wet blotting paper, and the eye is lost.

The pathology has been investigated by a number of writers.[3] In the centre of the cornea there is extensive and complete necrosis more marked in the deeper than in the superficial layers; the periphery is always vital. The epithelium and endothelium are both absent, and Bowman's and Descemet's membranes intact. Around the periphery there is a massive polymorphonuclear infiltration, usually more concentrated in the middle and deeper layers of the cornea (Fig. 352).

The prognosis is thoroughly bad once the process has become established; unless effective treatment is instituted at the onset it is the rarest thing for the eye to be retained and some vision saved (Fuchs, 1903; Hanke, 1903; Happe, 1907). In the majority of cases the cornea becomes quite opaque

[1] Vol. VIII, p. 854.

[2] Happe (1907), Kodama (1910), Kuffler (1911), Arisawa (1914), R. Schneider (1926), Jackson and Hartmann (1927), Hoffmann (1933).

[3] Collins (1893), Axenfeld (1894), Fuchs (1903), Hanke (1903–5), Morax (1904), Happe (1907), Stoewer (1907), Tertsch (1910), Stölting (1913), Attias (1914), Flieringa (1922), Gifford and Hunt (1929), and others.

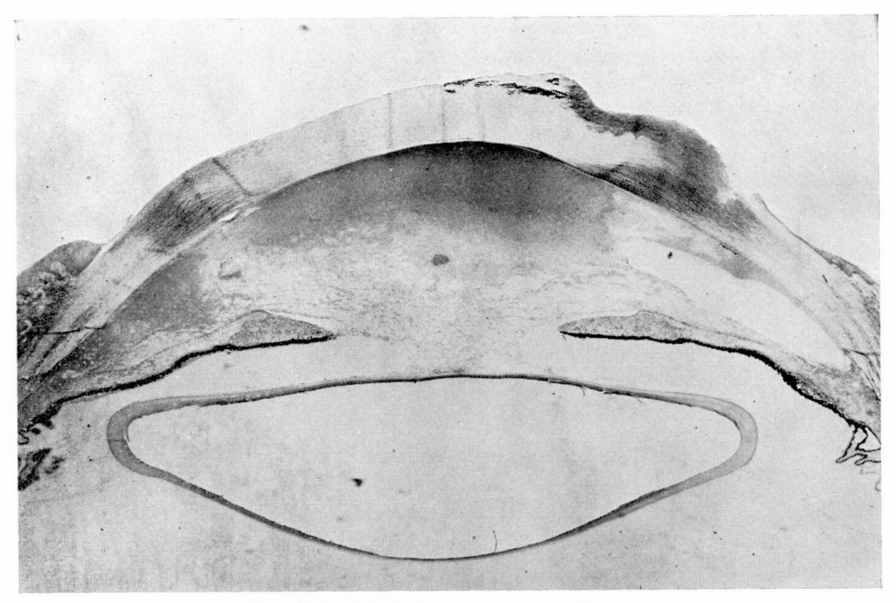

FIG. 352.—RING ABSCESS OF THE CORNEA.

The anterior chamber is full of purulent exudate (M. Hogan and L. Zimmerman's *Ophthalmic Pathology*, Saunders, Phila.).

and perception of light is abolished within 36 hours, and the eye must be eviscerated or enucleated.

The NECROTIC INFECTIVE SCLERITIS which follows acute infection of a scleral wound is less clinically evident since the picture is dominated by the associated panophthalmitis.

INFECTIONS OF THE INNER EYE

The catholicity of the objects which commonly cause perforating wounds and the multiplicity of organisms which inhabit the conjunctival (and lacrimal) sac would suggest that the resulting intra-ocular infection would have a very varied ætiology. Even although the precise organism involved is frequently difficult to determine, the literature shows this to be the case, for many have been isolated usually by culture from eyes which have been excised. The most common are the staphylococcus, streptococcus, pneumococcus, *C. xerosis*, *E. coli*, *Kl. pneumoniæ*, *Proteus*, *H. influenzæ*, *Ps. pyocyanea* and the diplobacillus of Morax-Axenfeld.

The *Bacillus subtilis* group of organisms is of particular importance owing to the fulminating character of the panophthalmitis which it initiates, usually between 6 and 24 hours after injury. It is to be noted that most members of this group are usually relatively innocuous in the conjunctival sac but extremely virulent when they obtain access into the eye, whether through a perforating wound, traumatic or operative, or as has occurred from an anterior chamber wash-out with saline contaminated by this organism in an operation for the extraction of cataract (Greenspon, 1918).

The first recorded series of cases of panophthalmitis due to the *Bacillus subtilis* was the eight cases following perforating injuries described by Poplawska (1891); 10 years later Römer (1901) described a case of post-operative infection. François (1934) was able to collect 40 cases from the literature, and others have been recorded by Motolese (1936), Reese and Khorazo (1943), and Davenport and Smith (1952). There is some doubt about the nature of the bacillus owing to the confusion that exists in the classification of this group of organisms, and Chu (1949) suggested that many of the organisms which give rise to this type of fulminating infection are in reality strains of *B. cereus*, the virulence of which is accounted for by the fact that it produces a toxin, lecithinase, similar to the toxin of *Cl. welchii*. In Davenport and Smith's case the organism isolated was identified as *B. cereus*. It must be added, however, that the organisms described by other authors correspond more closely to the classical *B. subtilis*.

PANOPHTHALMITIS following an infected wound provides one of the most dramatic and tragic clinical pictures in ophthalmology. There is usually acute pain in the eye associated with general malaise, an œdematous

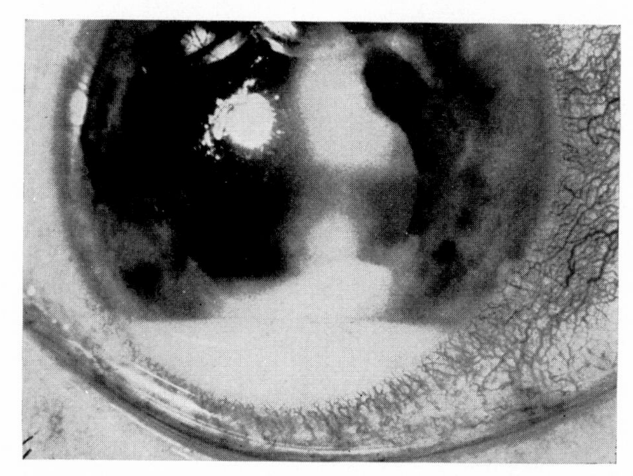

FIG. 353.—EXOGENOUS ENDOPHTHALMITIS DUE TO ASPERGILLOSIS.
Following a perforating injury. There is a considerable hypopyon (H. Tiburtius).

swelling of the lids, an intense conjunctival injection rapidly developing into chemosis, and the cornea becomes hazy and lustreless. If a view through the cornea is possible it is seen that from an early stage the iris is muddy and grey, the aqueous turbid, and the posterior surface of the cornea plastered with precipitates, a process which may soon develop into an ever-increasing hypopyon (Fig. 353). The vitreous becomes gradually more hazy until the posterior segment of the globe becomes obscured, while eventually a yellow reflex develops behind the pupil due to the accumulation of pus in the vitreous cavity. Depending on the virulence of the organism this stage may persist for some hours or days while the symptoms gradually become more violent; the tension rises, the eye becomes fixed and proptosed as the sclera becomes involved, systemic symptoms increase and the temperature rises, and the pain becomes more and more unbearable until relief is obtained by surgical measures or by a spontaneous perforation of the globe, usually through the wound, the lips of which become swollen and necrotic. Thereupon the pain immediately subsides, and after prolonged suppuration the end-result is a shrunken and completely disorganized eye. As a rule, such an eye shrinks to a condition of phthisis and then usually gives rise to very little trouble. In these cases the prognosis with regard to the eye and vision is almost invariably bad (Figs. 354–358).

A SUB-ACUTE FIBRINO-PLASTIC UVEITIS (Fuchs, 1904–5), presenting a less fulminating and generalized picture than panophthalmitis, may result if the infection is less virulent or is partially controlled. If the perforation involves the anterior part of the globe the lips of the wound become swollen, the cornea hazy and the conjunctiva chemotic; the iris is thickened, swollen

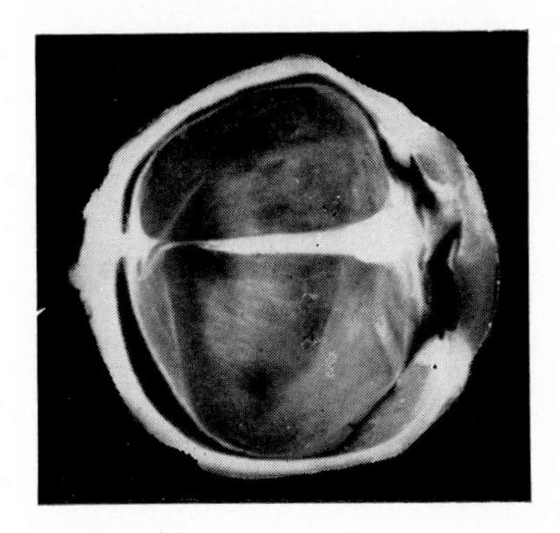

FIG. 354.—EARLY INFECTION OF A PERFORATING WOUND.

Perforating wound of the cornea and lens; the eye was excised $3\frac{1}{2}$ weeks later. The iris is seen to be adherent to the cornea, the lens is partially absorbed and from it a mass of inflammatory exudate passes posteriorly along Cloquet's canal to reach the optic disc (Museum, Inst. Ophthal.).

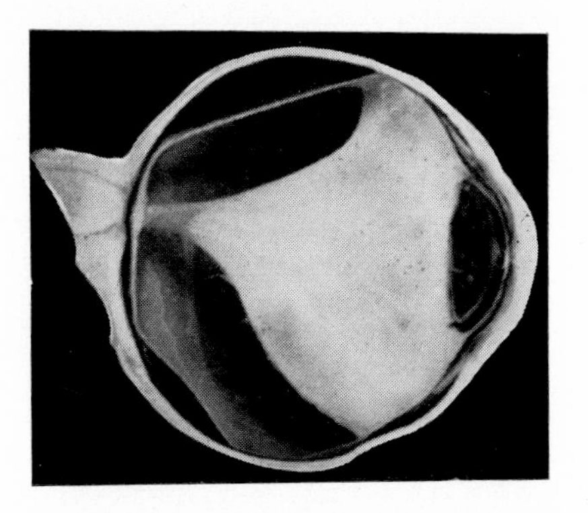

FIG. 355.—INFECTED PERFORATING WOUND.

Resulting in an abscess in the anterior segment of the eye and in the vitreous. The retina is detached (Museum, Inst. Ophthal.).

and intensely hyperæmic, its tissues being densely infiltrated, even in places becoming necrotic, and from them is poured out a copious inflammatory exudate, coagulating on the surface of the iris, spreading over the lens capsule to cover the pupillary area, coating the back of the cornea, filling up the anterior chamber to form a hypopyon or the posterior chamber to surround the lens, and spreading into the anterior part of the vitreous body.

If resolution sets in, macrophages invade the exudate and organization and fibrosis result (Fig. 359). The exudate in the anterior chamber may thus become converted into fibrous tissue in the consolidation of which new-formed vessels grow in from the iris. Sometimes the organized exudate spreads over the posterior surface of the cornea and envelops the lens so that the posterior chamber is obliterated. The iris habitually becomes adherent to

FIGS. 356 to 358.—PANOPHTHALMITIS FOLLOWING PERFORATING INJURIES (N. Ashton).

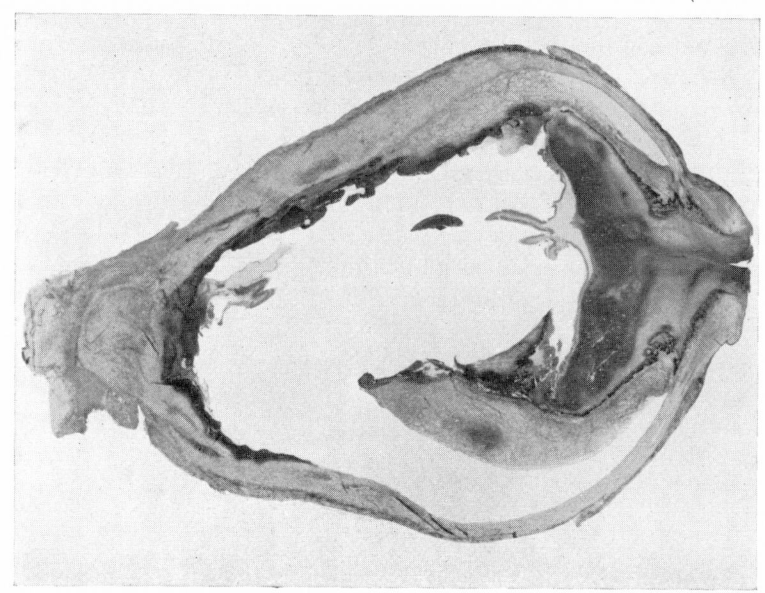

FIG. 356.—A corneal abscess followed the development of an ulcer due to injury. The iris is almost completely destroyed and both the anterior chamber and vitreous space are filled with purulent exudate. The lens has been extruded. The posterior uvea is densely infiltrated with pus cells and the totally detached retina is necrotic.

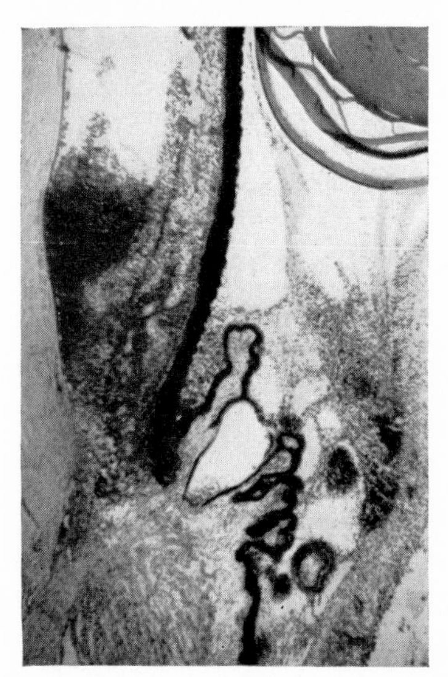

FIG. 357.

Note the purulent exudate in the anterior chamber, in the outer third of the iris and in the newly formed cyclitic membrane (H. and E.; × 32).

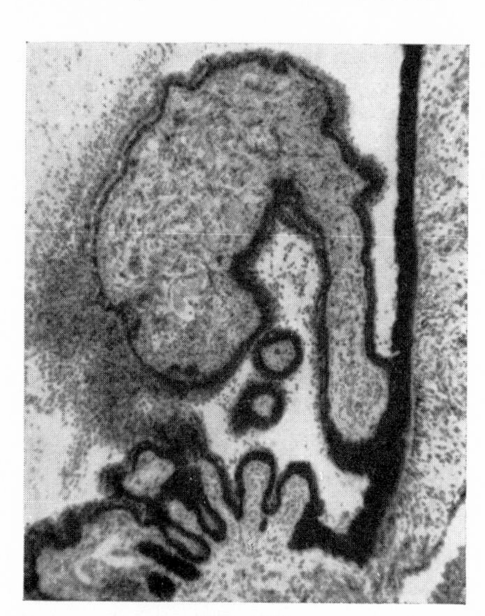

FIG. 358.

A case of panophthalmitis showing large numbers of polymorphonuclear leucocytes pouring out of the ciliary body (H. and E.; × 68).

the cornea at its periphery, and occasionally the cornea, the iris and the lens become welded together in an adherent staphyloma. Simultaneously, in the ciliary region the exudate organizes to form a cyclitic membrane which, strangulating the ciliary processes as it organizes and contracts, reduces them to a state of atrophy and draws them into the interior of the eye, while the epithelium, both pigmented and unpigmented, proliferates into the organized fibrous tissue as long finger-like processes. The lens also, encircled and pressed upon by fibrous tissue, becomes cataractous and shrinks, while if much exudate has escaped into the anterior vitreous, its subsequent contraction may result in atrophy of the globe.

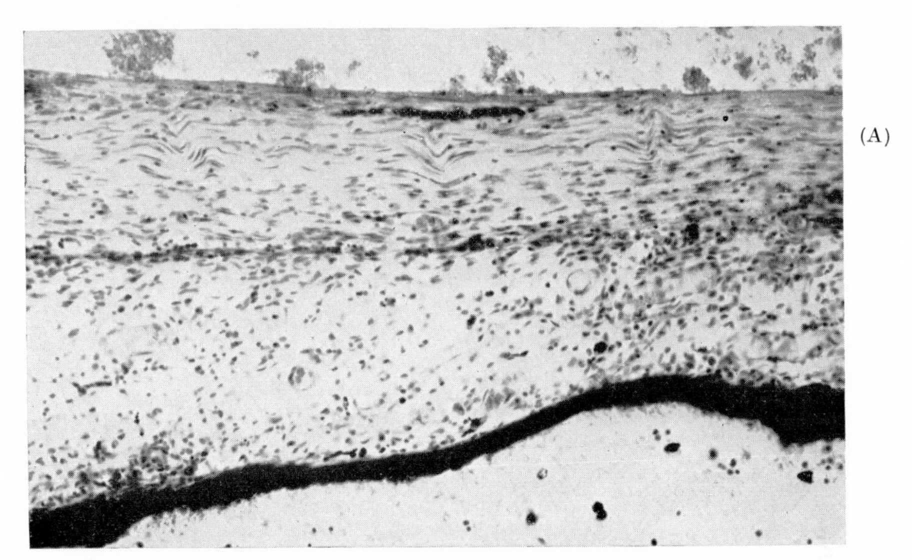

FIG. 359.—FIBROUS TISSUE ON THE IRIS.

In an old case of traumatic uveitis, showing a thick fibrous membrane (A) on the surface of the iris (H. & E.; ×120) (N. Ashton).

Infections of the lens form an important part of the clinical picture in such cases, since this tissue provides an ideal culture medium for the multiplication of organisms, although if the capsule is intact it offers excellent protection against the entrance of bacteria. For this reason, even in cases of panophthalmitis, pus cells are rarely found within this tissue (B. Samuels, 1942). Indeed, in experimental work carried out on rabbits, Busacca (1933) concluded that a rupture of this membrane was a necessary prelude to the infection of the lens, but von Szily (1938) found that in cases of abscess of the vitreous the pus may erode the capsule. Once its continuity has been broken, which usually occurs either as the result of a perforating injury or a foreign body, infection usually runs on apace, for not only pyogenic cocci and bacteria but also spore-bearing organisms grow luxuriantly within it, multiplying at a rapid rate before they are reached by pus cells or can be attacked by the immune defences of the body (Morax and Chiazzaro, 1927).

Although injuries to the lens are common in perforating wounds, infection of the lens is relatively rare (8 in 73 enucleated eyes, Rychener and Ellett, 1942), and a primary infection of the lens is still more rare (ABSCESS OF THE LENS). Such primary infections usually pursue a stormy clinical

FIGS. 360 to 363.—ABSCESS OF THE LENS FOLLOWING A PERFORATING INJURY.

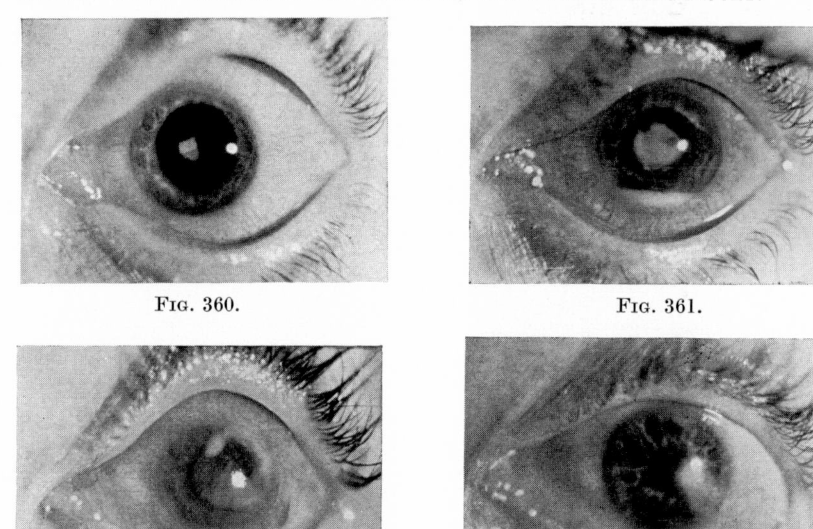

FIG. 360. FIG. 361.

FIG. 362. FIG. 363.

The cornea was perforated by a fragment of steel which lodged near the centre of the lens; this was extracted through a keratome incision by the hand magnet. Five weeks later a primary abscess of the lens developed (Fig. 360). Intravenous typhoid and sulphathiazole were administered ; 2 months after the original injury the abscess of the lens had increased and a hypopyon had formed (Fig. 361). Repeated paracenteses were done whereafter the eye began to show signs of improvement (Fig. 362). The end stage of the inflammation showed a clearing of the anterior chamber, seclusion of the pupil and a residual corneal opacity (Fig. 363). Secondary glaucoma developed subsequently which was successfully controlled by an iridectomy (R. O. Rychener and E. C. Ellett).

course, resulting in enucleation (Yver and Barrat, 1935; Hertel, 1938), but exceptionally the eye may survive with the development of cataract and a secluded pupil (Busacca, 1933, perforating injury with a pen; Rychener and Ellett, 1942, steel foreign body in the lens; S. L. Samuels, 1954, in a child pecked in the cornea by a cock). At this stage it is possible that the most effective measure to prevent destruction of the eye is early removal of the lens before the infection spreads; thus Mejer (1948) saved 4 out of 13 eyes infected in this way (Figs. 360–363).

The pathological reaction of a traumatized lens to infection is essentially passive.[1] Initially in acute infections it is invaded by swarms of leucocytes forming a localized abscess (Fig. 364) or, in the more subacute cases, by lymphocytes which insinuate themselves in long chains between the fibres, disintegrating the structure of the lens, breaking up the tissue and hastening its absorption. In older persons the nucleus may long withstand this invasion and may eventually be surrounded by a wall of infiltration containing giant cells as if it were a foreign body (von Szily, 1938). As time goes on this disintegrative process is replaced by reparative activity and the lens substance tends to become replaced by fibrous tissue to form a *fibrous-tissue cataract*, a change which has sometimes been followed by the development of bone, containing on occasion fully developed haversian systems (*cataracta ossea*).[2]

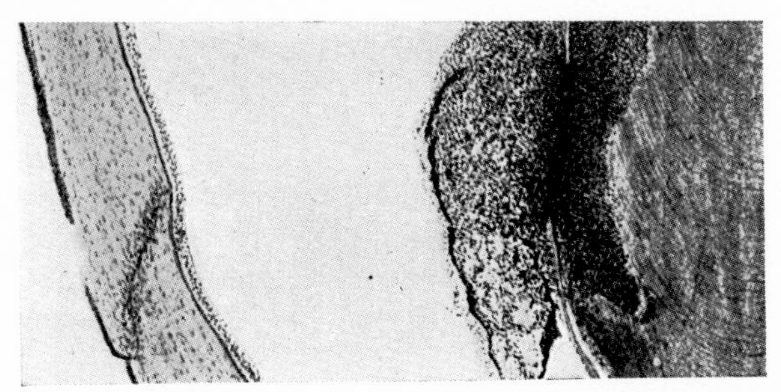

FIG. 364.—ABSCESS OF THE LENS AFTER A PERFORATING INJURY.

The perforating wound is seen through the cornea (left). There is an abscess in the superficial layers of the lens and the heavily infiltrated iris is seen adherent to the tear in the capsule (E. Hertel).

Infection of the vitreous body is the main feature if the wound involves the posterior part of the eye. The pathology of the process is analogous to that occurring in the anterior segment, but the results are usually more disastrous since, while a hypopyon in the anterior chamber can in favourable circumstances disappear to leave few traces behind, pus in the vitreous cavity invariably entails permanent and serious damage and usually loss of the eye. There is first an intense engorgement of the choroid, a leucocytic and histiocytic infiltration, a spread into and a disorganization of the retina, and a pouring of exudate into the vitreous to form an abscess in it (Fig. 365). If, on the other hand, the abscess starts in the vitreous, it spreads therefrom to the retina and then affects the choroid secondarily, the suppurative process usually establishing itself first at the periphery and near the optic disc and spreading thence towards the equator (Fig. 366). In either case the suppurative exudate in the vitreous becomes transformed into fibrous tissue

[1] Vol. XI, p. 4.

[2] Panas and Rémy (1879), Goldzieher (1880), Alt (1880), Dunn and Holden (1898), Aubineau (1904), Pitsch (1926), Meves (1929), and others.

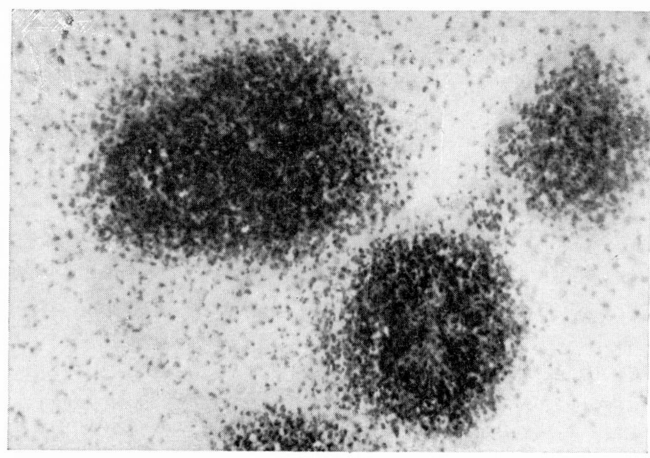

Fig. 365.

Panophthalmitis following a perforating injury. Aggregations of pus cells are seen in the vitreous (H. & E. ; ×160) (N. Ashton).

which, contracting and degenerating, detaches the retina and forms a pseudoglioma or more usually results in an atrophic globe. From the clinical point of view the absence of sensory nerves in the choroid allows a purulent inflammation of the posterior segment to be painless and symptomless, and, indeed, the eye may appear relatively normal until the yellow mass of purulent exudate behind the lens is seen through the dilated pupil (*amaurotic cat's eye*). At an early stage, of course, vision is rapidly reduced and ultimately is completely and irrevocably destroyed, the common result being atrophic degeneration of the globe with subsequent shrinkage.

It is to be remembered, however, that the subsidence of the acute inflammation and the development of atrophy do not by any means indicate

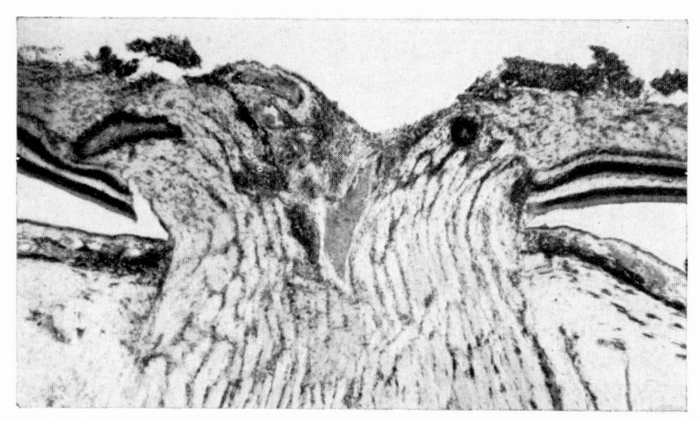

Fig. 366.—Post-traumatic Panophthalmitis.

The optic nerve-head showing infiltration with acute inflammatory cells in panophthalmitis following injury (H. & E. ; ×33) (N. Ashton).

the end of the patient's troubles since, in contradistinction to a phthisical eye which usually remains quiet since it is reduced to little more than a fibrotic mass, an atrophic eye tends to develop periodic attacks of irritation and inflammation. This condition of *relapsing atrophic uveitis* may, indeed, be associated with so much recurrent pain and discomfort that in many cases excision is preferable to the retention of the eye.

A CHRONIC SEPTIC ENDOPHTHALMITIS runs a much less turbulent course. Pain and photophobia are only moderate and the ciliary injection does not progress to the chemotic stage, so that the external appearance of the eye conforms somewhat to the picture presented by a post-traumatic, non-infective uveitis. In contradistinction, however, to this condition when unassociated with concussive trauma, the ciliary injection does not quieten and, although there is an aqueous flare with free-floating cells, corneal precipitates are rarely prominent. From the time of the injury the eye remains inflamed and the continued irritation usually calls for enucleation; in this event histological examination shows a localized focus of polymorphonuclear exudate somewhere along the path of the penetrating wound in the uvea or the lens, the abscess thus formed being walled off with fibrous tissue while the remainder of the eye shows a more chronic round-celled infiltration. The natural result of such a process is the gradual development of atrophy of the globe with retinal detachment, often associated with recurrent inflammatory exacerbations.

Treatment

The treatment of an eye thus infected if it is to be of any value must be immediate and drastic. It is true that antibiotic drugs are therapeutic agents of great efficacy, the introduction of which has altered a prognosis previously almost invariably gloomy, but it is to be remembered that the delicacy of the intra-ocular tissues makes them extremely susceptible to the toxins liberated by invading organisms so that once a suppurative process has started, even although it may be ultimately controlled, the end-result is frequently disappointing. Too often, although not excised, a useless eye is retained. The only satisfactory treatment for such cases is therefore prophylactic.

As soon as the presence of an infective process has been recognized the standard treatment for an acute uveitis should be instituted. The fullest possible mydriasis should be maintained with atropine, mydricaine or other mydriatics, and heat, either with hot bathings or medical diathermy or the application of ice-packs if heat is found intolerable in acutely congestive conditions, should be combined with such general measures as rest, sedatives and analgesics. Additional benefit may be obtained by the use of corticosteroids which block the acute and exudative phases of inflammation sometimes in a most dramatic manner. They may be administered systemically or topically, either by drops or more effectively by subconjunctival injection but, although the immediate results may be dramatic, reliance for a permanent cure must be placed on a specific attack on the invading organism itself.[1]

Because of the ability of the *sulphonamides* to traverse the blood-aqueous barrier, the greatest value of these drugs is by systemic administration and, since their toxicity depends on their concentration, and sensitization is specifically limited to the particular drug used, the simultaneous administration of several sulphonamides, by reducing the dose of each below the sensitization level, avoids toxic symptoms and at the same time allows a high total concentration to be given with safety; their effect, however, is by no means invariably dramatic. *Antibiotic* drugs are of considerably more therapeutic value and of these the prototype, penicillin, is still the most effective, particularly in streptococcal and pneumococcal infections. Local administration is necessary, however, since this drug cannot pass the blood-aqueous barrier in therapeutic quantities. Subconjunctival injections of penicillin up to 500,000 units in 0·5 ml. water can safely be given and thereby a therapeutic concentration can be maintained within the eye during the following 36 or 48 hours.[2] When a more wide-ranging antibiotic is required, framycetin (250–500 mg.) or neomycin (100–500 mg.) may be given subconjunctivally; when the infection is caused by *Pseudomonas pyocyanea* the most effective antibiotics are polymyxin (10 mg.) (Ainslie, 1953–65) and colistin (15 mg.) (Jones and Armenia, 1963), which should be given by subconjunctival injection. Although the subconjunctival injection of antibiotics is generally sufficient, it may be necessary to supplement this by systemic administration and in severe cases and in some mycotic infections their direct injection into the anterior chamber may be indicated.

The large number of the chemotherapeutic and antibiotic agents now available undoubtedly makes the ophthalmologist's choice of the treatment appropriate to each particular case increasingly more difficult. Technically the antibiotic employed should be suited to the appropriate organism, the susceptibility of which should theoretically be determined.[3] Occasionally the clinical appearance of the eye may suggest the type of infection while conjunctival swabs or epithelial smears may betray the presence of an organism which may be presumed to be the causal agent. As a rule in practice the effectivity of treatment depends almost entirely on the timeliness of its commencement, and the nature of an intra-ocular infection may be impossible to determine even by resorting to the technique of puncture of the anterior chamber and withdrawal of aqueous. Probably the best comprehensive therapy for immediate application is local penicillin or framycetin given by subconjunctival injection combined with the systemic administration of penicillin, tetracyclines, chloramphenicol or a sulphonamide mixture. If positive bacteriological findings can be obtained, as for example by aqueous puncture, and the sensitivities of the organism determined the treatment can be accordingly modified.

It is to be noted that if the infection has gained a foothold in the lens the prognosis is bad; if in the vitreous it is worse: in the former case if the lenticular infection is primary, immediate extraction or evacuation of the lens followed by the introduction of penicillin may on occasion save the eye. Extraction should preferably be performed by the intracapsular method but if this is impossible the maximum amount of lens matter should be removed.

[1] For a detailed description of the treatment of infective uveitis see Volume IX, pp. 167 and 218.

[2] Sorsby and Ungar (1946), Records (1966–67), Records and Ellis (1967), McPherson *et al.* (1968).

[3] Leopold (1967–68), Ellis (1968), Kanski (1969–70), and many others.

If medical and chemotherapeutic measures fail to control the infection recourse must be had to radical surgery. In subacute and chronic cases enucleation can be safely performed but in acute cases when the intra-ocular contents are purulent and the wound is likely to be reopened during the operative manipulations, evisceration of the globe is a safer procedure. Of the two alternatives an excision results in the more rapid healing but it involves two dangers—bursting of the eye during the operation with an escape of pus into the orbital tissues, and a spread of the infection along the severed optic nerve sheaths with the possible development of meningitis. Moreover, this operation should not be attempted if the surrounding orbital tissues are infected and probably should not be when a suppurative process which started in the posterior segment has reached a fulminating stage. The safer alternative is to open the cornea freely by cruciate incisions which leave the conjunctiva at the limbus intact, scoop out the contents of the globe, swab the interior of the sclera with some antiseptic and dust it with an antibiotic powder. If the orbital tissues are not infected this operation can be done without opening Tenon's capsule, but if they are also implicated more rapid healing would be obtained by removing most of the sclera, leaving only a frill around the optic nerve-head.

Infections by Specific Organisms

GAS GANGRENE. The infection of a perforating wound by the *Cl. welchii* (*perfringens*) is a very rare event generally associated with a wound involving the vitreous or the presence of a foreign body; Leavelle (1955) reviewed 53 cases from the literature since the original observation by Chaillous (1904) and added three more. Additional cases have been described by Oehring and Jütte (1963), Walsh (1965), McEntyre and Curran (1968), and Kurz and Weiss (1969). Contamination of traumatic wounds by Gram-positive anaerobic spore-forming organisms is common (10–30% of cases, MacLennan, 1962; Baker, 1964) yet they rarely produce this specific disease; *Cl. perfringens* is the organism most frequently isolated in true gas gangrene and is usually responsible for ocular clostridial infection. Its pathogenicity is due to the production of potent soluble exotoxins of which at least twelve are known (McHenry *et al.*, 1963), the most important being lecithinase which has a destructive action on the lipo-protein complex of the cell-wall. The avascularity of the vitreous may provide the clostridia with the most important requirement for growth, namely, an environment with a lowered oxidation-reduction potential. In every case, usually within 24 hours after the injury, a characteristic fulminating panophthalmitis develops with six distinctive clinical features, the recognition of which is important because of the necessity for urgent and radical treatment. These are, the rapid onset with unusually severe pain, a brawny swelling of the eyelids, an early rise of ocular tension, the appearance of blood or of a thin coffee-coloured discharge, the eventual formation of gas bubbles in the anterior chamber and the rapid development of total amaurosis. These clinical signs are sufficient to establish a diagnosis without waiting for bacterial confirmation. The pain is probably associated with ocular hypertension and the rapid loss of the perception of light is presumably due to the effect of the necrotizing toxins liberated by the organisms on the retinal tissues. Systemic manifestations include a moderate fever and leucocytosis, malaise, nausea and vomiting. In its clinical course the infection is unusually rapid and fulminating (Figs. 367–8); a ring abscess of the cornea may appear, the uveal tissue necrotizes, the eye fills with a mass of gelatinous blood-stained and eventually purulent material

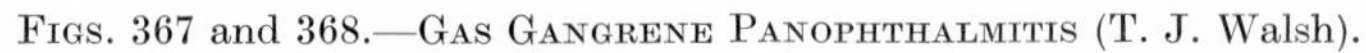

Figs. 367 and 368.—Gas Gangrene Panophthalmitis (T. J. Walsh).

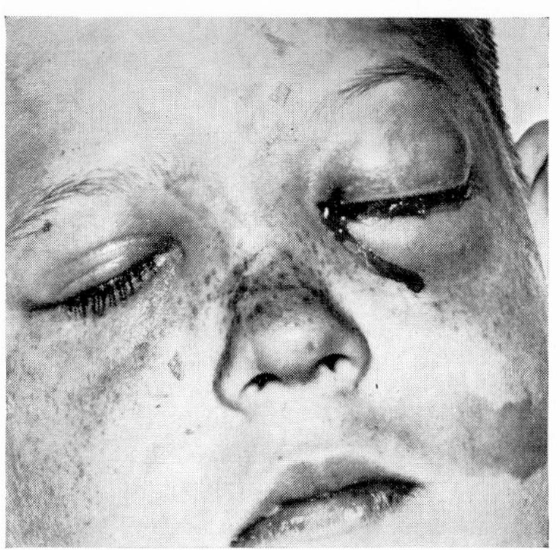

Fig. 367.—In a 9-year old boy whose left eye was perforated by a flying object while using a hammer and chisel. The lids are erythematous with brawny non-crepitous œdema.

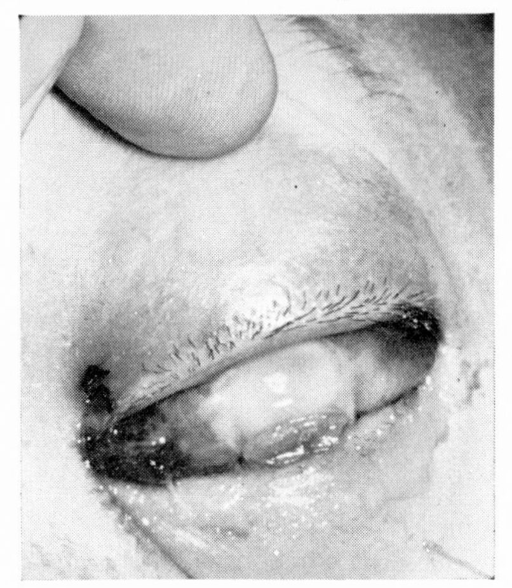

Fig. 368.—The eye, showing a fulminating panophthalmitis with hypopyon filling the anterior chamber. There were no visible gas bubbles. Owing to lack of response to any therapy the eye was eviscerated.

and perforation follows. In all cases described the vision has invariably been destroyed despite heroic therapeutic measures, even in those cases recognized and treated at a very early stage (Davidson and Burn, 1943; Capus, 1946; Leavelle, 1955). Treatment must consist of evisceration or enucleation, the former being preferred if retrobulbar infection is suspected, while exenteration of the orbit may rarely be required to control the infection (Davidson and Burn, 1943).

It is interesting that in intra-ocular infections the toxins are apparently confined within the globe so that all the reported cases have recovered uneventfully whether the eyes were eviscerated or enucleated, healing being usually as prompt and kindly as in uninfected cases. In no case was there any widespread infection and there was no mortality, a striking contrast to this type of infection in other parts of the body; thus in a heavily contaminated wound of a limb with much muscular damage if all infected tissue is not removed surgically death is likely, and uterine gas gangrene occurring as a post-abortal infection has a fatal outcome in many cases (Douglas, 1956; and others).

The organism is, however, sensitive to penicillin and this drug should certainly be given in adequate dosage; thus at least 10 million units daily are required, preferably by intravenous injection in the early stages; some workers, however, consider that tetracycline is more effective in the treatment of clostridial infections. Both these antibiotics were completely effective in the prophylaxis of experimental gas gangrene in sheep (Owen-Smith, 1968), and British soldiers involved in jungle warfare in Borneo were provided with tetracycline capsules for self-administration after wounding to reduce sepsis and the likelihood of gas gangrene (Wheatley, 1967). Tetracycline should be given initially by intravenous injection in a total daily dose of not more than 2 g. bearing in mind the risk of damage to the liver with this method of administration, and when improvement is obvious the drug should be continued in the same dose by mouth for about 10 to 14 days. Cephalothin has also been recommended as useful in the treatment of clostridial infections in a dose of up to 6 g. daily for 10 days (Goodman and Gilman, 1965). Although specific antitoxins are essential in the management of clostridial infections at other sites, their use in ocular infections does not have any definite beneficial effect on the course of the inflammation; nevertheless, the prophylactic administration of polyvalent gas gangrene antitoxin is a wise precaution. This mixture contains antibodies for the three most commonly found gas-forming anaerobes, each ampoule containing antitoxin to *Cl. welchii* (*perfringens*) 10,000 units, *Cl. septicum* 5,000 units and *Cl. œdematiens* 10,000 units. When a wound may have been exposed to clostridrial infection, especially if devitalized tissue is present, a protective dose of antitoxin is indicated, the actual dose required depending on the intensity of infection and the time elapsing before the patient is seen. When the patient is treated soon after injury one ampoule of mixed antitoxin should be given, preferably by intravenous injection; if there has been much delay two or even three ampoules may be required. When gas gangrene is clinically obvious the antitoxin should be given without waiting for identification of the causal organism. If, however, *Cl. welchii* alone is isolated the specific antitoxin to this organism is preferable. Following the initial intravenous dose, further doses should be given 4 or 6 hourly according to the response, regardless of the age of the patient. Slowing of the pulse is usually a sign of improvement.

In all cases the possibility of serum reactions should be borne in mind and measures for the treatment of such complications should be readily available (adrenaline 1 : 1,000 for hypodermic injection and intravenous hydrocortisone). In all cases a test-dose should be given before definitive treatment.

Finally, *hyperbaric oxygen* therapy, in which patients suffering from gas gangrene are exposed intermittently to oxygen at pressures of three atmospheres, has proved of considerable benefit in some cases of clostridial infection at other sites, possibly as a result of the inhibition of the production of alpha-exotoxin (Ledingham, 1969), but it is doubtful if this form of treatment has any application in the very rare cases of ocular infection.

Infection by TETANUS of a perforating wound of the globe although rare is a spectacular catastrophe which has occurred with sufficient frequency to make it desirable to use prophylactic measures when the circumstances of the accident suggest the possibility of its occurrence. In practically every reported case the causal agent has been an object associated with horses (10 cases were horsewhip injuries), or with ground contaminated by manure. It is interesting that in the majority of cases an infective endophthalmitis or panophthalmitis has followed the trauma, and since the experimental intra-ocular injection of *Cl. tetani* produces only a mild iridocyclitis in rabbits (Ulbrich, 1905), it would seem likely that the infection is more prone to develop in the presence of a mixed pyogenic infection (Fig. 369). It is to be remembered that contamination may occur not only at the time of the accident but subsequently, a sequence suggested in a case reported by Hagedoorn (1950) wherein tetanus developed through contamination from dirty fingers after a corneal burn from a firework.

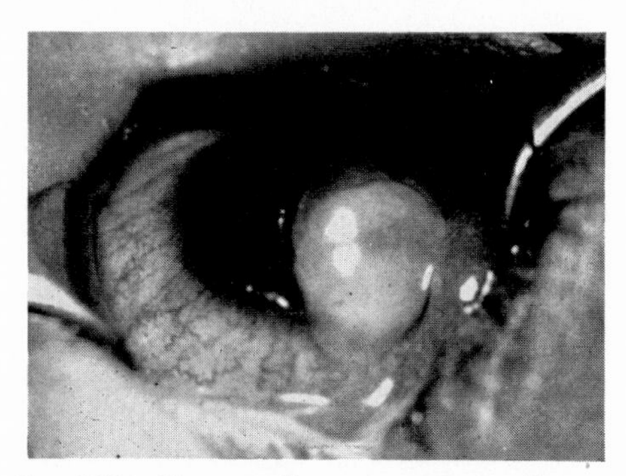

Fig. 369.—Tetanus Infection of the Cornea.

Occurring in a boy aged 4 after perforation of the conjunctiva into the orbit by a piece of wood (J. Tsutsui).

The literature on this subject is not large; since Pollock's (1847) first report from Dublin, Wagenmann (1910) collected 14 cases recorded up to the time of his monograph, E. R. Schneider (1916) brought the number up to 20, Collin (1921) to 23, Quentin (1937) and Cogan (1939) to 29. Subsequent cases have been reported by Jayme-Goyaz (1941) and Wetzel (1942), both of whom reviewed the literature extensively bringing the number of cases to 33, while further reports have been made by Wall (1948), Lenkiewicz and his colleagues (1963), and Czukrász (1963, following a pitch-fork wound of the conjunctiva and crushing of the inferior rectus), and tetanus following retained orbital foreign bodies has been reported by Dellaporta (1950) and Tsutsui (1957), both due to a piece of wood and by Damato (1966) due to a piece of broken reed. It is interesting that only 14 case reports were available in the world literature prior to the general introduction of tetanus prophylaxis during the first World War.

The tetanus which develops 6 to 8 days after the injury is usually of the cephalic type, characterized initially by trismus associated with ocular motor paralysis and a facial palsy of the peripheral type, but this initial localization is usually temporary and the generalized spasmodic contractions characteristic of the disease have usually supervened.

Prophylaxis. Active immunization against tetanus can be produced by injections of tetanus toxoid (the toxin of *Clostridium tetani* converted to toxoid by formalin and adsorbed onto aluminium hydroxide). This is now widely accepted as an essential part of immunization in childhood, frequently administered at the same time as vaccines for diphtheria and pertussis with boosters for patients who by reason of their occupation or environment are exposed to tetanus if they are injured. These include all agricultural, horticultural, veterinary, sewage and garbage workers, demolition workers and foundry men, athletes, those involved in road accidents and children in general. If the patient has a reliable history of tetanus immunization including adequate reinforcing doses, a dose of only 0·5 ml. of the toxoid need be given; when a patient has never been immunized against tetanus or there is doubt about this, active immunization should be ensured by the administration of 0·5 ml. of toxoid, a dose which should be repeated on two subsequent occasions. A reinforcing dose of toxoid 0·5 ml. should be repeated 6 to 12 months after the primary course and again after an interval of not more than five years; caution, however, should be exercised with patients who repeatedly present with minor injuries lest too frequent administrations of the toxoid lead to the development of hypersensitivity. When tetanic infection is clinically obvious, tetanus antitoxin should be given at the earliest possible moment but it should be remembered that the antitoxin neutralizes only circulating toxin and cannot influence that already fixed in the nervous system. As a general rule systemic antibiotic therapy is desirable; although this has no effect on the toxins in the nervous tissue it may help in the eradication of active organisms at the site of injury.

Where possible, antitetanic gamma globulin prepared from human patients carrying antibodies to tetanus should be used since this eliminates the problem of anaphylactic reactions. If this cannot be obtained recourse may be had to the administration of other antitetanic sera with due attention to precautions against the risk of anaphylaxis such as the administration of a test dose and the availability of adrenaline. The serum, however, should be reserved for patients who have not received such an injection within the last 10 years and present with heavily contaminated or infected wounds of several hours' duration. Indeed, the use of antitetanic serum is nowadays rarely indicated since, in an area of low tetanus incidence, the majority of wounds can be adequately treated with antibiotics and the initiation of a course of active immunization with tetanus toxoid.

Enucleation or evisceration of the eye does not alter the course of the disease for the infection spreads at an early stage. More general measures such as the use of muscle relaxants, barbiturates and other drugs for the control of muscular spasms, tracheotomy and intravenous feeding usually require that the patient should be transferred as soon as possible to a centre specializing in the care of such cases.

Ainslie. *Brit. J. Ophthal.*, **37**, 336 (1953); **49**, 98 (1965).
Alt. *Lectures on the Human Eye*, N.Y. (1880).
Arisawa. *Arch. vergl. Ophthal.*, **4**, 314 (1914).
Attias. *Arch. Ottal.*, **21**, 1 (1914).
Aubineau. *Ann. Oculist.* (Paris), **132**, 100 (1904).
Axenfeld. *v. Graefes Arch. Ophthal.*, **40** (3), 1; (4), 103, 128 (1894).
Bakteriologie in d. Augenheilkunde, Jena (1907).
Baker. *Amer. J. Surg.*, **107**, 689 (1964).
Busacca. *Boll. Oculist.*, **12**, 647 (1933).
Capus. *Arch. Ophthal.*, **36**, 226 (1946).
Chaillous. *Clin. Ophtal.*, **10**, 328 (1904).
Chu. *J. gen. Microbiol.*, **3**, 255 (1949).
Cogan. *Amer. J. Ophthal.*, **22**, 1365 (1939).
Collin. *A propos d'un cas de tétanus*, Paris (1921).
Collins. *Ophthal. Rev.*, **12**, 221 (1893).
Czukrász. *Klin. Mbl. Augenheilk.*, **143**, 375 (1963).
Damato. *St. Luke's Hosp. Gaz.*, **1**, 53 (1966).
Davenport and Smith. *Brit. J. Ophthal.*, **36**, 389 (1952).
Davidson and Burn. *Trans. ophthal. Soc. U.K.*, **63**, 375 (1943).
Dellaporta. *v. Graefes Arch. Ophthal.*, **150**, 614 (1950).
Deutschmann. *v. Graefes Arch. Ophthal.*, **30** (3), 77, 331 (1884).
Douglas. *N.Y. St. J. Med.*, **56**, 3673 (1956).

Dunn and Holden. *Arch. Ophthal.*, **27**, 499 (1898).
Ellis. *Surv. Ophthal.*, **13**, 157 (1968).
Flieringa. *Klin. Mbl. Augenheilk.*, **69**, 241 (1922).
François. *Bull. Soc. franç. Ophtal.*, **47**, 423 (1934).
Fuchs. *v. Graefes Arch. Ophthal.*, **56**, 1 (1903); **58**, 391 (1904); **61**, 365 (1905).
Gifford and Hunt. *Arch. Ophthal.*, **1**, 494 (1929).
Goldzieher. *Arch. Augenheilk.*, **9**, 322 (1880).
Goodman and Gilman. *The Pharmacological Basis of Therapeutics*, 3rd ed., N.Y. (1965).
Greenspon. *Amer. J. Ophthal.*, **1**, 316 (1918).
Hagedoorn. *Ophthalmologica*, **119**, 245 (1950).
Hanke. *Z. Augenheilk.*, **10**, 373 (1903).
Klin. Mbl. Augenheilk., **43** (1), 724 (1905).
Happe. *Ber. dtsch. ophthal. Ges.*, **34**, 343 (1907).
Hertel. *v. Graefes Arch. Ophthal.*, **139**, 1 (1938).
Hoffmann. *Z. Augenheilk.*, **80**, 124 (1933).
Jackson and Hartmann. *J. lab. clin. Med.*, **12**, 442 (1927).
Jayme-Goyaz. *Amer. J. Ophthal.*, **24**, 1281 (1941).
Jones, W. and Armenia. *Amer. J. Ophthal.*, **56**, 758 (1963).
Kanski. *Brit. J. Ophthal.*, **53**, 64 (1969); **54**, 316 (1970).
Kodama. *Klin. Mbl. Augenheilk.*, **48** (1), 624 (1910).
Kuffler. *v. Graefes Arch. Ophthal.*, **78**, 227 (1911).
Kurz and Weiss. *Brit. J. Ophthal.*, **53**, 323 (1969).
Leavelle. *Arch. Ophthal.*, **53**, 634 (1955).
Ledingham. *Recent Advances in Surgery*, 7th ed., London, 295 (1969).
Lenkiewicz, Bobrowski and Górlaski. *Klin. oczna*, **33**, 235 (1963).
Leopold. *Symposium on Ocular Therapy*, St. Louis, **2** (1967); **3** (1968).
McEntyre and Curran. *Amer. J. Ophthal.*, **65**, 109 (1968).
McHenry, Martin, Hargraves and Baggenstross. *Proc. Mayo Clin.*, **38**, 23 (1963).
MacLennan. *Bact. Rev.*, **26**, 177 (1962).
McPherson, Presley and Crawford. *Amer. J Ophthal.*, **66**, 430 (1968).
Mejer. *Klin. Mbl. Augenheilk.*, **113**, 366 (1948).
Wien. klin. Wschr., **62**, 34 (1950).
Meves. *Z. Augenheilk.*, **68**, 30 (1929).
Morax. *Ann. Oculist.* (Paris), **132**, 409 (1904).
Morax and Chiazzaro. *Ann. Oculist.* (Paris), **164**, 241, 641 (1927).
Motolese. *Boll. Oculist.*, **15**, 1023 (1936).
Oehring and Jütte. *Dtsch. med. Wschr.*, **88**, 2092 (1963).
Owen-Smith. *Brit. J. Surg.*, **55**, 43 (1968).
Panas. *Arch. Ophtal.*, **17**, 273 (1897).
Panas and Rémy. *Anat. pathologique de l'oeil*, Paris (1879).
Pitsch. *Klin. Mbl. Augenheilk.*, **77**, 636 (1926).
Pollock. *Dublin med. Press*, **17**, 372 (1847).
Poplawska. *Arch. Augenheilk.*, **22**, 337 (1891).
Quentin. *Bull. Soc. franç. Ophtal.*, **50**, 92 (1937).
Records. *Arch. Ophthal.*, **76**, 720 (1966); **78**, 380 (1967).
Records and Ellis. *Amer. J. Ophthal.*, **64**, 135 (1967).
Reese and Khorazo. *Amer. J. Ophthal.*, **26**, 1251 (1943).
Römer. *Ber. dtsch. ophthal. Ges.*, **29**, 209 (1901).
Rychener and Ellett. *Trans. Amer. ophthal. Soc.*, **40**, 285 (1942).
Safar. *Z. Augenheilk.*, **61**, 25 (1927).
Samuels, B. *Arch. Ophthal.*, **27**, 345 (1942).
Samuels, S. L. *Acta XVII int. Cong. Ophthal.*, Montreal-N.Y., **3**, 1841 (1954).
Schneider, E. R. *Ann. Oculist.* (Paris), **153**, 395 (1916).
Schneider, R. *Klin. Mbl. Augenheilk.*, **77**, 103 (1926).
Sorsby and Ungar. *Brit. med. J.*, **2**, 723 (1946).
Stoewer. *Klin. Mbl. Augenheilk.*, **45** (1), 372; (2), 560 (1907).
Stölting. *Klin. Mbl. Augenheilk.*, **51** (1), 5; (2), 304 (1913).
von Szily. *Trans. ophthal. Soc. U.K.*, **58**, 595 (1938).
Tertsch. *v. Graefes Arch. Ophthal.*, **73**, 314 (1910).
Tsutsui. *Amer. J. Ophthal.*, **43**, 772 (1957).
Ulbrich. *Ber. dtsch. ophthal. Ges.*, **32**, 256 (1905).
Wagenmann. *Graefe-Saemisch Hb. d. ges. Augenheilk.*, 2nd ed., Leipzig, **9** (17), 132 (1910).
Wall. *Eye, Ear, Nose Thr. Mthly.*, **27**, 179 (1948).
Walsh. *Brit. J. Ophthal.*, **49**, 472 (1965).
Wetzel. *Amer. J. Ophthal.*, **25**, 933 (1942).
Wheatley. *J. roy. Army med. Corps.*, **113**, 18 (1967).
Yver and Barrat. *Arch. Ophtal.*, **52**, 676 (1935).

SYMPATHETIC OPHTHALMITIS

The entire subject of SYMPATHETIC OPHTHALMITIS has already been discussed at length elsewhere in this *System*[1]—its ætiology, clinical picture, pathology and treatment—and need not be further elaborated here. It will

[1] Vol. IX, pp. 558–589.

be remembered that it is a rare disease, and that a perforating wound involving uveal tissue is the most common antecedent, particularly if the uveal tissue has prolapsed and has remained so for some time. Although a subacute inflammation in a soft eye with delayed or incomplete healing of the wound is the most common and suppuration in the injured eye the least common exciting condition, the greatest vagaries may occur, sometimes a minute and hardly noticeable puncture and at others a gross and extensive injury giving rise to the inflammation in the other eye. Sympathetic inflammation, however, is not typically the result of a profound ocular catastrophe, the minor injuries, limbal perforations and slight incarcerations of uveal tissue provide the greatest proportion of cases wherein this unfortunate complication occurs, while on very rare occasions it has been observed following contusion injuries without obvious perforation. A curious geographical incidence has been noted: thus, although perforating injuries with prolapse of the uveal tissue are common throughout the world, sympathetic ophthalmitis is very rare in Central Africa (Evans, 1963) and is virtually unknown amongst Australian aboriginals (Mann and Rountree, 1968). It will be remembered that while the onset of inflammation in the fellow eye usually appears within three weeks to two months after the injury, the latent period may vary from five days to many years, and that the inflammation which has a characteristic pathological picture tends to be progressive, running a chronic course with a decided tendency to relapse. Before control of the inflammation by corticosteroids was introduced the eye was unable to survive this ordeal and a high proportion of the patients lost useful vision. In addition to the use of these compounds, considerable success has been claimed with immuno-suppressive agents, such as methotrexate (Wong *et al.*, 1966) and azathioprine (Moore, 1968), and with anti-lymphocyte globulin (Fuchs, 1969). The previous somewhat grim prognosis has been considerably improved with these modern methods of treatment, but sympathetic ophthalmitis must still always be looked upon as a very serious disease.

Traumatic Cysts

The development of cysts within the eye after a perforating injury is a relatively rare event, the ultimate consequences of which, however, are usually serious. We have already discussed the epithelial "cysts," sometimes of enormous proportions, which may result from the ingrowth of corneal epithelium through the wound itself, and we shall see presently that an organized foreign body, particularly a cilium, retained within the eye frequently results in cystic formation.

In addition to these, EPITHELIAL IMPLANTATION CYSTS may occasionally result from a perforating wound. *In the cornea* their formation is determined by the active proliferation of the epithelium, and when these cells grow into the wound or when small fragments of the epithelium are detached and transposed to another layer, a cyst occasionally of considerable size may be formed at any part in the track, either on the surface of the cornea, in its substance or at its posterior aspect and, as we have seen, the epithelial proliferation may be of such an extent as to form a cyst of the anterior chamber. Several cysts may co-exist (one in the cornea, one in the anterior chamber and one between the ciliary body and the sclera—Clausnizer, 1911). A cyst of the anterior chamber may, indeed, communicate with the surface by a fistula (Kümmell, 1907). If the iris is incorporated in the scar, a cyst may be formed lined by pigmented epithelium (Claiborne, 1905). It is to be remembered that such cysts may appear with great rapidity after an injury; they have been produced experimentally by introducing a conjunctival flap into an artificially prepared corneal wound (Suzuki, 1934).

In the sclera traumatic implantation cysts are also rare. As in the cornea, they represent a proliferation of the surface epithelium within the deeper tissues. As a rule it is probable that the cyst is formed from conjunctival epithelium which has had an opportunity to grow in between the lips of a wound in which healing has been delayed, although it is possible that it may arise from cells transferred by trauma from the epithelial layers, maintaining no connection with them. The latter is probably the rarer mechanism; but it was experimentally demonstrated by Niwa (1930), and its clinical occurrence in one case has been suggested by the finding of foreign particles in the vicinity (Rubert, 1910). The rarity of these cysts may be explained by the inadequacy of the scleral tissue to act as a culture medium for epithelial cells owing to its avascularity, as well as by the mechanical inhibition caused by its dense consistency; probably for this last reason such cysts are usually seen in the young.

Such cysts are naturally found anteriorly in the exposed parts of the sclera near the limbus or underneath the bulbar conjunctiva. Some considerable time (months or years) after the injury, a small vesicular swelling appears which may remain stationary (Ischreyt, 1907). More usually, however, it slowly increases in size, its outer wall becoming thin, soft and fluctuating, and occasionally the posterior wall shows the dark tint of uveal pigment (Eisenstein, 1907); on the average it attains the size of a bean, but it may reach larger dimensions. Usually the limbus stops its anterior spread, and it may tend to encircle it (half or two-thirds of the circumference, Waldhauer, 1866; Gruening, 1901); but occasionally it has trespassed this boundary to insinuate itself between the lamellæ of the cornea and form a corneo-scleral cyst (Michel, 1901) (Fig. 370).

The cyst may be multilocular (Lagrange, 1901; Michel, 1901; Lauber, 1904; de Lapersonne, 1913); it may send large extensions into the cavity of the globe, a process which eventually causes a reaction and painful symptoms (Rados, 1919; Michaïl, 1933), or more than one cyst may exist (Früchte and Schürenberg, 1906; Goulden and Whiting, 1921). Occasionally a small communication has existed with the chambers of the eye (Lawrence, 1847; Lauber, 1904). Histologically the cyst is lined by surface epithelium, usually in several stratified layers, almost invariably conjunctival but on occasion resembling corneal epithelium (Velhagen, 1925; Weymann, 1930; Melanowski, 1938), and it contains a watery fluid and some cellular debris (Figs. 371 and 372); the surrounding sclera may show considerable hyaline degeneration (Grom, 1949). Such cysts are diagnosed from conjunctival cysts in that they are fixed to the sclera and the conjunctiva moves freely over them.

They have been noted in association with puncture wounds, as by scissors, (Melanowski, 1938), operation wounds (Gruening, 1901; Pravossud, 1907; Odinzov, 1910; Filatov, 1923), or after an evisceration (Potechina, 1929) or burn (de Vincentiis, 1887), or post-traumatically on a shrunken globe (Beigelman, 1934).

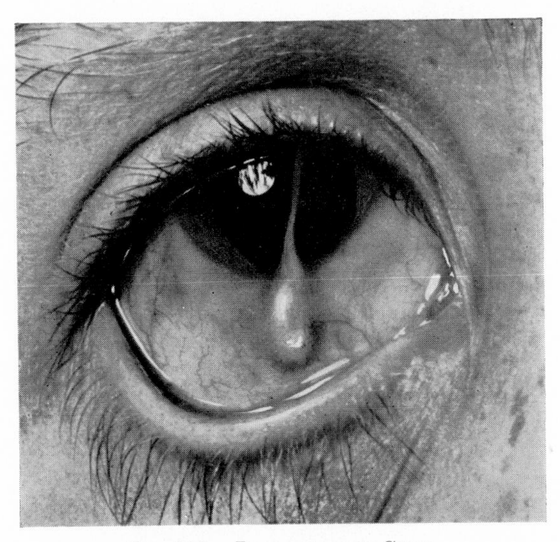

FIG. 370.—IMPLANTATION CYST.

Healed corneo-scleral perforating wound, complicated subsequently by an implantation cyst in the sclera (Inst. Ophthal.).

Within the globe implantation cysts are relatively rare, following an incised wound or in association with a retained foreign body. All kinds of wounds may be responsible for such a development, particularly accidental perforating wounds with steel instruments or glass (even a lead pencil, Roth and Geiger, 1925). Foreign bodies of all kinds entering the eye have been the transplanting agent, such as pieces of metal (Ahlström, 1903; Blaschek, 1905) or wood (Pickard, 1906). Operative wounds involving perforation have frequently figured in the ætiology. It is important when considering the origin of "spontaneous" cysts to realize how readily a small injury can be missed, for in several of the cases the occurrence of an accident has not been realized, or it has been dismissed as a triviality although the presence of a foreign body in the eye has provided proof of the ætiology.

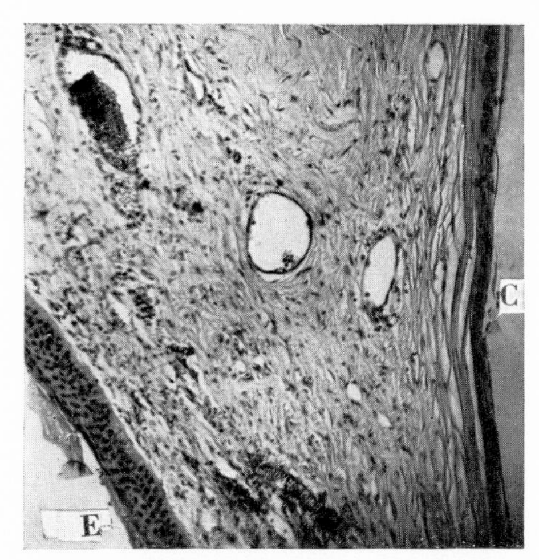

Fig. 371.—Traumatic Intrascleral Cyst.

The cyst appeared in a child of 6 after an injury by an arrow 6 months previously. E, conjunctival epithelium; C, the epithelium of the cyst which was about the size of a lentil formed of cubical and cylindrical cells. The fibrous tissue in the region of the cyst shows some hyaline degeneration. In the sclera itself there are large capillary vessels resembling an inflammatory infiltration (E. Grom).

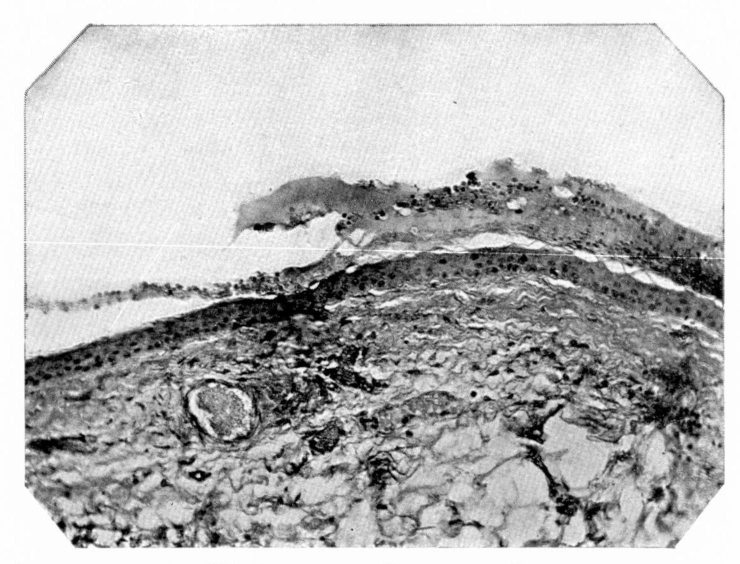

Fig. 372.—Epithelial Cyst of the Sclera.

A fixed implantation cyst. Note the wall of stratified epithelium and the epithelial debris in the cyst (C. Goulden and M. Whiting).

The implantation of an eyelash is a typical precedent, a subject which will be separately discussed.[1]

The literature contains a large number of such cases. Mackenzie (1830) described one in detail, and sporadic cases were recorded by Wharton Jones (1852), von Graefe (1857–64), Hulke (1869) and others, until the paper of Rothmund (1871–72) appeared which established the pathology of the condition. He collected 36 cases, of which 28 followed perforating wounds, two followed cataract operations, and three the inclusion of an eyelash, and established the theory of the mechanical transference of epithelial elements from the surface into the inner eye (see further Greeff, 1892; Meller, 1901; Streiff, 1904; Kümmell, 1907; Urmetzer, 1908; Collins, 1914; and others).

Such cysts have been produced experimentally on several occasions in animals by introducing into the anterior chamber foreign bodies, skin, mucous membrane or hairs.[2]

The implantation cysts thus formed may be of two distinct types: solid-looking round or oval pearl cysts, and translucent serous cysts with thin walls.

PEARL CYSTS (TUMOURS) appear as solid greyish-white round or oval bodies with a pearly lustre, usually situated in the peripheral parts of the iris stroma or in the angle of the anterior chamber. Their nature was first clearly demonstrated by Monoyer (1872); they may become evident a few months (Silva, 1905) or a few years (Früchte, 1906) or a very considerable time after injury (14 years, Villard and Dejean, 1933; 37 years, Horay, 1928), and frequently they are associated with an eyelash or a foreign body. The walls are formed of stratified or cubical epithelium, sometimes closely resembling that of the cornea or conjunctiva, and these cells may be continued throughout the entire mass arranged in concentric lamellæ like the layers of an onion. Frequently, however, the central cells undergo degeneration, the nuclei disappear, globules of fat or cholesterol crystals are deposited often in considerable quantity, together with indeterminate granular material. Finally, the degeneration may progress to the formation of cystic spaces, so that an actual cyst may eventually be formed.[3]

SEROUS CYSTS are more common; they may arise within a few weeks (Blaschek, 1905) or may not be noted for many years after an injury (44, Klien, 1945) (Figs. 373 and 376). The cyst is composed of a relatively thin wall, often of ill-developed or irregular epithelium, and contains a yellowish or slightly turbid fluid. The wall may, indeed, be so thin as to be readily transparent clinically, and in one case von Hippel (1913) saw a hypopyon-like deposit which kept a horizontal level when the head was moved. The cyst usually occurs in the periphery of the iris stroma, the anterior layers of which are stretched over it to become thin and atrophic; as growth proceeds it advances into the anterior chamber and may become adherent to the cornea,

[1] p. 553.

[2] van Dooremaal (1873), Goldzieher (1874), Masse (1881–85), Hosch (1885), Corrado (1931), Suzuki (1934), Accardi and Rossi (1936), Perera (1938), and others.

[3] Strawbridge (1878), Snell (1881), Cross and Collins (1893), Wintersteiner (1900), Wallner (1905), Silva (1905), Früchte (1906), Pickard (1906), and many others.

FIGS. 373 and 374.—CYST OF THE IRIS (E. F. Krug).

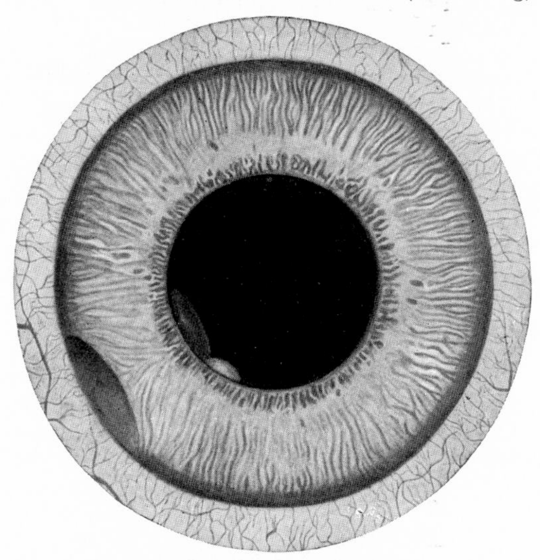

FIG. 373.—Cyst of the posterior chamber following a perforating injury 9 years previously.

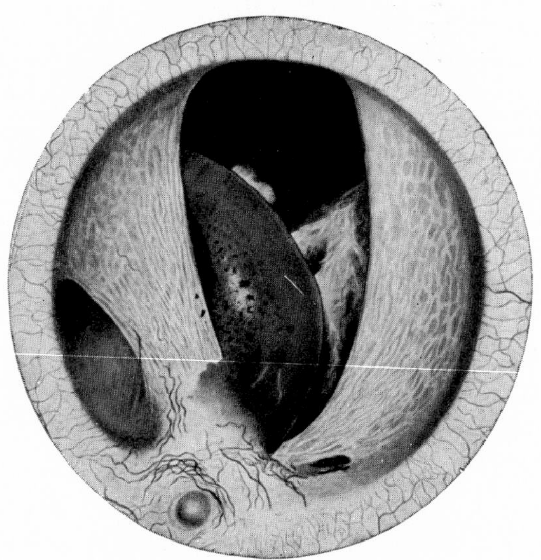

FIG. 374.—The same case, showing recurrence after operation.

while the stretched tissues of the iris anteriorly or the pigmented epithelium posteriorly may seem to take part in the formation of its walls (Stölting, 1885; Claiborne, 1905). Alternatively, it may be more deeply placed and bulge into the posterior chamber, appearing eventually as a dark mass in the pupil; or it may develop deeply situated in the ciliary region[1] (Figs. 373–375).

[1] Früchte (1906), Chance (1909), Marbourg (1925), Tooker (1933), Krug (1938), and others.

Much more rarely cysts of this type appear between the two epithelial layers of the iris some considerable time after an injury (Fig. 377).

Occasionally these intra-ocular cysts cease to grow and may remain unchanged for an indefinite period. In exceptional cases they may even become smaller or disappear (Fehr, 1902; Früchte, 1906; Wolfrum, 1914);

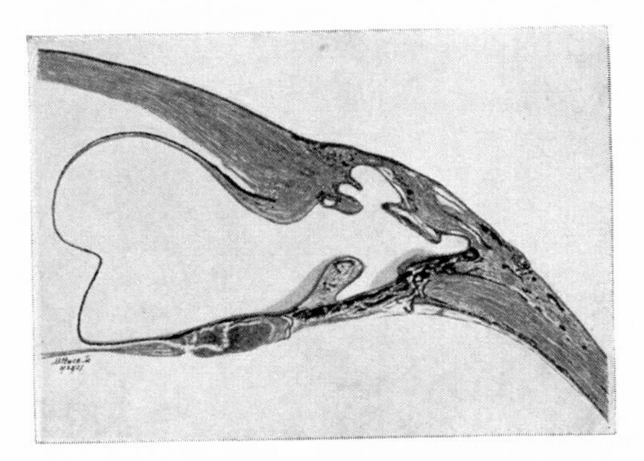

Fig. 375.—Cyst of the Posterior Chamber.

The same case as Figs. 373 and 374 in section (E. F. Krug).

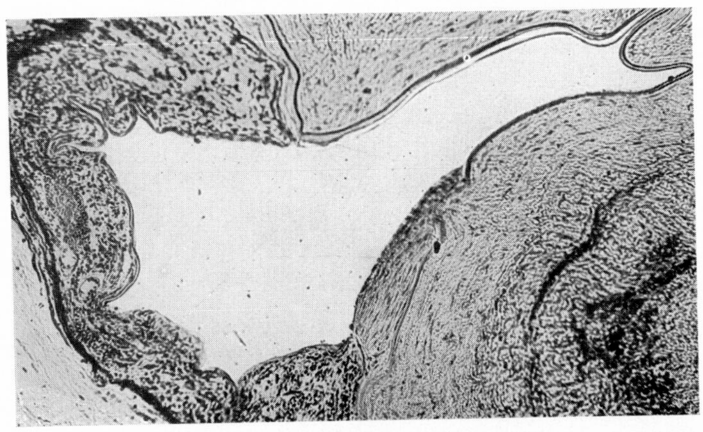

Fig. 376.—Epithelial Cyst.

In a woman of 48 whose eye was perforated by a piece of wood at the age of 4. The eye was quiet until 7 weeks prior to enucleation. There was a cyst in the anterior chamber, the nasal wall being formed of epithelium and the temporal wall by partly detached and partly new-formed Descemet's membrane. The cyst was almost embedded in the iris, surrounded by foci of lymphocytic infiltration (Bertha Klien).

but if they do rupture they almost invariably fill up again, and the more usual course is that of a slow and steady increase in size. In this growth three typical stages occur: first, a symptom-free period when no discomfort or visual disturbance arises; second, an irritative period when an irido-cyclitis may develop; third, a period of raised tension which results in absolute glaucoma, vision being completely destroyed and excision of the eye usually being necessary because of pain. In at least one case the phase of iridocyclitis has given rise to an inflammation in the other eye, simulating sympathetic ophthalmitis (Fields, 1943). It is important, therefore, as soon as the diagnosis of an intra-ocular cyst is made, to arrange for adequate treatment while it is yet small, especially if it is seen to be growing in size, since the only ultimate result which can be legitimately expected if events are allowed to take their course is loss of the eye.

The *diagnosis* of these intra-ocular cysts is not always easy; and in few conditions are care in taking the history and scrupulous exactitude in making the clinical examination of more importance. It is to be remembered that a cyst can itself cause an iridocyclitis, and consequently, in the case of cysts of the iris stroma, nodular inflammations such as tuberculosis, syphilis, and so on, must be eliminated. The most important differential diagnosis, however, concerns a neoplasm, which almost invariably means a malignant tumour, a problem which is most difficult to clear up in the case of cysts in the posterior chamber.

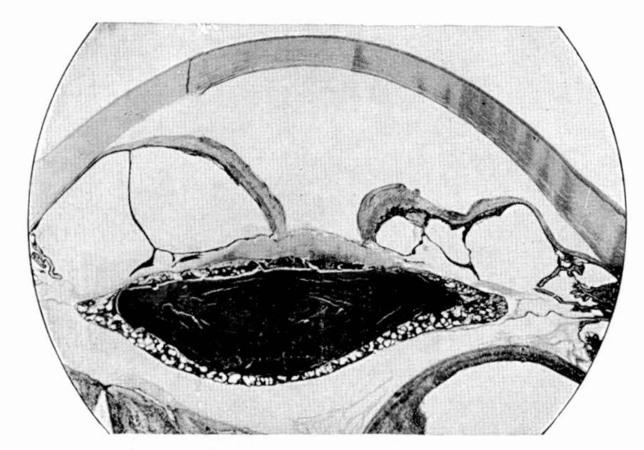

Fig. 377.—Cyst of the Pigmented Epithelium of the Iris.

Five years after injury. Seclusion and occlusion of the pupil; separation of the two epithelial layers of the iris with the formation of numerous cysts. Anterior capsular cataract and detached retina (×7) (J. H. Parsons).

The history should sift the question of trauma, how long the cyst has been present, whether other people have noted it, and if it has been observed to grow. The clinical examination should include a minute search for a perforating wound, a determination of the mobility of the pupil and any question of infiltration of the tissues, the presence of new blood vessels or unusual pigment proliferation and, above all, the transparency. This last should be investigated by diascleral illumination and with the direct beam of the slit-lamp. In summary, the features which may indicate the diagnosis of a cyst in contradistinction to a tumour are therefore—multiplicity, tremulousness, mobility, the presence of a notched margin and, particularly, translucency. The difficulties may be considerably aggravated by the fact that a cyst in this position may have walls so thick that transillumination is impossible, but it is to be remembered that translucency can be obtained with the slit-lamp even when diascleral illumination would indicate a solid growth. If doubt is felt as to the presence of a neoplasm, an iridectomy should be done if the mass is excisable, and if not a diagnostic puncture may be performed which, if negative, should be followed by removal of the eye.

The *treatment* of superficial cysts in the cornea or sclera is dictated by the state of the eye. If the cyst is large and the eye blind, enucleation is the easiest course; but if vision is retained the experience in the literature shows that removal of the anterior wall, an operation first performed by Lawrence (1847), is usually an adequate measure.

The treatment of intra-ocular implantation cysts presents larger problems which are fully discussed elsewhere in this *System*[1]; briefly the methods available include excision or destruction of the lesion by electrolysis, diathermy, light-coagulation, cryotherapy or radiation or (less effectively) by chemical means as by the application of carbolic acid, iodine or trichloracetic acid.

While surgical removal should be attempted and is sometimes successful, the prognosis is frequently bad. At the same time, complications may be long delayed; thus Cohen (1951) reported a case of an implantation cyst in the anterior chamber wherein glaucoma did not develop until 45 years after the occurrence of a penetrating wound at the limbus, complicated by the retention of a piece of glass.

In addition to these cysts of epithelial origin, *pseudo-cysts* may be formed when the portions of the anterior and posterior chambers are shut off by inflammatory adhesions, while similar cystic formations may arise from *endothelial* elements, frequently associated with extensions of Descemet's membrane (Klien, 1945).

Degenerative cysts in the corneal stroma resulting from colliquative necrosis are rare events after a perforating wound; such a cystic formation was reported by Engel (1950) wherein the affected area was surrounded by opaque and highly vascularized corneal tissue.

Accardi and Rossi. *Rass. ital. Ottal.*, **5**, 3 (1936).
Ahlström. *Zbl. prakt. Augenheilk.*, **27**, 257 (1903).
Beigelman. *Arch. Ophthal.*, **12**, 188 (1934).
Blaschek. *Z. Augenheilk.*, **13**, 804 (1905).
Chance. *Ophthal. Rec.*, **18**, 209 (1909).
Claiborne. *Trans. Amer. ophthal. Soc.*, **10**, 588 (1905).
Clausnizer. *Klin. Mbl. Augenheilk.*, **49** (2), 434 (1911).
Cohen. *Arch. Ophthal.*, **45**, 413 (1951).
Collins. *Trans. ophthal. Soc. U.K.*, **34**, 21 (1914).
Corrado. *Ann. Ottal.*, **59**, 706 (1931).
Cross and Collins. *Trans. ophthal. Soc. U.K.*, **13**, 199 (1893).
van Dooremaal. *v. Graefes Arch. Ophthal.*, **19** (3), 359 (1873).
Eisenstein. *Z. Augenheilk.*, **18**, 92 (1907).
Engel. *Klin. Mbl. Augenheilk.*, **116**, 515 (1950).
Evans. *Brit. J. Ophthal.*, **47**, 694 (1963).
Fehr. *Zbl. prakt. Augenheilk.*, **26**, 233 (1902).
Fields. *Amer. J. Ophthal.*, **26**, 193 (1943).
Filatov. *Russ. oftal. J.*, **2**, 122 (1923).
Früchte. *Klin. Mbl. Augenheilk.*, **44** (2), 42 (1906).
Früchte and Schürenberg. *Klin. Mbl. Augenheilk.*, **44** (2), 404 (1906).
Fuchs. *Klin. Mbl. Augenheilk.*, **154**, 777 (1969).
Goldzieher. *Arch. exp. Path. Pharm.*, **2**, 388 (1874).
Goulden and Whiting. *Trans. ophthal. Soc. U.K.*, **41**, 316 (1921).
von Graefe. *v. Graefes Arch. Ophthal.*, **3** (2), 412 (1857); **7** (2), 39, 139 (1860); **10** (1), 211 (1864).
Greeff. *Arch. Augenheilk.*, **25**, 395 (1892).
Griscom. *Amer. J. Ophthal.*, **12**, 400 (1929).
Grom. *Ann. Oculist.* (Paris), **182**, 52 (1949).
Gruening. *Trans. Amer. ophthal. Soc.*, **9**, 339 (1901).
von Hippel. *Klin. Mbl. Augenheilk.*, **51** (1), 520 (1913).
Horay. *Klin. Mbl. Augenheilk.*, **80**, 202 (1928).
Hosch. *Virchows Arch. path. Anat.*, **99**, 446 (1885).
Hulke. *Roy. Lond. ophthal. Hosp. Rep.*, **6**, 12 (1869).
Ischreyt. *Klin. Mbl. Augenheilk.*, **45** (1), 59 (1907).

[1] Vol. IX, p. 772.

Jones, Wharton. *Lancet*, **1,** 568 (1852).
Klien. *Amer. J. Ophthal.*, **28,** 1193 (1945).
Krug. *Amer. J. Ophthal.*, **21,** 413 (1938).
Kümmell. *Klin. Mbl. Augenheilk.*, **45** (2), 421 (1907).
Lagrange. *Tumeurs de l'oeil*, Paris, **1** (1901).
de Lapersonne. *Zbl. prakt. Augenheilk.*, **37,** 265 (1913).
Lauber. *v. Graefes Arch. Ophthal.*, **58,** 220 (1904).
Lawrence. *Treatise on Diseases of the Eye*, London (1847).
Mackenzie. *A Practical Treatise on the Diseases of the Eye*, London (1830).
Mann and Rountree. *Amer. J. Ophthal.*, **66,** 1020 (1968).
Marbourg. *Amer. J. Ophthal.*, **8,** 147 (1925).
Masse. *C. R. Acad. Sci.* (Paris), **92,** 797 (1881); **96,** 202 (1883).
Kystes, tumeurs perlés et tumeurs dermoides de l'iris, Paris (1885).
Melanowski. *Klin. oczna*, **16,** 739 (1938).
Meller. *v. Graefes Arch. Ophthal.*, **52,** 436 (1901).
Michaïl. *Arch. Ophtal.*, **50,** 385 (1933).
Michel. *Z. Augenheilk.*, **6,** 1 (1901).
Monoyer. *Ann. Oculist.* (Paris), **67,** 249 (1872).
Moore. *Brit. J. Ophthal.*, **52,** 688 (1968).
Niwa. *Acta Soc. ophthal. jap.*, **34,** 80 (1930).
Odinzov. *Vestn. oftal.*, **27,** 996 (1910).
Perera. *Amer. J. Ophthal.*, **21,** 605 (1938).
Pickard. *Trans. ophthal. Soc. U.K.*, **26,** 62 (1906).
Potechina. *Russ. oftal. J.*, **9,** 485 (1929).
Pravossud. *Vestn. oftal.*, **24,** 260 (1907).
Rados. *v. Graefes Arch. Ophthal.*, **99,** 152 (1919).
Roth and Geiger. *Amer. J. Ophthal.*, **8,** 870 (1925).
Rothmund. *Klin. Mbl. Augenheilk.*, **9,** 397 (1871); **10,** 189 (1872).
Rubert. *Klin. Mbl. Augenheilk.*, **48,** Beil., 145 (1910).
Silva. *Klin. Mbl. Augenheilk.*, **43** (2), 450 (1905).
Snell. *Roy. Lond. ophthal. Hosp. Rep.*, **10,** 208 (1881).
Stölting. *v. Graefes Arch. Ophthal.*, **31** (3), 99 (1885).
Strawbridge. *Trans. Amer. ophthal. Soc.*, **2,** 385 (1878).
Streiff. *Arch. Augenheilk.*, **50,** 56 (1904).
Suzuki. *Acta Soc. ophthal. jap.*, **38,** 553 (1934).
Tooker. *Trans. Amer. ophthal. Soc.*, **31,** 187 (1933).
Urmetzer. *v. Graefes Arch. Ophthal.*, **68,** 494 (1908).
Velhagen. *Klin. Mbl. Augenheilk.*, **74,** 763 (1925).
Villard and Dejean. *Arch. Ophtal.*, **50,** 91, 194, 272 (1933).
de Vincentiis. *Zbl. prakt. Augenheilk.*, **11,** 340 (1887).
Waldhauer. *Petersburger med. Arch.*, **11,** 337 (1866)
Wallner. *Ein klinisch-pathologisch-anatomischer Beitr. z. Lehre v. d. Cysten d. Regenbogenhaut* (Diss.), München (1905).
Weymann. *Amer. J. Ophthal.*, **13,** 314 (1930).
Wintersteiner. *Ber. dtsch. ophthal. Ges.*, **28,** 4 (1900).
Wolfrum. Lubarsch-Ostertag's *Ergebn. d. allg. Path. u. path. Anat. d. Menschen u. d. Tiere*, Wiesbaden, **16,** Erg., 757 (1914).
Wong, Hersh and McMaster. *Arch. Ophthal.*, **76,** 66 (1966).

The General Prognosis of Perforating Wounds

To give a general prognosis of perforating injuries of the eye is an impossibility in view of the variations in severity of the wound itself and of the intra-ocular damage as well as the great diversity of complications which may arise. Some instructive and important conclusions, however, can be drawn. It is interesting to compare the fate of such eyes injured in civilian life (usually with a better prognosis than war injuries) in 1904 with those in 1968. Taking series sufficiently large to give statistically valuable results, we have chosen those of Kaufmann (1904; 185 cases at Jena) and Theopold (1907; 251 cases at Göttingen) and compared them with those of Snell (1945; 275 cases at Baltimore), and Moncreiff and Scheribel (1945; 133 cases at Chicago). In Table XVII are the figures of the earlier authors which show no significant difference from those of the later writers.

Of Snell's cases 17% were enucleated immediately and a further 15% subsequently while 2% retained a blind eye; 34% thus lost the eye or vision. Of 172 cases in which immediate enucleation was not practised 8% had light perception, 35% had reduced and 30% normal vision. Of Moncreiff and Scheribel's cases 46% lost the eye, while in 54% it was retained. In recent years the overall position has improved slightly as shown by the figures from a study of 1,000 cases of perforating injury dealt with at the Munich University Eye Clinic between 1959 and 1963 (Remky *et al.*, 1967): vision better than 5/12 was retained in 59·9% of cases while enucleation was required in 15%. At present the enucleation rate following perforating wounds of the eye in adults is of the order of 15–20% of cases (Roper-Hall, 1967; Remky *et al.*, 1967; Edmund 1968; Jensen, 1968; and others), but in children in whom the incidence of such wounds is high, enucleation may be required in 25–30% of cases.[1] Although the actual incidence of severe ocular injury seems to be continuously on the increase the results have improved slightly over the years, probably due to earlier treatment, improved surgical technique and more effective measures for the prevention and control of infection and post-traumatic inflammation.

TABLE XVII

THE PROGNOSIS OF PERFORATING WOUNDS

	Kaufmann (1904)	*Theopold* (1907)
Eyes lost by enucleation or evisceration	27%	25%
Vision absent	10%	7%
Loss of the eye or total blindness . .	37%	32%
Less than one tenth vision	18%	30%
More than one tenth vision	34%	38%
Undetermined vision	11%	—

It is important that the prognosis of an incised perforating wound is in general much better than that of a rupture of the globe caused by blunt force. In the former type of injury Moncreiff and Scheribel (1945) found that at least 55% of eyes were saved, in the latter only 25%. Moreover in perforating wounds a clean cut, as by glass, has a better prognosis than an injury also involving a concussive effect. A double perforation of the globe has on the whole a worse prognosis than a single wound. The site of the wound is not the main influence in the prognosis provided that the factor of prolapse of the intra-ocular contents does not complicate matters; since it frequently does, the general prognosis of a corneal is better than a corneo-scleral or a scleral wound. Prolapse of iris tissue, if adequately treated, is not of serious prognostic import but the prolapse of other tissues, particularly the choroid or vitreous, is. Injury to the lens is a grave incident not because of the lenticular damage but owing to the tendency for an irritative inflammation or infection to become established; similarly, severe intra-ocular hæmorrhage is a serious prognostic factor. Several studies have confirmed that damage to the lens, prolapse of the uveal tissues, particularly of the choroid, and the loss of vitreous are the main factors responsible for a bad result[2] (Table XVIII).

[1] For an extensive bibliography on this subject see p. 7.

[2] Page and Stonehill (1959), George and Slack (1962), Roper-Hall (1967), Remky *et al.* (1967), Edmund (1968).

TABLE XVIII

ENUCLEATION IN PERFORATING WOUNDS RELATED TO EXTENT OF INJURY
(Roper-Hall, 1967)

EXTENT OF INJURY	PROPORTION OF ENUCLEATIONS
Corneal Wounds less than half diameter . . .	1 in 15
Corneal Wounds more than half diameter . .	1 in 3
Limbal Wounds without Uveal Prolapse . . .	1 in 9
Limbal Wounds with Uveal Prolapse . . .	1 in 3
Perforations with Lens Damage	1 in 4
Perforations with Vitreous Loss	1 in 2
Limbal Wounds with Vitreous Loss . . .	1 in 1·5
Overall Enucleation Rate 17%	1 in 6

If infection becomes established the outlook, so far as vision is concerned, is poor, even with the best therapeutics available today, although with antibiotic treatment more (comparatively useless) eyes may be retained. Thus at Munich between 1947 and 1953 of 996 cases of infected wounds, 29% retained a visual acuity of at least 5/12, a proportion which had improved between 1954 and 1961 to 55·7% of 1,371 cases, no doubt due to improved prophylaxis and the control of intra-ocular infection (Remky *et al.*, 1967). It is interesting that if reasonably good vision is present in the eye immediately after the accident the prognosis is usually good, but if perception of light is lost the eye nearly always has to be removed in the end. With such an eye no risks should therefore be taken.

The value of the *electroretinogram* in the assessment of the prognosis following severe trauma to the eye including perforating wounds, wherein opacification of the media prevented observation of the fundus, was studied by Jayle and Tassy (1970) in 61 cases within a few days of the injury: those cases in which the ERG was extremely small or absent failed to recover their sight; on the other hand, in almost every case with a normal or slightly subnormal ERG useful vision was regained, even when the causative injury was severe.

Sympathetic ophthalmitis is now a rare complication, the overall incidence in perforating wounds of the globe being in the region of about 2%. Improved early management, careful assessment in the second week following the injury and the appropriate use of corticosteroids seem to have contributed to its lower incidence. Nevertheless, if the post-traumatic inflammation in a severely damaged eye does not show evident signs of subsidence within 2 to 3 weeks of the injury, it should be removed unless the reasons for its retention are cogent as when it is the only eye with some prospect of vision.

The difficult problem of whether and when to remove an eye with a perforating injury has already been discussed[1]; the reasons for enucleation in 16·4% of 1,000 perforating wounds at the Munich Clinic (Remky

[1] p. 362.

et al., 1967) are indicated in Table XIX; 69% of the enucleations were carried out within three weeks of the injury. Early enucleation is still occasionally required when the eye is so badly damaged as to be unlikely ever to regain satisfactory vision or when it is considered to be potentially dangerous. Subsequent hæmorrhage or infection may necessitate this course and at a later stage enucleation may be required because the eye has become painful as well as blind as a result of glaucoma or prolonged intra-ocular inflammation leading to shrinkage of the globe. At a still later stage removal of an unsightly blind eye from disorganization, corneal scarring, staphyloma or shrinkage may be advisable.

TABLE XIX

REASONS FOR ENUCLEATION IN CASES OF PERFORATING WOUNDS IN MUNICH, 1959–63

(Remky, Kobor and Pfeiffer, 1967)

Severe Injury	22·5%	Vitreous Abscess	17·7%
Hæmophthalmitis	19·0%	Infection	11·2%
Chronic Inflammation	19·0%	Phthisis Bulbi	10·6%

The end-result of a perforating injury can be assessed in two ways: the retention of the eye as a cosmetically satisfactory and safe organ, and the retention of useful vision (Roper-Hall, 1967). The prognosis for the safe retention of an eye with a perforating injury depends on whether wound re-apposition can be accurate and secure and whether the eye can regain and maintain normal intra-ocular pressure within a reasonable time. The final vision of the retained eye depends upon the control of intra-ocular pressure, the transparency of the media, the ability to correct a resultant refractive error soon enough to maintain binocular vision and the intact functioning of the central retina. Damage to the cornea or lens deprives many eyes of useful vision, since both may result in an irregular and variable astigmatism which stabilizes only after a considerable period of time. All patients who have sustained a perforating wound of the eye should be examined at regular intervals. If there has been damage to the retina careful examination is desirable so that prophylactic treatment may be applied in sufficient time to prevent its detachment. Those with significant damage to the anterior segment particularly in the region of the angle of the anterior chamber should be carefully assessed for the presence of post-traumatic glaucoma, so that appropriate treatment can be instituted before it becomes established. Those with traumatic cataract may require further surgical treatment or it may be opportune to fit them with spectacles or contact lenses, while corneal scarring, if contact lenses are inappropriate, may suggest keratoplasty.

The prognostic significance of the presence of an intra-ocular foreign body will be considered in the next chapter.[1]

[1] p. 645.

Edmund. *Acta ophthal.* (Kbh.), **46,** 1165 (1968).
George and Slack. *Amer. J. Ophthal.*, **54,** 119 (1962).
Jayle and Tassy. *Brit. J. Ophthal.*, **54,** 51 (1970).
Jensen. *Acta ophthal.* (Kbh.), **46,** 1194 (1968).
Kaufmann. *Klin. statistische Zusammenstellung d. perf. Verwundungen d. Augapfels*, Jena (1904).
Moncreiff and Scheribel. *Amer. J. Ophthal.*, **28,** 1212 (1945).
Page and Stonehill. *Amer. J. Ophthal.*, **47,** 399 (1959).
Remky, Kobor and Pfeiffer. *An. Inst. Barraquer*, **7,** 487 (1967).
Roper-Hall. *Proc. roy. Soc. Med.*, **60,** 597 (1967).
Snell. *Amer. J. Ophthal.*, **28,** 263 (1945).
Theopold. *Statistische Erhebungen über d. . . . . perforierenden Augenerkrankungen* (Diss.), Göttingen (1907).

PERFORATING WOUNDS OF THE ADNEXA

Perforating wounds of the lids, often involving the orbit and lacrimal apparatus, are common and may be due to all sorts of sharp instruments used in work or play or encountered in accidents or assaults, and may also be caused by blunt bodies driven in with great force; the consequent injuries are of all degrees of severity, varying from superficial punctures or incised wounds to those causing gross ocular or cerebral damage and sometimes death.

Perforating Wounds of the Lids

PERFORATING WOUNDS OF THE LIDS include abrasions of the skin, punctured or incised wounds caused by sharp instruments, or lacerated wounds inflicted by blunt objects.

ABRASIONS OF THE SKIN are relatively unimportant; despite their somewhat serious clinical appearance owing to the associated œdema and swelling, they heal up rapidly without ill-effects provided they do not become infected.

INCISED WOUNDS are of importance if they are sufficiently deep to involve the orbicularis muscle, the tarsus or the structures underneath. As a rule, cuts running horizontally in the lids gape little, but vertical wounds cutting the fibres of the orbicularis muscle transversely tend to gape widely; and in them all hæmorrhage is profuse (Figs. 378–380). So far as the lids themselves are concerned, consequential damage may be done to two structures—the tendon of the levator palpebræ superioris, the cutting of which leads to a complete traumatic ptosis (Fig. 381), and the lid-margin, injury to which may involve an immediate disalignment of the cilia which may be carried into the wound, or a subsequent distortion of the lid-margin leading to the development of entropion or a coloboma, with the eventual dangers of trichiasis and exposure of the globe. The latter complication, of course, becomes important in the severe types of wound, when a large portion of the lid may be amputated. More rarely a wound above the eyebrow may induce a paralysis of the frontalis muscle (Fig. 382).

PUNCTURED OR STAB WOUNDS are usually of less consequence so far as the lids are concerned: their danger arises from damage to the deeper

FIGS. 378 to 380.—WOUNDS OF THE UPPER LID.

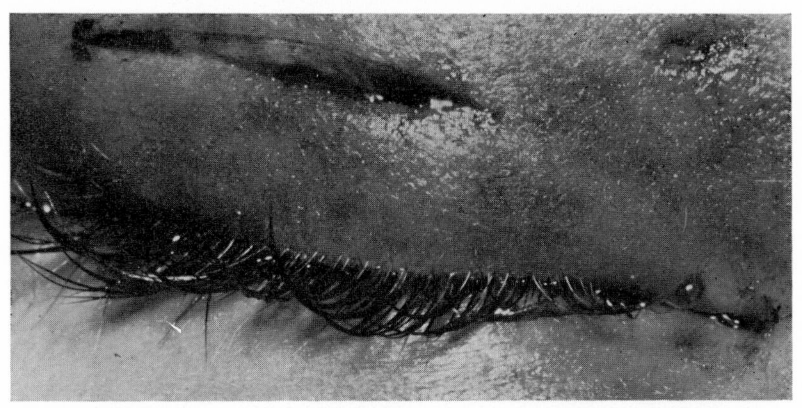

FIG. 378.—In a child, caused by the bite of a dog. There is a long laceration and (on the right) a small punctured wound (see also Fig. 390).

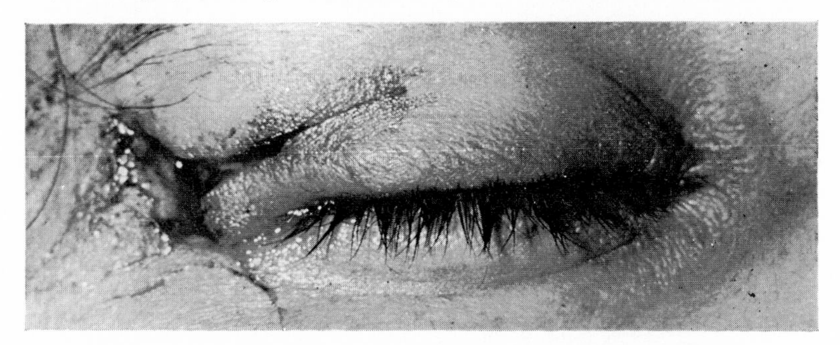

FIG. 379.—There is a laceration of the outer third of the upper eyelid and the external canthus from a broken driving mirror in a road accident.

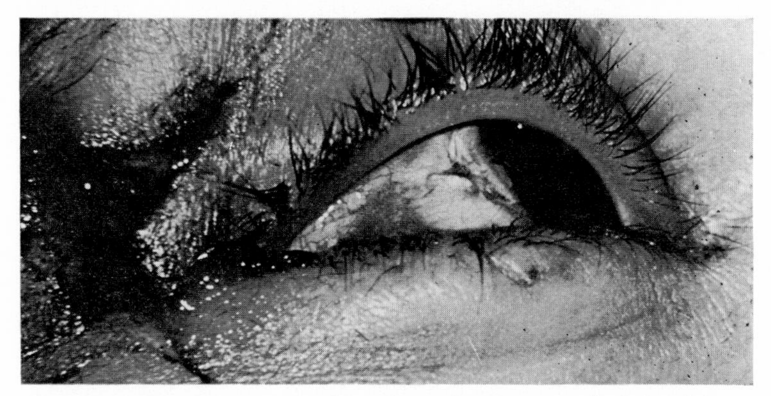

FIG. 380.—The same case, to show the perforating wound of the globe at the limbus extending some millimetres back on the temporal side.

structures (Fig. 378), and the possibility of intracranial extension of the wound must be remembered.

LACERATED WOUNDS are usually of more serious import. We have already seen that such a wound may arise from a severe contusion which involves no perforation when the soft tissues are ruptured as they are suddenly compressed between an impinging force and the underlying bone.

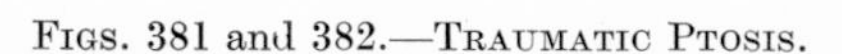

FIGS. 381 and 382.—TRAUMATIC PTOSIS.

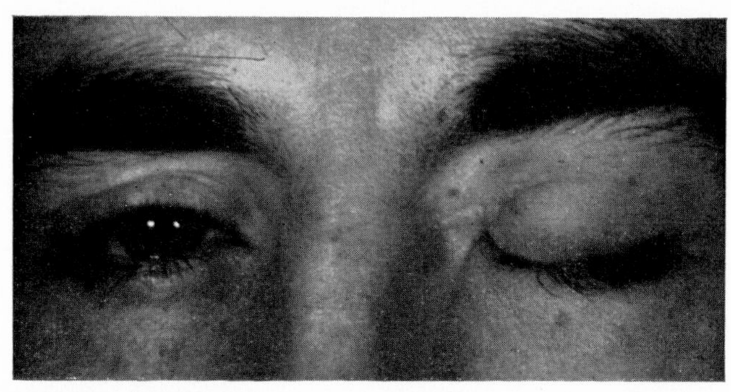

FIG. 381.—Ptosis following an incised wound of the left upper lid involving the levator palpebræ (A. McIndoe).

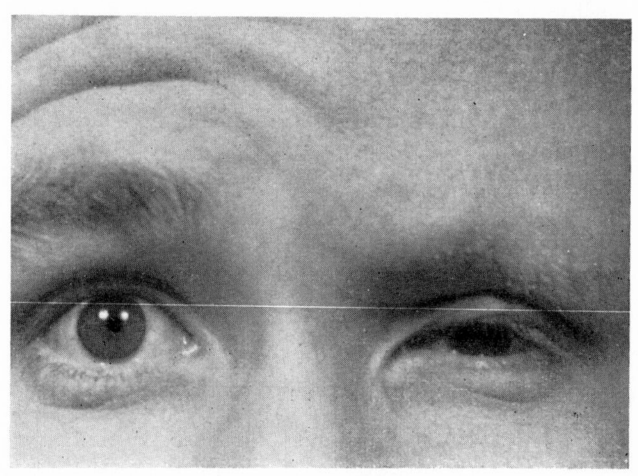

FIG. 382.—A deep incised wound was inflicted above the left eyebrow with a broken beer mug. There is a sag in the left brow due to paralysis of the left half of the frontalis muscle with consequent ptosis (Byron Smith).

The same type of wound with torn, bruised and ragged edges, involving extensive tearing of the tissues and frequently heavily impregnated with dirt, may result from a laceration in an accident such as a road injury (Fig. 383), or the impact of a blunt body driven into the tissues with great force—a foreign body, a broken piece of wood, the handle of an implement, a clothes hook or a meat hook, the horn of a cow, and a hundred and one other things. As a rule the damage thus caused to the lid is small compared with that sustained by the globe or the orbital tissues, and in wounds of this type it is to be remembered that infection is a common sequel. Kicks may produce the most bizarre effects; the skin and orbicularis muscle, for example, may be torn away from the outer part of the tarsal plate, which itself may be split vertically without injury to the eye (Stallard, 1965). Lacerated injuries of a similarly extensive type may be caused by the claws of animals (a bear, Würdemann, 1932), the beak of a bird (owl, Rodewald, 1896) or the teeth of an animal (commonly a dog) (Silverman and Obear, 1970) or a human being, the latter in circumstances as different as assault (Morel-Lavallée, 1886) or the ecstasies of love (Callahan, 1956).

One of us has seen a woman of Uganda the outer half of whose eyebrow and upper lid were thus bitten off; proud of her capacity for exciting passion, she refused treatment apart from hæmostasis. It is to be noted that the female has also been reported as being equally violent in the demonstration of her affections (Würdemann, 1932).

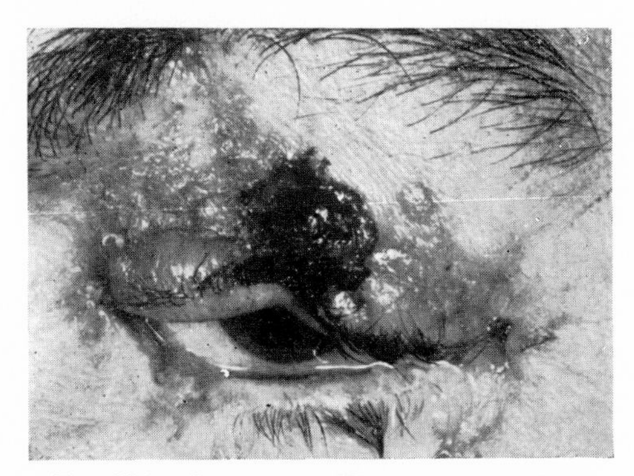

FIG. 383.—LACERATED WOUND OF THE LID.

After a road accident, showing the early stage with œdema, distortion and scab formation (Inst. Ophthal.).

Complications. The *immediate complication* of serious importance of palpebral wounds is the introduction of infection which, apart from causing delay in healing and ultimately resulting in extensive cicatricial deformities of the lids themselves, involves severe local damage leading on occasion to gangrene of the lids, orbital cellulitis with loss of the eye or, indeed, intracerebral infection and death. On the whole, however, the rich blood supply of the palpebral area makes the incidence of infection more rare and its duration less than in most other regions of the body.

Even relatively small and superficial wounds, however, may involve infective sequels for which pyogenic organisms are most frequently responsible. A staphylococcal infection usually leads to cellulitis or the formation of an abscess (Fig. 384) but may also result in acute eczematoid dermatitis or much more rarely give rise to the formation of a pyogenic granuloma. In the same way a streptococcal infection may lead to the development of an abscess or a virulent erysipelas. In addition to these common infections, however, an avenue may on rare occasions be created for such organisms as those of diphtheria, anthrax, vaccinia or the many fungi which may find lodgment in the lids. Similarly a scratch (Alexander, 1888; Marlow, 1890) or a bite on the lids has conveyed syphilis (Morel-Lavallée, 1886; Fox and Machlis, 1924) and tuberculosis (Stutzer, 1898).

Tetanus is a complication greatly to be feared, particularly in accidents involving contamination with agricultural soil or associated with horses. Cases of this disease which have arisen as a result of palpebral injury are not common but over 200 have been periodically recorded since Biermayer (1816) noted such a sequel following an injury to the eyebrow with a stone.[1] Generally the tetanus conforms to the usual type of the disease but, as may occur in similarly infected injuries involving the globe, the

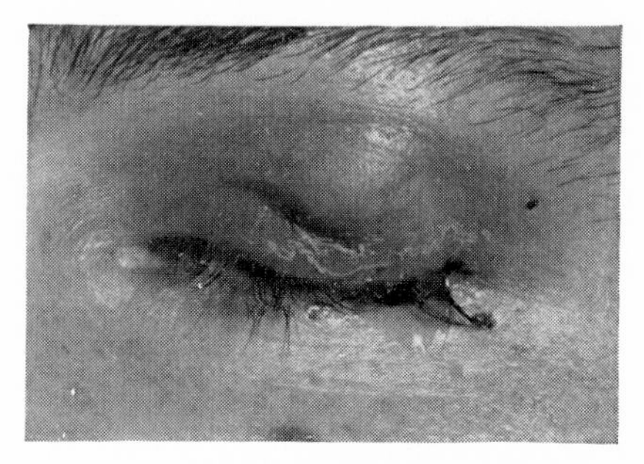

Fig. 384.—Abscess of the Lid after a Superficial Injury.

orbit and the region around the orbital rim, the cephalic type of tetanus has also been observed wherein the initial trismus may be associated with facial palsy of the peripheral type and various degrees of ophthalmoplegia (Fig. 385) (Jayme-Goyaz, 1941; Wetzel, 1942; Bagratuni, 1952).

The *late complications* of palpebral wounds include the development of a number of sequels, some of them of considerable danger to the eye and most of them involving much cosmetic deformity. Section of the levator muscle may result in a complete traumatic ptosis (Fig. 381), injury to the frontalis in a partial ptosis (Fig. 382), and cutting of either of the palpebral ligaments to a disfiguring shortening of the palpebral fissure (Fig. 270). Bad coaptation of a wound at the inner canthus may result in the deformity of a traumatic epicanthus. The small unsightly notch which often marks the edge of a maladjusted palpebral wound may cause trichiasis in its immediate neighbourhood, and in the lower lid almost invariably leads to constant epiphora, since it serves as a spout from which the tears fall over the cheek (Fig. 386). For the most part, however, the deformity depends on the contraction of cicatricial tissue which shortens and deforms the lid as a whole resulting, on the one hand, in traumatic ectropion whereby the lid may even be anchored to the tissues of the orbital margin with the

[1] Rose (1869), Roberts and Williamson (1891), van Spanje (1891), Keiper (1895), Pes (1903), Ramsay (1904), Brown (1912) with a review of 94 cases, van der Hoeve (1920), Bonnet *et al.* (1933), Jebavy (1937), Littwin (1947), Roger and Alliez (1948), Hudelo and Lallemond (1950), Bagratuni (1952), and others.

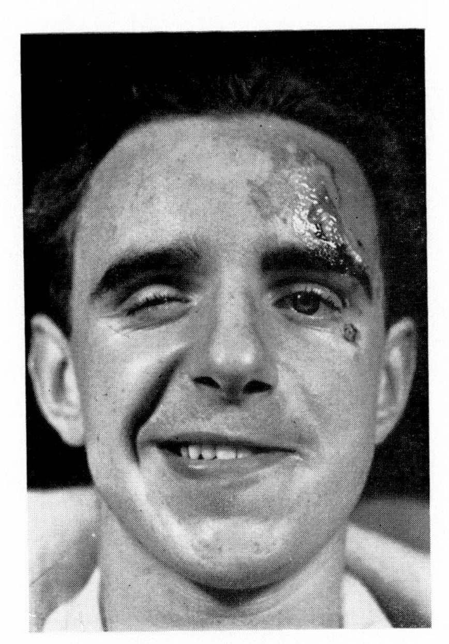

FIG. 385.—CEPHALIC TETANUS.

A 19-year-old patient who had an accident riding a bicycle along a road strewn with hay. There was an extensive cut over the left eyebrow. Eleven days later the left side of the face became immobile: there was a complete left facial palsy and trismus without other symptoms. Diplopia, right-sided ptosis and stiffness of the left side of the neck developed later. With sedatives and anti-tetanic serum intravenously and intramuscularly the condition improved during the subsequent 8 weeks; 18 months after the initial injury the patient was well and symptomless without facial weakness but with a minimal degree of facial asymmetry at rest, the left naso-labial fold being less marked than the right (L. Bagratuni).

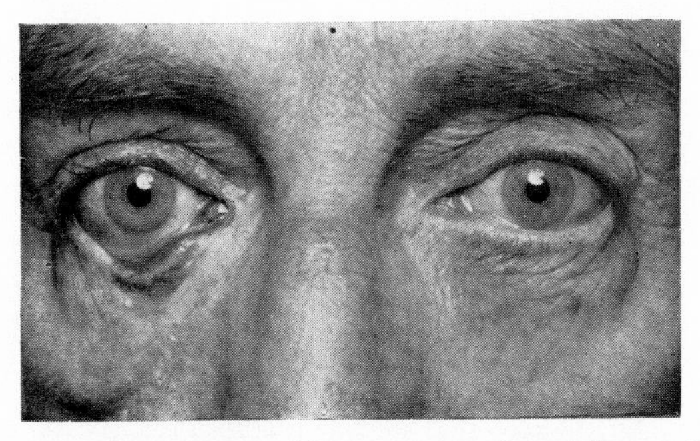

FIG. 386.—PENETRATING WOUND OF THE RIGHT LOWER LID.

It was cut by his broken spectacle glass. The illustration shows the result of mal-apposition of the lower lid in its surgical repair; there is gross deformity with cicatricial ectropion. A less degree of the same deformity is a common result of mal-apposition of the lid border.

FIGS. 387 and 388.—CICATRICIAL ECTROPION AND SYMBLEPHARON

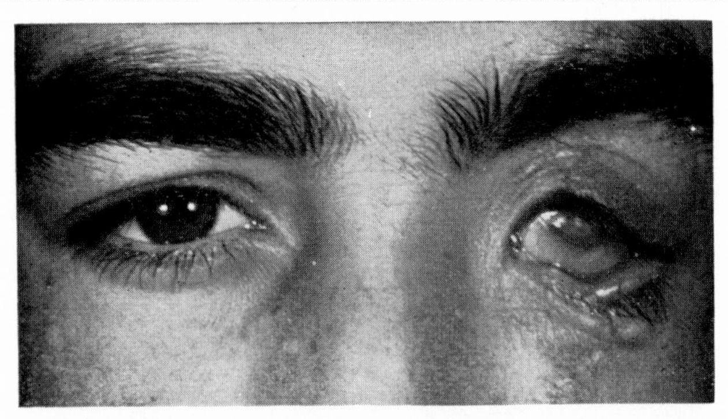

FIG. 387.—From an injury due to an aircraft propeller blade (A. McIndoe).

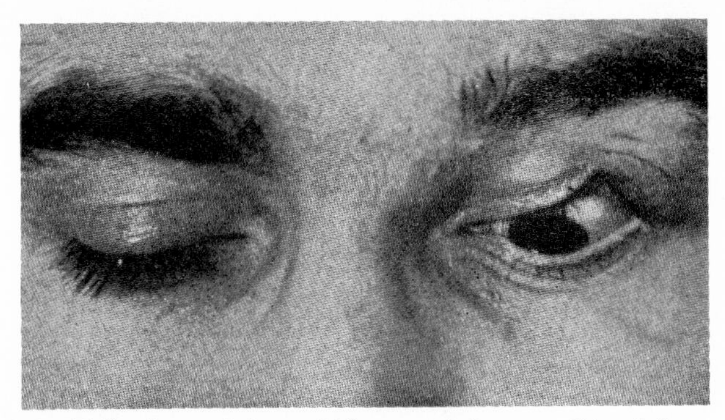

FIG. 388.—Following an injury which severed the upper lid and the region of the outer canthus (D. B. Kirby).

attendant dangers of lagophthalmos or, on the other hand, to entropion with resultant damage to the cornea from trichiasis (Figs. 387 and 388). In deeply penetrating wounds symblepharon may result. Actual loss of tissue, apart from the cosmetic defect of the coloboma, may also lead to ocular damage owing to exposure of the cornea (Fig. 389).

A rare complication which may become apparent many years after the original wound is the development of an *implantation cyst* when epithelial structures become

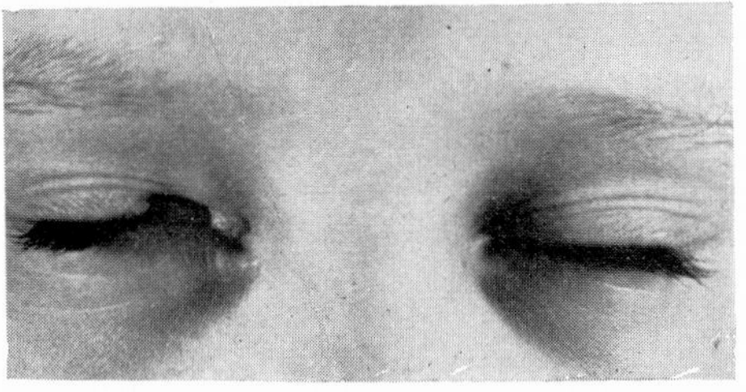

FIG. 389.—TRAUMATIC COLOBOMA OF THE LIDS.
Following an injury in early life (A. McIndoe).

buried in the depths of a wound; we have already seen that a similar cystic formation may develop in the conjunctiva. Such a cyst grows slowly and painlessly and on occasion may reach a considerable size; excision, which must be total to be effective, is the only satisfactory treatment.

A further rare complication is the development of large *varices* in the lids due to venous obstruction caused by cicatricial tissue. Occasionally such varices grow to a considerable size and may bleed spontaneously, in which case their removal is desirable (Reeh and Swan, 1950).

An interesting and rare complication of a wound of the forehead which involved section of the supra-orbital nerve is the occurrence of anæsthesia dolorosa with chromidrosis in the area of the sectioned nerve (Bonnet, 1952).

Treatment. In general terms, if properly handled, wounds of the lids heal well and rapidly; if, however, they are improperly treated, a number of complications may arise involving, as an immediate event, blindness or even death resulting from infection or, as a remote event, cicatricial deformities requiring a whole series of reparative surgical procedures for their correction. After attention to prophylaxis against tetanus[1] in all cases wherein there is the slightest suspicion that such infection may have been incurred, the immediate treatment involves, first, the control of hæmorrhage; second, an attempt to clean the wound and eliminate infection; and third, its repair so that functional integrity and cosmetic appearance are retained. Repair should be undertaken early, during the first few days after the injury; within a week muscle fibres fibrose and retract, and a relatively easy procedure becomes converted into a difficult task involving much time, considerable incapacity and the need for the extensive correction of cicatricial deformities.

Hæmorrhage may be profuse if one of the larger vessels is involved, but is usually readily controlled by pressure; at the time of repair the application of a clamp for a few moments or cauterization by diathermy is usually effective, and as a general rule ligatures need to be used sparingly lest they excite an irritant foreign-body reaction. If a hæmatoma has developed it is best left alone, since it will disappear in 10 to 14 days; only if it is very large should it be opened, and then with the most stringent aseptic precautions. Cold compresses may help to reduce œdema and swelling.

The cleansing and general toilet of the wound next come under consideration. The wound should be thoroughly cleaned, any foreign material being removed by a stream of warm saline (43° C) from a syringe or by a soft brush with soap and water; foreign particles which cannot be seen may often be felt by palpation in the thin lids, and these are best removed by seizing them with forceps and cutting them out. In lacerated wounds in this region little debridement of the edges is usually required; the abundant blood supply maintains the vitality of apparently crushed tissue to a surprising extent, allowing healing without necrosis; and conservatism in this regard lessens the need for subsequent plastic repair. It is to be

[1] p. 408.

remembered that every fragment of the lid is valuable, particularly any portion of the ciliary margin or any tissue remaining at the canthi, for the fashioning of a new canthal angle is a difficult problem; especially is this so in the case of the inner canthus, and the salvaging of a small portion of the lower lid at this point may preserve the lacrimal passages. Even the tarsus should be retained if badly torn; if it has been altogether detached it may be transplanted subcutaneously into some other area and restored at a later date when the lid is reconstructed. The excellence of the blood supply, as we have seen, is also a most efficient safeguard against infection and, unless this has already developed, most such wounds can be closed immediately, a preliminary dusting with such preparations as sulphathiazole-penicillin powder being often a suitable prophylactic. If, however, infection is already established, the wound must be opened widely and allowed to granulate, while the organisms involved are suitably dealt with by antibiotics or other means, repair being eventually accomplished by plastic reconstruction.

If the wound is deep its full extent should be explored before suturing, and in so doing particular attention should be paid to possible trauma to the levator tendon; inability to raise the lid voluntarily indicates a lesion of this type. Such an injury is best immediately repaired by locating the cut muscle and suturing it to Müller's muscle and the tarsal plate. A similar immediate repair of the tarsal ligaments by suturing to the periosteum is advisable if either of these structures has been cut.

In repairing cuts of the lids which do not involve serious loss of tissue but implicate the lid-margin, this latter part must first be brought into alignment with scrupulous accuracy. The cut margins should be brought together and supported by hooks, the grey intermarginal line being taken as a useful landmark; with this as a basis, the edges should be sewn together with fine silk sutures so that the sharp posterior margins are accurately coapted by one stitch in order to preserve the continuity of the muscle of Riolan, whereafter the lashes are properly positioned and correctly aligned by a second suture. The lid may then be everted with the aid of these sutures and any wound on the posterior surface coapted. The anterior part of the wound is then closed in layers, buried catgut sutures being used in the deeper tissues to withstand tension, a point of particular importance if the orbicularis muscle is cut transversely, for retraction of its fibres always tends to cause tension and gaping; finally, fine silk sutures, which may be removed in 48 hours, are used to secure accurate coaptation of the skin. If such immediate repair is possible, deformity is minimized and late plastic procedures for cosmetic or functional correction are rarely necessary.

When a linear wound traverses the lid completely Wheeler's (1939) technique was widely used to obviate the unsightly notch which so frequently develops on subsequent cicatrization at the lid-margin. In this technique the substance of the lid is split into its two constituent laminæ a short distance on either side of the wound; two sectors of triangular shape with their bases towards the lid-margin are then removed, one from the superficial lamina of skin and muscular tissue on one side of the wound, and the other from the deep lamina of tarsus and conjunctiva on the other side. It follows that when each is sutured to its fellow the one slightly overlaps the other, thus offsetting the lines of junction so that the tendency for linear contraction is obviated.

This technique suffers from the defect of sacrificing normal tissue. Another procedure is the " tongue and groove joint " of Hughes (1951). The cut margins of the lid are trimmed, one side in a convex (the tongue) and the other in a concave form (the groove), so that the one fits into the other. On the outside of the lid a flap of skin and subcutaneous tissue is undermined so that it fits into a denuded area on the other side of the laceration, thus supporting the lid-margin. For most wounds, however, the best technique is the direct suturing of the tarsal edges with catgut and the orbicularis and skin with silk, a procedure possible with fine atraumatic needles (Mustardé, 1966).

If the wound is more extensive and involves considerable loss of tissue, protection of the eye (if it is still present) becomes the primary consideration and effective plastic repair can be left until a later date. If the defect is too great to allow approximation of its edges, the lid may be reconstructed immediately by lining its inner part with reflected conjunctiva or grafted buccal mucosa, and its outer portion with a skin graft; the whole upper lid may be reconstructed in this way, support being attained by a graft of auricular cartilage at a later date. If the lower lid is lacking the most convenient method of protecting the eye as a temporary measure until plastic reconstruction can be effected is to suture the margin of the upper lid to the tissue that remains on the lower orbital margin. In most cases sufficient skin can be obtained at any early stage after the injury, before contractures develop, by undermining and mobilizing the skin of the temporal region. Finally, if the superficial tissues only are torn away, the deep tissues can be sutured to the lower lid and the raw surface covered immediately by a free skin graft. Even if these preliminary grafts are lost or require subsequent replacement, they have served their purpose if they afford protection to the eye. If the eye has also been destroyed the lids should similarly be reconstructed, since the groundwork is thus laid for providing a socket which will retain a prosthesis.

The *late treatment* of deformities following palpebral wounds involves a number of plastic procedures which may require multiple and extensive operations, particularly when infection or sloughing of the tissues has led to extensive cicatrization or when considerable portions of the lids have been lost; nevertheless, even the most extensive deformities can usually be satisfactorily repaired and it is relatively easy to reconstitute entirely one or both lids.

Isolated deformities demand appropriate treatment. Traumatic ptosis may be repaired by the recovery and re-insertion of the levator muscle, the surgical approach being made externally (Eversbusch) or internally (Blaskovics); if that is impossible, attachment of the lid is made to the superior rectus muscle by Motais's procedure or one of its many modifications or, if necessary, to the frontalis muscle. Canthal deformities require reconstruction, notches on the lid-margin, entropion or ectropion require repair, but for the most part the surgery necessary is a wide excision of scar-tissue, the repair of the mucous membrane by conjunctival or oral mucosa, the replacement of the tarsal plate by auricular cartilage and the ample renewal of skin by whole-skin grafts from such localities as the opposite upper lid, the retro-auricular area or the inner aspect of the upper arm, or in more extensive reconstructions by pedicle flaps from surrounding areas or tube flaps from a distance.

The literature on the technique of plastic procedures on the lids is vast and extensive; see particularly the treatises of Gillies (1920–29), Imre (1928), Wheeler (1939), Hughes (1943), Malbran and Nocito (1947), Lagrot and Py (1951), Fox (1963), Stallard (1965), Callahan (1966), Mustardé (1966), and others.

Perforating Wounds of the Lacrimal Passages

One of the most unfortunate complications of perforating wounds involving the inner canthus or the neighbouring part of the lower lid is damage to the lacrimal passages with consequent epiphora, a distressing inconvenience to which is frequently added the development of a chronic infective dacryocystitis. Post-traumatic epiphora after such wounds may, of course, be due to other causes such as the development of a colobomatous notch on the lower lid-margin out of which the tears fall, a failure in the accurate apposition of the sharp posterior border of the lid-margin to the globe so that the tears are not conducted to the lacus lacrimalis, or an eversion of the punctum due to cicatricial ectropion which need not be marked in degree to cause persistent weeping by abolishing the mechanism of capillarity by which the lacrimal fluid enters the canaliculus. We have seen that the first two of these can be remedied by plastic procedures; in the case of the last deformity, the punctum may occasionally be brought into its proper place by inducing contraction of the conjunctival surface of the lid by cauterization, but a more satisfactory result is usually obtained by the reverse process of counteracting the cicatricial contraction on the skin surface by transferring a small skin flap from the horizontal to the vertical position below and medial to the canthus. A further expedient is the transformation of the punctum into a gutter.[1] On the whole, successful lacrimal conduction depends on the accuracy of the reposition of the lids, and its continued presence is one of the most important criteria in evaluating the results of the post-traumatic surgery of these structures.

Direct injury to the canaliculi is generally associated with an incised wound or an avulsion injury involving the medial portion of the lower lid, in which case these structures are transected and, the two ends being lost in the subsequent scar, the continuity of the channels is abolished (Fig. 390). Damage to the lacrimal passages below this level does not follow simple incised wounds which leave the bony structures unaffected; the gross damage

[1] Vol. XIII.

which follows fractures in this region and its repair have already been discussed. A rarity is an internal penetration of the lacrimal sac; such an injury caused by a splinter of wood has led to stenosis and a fistula into the tissues of the lid (Posthumus, 1940); further rare complications of injury are the subsequent development of granulomatous proliferations from the mucosa of the sac (Wagenmann, 1906; Spoto, 1910) and the development of cysts or diverticula.[1]

Surgical treatment for all injuries to the upper lacrimal passages should be immediate and every endeavour should be made to re-establish continuity at the time of primary repair; if this can be accomplished, the prognosis for restoration of function is generally good.

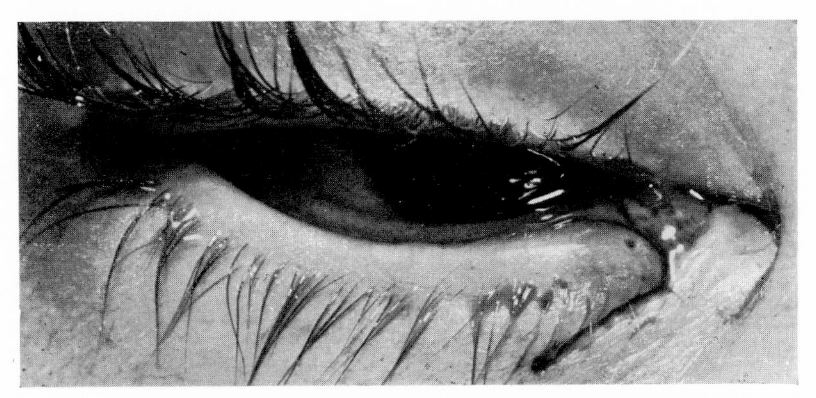

FIG. 390.—LACERATION OF THE LACRIMAL PASSAGES.
A wound of the lacrimal passages caused by the bite of a dog (see also Fig. 378).

Many procedures have been suggested for finding and joining together the lateral and medial ends of a severed canaliculus. If the break is close to the punctum the two ends can be found easily; the more medial to the punctum the injury lies, the more difficult it becomes to find the nasal end of the canaliculus which, it will be recalled, sinks deeper into the tissues as it passes towards the lacrimal fascia. If the two ends can be easily seen then all that is required is to thread them together over a splint such as a suture or plastic tube inserted through the punctum into the canaliculus followed by repair of the laceration of the eyelid. If the medial end cannot be seen then the following procedures may be tried:—

1. With the two ends of the eyelid held in accurate apposition a probe or cannula should be passed through the lower punctum and may well find its way into the medial end of the severed canaliculus.

2. A coloured fluid such as boiled milk or methylene blue may be injected through the intact upper canaliculus, or if this is also damaged through the lacrimal sac, in the hope that it will emerge from the medial end of the lower canaliculus.

3. A lacrimal cannula may be passed through the upper canaliculus and manipu-

[1] Vol. XIII.

lated so that it emerges through the medial end of the lower canaliculus, although this is frequently a difficult procedure. Alternatively, the pigtail probe recommended by Worst (1962) may facilitate the location of the medial end of the severed canaliculus. Whichever method is used a nylon suture or fine polythene tube is then threaded through to act as a splint.

4. A cannula or tube may be passed into the lower canaliculus through an incision into the lacrimal sac.

5. If there is much swelling of the tissues it may be advisable to delay exploration for 24 to 48 hours after which time the severed ends of the canaliculus are usually more easily identified by their whitish pouting appearance.

When the canalicular ends have been identified a splint should be inserted along the canaliculus into the sac: a Bowman's probe, a fine polythene tube, a silk suture, a Veirs's needle (1962), or the straightened-out end of a blunt needle carrying a 4·0 black silk suture have all had their advocates. Alternatively, a polythene tube or nylon suture may be passed via the upper canaliculus through the lacrimal sac and along the lower canaliculus as previously described and left *in situ* for at least two weeks. This is, however, a somewhat complicated method of splinting, and pressure necrosis of the puncta may result. The simplest method is certainly the use of a polythene tube or a sling suture inserted along the canaliculus into the sac and through the skin at the inner canthus while the outer end can be secured onto the cheek by strapping for at least two weeks. With the splint in place the canaliculus should be repaired by one or two carefully placed sutures followed by repair of the eyelid in the usual way. Silk sutures in the vicinity of the inner canthus may be left long to prevent their ends from rubbing on the eye. Good illumination and magnification are essential for these procedures and if there is considerable hæmorrhage and œdema it is probably wise to delay the primary repair for a day or so until the swelling of the soft tissue has subsided. These methods may be successful in the case of a recent injury; but if the wound of the eyelid has been allowed to heal with scarring so that the lumen of the canaliculus is obstructed by a stricture, more complex procedures are required which are dealt with in detail elsewhere in this *System*.[1]

A stricture of the punctum may be dealt with by repeated dilatation or canaliculotomy. If such procedures are unsuccessful an alternative approach is to create an entirely new communication between the conjunctival and lacrimal sacs—a conjunctivo-dacryocystostomy—or between the conjunctival sac and the nose—a conjunctivo-rhinostomy. Stenosis of the canaliculus itself may be treated by division of the stricture followed by splinting until epithelialization occurs or by the excision of the scar-tissue and its replacement by a segment of vein or of plastic tube. If the lower canaliculus has been completely destroyed and the upper canaliculus remains patent a waiting period is advisable before attempting any lacrimal surgery. If both canaliculi have been irreparably damaged the primary procedure may well consist of a canthoplasty, dacryocystorhinostomy and the insertion of a polythene tube between the medial canthus and the nasal cavity.[2]

Alexander. *Syphilis und Auge*, Wiesbaden (1888).
Bagratuni. *Brit. med. J.*, **1**, 461 (1952).
Beard. *Plastic and Reconstructive Surgery of the Eye and Adnexa* (ed. Smith and Converse), St. Louis, 171 (1967).
Biermayer. *Musœum nosocomii Vindobonensis*, 45 (1816).
Bonnet. *Bull. Soc. Ophtal. Fr.*, 109 (1952).
Bonnet, Paufique and Perron. *Bull. Soc. Ophtal. Paris*, 698 (1933).
Brown. *Ann. Surg.*, **55**, 473 (1912).

[1] Vol. XIII.

[2] Converse and Smith (1952), Henderson (1953), B. R. Jones (1960), L. T. Jones (1961–69), Worst (1962), Veirs (1962–66), Griffith (1963), Fox (1963), Fasanella (1965), Stallard (1965), Shannon and Hamdi (1966), Mustardé (1966), Beard (1967), Keith (1968), Sisler (1968), Smith and Dodick (1968), B. R. Jones and Corrigan (1969), Werb (1969).

Callahan. *Surgery of the Eye: Diseases,* Springfield, 413 (1956).
Reconstructive Surgery of the Eyelids and Ocular Adnexa, Bgham., Ala. (1966).
Converse and Smith. *Amer. J. Ophthal.,* **35,** 1103 (1952).
Fasanella. *Complications in Eye Surgery,* Phila., 133 (1965).
Fox. *Ophthalmic Plastic Surgery,* 3rd ed., N.Y., 450 (1963).
Fox and Machlis. *Amer. J. Ophthal.,* **7,** 701 (1924).
Griffith. *Brit. J. Ophthal.,* **47,** 203 (1963).
Gillies. *Plastic Surgery of the Face,* London (1920–29).
Henderson. *Arch. Ophthal.,* **49,** 182 (1953).
van der Hoeve. *Ned. T. Geneesk.,* **64,** 1173 (1920).
Hudelo and Lallemond. *Ann. Oculist.* (Paris), **183,** 787 (1950).
Hughes. *Reconstructive Surgery of the Eyelids,* London (1943).
Plastic reconst. Surg., **8,** 281 (1951).
Imre. *Lidplastic,* Budapest (1928).
Jayme-Goyaz. *Amer. J. Ophthal.,* **24,** 1281 (1941).
Jebavy. *Cs. oftal.,* **3,** 126 (1937).
Jones, B. R. *Trans. ophthal. Soc. U.K.,* **80,** 343 (1960).
Jones, B. R. and Corrigan. *Corneo-Plastic Surgery* (ed. Rycroft), Oxford, 101 (1969).
Jones, L. T. *Arch. Ophthal.,* **66,** 111 (1961).
Trans. Amer. Acad. Ophthal., **66,** 506 (1962).
Plastic and Reconstructive Surgery of the Eye and Adnexa (ed. Smith and Converse), St. Louis, 148 (1967).
Corneo-Plastic Surgery (ed. Rycroft), Oxford, 113 (1969).
Keiper. *Ann. Ophthal. Otol.,* **4,** 366 (1895).
Keith. *Amer. J. Ophthal.,* **65,** 70 (1968).
Lagrot and Py. *Bull. Soc. Ophtal. Fr.,* 231 (1951).
Littwin. *Amer. J. Ophthal.,* **30,** 201 (1947).
Malbran and Nocito. *Plásticas palpebrales y conjuntivales,* Buenos Aires (1947).
Marlow. *N.Y. med. J.,* **51,** 237 (1890).
Morel-Lavallée. *Ann. Derm. Syph.,* **7,** 85 (1886).
Mustardé. *Repair and Reconstruction in the Orbital Region,* Edinburgh, 228 (1966).
Pes. *Progresso Med.,* Torino, **2,** 157 (1903).
Posthumus. *Ophthalmologica,* **99,** 476 (1940).
Ramsay. *Ophthal. Rec.,* **13,** 537 (1904).
Reeh and Swan. *Trans. Amer. Acad. Ophthal.,* **54,** 312 (1950).
Roberts and Williamson. *Lancet,* **2,** 61 (1891).
Rodewald. *Drei Fälle v. Bissverletzungen d. Auges* (Diss.), Kiel (1896).
Roger and Alliez. *Rev. Oto-neuro-oftal.,* **20,** 296 (1948).
Rose. Billroth's *Hb. d. allg. spec. Chir.,* Stuttgart (1869).
Shannon and Hamdi. *Amer. J. Ophthal.,* **62,** 974 (1966).
Silverman and Obear. *Amer. J. Ophthal.,* **70,** 230 (1970).
Sisler. *Arch. Ophthal.,* **79,** 54 (1968).
Smith and Dodick. *Canad. J. Ophthal.,* **3,** 263 (1968).
van Spanje. *Ned. T. Geneesk.,* **27,** 397 (1891).
Spoto. *Progresso Oftal.,* **5,** 79 (1910).
Stallard. *Eye Surgery,* 4th ed., Bristol (1965).
Stutzer. *Beitr. Augenheilk.,* **3** (30), 884 (1898).
Veirs. *Trans. Amer. Acad. Ophthal.,* **66,** 263 (1962).
Arch. Ophthal., **73,** 89 (1965).
Symposium on Surgery of the Ocular Adnexa, St. Louis, 113 (1966).
Wagenmann. *Ber. dtsch. ophthal. Ges.,* **33,** 296 (1906).
Werb. In *Corneo-Plastic Surgery* (ed. Rycroft), Oxford, 87 (1969).
Wetzel. *Amer. J. Ophthal.,* **25,** 933 (1942).
Wheeler. *Collected Papers,* N.Y. (1939).
Worst. *Amer. J. Ophthal.,* **53,** 520 (1962).
Würdemann. *Injuries of the Eye,* 2nd ed., London, 689 (1932).

Penetrating Wounds of the Orbit

INCISED WOUNDS which penetrate into the orbit are relatively rare except in the gross injuries associated with war; PUNCTURED WOUNDS acquired in personal assault or in war are more common. These may be either STAB WOUNDS caused by a sharp object (knife, hook, pen, pointed pieces of wood or an implement) or LACERATED WOUNDS caused by blunt objects driven forcibly inwards.

As a rule a sharp instrument does comparatively little damage to the orbital tissues unless, indeed, the bone is fractured and the cranial cavity penetrated; the eyeball is usually pushed aside and only the soft tissues between it and the orbital wall injured. Hæmorrhage is often immediate, producing a proptosis; but compression of the hæmatoma between the orbital wall and the globe usually stops the bleeding. The lacrimal gland, any of the extra-ocular muscles or the orbital nerves may be injured, and occasionally, and with catastrophic results, the optic nerve.

The diagnosis of such a penetrating wound is usually obvious even although the clinical picture may be obscured by massive swelling of the lids, ecchymosis and chemosis. A change in the position of the globe, its immobility or a restriction in its movement, or the protrusion of orbital fat in the depths of the wound are pathognomonic signs, while blindness indicates damage to the optic nerve. Occasionally, however, the diagnosis is more difficult if a puncture is small or if the external injury is not obvious but is hidden in the fornix or canthi.

Blunt objects entering the orbit, on the other hand, habitually do considerable damage. The lids are usually extensively lacerated, injury to the globe is common and involves rupture, luxation or avulsion; the optic nerve is crushed, the muscles torn, the lacrimal gland dislocated and extensive fractures may occur involving injury to the cranial cavity or the nasal sinuses.

The various types of injury which have been reported in the literature are legion and many of them bizarre (Figs. 391–397). The most common objects are the ends of umbrellas, canes, or implements used in work, blunt hooks, the shafts of vehicles or the horns of cattle. Even small objects can cause great damage; thus a twig penetrating the upper lid has been reported to traverse the orbit and enter the skull to come to rest in the interpeduncular space whence it was removed by forceps; the IIIrd, IVth and VIth nerves, the first division of the Vth and the optic nerve were damaged, the eyeball being rendered immobile, anæsthetic and blind (Rees, 1947). A spicule of chopped ice passing through the eye and the optic foramen has caused sudden death (Palin, 1948). On the other hand, gross injury may cause astonishingly little damage and often leaves the globe intact (Schmidt and Frowein, 1971) (Figs. 391–2); thus Thomas (1942) saw a case wherein a knife-blade had entered the plica without injury to the lid-margins or the eyeball, passed through the orbit without damaging any important structure, traversed the nasal cavity and entered the antrum on the other side; recovery was uneventful and function unimpaired (Figs. 393 and 394); alternatively, an injury such as this may lead to enucleation (Viallefont *et al.*, 1967) (Fig. 397). Again, Svoboda (1948) reported a sword thrust which penetrated the cavernous sinus without damaging the eye or vision although it eventually proved fatal owing to delayed intracranial hæmorrhage. A similarly astonishing incident concerned a curtain rod, ¼ inch in diameter, which entered the orbit and was forced through the pharynx into the neck of a 7-year-old child who recovered completely without visual disturbances after the rod was removed with counter-traction against the head (Field, 1951); or the handle of a spoon which penetrated 2·5 in. into the lower part of the orbit of a 19-month-old baby, leaving no permanent ill-effects (Le Win, 1952). Again, the penetration of the orbit by the handle of a bicycle has led to the subluxation of the eyeball backwards and downwards where it lay intact (when light could be perceived through the lid), a luxation subsequently replaced by operation (Bailliart, 1950).

In such injuries any of the orbital structures may be damaged, often irreparably; complications to the globe, which may include perforation, concussion injuries and rupture, have already been considered.

The OPTIC NERVE is obviously of great importance in this respect, for

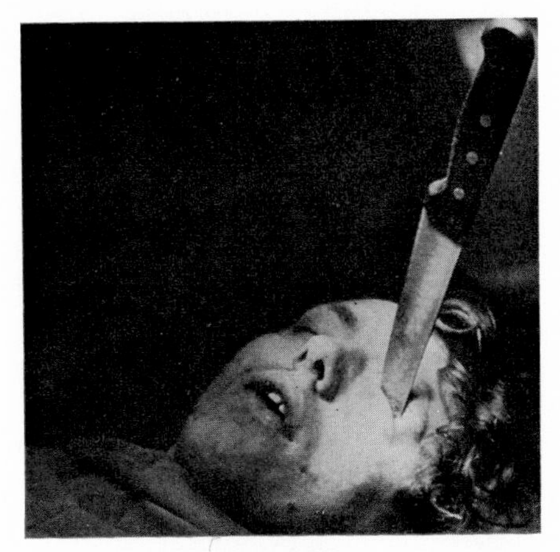

Fig. 391.

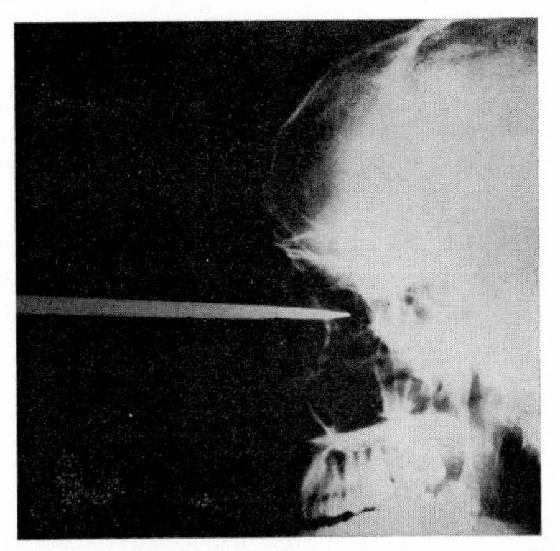

Fig. 392.

Figs. 391 and 392.—Penetrating Injury of the Orbit (J. G. H. Schmidt and R. A. Frowein).

The man's left orbit was penetrated by a butcher's knife causing an orbito-fronto-basal injury.

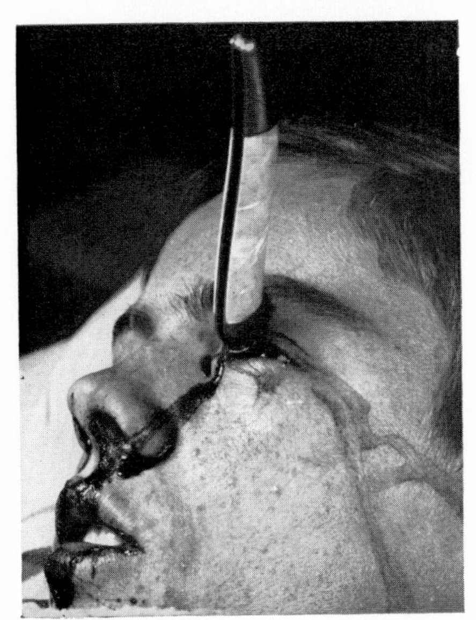

Fig. 393.

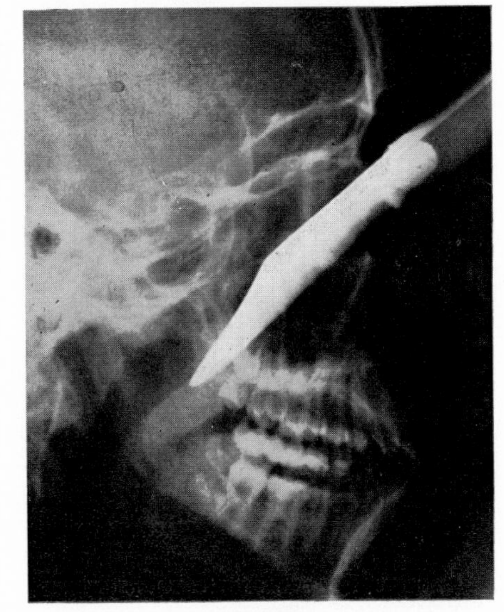

Fig. 394.

Figs. 393 and 394.—Penetrating Wound of the Orbit.

The knife penetrated the left orbit at the inner canthus and traversed both sides of the nasal cavity, the tip finally resting in the wall of the right maxillary sinus. There was no apparent injury to the eye or the lacrimal sac (Maxwell Thomas).

an injury thereto is functionally irreparable and results in blindness. Penetrating injuries by sharp objects such as knives may result in its severance.[1] If the nerve is cut anterior to the entrance of the retinal vessels the ophthalmoscopic picture resembles that of embolism of the central retinal artery with œdema of the posterior region of the retina; when cut more posteriorly optic atrophy develops.[2] Lacerating wounds by blunt objects may cause its avulsion from the globe at its weakest point at the nerve-head; the clinical picture and pathology of this lesion have already been described. Finally, in cases of severe intra-orbital hæmorrhage or incomplete avulsion of the globe, a post-traumatic atrophy of the optic nerve may develop resulting in defects of the visual field or blindness (Michaelson, 1944).

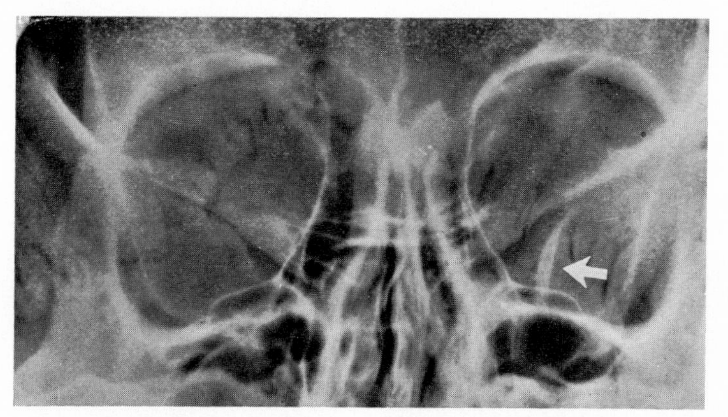

FIG. 395.—PENETRATING INJURY TO THE ORBIT.

In a woman aged 23. The tip of an umbrella penetrated the left orbit causing a fracture of the lateral portion of the superior orbital fissure (arrowed). There was a temporary palsy of the IIIrd nerve (S. L. Trokel).

In the case of a seaman struck over the left eye by a steel wire, described by Rafalovich and Belyaev (1958), the upper eyelid was penetrated and the optic nerve completely transected, resulting in a traumatic dislocation of the globe which had to be enucleated. Four cases of optic atrophy with complete unilateral blindness following wounds of the lower eyelid in young people were reported by Levy and Chatfield (1969), all the result of a fall onto a semi-sharp object; the characteristic clinical picture is that of an injury to the lower eyelid followed in a few weeks by the development of a squint. Young children rarely complain of unilateral blindness and until the optic disc becomes pale the only objective sign of this is the amaurotic pupillary reaction; it seems that in these cases damage to the optic nerve is indirect, in the nature of a tearing of the intra-vaginal blood vessels at the orbital apex or a concussion necrosis rather than a direct laceration of the nerve. *Treatment* is impossible.

[1] Steindorff (1898), Parsons (1903), Distler (1905), Adam (1908), Rafalovich and Belyaev (1958), and many others.

[2] von Graefe (1859), Pagenstecher (1869), Hirschberg (1879), Steindorff (1898), Parsons (1903), Distler (1905), Adam (1908), and others.

FIGS. 396 and 397.—PENETRATING WOUNDS OF THE ORBIT.

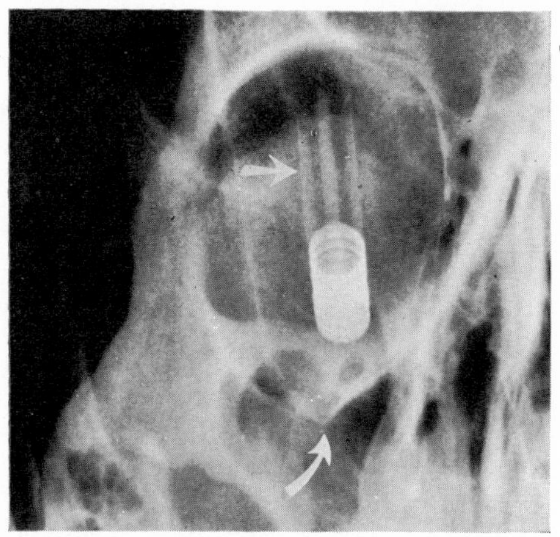

FIG. 396.—The driver of a taxi was thrown forwards in a road accident and a pencil protruding from the dashboard entered the right orbit above the globe without damage to the eye. There is a small fracture of the orbital floor (curved arrow), while the position of the pencil, paint-coat and the graphite core can be seen in the x-ray (straight arrow) (S. L. Trokel).

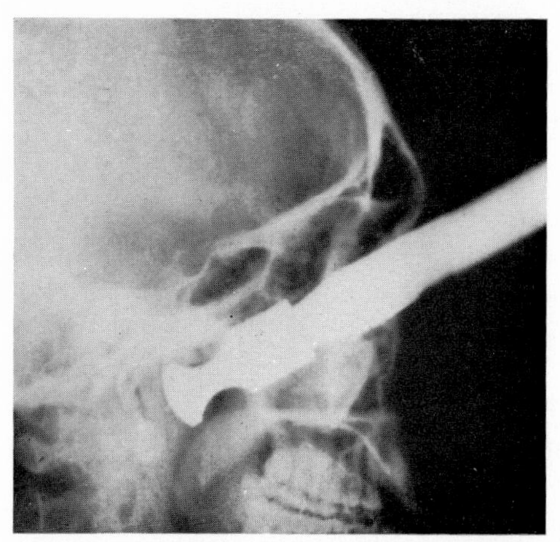

FIG. 397.—ORBITO-CRANIAL INJURY DUE TO IMPALEMENT BY A RIFLE BOLT.

The bolt penetrated the maxillary sinus and the pterygo-maxillary fossa and was arrested at the temporo-mandibular joint. The eye was completely destroyed and had to be enucleated. Otherwise recovery was complete (H. Viallefont *et al.*).

The OCULAR MUSCLES are frequently injured, although the incidence of this complication in perforating wounds is much less than that of the occurrence of muscular palsies after concussion injuries. The ecchymosis and chemosis combined with swelling of the lids may mask the damage at the time although a failure of the mobility of the globe may be remarked; limitation of movement and distressing diplopia are constant developments at a later date unless the muscle is only partially severed, in which case adequate function may return as after an incomplete tenotomy. The injury may involve a traumatic disinsertion of the muscular tendon, in which case scraps of the tendon may be seen in the wound, or the muscle belly itself may be cut or torn across in part or completely.

Many varied accidents may involve such an injury—perforation by a knife (Berlin, 1880; van der Hoeve, 1914), scissors (A. Graefe, 1887), a nail (Philipsen, 1887), a piece of china (Chevalier, 1884), wire (de Britto, 1887; Berger, 1905), a sharp stick (Berlin, 1880; Steiner, 1951), a fencing foil (Weeks, 1903), a meat hook (Würdemann, 1932), an iron bar (Dimmer, 1903), the horn of a goat (Gutmann, 1883) or cow (Corrado, 1951), and a host of others. Any of the extra-ocular muscles may be injured in such perforations, singly or in groups—the levator palpebræ (Dürr, 1879; and others), the superior rectus (Terson, 1890; Panas, 1902), the medial rectus (von Graefe, 1859; Terson, 1890; and many others), the inferior rectus (Gutmann, 1883–95; A. Graefe, 1887; Berger, 1905; Steiner, 1951; Corrado, 1951; and others), the lateral rectus (Zander and Geissler, 1864; and others), the inferior (Berlin, 1880; Roche, 1905) or the superior oblique (Zander and Geissler, 1864) or its trochlea (Bettrémieux, 1903). Involvement of the inferior oblique without injury to the inferior rectus in a penetrating wound of the lower lid is a rarity (Bonamour and Hugonnier, 1952, a piece of wire). Combinations of muscles may also be injured—the levator and the superior rectus (Berlin, 1880; Viciano, 1889; Hubbell, 1905), and the same two together with the superior oblique (Kempner, 1903), the superior rectus and the superior oblique (Wertheim, 1908), the levator, the superior and medial recti (Dimmer, 1903), the medial and inferior recti (Valude, 1902), and so on. Each of these injuries may be complicated by a simultaneous lesion of the optic nerve.

The ORBITAL NERVES are more rarely injured in stab wounds.[1] An isolated palsy of the oculomotor is typically associated with section of the optic nerve (Garrard and Snell, 1888; Snell, 1897; and others); a direct lesion of the abducens in the orbit is not common (Donkin, 1882–83; Leplace, 1891); but the more usual lesion involves most of the structures entering the orbital apex when damage occurs to all the ocular motor nerves, the first division of the trigeminal and, usually, section of the optic nerve, resulting in an immobile, anæsthetic and blind eye (van der Hoeve, 1914; Rees, 1947; Agnello, 1952; and others); the last nerve, however, may be spared in a wound of this type (Pfalz, 1892; and others). Such an injury, of course, in addition to causing widespread paralyses, internal ophthalmoplegia and blindness if the optic nerve is injured, involves anæsthesia of the cornea and conjunctiva with the consequent danger of neuroparalytic keratopathy (Steindorff, 1901; Goldzieher, 1903; and others).

In this connection an injury to the CILIARY GANGLION is of interest in causing a traumatic Argyll Robertson pupil, wherein the direct reaction to light is absent and the convergence reaction retained (Nathan and Turner, 1942; Bender, 1945).[2]

[1] For the disturbance of motility and the symptoms following paralysis of the various muscles, see Vol. VI.

[2] Vol. XII, p. 657.

The LACRIMAL GLAND may occasionally suffer direct injury. If the gland is perforated, a secondary dacryoadenitis may ensue which in the presence of infection may assume suppurative characteristics (Bock, 1896), while if foreign material is retained complete necrosis may result (Laval, 1938). Moreover, in the event of its laceration a fistula may form (Jarjavay, 1855; Ahlström, 1895).[1] An alternative sequel when the tarso-orbital fascia is severed is a dislocation of the gland or its prolapse out of the wound, an event which occurs almost exclusively in children owing to the slight development of the orbital margin (von Graefe, 1866; Ahlström, 1898; Jackson, 1904; Oloff, 1910; El-Kinani, 1945; and others).

Apart from damage to the contents of the orbit, other injuries may be sustained; a fracture of the orbital wall is a common occurrence and the wound may penetrate into the surrounding structures—the nasal sinuses, the nasal cavity and the cranium. The first two events are relatively unimportant, but the third always involves serious complications which may be fatal, such as leakage of cerebro-spinal fluid, infection of the meninges, the development of a cerebral abscess, or perforation of the great blood-vessels or the cavernous sinus. These vascular injuries may cause a carotico-cavernous aneurysm or profuse hæmorrhage, externally through the nose and internally into the cranium, in the latter case with the production of the symptoms of cerebral compression (Dejean, 1951; Schneider and Henderson, 1952; and others).[2]

The INTRACRANIAL EXTENSION of a penetrating wound of the orbit may not be suspected when a patient with such an injury is first seen. The wound of entry may be small and it may be entirely overlooked or dismissed as trivial; on the other hand, the depth and direction of penetration may be difficult to determine if the weapon or other object has already been removed. In wartime high velocity missiles commonly and easily pass through the orbit into the cranial cavity (Small and Turner, 1947); in civilian life penetrating wounds of the orbit are less common and are usually caused by missiles with a low velocity, occurring frequently in children as a result of an accident which is often regarded as trivial. The fact that intracranial penetration has occurred may not be recognized until the onset of cerebral complications which may be delayed for several days or weeks, although occasionally the signs may develop with aggressive rapidity, running a fulminating course which ends in death within a relatively short time. Penetration into the intracranial cavity may occur either through the orbital plate of the frontal bone or via the region of the optic foramen, depending on the angle at which the penetrating object enters the orbit. Usually in these cases the globe itself is not injured and because of its resilience may play a part in directing the course of the penetrating object (Klug, 1968).

[1] Vol. XIII. [2] Vol. XIII.

The consequences of intracranial extension of a penetrating wound of the orbit can be divided into three groups. Firstly, the immediate and obvious effect of intracranial damage consisting of cerebral lacerations, intracerebral and intraventricular hæmatomata and cerebral œdema; treatment in this group is obviously urgently required but the results are in general not satisfactory; secondly, delayed vascular complications such as the development of a carotico-cavernous fistula or an aneurysm (Fig. 398); and, thirdly, infection. Radiological examination soon after injury does not always reveal a fracture but it should be remembered that the bone of the roof of the orbit is thin and easily fractured particularly in children in whom the relative under-development of the superciliary arch renders it vulnerable to a penetrating wound in an upward direction. Even if a fracture is not seen on the

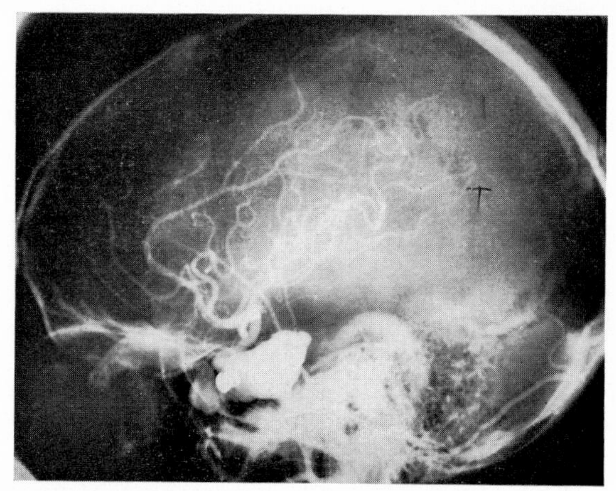

FIG. 398.—CAROTID ANEURYSM.
The aneurysm was caused by a perforation of the orbit by a pellet (G. P. Duffy).

radiograph the presence of pneumocephalus is proof that such an injury is present while the persistence of an unexplained swelling of the lid after the subsidence of a hæmatoma should lead to the suspicion that it represents an accumulation of cerebro-spinal fluid.

It is difficult to assess the incidence of intracranial damage associated with penetrating injuries of the orbit. Birch-Hirschfeld (1930) collected 172 cases of stab wounds from the literature and found involvement of the optic nerve in 125; McClure and Gardner (1949) added 4 more cases. Isolated examples of penetrating wounds of the orbit with intracranial complications have been reported by Murphree and Broussard (1965), Albert *et al.* (1965), Gossman (1966) and Hamilton (1966) (Fig. 33). Serious intracranial damage associated with apparently trivial wounds of the eyelids occurred in 6 children reported by Guthkelch (1960): one child sustained severe bilateral damage to the brain, intracranial suppuration developed in 4 others with one fatality, while the other 3 underwent numerous operations with a residue of post-traumatic epilepsy and change of personality; in each a small perforating wound of the upper eyelid had been caused by an arrow, a pencil or sharp stick or a chisel. Nine out of 15 cases of trans-orbital stab-wounds observed by Kjer (1954) developed cerebral complications including infection by tetanus and gas gangrene in 2 cases. Bard and Jarrett (1964) reviewed 44 cases from the literature adding 9 cases of their own: in only 1 of 8 cases examined radiologically soon after the injury was a fracture demonstrated while in a further 2 the bony injury was seen at operation; meningitis developed in 4, brain abscess in a further case in which there had been only a very trivial eyelid injury, and 2 patients died from unrecognized intracranial injury with laceration of the vessels and intracerebral hæmorrhage; 4 of the 7 survivors lost the sight of one eye. A further 6 cases were reviewed by Klug (1968) and 9 cases including 5 children between the ages of 2 and 15 years were described by Duffy and Bhandari (1969).

The possibility of intracranial injury should always be considered whenever there has been a wound in the region of the orbit associated with a sharp object, especially in children; however slight the local symptoms and signs may therefore seem to be, all cases with penetrating wounds of the eyelids and orbit should be admitted to hospital for observation. Even if there is no history of loss of consciousness or other neurological signs, immediate radiological examination of the skull with particular reference to the state of the roof of the orbit is essential. If the cranium has been penetrated, early and complete exploration of the wound should be undertaken; antibiotic therapy, although essential, is not an adequate substitute for timely surgical intervention which should be instituted preferably before the onset of cerebral œdema.[1]

Complications in the Orbit. Of the *immediate complications* which follow a penetrating orbital wound, *hæmorrhage* is often sufficiently profuse to cause a considerable degree of proptosis, although it is usually controlled by pressure; but *infection* may assume much more serious importance. Pyogenic infection introduced into the wound is the most common event, and a number of cases is on record wherein this has led to the development of orbital cellulitis and blindness (Knapp, 1906; Talkovskii, 1940; and others), purulent tenonitis (Puech, 1902) and even death from septicæmia or thrombophlebitis of the cavernous sinus. Less fulminating infections may produce a more chronic type of granulomatous inflammation, while if the nasal sinuses have been opened, infection may eventually find its way secondarily from these into the orbit.

Two relatively rare but important types of infection should be noted—gas gangrene and tetanus. GAS GANGRENE infection of the orbit is rare and is associated with heavily contaminated wounds, and if the eye is also perforated, may be accompanied by a similar intra-ocular involvement.[2] This complication is distinguished by the great brawny swelling of the lids, the foul, bloody or coffee-coloured discharge and the appearance of gas bubbles with the characteristic odour; these can be detected radiographically in the orbit.[3] If the infection is recognized early, polyvalent anti-gas gangrene antitoxin may be given as well as massive doses of penicillin or injections

[1] Carver and Patterson (1954), Guthkelch (1960), Bard and Jarrett (1964), Duffy and Bhandari (1969).

[2] p. 405.

[3] Compare emphysema, Fig. 258, p. 293.

of tetracycline.[1] Occasionally after such treatment the infection has cleared, but the eye remains blind with optic atrophy (McGregor, 1941). As a rule, however, enucleation of the eye with the establishment of the freest drainage is the minimal, and exenteration of the orbit the optimal treatment (Davidson and Burn, 1943; Kjer, 1954).

TETANUS may be associated with orbital wounds particularly when a contaminated foreign body is retained (Wagenmann, 1905; Collins, 1918; Kjer, 1954; and others). The manifestations of such an infection resemble those seen in wounds of the lids[2].

Late complications in the orbit after perforating wounds include the development of encysted abscesses, chronic osteoperiostitis, granulomatous masses (Fig. 399), blood cysts or implantation cysts (Critchett and Griffith, 1897). Injury to vessels of some size may lead to the development of an arterio-venous aneurysm (Terry and Mysel, 1934; Sugar and Meyer,

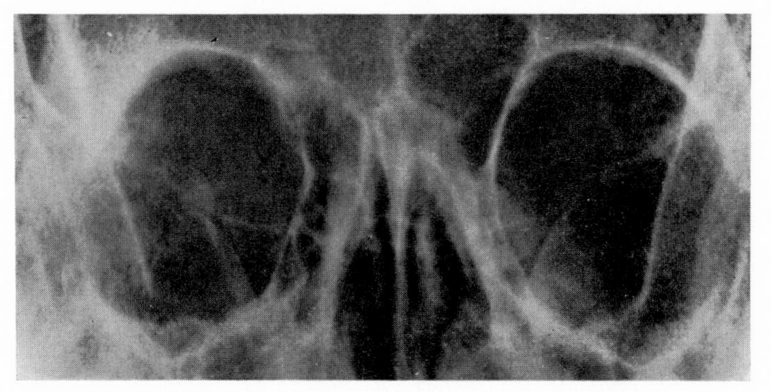

FIG. 399.—FOREIGN-BODY GRANULOMA.

In a man aged 24. A firm palpable mass was present in the upper and outer quadrant of the right orbit. The mass was found to be a granuloma containing a sliver of wood and the X-ray shows hyperostosis in this region (S. L. Trokel).

1940) or a cirsoid aneurysm in the orbit (Sniderman, 1940). These vascular lesions, if progressive, may require extensive surgical interference—ligation of the carotid (sometimes both external and internal) as well as extirpation of the more prominent vessels appearing in the lids. Wounds which have penetrated beyond the orbit may be followed by late complications such as a chronic sinusitis or a mucocele if the nasal sinuses are involved, chronic intracranial arachnoid infection or an intracranial aneurysm, particularly if the cavernous sinus has been implicated (Schmidt and Frowein, 1971) (Fig. 400).

Cases of infective meningitis are rare after orbital injuries but a hæmorrhagic lesion is exceptional. Muscas (1952) reported two cases of leptomeningeal hæmorrhage observed 48 hours after orbital injuries. In one of these, symptoms of an infective meningitis appeared 15 days after the initial meningeal disturbance seemed to have subsided.

[1] p. 407. [2] p. 428.

The *treatment* of penetrating wounds of the orbit consists of such exploration of the wound as can reasonably be undertaken, particularly if there is any question of the retention of a foreign body or of intracranial extension, its cleansing so far as possible, dusting with antibiotic powder, and its closure in layers as has already been indicated in wounds of the lids. If the wound is very extensive a drain may be inserted and removed after 24 hours, whereafter healing by first intention usually occurs. Prophylaxis against tetanus[1] is a wise precaution in every case in which such an infection

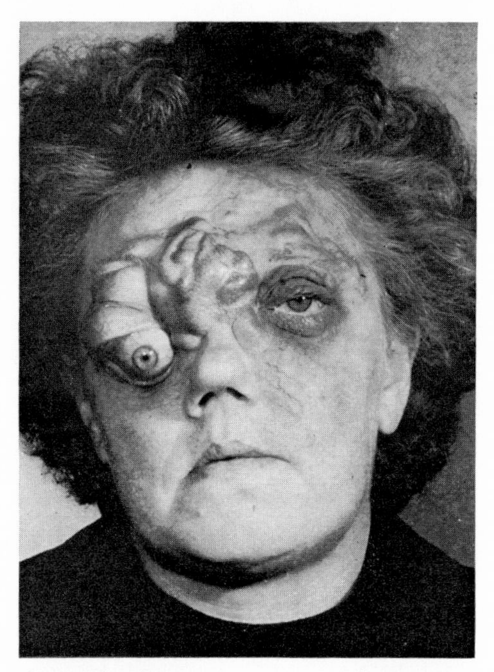

FIG. 400.—CAROTICO-CAVERNOUS ANEURYSM.

In a woman aged 40. A hay fork penetrated the left orbit 22 years previously with a resultant carotico-cavernous aneurysm and pulsatory exophthalmos on the left side. One year later there was marked exophthalmos and displacement of the globe on the right side with the development of gross clusters of dilated vessels (J. G. H. Schmidt and R. A. Frowein).

is possible and, unless the wound is obviously clean, prophylactic treatment by antibiotics given systemically is indicated.

So far as technical surgery is concerned, any prolapse of orbital fat should be excised; injury to or prolapse of the lacrimal gland is best treated by the excision of this structure, and if the torn ends of muscles are obvious in the wound, these should be sutured at the time of primary closure. When, however, muscles have been damaged in the depths of the wound, it is usually well to delay surgical treatment until the swelling and ecchymosis have died

[1] p. 408.

down so that the full extent of the damage can be ascertained, but functional restoration should be attempted before the severed muscle belly has retracted and perhaps has become fixed in scar-tissue, and before contractions of the antagonistic muscles have added complications to the surgical correction of the diplopia. If it can be found, the muscle should be isolated and re-sutured in place, and if this is possible and widespread laceration has not occurred the functional result may be excellent. In the more common event of a permanent residual weakness, surgical treatment should be directed to the readjustment of the remaining muscles of both eyes so that binocularity is attained, in any event in the primary position, by the procedures already described in the treatment of residual palsies after concussion injuries.[1] Injuries to the nerves (including the optic nerve) are not, of course, amenable to reparative surgery.

The treatment of the general condition of the patient, who may be considerably shocked, and of intracranial or nasal complications, must follow general lines.

Adam. *Klin. Mbl. Augenheilk.*, **46,** 483 (1908).
Agnello. *Riv. Oto-neuro-oftal.*, **27,** 511 (1952).
Ahlström. *Zbl. prakt. Augenheilk.*, **19,** 193 (1895); **22,** 300 (1898).
Albert, Burns and Scheie. *Amer. J. Ophthal.*, **60,** 1109 (1965).
Bailliart. *Bull. Soc. Ophtal. Fr.*, 90 (1950).
Bard and Jarrett. *Arch. Ophthal.*, **71,** 332 (1964).
Bender. *Arch. Neurol. Psychiat.*, **53,** 418 (1945).
Berger. *Klin. Mbl. Augenheilk.*, **43** (2), 480 (1905).
Berlin. *Graefe-Saemisch Hb. d. ges. Augenheilk.*, 1st ed., Leipzig, **6,** 640 (1880).
Bettrémieux. *Zbl. prakt. Augenheilk.*, **27,** 362 (1903).
Birch-Hirschfeld. *Graefe-Saemisch Hb. d. ges Augenheilk.*, 2nd ed., Berlin, **9** (1), 998 (1930).
Bock. *Zur Kenntnis d. gesunden u. kranken Tränendrüse*, Wien (1896).
Bonamour and Hugonnier. *Bull. Soc. Ophtal. Fr.*, 153 (1952).
de Britto. *Arch. Ophtal.*, **7,** 83 (1887).
Carver and Patterson. *Surgery*, **35,** 475 (1954).
Chevalier. *J. méd. Bordeaux*, **14,** 79 (1884).
Collins. *Trans. ophthal. Soc. U.K.*, **38,** 292 (1918).
Corrado. *Rass. ital. Ottal.*, **20,** 185 (1951).
Critchett and Griffith. *Trans. ophthal. Soc. U.K.*, **17,** 242 (1897).
Davidson and Burn. *Trans. ophthal. Soc. U.K.*, **63,** 375 (1943).
Dejean. *Arq. port. Oftal.*, **3,** 9 (1951).
Dimmer. *Z. Augenheilk.*, **9,** 337 (1903).
Distler. *Aus der Stuttgarter Augenheilanstalt für Unbemittelte*, Stuttgart (1905).
Donkin. *Brain*, **5,** 554 (1882–83).
Dürr. *Klin. Mbl. Augenheilk.*, **17,** 332 (1879).
Duffy and Bhandari. *Brit. J. Surg.*, **56,** 685 (1969).
El-Kinani. *Bull. ophthal. Soc. Egypt*, **38,** 137 (1945).
Field. *Arch. Ophthal.*, **46,** 157 (1951).
Garrard and Snell. *Trans. ophthal. Soc. U.K.*, **8,** 277 (1888).
Goldzieher. *Zbl. prakt. Augenheilk.*, **27,** 169 (1903).
Gossman. *J. Neurol. Neurosurg. Psychiat.*, **29,** 476 (1966).
Graefe, A. v. *Graefes Arch. Ophthal.*, **33** (3), 206 (1887).
von Graefe. *v. Graefes Arch. Ophthal.*, **2** (1), 227 (1855); **5** (1), 136 (1859); **12** (2), 224 (1866).
Guthkelch. *Brit. med. J.*, **2,** 842 (1960).
Gutmann. *Zbl. prakt. Augenheilk.*, **7,** 36 (1883).
Berl. klin. Wschr., **32,** 1114, 1138 (1895).
Hamilton. *J. Neurol. Neurosurg. Psychiat.*, **29,** 476 (1966).
Hirschberg. *Arch. Augenheilk.*, **8,** 169 (1879).
van der Hoeve. *Klin. Mbl. Augenheilk.*, **53,** 584 (1914).
Hubbell. *J. Amer. med. Ass.*, **44,** 4 (1905).
Jackson. *Ophthal. Rec.*, **13,** 345 (1904).
Jarjavay. *Ann. Oculist.* (Paris), **34,** 281 (1855).
Kempner. *Klin. Mbl. Augenheilk.*, **41** (1), 160 (1903).
Kjer. *Arch. Ophthal.*, **51,** 811 (1954).
Klug. *Zbl. Neurochir.*, **29,** 45 (1968).
Knapp. *Arch. Ophthal.*, **35,** 524 (1906).
Laval. *Arch. Ophthal.*, **19,** 762 (1938).
Leplace. *Med. News*, Phila., **59,** 657 (1891).
Levy and Chatfield. *Brit. J. Ophthal.*, **53,** 49 (1969).
Le Win. *Arch. Ophthal.*, **47,** 515 (1952).

[1] p. 304.

McClure and Gardner. *Cleveland Clin. Quart.*, **16**, 118 (1949).
McGregor. *Brit. med. J.*, **1**, 292 (1941).
Michaelson. *Brit. J. Ophthal.*, **28**, 458 (1944).
Murphree and Broussard. *J. Neurosurg.*, **23**, 450 (1965).
Muscas. *Boll. Oculist.*, **31**, 703 (1952).
Nathan and Turner. *Brain*, **65**, 343 (1942).
Oloff. *Klin. Mbl. Augenheilk.*, **48** (2), 472 (1910).
Pagenstecher. *v. Graefes Arch. Ophthal.*, **15** (1), 223 (1869).
Palin. *Trans. ophthal. Soc. U.K.*, **68**, 351 (1948).
Panas. *Arch. Ophtal.*, **22**, 229 (1902).
Parsons. *Roy. Lond. ophthal. Hosp. Rep.*, **15**, 362 (1903).
Pfalz. *Klin. Mbl. Augenheilk.*, **30**, 62 (1892).
Philipsen. *Hospitalstidende*, **5**, 601 (1887).
Puech. *Bull. Soc. franç. Ophtal.*, **19**, 117 (1902).
Rafalovich and Belyaev. *Vestn. oftal.*, No. 3, 34 (1958).
Rees. *Med. Ann. Dist. Columbia*, **16**, 548 (1947).
Roche. *Recueil Ophtal.*, **27**, 73 (1905).
Schmidt and Frowein. *Klin. Mbl. Augenheilk.*, **159**, No. 5 (1971).
Schneider and Henderson. *Arch. Ophthal.*, **47**, 81 (1952).
Small and Turner. *Brit. J. Surg., War Surg. Suppl.*, **1**, 62 (1947).
Snell. *Trans. ophthal. Soc. U.K.*, **17**, 81 (1897).
Sniderman. *Arch. Ophthal.*, **24**, 1190 (1940).
Steindorff. *Die isolierten, direkten Verletzungen d. Sehnerven innerhalb d. Augenhöhle* (Diss.), Halle (1898).
Zbl. prakt. Augenheilk., **25**, 19 (1901).
Steiner. *Amer. J. Ophthal.*, **34**, 100 (1951).
Sugar and Meyer. *Arch. Ophthal.*, **23**, 1288 (1940).
Svoboda. *Cs. oftal.*, **4**, 72 (1948).
Talkovskii. *Pub. Helmholtz Inst. Ophthal.* (Russia), 89 (1940).
Terry and Mysel. *J. Amer. med. Ass.*, **103**, 1036 (1934).
Terson. *Prog. Méd.*, **12**, 264 (1890).
Thomas. *Amer. J. Ophthal.*, **25**, 210 (1942).
Valude. *Ann. Oculist.* (Paris), **127**, 133 (1902).
Viallefont, Boudet and Philippot. *Bull. Soc. franç. Ophtal.*, **80**, 601 (1967).
Viciano. *Arch. Ophtal.*, **9**, 508 (1889).
Wagenmann. *Ber. dtsch. ophthal. Ges.*, **32**, 260 (1905).
Weeks. *Trans. Sect. Ophthal., Amer. med. Ass.*, 218 (1903).
Wertheim. *Klin. Mbl. Augenheilk.*, **46** (1), 425 (1908).
Würdemann. *Injuries of the Eyes*, 2nd ed., London (1932).
Zander and Geissler. *Die Verletzungen d. Auges*, Leipzig (1864).

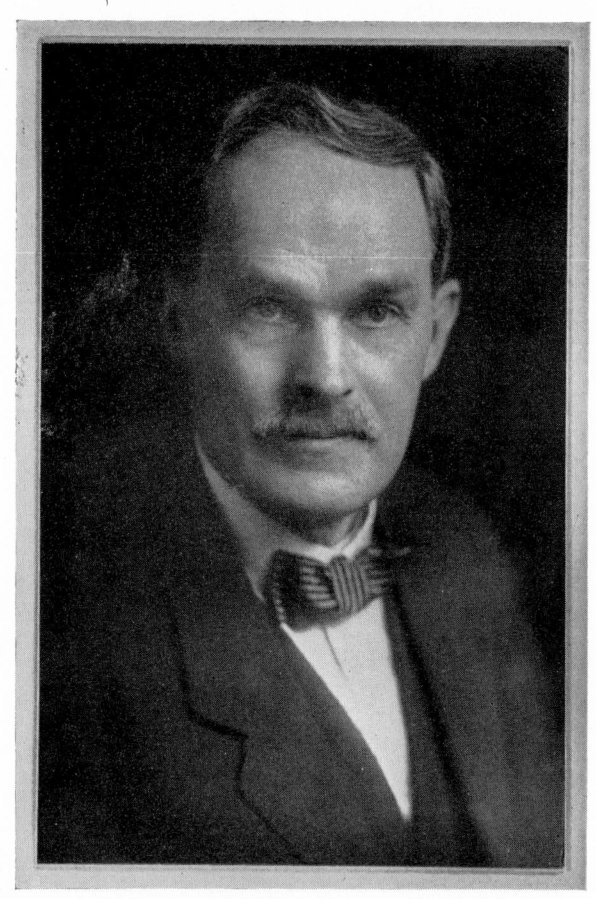

Fig. 401.—Sir William Tindall Lister [1868–1944].

CHAPTER IV

RETAINED FOREIGN BODIES

As WOULD be expected a retained extra-ocular foreign body is no modern accident. When Rameses II built his tomb at Thebes in the Valley of the Nile about 1200 B.C., the artist, Ipuy, broke with convention and decorated the walls with the incidents that accompanied its building; one of these is the picture of a workman having a foreign body removed from his eye, another depicts the agony of a man on whose foot an axe-head had fallen, while a third shows a man lying on the ground having his dislocated shoulder reduced by Kocher's modern method.

Retained intra-ocular foreign bodies must have had an equally long history but it has been less fully documented. As an introduction to this Chapter we are therefore inserting the photograph of SIR WILLIAM TINDALL LISTER [1868–1944] (Fig. 401) who was one of those who contributed most richly to our knowledge of ocular injuries. A kindly physician and a great surgeon with a sound knowledge of the fundamentals of pathology acquired as curator at Moorfields Eye Hospital, he was the ideal person to be chosen as Ophthalmic Consultant to the British Army in the first World War—the first occasion that such an appointment was made. War is the ideal school in which to observe and learn traumatic surgery; and the Army—and ophthalmology—gained much from Lister's experience, for his unbounded enthusiasm, scrupulous accuracy and unusual conscientiousness made it inevitable that the behaviour of the injured eye should be studied as seldom before. His name appears in most chapters in this book for his observations on concussion injuries and wounds, particularly those affecting the retina, were fundamental and will always be classical. The debt to Lister of the senior author is unusually great, not only because of the memory of his friendship but also for the lessons and example from which he profited when it was his privilege to follow in the footsteps of his predecessor in the second World War.

EXTRA-OCULAR FOREIGN BODIES

The most common accident encountered in ophthalmology is the retention of a foreign body on the surface of the eye; this is a constantly recurring incident in domestic, industrial or agricultural life and, although often a trivial matter, it is not always so, for if the foreign material is not automatically removed by the tears it frequently incapacitates the patient so long as it remains, while the trauma involved by injudicious and awkward attempts at removal or the introduction of infection may cause permanent damage to vision and even on occasion the loss of the eye.

The catalogue of such foreign bodies which may enter the eye is endless—the ordinary " motes " of organic matter or dust, textile material, ashes, coal-dust, pieces of tobacco, eyelashes and innumerable other particles, including a piece of finger-nail (Critchett, 1891) or a fragment of a gramophone record (Velicky, 1951), are commonplace in domestic surroundings (Fig. 402); pieces of metal, emery or stone give rise to the most common accidents in industry; fragments of missiles, the debris of explosions, even splinters of bone from mutilated fellow-soldiers (Cunningham, 1916) are typical of war; while seeds, husks, pieces of chaff, straw or grain, thorns, leaves or flowers, insects or their wings, legs or spines are common intruders in agricultural surroundings, the visitants varying with the locality and the season.

Thus in tropical jungles, leeches which may be minute and present in myriads occasionally enter the eyes and, having entered, their bites may cause considerable conjunctival reactions and leucomata of the cornea (Kuwahara, 1903; Coburn, 1911; van Hoorn, 1948). Other examples are the green bugs (*Jassidæ*), the thrips (*Thysanoptera*) and the locusts of India (Elliot, 1920), the "fumuski" (*Scotinophora vermiculata*) which are abundant during the rice harvest in Japan (Takashima, 1912) or the cochineal insect (*Coccus cacti*) of tropical America. The tail of a 5-inch-long scorpion deeply embedded in the cornea is a unique foreign body (True, 1951). The larvæ of insects, however, are not unusual visitors (*external myiasis*), an entire louse is more

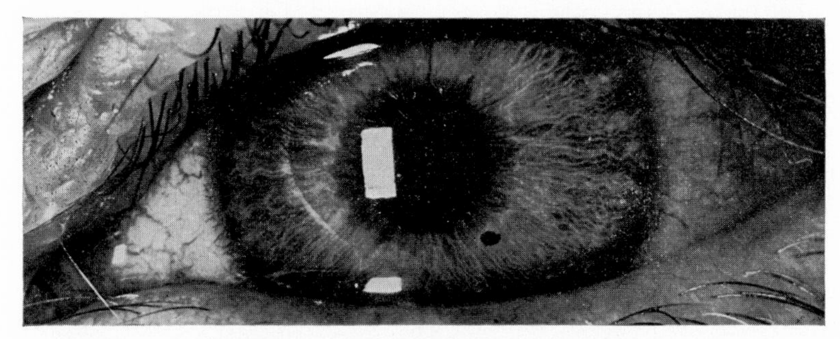

Fig. 402.—Foreign Body in the Cornea.
A metallic foreign body is seen at 5 o'clock (Inst. Ophthal.).

rare (Cohen, 1892; Fischer, 1897) or a tick (Scott, 1883); even a crab (Batten, 1900) and a snail have been unsuspected foreign bodies, the latter of which eventually burrowed subconjunctivally (Ghose, 1949, in India), while the entrance of the *Sarcoptes* has produced the lesions of scabies of the cornea (Saemisch, 1898).

The *size* of the foreign body which may be thus retained in the conjunctival sac, particularly in the upper fornix, has sometimes been remarkable—a piece of slag the size of a hazel nut retained for six weeks (Thilliez, 1899), a piece of iron 2 × 1 cm., weighing 6 gm. (de Micas, 1904), a fragment of a shell 1 × 0·5 × 0·5 cm. (Cunningham, 1916), a brass ring 22 mm. in diameter and 2·5 mm. thick (Lederer, 1900), or a splinter of wood 18 × 6 × 3 mm. (Croskey, 1898); and the length of time over which they have on occasion been allowed to remain there seems incredible—a thorn under the upper lid for two years (Swan, 1889) or a twig (15 × 1·5 mm.) in the outer canthus for 12 years (Fränkel, 1891), a portion of a knitting needle (22 × 3 mm.) in a highly oxidized state for 22 years (Sexe, 1905) or a piece of slate-pencil 17 mm. long for 29 years (Schoute, 1911). Even a contact lens has been lost in this way.[1]

Multiple foreign bodies, such as are typically caused by an explosion, produce a characteristic problem which will be dealt with subsequently.[2]

As it impinges upon the eye, the foreign body most usually hits the cornea but may land upon the bulbar conjunctiva; in either of these two

[1] p. 23. [2] p. 671.

places it may remain, particularly if it is sharp and angular or adherent, or if it is hot as are many metal splinters. Some merely adhere to the surface, but this they may do with extraordinary tenacity—the calyces of flowers and seeds and the wings of insects; others, such as the ordinary mote or cinder or pieces of metal flying with a small velocity, embed themselves superficially in the epithelium; others are washed by the reflex flow of tears excited by the sudden irritation into the lower conjunctival cul-de-sac and may eventually find their way to the inner canthus, and occasionally into the lacrimal passages; much more commonly a small foreign body is swept up by the upper lid in the violent movements of blinking excited by its impact and finds lodgment about the middle of the upper subtarsal sulcus, the groove running a little above and parallel to the ciliary margin which marks the transition between the stratified and columnar epithelium of the onjunctiva; while others, usually more bulky, work their way up with the novements of the lids into the recesses of the upper fornix. In domestic fe, where motes and particles of relatively soft consistency contribute the ıajority of such intruders, the lower fornix is a frequent resting place; in dustrial surroundings, where flying pieces of metal form the commonest reign bodies, most impinge upon and remain adherent to the cornea, ıile the majority of those lodging in the upper fornix is made up of the ces of chaff or other vegetable matter met with in rural surroundings.

Other foreign bodies, particularly if sharp and metallic and travelling speed, embed themselves more deeply in the tissues of the cornea or the sclera or sclera; while others, endowed with sufficient momentum, etrate the coats of the eye and enter the globe. It is interesting that, e metallic particles bury themselves in the corneal tissues or traverse ı directly, vegetable materials such as pieces of grain or straw, being more 1 le and travelling with less velocity, tend to take the path of least r ance and, running between the corneal lamellæ, bury themselves radially.

s would be expected because of its exposed position, the most usual site of impact is ɔw and somewhat nasally to the corneal vertex, a predilection verified by an an is of 2,000 cases by Grönvall and Ohlsson (1951). This is particularly so in in ial conditions where most of the foreign bodies are small pieces of metal which adl at the site of impact: in an industrial plant, for example, Callahan (1944) fou hat 77% involved the cornea. Those commonly met with in domestic circum-sta (grit, dust, motes) are more frequently caught up in the subtarsal sulcus of the upp d.

s interesting and beyond doubt that if the vision of the two eyes is unequal eith ırough amblyopia or anisometropia, foreign bodies tend to enter the better eye. is is explained by the fact that if dominance of one eye is established in child-hood eferential unilateral winking tends to develop in the eye with the poorer acuit Some 60% of people wink preferentially with one eye, and since the weaker eye is more facile winker, it is protected more efficiently and rapidly on the approach of an uder.[1]

[1] See Vol. XIII.

The clinical pictures produced by such foreign bodies are known to everyone. The symptoms vary in intensity with the type of particle and more widely with the site of lodgment.

The Mechanical Effects of Foreign Bodies

If the *cornea* is struck by a gritty foreign body which does not penetrate, at the moment of impact there is a sharp burning pain, a reflex gush of tears with momentary blindness, and the lids close in blepharospasm; the patient thereupon rubs the eye violently and thereby often succeeds in impacting the foreign body securely into the corneal epithelium whereas, if left alone, it might well have been safely washed down into the conjunctival cul-de-sac. So long as the foreign body remains these symptoms of irritation persist, continuously accentuated by the act of blinking, gradually ameliorating, however, as the epithelium with the associated particle sloughs away or until it penetrates the cornea more deeply. These symptoms are always most pronounced in the upper or middle parts of the cornea; in the lower part, which is not so actively involved in the act of blinking, they are considerably less. On the other hand, particles which penetrate deeply and remain impacted or perforate the globe cause much less annoyance; these may, indeed, be considered trivial at the time or pass unnoticed and remain practically without symptoms, since no sharp edges rub against the conjunctiva of the lid; it is only later, after some days or occasionally weeks, when the epithelium sloughs away, that the projecting foreign body gives rise to symptoms or the reaction in the corneal tissues draws attention to the accident. In all these cases, apart from the incapacitating reaction of the subjective symptoms, there is evidence of uveal irritation as shown by circumcorneal injection and miosis. Even from the first, if the foreign body is central, a considerable diminution of vision may result, due not only to the lacrimation and the irregularity produced on the corneal surface, but also, perhaps, to the disturbing shadow thrown on the retina due to the stresses and distortion of the corneal tissues and the optical effects of variations in refraction thus caused (Stewart and Lloyd, 1943; Lenggenhager, 1950).

The subsequent fate of such buried foreign bodies depends partly upon their ability to excite irritation in the tissues and partly upon the complication of infection. If the foreign material is chemically indifferent (coal, glass, etc.) it is usually incorporated in the corneal tissues, where it is permanently embedded and may be tolerated indefinitely without ill-effects. On the other hand, if it is irritative or excites chemical reactions in the tissues (iron, copper, etc.) an inflammatory infiltration gathers around it, usually appearing clinically as a grey ring; here the corneal tissues break down so that the foreign body becomes loose and is eventually extruded with the slough. At this time serious irritative symptoms may first become evident and the process of elimination is accompanied by an iritis which may be severe, the distressing symptoms of which may persist for some time after the extrusion of the particle; generally, however, the resulting ulcer heals, but unless the epithelium alone is involved, the site is invariably marked by a permanent opacity, sometimes minute in size but sometimes developing into a leucoma of considerable extent. Frequently this process is complicated by infection, in which case the resulting ulceration, the associated intra-ocular inflammation and the residual scarring are all accentuated and may persist long after expulsion of the foreign body by suppuration has occurred.

Exceptional incidents have been related. Thus Voisin and his colleagues (1950) reported a case wherein a foreign body, deeply embedded in the cornea, remained quiet for three months after unsuccessful attacks at removal; thereupon a fistula developed, the anterior chamber collapsed and the foreign body was washed away—all without sequelæ.

Organic foreign bodies of a non-gritty nature, on the other hand, cause much less immediate trouble. Chaff and the husks and calyces of flowers or seeds or the wings of insects, for example, may adhere firmly to the cornea and stick for days, giving rise to surprisingly few symptoms; eventually however, if allowed to remain, the tendency is for ulceration to develop, when the macerated organic material may be found, sometimes unexpectedly, at the bottom of the crater.

An interesting case of this nature was reported by Sédan and Sédan-Bauby (1950). A husk of grain embedded itself in this way on the periphery of the cornea of a girl, who remained with a quiet eye showing no reaction for 15 years; thereafter, removal of the foreign body revealed a perforation of the cornea with incarceration therein of a knuckle of iris.

In the conjunctiva the clinical picture is more varied. Sharp gritty particles adherent to the inner surface of the upper lid, particularly those lying in the subtarsal fold, continuously abrade the cornea in the movements of blinking and thereby cause symptoms as or more severe than result from those impacted on the corneal surface; and so long as they are allowed to remain these acutely irritative symptoms persist. Much less irritation results from superficial foreign bodies resting elsewhere on the conjunctiva; indeed, the upper fornix or the semilunar fold may remain the secret hiding-place of a foreign body of considerable size until the development of irritative inflammatory symptoms draws attention to it; while those embedded in the subconjunctival tissues may give rise to transient symptoms only, so that they remain without annoyance after the initial irritation has passed off.

In the sclera the impaction of foreign bodies is rare—according to Praun (1899) 200 times less frequently than in the cornea. They are usually found in the palpebral aperture, since elsewhere the lids provide adequate protection and it is a very remote chance that a missile which has traversed their tissues lodges in the sclera and does not penetrate into the inner eye

(Cramer, 1907); a particle which has penetrated the globe, however, often becomes embedded in the sclera on the opposite side. The most common incident is the rain of multiple debris thrown up in an explosion, when the whole eye is bespattered with pieces of sand, dust, powder and other particles, many of which may traverse the conjunctiva to rest in the sclera: this problem will be considered separately.[1] Isolated foreign bodies consist mainly of pieces of metal or glass, splinters of wood or fragments of stone flying with sufficient force to pierce the conjunctiva and lodge in the sclera, but without the energy to traverse its thickness.

At the time of the accident the injury is generally obscured by a small hæmorrhage; thereafter the foreign body may become visible or lie buried out of sight. There it usually lies indefinitely, giving rise to no symptoms (iron splinters for 21 years, Strawbridge, 1875; 7 years, Roulet, 1877; Praun, 1899; a piece of wood for 17½ years, Oeller, 1882); occasionally a granuloma may arise at the site or irritation and infection may ultimately develop. It is to be remembered, however, that pieces of copper[2] may give rise to a localized abscess.

Multiple Minute Foreign Bodies

In many industries dusts of finely powdered particles abound, and these tend to become deposited on the brows and lashes, clog the depressions on the skin of the lids and collect in the lower part of the conjunctival sac, particularly in the recesses of the caruncle and plica at the inner angle. The same powdering of the eye and its adnexa occurs in dry windy climates and is seen in its most severe forms in desert conditions, particularly during sand-storms. Some of these materials are inert and act mechanically as minute foreign bodies (Fig. 403); others are chemically active either at the time or subsequently—these will be discussed at a later stage.[3]

Inert or indifferent powdered materials which act upon the eye passively are as a rule too minute to give rise to the acute symptoms characteristic of a foreign body, and their ill-effects depend on the cumulative action of their numbers and the constancy or frequency of their entrance. If the particles are soft they are usually washed out by the tears without harm; but if they are hard, particularly with gritty, irregular surfaces, they may adhere to the tissues and even penetrate them, occasionally acting as a tattoo. This is seen in its most dramatic form among charcoal workers, in whom the lids, conjunctiva and in some cases even the cornea may be indelibly tattooed in this way.

On the *lids* repeated minute traumata of this type may give rise to a chronic blepharo-conjunctivitis, usually of the hyperæmic type, a condition which may be called BLEPHAROCONIOSIS (βλέφαρον, lid; κονία, dust). In many occupational dermatoses of this type the effect is enhanced by heat

[1] p. 671. [2] p. 512. [3] Chap. XI.

and chemical irritation (wood-dust, alkalis, arsenicals, etc.)[1] when a furuncular or ulcerative blepharitis may occur, but in the case of inert powdered material with which a mechanical effect only is operative, the disease does not usually assume such proportions. In the conjunctiva the usual result is a hyperæmic conjunctivitis which tends to become hypertrophic and follicular in type.

A pinguecula possibly, and a pterygium certainly, should be included in pathological manifestations of this type, for these degenerative changes are hastened by exposure to wind and dust in countries where these are common; these lesions are said to occur preferentially in employments wherein similar conditions exist, such as among brakesmen on railways (Fuchs, 1891–92; Hübner, 1898; de Lantsheere, 1901; Mérigot de Treigny and Coirre, 1933; and others).

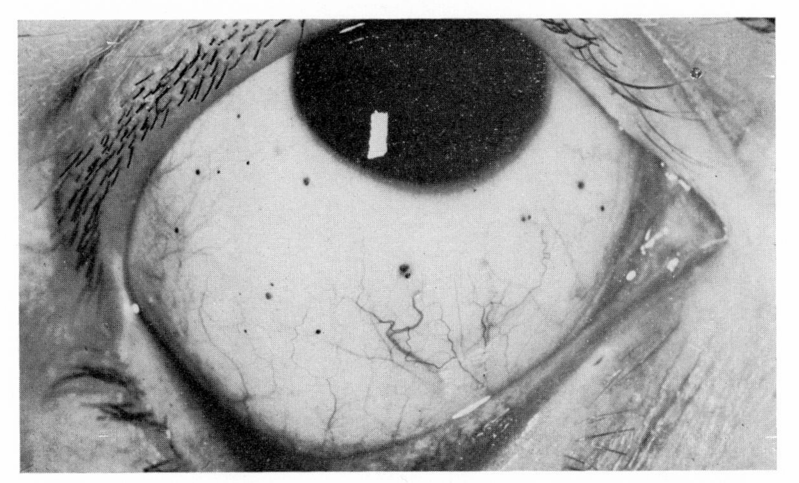

Fig. 403.—Multiple Subconjunctival Foreign Bodies (Inst. Ophthal.).

On the *cornea* innumerable abrasions may be caused, so minute that their clinical detection, even on staining with fluorescein, may be difficult; their presence is rendered evident by the symptoms of chronic irritation, mild photophobia and lacrimination to which they give rise. Occasionally a veritable encrustation of the cornea occurs wherein the particles collect usually under the epithelium and upon Bowman's membrane, a bilateral affection most pronounced in the central areas of the cornea which may involve a considerable diminution of vision. KERATOCONIOSIS is a suitable name to apply to the state of the corneæ in workers constantly exposed to a rain of sharp inert particles—stone-workers (Wood, 1925; Lebas, 1929), marble workers (marmoroconiosis) (Trantas, 1909; Coutela, 1939), grinders and sandblasters (Davidson, 1936–39; Biernacka-Biesiekierska, 1952), lathe workers (Samoilov, 1929) and others (Fig. 404.) The corneæ may be covered with innumerable minute, sharp-angled lesions, occasionally with glistening

[1] Chap. XI.

foreign bodies embedded in them. Such eyes may show signs of persistent irritability; on other occasions they may be symptomless and, indeed, it is not uncommon for hypoæsthesia to occur so that further damage by minute particles is unremarked. Samoilov (1929) found on intravital staining with methylene blue that this loss of sensation was associated with the presence of necrotic points in the corneal epithelium and damage to the terminal plexus of the corneal nerves.

SILICON in minute particles may have this typical effect. Thus the fine dust of MICA, a natural silicate varying widely in composition, which is a prominent constituent of many igneous and metamorphic rocks, may give rise to lesions of this type among workers (Minton, 1946). A somewhat similar keratitis has been recorded in the eyes of men exposed to peat dust, a condition which Powell (1934) considered to be due essentially to traumata from minute spicules of silica.

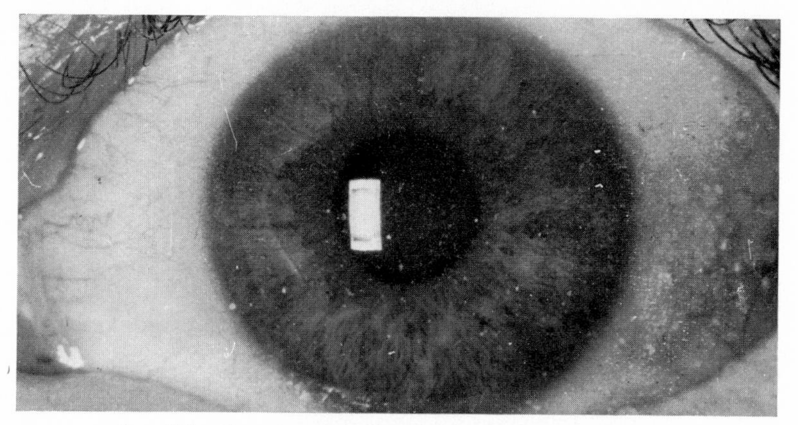

FIG. 404.—CORNEAL AND CONJUNCTIVAL FOREIGN BODIES.
Multiple minute foreign bodies of stone (Inst. Ophthal.).

The same phenomenon has been observed in hatters working with skins, in whom a band-shaped keratitis may occur in which there is incorporated a felt-like encrustation of minute pieces of fine hairs (Topolanski, 1894).

STONE in small fragments, on the other hand, may lodge in the cornea and conjunctiva and in so doing usually causes remarkably little reaction. Thus the stone-cutters in Jerusalem who spend their lives squatting before pieces of stone, cutting them into shape with a hammer and chisel, complain of dimness of vision in their old age due to a haziness of the cornea from a cloud of particles of stone which excites neither pain nor reaction.

The specific staining of the tissues of the eye by metals such as silver will be discussed at a later stage.[1]

Batten. *Lancet*, **1,** 1002 (1900).
Biernacka-Biesiekierska. *Klin. oczna*, **22,** 89 (1952).
Callahan. *J. med. Ass. Georgia*, **33,** 312 (1944).
Coburn. *Ophthal. Rec.*, **20,** 234 (1911).
Cohen. *Lhb. d. Hyg. d. Auges*, Wien (1892).
Coutela. *L'oeil et les maladies professionelles*, Paris (1939).
Cramer. *Mschr. Unfallheilk.*, **14,** 333 (1907).
Critchett. *Brit. med. J.*, **2,** 1196 (1891).

[1] Chap. XI.

Croskey. *Ophthal. Rec.*, **7**, 33 (1898).
Cunningham. *Ophthalmoscope*, **14**, 412 (1916).
Davidson. *Amer. J. Ophthal.*, **19**, 896 (1936). *Arch. Ophthal.*, **21**, 673 (1939).
Elliot. *Tropical Ophthalmology*, London (1920).
Fischer. *Münch. med. Wschr.*, **44**, 112 (1897).
Fränkel. *Klin. Mbl. Augenheilk.*, **29**, 92 (1891).
Fuchs. *v. Graefes Arch. Ophthal.*, **37** (3), 143 (1891); **38** (2), 1 (1892).
Ghose. *Brit. J. Ophthal.*, **33**, 520 (1949).
Grönvall and Ohlsson. *Acta ophthal.* (Kbh.), **29**, 169 (1951).
van Hoorn. *Ned. T. Geneesk.*, **92**, 3748 (1948).
Hübner. *Arch. Augenheilk.*, **36**, 70 (1898).
Kuwahara. *Zbl. prakt. Augenheilk.*, **27**, 262 (1903).
de Lantsheere. *Presse méd. belge*, **53**, 326 (1901).
Lebas. *Bull. Soc. belge Ophtal.*, No. 58, 23 (1929).
Lederer. *Clin. Ophtal.*, **6**, 13 (1900).
Lenggenhager. *Schweiz. med. Wschr.*, **80**, 75 (1950).
Mérigot de Treigny and Coirre. *Bull. Soc. Ophtal. Paris*, 48 (1933).
de Micas. *Clin. Ophtal.*, **10**, 91 (1904).
Minton. *Brit. med. J.*, **1**, 211 (1946).
Oeller. *Zbl. prakt. Augenheilk.*, **6**, 18 (1882).
Powell. *Amer. J. Ophthal.*, **17**, 206 (1934).
Praun. *Die Verletzungen der Auges*, Wiesbaden (1899).
Roulet. *Korresp.-Bl. schweiz. Aerz.*, **7**, 81, 112 (1877).
Saemisch. *Klin. Mbl. Augenheilk.*, **36**, 449 (1898).
Samoilov. *Professionalnaya Patologia Glaza*, Moscow (1929).
Schoute. *Ned. T. Geneesk.*, **1**, 492 (1911).
Scott. *Brit. med. J.*, **2**, 582 (1883).
Sédan and Sédan-Bauby. *Bull. Soc. Ophtal. Fr.*, 852 (1950).
Sexe. *Bull. Soc. franç. Ophtal.*, **22**, 441 (1905).
Stewart and Lloyd. *Brit. J. Ophthal.*, **27**, 483 (1943).
Strawbridge. *Trans. Amer. ophthal. Soc.*, **2**, 302 (1875).
Swan. *Lancet*, **2**, 69 (1889).
Takashima. *Klin. Mbl. Augenheilk.*, **50** (2), 685 (1912); **51** (1), 776 (1913).
Thilliez. *Recueil Ophtal.*, **21**, 311 (1899).
Topolanski. *Wien. klin. Wschr.*, **7**, 98 (1894).
Trantas. *XI int. Cong. Ophthal.*, Naples, 339 (1909).
True. *U.S. armed Forces med. J.*, **11**, 1741 (1951).
Velicky. *Prakt. Lék.* (Praha), **3**, 145 (1951).
Voisin, Reboul, Bismut and Cottenot. *Bull. Soc. Ophtal. Fr.*, 159 (1950).
Wood. *Trans. ophthal. Soc. U.K.*, **45**, 724 (1925).

Specific Effects of Extra-ocular Foreign Bodies

Apart from these mechanical effects, the specific action of certain types of foreign body should be noted.

UNORGANIZED MATERIAL, if allowed to remain in the eye, produces irritative effects depending on the tendency of the substance concerned to interact with the ocular tissues and produce decomposition products which cause irritation. Some materials are chemically inert in this respect and are well tolerated, lying quietly in the tissues and exciting no specific irritation—glass, plastics, coal and stone are examples, while inert metals such as gold may be retained indefinitely in the cornea without reaction (9 years, McDannald, 1936).

Glass and *plastics* provide good examples of the tolerance of the corneal tissues to inert material. Fragments of glass, even in considerable number, may remain deeply embedded in the cornea without ill-effects after the initial irritation of the injury has subsided (Mann, 1941)(Fig. 405). Thus Elkington (1949) reported a case wherein both corneæ were bespattered with innumerable spicules of glass from the smashed windscreen of an automobile. The immediate reaction and blepharospasm were marked and a few of the superficial spicules were removed. When slit-lamp examination became possible the corneæ were found to glitter with minute glass particles too numerous to count, vision being considerably reduced owing to the associated corneal œdema. Although a few of these were extruded in succeeding weeks, each incident being accompanied by a slight flare-up of the eyes, normal vision was recovered and the eyes were asymptomatic when seen three years later, although innumerable spicules remained lying inert in the corneal stroma. Such is not an isolated case. A particle of glass has been seen to lie inert in the corneal tissue for 15 years (Sédan and Sédan-Bauby, 1950).

It is interesting that *cordite,* occasionally blown into the corneal tissues in an explosion, lies inert within the cornea: it may be easily extracted (Cunningham, 1916) or may even disappear spontaneously (Unsworth, 1944).

Certain metals, on the other hand, are not chemically indifferent in this way but participate in a chemical reaction with the tissues, impregnating them with decomposition products and thereby exciting irritative symptoms and degenerative changes which are of considerable importance. The whole question of the chemical effects of such materials upon the tissues of the eye will be fully discussed when we deal with intra-ocular foreign bodies, so

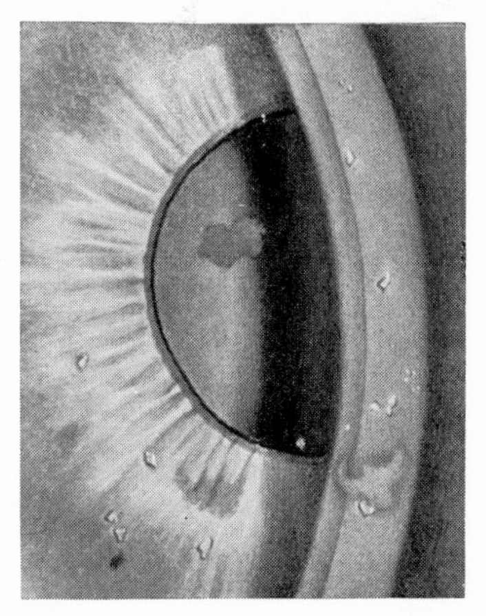

FIG. 405.—SPICULES OF GLASS IN THE CORNEA AND IRIS.

Injury in a car, the windscreen of which was shattered by the explosion of a bomb. Six weeks after the injury there was no pain and the eyes were quiet without injection or vascularization but the cornea and iris were densely bespattered with small dust-like crystals of glass, appearing like granulated sugar (Ida Mann).

that a short note at this stage will be sufficient. It is interesting, however, that rapid extrusion of the foreign material, even although it is highly irritant, may occur with complete resolution if Bowman's membrane has not been perforated, as in a case in which mercury globules impregnated the corneal epithelium after a laboratory explosion (Fleischanderl, 1940).

LEAD. Lead as a foreign body in the cornea is relatively rare and although molten lead may find its way into the eye in civilian life (Clark, 1851; Aguirre, 1943; and others), most of the reported cases have been wounds received in war.[1] There is usually remarkably little reaction and particles have remained quietly in the corneal tissue for long periods (22 years, Thompson, 1898), even although they are deeply situated (Rademacher, 1909). Extensive encrustations are sometimes apt to develop from the superficial layers of the particle and the eventual result may be the formation of a bluish-white leucomatous opacity (Plate XV, Fig. 1). Such an event used to be

[1] Oguchi (1913), Handmann (1915), Uhthoff (1916), Brenske (1916), Böhm (1916), Weigelin (1917), Pichler (1918), Winkler (1919), and others.

PLATE XV

FOREIGN BODIES IN THE CORNEA.

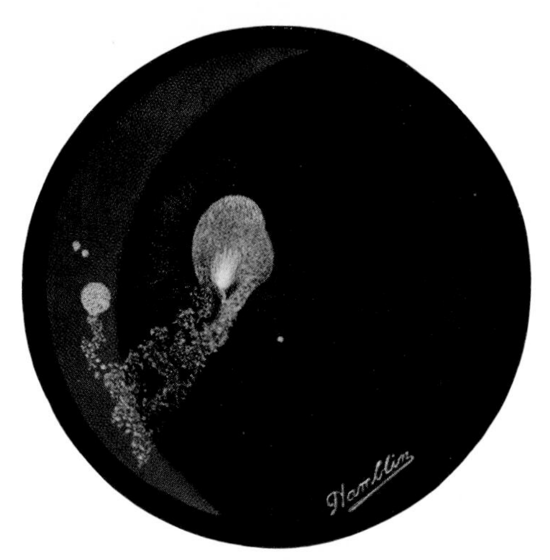

FIG. 1.—LEAD.

A piece of lead resulting from a war wound was buried deep in the cornea and covered by epithelium. Extending from it was a widespread encrustation in crystalline form, deep in the cornea. When the central area was opened with a needle a large quantity of the material escaped.

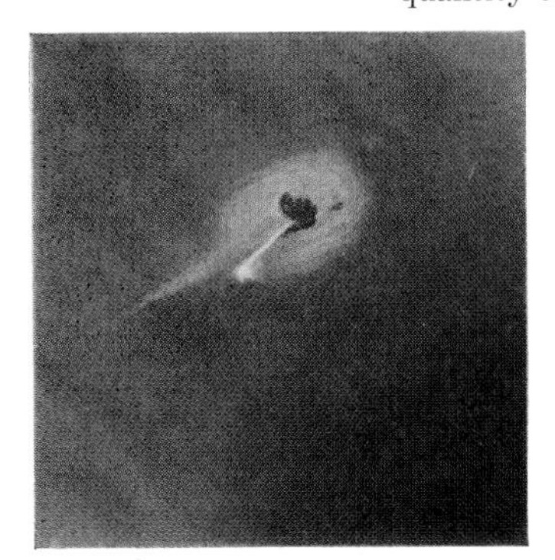

FIG. 2.

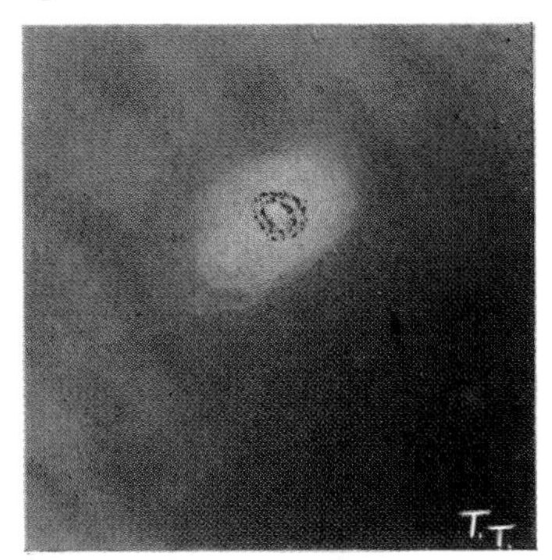

FIG. 3.

FIGS. 2 and 3.—IRON.

FIG. 2.—A particle of iron buried deeply in the cornea. FIG. 3.—The rust ring left after removal of the foreign body.

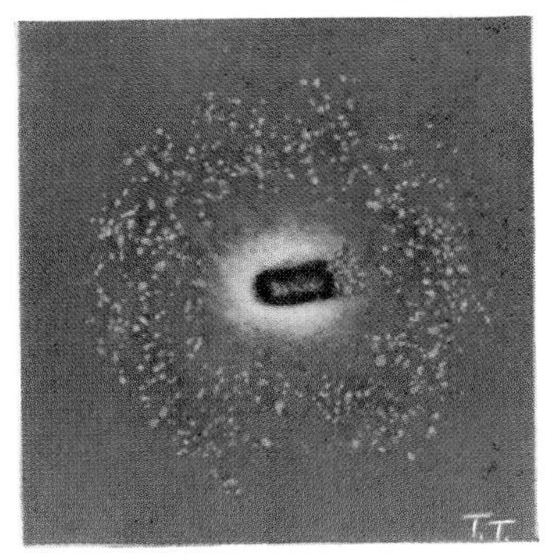

FIG. 4.—DIRECT CHALCOSIS OF THE CORNEA.

In the centre is a copper foreign body surrounded by dense infiltration and around this is a cloud of brownish-yellow deposits arranged generally in a ring shape.

more common in the days when lead acetate was frequently employed as a collyrium, when a similar encrustation developed in the presence of any epithelial defect such as an abrasion or an ulcer, but it may also occur in industry (Bellouard, 1882). The encrustation is mainly due to the deposition of an albuminate of lead (Santos Fernandez, 1906).[1] It is sometimes possible to dissolve these deposits by the application of a solution of potassium iodide (3 to 5%) on cotton pledgets, followed by iodic acid (3 to 5%), thus forming a soluble iodate of lead (Schiele, 1904); ammonium tartrate has been advised (Michtner, 1948); but mechanical curettage is usually required in addition.

SOLDER (2/3 lead, 1/3 tin) forms an inert foreign body exciting no tissue-reaction (Kamel, 1949); in the superficial layers of the cornea or conjunctiva it changes its appearance into an ashy grey hue, while in the deeper layers it retains its lustre.

COPPER. Copper, on the other hand, may excite much more widespread damage. It is true that pieces of metallic copper may occasionally remain embedded in the cornea without exciting a reaction (Bowen, 1887); but if the metal is in relatively pure form and not heavily alloyed, a localized purulent infiltration may occur associated with necrosis of the surrounding tissue and accompanied by an iritis (Hornstein, 1905; Rust, 1908). In such cases the foreign body may well be extruded. If the fragment contains a low content of copper, on the other hand, it may remain for some years surrounded by a halo of infiltration, but eventually diffusion of the metal may take place as occurs with iron, producing a DIRECT CHALCOSIS OF THE CORNEA. Therein the epithelium, Bowman's membrane and parts of the stroma may be peppered with a deposit of reddish-gold particles producing a striking picture as seen with the slit-lamp; occasionally the endothelium becomes impregnated with a reddish colour (Vogt, 1921–30; Knüsel, 1924) (Plate XV, Fig. 4). More rarely diffusion may also take place into the eye, where it has been observed to give rise to the typical sunflower cataract of GENERALIZED OCULAR CHALCOSIS,[2] a complication which results particularly if the corneal foreign body penetrates into the anterior chamber (Urbanek, 1927; King, 1948).

The impregnation of the cornea with copper after its therapeutic use or in industrial conditions will be noted subsequently.[3]

In the sclera the reaction of a copper particle may also be intense. Although it may remain quietly *in situ*, a localized abscess with necrosis of the surrounding tissue may be formed, and this on occasion may lead to iridocyclitis, choroiditis and retinal detachment, so that the eye may ultimately be lost (Rampoldi, 1891; Hornstein, 1905). Kleczkowski (1913) reported an interesting case wherein such a foreign body remained in the subconjunctival tissues for 17 years, whereafter an abscess developed, the incision of which released the particle.

A common type of injury results from a foreign body of copper oxide, formed when a particle of metallic copper suffers immediate oxidation as it is cast off as a spark from the plates of the hangers and switches of an overhead electric trolley-wire

[1] See further Chap. XI. [2] p. 518. [3] Chap. XI.

such as is commonly employed with electric tramcars or cranes (25 out of 26 copper foreign bodies, Rust, 1908). Such a foreign body has the consistency of rotted rubber and may be difficult to remove.

IRON. When a particle of iron is embedded in the *cornea* it undergoes partial disintegration[1] and is deposited in the tissues in the neighbourhood of the foreign body (DIRECT SIDEROSIS OF THE CORNEA); there it appears as a particulate brown deposit resembling a " rust ring ", which is especially evident in the epithelium, Bowman's membrane and the neighbouring corneal stroma around the edges of the wound, particularly around the keratocytes (Mayou, 1925; Zuckerman and Lieberman, 1960). Such an appearance is a commonplace and exceptionally, if the foreign body has remained *in situ* for a long period, a double concentric ring is deposited (Praun,

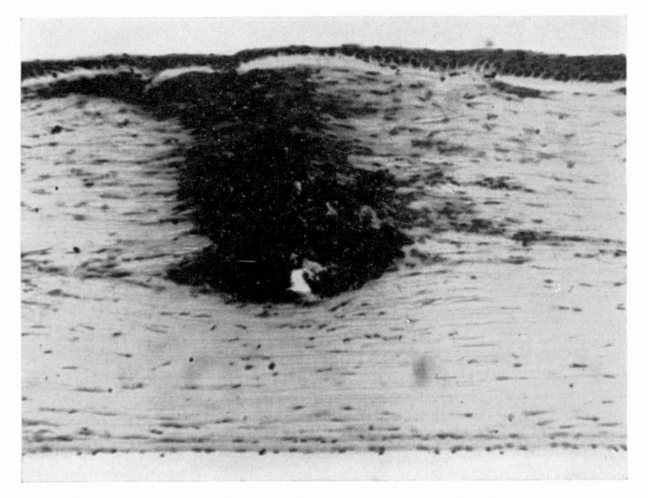

FIG. 406.—Fragments of a foreign body embedded in the corneal stroma. Note the breaks in Bowman's membrane and the dense inflammatory reaction. The eye was injured in an explosion in a steel works (H. & E.; × 132) (N. Ashton).

1899, after one year). Microscopic and chemical examinations of the deposit in excised pieces of tissue were first reported by Bunge (1890). These deposits may give rise to considerable irritation and lead to the formation of some opacity; but, although their removal is advisable, their retention leads to no catastrophic results (Plate XV, Figs. 2 and 3; Fig. 406).

In the *conjunctiva and sclera* a similar breakdown of a particle of iron may occur with a local area of rusty coloration which, if the foreign body lies near the limbus, may spread into the cornea (Dodd, 1901). This condition of SIDEROSIS CONJUNCTIVÆ has long been known and was first described by Reich (1881) in a soldier who suffered from a self-inflicted injury with iron sulphate. The condition is well seen with the slit-lamp, when tiny particles with a metallic lustre can be observed in the conjunctiva

[1] p. 529.

Figs. 407 to 409.—Direct Siderosis of the Conjunctiva (J. F. Chisholm).

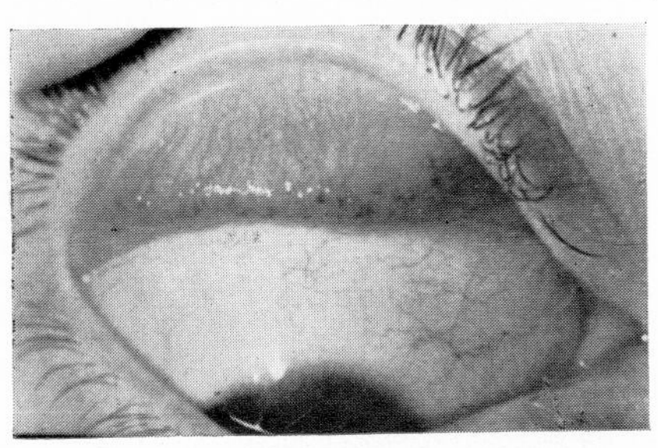

Fig. 407.—Resulting from constant exposure to dust rich in iron oxide. There is a hypertrophic folliculosis of the tarsal conjunctiva of the upper lid which is seen everted; numerous pigmented spots are visible particularly on the medial aspect.

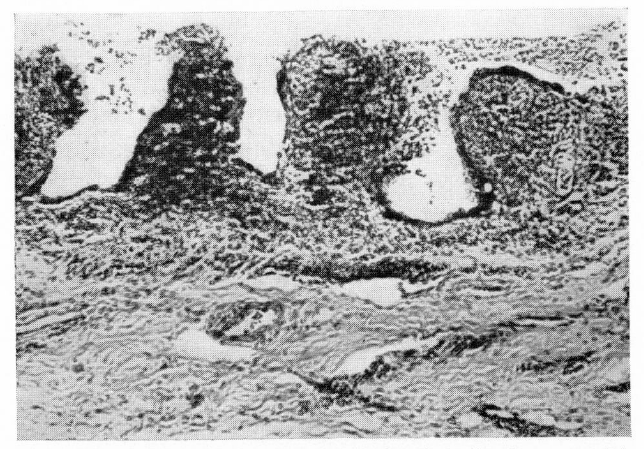

Fig. 408.—The same case as Fig. 407 showing the hypertrophic follicular concentration on the palpebral conjunctiva (H. and E.).

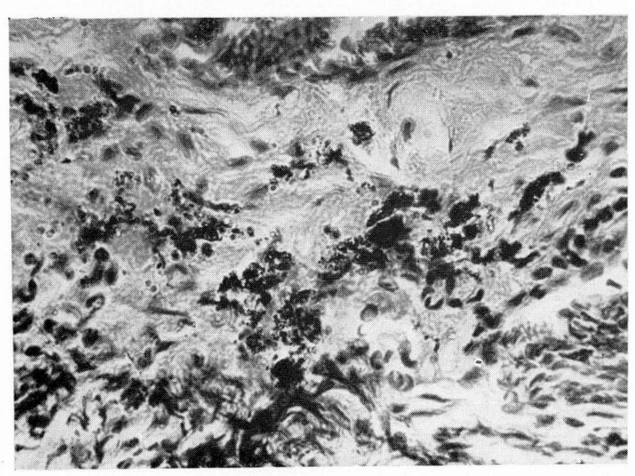

Fig. 409.—Showing the amorphous deposits of iron in the subfollicular stroma stained Prussian blue in Perls's reaction.

and sclera, while around them is a diffuse deposition of rust-brown spots (Koeppe, 1918).

Chisholm (1950) reported an unusual case which showed siderosis of the conjunctiva after prolonged exposure to the volcanic dust of the Philippine Islands, which is rich in iron oxide. A follicular hypertrophy developed in the tarsal conjunctiva with a fine dusting of pigment granules (Fig. 407). Histological examination showed a chronic inflammation with deposits of brown amorphous pigment granules, especially in the subfollicular stroma, which gave a positive response to Perls's reaction for iron[1] (Figs. 408 and 409).

The injuries caused by foreign bodies impregnated with irritative chemicals (such as the aniline dyes in indelible pencils) are more appropriately discussed in the section on chemical injuries.[2]

ORGANIZED MATERIAL, if allowed to remain, usually causes considerable irritation. *Vegetable matter* such as a piece of chaff or a grain of corn in the upper fornix, for example, may eventually excite an irritative inflammatory reaction associated with much œdema and discharge, and characterized by the formation of granulation tissue containing numerous giant cells which may proliferate eventually to form great cockscomb masses simulating the picture of a tuberculous lesion; when such a granuloma springs from the relatively inaccessible recesses of the upper fornix, covering and obscuring the foreign body and exciting an œdematous reaction which makes eversion of the lid a matter of extreme difficulty, it is easy to understand that the diagnosis may be missed. Grains of barley or oats may excite a proliferation of this nature (de Lantsheere, 1899; Terson, 1909), while a piece of barley straw retained in the upper fornix has given rise to a reaction so violent that it eventually ulcerated into the orbital tissue to become embedded in the lacrimal gland (Colley, 1930). The formation of a pseudo-epitarsus has been reported as the end-result of the long retention of a piece of straw in this region (Fronimopoulos and Vlachos, 1950). The introduction of flax-seeds into the eye, an old-fashioned therapeutic measure, may give rise to a considerable inflammatory reaction (Humphrey, 1970). Other vegetable material, such as wood, may produce a less severe reaction (Zander and Geissler, 1864; Roure, 1900; and others); the retention of a splinter in the upper fornix for 8 months has been reported as giving rise to a proliferative granular conjunctivitis affecting the entire upper lid and a haziness of the upper part of the cornea (Croskey, 1898). As we have already noted, a similar ulcerative reaction may occur in the cornea, while if vegetable matter is driven into its substance the reactive proliferation may be marked (Figs. 410 and 411).

This reaction to organized material is by no means invariable. Thus the half-section of a twig of an elder bush (9 × 5 × 1 mm.) has been retained deeply hidden in the upper conjunctival fornix for 4½ years, exciting only occasional attacks of irritation

[1] p. 533. [2] Chap. XI.

FIGS. 410 and 411.—VEGETABLE MATTER IN THE CORNEA.

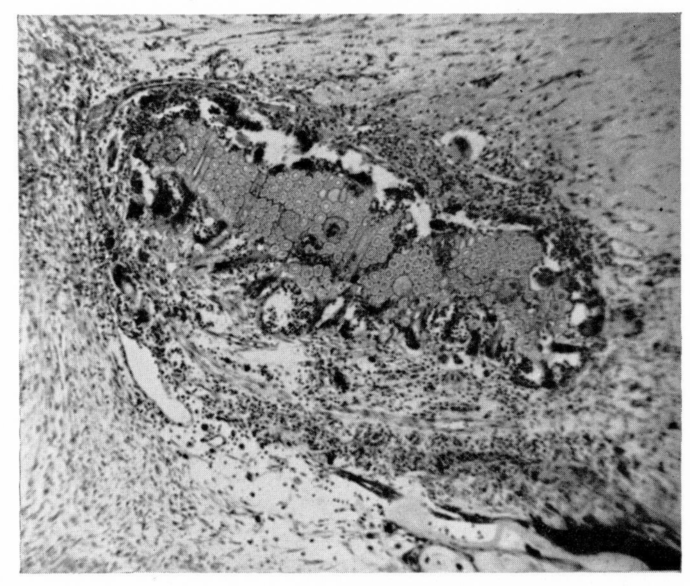

FIG. 410.

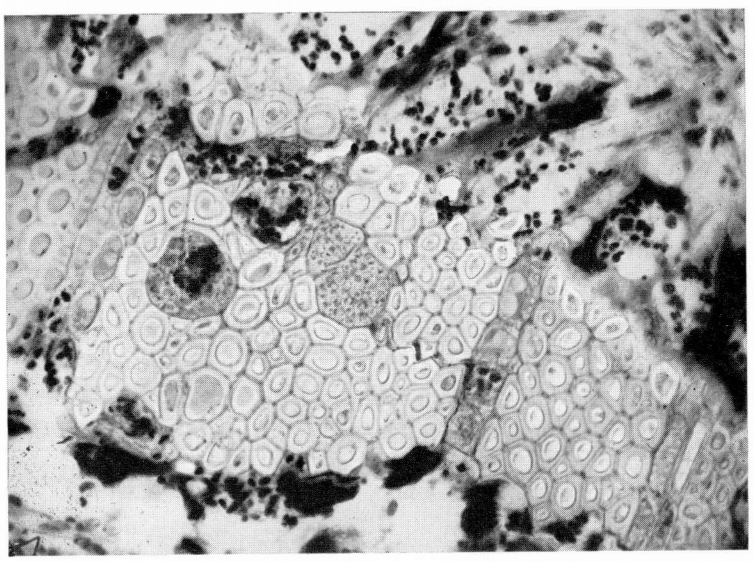

FIG. 411.

Perforating injury of the cornea with a twig. Embedded in granulation tissue in the inner aspect of the wound there is a piece of vegetable matter surrounded by phagocytic giant cells (Fig. 410, × 106; Fig. 411, × 390) (N. Ashton).

and infection which were interpreted as a mild conjunctivitis and each time cleared up under local treatment (Elkington, 1949).

The proliferative reaction which results if *talc powder* used to dust surgical gloves, or pieces of *lint* or *cotton*—often of microscopic size—are buried underneath the conjunctiva, will be discussed at a later stage.[1] Such a reaction may be long delayed: thus a granuloma arising from the irritation of talc has been reported to occur 14 years after muscle surgery (McCormick *et al.*, 1949).

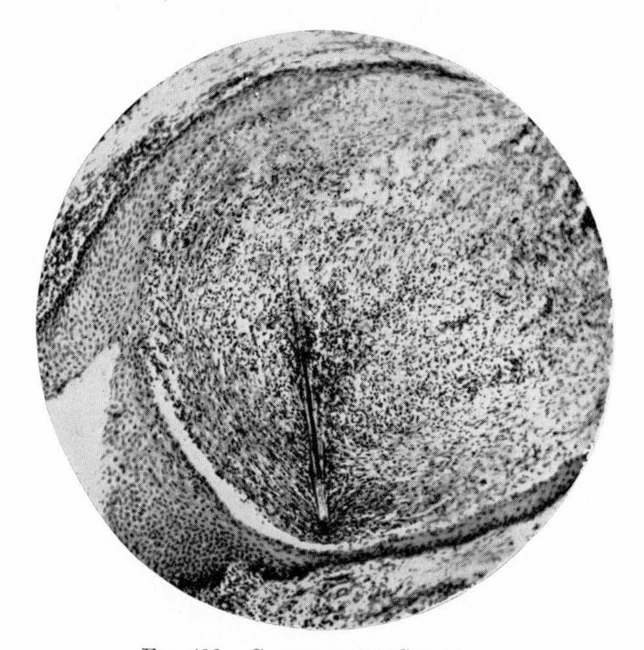

FIG. 412.—CILIUM IN THE CORNEA.

Perforating corneal wound showing ingrowth of epithelium and a mass of granulation tissue in which an eyelash is embedded (H. & E.) (N. Ashton).

Animal tissues frequently tend to excite a somewhat similar reaction. An eyelash driven into the cornea may give rise to a granulomatous reaction of the same type (Fig. 412), a proliferation which may also appear in the conjunctiva (Smith, 1936); a similar reaction has been reported as the result of the bristles of brushes working themselves into this membrane (Barrie, 1933). The entry into the eye of such substances as pieces of oyster shell or minute animals—insects, leeches and others—may cause severe irritative symptoms, often aggravated by the poisonous effects of their body juices, stings or bites.[2]

A peculiar nodular reaction which may entail a serious and incapacitating iridocyclitis and a violent keratitis may follow the entry into the eye of the hairs of cater-

[1] pp. 505, 545. [2] Chap. XI.

pillars, grasshoppers and certain plants; the clinical picture of OPHTHALMIA NODOSA thus caused which, although partly due to mechanical injury, is largely the result of chemical irritation, will be discussed in the section on chemical injuries.[1]

Aguirre. *Pren. méd.* (La Paz), **3**, 67 (1943).
Barrie. *Glasg. med. J.*, **119**, 33 (1933).
Bellouard. *Arch. Ophtal.*, **2**, 1 (1882).
Böhm. *Klin. Mbl. Augenheilk.*, **57**, 82 (1916).
Bowen. *Arch. Augenheilk.*, **17**, 406 (1887).
Brenske. *Ber. dtsch. ophthal. Ges.*, **40**, 129 (1916).
Bunge. *X int. Cong. Med.*, Berlin, **4** (10), 151 (1890).
Chisholm. *Amer. J. Ophthal.*, **33**, 1108 (1950).
Clark. *New Jersey med. Rep.*, **5**, 303 (1851).
Colley. *Brit. med. J.*, **2**, 600 (1930).
Croskey. *Ophthal. Rec.*, **7**, 33 (1898).
Cunningham. *Trans. ophthal. Soc. U.K.*, **36**, 147 (1916).
Dodd. *Ophthal. Rec.*, **10**, 256 (1901).
Elkington. *Trans. Canad. ophthal. Soc.*, **12**, 100 (1949).
Fleischanderl. *Klin. Mbl. Augenheilk.*, **104**, 423 (1940).
Fronimopoulos and Vlachos. *Bull. Greek ophthal. Soc.*, **18**, 449 (1950).
Handmann. *Z. Augenheilk.*, **34**, 81 (1915).
Hornstein. *Verletzungen d. Auges durch Kupfer- u. Messingsplitter* (Diss.), Tübingen (1905).
Humphrey. *Amer. J. Ophthal.*, **70**, 287 (1970).
Kamel. *Bull. ophthal. Soc. Egypt*, **42**, 285 (1949).
King. *Proc. roy. Soc. Med.*, **41**, 267 (1948).
Kleczkowski. *Postep Okul.*, Nos. 7 and 8 (1913). See *Jber. ges. Ophthal.*, **44**, 705 (1913).
Knüsel. *v. Graefes Arch. Ophthal.*, **113**, 282 (1924).
Koeppe. *v. Graefes Arch. Ophthal.*, **97**, 1, 27 (1918).
de Lantsheere. *Presse méd. belge.*, **51**, 61 (1899).
McCormick, Macaulay and Miller. *Amer. J. Ophthal.*, **32**, 1252 (1949).
McDannald. *Arch. Ophthal.*, **16**, 462 (1936).
Mann. *Trans. ophthal. Soc. U.K.*, **61**, 58 (1941.)
Mayou. *Trans. ophthal. Soc. U.K.*, **45**, 274 (1925).
Michtner. *Wien. klin. Wschr.*, **60**, 538 (1948).
Oguchi. *Beitr. Augenheilk.*, **9** (83), 75 (1913).
Pichler. *Z. Augenheilk.*, **39**, 37 (1918).
Praun. *Die Verletzungen des Auges*, Wiesbaden (1899).
Rademacher. *Ueber einige seltene Fremdkörperverletzungen im vorderen Augenabschnitt* (Diss.), Jena (1909).
Rampoldi. *Ann. Ottal.*, **20**, 538 (1891).
Reich. *Zbl. prakt. Augenheilk.*, **5**, 133 (1881).
Roure. *Recueil Ophtal.*, **22**, 286 (1900).
Rust. *Arch. Ophthal.*, **37**, 174 (1908).
Santos Fernandez. *Arch. Oftal. hisp.-amer.*, **6**, 549 (1906).
Schiele. *Wschr. Therap. Hyg. Auges*, **7**, 265 (1904).
Sédan and Sédan-Bauby. *Bull. Soc. Ophtal. Fr.*, 852 (1950).
Smith. *Brit. J. Ophthal.*, **20**, 455 (1936).
Terson. *Klin. Mbl. Augenheilk.*, **47** (2), 347 (1909).
Thompson. *Brit. med. J.*, **1**, 368 (1898).
Uhthoff. *Berl. klin. Wschr.*, **53**, 5 (1916).
Unsworth. *Arch. Ophthal.*, **32**, 414 (1944).
Urbanek. *Z. Augenheilk.*, **62**, 174 (1927).
Vogt. *v. Graefes Arch. Ophthal.*, **106**, 80 (1921).
Lhb. u. Atlas d. Spaltlampenmikroskopie d. lebenden Auges, 2nd ed., Berlin, **1**, 255 (1930).
Weigelin. *Klin. Mbl. Augenheilk.*, **59**, 84 (1917).
Winkler. *Z. Augenheilk.*, **41**, 60 (1919).
Zander and Geissler. *Die Verletzungen des Auges*, Leipzig (1864).
Zuckerman and Lieberman. *Arch. Ophthal.*, **63**, 254 (1960).

COMPLICATIONS OF EXTRA-OCULAR FOREIGN BODIES

Apart from the results of the specific irritations just described, the important complications of extra-ocular foreign bodies are the introduction of infection at the time of the injury and, at a later date, the formation of corneal opacities and traumatic implantation cysts.

INFECTION

Wherever the corneal epithelium is abraded, and much more so if the substantia propria is involved, infection is always a possibility; even a minute break in the continuity of the surface cells may lead to the development of an ulcer which may incapacitate the patient for a long period,

[1] Chap. XI.

resulting, at the best, in a scar which permanently affects vision and, at the worst, if the infection is of a fulminating character, in panophthalmitis and loss of the eye, sometimes with dramatic rapidity. It will be remembered that foreign bodies are the commonest cause of infective corneal ulcers, the majority of which start in those minute abrasions due to dust or particles so small that the symptoms to which they give rise are transitory and virtually unnoticed; indeed, it is frequently only at the stage of ulceration that the patient's attention is drawn for the first time to the accident that has befallen him. It is to be remembered that organisms even of the virulence of the pneumococcus are unable to penetrate the intact epithelium but can readily do so if the superficial layer of cells has been desquamated. If this occurs, an infection of any degree of severity may develop varying from a superficial ulcer to a corneal abscess or a hypopyon iridocyclitis.

The infection in such cases may be due to three causes. In the first place, it may be introduced by the foreign body itself. It is true that many foreign bodies, particularly those of metal which are detached by hammering or other forces and travel with a high velocity, are sterilized by the heat which is thus generated; others, however, such as chips of stone or coal, particles of dust or pieces of vegetable matter, are frequently contaminated by micro-organisms or fungi. For this reason severe infection due to a foreign body resulting, for example, in a hypopyon ulcer is more common in agricultural, mining and quarrying communities than it is in the engineering or other industrial trades. The second source of infection is the use of dirty instruments to remove the foreign body, a commonplace not only in the factory or the field but also, unfortunately, in the surgery of the irresponsible medical man. The final source, and perhaps the most common, is the conjunctival sac which, it will be remembered, is rarely sterile and may contain germs of considerable potential virulence. Fortunately if proper care is taken prophylactically, most of the ill-effects of such infection can be successfully controlled by scrupulous surgical care at the time of the removal of the foreign body and adequate treatment immediately thereafter, provided the patient seeks skilled advice at a sufficiently early date after his accident.

The prognosis of corneal foreign bodies in this respect was completely revolutionized by the introduction of the anti-bacterial drugs. Among coal or shale miners, for example, the incidence of severe hypopyon ulcers used to assume the proportions of a medical and economic tragedy. Thus in Scotland, Paterson (1931) found that among 223 cases of traumatic infected corneal ulcers, 182 required hospitalization for an average duration of 30 days; in 10% of the cases the eye was lost; in over 50% vision was less than 6/60; and in only 20% was useful vision (6/12) retained. Following the introduction of sodium sulphacetamide (used as a 30% solution or in powder form) Cameron (1949) found that during the previous seven years, among the same mining population, no eye was lost from a similar accident, while in only 20% of cases was vision reduced to 6/60. The more recent and more effective antibiotics have fully consolidated this transformation (Scott, 1954; Ainslie, 1965).

It is noteworthy that an attack of zoster has followed the removal of a foreign body from the cornea (Klauder, 1947; Giroire *et al.*, 1960; Sédan and Farnarier, 1963).

Conjunctival infection owing to the presence of a foreign body in this tissue is much less common, but not only may pyogenic infection occasionally occur, particularly if the foreign body becomes embedded or penetrates the deeper tissues (Colley, 1930), but as an exceptional event specific infections such as glanders (Nicolle and Dubos, 1902) may be introduced thereby.

CORNEAL OPACIFICATION

It is, of course, obvious that whenever Bowman's membrane is perforated by a foreign body a permanent opacity must remain,[1] varying in extent with the immediate trauma caused, the amount of manipulation employed in its removal and the subsequent incidence of infection. The resultant scar is usually small and incidental as far as the visual function is concerned if it is not central, but occasionally, particularly when infection has become established, an extensive leucoma may result which may not only cause permanent visual loss but may eventually give rise to persistent trouble if degenerative changes take place. Long after an injury which may at the time have appeared to be trivial, degenerative changes occasionally result in the clinical picture of *white rings in the cornea.*[2]

IMPLANTATION CYSTS

We have seen that the formation of an implantation cyst is not an uncommon sequel to a conjunctival wound. If such a wound is complicated by the presence of a foreign body (such as a piece of wood, Mayou, 1905,

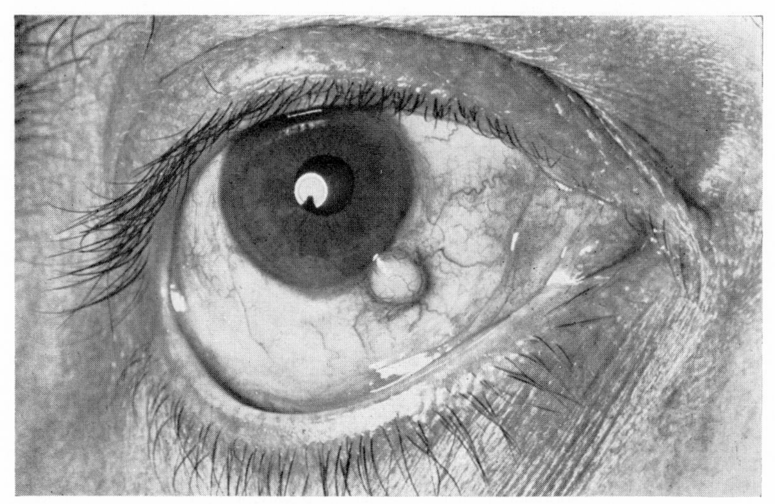

FIG. 413.—TRAUMATIC IMPLANTATION CYST.

Implantation cyst of the conjunctiva, associated with a foreign body retained for 15 years near the limbus (Inst. Ophthal.).

[1] Vol. VIII, p. 632. [2] Vol. VIII, p. 883.

or cotton-wool, Passera, 1910) a cyst is more likely to arise (Fig. 413), and it is particularly prone to occur in the event of an eyelash being incarcerated in the scar (Uhthoff, 1879; Baudry, 1882; Nuyts, 1896; and others). The pathology, symptomatology and treatment of the cysts thus formed are the same as have been described in connection with similar cysts uncomplicated by the presence of foreign bodies.

Diagnosis of Extra-ocular Foreign Bodies

The diagnosis of an extra-ocular foreign body is usually easy but may be fraught with considerable difficulties, particularly if the particle itself is minute in size or if the patient is in such distress that the associated photophobia and blepharospasm make the requisite manipulations of his eye difficult or impossible. Since a thorough scrutiny is always necessary in such cases, it is well in this latter event to instil an analgesic before any attempt is made at investigation, a course which is frequently essential in dealing with children. In all cases it must be remembered that the discovery of one foreign body does not eliminate the presence of others, so that not only the cornea and bulbar conjunctiva but also the lids and fornices should be scrutinized. In such an examination the essential requirements are good focal illumination and adequate magnification by an ophthalmic loupe or, if necessary, the slit-lamp.

In such cases a routine should be adopted of examining first the lower fornix by pulling down the lower lid, then the surface of the cornea and the bulbar conjunctiva, where a small leash of blood vessels may indicate the position of the foreign body if it is on the cornea near the limbus; the upper lid should then be everted and its under surface examined, particularly the favourite site of lodgment in the subtarsal fold and, if necessary, the recesses of the upper fornix should be explored after double eversion of the lid. Nor should the region of the inner canthus and the recess beneath the plica be neglected, while it must be remembered that a foreign body, particularly a bristle or an eyelash, may protrude from the lacrimal punctum and cause symptoms by excoriating the eye.

If the foreign body is not immediately obvious in this general examination, it is well to stain the cornea with a solution of fluorescein; not only does this dye frequently demonstrate the presence of a minute particle sharply contrasted on a background of brilliant green, but it also reveals an abrasion made by a corneal foreign body which has disappeared spontaneously or as a result of the patient's efforts, or the excoriations on the corneal surface made by a particle which may have disappeared from beneath the upper lid, for these epithelial injuries give rise to the same symptoms as if the foreign body itself were still present.

If no diagnostic clues become evident at this preliminary examination, resort should be had to the slit-lamp, an instrument which is essential for the discovery and accurate localization of minute and colourless foreign bodies lying deeply in the corneal stroma. It is only thus, for example, that small spicules of glass may be recognized; these are not seen by the naked eye and usually not by a magnifying loupe, but are rendered evident with the slit-lamp using oscillatory illumination by the play of glinting light reflexes and shadows in the change from direct to trans-illumination.

The localization of a foreign body in the corneal substance can usually be accurately accomplished with the use of this instrument, for if the particle is examined in the side of the beam nearer the observer, its distance from the anterior band of the cornea indicates its relative depth; it is to be remembered that, as it is thus seen, its apparent depth is about two-thirds of the real depth (Fig. 414). At the same time this examination will reveal the amount of damage done to the tissues of the cornea—folds in Bowman's membrane, wrinkles in Descemet's membrane which appear if the foreign body has remained for some time, and the earliest traces of infiltration in the corneal stroma which may indicate the onset of complications. In this connection, also, the absence of interruptions in the continuity of the endothelial mosaic establishes without doubt that a recent perforation has not taken place.

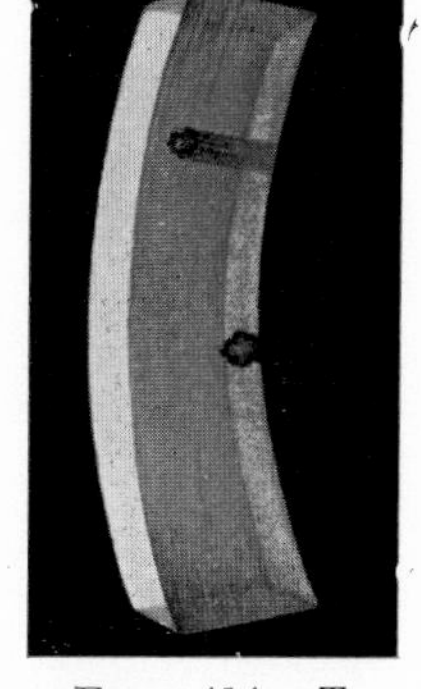

FIG. 414.—THE LOCALIZATION OF DEPTH IN THE CORNEA.

In the beam of the slit-lamp an object in the substance of the cornea projects a shadow, while one on the posterior surface is seen in the posterior band.

The Treatment of Extra-ocular Foreign Bodies

Although the lodgment of a foreign body upon the eye would appear to be an event of no great dignity, it is a condition often requiring a considerable degree of skill in treatment if the particle is to be removed without visual damage and without running a risk of complications which may be of grave importance.

In all cases the lighting must be good, the visual magnification of the operator sufficient and the control of the patient adequate; the maintenance of immobility of the eye usually requires a local analgesic and may be considerably aided if the patient is lying down or the head is supported against the back of a chair or the wall or by an assistant, while the patient himself fixates a light or other object in the direction affording the best view of the particle. The assistant may hold the patient's lids apart or alternatively a speculum may be used. The slit-lamp is an ideal adjunct, particularly in the removal of deep foreign bodies, in which case the patient's chin and forehead should be firmly pressed on the appropriate supports while the surgeon ensures steadiness and delicacy of touch by resting his elbow on the table or on a box thereon, and his little finger on the patient's cheek. The immobility of the eye is greatly aided by attaching a spotlight as a fixation point to the slit-lamp. The surgeon, looking through the microscope, then locates the instrument with which he is to do the extraction and moves it towards the foreign body, which is then removed. In all cases, every instrument touching the eye should be sterilized.

These ideal conditions, of course, are not available in the usual industrial workshop or in rural surroundings. In these it is certainly well to dispense with the peculiar but handy implements such as pins, knife-blades and nails which are commonly used by those who attempt to do first-aid, and confine the efforts of the uninitiated only to those superficial foreign bodies which can be removed with the aid of cotton wool twisted on a stick or, perhaps preferably, by irrigation, if necessary under pressure with a syringe. This limitation probably wisely includes even the general practitioner who is unskilled in this type of work and whose vision and manual dexterity may be inadequate and may lead to the infliction of greater trauma than would arise if the foreign body were left alone until adequate help is available.

The old and most unhygienic habit of removing foreign bodies from under the lid with the tongue occasionally survives; it is interesting that thereby syphilis has been communicated and a primary conjunctival chancre has resulted.[1]

Superficial Foreign Bodies

The removal of these from the corneal or conjunctival surface is simple and can frequently be accomplished without an analgesic, but if there is any fear that the patient will be unable to hold his eye steady during

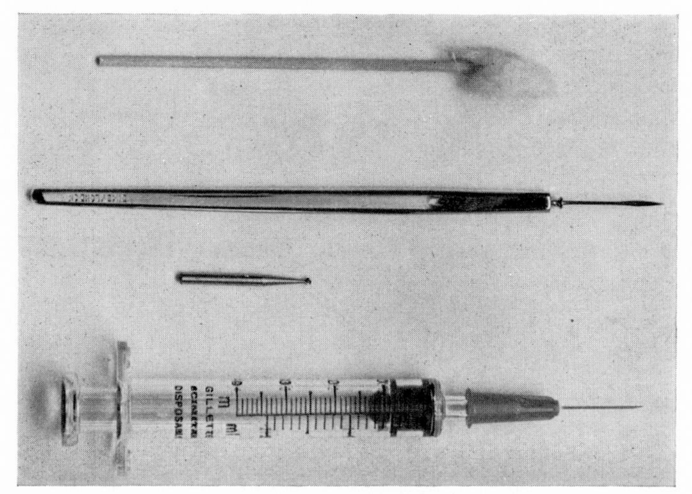

FIG. 415. A SELECTION OF INSTRUMENTS FOR THE REMOVAL OF SUPERFICIAL FOREIGN BODIES.

A cotton-wool pledget, a corneal needle, a dental burr a disposable syringe and sharp needle.

the manipulations, particularly when the cornea is implicated, one of the substitutes of cocaine should be instilled. A superficial foreign body is usually readily removed by a moist sterile cotton-tipped applicator (Fig. 415), extreme care being taken to touch as little other than the foreign body as possible so that the corneal surface is not damaged. Thereafter the cornea should be stained with fluorescein to reveal any small abrasion. If this is not present the eye need only be padded for such time as the analgesic requires to wear off; but if a corneal abrasion is present, it is as well to take

[1] de Beck (1886), Tepljaschin (1887), Bourgeois (1894), Alexander (1895), Ernrot (1898), Dagilaiski (1898), Janpolski (1901), and others.

the precaution of instilling a lubricant and an antibiotic (such as chloramphenicol ointment) and applying a pad and bandage for 24 hours so that epithelialization may be prompt, firm and lasting.

Embedded Foreign Bodies

Foreign bodies buried in the epithelium are usually relatively easily removed with the ordinary stainless steel hypodermic needle supported on the syringe (Fig. 415) (Harding, 1943; Fox, 1963). In all such cases surgical cleanliness is essential, the whole of the particle should be removed and at the end of the operation its site should be clean-cut so that no ragged edges remain; the greatest enticement for infection is a frayed-out area of injury, and a clean cut, even although larger than a ragged injury, will heal up more quickly and usually much more satisfactorily. The same principle applies to the treatment of the site of a foreign body which has already sloughed off; the injured area should be stained with fluorescein and all the diseased tissue cleanly removed.

If the foreign body lies at an appreciable depth in the cornea a sharp, knife-edged needle is the ideal instrument for its extraction. In the manipulations the corneal tissue should be touched only to the minimum degree that is necessary and care taken to insert the point only to the depth that is required, making as clean a wound as possible; when the particle is reached the blade of the needle is then used to cut directly forward; this exposes the foreign body so that it may be removed with the point of the needle or with a spud. In all cases the excision should be purposeful and clean, for repeated attempts at "picking" at the foreign body result in mutilation of the corneal stroma, open up potential avenues for infection and lead to a more pronounced residual opacity.

Many instruments have been devised for this purpose; they are generally sharp needles, somewhat broad at the end and provided with a cutting edge (Fig. 415), but alternatives are constantly appearing[1]; a canaliculus knife or a discission knife serves well (Gundersen, 1947), while a sewing needle sterilized in a flame will suffice in an emergency. A useful forceps with the serrations pointing backwards for grasping a foreign body so that it does not easily slip was devised by Thorpe (1944–45). Finally, the erisophake has been employed to extract a deeply placed foreign body by suction, aided if necessary by a dissection through the corneal stroma down to the particle (Jones and Goldman, 1952).

The *rust ring* left by an iron foreign body merits special consideration; there is little doubt that if it is completely and cleanly removed, healing is more rapid and the resultant irritation and scar less than if it is left *in situ*; on the other hand, there is no doubt that if excessive trauma has to be employed in its removal, the rust ring is best left alone. In all cases the process of debridement must be undertaken with extreme care, limiting the

[1] Dessauer (1889), Levinsohn (1899), Haas (1902), Todd (1906), Haase (1912), Pelner (1942), Harding (1943), Huwaert (1948), Howard (1950), Loos (1952), and a host of others.

curettage to the affected area itself, a precaution which applies particularly to the central area of the cornea where the manipulation should be done with delicate precision and the least possible trauma. If complete removal of the stain is difficult, it is well to leave it for 24 or even 48 hours when further removal is usually much more easy in the softened tissues; but if it appears that trauma is to be in any way excessive the rust ring should be left, for over-zealous manipulation may well result in greater embarrassment to vision than if the ring were left alone.

Several expedients have been adopted for this purpose in cases wherein the ring cannot be readily removed by a spud or curette. Complete excision of the ring by dissection with a Graefe knife under the magnification afforded by the corneal microscope was advocated by Kadin (1950); a small corneal burr (0·5 mm. in diameter) or dental drill manipulated by hand has been widely employed (Arruga, 1946; Colenbrander, 1947; Callahan, 1950; Worst, 1961), while special instruments, such as the brush-like arrangement of fine needles used by Howard (1950), have been described.

Chemical methods for the removal of a corneal rust ring have been tried by several investigators. Desferrioxamine is an iron-free compound isolated from a strain of *Streptomyces pilosus* which binds ferric ions to form an octahedral complex—ferrioxamine; theoretically 100 parts by weight of desferrioxamine can bind 8·5 parts of ferric ion. This has been used with some success in the removal of experimental corneal rust rings in rabbits by Galin and his colleagues (1965) and in traumatic corneal rust rings in man by Valvo (1967). On the other hand, Wise (1966) found that this substance was of no value in the treatment of experimental siderosis bulbi, vitreous hæmorrhages and corneal blood-staining, while McGuinness and Knight-Jones (1968) concluded that treatment with 5% desferrioxamine ointment was less effective than surgical removal of the rust ring.

Deeply embedded foreign bodies provide a more difficult problem and their removal should be undertaken in the operating theatre as a major surgical procedure since complications are to be anticipated; clumsy or over-zealous efforts at removal may result in pushing the particle further in, an inadequately controlled instrument may perforate the cornea, while the danger of pushing the particle into the anterior chamber is considerable, in which case the seriousness of the condition is augmented (Summers and Hobbs, 1942; Thorpe, 1965; Stallard, 1965; and others).[1] If the foreign body is in the periphery of the cornea the easiest method of approach is to evert this tissue after a large limbal section as for a cataract extraction and remove the particle from the under side. If the foreign body is centrally placed, the classical method of approach is to transfix the lamellæ with a broad needle until the blade is behind the particle when an extraction needle may be used to cut it out in the usual way. Should the foreign body have penetrated so deeply that this appears impossible, a broad needle or a keratome may be passed into the anterior chamber so that the blade lies as a support beneath the foreign body, the point, if necessary, finding anchorage by entering the inner surface of the cornea (Desmarres, 1855; Lawson, 1867). Alternatively, after a keratome incision has been made, a

[1] p. 487.

spatula designed to fit the back of the cornea can be introduced into the anterior chamber for the same purpose (von Arlt, 1875); the spatula can be inserted and withdrawn without collapse of the chamber (with luck!). On the other hand, Rinaldi (1950) introduced a Daviel spoon into the anterior chamber and thrust the foreign body through the cornea with a needle so that it fell into the spoon. The alternative method of approach is to cut a triangular flap in the cornea to the requisite depth by two bevelled incisions meeting at an apex pointing towards the centre of the cornea and containing the foreign body between them; this flap is folded back on its base exposing the foreign body which can be freed and removed by the point of the knife (Fox, 1947); Vasserman (1948) achieved the same object by cutting a trephine disc to the requisite depth into the cornea, leaving a connecting bridge so that it could be raised up with a knife and reposed when the foreign body had been removed.

If the foreign body is magnetic the use of the electro-magnet[1] by itself in these cases is frequently not very effective, since it is usually unable to draw a particle through the dense corneal tissue; moreover, the particle is often so small that sufficient lines of force do not traverse it to make it respond. The magnet, however, may be of value in the final extraction of a foreign body if a clean cut is made through the corneal tissue onto it, as was originally done in 1624 by the surgeon Fabricius Hildanus (Fabry) and his wife Marie Colinet in Berne by means of a lodestone. A similar feat was recorded by Dawbigney Turberville of Salisbury in 1684; having failed to remove a foreign body embedded at the limbus with a spatula he applied a lodestone whereupon " it immediately jumped out ".[2]

Foreign bodies which have penetrated the cornea and project into the anterior chamber provide a special problem, for in addition to the danger of pushing in the particle still further so that it falls into the anterior chamber, its point may injure the capsule of the lens. It is sometimes possible, after making a corneal incision near the limbus with a keratome, to introduce forceps or a broad needle into the anterior chamber and to press the foreign body from behind forwards so that it can be grasped by its anterior extremity and extracted (Thorpe, 1947). If the foreign body is long so that it runs through the whole thickness of the cornea (such as a thorn which frequently breaks off flush with the surface) two needles may be inserted into its opposite sides in the substance of the cornea and used to lever it out; successful cases have been reported of removal in this way even although the point of the thorn has scratched (but not penetrated) the anterior capsule of the lens (de Beck, 1900; Weber, 1949). An alternative method is to evert the cornea after a large limbal incision and pick the particle out directly.

A special lancet-cannula was devised by Neubauer (1963) to facilitate the removal of a foreign body penetrating into the anterior chamber; through the cannula saline is injected into the anterior chamber to prevent the foreign body from touching the lens

[1] p. 620.
[2] Letter to W. Musgrave, *Phil. Trans.*, **14,** 736 (1684).

capsule, while manoeuvres are carried out with the aim of dislodging the foreign body into the angle of the anterior chamber whence it may be removed with forceps via a small limbal incision.

After the removal of any foreign body which has penetrated the corneal tissue, even although the epithelium only has been involved, the eye should be closed with a pad and bandage or strapping; if the trauma has been considerable both eyes should be thus occluded; a period of 24 hours is sufficient to allow epithelialization unless the abraded area is large. Prior to bandaging it is well to instil a drop of a lubricant and an antibiotic preparation; the purpose of the two can well be combined by using an ointment of an appropriate antibiotic. Atropine need not be employed as a routine, but only if infiltration of the cornea has already developed or if the trauma has been considerable; its routine instillation in every case involves unnecessary inconvenience or economic loss. When it is employed it is wise to exclude undue narrowness of the angle of the anterior chamber in an eye wherein pupillary dilatation is likely to induce an attack of glaucoma.

Foreign Bodies embedded in the Conjunctiva and Sclera

These present a much less acute problem. Those embedded in the conjunctiva itself can often be picked off with a sharp needle; in the many cases wherein this is difficult, it is easy to snip off the portion of conjunctiva involved. If the particle is embedded in the subconjunctiva or superficially in the sclera, it is usually wise to leave it alone unless it is large and unsightly or liable to cause irritation, in which case it can be removed after incision. In this event if the particle is deeply embedded in the sclera, care must be exercised lest it be pushed into the eye; if it is magnetizable, the hand-magnet is usually a valuable aid in its withdrawal after a route of exit has been opened with a knife.

Ainslie. *Brit. J. Ophthal.*, **49,** 98 (1965).
Alexander. *Neue Erfahrungen ü. luetische Augen-Erkrankungen*, Wiesbaden (1895).
von Arlt. *Ueber d. Verletzungen d. Auges*, Wien (1875).
Arruga. *Cirurgía ocular*, Barcelona (1946).
Ocular Surgery, Barcelona (1956).
Baudry. *Bull. méd. Nord.*, **21,** 243 (1882).
de Beck. *Ophthal. Rev.*, **5,** 298 (1886).
Cincinnati-Lancet-Clin., **44,** 377 (1900).
Bourgeois. *Recueil Ophtal.*, **16,** 79 (1894).
Callahan. *J. Amer. med. Ass.*, **142,** 249 (1950).
Cameron. *Brit. J. Ophthal.*, **33,** 368 (1949).
Colenbrander. *Ophthalmologica*, **113,** 247 (1947).
Colley. *Brit. med. J.*, **2,** 600 (1930).
Dagilaiski. *Klin. Mbl. Augenheilk.*, **36,** 11 (1898).
Desmarres. *Traité des maladies des yeux*, Paris, **2,** 312 (1855).
Dessauer. *Klin. Mbl. Augenheilk.*, **27,** 25 (1889).
Ernrot. *Vestn. Oftal.*, **15,** 213 (1898).
Fox. *Arch. Ophthal.*, **37,** 189 (1947).
Amer. J. Ophthal., **55,** 611 (1963).
Galin, Harris and Papariello. *Arch. Ophthal.*, **74,** 674 (1965).
Giroire, Charbonnel and Vercelletto. *Rev. Oto-neuro-ophtal.*, **32,** 38 (1960).
Gundersen. *Trans. Amer. Acad. Ophthal.*, **51,** 604 (1947).
Haas. *Wschr. Therap. Hyg. Auges*, **6,** 89 (1902).
Haase. *Klin. Mbl. Augenheilk.*, **50** (1), 569 (1912).
Harding. *Arch. Ophthal.*, **29,** 134 (1943).
Howard. *Arch. Ophthal.*, **43,** 92 (1950).
Huwaert. *Bull. Soc. belge Ophtal.*, No. 89, 436 (1948).
Janpolski. *Wratsch. Gaz.*, **8,** 828 (1901).
Jones and Goldman. *Arch. Ophthal.*, **48,** 48 (1952).
Kadin. *Trans. Amer. Acad. Ophthal.*, **54,** 392 (1950).
Klauder. *J. Amer. med. Ass.*, **134,** 245 (1947).

Lawson. *Roy. Lond. ophthal. Hosp. Rep.*, **6,** 36 (1867).
Levinsohn. *Berl. klin. Wschr.*, **36,** 813 (1899).
Loos. *Ned. T. Geneesk.*, **96,** 1653 (1952).
Mayou. *Roy. Lond. ophthal. Hosp. Rep.*, **16,** 318 (1905).
McGuinness and Knight-Jones. *Brit. J. Ophthal.*, **52,** 777 (1968).
Neubauer. *Trans. ophthal. Soc. U.K.*, **83,** 143 (1963).
Nicolle and Dubos. *Presse méd.*, **2,** 477 (1902).
Nuyts. *Recueil Ophtal.*, **18,** 276 (1896).
Passera. *Cisti di congiuntiva*, Gaddi-Novara (1910).
Paterson. *Trans. ophthal. Soc. U.K.*, **51,** 341, 354 (1931).
Pelner. *Amer. J. Ophthal.*, **25,** 456 (1942).
Rinaldi. *Atti Soc. Oftal. ital.*, **12,** 16 (1950).
Scott. *Trans. ophthal Soc. U.K.*, **74,** 105 (1954).
Sédan and Farnarier. *Bull. Soc. Ophtal. Fr.*, **63,** 563 (1963).
Stallard. *Eye Surgery*, 4th ed., Bristol (1965).
Summers and Hobbs. *Brit. J. Ophthal.*, **26,** 54 (1942).
Tepljaschin. *Wratsch.*, No. 17, 348 (1887).
Thorpe. *Arch. Ophthal.*, **32,** 497 (1944).
J. Amer. med. Ass., **127,** 197 (1945).
Surg. Gyn. Obstet., **84,** 809 (1947).
Complications in Eye Surgery (ed. Fasanella), Phila., 51 (1965).
Todd. *Ophthal. Rec.*, **15,** 208 (1906).
Uhthoff. *Berl. klin. Wschr.*, **16,** 729 (1879).
Valvo. *Amer. J. Ophthal.*, **63,** 98 (1967).
Vasserman. *Vestn. oftal.*, **27** (4), 45 (1948).
Weber. *Ophthalmologica*, **117,** 238 (1949).
Wise. *Arch. Ophthal.*, **75,** 698 (1966).
Worst. *Amer. J. Ophthal.*, **52,** 122 (1961).

INTRA-OCULAR FOREIGN BODIES

The retention of a foreign body within the eye is not a very common injury. Thus taking an overall percentage of approximately one million new ophthalmic cases seen in highly industrialized cities in England[1] Cridland (1933) found that the incidence of such an accident was about 1 in 1,000; the proportion of foreign bodies in all accident cases was 1 in 300; outside the centres of heavy metallurgical industry the frequency of these injuries is, of course, very much less. It is not easy to assess the general incidence of intra-ocular foreign bodies from national statistical records because injuries are not usually sub-divided in this way. Moreover, a study of reports from individual hospitals shows that the number of such injuries is related to the type of industrial process dominant in the locality served by that hospital.

Thus in the heavily industrialized city of Birmingham where motor car manufacture and other types of heavy engineering are particularly well represented, Roper-Hall (1954) found 555 cases between 1932 and 1951; at the same hospital between 1952 and 1966 there were 495 cases with a yearly average of 33 while in the quiet market town of Shrewsbury between 1958 and 1966 an average of only 5 cases of intra-ocular foreign body was seen each year (V. Smith, 1968). Of many individual series of cases the figures of the Munich Clinic are representative; thus amongst 1,028 cases of perforating wounds of the globe a retained intra-ocular foreign body was present in 403 (39·2%), two-thirds being in the posterior segment (Remky *et al.*, 1967).

Without any doubt, however, the lodgment of a foreign particle within the globe must often rank among ocular injuries as causing great anxiety; not only is there often much mechanical damage caused at the time of the accident but every complication of a perforating ocular injury may arise, while the immediate risk of infection—a common hazard—and the danger of the subsequent development of sympathetic ophthalmitis—a relatively rare

[1] Manchester, Wolverhampton, London.

hazard—are thereby increased. To these untoward effects must be added not only the irritative local reaction caused by most foreign bodies but also in the case of certain metals the possibility of the slow destruction of vision by chemical changes initiated within the eye. There is no doubt that innumerable foreign bodies have been left within the globe indefinitely without ill-effects, but it is equally true that many which were presumably inert have given rise to serious trouble; it is thus always wise to consider every such injury as potentially dangerous, for in every eye in which there is a retained foreign body, even although it is a particle of minute size, whether the eye is still of functional value or is blind and useless, there lurk dangers the assessment of which is difficult and often impossible.

The clinical effects of a foreign body are largely determined by the momentum with which it travels. A large foreign body, of course, travelling with sufficient velocity to enter the eye, usually disrupts the whole organ and the only course to adopt is enucleation; the typical example of this type of injury is that caused by a bullet or other missile met with in war wounds. Small foreign bodies, on the other hand, may leave the main structure of the globe relatively intact. If it is to traverse the corneo-scleral envelope such a foreign body must either be carried passively into the wound of a perforating injury or, alternatively, it must be travelling with sufficient velocity to pierce the tough envelope by its own momentum. By the first mechanism, organized substances such as vegetable matter or a cilium find entry into the globe; hard foreign bodies with sharp edges such as pieces of metal, stone or glass form the majority of the second class. If its velocity is sufficiently great, the particle may traverse the structures of the eye causing a double perforation and come to rest in the orbital tissues, but frequently the velocity is such that most of the available energy is expended in boring the wound of entrance through the outer coats of the eye and the particle is retained somewhere within the globe.

The relation between energy, mass and velocity is given by the equation $E = mv^2/2g$, where m is the weight in pounds, v the velocity in ft./sec., and g the acceleration of gravity (32 ft./sec.). It will thus be seen that velocity is more important than mass in endowing a foreign body with kinetic energy, for this is increased arithmetically with the latter but geometrically with the former; if the weight of a foreign body is doubled, the kinetic energy is also doubled, but if the velocity is doubled the kinetic energy is increased four times.

In addition to the kinetic energy of forward motion, a flying body may possess energy by virtue of rotatory motion around its own axes; such energy frequently adds considerably to its penetrative power. This energy depends primarily upon the rotatory inertia which is given by the formula $mr^2/2$, where m is the weight, and r the radius of the cross-section of the body. If this rotatory energy is represented by I, the extra energy imparted to the body by virtue of its rotation is computed from the formula $IW^2/2g$, where W is the angular velocity in radians per sec. ($2\pi \times$ number of rotations per sec.) and g the acceleration of gravity (32 ft./sec.).

One further method of entry of foreign bodies into the eye, fortunately rare, is of considerable interest—the inadvertent insertion of a foreign substance into the eye by the surgeon during an intra-ocular operation. A surprising number of things has been introduced into the eye in this way. The entrance of CILIA which have become detached or cut is rare. Ophthalmic OINTMENTS used as antiseptics immediately after an operation have found their way into the anterior chamber where they float like drops of oil; occasionally a mild temporary iritis ensues (Tietze, 1943), to avoid which the material has been evacuated (D. Binder, 1947), but more usually the ointment has disappeared without causing irritation (J. W. Smith, 1948; Sykowski, 1950; Olehla, 1954; Scheie *et al.*, 1965). Sykowski (1952) found that a water-soluble ointment (neobase) was completely absorbed from the anterior chamber of the rabbit, while a water-insoluble ointment (petrolatum) was not; in either case a small quantity was well tolerated, but a large amount excited a violent iritis. A piece of GLASS broken from an irrigator and retained in the anterior chamber was observed by J. W. Smith (1948) to give rise to a low-grade inflammation, while pieces of RUBBER, also from irrigators, were noted by Doherty (1928) and Brockhurst (1952) to lie embedded in the crypts of the iris without exciting a reaction for 11 years; SILK SUTURES are similarly inert (Plate XVIII, Figs. 2 and 5). TALC POWDER from surgical rubber gloves may enter the eye and give rise to a granulomatous reaction[1] (Chamlin, 1945; McCormick *et al.*, 1949; Duszynski, 1950). Finally—most common of all—COTTON FIBRES from swabs and sponges or the minute pieces of lint which float in the air in surprising quantities in the neighbourhood of the operating table may find their way into the eye (Duszynski, 1950); sometimes these have caused no irritation (Mukai, 1926, 3 cases), sometimes a corneal œdema (Brown, 1968) or a mild and transient congestion and hyperæmia (Purtscher, 1939; Vogt, 1942; Gürtler, 1949), and occasionally a moderately severe iritis (Vail, 1950).

On the whole, in contrast with the multiplicity of things which light upon the cornea or find their way into the conjunctival sac, the *types of intra-ocular foreign body* are fairly restricted. Of the organized materials which are carried passively into a perforating wound, the commonest are cilia or small pieces of vegetable matter; bits of twig or slivers of wood may enter the eye on their own momentum, the first usually when the face is swept by the branch of a tree and the eye is perforated by a sharp thorn which breaks off, and the second almost invariably by a piece of wood flying upwards when it is being chopped. A further type of organized foreign body is represented by sharp vegetable spines or the hairs of caterpillars which may work their way into the eye after being deposited on the cornea or in the conjunctival sac.[2]

More commonly, however, the foreign body is a flying particle, usually metallic in nature. Iron and steel come first in this respect and form the majority of the foreign bodies causing such injuries in the workshop or in war; in British industry they comprise approximately 90% of intra-ocular foreign bodies.[3] With the advancement of metallurgy, however, alloys are becoming more common than the pure metal; in order to increase tensile strength and hardness as well as resistance to corrosion, steel is frequently combined with such substances as tungsten, nickel, manganese, tantalum, molybdenum, chromium, cobalt or columbium. Copper, bronze and brass,

[1] p. 505. [2] Chap. XI.
[3] 85%, Whitehead (1916, in Manchester); 92%, Cridland (1916, in Wolverhampton); in New York Gulliver (1942) reported 98%.

the latter particularly from percussion caps, are also common, while lead frequently from shot pellets and less commonly zinc, may be encountered. Tungsten-wire from a burst incandescent lamp is a rarity (Sherman, 1939). In recent years foreign bodies composed of aluminium are met with more and more frequently, often combined with alloying elements such as copper, magnesium, manganese, nickel, silicon and zinc. Pieces of stone, rock or coal in industrial accidents, sand, clay or brick dust from explosions, as well as particles of powder and cordite are also occasionally found, while as a rarity such oddities as pieces of whiplash (Hutchinson, 1889; and others), a portion of a tobacco pipe (Smyly, 1876), a nutshell (Dodd, 1902), a piece of eggshell (Sachsalber, 1900), fibreglass (Gaines, 1958; Kavka, 1968, 13 cases) and in severe head-wounds pieces of bone and skin (Wilder, 1948) have found their way into the eye. Glass fragments are occasionally propelled into the eye as a result of a broken spectacle lens but increasingly this is the result of a shattered windscreen or a broken driving-mirror in traffic accidents (Draeger, 1966; Müller-Jensen and Allmaras, 1968; D. Archer *et al.*, 1969; and others).

There is no doubt that the use of the hand-hammer is the major cause of an intra-ocular foreign body[1]; at least 70% of cases arise in this way (Table XX) mostly among workers in the engineering industry but also in stone-masons, for whom it is a particular occupational hazard. It is noteworthy that even in the circumstances of war the most frequent single cause of an accidental intra-ocular foreign body has been found to be the use of a hammer and chisel (Stallard, 1944–47). Intra-ocular foreign bodies resulting from machining or the operation of power-driven tools are less common, while occasional injuries result in agricultural districts from splinters arising from the use of a plough or hoe striking stones or rocks in the ground (Frenkel, 1932; Villard, 1932). It should be remembered, however, that not all cases of intra-ocular foreign body result from occupational activities or are entirely confined to adult males of working age although, indeed, the majority is seen between the ages of 20 and 40; these injuries occasionally occur as a result of domestic or sporting activities and are not infrequently met with occurring in childhood (14% of perforating wounds in children, Remky *et al.*, 1967). It might be thought that the increasing use of non-metallic materials such as plastics would be expected to result in a rise in the proportion of intra-ocular foreign bodies of this type but this does not seem to be the case to judge from a study of the available figures, although it must be remembered that analysis of the information from different centres is complicated by the varying types of industrial process in each individual locality. Over the years the proportion of non-magnetic intra-ocular foreign bodies has varied between 5 and 15% of cases when industrial injuries are considered.[2] On

[1] Goulden (1908), Parsons (1916), Garrow (1923), Allport (1925), Cridland (1933), Gulliver (1942), McBride (1949), Minton (1949), Roper-Hall (1954), Rubinstein (1954), Stevens (1956), W. Levy (1958), Grönvall and Hultgren (1959), Chisholm (1964), V. Smith (1968); and others.

[2] Thus in Manchester 16% (Clegg, 1916) and 14·9% (Stevens, 1956), whereas in Birmingham 8% (Roper-Hall, 1954) and 6% (V. Smith, 1968).

TABLE XX

PERCENTAGE OF INTRA-OCULAR FOREIGN BODIES CAUSED BY THE USE OF A HAMMER

Allport (1925)	84	Mazur (1957)	78
Sherman (1939)	61	Grönvall (1958)	60
Roper-Hall (1954)	73	Chisholm (1964)	78
Rubinstein (1954)	77	V. Smith (1968)	70
Stevens (1956)	64		

the other hand, as we have seen, in war injuries the proportion is considerably higher.

The *size* of a retained foreign body varies but as a general rule, if the eye is not disorganized the particle is small, rarely less than 0·25 mm. or more than 2 mm. in diameter and 500 mg. in weight; smaller particles have rarely the momentum to traverse the sclera, while in the usual civilian accident the velocity attained by larger bodies is rarely sufficient for them to overcome the resistance of the ocular coats; if they do, as frequently occurs in battle casualties, the eye is usually hopelessly destroyed. Larger foreign bodies have usually been elongated and several of these of surprising length have been safely extracted leaving good vision—a piece of wire 15 mm. long (Wassef, 1950), a steel needle 24 mm. long, which pierced the limbus and traversed the zonule without damaging the lens and was happily extracted (Krückow, 1884), and a crochet needle which caused a double perforation of the globe (Feilke, 1905).

The damage done by more bulky objects is greater and their extraction has proved more difficult (a piece of steel 8 × 3·5 mm., Sherman, 1939; a metal plate 6·5 × 6·5 mm., Peleska, 1951), but in most cases foreign bodies of greater bulk have caused sufficient damage to produce gross and irrecoverable injury although the globe has not been pulped (irregular pieces of metal—20 mm. long, 2·5 g., Busse, 1873; 21 × 10·5 × 3·5 mm., weighing 20 g., Keyser, 1874; 23 × 10 mm., Hirschberg and Vogler, 1880; 15 × 10 mm., Binder, 1905; 18 × 10 mm., Wagenmann, 1921; arrow-heads 32 mm. long, Hirschberg, 1874, 25 mm. long, Steindorff, 1900, and others; a coil of

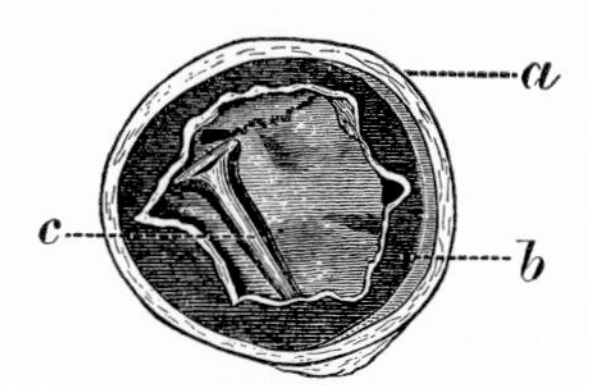

FIG. 416.—FOREIGN BODY IN THE EYE.

A classical woodcut from the *Royal London Ophthalmic Hospital Reports*, showing the retention of an unusually large foreign body in the eye without disruption of the globe. *a*, the sclera; *b*, a large subretinal hæmorrhage; *c*, a nail of considerable size retained in the globe (Jonathan Hutchinson, 1889).

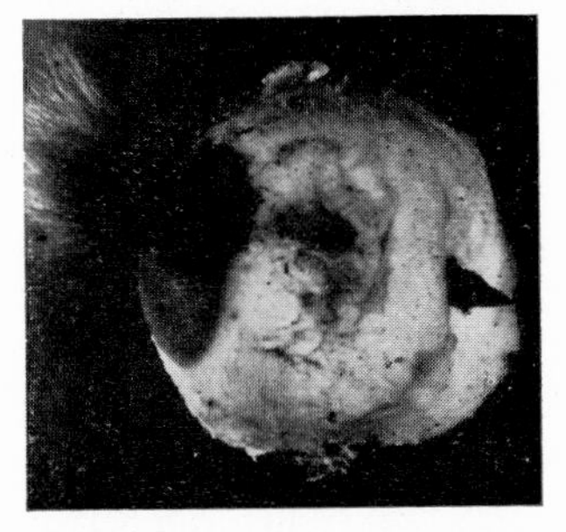

FIG. 417.—TRANSFIXION OF THE EYE BY A DART FROM AN AIRGUN

A domestic way—unfortunately not unique—of destroying the eye (Museum, Inst. Ophthal.).

fuse-wire 35 mm. long, Collins, 1918; an entire pistol bullet, Planten, 1952; a nail 1 cm. long, the head being 6 mm. wide, Hutchinson, 1889) (Fig. 416), or the feathered dart from an airgun (Fig. 417). Roper-Hall (1954) noted a gradual swing in preponderance from the right to the left eye as the foreign bodies increased in size, an observation subsequently confirmed in a series of 190 cases of metallic splinters reviewed by Grönvall and Hultgren (1959).

Multiple foreign bodies are often retained within the eye. Of these the most common and dramatic instances result from explosive wounds when quantities of sand, dust, clay, glass and other debris may lodge within the globe; these will be discussed subsequently.[1] In the ordinary industrial or domestic accident the entrance of more than one particle (generally of metal) is not unusual (3 of iron, von Hippel, 1896; 4 of lead, Schneider, 1877; 4 of copper, van der Hoeve, 1913; and many others). As would be expected, this multiplicity is not uncommon in war wounds.

From the clinical point of view the most important characteristic of a foreign body is its *magnetic properties*, since upon this largely depends the ease of its removal. In industrial accidents many of the foreign bodies which used to be retained within the eye (90%, Löwenstein, 1939, in Europe; 93%, Sherman, 1939, in the United States) had a high content of iron and were therefore magnetizable, but as the science of metallurgy advances and more and more alloys each with specific properties are introduced in industrial processes, and as non-ferrous metals are finding increasing scope in industry, fewer fall into this category. Even different types of steel differ very considerably in their magnetizability, stainless steel, for example, requiring a pull 30 times greater than carbon steel for its removal (Barling, 1953).

This tendency is particularly seen in the missiles used in war: in previous wars a majority of these had a high iron content and were magnetizable; in the second World War, a minority. Thus during the Spanish Civil War magnetizable foreign bodies were rare (Battignani, 1939), and in the second World War, Savin (1943–45) in England, found the low incidence of 1 magnetizable intra-ocular foreign body in every 6; Stallard (1944), in the Middle East campaign, found approximately 1 in 3; in the German army they were similarly rare (Gasteiger and Schmidt, 1940; Schlichting, 1943; Pokrowsky, 1943). In America, Cordes (1943) found no magnetizable foreign bodies in the early part of the Pacific campaign, Bellows (1947) found 1 in 2·5, while out of 150 enucleated eyes examined at the Armed Forces Institute of Pathology by Wilder (1945), 89 contained foreign bodies which were non-magnetizable, and the response in the other 61 cases was frequently weak and equivocal. A similar trend was noted in the Korean War (Hull, 1951) and in Vietnam (Hoefle, 1968).

The *site* whereat a foreign body comes to rest within the eye varies with its point of entry and velocity. As a general rule organized materials (cilia, etc.) do not travel far and when they enter the anterior segment, remain in the anterior chamber. Of 1,028 perforating injuries reported by Remky and his colleagues (1967), 403 had an intra-ocular foreign body of which 32% came to rest in the anterior segment. Metallic particles, on the other hand, if they have sufficient energy to pierce the ocular coats, usually

[1] p. 671.

traverse the relatively non-resistant tissues of the eye and pass to the posterior segment, sometimes even traversing the opposite wall. The average distribution of these is approximately as follows: in the anterior chamber, 15%, in the lens, 8%, in the posterior segment, 70%, in the orbit (having caused a double perforation), 7%.

Clinical Picture

The clinical picture following the entrance of a foreign body into the eye varies, of course, with the size of the particle concerned but if, as is usual, it is relatively small and the globe is not disorganized, little or no pain may be experienced at the time of impact; this is in striking contrast to the severe pain and immediate disability caused by a foreign body lying on or becoming impacted in the cornea. Usually there is a transient stinging sensation, occasionally a temporary " sick feeling in the stomach ", but quite often the incident is hardly noticed or even neglected altogether. As a rule there is some reduction of vision at the time of the accident and frequently, particularly if the particle is of any size, vision may be immediately blurred owing to the collapse of the anterior chamber, or lost owing to an intra-ocular hæmorrhage either into the anterior chamber or the vitreous. In the last event the clinical picture may be obscured and clinical examination rendered difficult so that the damage can only be assessed inferentially by the indirect evidence provided by the ability of the patient to project light accurately or perhaps even to perceive it. On the other hand, if the particle is small, apart from the immediate slight embarrassment on its entry, no further symptoms may arise and the vision may remain normal for weeks or years or sometimes indefinitely, the foreign body being eventually discovered on routine examination or after suspicion has been excited and special examinations undertaken by the chance remark of the wound of entry, a hole in the iris, the subsequent development of cataract, or the onset and persistence of an unexplained uveitis. If complications arise, however, such as the prolapse of the uveal tissues, tearing of the intra-ocular structures as occurs in perforating wounds, the onset of infection or the development of sympathetic ophthalmitis, the clinical picture becomes more obvious and dramatic; this aspect of the subject will be considered at a later stage.

Once the eye has been entered in the absence of infection, in addition to the more obvious mechanical effects produced by the momentum and the direction of the path of the foreign body, the ocular reaction varies with the particular tissues of the eye which are involved, the presence or absence of mechanical irritation set up at the site of lodgment and with the nature and composition of the foreign body itself.

The *tolerance of the separate tissues of the eye* towards the presence of a foreign body varies considerably. An intruder of this type may remain in the anterior chamber or enmeshed in the crypts of the iris indefinitely without exciting symptoms. The uveal tissues, especially the ciliary body, show the greatest reaction to injury of any kind and even although the particle is inert, this reaction frequently develops into a plastic iridocyclitis as we have seen to occur after perforating injuries. The lens, on the other hand, with its slow metabolic activity tends to show little reaction unless the rupture in the capsule allows the free entrance of aqueous into its tissues; even highly toxic substances may remain here without exciting a reaction for many years (steel, 32 years, Nottage, 1899; copper, 8 years, Würdemann, 1932). In the vitreous some degenerative changes always appear, but in favourable circumstances an inert foreign body may sometimes remain quietly in the posterior segment of the eye for an indefinite time.

The *presence or absence of mechanical irritation* set up at the site depends on the shape of the particle and the sharpness of its edges. A sliver of glass, for example, may set up continuous mechanical irritation, while a smoothly rounded piece of stone retained at the same site may be well tolerated. The nature and composition of the foreign body are also of extreme importance. Most organized materials set up a considerable tissue-reaction of the foreign-body granulomatous type. The usual unorganized particle, however, which does not decompose after a short time, either remains free or becomes encapsulated by organized exudate, depending on whether it has come to rest in a tissue which is capable of reacting to its presence. Metallic foreign bodies, however, which become electrolytically dissociated or react with the tissue-fluids to form decomposition products usually by oxidation, tend to set up specific toxic reactions which may eventually cause sufficient damage to destroy vision.

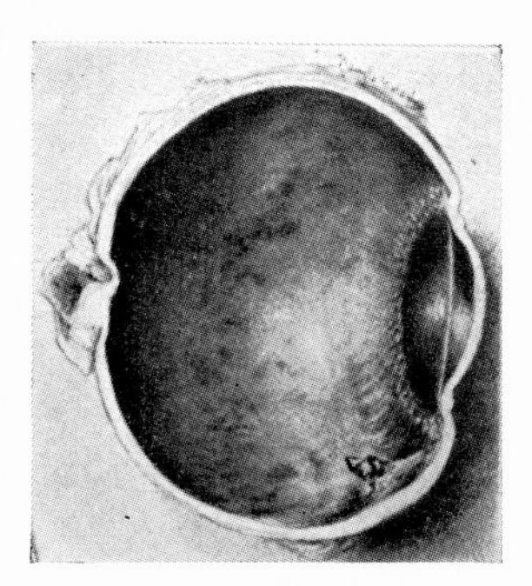

FIG. 418.—RETAINED FOREIGN BODY.

An iron foreign body covered by a layer of oxide retained in the eye for 67 years. The foreign body is embedded in the ciliary region. The eye showed no irritation, the lens had completely absorbed, the tissues of the eye were atrophic; vision was perception of light. The other eye was normal (C. Spratt).

Even although the material is inert, however, and apparently excites little reaction at the time so that the eye rapidly quietens after the accident, its presence often leads eventually to trouble, and the tissue-reaction may slowly and cumulatively develop into a recalcitrant traumatic uveitis which eventually leads to atrophy and shrinkage of the globe with complete loss of function. The tolerance which an eye may on occasion show to a retained encapsulated foreign body, however, is frequently remarkable and, indeed, its presence may first be noted many years after the original accident. This possibility, of course, raises the difficult therapeutic question as to whether more damage may sometimes be done in attempting the immediate removal of a foreign body in an inaccessible position, particularly if it is non-magnetizable, than by accepting the risk of leaving it alone (Bulson, 1926; Löhlein, 1951; and many others).

A foreign body may thus remain without exciting any inflammatory reaction almost indefinitely. Thus in a case recorded by Fejer (1932), even although the eye had been badly damaged at the time, the first evidence of inflammation arose 20 years after the injury; Dodd (1902) observed a piece of nut-shell in the posterior segment, and Doyne (1894) a foreign body in the lens for 30 years; a case was described by Spratt (1933) wherein a piece of iron remained quietly embedded in the ciliary body for 67 years in a blind eye, the specimen being obtained only after the patient's death (Fig. 418). This tolerance may sometimes be extended even to copper (10 years, Goldzieher, 1895; 46 years, Franklin and Cordes, 1922; 56 years with normal vision, Lewis, 1946).

The Mechanical Effects of Foreign Bodies

Most foreign bodies penetrate the eye in a general sense from before backwards, and the wound of entry is usually in the cornea, at the limbus or in the anterior part of the sclera. The bony orbit adequately protects the posterior part of the sclera, but occasionally a bizarre track has been found to traverse the anterior segment of the globe tangentially.

In a case recorded by Fox (1930), for example, a piece of small shot entered the eye at the temporal limbus, traversed the anterior chamber which it left anterior to the limbus at a point diagonally opposite the wound of entry and, after passing through the ciliary edge of the upper tarsus, it was lost. A more dramatic case was recorded by Lotin (1947) wherein a bullet striking the eye tangentially produced a trauma as if an iridectomy had been performed; the resultant vision in both these cases was good.

Unless the wound of entry is extensive it usually heals rapidly, and since the perforation is relatively small, the anterior chamber is frequently retained and the iris, pushed backwards by the particle itself, is rarely prolapsed into the wound. A corneal wound, however, always leaves a permanent track which, although it may eventually become inconspicuous, can always be seen by the slit-lamp; but a conjunctivo-scleral wound tends to become invisible unless it has been of considerable size when its presence may be betrayed by the migration of uveal pigment to the surface. Having entered the anterior chamber the particle often becomes entangled in the iris or sometimes falls to the bottom of the chamber where it frequently lies hidden in the angle by the scleral rim.

Alternatively, the velocity may be sufficient for the particle to traverse the anterior chamber and enter the lens, or to bore a hole through the iris and pass into the lens or through the zonule. A hole in the iris formed in this way remains as a permanent legacy of the accident and in this respect is an important diagnostic point; it appears black by oblique illumination and red by transillumination with the ophthalmoscope if the lens behind it is not cataractous (Figs. 419–420). The foreign body is frequently retained in the lens, coming to rest usually in the dense nucleus, causing in its transit damage which may vary from a localized opacity to a complete opacification of the entire tissue. If the particle traverses the lens it may come to rest in the vitreous body, but owing to the lack of resistance offered by the gel, its remaining energy is usually sufficient to carry it to the retina. Here, unless it is able to pierce the coats of the eye a second time and lose itself in the orbit, it may become embedded, damaging to a greater or less extent the tissues in the immediate vicinity, or alternatively it ricochets off the posterior wall of the globe and sometimes rebounds more than once before it finally comes to rest at the bottom of the vitreous cavity.

Apart from the descent of a foreign body in the vitreous cavity when its energy is spent or the angular course of a ricochet from the posterior wall, the track of a foreign body is usually a straight line from the wound of entry to the spot where it comes to rest. Occasionally, however, *migration of the particle* may occur after it has been in the eye for some time (de Wecker, 1896; Goldsmith, 1965; and many others). Thus a shot-pellet was found by

Figs. 419 and 420.—Hole in the Iris caused by Perforation by a Foreign Body.

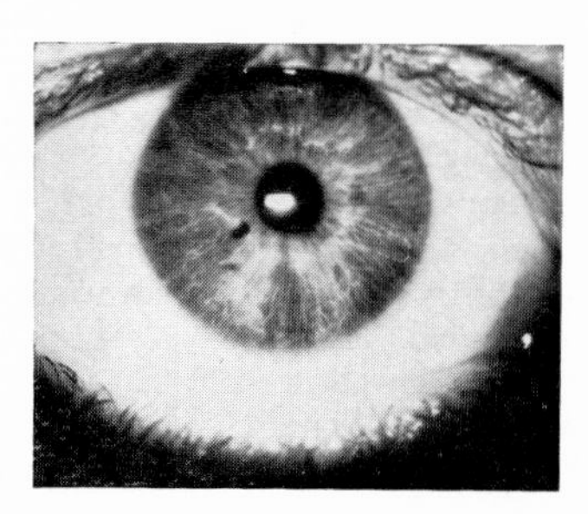

Fig. 419.—Photograph of the iris showing the small black permanent hole (at 8 o'clock) caused by the passage of a foreign body, seen by direct light.

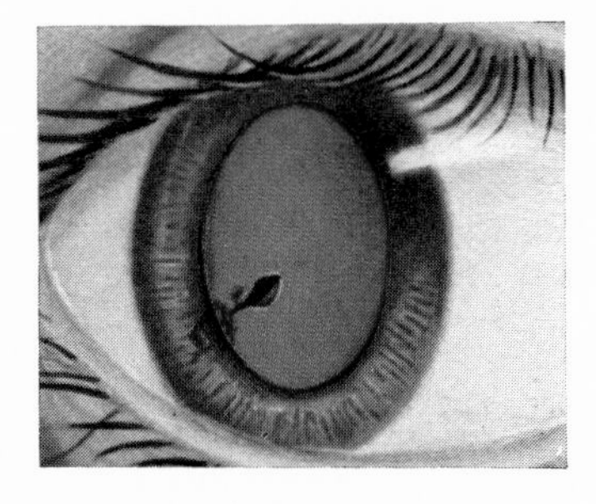

Fig. 420.—Drawing of the same case, seen ophthalmoscopically by transmitted light with a dilated pupil. Note that the hole at 8 o'clock shows the red reflex. There is a track in the lens caused by the foreign body.

Kümmell (1908) to have migrated from the interior of the eye to the angle of the anterior chamber after a year and a quarter, whence it was successfully extracted. A similar case was reported by Tulloh (1956) wherein a piece of brass moved from the pars plana to the angle of the anterior chamber. According to Tulloh such migration of intra-ocular foreign bodies may be related to the compression of the globe by the extra-ocular muscles, the pull of the ciliary muscle on the choroid during accommodation and the influence of the intra-ocular fluid. In another case a large particle of glass which had remained asymptomatic in the vitreous for five years came forward into the anterior chamber to rest against the corneal endothelium, causing corneal œdema and cataract; removal of the foreign body and of the cataractous lens resulted in satisfactory aphakic vision (Mitchell and Wolkowicz, 1968). This habit may be particularly unfortunate in the case of a sharp particle; thus a piece of glass which had remained quietly in the eye for 10 years eventually moved against the lens to form a cataract (Gandolfi, 1947).

Occurrences like this, of course, have considerable medico-legal implications. Occasionally the result is happier, for in this way after a long residence the foreign body may be eventually extruded from the globe although by that time the eye may have become atrophic, a phenomenon first described by Castelnau (1842) and subsequently reported by several observers.[1] Such spontaneous extrusion is most commonly seen with copper.[2]

The reaction within the eye largely depends, both from the clinical and the therapeutic points of view, on whether the foreign body comes to rest in the anterior or posterior segment of the globe or lies within the lens.

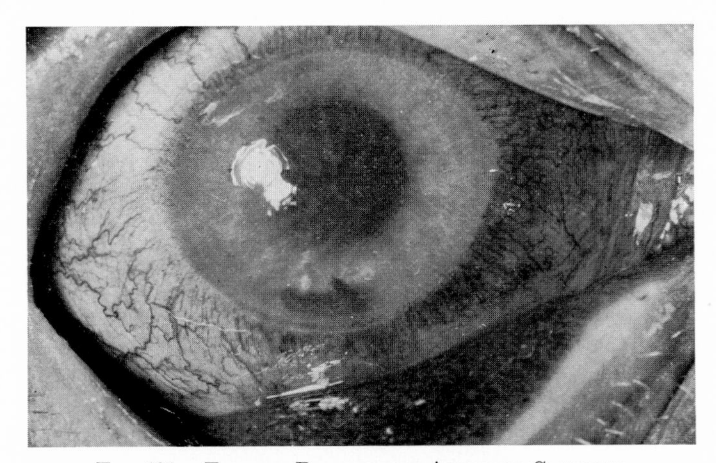

Fig. 421.—Foreign Body in the Anterior Chamber.

The foreign body, a fragment of metal, lies in the anterior chamber at 6 o'clock. The cornea is grossly œdematous (Inst. Ophthal.).

In the anterior chamber a foreign body naturally falls to the bottom of the chamber and if it is small it is usually hidden from view lying deep in the recess of the angle underneath the scleral rim where it may be seen only with the gonioscope (Plate XVIII, Figs. 3, 4 and 6). If the particle is chemically inert it may lie there quietly for an indefinite time, sometimes becoming encapsulated (14 years, Reeh, 1948; 15 years, Trantas, 1938; 20 years, D. Archer *et al.*, 1969), but if its edges are sharp or jagged it may cause irritation, as sometimes occurs, for example, with pieces of glass (Bruce, 1933; Doherty, 1947; Papmatheakis, 1947). If, on the other hand, the particle is irritative, an iridocyclitis or a persistent localized corneal œdema may be excited, the cause of which may only be revealed by gonioscopic examination, sometimes after the application of glycerol to clear the cornea[3] (Fig. 421).

[1] Wicherkiewicz (1904); iron, Scalinci (1905), Gesang (1905); glass, Azarova (1943), Cordes (1943); wood, Bochever (1947).

[2] p. 517.

[3] François (1950), Moskowitz (1953), Vannini (1953). Laibson (1965), Thorpe (1966).

Similarly, if caught on the surface of the iris, fragments of inert material and metal may remain indefinitely without causing irritation or degeneration (Shapland, 1945; and others); occasionally this immunity is extended to even the most toxic metals, as in Lewis's (1946) case, already noted, wherein a piece of brass was impacted on the iris with the retention of normal vision for 56 years. If the iris is torn, however, a small exudation of blood may appear in the tissues around the foreign body as well as a hyphæma in the anterior chamber, while a traumatic iritis is usual. In the ciliary body this reaction is always greater and a traumatic iridocyclitis which leads eventually to atrophy of the globe is prone to occur, the onset of which, however, after the initial traumatic reaction, may be delayed for many years.

In the lens all types of foreign body have been found to be impacted as well as the common fragments of various metals (Fig. 422).[1] An extraordinary case was described by Payrau and Guyard (1956) wherein, as a

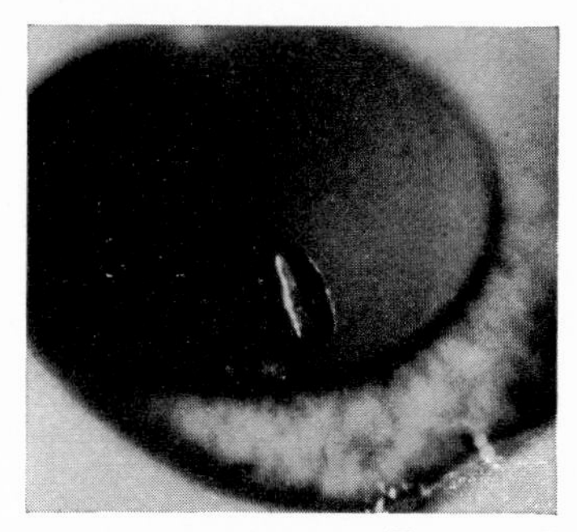

FIG. 422.—INTRALENTICULAR METALLIC FOREIGN BODY (H. Thorpe).

result of blast, six eyelashes were propelled through the cornea into the lens. The reaction of such a perforating injury, as we have seen,[2] may be varied. If the particle is of any size, a universal clouding of the whole tissue tends to develop rapidly, forming a complete traumatic cataract. On the other hand, if the wound in the capsule is small so that it is quickly closed with a coating of fibrin, and particularly if it is behind the iris so that the impaction of this tissue helps in the rapid closure of the wound, the capsular epithelium covers the defect and the opacity may be localized, an event which may occur even although the foreign body traverses the entire structure, piercing the capsule both anteriorly and posteriorly (Bondi, 1898; and others). Such an occurrence is rare, but a particle may occasionally be retained in the substance of the lens, causing only a small circumscribed zone of opacity, sometimes with fine linear streaks extending to the capsular perforation, and there it may

[1] Gunpowder, Millikin (1892); glass, Post (1896), Laqueur (1905); bone, Spierer (1891); coal, Knabe (1895), Zimmermann (1911), Castroviejo (1931); wood, Weidmann (1888); cilia, Samelsohn (1885), Lindner (1889); a piece of bodkin (Donaldson, 1965), and so on.

[2] p. 251.

PLATES XVI AND XVII

FOREIGN BODIES IN THE RETINA

PLATE XVI

FOREIGN BODIES IN THE RETINA.

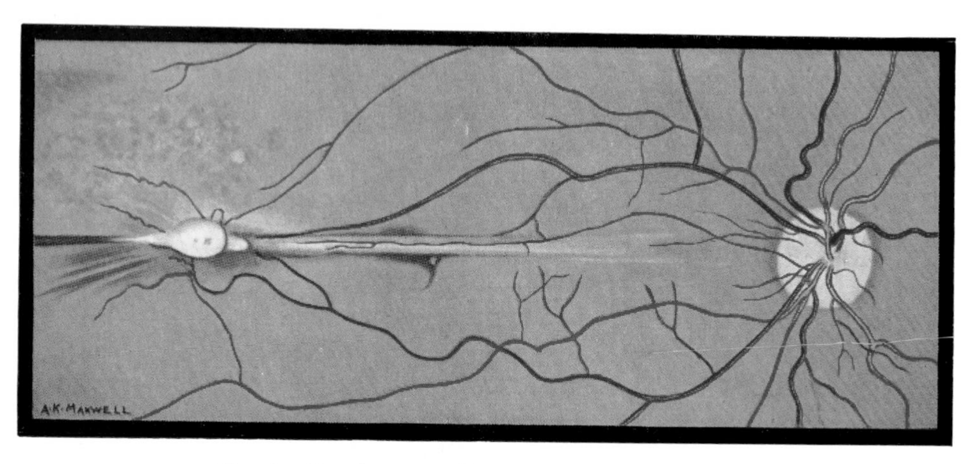

FIG. 1.—THE SCAR OF A PENETRATING FOREIGN BODY.

To the oval opalescent swelling is attached a band of fibrous tissue in the vitreous, indicating the track of the foreign body, and around the scar the retina is puckered. For visual field, see Fig. 433 (W. Lister).

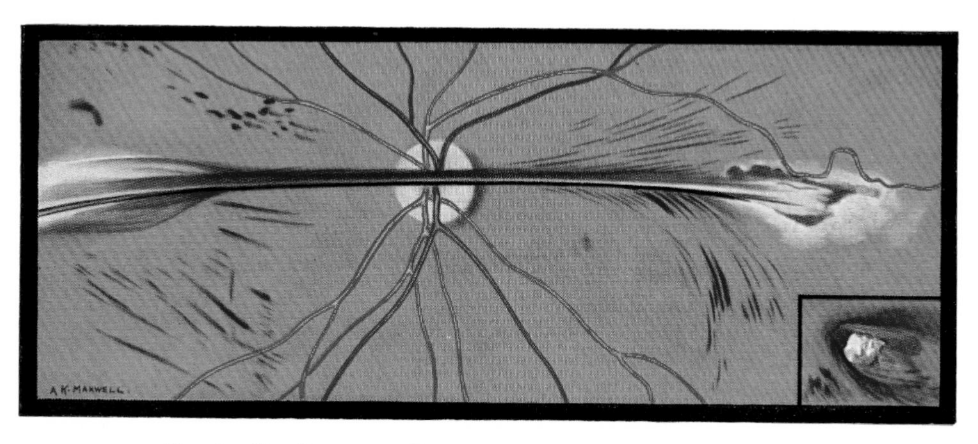

FIG. 2.—THE PATH OF A FOREIGN BODY THROUGH THE VITREOUS.

A foreign body had ricocheted twice within the eye. Two scars are seen on the retina, one on each side of the disc, bridged across by a fan of hæmorrhagic tissue. The inset shows the foreign body lying far forward in the vitreous which was blood-stained. The field defect is seen in Fig. 434 (W. Lister).

PLATE XVII

FOREIGN BODIES IN THE RETINA.

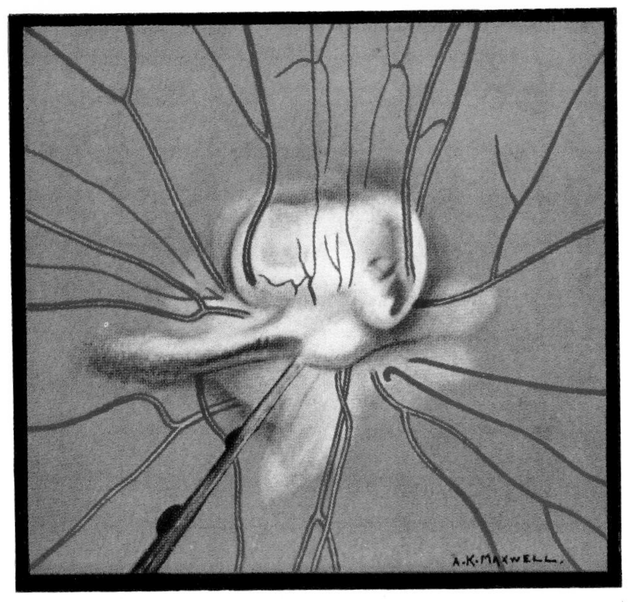

FIG. 1.—IMPACTION OF A FOREIGN BODY ON THE OPTIC DISC.

The track of the foreign body forming a fibrous band through the vitreous is seen below and to the left. The disc is covered by a mass of fibrous tissue through which the retinal vessels emerge. The field defect is seen in Fig. 435 (W. Lister).

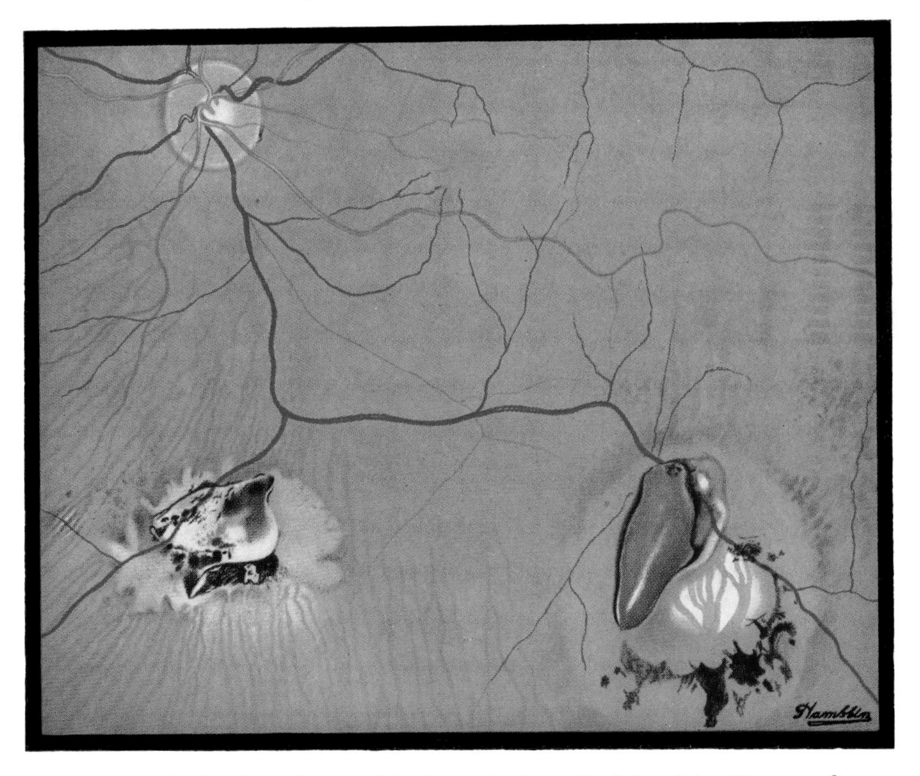

FIG. 2.—A foreign body impacted in the posterior wall of the globe, 18 years after injury. The area of choroidal atrophy directly below the disc marks the first point of impact from which the fragment of metal ricocheted to its final position on the right (A. B. Cridland).

remain for years without causing any optical or physiological disturbance to the function of the lens[1]; this may occur even although the foreign body itself is potentially toxic.[2]

The subsequent history of the traumatic cataract thus formed varies. If a total opacification of the lens occurs the eye may eventually quieten; rapid tumescence or the later onset of degenerative changes may require surgical extraction; and occasionally the cataract, even although complete, may spontaneously absorb (Topolanski, 1895; Cramer, 1899; and others), sometimes leaving a small circumscribed opacity on the capsule marking the wound of entry (Sédan and Farnarier, 1947). In this event the foreign body falls into the anterior or posterior chamber or backwards into the vitreous. If the opacity formed at the time of injury is localized, it occasionally clears up to a considerable extent (Desmarres, 1847; Berger, 1887; Ischreyt, 1907; Blatt, 1930); at other times there is a slow increase of opacification some months or years after the injury (Laqueur, 1905, glass; François, 1951, iron); occasionally hypertension develops at a later date sometimes associated with uveitis (after 29 years, steel, Tromeur, 1938); and finally, if the foreign body is removed, the operative trauma usually results in the opacification of the whole lens (Monsilla Sinforiano, 1920) or its absorption (Lampert, 1921; Abrahamson, 1923), although occasionally a delicate localized opacity remains unchanged after this manipulation.[3]

An epithelial implantation into the lens is an exceptional rarity (Früchte, 1906).

The posterior segment of the globe may be entered either through the cornea, pupil and lens, through the cornea, iris and lens, through the cornea, iris and zonule or directly through the sclera; in 43 cases Hildebrand (1891) found that the frequency of these four routes had the proportion of 6, 16, 6 and 15. Most fragments which travel so far are metallic splinters, usually elongated in shape (75%, Weidmann, 1888), but occasionally unusual materials are found—fragments of bone (Rémy, 1874; Hertel, 1916–22; von Szily, 1918), whip-lash (Hutchinson, 1889; Bryant, 1895; Nöldecke, 1904; Vigier, 1907), nut-shell (Dodd, 1902), coal (Stewart, 1894) and cilia (Deutschmann, 1890; Wintersteiner, 1894; and others). In this situation serious complications are prone to arise. If the force involved is considerable, massive hæmorrhages are likely to occur at the time of the injury, obscuring the whole picture; moreover, if the eye becomes infected, the consequences are particularly disastrous. Excluding these major complications, if the particle is small and sterile and enters the vitreous but does not travel to the posterior pole, it may remain there for some time, appearing in the light

[1] Whitehead (1916), Lampert (1921), Blatt (1930), Cordes (1943).

[2] Iron, 16 years, T. B. Archer (1897); 32 years, Nottage (1899); 10 years, Blatt (1930); copper, 30 years, Doyne (1894); 27 years, Wagenmann (1897); 8 years, Würdemann (1932).

[3] Vossius (1880–1909), Sacher (1901), Morax (1905), Bruner (1907), Marx (1909), Paderstein (1910), Elschnig (1911–13), Mellinghoff (1913), Wibaut (1913), Lacompte (1914), Bell (1924), Dollfus and Halbron (1934), Stokes (1938), Kronenberg (1944), and others.

of the ophthalmoscope to shine and scintillate like a jewel; eventually, however, it sinks to the bottom of the vitreous chamber, for in these circumstances the gel degenerates and turns fluid. More frequently, however, the foreign body traverses the vitreous and buries itself in the posterior wall of the globe or ricochets off once or twice from the surface of the retina before it falls spent to the bottom of the chamber.

This phenomenon of the rebounding of a foreign body from the posterior wall of the eye is common and was first demonstrated by Berlin (1867–68), who found in 19 enucleated eyes that 14 foreign bodies had thus rebounded, 4 had become impacted directly in the posterior wall and 1 had passed through into the orbit (Fig. 423).

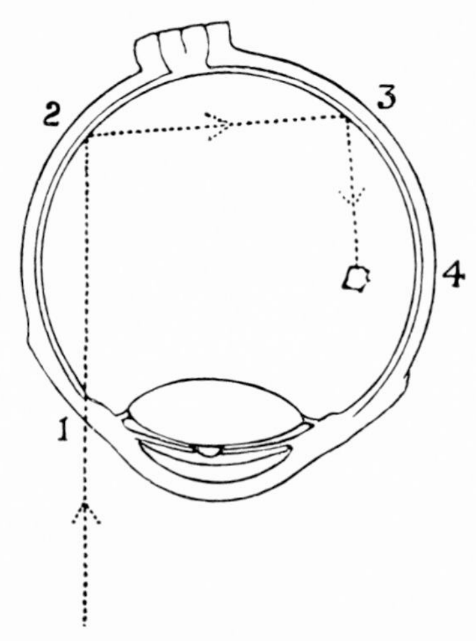

FIG. 423.—THE RICOCHETING OF A FOREIGN BODY WITHIN THE EYE.

Diagram of the path of the foreign body seen in Plate XVI, Fig. 2. It entered through the anterior part of the sclera (1), struck the retina immediately behind (2), ricocheted across the vitreous to strike the retina again (3), and finally came to rest in the vitreous (4) (W. Lister).

In all these cases the track of the particle through the humour may appear first as an indefinite grey line. Occasionally bubbles of air are carried in with it, and although they rapidly become absorbed, these may be seen clinically for some time as small, sharply defined spheres with bright centres and dark rims; this appearance was first described by Jacobi (1868) as being due to blood but was properly interpreted as air by Morton (1876), an observation subsequently confirmed by many other writers.[1] Quite often, also, the track is marked by small hæmorrhages which eventually become organized into fibrous bands; in time, of course, if these are of any size, their contraction may eventually lead to a detachment of the retina and

[1] Hirschberg (1885), Pfalz (1887), Meesmann (1893), Blessig (1893), and many others. Very occasionally similar air bubbles are found in the anterior chamber associated with a foreign body (Hirschberg, 1894); they are more common in extensive perforating wounds. Exceptionally a bubble has been seen in the lens associated with a foreign body (A. Levy, 1900). In the vitreous they are commonly seen.

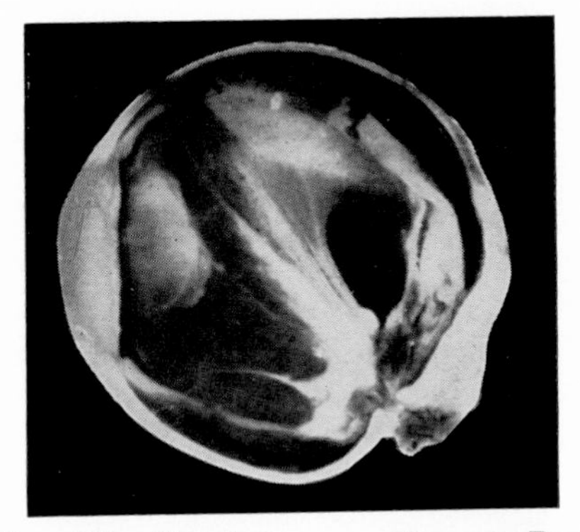

FIG. 424.—THE PATH OF A FOREIGN BODY THROUGH THE VITREOUS.

A deeply penetrating foreign body which entered the eye above the cornea and left below the disc. The streaks of infiltration in the vitreous are seen to radiate from the point of exit.

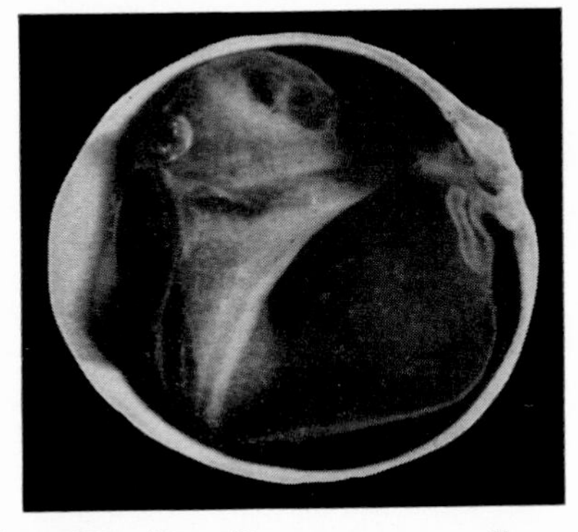

FIG. 425.—THE RICOCHET OF A FOREIGN BODY ON THE RETINA.

The track of the foreign body through the vitreous is marked out by hæmorrhage. It struck the retina close to the disc where the marked wrinkling is clearly seen.

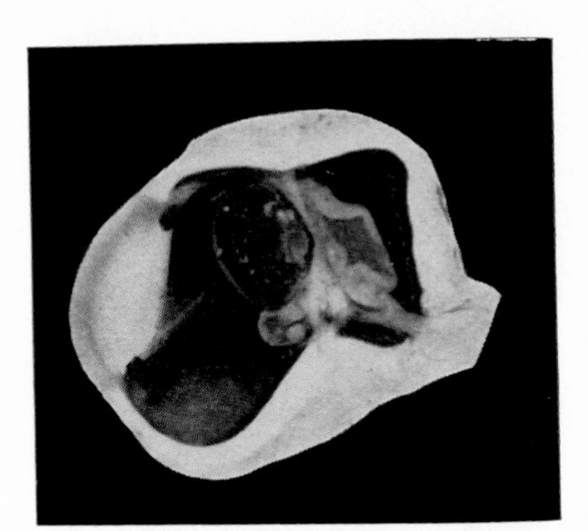

FIG. 426.—THE TRAVERSAL OF A FOREIGN BODY THROUGH THE GLOBE.

The foreign body has passed obliquely down through the middle of the globe. Its track through the vitreous has become marked out by fibrous tissue which, on contraction, has deformed the eyeball, pulled the iris and lens backwards, and caused a total detachment of the retina.

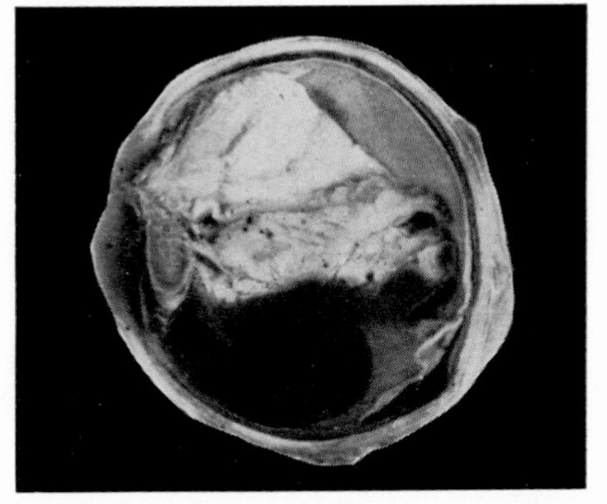

FIG. 427.—DISORGANIZATION OF THE GLOBE BY A FOREIGN BODY.

The foreign body has entered in the upper part of the cornea, traversed the lens causing a traumatic cataract, and come to rest at the bottom of the vitreous chamber. The lens capsule is incarcerated in the wound, the whole of the inner eye is disorganized and the foreign body (a piece of stone) lies in blood clot in the vitreous chamber.

(Museum, Institute of Ophthalmology.)

choroid or be ultimately responsible for general distortion, disorganization and atrophy of the globe (Figs. 424–427).

When a foreign body strikes the retina it bruises it and in most cases cuts into it (Figs. 428 and 429). At the point of impact it may remain a little while and then migrate to come to rest at a new site, leaving a damaged area behind (Plates XVI–XVII). If it buries itself deeply, the retina and sometimes the choroid, are torn, the vitreous usually becomes adherent to the wound and the gap thus caused is rapidly filled by a plug of newly formed fibrous tissue which becomes continuous with the organizing tissue that begins to fill the track through the vitreous. At the point where the particle becomes impacted into the retina the tissue-reaction excited in the neighbouring retina and choroid is usually considerable so that the intruder rapidly becomes partially or completely encapsulated. The resulting ophthalmoscopic picture, first described by Jäger (1857) and von Graefe (1857), is frequently beautiful; the foreign body appears boldly outlined, usually as a black or lustrous object, often shining and glinting with a

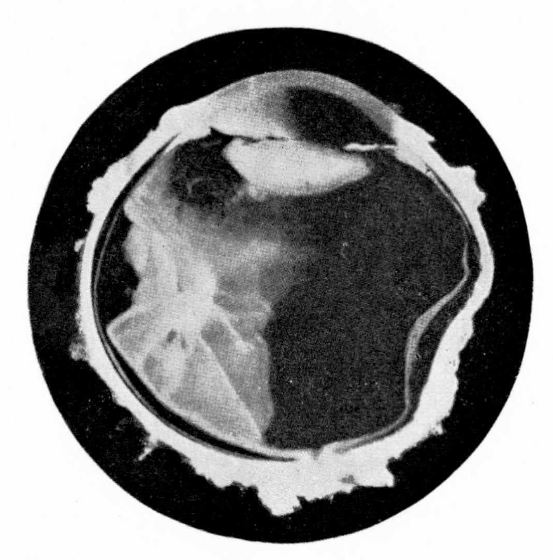

Fig. 428.—Damage to the Retina by an Intra-ocular Foreign Body.

The foreign body has struck the retina towards the left part of the figure and has remained embedded therein. The section shows the intense puckering which may occasionally occur in such circumstances (W. Lister).

metallic sheen, surrounded at first by white exudate and blood clot and eventually by a small encircling mass of white fibrous tissue round which pigment tends to accumulate (Plate XVII). With the passage of time this new-formed tissue may completely bury and obscure it, and in favourable circumstances it may thus remain encapsulated indefinitely (Plate XVI).

As occurs at the point of ricochet, the proliferation of fibrous tissue tends to extend from the site of impaction along the track of the foreign body in the vitreous, so that the complicated course of the particle may be permanently outlined from its point of entrance into the posterior segment of the eye to the site of its rebound, and finally to its resting place, occasionally producing a most dramatic ophthalmoscopic appearance (Plate XVI) (Hirschberg, 1907; Lister, 1924). A similar picture is often apparent at the site of exit from the eye if a double perforation occurs. At this point a massive proliferative choroiditis tends to develop wherein the newly formed tissue herniates without restraint through the opening in Bruch's membrane and the retina, a reaction which in many instances may be not without value in sealing the retinal hole and preventing detachment of this tissue.[1]

Occasionally the foreign body may rest by chance upon the optic disc, where it may lie ophthalmoscopically visible on the surface[2] (Fig. 430); at other times it buries itself into the disc and travels some distance up the nerve, where it is found only on enucleation (Fig. 431) (Power, 1892)[3] or histological examination[4]; occasionally it happens that it buries itself

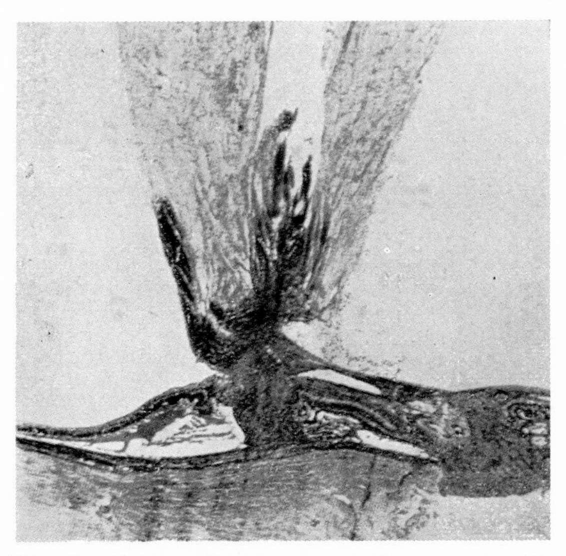

Fig. 429.—The Retinal Reaction at the Spot where a Foreign Body Ricocheted.

The retina is divided and the gap thus caused is occupied by a plug of fibrous tissue continuous with the shrunken and hæmorrhagic vitreous which has become attached to the wounded area and in which fibrous tissue is beginning to replace the blood (W. Lister).

alongside the nerve (Fig. 432) (Marin Amat, 1947). In such an event a considerable amount of damage may occur in the nerve-head accompanied by much inflammatory reaction involving the disc and the parts immediately around it, whereon an exuberant proliferation of fibrous tissue may occur showing the same tendency to organization along the track of the missile

[1] Wagenmann (1900), Krückow (1901), Genth (1903), Oleynick (1915), Michaelson and Kraus (1943), and others.

[2] Noyes (1886), Krüger (1887), Oeller (1896), Hirschberg (1904), Lange (1912), Exnerova (1950), and many others.

[3] Power's case is interesting. At enucleation, section of the optic nerve proved difficult owing to the presence of a large elongated piece of iron which had buried itself deeply in the nerve 12 years previously.

[4] Eschenauer (1891), Oliver (1899), Wagenmann (1900), Gradle (1908), Butler (1909), Law (1948), and many others.

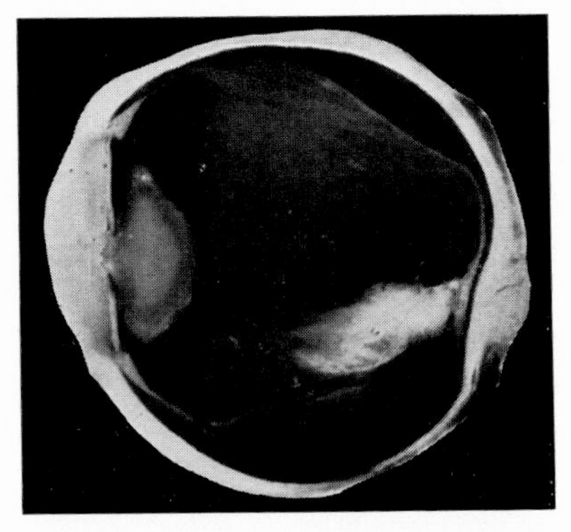

FIG. 430.—THE IMPACTION OF A FOREIGN BODY ON THE RETINA NEAR THE DISC.

The foreign body traversed the cornea and lens and a tongue of infiltration protrudes into the vitreous from the site of its impaction (Museum, Inst. Ophthal.).

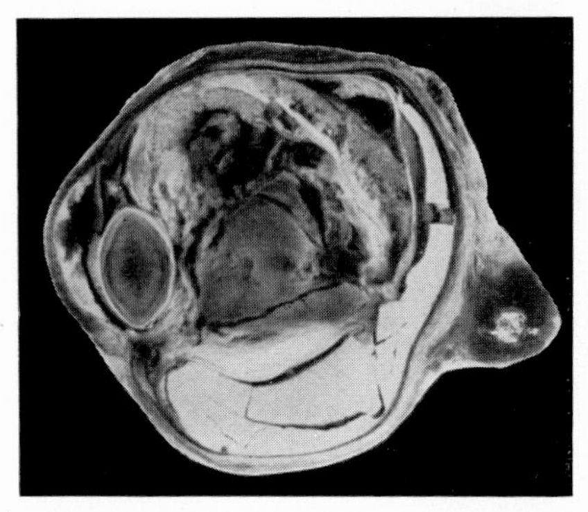

FIG. 431.—FOREIGN BODY IN THE OPTIC NERVE.

The foreign body has traversed the globe and come to rest in the optic nerve behind the disc. The globe is disorganized. There is exudate in the anterior chamber, a traumatic cataract, the retina is completely detached, and hæmorrhage and exudate fill the inner eye (Museum, Inst. Ophthal.).

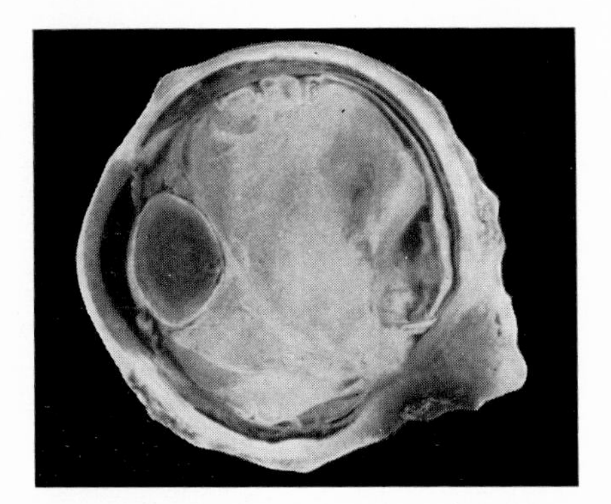

FIG. 432.—LODGMENT OF A FOREIGN BODY ALONGSIDE THE OPTIC NERVE.

A piece of steel passed through the lid, cornea, iris, suspensory ligament (above the lens), the vitreous and sclera and came to rest just outside the globe by the optic nerve. The whole of the inner eye is filled with exudates (Museum, Inst. Ophthal.).

as occurs if the particle had embedded itself elsewhere in the fundus (Plate XVII, Fig. 1) (Lister, 1924).

These injuries cause striking defects in the visual field corresponding to their site. If the wound is located near the centre of the retina above or below the horizontal plane, the defect in the visual field is out of all proportion to the apparent retinal disturbance, a large nerve-fibre defect being evident in addition to the local damage caused to the sentient elements at the point where the retina is struck; indeed, a defect in the field running fan-shaped outwards from the point corresponding to the lesion, extending from the periphery and ending at the median raphe, may demonstrate that

FIGS. 433 to 435.—VISUAL FIELDS IN CASES OF FOREIGN BODIES IMPACTED IN THE RETINA.

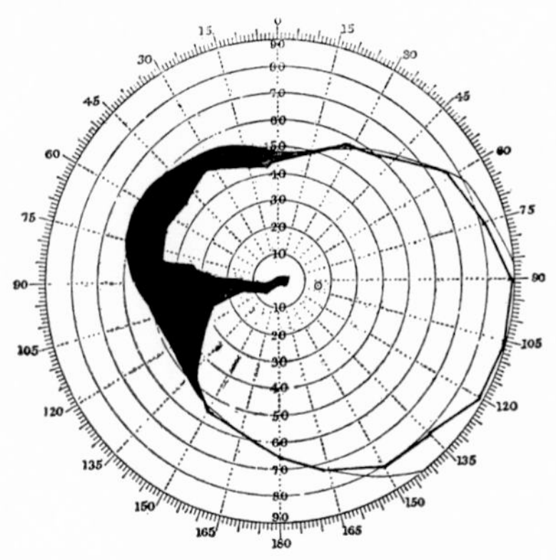

FIG. 433.—The case seen in Plate XVI, Fig. 1, where the foreign body was impacted in the retina. The defect extends towards the periphery owing to division of the nerve fibres at the point of injury.

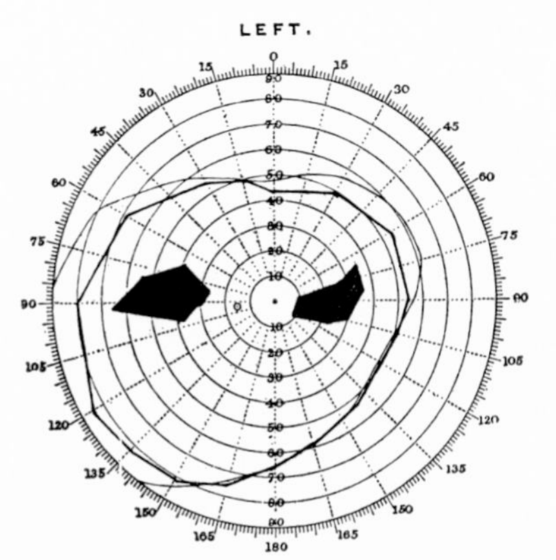

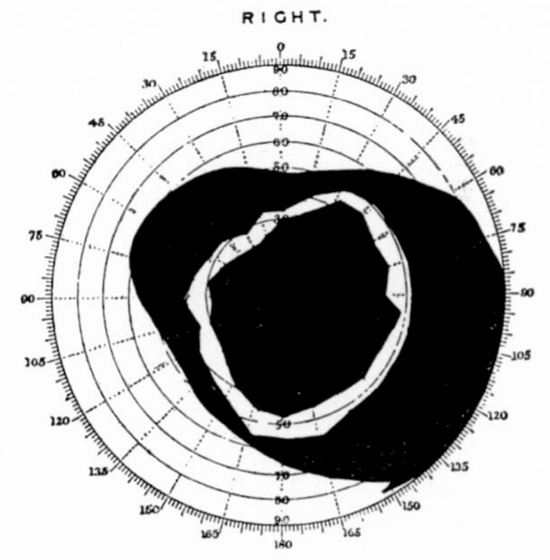

FIG. 434.—The foreign body injured the retina at the horizontal raphe and ricocheted across to the opposite side of the disc, affecting the terminal region of the nerve fibres (the case seen in Plate XVI, Fig. 2).

FIG. 435.—The bizarre effects caused by a foreign body lodged in the disc. The retinal periphery is scotomatous and there is a large central defect leaving a circular ring corresponding (presumably) to a circular zone of nerve fibres which had been left intact (the case seen in Plate XVII, Fig. 1) (W. Lister).

the nerve fibres passing on to the more peripheral portions of the retina have been divided. The nearer the lesion to the disc the greater the section of the field thus destroyed (Fig. 433). On the other hand, if it is situated in the horizontal meridian the scotoma may well correspond to the actual lesion itself, a limitation to be expected since the median horizontal raphe is the terminus for nerve fibres along this line (Fig. 434). If the optic disc is struck and deeply wounded, irregular and apparently bizarre scotomata may be found, depending on the extent of the damage done to the nerve fibres. The curious clinical phenomena which may be observed in this type of injury

FIGS. 436 and 437.—DEGENERATIVE CHANGES FOLLOWING THE LODGMENT OF A METALLIC FOREIGN BODY IN THE FUNDUS.

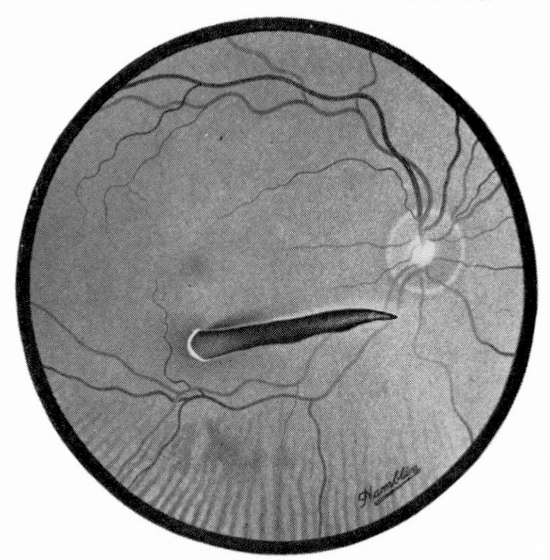

FIG. 436.—The foreign body pierced the eye of a hammerman who was punching a steel plate; three weeks after the accident. The fragment of steel was 1 cm. long.

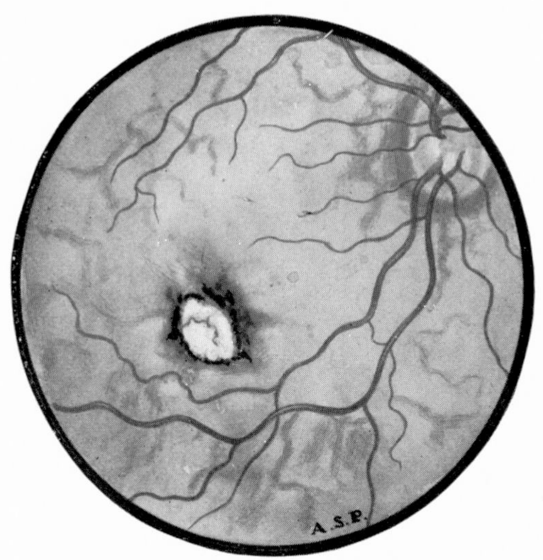

FIG. 437.—The appearance of the fundus 2 years after the piece of steel was extracted by the posterior route (A. S. Philps) (see also Figs. 608 and 609).

are well exemplified in the astonishing case reported by Lister (1924), wherein the field was reduced to a narrow ring in the middle periphery (Plate XVII, Fig. 1; Fig. 435). Such scotomata are, of course, permanent.

A comparatively rare and interesting sign of some significance, occurring usually some 3 to 6 weeks after the lodgment of a foreign body in the posterior segment of the

Knabe. *Beiträge z. Statistik u. Kasuistik d. Augenverletzungen* (Diss.), Halle (1895).
Kronenberg. *Amer. J. Ophthal.*, **27**, 1427 (1944).
Krückow. *Vestn. oftal.*, **1**, 526 (1884). *Wratsch.*, **22**, 1600 (1901).
Krüger. *Ber. dtsch. ophthal. Ges.*, **19**, 180 (1887).
Kümmell. *Z. Augenheilk.*, **19**, 36 (1908).
Lacompte. *Ann. Oculist.* (Paris), **152**, 171 (1914).
Laibson. *Arch. Ophthal.*, **74**, 191 (1965).
Lampert. *Arch. Ophtal.*, **38**, 745 (1921).
Lange. *Klin. Mbl. Augenheilk.*, **50** (2), 553 (1912).
Laqueur. *Arch. Augenheilk.*, **53**, 97 (1905).
Law. *Trans. ophthal. Soc. U.K.*, **68**, 351 (1948).
Lesenne and Béal. *Bull. Soc. Ophtal. Fr.*, 607 (1950).
Levy, A. *Klin. Mbl. Augenheilk.*, **38**, 837 (1900).
Levy, W. J. *Brit. J. Ophthal.*, **42**, 610 (1958).
Lewis. *Amer. J. Ophthal.*, **29**, 1164 (1946).
Lindner. *Wien. med. Wschr.*, **39**, 1433, 1479 (1889).
Lister. *Brit. J. Ophthal.*, **8**, 305 (1924).
Löhlein. *Klin. Mbl. Augenheilk.*, **119**, 113 (1951).
Löwenstein. *Glasg. med. J.*, **132**, 169 (1939).
Lotin. *Vestn. oftal.*, **26** (1), 70 (1947).
McBride. *Amer. J. Ophthal.*, **32**, 1255 (1949).
McCormick, Macaulay and Miller. *Amer. J. Ophthal.*, **32**, 1252 (1949).
Marin Amat. *Arch. Soc. oftal. hisp.-amer.*, **7**, 375 (1947).
Marx. *Klin. Mbl. Augenheilk.*, **47** (2), 178 (1909).
Mazur. *Klin. oczna*, **27**, 293 (1957).
Meesmann. *Ueber d. reaktionslose Einheilen v. Fremdkörpern in Augenhintergrunde* (Diss.), Berlin (1893).
Mellinghoff. *Klin. Mbl. Augenheilk.*, **51** (2), 687 (1913).
Michaelson and Kraus. *Brit. J. Ophthal.*, **27**, 449 (1943).
Millikin. *Ophthal. Rev.*, **11**, 285 (1892).
Minton. *Occupational Eye Diseases and Injuries*, London (1949).
Mitchell and Wolkowicz. *Amer. J. Ophthal.*, **65**, 620 (1968).
Monsilla Sinforiano. *Rev. med. Cir. pract.*, **126**, 169 (1920).
Morax. *Ann. Oculist.* (Paris), **133**, 127 (1905).
Morton. *Roy. Lond. ophthal. Hosp. Rep.*, **9**, 38 (1876).
Moskowitz. *Arch. Ophthal.*, **50**, 319 (1953).
Mukai. *Klin. Mbl. Augenheilk.*, **76**, 88 (1926).
Müller-Jensen and Allmaras. *Klin. Mbl. Augenheilk.*, **153**, 803 (1968).
Nöldecke. *Münch. med. Wschr.*, **51**, 1391 (1904).
Nottage. *Ophthal. Rec.*, **8**, 78 (1899).
Noyes. *Ophthal. Rev.*, **5**, 274 (1886).
Oeller. *Atlas d. Ophthalmoscopie*, Wiesbaden (1896).
Olehla. *Cs. Oftal.*, **10**, 190 (1954)
Oleynick. *Z. Augenheilk.*, **34**, 301 (1915).
Oliver. *Ophthal. Rec.*, **8**, 142 (1899).
Paderstein. *Klin. Mbl. Augenheilk.*, **48** (2), 105 (1910).
Papmatheakis. *Wien. klin. Wschr.*, **59**, 818 (1947).
Parsons. *Trans. ophthal. Soc. U.K.*, **36**, 69 (1916).
Payrau and Guyard. *Bull. Soc. Ophtal. Fr.*, 485 (1956).
Peleska. *Cs. Oftal.*, **7**, 292 (1951).
Pfalz. *Klin. Mbl. Augenheilk.*, **25**, 239 (1887).
Planten. *Ned. T. Geneesk.*, **96**, 94 (1952).
Pokrowsky. *Vestn. oftal.*, **22**, 5 (1943).
Post. *Ophthal. Rev.*, **15**, 311 (1896).
Power. *Trans. ophthal. Soc. U.K.*, **12**, 196 (1892).
Purtscher. *Klin. Mbl. Augenheilk.*, **102**, 844 (1939).
Reeh. *Amer. J. Ophthal.*, **31**, 336 (1948).
Remky, Kobor and Pfeiffer. *An. Inst. Barraquer*, **7**, 487 (1967).
Rémy. *Bull. Soc. Anat. Paris*, **9**, 127 (1874).
Roper-Hall. *Brit. J. Ophthal.*, **38**, 65 (1954).
Rubinstein. *Brit. J. Ophthal.*, **38**, 369 (1954).
Sacher. *Z. Augenheilk.*, **6**, 292 (1901).
Sachsalber. *Zbl. prakt. Augenheilk.*, **24**, 9 (1900).
Samelsohn. *Zbl. prakt. Augenheilk.*, **9**, 363 (1885).
Savin. *Med. Press Circ.*, **209**, 134 (1943). *Proc. roy. Soc. Med.*, **38**, 471 (1945).
Scalinci. *Progr. Ottal.*, **1**, 106 (1905).
Scheie, Rubenstein and Katowitz. *Arch. Ophthal.*, **73**, 36 (1965).
Schlichting. *Klin. Mbl. Augenheilk.*, Beil., 15 (1943).
Schneider. *Klin. Mbl. Augenheilk.*, **15**, 292 (1877).
de Schweinitz. *Ophthal. Rec.*, **9**, 387 (1900).
Sédan and Farnarier. *Bull. Soc. franç. Ophtal.*, **60**, 140 (1947).
Shapland. *Proc. roy. Soc. Med.*, **38**, 663 (1945). *Trans. ophthal. Soc. U.K.*, **66**, 371, 375, 376 (1946).
Sherman. *Amer. J. Ophthal.*, **22**, 1368 (1939).
Smith, J. W. *Arch. Ophthal.*, **39**, 390 (1948).
Smith, Priestley. *Trans. ophthal. Soc. U.K.*, **12**, 191 (1892).
Smith, V. *Int. Ophthal. Clin.*, **8**, 137 (1968).
Smyly. *Dublin J. med. Sci.*, **62**, 181 (1876).
Spierer. *Klin. Mbl. Augenheilk.*, **29**, 224 (1891).
Spratt. *Arch. Ophthal.*, **9**, 102 (1933).
Stallard. *Brit. J. Ophthal.*, **28**, 261 (1944); **31**, 12 (1947).
Steindorff. *Zbl. prakt. Augenheilk.*, **24**, 165 (1900).
Stevens. *Brit. J. Ophthal.*, **40**, 622 (1956).
Stewart. *Med. Rec.* (N.Y.), **46**, 380 (1894).
Stokes. *Arch. Ophthal.*, **19**, 205 (1938).
Sykowski. *Amer. J. Ophthal.*, **33**, 800 (1950); **35**, 1030 (1952).

von Szily. *Atlas d. Kriegsaugenheilkunde*, Stuttgart (1918).
Thorpe. *J. Amer. med. Ass.*, **127**, 197 (1945).
Amer. J. Ophthal., **61**, 1339 (1966).
Tietze. *Brit. med. J.*, **1**, 665 (1943).
Topolanski. *Wien. med. Wschr.*, **45**, 1894 (1895).
Trantas. *Bull. Soc. hellen. Ophtal.*, **7**, 166, 207 (1938).
Tromeur. *Arch. Ophtal.*, **2**, 124 (1938).
Tulloh. *Brit. J. Ophthal.*, **40**, 173 (1956).
Vail. *Trans. Amer. ophthal. Soc.*, **48**, 243 (1950).
Vannini. *Rass. ital. Ottal.*, **22**, 125 (1953).
Vigier. *Ann. Oculist.* (Paris), **137**, 126 (1907).
Villard. *Bull. Acad. méd. Paris*, **107**, 427 (1932).
Vogt. *Lhb. u. Atlas d. Spaltlampenmikroskopie d. lebenden Auges*, Berlin, **3** (1942).
Vossius. *Klin. Mbl. Augenheilk.*, **18**, 261 (1880).
Dtsch. med. Wschr., **35**, 21 (1909).
Wagenmann. *v. Graefes Arch. Ophthal.*, **44**, 272 (1897).
Ber. dtsch. ophthal. Ges., **28**, 170 (1900).
Graefe-Saemisch Hb. d. ges. Augenheilk., 3rd ed., Berlin, **2**, 1244 (1921).
Wassef. *Bull. ophthal. Soc. Egypt*, **41**, 146 (1950).
de Wecker. *Progr. méd.* (Paris), **4**, 153 (1896).
Weidmann. *Ueber die Verletzungen d. Auges durch Fremdkörper* (Diss.), Zürich (1888).
Whitehead. *Trans. ophthal. Soc. U.K.*, **36**, 63 (1916).
Wibaut. *Ned. T. Geneesk*, **2**, 1300 (1913).
Wicherkiewicz. *Klin. Mbl. Augenheilk.*, **42** (2), 559 (1904).
Wilder. *Bull. U.S. Army med. Dept.*, **4**, 9 (1945).
Trans. Amer. Acad. Ophthal., **52**, 585 (1947).
Amer. J. Ophthal., **31**, 57 (1948).
Wintersteiner. *v. Graefes Arch. Ophthal.*, **40** (2), 1 (1894).
Würdemann. *Injuries of the Eyes*, 2nd ed., London (1932).
Zander and Geissler. *Die Verletzungen des Auges*, Leipzig (1864).
Zimmermann. *Klin. Mbl. Augenheilk.*, **49** (2), 30 (1911).

Specific Effects of Retained Foreign Bodies

The reaction of the eye to a retained foreign body varies within wide limits with the composition of the particle. Some are inert and excite no specific irritation; others, which enter into combination with the tissue fluids, set up a reaction even when sterile, sometimes of great severity and occasionally purulent in type. In general terms it may be said that only if the foreign body is chemically indifferent and aseptic can it be tolerated within the eye without exciting irritation and inflammation. Moreover, as we have seen, the same foreign body in different locations in the eye excites a very different reaction—that in the anterior chamber is much less than in the posterior segment, while in the lens, owing to the torpidity of the metabolism in this tissue, particularly of its nucleus, the reaction is least of all, so that even the most virulent and chemically active particles may occasionally be retained for an indefinite time.

For descriptive purposes the ocular reaction may be of three types. In the first place, certain non-organized substances cause no specific reaction beyond the response to the mechanical irritation caused by their presence if they lie in a tissue which is wont to respond in this way to any intruder. This reaction is essentially exudative and fibroblastic in type, its function being to isolate and encapsulate the foreign body. In the second place, in addition to this exudative reaction, several non-organized materials which are not chemically indifferent but interact with the tissues of the eye set up chemical reactions which may produce non-specific or, occasionally, specific damage. In the third place, organized material tends to set up a proliferative response characterized by the formation of granulation tissue with giant cells, a completely different method of achieving isolation.

Our knowledge of these pathological reactions has been based largely on the study of clinical cases, the literature on which is now voluminous. In many cases, of course, the clinical picture is complicated by the effects of mechanical damage to the tissues, the organization of hæmorrhage and the introduction of infection, and to this extent more scientifically exact information has been obtained from experimental work on animals wherein pieces of different materials have been introduced into the eye under controlled conditions. On this subject much research has been done, all of which emanates from Leber's classical work undertaken at Leipzig, which was first communicated to the International Congress of Medicine in London in 1881, and later summarized in his monograph in 1891.

INERT SUBSTANCES

Of the chemically indifferent substances which excite no reaction within the eye, apart from that due to their mechanical presence, the most common are the chemically inert and precious metals (gold, silver, platinum, tantalum, etc.); such substances as stone, rock, sand, clay, coal and carbon; glass, quartz, porcelain and plastics; and organic materials such as rubber. In general terms the response of the ocular tissues to their introduction is non-specific and depends in its severity on their location; in the anterior chamber they lie quietly for an indefinite time without signs of irritation, but if introduced in the posterior segment, although there is little evidence of an inflammatory response, the ultimate development of degenerative changes is the rule. There is opacification, liquefaction and shrinkage of the vitreous gel, some exudative and proliferative activity in the retina which may become detached, and degenerative changes in this tissue and the optic nerve essentially characterized by an atrophy of the nervous elements and an overgrowth of neuroglia.

STONE, SAND, CLAY, CONCRETE, ETC.

The intra-ocular reaction to different types of STONE was explored experimentally by Speciale Cirincione (1907) who introduced limestone, sandstone, marble, brick and other material into the eyes of rabbits. In no case were any marked disturbances seen beyond the mechanical effects of their presence and the exudative response already noted, a negative experimental result confirmed by Choutko (1948–51). It may be that there is some difference of reaction varying with the calcium content of the material involved, but this is questionable and, in any event, is negligible, although materials such as chalk may be completely absorbed (Schnaudigel, 1916).

Clinical cases, of which there are a considerable number, bear this out, for small particles of stone may be retained without more than the usual mechanical irritative reaction, although a chronic plastic iridocyclitis is not uncommon (Plate XVIII, Fig. 1).

The early cases in the literature have been summarized by Franke (1884), Praun (1899) and Speciale Cirincione (1907), and the considerable number of cases reported in more recent years, wherein stone, sand, clay and other debris have been blown into the eye in explosions in war, reinforces the same conclusion (Löwenstein, 1916, 73 cases in 98 intra-ocular foreign bodies; von Szily, 1918; Shapland, 1946; Savin, 1946; Wilder, 1948; and many others). The subsequent history of these cases varies. In quite a number a small particle of stone in the anterior chamber, particularly if it is entangled in the iris, has remained indefinitely without apparent ill-effects (14 years, de Wecker, 1866; 19 years, Bicknell, 1899; 20 years, Knabe, 1895; 25 years, Berger, 1885; 32 years, Rieke, 1890, Jay, 1899; 54 years, Dickey, 1909); a similar long inactivity may occur if the particle is lodged in the lens, wherein a total cataract does not necessarily develop (Rademacher, 1909), and even in the vitreous cavity the exudative reaction may be small (Jacobson, 1865; Burchardt, 1895; van der Hoeve, 1918). The state of the eye, however, even in these cases is not necessarily secure, for a delayed inflammatory reaction not uncommonly occurs after many years of immunity (8 years, Mendelssohn, 1917; 12 years, Saemisch, 1865, Zirm, 1901; 13 years, Tooke, 1934; 14 years, Martin, 1876, Lindner, 1889; 17 years, Yvert, 1880; or 19 years, Friedinger, 1878). Eventually it may happen that the piece of stone is spontaneously extruded from the globe (Cooper, 1859; Jeaffreson, 1874; Kümmell, 1908).

It is to be remembered, however, that infection is frequently introduced into the eye with a particle of stone, in which case a destructive purulent reaction is to be expected; and from the clinical point of view it is noteworthy that in the ordinary accident received on chipping stone it is more frequently a fragment of iron from the hammer or chisel which reaches the eye than of the stone itself.

CONCRETE reacts similarly to stone, although irritation may be set up by its disintegration. Thus Tooke (1934) reported a case wherein a piece of concrete was retained in the anterior chamber for 13 years with recurrent attacks of iritis without serious sequelæ.

COAL AND CARBON

COAL is similarly inactive. The cases on record with this substance as an intra-ocular foreign body are few. In the anterior part of the eye the reaction is minimal—in the anterior chamber (Prokopenko, 1898); in the iris (Bock, 1907); in the lens (Knabe, 1895; Zimmermann, 1911; Castroviejo, 1931); but in the vitreous it may lead to recurrent inflammation (necessitating enucleation after 6 years (Stewart, 1894).

Particles of CARBON have been found to lie without reaction in a post-traumatic cyclitic membrane (Wilder, 1948) (Fig. 438).

GUNPOWDER, CORDITE

POWDER from firearms, which is aseptic, also forms an inert material within the eye whether, after an explosive injury, it lies upon the iris (van Lint, 1913) or the lens capsule or within the lens, wherein localized opacities may result[1]; even in the posterior segment it may cause only vitreous opacities and a localized chorioretinitis which need not impair the vision (Ballias, 1865; Wagenmann, 1901). Only when there is contamination with other foreign material which may itself be irritable or is infected does a

[1] Pooley (1871), Oliver (1892), Terson (1892), Millikin (1892), Mihalyhegyi (1946), and others.

PLATE XVIII

INERT INTRA-OCULAR FOREIGN BODIES.

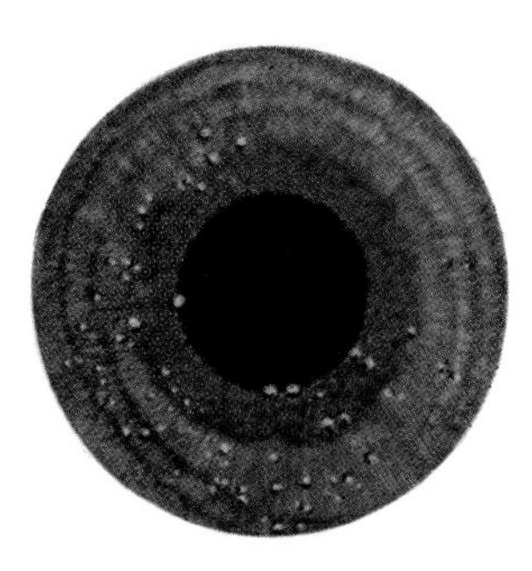

FIG. 1.—Numerous pieces of stone impacted in the iris (A. Loewenstein).

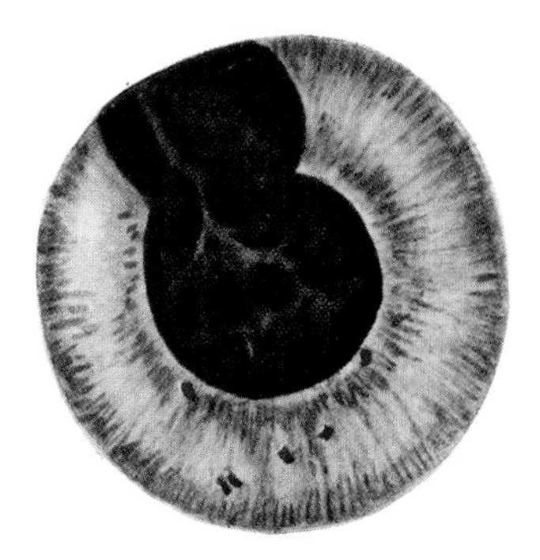

FIG. 2.—Small pieces of rubber lying on the iris, introduced 11 years previously during irrigation of the anterior chamber in a cataract operation (W. B. Doherty).

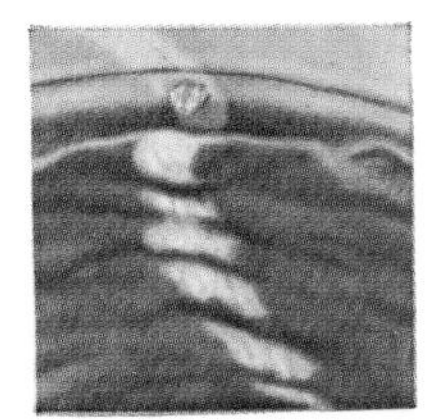

FIG. 3.

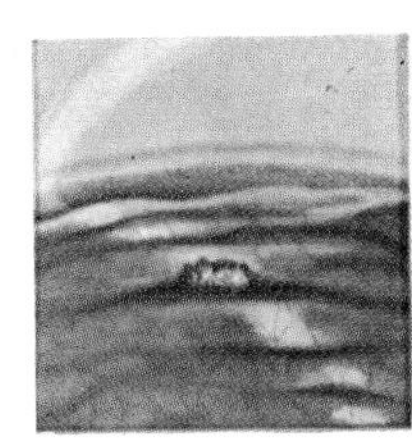

FIG. 4.

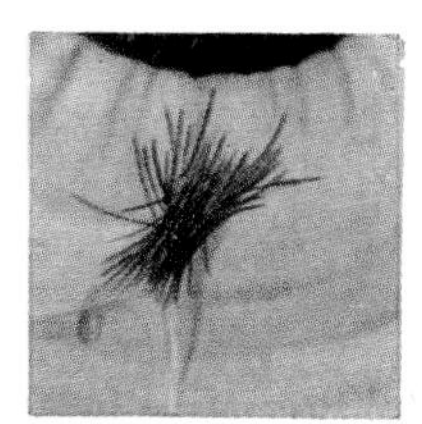

FIG. 5.

FIGS. 3 AND 4.—A foreign body entangled in the angle of the anterior chamber (Fig. 3) and near the root of the iris (Fig. 4). Gonioscopic appearance.

FIG. 5.—Pieces of silk suture left in the eye without reaction for 3 years.

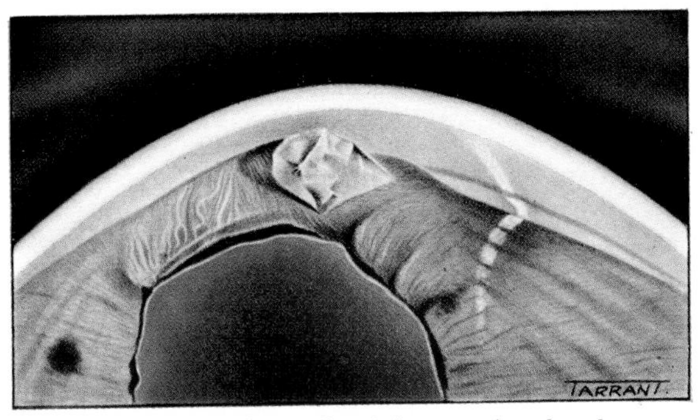

FIG. 6.—A piece of glass lying in the angle of the anterior chamber, seen gonioscopically.

destructive inflammation arise (a vitreous abscess when contaminated with vegetable material, Hirschberg, 1890). CORDITE is similarly inert, and its retention in the vitreous is also compatible with normal vision (Unsworth, 1944; Philps, 1946). In all these cases conservative treatment is indicated.

GLASS, QUARTZ, PORCELAIN AND PLASTICS

Glass, quartz and porcelain are also inert, but the response due to the presence of the foreign material is frequently intensified by the mechanical trauma produced by the sharp edges characteristic of such materials.

The quiescence of GLASS within the eye was originally verified experimentally by Leber (1881–91) whose findings were confirmed by Choutko

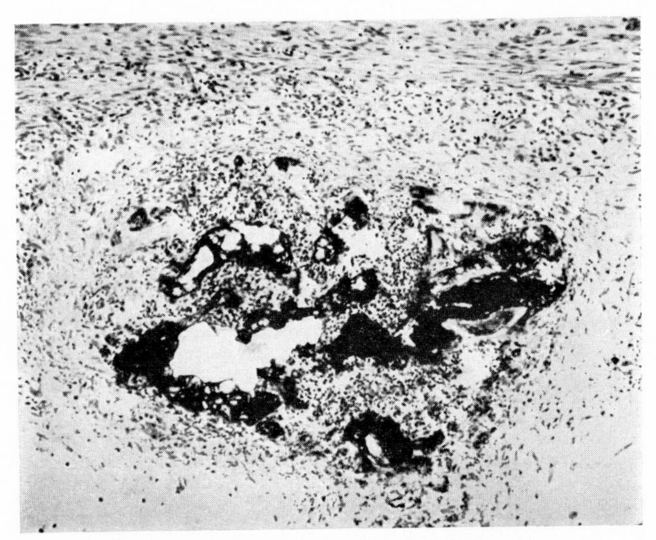

FIG. 438.—INTRA-OCULAR CARBON PARTICLES.

Carbon particles lying in the cyclitic membrane without specific or giant-cell reaction. Enucleation 6 weeks after a dynamite explosion (Helenor Wilder).

(1948–51) and Eggenschwyler (1949): this is to be expected as it is almost entirely composed of neutral sodium silicate (98%) and is thus completely inert. A large number of clinical cases has been reported. In the anterior chamber spicules of glass may remain quiet indefinitely even although they are of considerable size and multiple in number (Landmann, 1882; Bickerton, 1888; Burke, 1930; Mann, 1941; and many others) and even if the lens has been wounded (Ferguson, 1885; Claiborne, 1912–22) (Fig. 405); in a case reported by Cohen (1951), after 45 years' quiescence an implantation cyst developed at the site of the old wound. Corneal œdema is the commonest complication and may not appear until some considerable time after the injury (11 months and 20 years, Archer *et al.*, 1969); in some cases a bullous keratopathy may develop. Careful slit-lamp examination and gonioscopy after the instillation of 30% glycerol drops to clear the œdema is often required to demonstrate these foreign bodies. If it is free in the anterior chamber, however, and moves with movements of the eye, although it may occasionally do no apparent damage in its excursions (Critchett, 1857, during 16 years), it may injure the corneal endothelium, thus causing a progressive opacification of the corneal stroma which after some years may considerably reduce the vision (Wagenmann, 1900; Brandenburg, 1903; Juler, 1930); the migrations of a spicule of glass may be astonishing, for the particle may appear and disappear at intervals of weeks or months, and occasionally, if it is sharp, it may injure the lens and produce a cataract, an event which has occurred 12 years after the original injury (Gandolfi, 1947). On the other hand, if it is hiding deeply in the angle of the anterior chamber, the irritation caused to the tissues by its sharp edges may provoke repeated

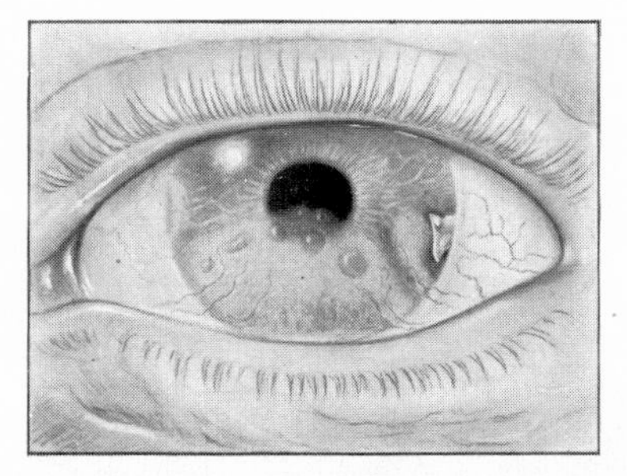

Fig. 439.—Glass in the Anterior Chamber.

A piece of glass seen near the angle of the anterior chamber at half past 3 o'clock was present for 4 years in the eye of a youth aged 17 who was involved in a laboratory explosion. There is considerable reaction with a marked bullous keratopathy (W. B. Doherty).

attacks of iridocyclitis, sometimes accompanied by corneal degeneration and bullous keratitis, an irritative condition which usually resolves rapidly on removal of the foreign body (Bruce, 1933; Summers and Hobbs, 1942; 4 years, Doherty, 1947; 13 years, Papmatheakis, 1947; 10 years, Meyer, 1957; 3 years 10 months (Fiberglas), Gaines, 1958) (Plate XVIII, Fig. 6; Fig. 439); if allowed to persist, however, such an inflammatory reaction has resulted in the development of sympathetic ophthalmitis (van der Hoeve, 1918, after 12½ years). If the piece of glass is embedded deeply in the ciliary body itself, it may occasionally be innocuous (Sweet, 1900), but frequently excites a violent iridocyclitis (Azarova, 1943). In the lens a fragment has remained in the capsule for 15 years, the lens remaining transparent and the eye free from irritation with perfect vision (Whitehead, 1916), but more usually a partial or complete cataract is formed (Post, 1896; Laqueur, 1905). In the vitreous chamber the particle may sometimes lie without exciting irritation for months or years (Grünthal, 1895; Tweedy,

1896; 28 years, Cohen, 1929); at other times the inflammatory reaction is considerable (von Graefe, 1854; Weinstein, 1908). Occasionally the glass has been extruded from the globe altogether (Azarova, 1943; Cordes, 1943; Nicolas, 1952). The occasional migration of a particle of glass has already been mentioned (Tulloh, 1956).

QUARTZ and PORCELAIN have the same effect as glass.

PLASTIC MATERIALS usually behave indifferently in the same way as glass; injuries caused by " Perspex " and other plastics have been relatively common particularly in airplanes in war, since they have been widely employed in the making of windows liable to be shattered by bullets. If no irritation is caused there is no need to extract such foreign bodies, whether of glass or of the plastic materials commonly in use. Several thermoplastic substances have been buried in the tissues of the body in surgery for many purposes, the most common of which belong to the polymethyl methacrylate group (Perspex, lucite, etc.), the polyethylene group (polythene, etc.) and the super-polyamides (nylon, etc.). It has been found, however, that their presence is rarely completely tolerated although the reaction may be slight and, even although a plastic may be a pure chemical substance, other chemicals added to it during the course of manufacture may sweat out and cause a tissue-reaction of some severity. On the other hand, the thermo-setting plastics such as bakelite and the casein plastics usually cause a violent inflammatory reaction.[1]

INDIA-RUBBER

INDIA-RUBBER has been found to remain quietly in the anterior chamber or impacted in the crypts of the iris without exciting a reaction for periods up to many years (Doherty, 1928; Brockhurst, 1952); so also have SILK strands derived from sutures (Plate XVIII, Figs. 2 and 5).

TALC

TALC POWDER (largely silica and magnesium oxide), commonly used as a dusting powder for surgical gloves, is generally considered to be an innocuous contaminant of wounds. It is interesting, however, that in a considerable number of cases minute particles have been found, when especially looked for, after surgical procedures in practically every organ of the body, including the eye; the search is aided histologically by the use of polarized light. The typical reaction to the presence of such particles is a chronic proliferative inflammation with giant cells which may go on to the formation of destructive granulomata (McCormick *et al.*, 1949; Duszynski, 1950), a reaction which has been verified experimentally in rabbits by the introduction of this material as well as modified starch powders into the anterior chamber (Chamlin, 1945; Schwartz and Linn, 1951) (Figs. 440–442).

Foreign bodies of other constitution have entered the eye so rarely as to make it difficult to form a considered judgment of their effect or analyse the difference between the reaction to the substance itself and other incidental complications, such as the degree of trauma and the introduction of infection. Such foreign bodies are varied and their effects may be surprising. Thus Sachsalber (1900) recorded that a piece of EGG-SHELL, 5 mm. long, in the anterior chamber resulted in a severe inflammation, while Dodd (1902) reported a case in which a piece of NUT-SHELL remained in the vitreous for 30 years before a deleterious effect became evident.

[1] See *Brit. med. J.*, **1**, 750 (1952), with bibliography.

FIGS. 440 to 442.—FOREIGN-BODY GRANULOMA IN THE ANGLE OF THE ANTERIOR CHAMBER (M. Chamlin).

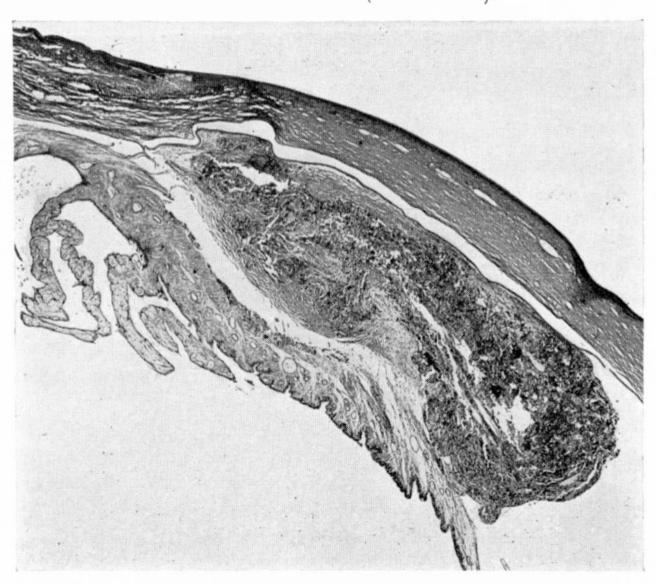

FIG. 440.—Produced in the rabbit by the injection of talc into the chamber. The large granulomatous mass is seen lying between the cornea and the iris with fibrotic adhesions to Descemet's membrane.

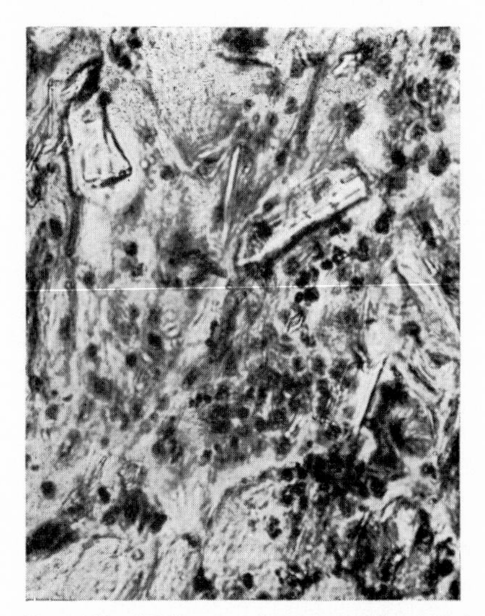

FIG. 441.—Talc crystals, seen in Fig. 440, in the foreign-body granuloma in the anterior chamber surrounded by polymorphonuclear cells.

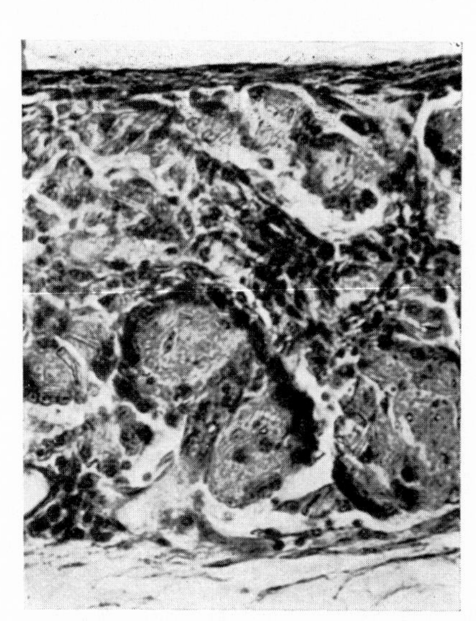

FIG. 442.—Foreign-body granuloma in the orbit caused by an injection of talc. The large multinucleated foreign-body giant cells are very obvious with disintegrated talc within them.

Archer, Davies and Kanski. *Brit. J. Ophthal.*, **53**, 453 (1969).
Azarova. *Vestn. oftal.*, **22**, 38 (1943).
Ballias. *Des corps étrangers du corps vitré* (Thèse), Paris (1865).
Berger. *Wien. med. Blätter*, No. 6, 161 (1885).
Bickerton. *Brit. med. J.*, **1**, 896 (1888).
Bicknell. *Ophthal. Rec.*, **8**, 337 (1899).
Bock. *Zbl. prakt. Augenheilk.*, **31**, 65 (1907).
Brandenburg. *Klin. Mbl. Augenheilk.*, **41** (2), 142 (1903).
Brockhurst. *Arch. Ophthal.*, **47**, 465 (1952).
Bruce. *Arch. Ophthal.*, **10**, 615 (1933).
Burchardt. *Charité Ann.*, **19**, 244 (1895).
Burke. *Trans. Amer. ophthal. Soc.*, **28**, 53 (1930).
Castroviejo. *Amer. J. Ophthal.*, **14**, 537 (1931).
Chamlin. *Arch. Ophthal.*, **34**, 369 (1945).
Choutko. *Vestn. oftal.*, **27** (2), 12 (1948); **30** (4), 37 (1951).
Claiborne. *Ophthal. Rec.*, **21**, 491 (1912).
Amer. J. Surg., **36**, 228 (1922).
Cohen. *Arch. Ophthal.*, **1**, 528 (1929); **45**, 413 (1951).
Cooper. *Injuries of the Eye*, London (1859).
Cordes. *Amer. J. Ophthal.*, **26**, 1062 (1943).
Critchett. *Roy. Lond. ophthal. Hosp. Rep.*, **1**, 264 (1857).
Dickey. *West Virgin. med. J.*, **4**, 91 (1909).
Dodd. *Ophthal. Rec.*, **11**, 220 (1902).
Doherty. *Amer. J. Ophthal.*, **11**, 16 (1928); **30**, 177 (1947).
Duszynski. *Trans. Amer. Acad. Ophthal.*, **55**, 110 (1950).
Eggenschwyler. *Z. Unfallmed. Berufsk.*, **42**, 287 (1949).
Ferguson. *Ophthal. Rev.*, **4**, 293 (1885).
Franke. *v. Graefes Arch. Ophthal.*, **30** (1), 211 (1884).
Friedinger. *Wien. med. Wschr.*, **28**, 352 (1878).
Gaines. *Arch. Ophthal.*, **60**, 941 (1958).
Gandolfi. *Atti Soc. Oftal. Lombarda*, **2**, 328 (1947).
von Graefe. *v. Graefes Arch. Ophthal.*, **1** (1), 405 (1854).
Grünthal. *Berl. klin. Wschr.*, **32**, 78 (1895).
Hirschberg. *Zbl. prakt. Augenheilk.*, **14**, 8 (1890).
van der Hoeve. *Z. Augenheilk.*, **39**, 20 (1918).
Jacobson. *v. Graefes Arch. Ophthal.*, **11** (1), 129 (1865).
Jay. *Ophthal. Rec.*, **8**, 233 (1899).
Jeaffreson. *Med. Times Gaz.*, **1**, 340 (1874).
Juler. *Trans. ophthal. Soc. U.K.*, **50**, 118 (1930).
Knabe. *Beiträge z. Statistik u. Kasuistik d. Augenverletzungen* (Diss.), Halle (1895).
Kümmell. *Z. Augenheilk.*, **19**, 36 (1908).
Landmann. *v. Graefes Arch. Ophthal.*, **28** (2), 153 (1882).
Laqueur. *Arch. Augenheilk.*, **53**, 97 (1905).
Leber. *Proc. VII int. Med. Cong.*, London, **3**, 15 (1881).
v. Graefes Arch. Ophthal., **28** (2), 237 (1882); **30** (1), 243 (1884).
Die Entstehung. d. Entzündung, Leipzig (1891).
Lindner. *Wien. med. Wschr.*, **39**, 1433, 1479 (1889).
van Lint. *Clin. Ophtal.*, **5**, 564 (1913).
Löwenstein. *Ber. dtsch. ophthal. Ges.*, **40**, 313 (1916).
McCormick, Macaulay and Miller. *Amer. J. Ophthal.*, **32**, 1252 (1949).
Mann. *Trans. ophthal. Soc. U.K.*, **61**, 58 (1941).
Martin. *Recueil Ophtal.*, **3**, 328 (1876).
Mendelssohn. *Zwei Fälle von Fremdkörperverletzung in d. vorderen Kammer d. Auges* (Diss.), Heidelberg (1917).
Meyer. *Klin. Mbl. Augenheilk.*, **130**, 59 (1957).
Mihalyhegyi. *Ophthalmologica*, **109**, 159 (1946).
Millikin. *Ophthal. Rev.*, **11**, 285 (1892).
Nicolas. *Bull. Soc. Ophtal. Fr.*, 834 (1952).
Oliver. *Trans. Amer. ophthal. Soc.*, **6**, 323 (1892).
Papmatheakis. *Wien. klin. Wschr.*, **59**, 818 (1947).
Philps. *Trans. ophthal. Soc. U.K.*, **66**, 371 (1946).
Pooley. *N.Y. med. J.*, **14**, 237 (1871).
Post. *Ophthal. Rev.*, **15**, 311 (1896).
Praun. *Die Verletzungen d. Auges*, Wiesbaden (1899).
Prokopenko. *Vestn. oftal.*, **15**, 369 (1898).
Rademacher. *Ueber einige seltene Fremdkörperverletzungen im vorderer Augenabschnitt* (Diss.), Jena (1909).
Rieke. *Klin. Mbl. Augenheilk.*, **28**, 375 (1890).
Sachsalber. *Zbl. prakt. Augenheilk.*, **24**, 9 (1900).
Saemisch. *Klin. Mbl. Augenheilk.*, **3**, 46 (1865).
Savin. *Trans. ophthal. Soc. U.K.*, **66**, 379 (1946).
Schnaudigel. *Ber. dtsch. ophthal. Ges.*, **40**, 130 (1916).
Schwartz and Linn. *Amer. J. Ophthal.*, **34**, 585 (1951).
Shapland. *Trans. ophthal. Soc. U.K.*, **66**, 371, 375 (1946).
Speciale Cirincione. *Z. Augenheilk.*, **17**, 143 (1907).
Stewart. *Med. Rec.* (*N.Y.*), **46**, 380 (1894).
Summers and Hobbs. *Brit. J. Ophthal.*, **26**, 54 (1942).
Sweet. *Ophthal. Rec.*, **9**, 627 (1900).
von Szily. *Atlas d. Kriegsaugenheilkunde*, Stuttgart (1918).
Terson. *Arch. Ophtal.*, **12**, 156 (1892).
Tooke. *Brit. J. Ophthal.*, **18**, 695 (1934).
Tulloh. *Brit. J. Ophthal.*, **40**, 173 (1956).
Tweedy. *Trans. ophthal. Soc. U.K.*, **16**, 360 (1896).
Unsworth. *Arch. Ophthal.*, **32**, 414 (1944).
Wagenmann. *Korresp.-Bl. allg. ärztl. Vereins v. Thuringen*, No. 1 (1900).
Ophthal. Klin., **5**, 129 (1901).
de Wecker. *Gaz. Hôp.* (Paris), **39**, 363 (1866).

Weinstein. *Klin. Mbl. Augenheilk.*, **46** (1), 204 (1908).
Whitehead. *Trans. ophthal. Soc. U.K.*, **36,** 63 (1916).
Wilder. *Amer. J. Ophthal.*, **31,** 57 (1948).
Yvert. *Traité prat. et clin. des blessures de globe de l'oeil*, Paris, 89 (1880).
Zimmermann. *Klin. Mbl. Augenheilk.*, **49** (2), 30 (1911).
Zirm. *Zbl. prakt. Augenheilk.*, **25,** 86 (1901).

THE INERT METALS

Leber (1881–91) found that a piece of GOLD WIRE, 2 cm. long, remained without reaction for 269 days in the anterior chamber of the rabbit, but that the degenerative changes already described followed the introduction of such a foreign body into the vitreous cavity; Savin (1947) found PLATINUM wire similarly inactive. The few clinical cases which have been reported wherein a foreign body of this type has been retained within the eye conform to this picture, although in those cases wherein the pure metal has been contaminated by other elements, such as copper or zinc, a considerable amount of irritation may follow their introduction into the globe (gold, Wardrop, 1826; Stellwag, 1853; silver, Kipp, 1884; and others). The lack of reaction on the introduction of such metals as gold and tantalum after the manner of a seton in an attempt to ensure permanent drainage in recalcitrant cases of glaucoma is evidence of this inactivity in the anterior segment of the eye (Weekers, 1922; Stefansson, 1925; Harbridge, 1950; and others).

THE IRRITATIVE METALS

LEAD

Apart from the precious metals we have just discussed, lead is the most inert of the metals which commonly form intra-ocular foreign bodies; this is presumably because it is rapidly covered with a layer of insoluble carbonate which prevents diffusion and any chemical reactivity. In the anterior chamber there are few reactive changes, in the lens there are none, and in the vitreous the sequence of events follows closely those found with completely inert substances—liquefaction and opacification of the gel, exudative changes in which the metal may become encapsulated, and retinal degeneration involving atrophy of the neural and overgrowth of the neuroglial elements. If the metal lies in the retina or choroid, however, there is usually an exudation, partly fibrinous and partly purulent, with a considerable amount of connective-tissue reaction.

Experimental studies on the action of lead on the eye have been thoroughly undertaken by several investigators.[1] Clinically the most common foreign bodies are shot-pellets from sporting rifles and fragments of the metal derived from bullets and other missiles in war. In the anterior chamber, whether lying freely or impacted on the surface of the iris, such bodies may remain for a long time without causing inflammatory symptoms.[2] In the posterior segment, also, small pieces may remain indefinitely without exciting much tissue-reaction even although they are multiple[3]; on the other hand, the reaction may be considerable and on enucleation it may be found that the

[1] Leber (1881–91), Rolland (1887), Tornatola (1894), Ovio (1895), Valois (1902), Okabe (1931), and others.
[2] Gotti (1892), Handmann (1915), Böhm (1916), Winkler (1919).
[3] Schneider (1877, 2 years), Uhthoff (1916), Schlichting (1943), and others.

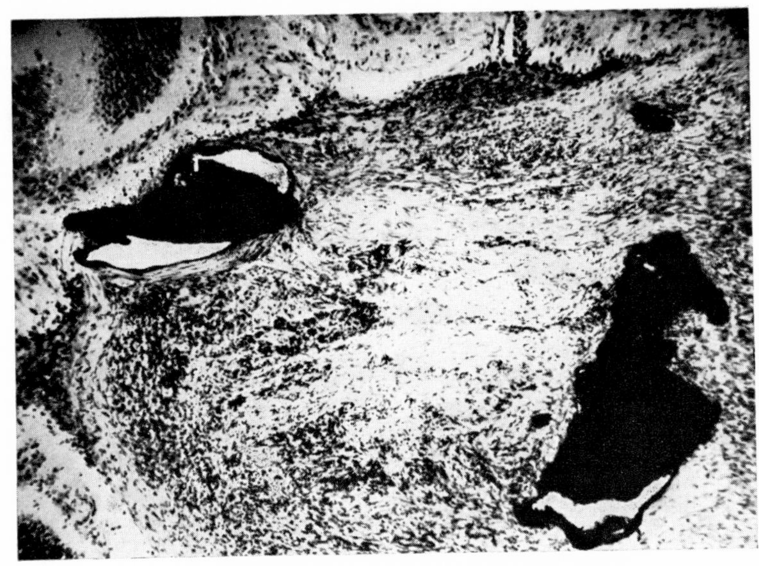

FIG. 443.—INTRA-OCULAR LEAD.

Lead lying in inflammatory tissue in the vitreous chamber. Enucleation 5 months after injury (Helenor Wilder).

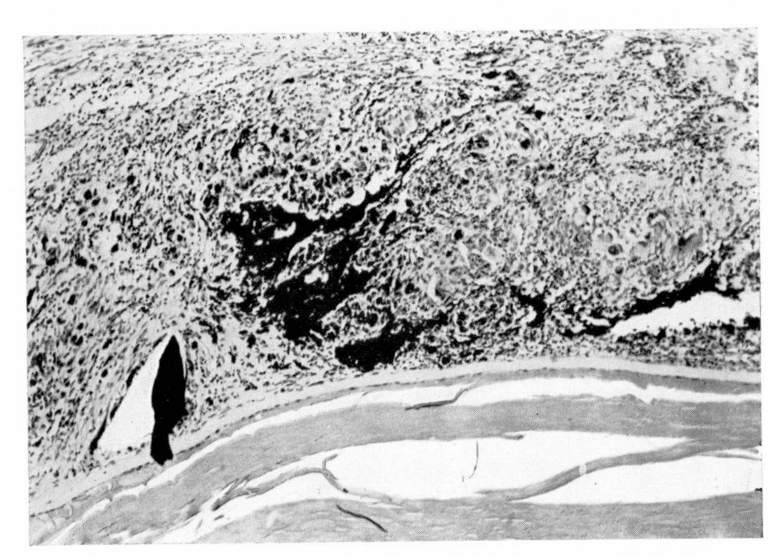

FIG. 444.—SYMPATHETIC OPHTHALMITIS CAUSED BY A LEAD INTRA-OCULAR FOREIGN BODY.

The lead foreign body is in the iris. There is well developed sympathetic uveitis with a granulomatous inflammation of the iris and the whole uveal tract with posterior synechiæ. Enucleation 2 months after injury (Helenor Wilder).

particle of lead lies in a mass of inflammatory tissue of a non-specific exudative type[1] (Fig. 443). It is to be remembered that shot-pellets may migrate after some time from one part of the eye to another, as from the posterior segment into the anterior chamber (Kümmell, 1908, after $1\frac{1}{4}$ years; Kauders, 1909, after 25 years; Hinken, 1965, after 1 year), and sympathetic ophthalmitis may follow the retention of lead foreign bodies (Wilder, 1948) (Fig. 444).

As would be expected, SOLDER (two-thirds lead, one-third tin) is completely inert as an intra-ocular foreign body (Kamel, 1949).

ZINC

ZINC, somewhat like lead, has a slight reaction if retained within the eye, provided it is pure and sterile, a change which becomes particularly evident in the posterior segment where the typical inflammatory exudation is accompanied by some degree of retinal atrophy. This has been shown experimentally in rabbits by Leber (1881–91) and Vollert (1898). Clinical cases have been few. Ginestous (1912) reported a case wherein a particle of zinc lodged in the lens; Lauber (1913) a second wherein the metal was impacted in the retina; and Vollert (1898), a case wherein a particle in the vitreous was heavily enshrouded in exudation and fibrous tissue in an eye in which the vision progressively deteriorated. Shipman (1949), on the other hand, observed a foreign body of zinc which remained embedded in the retina for 16 years without giving evidence of irritation.

NICKEL

Particles of NICKEL in the posterior segment of the eye produce a purulent inflammation which results in widespread degeneration of the neural elements of the retina. Ultimately, however, the particle of nickel tends to become encapsulated with a firm coating of connective tissue (Okabe, 1931).

ALUMINIUM

As would be expected, the history of ALUMINIUM as an intra-ocular foreign body is shorter than that of most other metals, for the first clinical references to the possibility of such an occurrence date from the first World War (Weigelin, 1917; Cords, 1917; Hertel, 1924). Experimental findings are somewhat contradictory. Among the several observers who have introduced fragments of the metal into the eyes of rabbits, Jess (1924), Fontana (1938), Mielke (1941) and Celotti (1947) found few resulting effects, but Savin (1947), using larger implants and carrying out his observations over a longer period, found a considerable reaction which applied without significant difference to aluminium and its various alloys.

As a rule, within the first few days or weeks after implantation, the metal was observed to become coated with a white crust of powder and sometimes was partially encased in exudate. This tendency to disintegration increased until, after about six weeks, the pieces of aluminium began to fragment and occasionally showed complete absorption. Wherever the

[1] Salva (1909), Oguchi (1913), Weigelin (1917), von Szily (1918), Winkler (1919) and Wilder (1948).

PLATE XIX

ALUMINIUM IN THE EYE OF THE RABBIT.

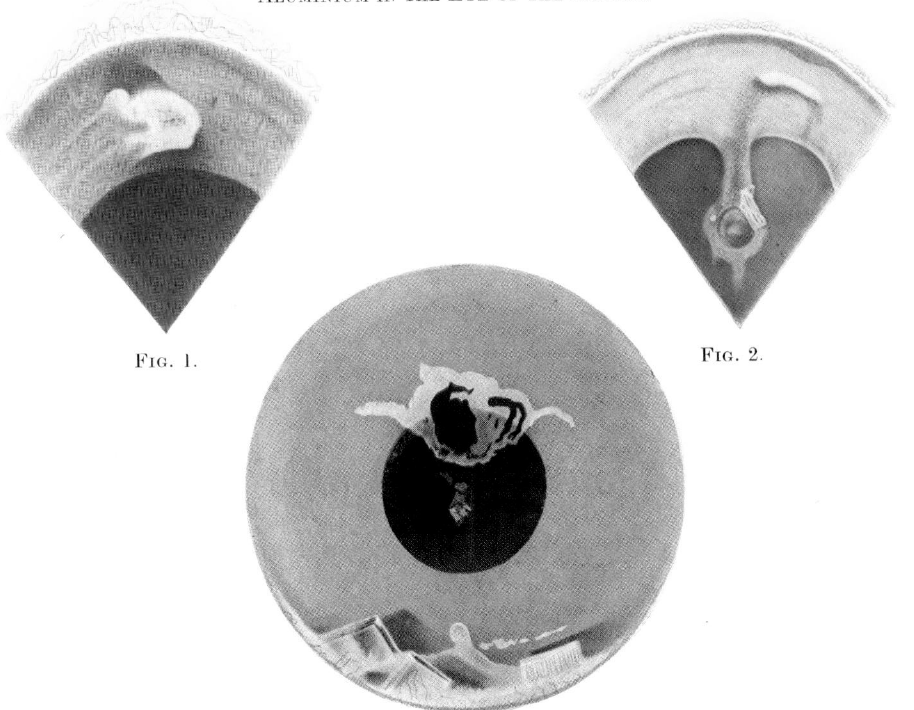

FIG. 1.

FIG. 2.

FIG. 3.

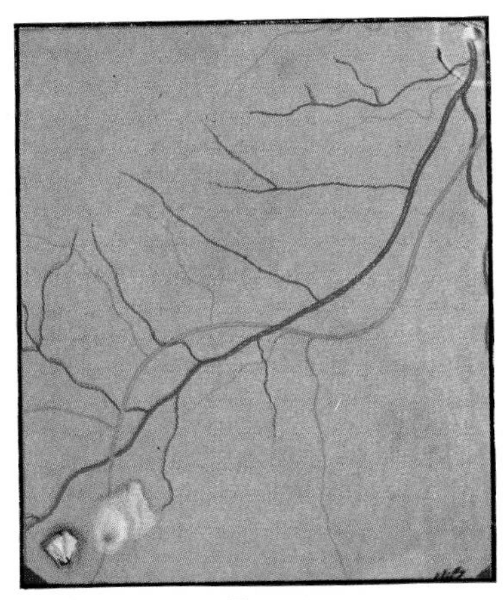

FIG. 4.

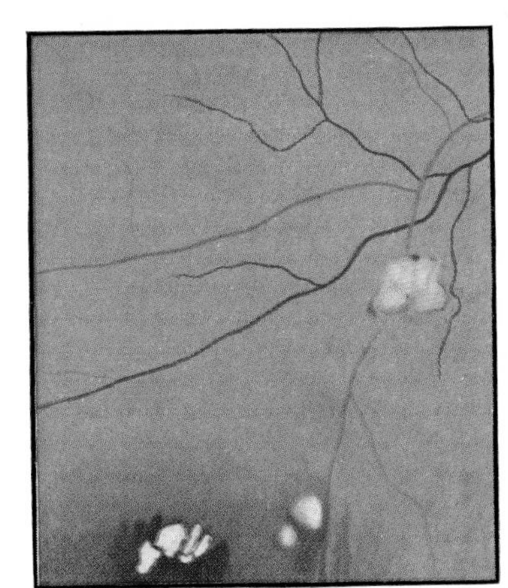

FIG. 5.

FIGS. 1 AND 2.—5 months after insertion. An iris imprint with small fragments of powdered metal.

FIG. 2.—The fragment partly absorbed and coated white had fallen from the iris upon the anterior lens capsule producing an opacity.

FIG. 3.—10 months later. Pieces of metal covered with exudate in the angle of the A.C. where the cornea is vascularized. A central corneal " imprint " is seen.

FIG. 4.—11 months after injury. The fragment is seen with an " imprint " indicating its previous site just above it.

FIG. 5.—The same eye 14 months later. The foreign body has shifted twice further down in the retina so that two imprints are seen. The fragment itself (lower left corner) is seen to be breaking up into powdery white debris (L. H. Savin).

metal was in contact with tissue, whether it was the posterior surface of the cornea, the iris or the fundus, there tended to develop a grey necrotic imprint where the powdery metal bespattered an atrophic area. General effects in the eye included the occurrence of lenticular opacities, sometimes striate, sometimes punctate and often irregular, and occasionally accompanied by a polychromatic lustre. Quiet inflammatory changes were frequently present in the uveal tract, the uveitis being milder if the metal were in the anterior than if it were in the posterior segment, and these were followed by degenerative changes (Plate XIX). Experimentally in rabbits the ERG has been found to be reduced (Knave, 1970).

Clinical cases are few and in general show less changes than are apparent in animal experiments. Similar powdering and fragmentation of the metal have been observed with the production of corneal opacification and iridocyclitis if it were in the anterior chamber,[1] and localized imprints with pigmentary degeneration associated with vitreous opacities and mild iridocyclitis if the metal were in the posterior segment (Savin, 1947). On the other hand, a number of cases has been reported wherein the tolerance of the eye has been good (Bellows, 1947) even although observation has been continued for periods up to six (Marisi, 1950) or twelve years (May, 1957).

MERCURY

MERCURY tends to excite an active purulent inflammation in the eye whether it lies in the anterior chamber or the posterior segment; in the latter, Leber (1881–91) found experimentally that phthisis bulbi rapidly developed. The reaction is analogous to the necrosis which occurs in the cornea after mercury, its yellow oxide or calomel is injected into this tissue. Clinical cases involving mercury as a foreign body have been rare and have resulted from explosions. Such a case was reported by Gifford (1942): the explosion of a neon light shattered a man's spectacles, the glass from which penetrated the anterior chamber carrying with it three globules of mercury from the lamp; the subsequent inflammation proved intractable to treatment. Wagenmann (1907) also observed that the presence of mercury as a foreign body excited a severe purulent inflammation in the vitreous cavity for which enucleation was necessary, but Fujita (1913) found a globule of pure mercury encysted in fibrous tissue 14 years after the explosion of a mine.

Bellows. *Amer. J. Ophthal.*, **30**, 309 (1947).
Böhm. *Klin. Mbl. Augenheilk.*, **57**, 82 (1916).
Celotti. *Atti Soc. Oftal. Lombarda*, **2**, 13 (1947).
Cords. *Z. Augenheilk.*, **37**, 67 (1917).
Fontana. *Rass. ital. Ottal.*, **7**, 695 (1938).
Fricke. *Klin. Mbl. Augenheilk.*, **74**, 209 (1925).
Fujita. *Arch. Augenheilk.*, **75**, 99 (1913).
Gifford. *Trans. Amer. ophthal. Soc.*, **40**, 259 (1942).
Ginestous. *Ophtal. Provinc.*, **9**, 149 (1912).
Gotti. *Recueil Ophtal.*, **14**, 445 (1892).
Handmann. *Z. Augenheilk.*, **34**, 81 (1915).
Harbridge. *Trans. Amer. ophthal. Soc.*, **48**, 256 (1950).
Hertel. *Hb. d. ärztl. Erfahrungen im Weltkrieg 1914–18*, Leipzig, **5**, 364 (1924).
Hesky. *Boll. Oculist.*, **12**, 832 (1933).
Hinken. *Arch. Ophthal.*, **74**, 485 (1965).
Jess. *Klin. Mbl. Augenheilk.*, **72**, 133 (1924).
Ber. dtsch. ophthal. Ges., **53**, 122 (1940).
Kamel. *Bull. ophthal. Soc. Egypt*, **42**, 285 (1949).
Kauders. *Wien. med. Wschr.*, **59**, 255 (1909).
Kipp. *Amer. J. Ophthal.*, **1**, 103 (1884).
Knave. *Acta ophthal.* (Kbh.), **48**, 159 (1970).
Kümmell. *Z. Augenheilk.*, **19**, 36 (1908).
Lauber. *Klin. Mbl. Augenheilk.*, **51** (1), 239 (1913).
Leber. *Proc. VII int. Cong. Med.*, London, **3**, 15 (1881).

[1] Jess (1924–40), Fricke (1925), Hesky (1933), Stock (1940), Schlichting (1943).

v. *Graefes Arch. Ophthal.*, **28** (2), 237 (1882); **30** (1), 243 (1884).
Die Entstehung d. Entzündung, Leipzig (1891).
Marisi. *Boll. Oculist.*, **29**, 661 (1950).
May. *Brit. J. Ophthal.*, **41**, 574 (1957).
Mielke. *Dtsch. med. Wschr.*, **67**, 350 (1941).
Oguchi. *Beitr. Augenheilk.*, **9** (83), 75 (1913).
Okabe. *Acta Soc. ophthal. jap.*, **35**, 1092 (1931).
Ovio. *Ann. Ottal.*, **24**, Suppl. 14 (1895).
Rolland. *Recueil Ophtal.*, **9**, 530 (1887).
Salva. *Clin. Ophtal.*, **15**, 373 (1909).
Savin. *Brit. J. Ophthal.*, **31**, 449 (1947).
Schlichting. *Klin. Mbl. Augenheilk.*, Beih., 15 (1943).
Schneider. *Klin. Mbl. Augenheilk.*, **15**, 292 (1877).
Shipman. *Amer. J. Ophthal.*, **32**, 815 (1949).
Stefansson. *Amer. J. Ophthal.*, **8**, 681 (1925).
Stellwag. *Die Ophthalmologie v. naturwiss. Standpunkte*, Freiburg, **1**, 327 (1853).
Stock. *Ber. dtsch. ophthal. Ges.*, **53**, 123 (1940).
von Szily. *Atlas d. Kriegsaugenheilkunde*, Stuttgart (1918).
Tornatola. *Rev. gén. Ophtal.*, **13**, 206 (1894).
Uhthoff. *Berl. klin. Wschr.*, **53**, 5 (1916).
Valois. *Recueil Ophtal.*, **24**, 401, 475 (1902).
Vollert. *v. Graefes Arch. Ophthal.*, **46**, 656 (1898).
Wagenmann. *Ber. dtsch. ophthal. Ges.*, **34**, 272 (1907).
Wardrop. *Lancet*, **10**, 475 (1826).
Weekers. *Arch. Ophtal.*, **39**, 279 (1922).
Weigelin. *Klin. Mbl. Augenheilk.*, **59**, 84 (1917).
Wilder. *Amer. J. Ophthal.*, **31**, 57 (1948).
Winkler. *Z. Augenheilk.*, **41**, 60 (1919).

COPPER

COPPER, as well as its alloys which are rich in this metal such as brass and bronze, has frequently been found in the eye as a foreign body, the particle usually being derived from a percussion-cap shattered by an explosion but occasionally arising from the retention of a piece of copper wire or other material in the globe. In British industry foreign bodies composed of brass used to constitute about 4% of the total (Whitehead, 1916). Exceptionally a bilateral injury of this type has been reported (a piece of copper lying on each iris, Granström, 1949).

As with other foreign bodies, unusual cases arise such as that reported by Berendes (1907), which followed a blow with a whip-lash loaded with pieces of copper wire whereof one, 19 mm. long, remained for five months in the eye with its anterior end lying at the inner corneal surface and its posterior end protruding through the globe into the orbital fat. Jess (1918) reported a somewhat similar case with telephone wire.

Within the eye the metal excites a reaction which varies very widely with the degree to which the pure metal is combined with other materials to form alloys. If it is present in a relatively pure state the reaction (with somewhat curiously inexplicable exceptions) is turbulent in type, suppurative in nature and catastrophic in its consequences; if, on the other hand, it is present in the form of a dilute alloy containing less than 85% of copper, the virulence of the immediate reaction is less, but the metal tends to be disseminated and deposited widely throughout the tissues of the eye, producing the characteristic picture of CHALCOSIS, the prognosis in this case being much less gloomy. In view of the fact that scarcity of the metal in the last few decades has stimulated the widespread use of alloys, it follows that the reports in the earlier literature are largely a record of disaster, while in more recent years the less acute changes of chalcosis have been more common.

Experimental observations on the effects of *copper in a relatively pure state* as an intra-ocular foreign body were first conducted in rabbits by

Leber (1891), whose researches were followed by many others.[1] Leber established the fact that the reaction was much more intense following the insertion of pure copper than when a copper alloy was used. Whether the former is inserted into the anterior chamber or the posterior segment the result is essentially the same: even in experiments conducted aseptically the immediate reaction is one of a violent uveitis with profuse leucocytosis and the rapid accumulation of pus. This is the result of chemical irritation and is not progressive, so that instead of resulting in a perforation of the globe as occurs normally in pyogenic infections, the suppuration is self-limited and tends to result in phthisis bulbi. In the anterior chamber this reaction becomes evident as an acute iridocyclitis with a hypopyon; in the posterior segment it leads to shrinkage of the vitreous, detachment and degeneration of the retina and rapid phthisis; only when the foreign body

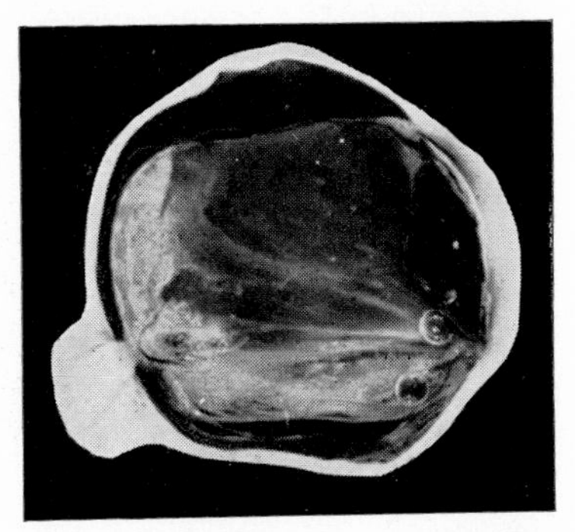

FIG. 445.—PERFORATION OF THE EYE BY A COPPER FOREIGN BODY WHICH LODGED UPON THE DISC.

The eye shows the early stages of panophthalmitis (Museum, Inst. Ophthal.).

is embedded in the lens is the intense leucocytosis absent, but a partia cataract, sometimes associated with a dull yellowish coloration of the surrounding lens substance, is the most frequent result.

Clinical experiences confirming this violent response of the eye to relatively pure particles of copper are numerous. In general terms, in the anterior chamber the same picture of acute iridocyclitis with hypopyon tends to develop. In the posterior segment detachment of the retina, abscesses in the choroid and phthisis bulbi are the rule, but in the lens the leucocytic reaction is absent and a partial or complete traumatic cataract tends to develop.

The early clinical literature has been summarized by Franke (1884), Praun (1899) and Plitt (1906). Hornstein (1905) discussed 66 cases (57 of copper and 9 of brass) observed at the Tübingen clinic, many of the injuries being inflicted on young children

[1] Denig (1896), on brass, Schmidt (1898), Bär (1923), Loddoni (1929), Sená (1930), Okabe (1931), Duc (1936), Sala and Borsellino (1936), Takahaschi (1936), Fontana (1938), Mielke (1940), Newell *et al.* (1949) and Tichomirov (1950).

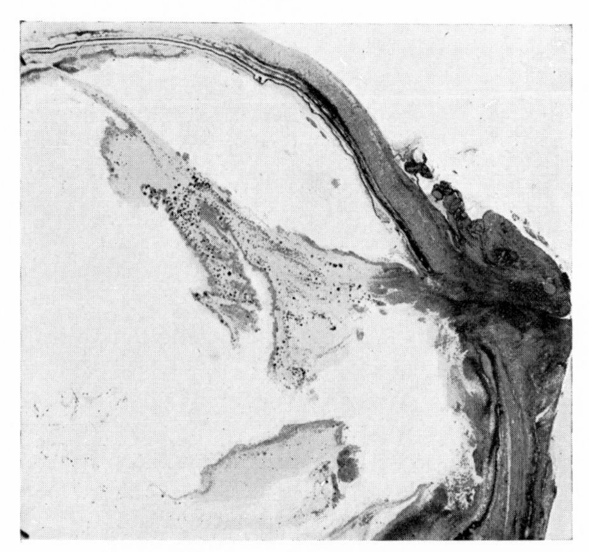

Fig. 446.—Early Suppuration with a Copper Intra-ocular Foreign Body.

The sclera was perforated by a copper fragment which lodged in the vitreous. Colonies of cocci are seen in a vitreous abscess. Enucleation 2 weeks after the explosion of a dynamite cap (Helenor Wilder).

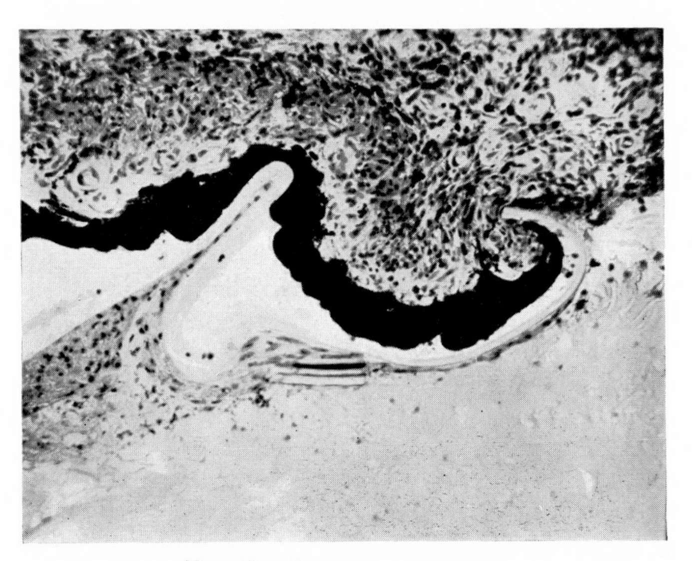

Fig. 447.—Intra-ocular Copper.

The beginning of the inflammatory reaction. A piece of copper wire is embedded in an early anterior capsular cataract. The lens capsule has recoiled outwards at the site of entrance. There is iridocyclitis with posterior synechiæ. Enucleation 6 days after injury (Helenor Wilder).

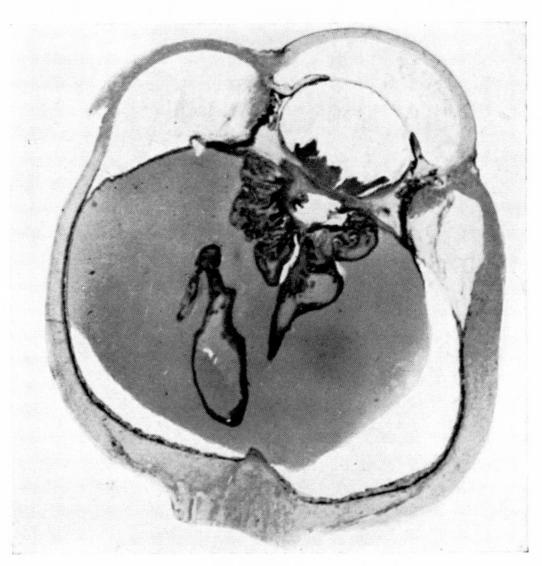

FIG. 448.—INTRA-OCULAR COPPER.

A later stage of intra-ocular suppuration. There is a vitreous abscess at the site of a brass foreign body and detachment of the retina by a pyogenic cyclitic membrane. Early phthisis bulbi. Enucleation 2 weeks after injury (Helenor Wilder).

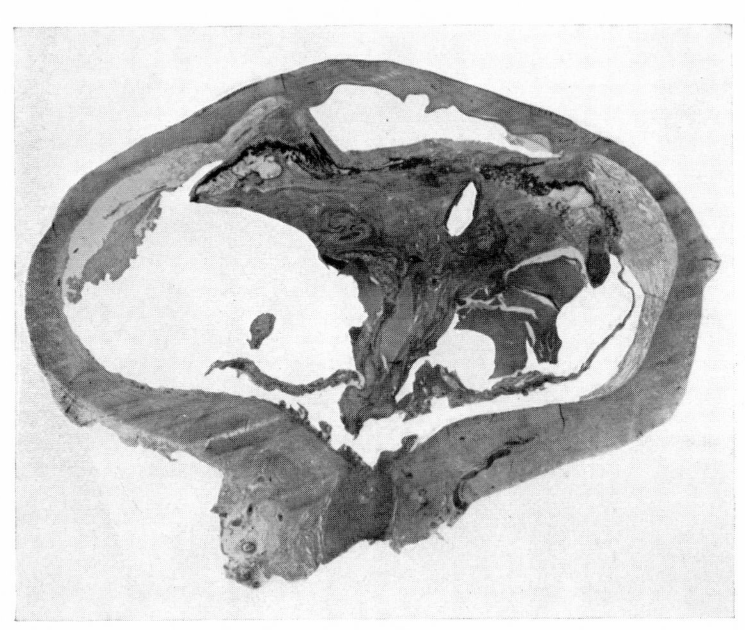

FIG. 449.—THE SUPPURATIVE EFFECTS OF A PURE COPPER INTRA-OCULAR FOREIGN BODY.

The globe is shrunken and degenerate and the lens is missing. The totally detached retina is folded and adherent to a dense cyclitic membrane within which two copper foreign bodies were embedded. Perls's reaction for copper showed evidence of chalcosis involving the tissue immediately surrounding the foreign body (H. and E.) (N. Ashton).

FIGS. 450 and 451.—A COPPER FOREIGN BODY WITHIN THE EYE
(J. Mishler and R. Harley).

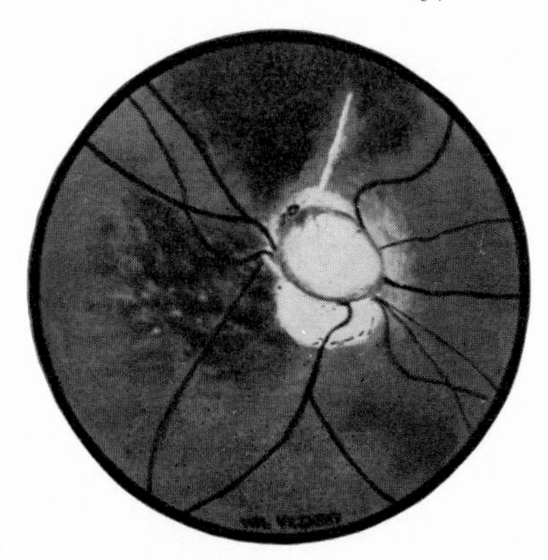

FIG. 450.—The encapsulation of a piece of a percussion cap, assumed to be 85% copper, after 30 years' retention in the eye. In the final 8 months' period of observation the lesion simulated a growing intra-ocular tumour, 2·5 mm. in diameter, adjacent to and partly overlapping the nerve-head, to the extent of 5 to 6 dioptres. The optic nerve was atrophic but there was no demonstrable evidence of chalcosis.

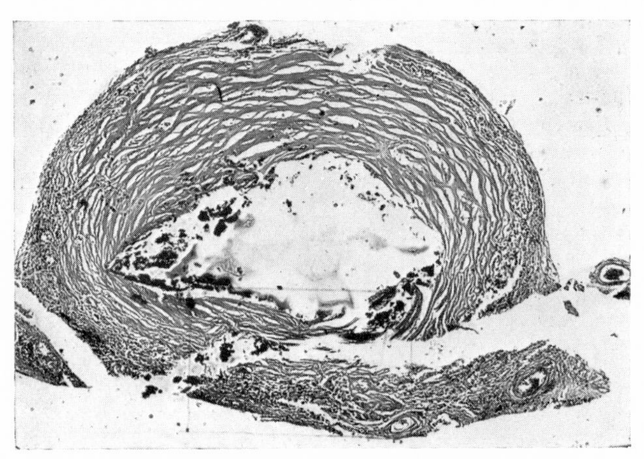

FIG. 451.—The encapsulated mass in a choroidal scar, containing the foreign body (1 mm. in diameter) which dropped out of the section.

owing to explosions; later cases were described by von Hippel (1912), van der Hoeve (1913) and Jacqueau (1913). After this period and during the first World War the extensive use of alloys containing less amounts of copper began to change the clinical picture.

Pathological studies are equally numerous.[1] The pathological picture is typical and characteristic: necrosis of the tissues in the region of the foreign body is frequently rapid; occasionally the particle is quickly encapsulated, sometimes with the formation

[1] Berlin (1867–68), Reuling (1881), Kostenitsch (1891), Hirschberg (1894), Wagenmann (1896–97), Schmidt (1898), Stein (1902), Bär (1903), Greeff (1905), Hornstein (1905), Hahn (1907), Blascheck (1903), Berendes (1907), Cohen (1908), Posern (1913), Maas (1917), Weigelin (1917), von Szily (1918), Winkler (1919), and others.

of a localized abscess; more usually, however, the reaction is more widespread and the intense leucocytosis forms large quantities of pus, sometimes golden-brown in colour, and the subsequent fibrosis is considerable in extent and dense in consistency (Figs. 445–449). Occasionally masses of granulation and fibrous tissue appear which after a long period may assume massive proportions and even simulate an intra-ocular tumour (after 12 years, Velhagen, 1930; after 30 years, Mishler and Harley, 1952) (Figs. 450–451). There is much retinal degeneration and even necrosis, while in the cases of longest duration calcareous and bony changes may be seen in the phthisical globe (Bruns, 1897; Hahn, 1907). Experimentally in rabbits the ERG has been found to be reduced (Knave, 1970).

The clinical picture, if the particle is in the anterior chamber, is typical of an acute iridocyclitis with hypopyon, the virulence of which is sometimes indicated by the development of an associated toxic papillitis (Franke, 1901); only occasionally is a granulomatous reaction seen (Bocchi, 1910). In the posterior segment a similar reaction occurs, sometimes associated with localized abscesses in the choroid (Cohen, 1908; Neubauer and Heimann, 1968). In the lens, although the usual result has been a total cataract, the particle of copper may remain quietly for a very long time, causing only a localized opacity.[1]

Occasionally, however, anomalous reactions occur. Sometimes there is little or no disturbance in the eye, an event possibly due to rapid and secure encapsulation[2]; on the other hand, after remaining quietly in this way for some time the particle may migrate and suddenly set up a purulent inflammation (after 3½ years, Kümmell, 1908). This relative quiescence may occasionally be observed even although the particle is in the posterior chamber, but as a rule degenerative changes occur which slowly destroy the vision by the development of such conditions as macular degeneration (after 3 years, Barten, 1908), changes resembling pigmentary retinal dystrophy (Adamük, 1897; after 12 years, Siegfried, 1898) or retino-choroidal atrophy (after 4 years, Tobias, 1919; after 20 years, Ruhberg, 1889). Occasionally also, after a long period of quietude, inflammatory symptoms may suddenly appear which may sometimes involve the loss of the eye.[3] Sometimes the suppurative reaction may cause softening and necrosis of the sclera and the particle is eventually spontaneously expelled from the eye; this phenomenon, first observed by Castelnau (1842), may occur at a very variable time after the original injury.[4] Finally, owing to chemical changes, the particle may

[1] Leber (1891, 25 years), Wagenmann (1897, 27 years), Doyne (1894, 30 years), Würdemann (1932, 8 years), Fejer (1932, 3 years).

[2] Hotz (1881), Decker (1890, 6 years with normal vision but spasm of accommodation), Kipp (1901, 30 years), Mishler and Harley (1952, 30 years), P. M. Lewis (1946, 56 years, with brass).

[3] After 8 years (Fortunati, 1889), 20 years (Hahn, 1907), 25 years (Meyerhöfer, 1877; D'Oench, 1889), 34 years (Valude, 1885), 45 years (Franklin and Cordes, 1922).

[4] Some days (3, Brandenburg, 1899), weeks (3, Roulet, 1877; 6, Weigelin, 1917), months (2, Hoor, 1896; 3, Rolland, 1886) or a period of years varying from 1 or 2 (Rampoldi, 1891; Meyer, 1894; Hoesch, 1895), 4 or 5 (Kipp, 1884; Erb, 1899; Blake, 1931), 7 to 10 (Hartley, 1883; Spechtenhauser, 1894), 18 (G. Lewis, 1897), 19 (Hartley, 1883) up to 21 years (Raulin, 1897).

become totally absorbed and disappear, a somewhat unusual event shown to occur by Leber (1891) experimentally and verified clinically by the sequence of a positive x-ray followed at a later date by a negative picture (Hirschberg, 1901; Franke, 1901).

Sympathetic ophthalmitis following the introduction of a copper foreign body into the eye is rare, an immunity possibly depending on the violent purulent reaction which it excites; such a sequence, however, has been reported (Blascheck, 1903; Franklin and Cordes, 1922, after 45 years).

CHALCOSIS. When the intra-ocular foreign body is in the form of an alloy containing relatively little pure copper, the reaction in the eye is much less dramatic, losing the suppurative character so typical of the response of the ocular tissues to the pure metal. Instead, a slow diffusion of copper occurs, occasionally with complete disappearance of the particle, so that the metal is deposited preferentially in the limiting membranes of the eye, producing the picture of CHALCOSIS (χαλκός, copper) (Plate XX). The complete picture, which is one of unusual beauty, is characterized by:

(1) a greenish-blue ring in the peripheral cornea located mainly in Descemet's membrane;

(2) a sunflower cataract in the anterior capsule of the lens and, exceptionally, a deposit on its posterior surface;

(3) an impregnation of the zonular fibres;

(4) the appearance of a multitude of metallic particles in the aqueous humour;

(5) occasionally a greenish coloration of the iris;

and if the particle is in the posterior segment (6) a deposition of copper on the framework of the disorganized vitreous;

(7) a brilliant and highly refractile deposit on the surface of the retina.

The earliest description of such changes dates back for a considerable time. The first mention in the literature is that of Priestley Smith (1892), who noted the peculiar retinal appearances following the long retention of a minute foreign body in the posterior segment of the eye; his observation of retinal chalcosis was followed by those of Goldzieher (1895), Ertl (1907), Haab (1919), Coppez (1927), Vogt (1931), Belz and Bonnet (1948) and others. The discoloration of the iris was noted about the same time (von Gonzenbach, 1892; Hirschberg, 1899; Caspar, 1908; Barten, 1908). The peculiar iridescent greenish-yellow sheen in the lens which forms the most striking part of the clinical picture was remarked first by Hillemanns (1896), zur Nedden (1903) and Ertl (1907), but the full picture did not excite general interest until the slit-lamp became available and the widespread use of copper alloys was stimulated in the first World War. Since German industry felt the pinch of the scarcity of copper most severely and turned wholesale to the use of alloys, the early observations came from that country, and Purtscher (1918) was the first to give a detailed description of the slit-lamp appearance of *sunflower cataract* (*Sonnenblumenstar*). About the same time other observations[1] appeared and the clinical picture was finally consolidated by the extensive

[1] Kümmell (1918), Esser (1918), Klauber (1918), Wirths (1918), Bleisch (1919), Pichler (1919), Haab (1919), Uhthoff (1919) and Rumbaur (1919–20).

PLATE XX

CHALCOSIS.

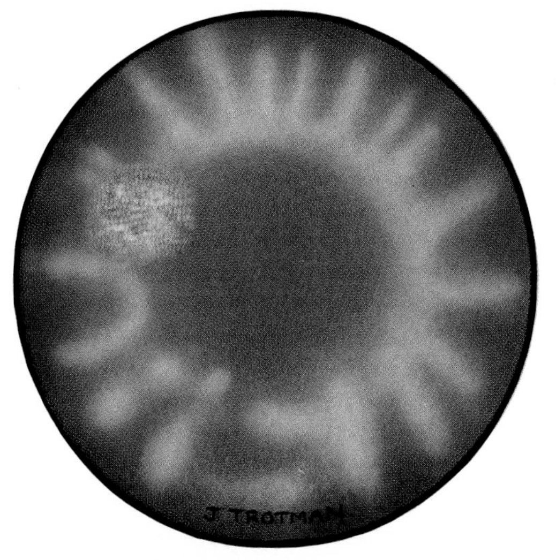

FIG. 1.—Sunflower cataract.

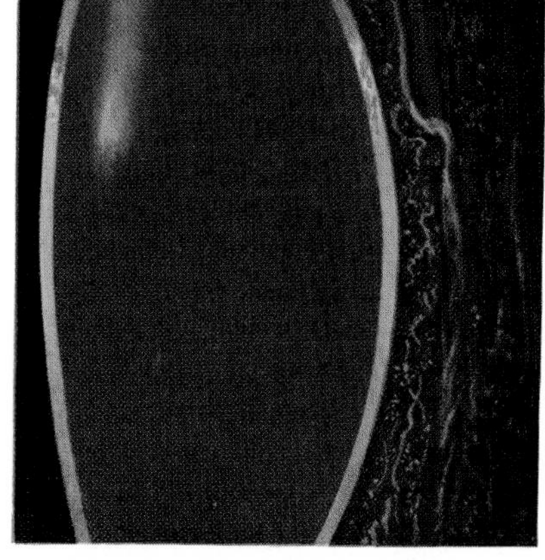

FIG. 2.—The lens and vitreous.

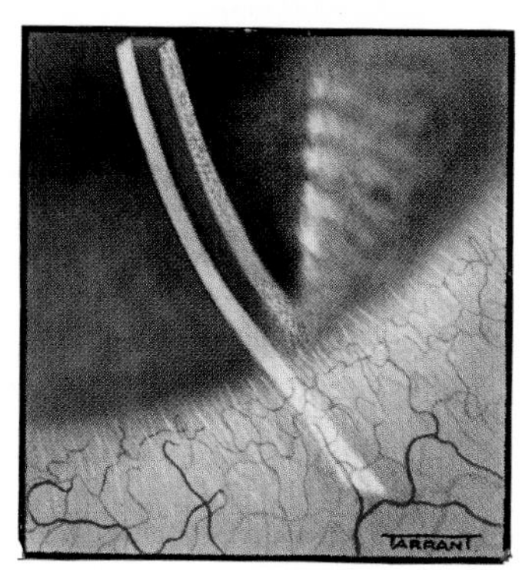

FIG. 3.—The cornea.

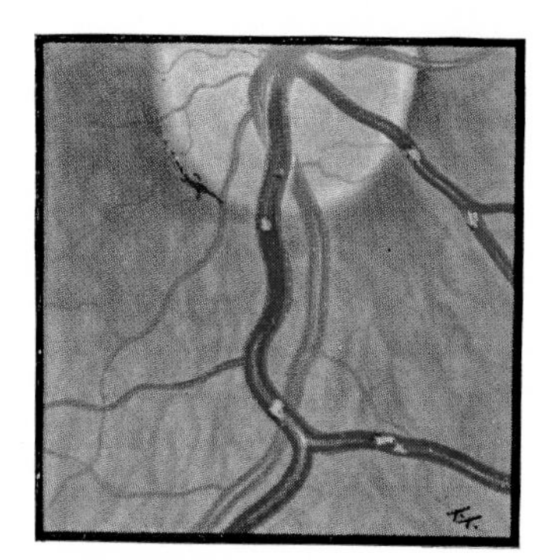

FIG. 4.—Metallic deposits on retinal veins.

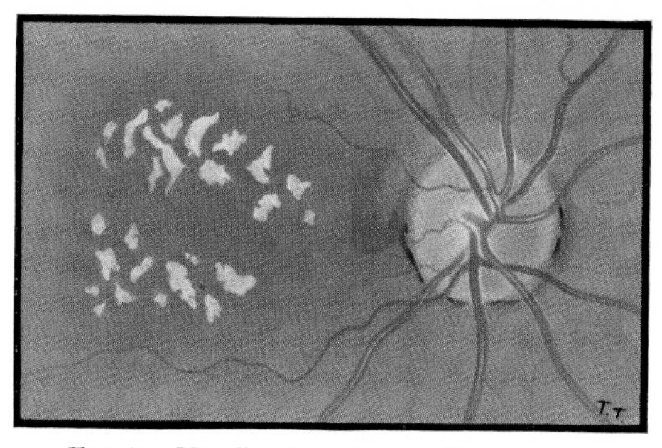

FIG. 5.—Metallic deposits near the macula.

observations of Jess (1919–30) and Vogt (1921–31). Since this time few fundamental facts have been added to our knowledge of the subject.

It is interesting that a similar picture is not uncommon in the ENDOGENOUS CHALCOSIS which occurs in *hepato-lenticular degeneration*. In the cornea the Kayser-Fleischer ring is well known; there was considerable controversy on the nature of this ring, which Fleischer (1910–22) originally thought was hæmatogenous in origin, and discussions have taken place as to whether the pigmentation is due to silver, urobilin or a lipochrome. The opinion of Kubik (1930) that it was due to a deposition of copper has, however, been confirmed by subsequent histo-spectrographic researches.[1] Similarly, the occurrence of a typical sunflower cataract in this disease has been widely observed.[2] It is also interesting that Vogt (1931) reported a typical case of this form of cataract in a man without a history of injury or signs of hepato-lenticular degeneration, who appeared to be suffering from chronic copper poisoning owing to the use of cooking utensils made of this metal.

In the cornea, chalcosis becomes evident by the deposition of an infinity of tiny granules packed closely together in the plane of Descemet's membrane and the deepest layers of the stroma (Jess, 1922; Knüsel, 1924; Loddoni, 1929); Knüsel considered that the deposit occurred also in the endothelium, but this is questionable. In reflected light this deposit produces a typical and beautiful appearance of a brilliant, glittering brownish-yellow colour which, however, is almost invisible and difficult to see by direct light. The ring starts at the periphery of Descemet's membrane, so that it is separated from the limbus itself by a clear zone with the distribution characteristic of a gerontoxon; it usually runs round the entire circumference of the cornea but may be segmental in its distribution, forming, for example, two semicircles superiorly and inferiorly (Plate XX, Fig. 3).

In the lens the appearance of SUNFLOWER CATARACT, which is pathognomonic of the deposition of copper, is one of peculiar beauty. The pupillary area is occupied by a thick powdery deposit located in and underneath the anterior lens capsule; this assumes a disc shape in the pupillary aperture, but when the pupil is dilated, spokes are seen to run from it like the petals of a flower, diverging towards the periphery of the lens and fading out before they reach the equator. Very occasionally a second ring concentric with the central disc appears nearer the periphery. On clinical examination by reflected light the deposition is invisible, so that the condition may be termed a " pseudo-cataract "; it is thus not seen ophthalmoscopically, nor does it seriously impair vision. On focal illumination, however, it presents one of the most beautiful pictures in ophthalmology. The deposit is of a delicate and brilliant colour, varying from greyish green or olive green to brown or brownish red, and the anterior shagreen of the lens emits a lively display of variegated and shimmering colours comprising all shades of the rainbow, among which reds and blue-greens predominate. On high magnification a light spattering of greyish-white and blue and green dots is visible over the entire anterior capsule, and it is evident that the sunflower

[1] Vol. VIII, p. 988. [2] Vol. XI, p. 195.

appearance is merely an intensification of this diffuse peppering with particles so numerous that they cannot be individually resolved. So thick is the deposit in the areas preferentially involved that the capsule appears to have a soft velvety surface (Plate XX, Figs. 1 and 2).

Although Loddoni (1929) thought that the radial arrangement of the opacities forming the petals of the sunflower was determined by folds in the anterior capsule of the lens, it would seem that the peculiar pattern is related to the radial folds on the posterior surface of the iris and that the movement of this tissue aggregates the particles in their peculiar configuration (Vogt, 1923). Thus Jess (1929–30) showed that, if mydriasis were maintained, the peripheral rays were replaced by an extension of the central disc, and Hillemanns (1896) found that the opacity took the shape of a deformed pupil. In an interesting case reported by Belz and Bonnet (1948), wherein a second traumatic " pupil " was present, two green circles appeared on the anterior capsule; moreover, it is significant that on the rare occasions when there is a deposition on the posterior surface of the lens no such configuration is evident.

A *posterior copper cataract* is a rarity. Such an appearance was described by Müller (1937) in a case wherein a minute particle of copper lay in the vitreous just behind the lens; in this case the posterior surface of the lens and the cornea, but not the anterior capsule, developed a typical greenish-blue colour. Rosen (1949) also described a case wherein a small particle was encapsulated on the retina. When the deposition occurs on the posterior capsule the iridescence is light and uniformly distributed without showing any pattern, while the particles of deposit appear to be finer.

Pathological investigations of sunflower cataract have been carried out by Ertl (1907), Jess (1922) and Vogt (1931). Jess considered that copper was deposited in the deeper layers of the capsule and between it and the epithelial cells in a layer 0·2 to 0·5μ thick, from which delicate linear extensions ran between the fibres of the anterior cortex for a short distance. A less dense deposition of copper was also seen in the substance of the lens near the equator and the posterior pole (Figs. 452 and 453). Only rarely does the entire lens become impregnated (Belz and Bonnet, 1948). Histologically the deposit is seen as round or flaky particles which, when stained with potassium ferrocyanide and acetic acid, assume the characteristic brownish-red colour of copper ferrocyanide (*Perls's reaction for copper*). This stains the epithelial cells themselves, a circumstance which Jess considered accidental; Vogt, however, took the opposite view and contended that the epithelial cells formed the real substrate for the opacity.

The changes in the other tissues are much less dramatic than the striking picture in the lens. Occasionally in the beam of the slit-lamp the *aqueous humour* is seen to be packed with microscopic particles, brightly refringent and greenish-brown in colour, continually dancing with a Tyndall movement (Belz and Bonnet, 1948); in these circumstances the aqueous removed by puncture of the anterior chamber eight days or later after the accident may give a positive chemical reaction for copper (Tichomirov, 1950). The *iris* occasionally may take on a greenish tinge and shows sluggishness in dilatation with mydriatics. The *vitreous* is always totally disorganized if the copper lies in the posterior segment and its framework is liberally bespangled with brilliant brownish-red particles; these are especially numerous in the retrolental space where their presence gives a red coppery tint immediately behind the lens to the beam of the slit-lamp. The *zonular fibres* are similarly heavily festooned with a multitude of refringent dots.

Chalcosis of the retina has rarely been observed, but when the foreign body is located in the posterior segment of the globe the appearance may be very striking. Priestley Smith's (1892) early description of the commonest appearance cannot be bettered: shining lustrous points like tiny pieces of gold leaf are seen to be arranged down the main trunks of both arteries and

FIGS. 452 and 453.—CHALCOSIS LENTIS (after A. Jess).

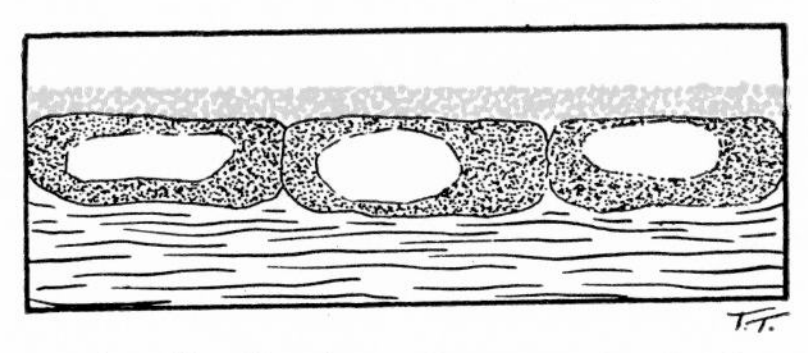

FIG. 452.—To show the distribution of copper in the lens capsule and between it and the epithelium as demonstrated by the precipitation of copper ferrocyanide (× 1,500).

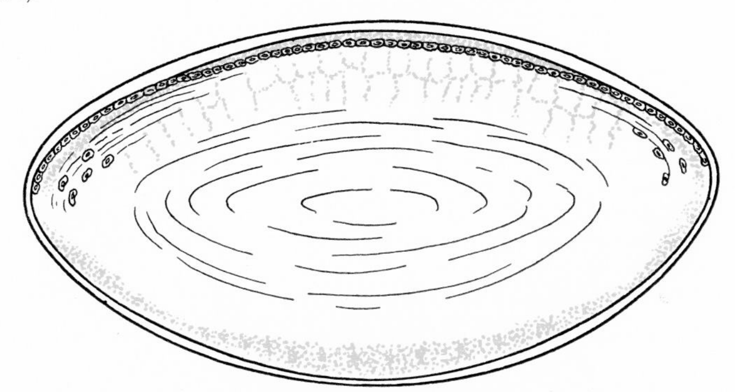

FIG. 453.—The distribution of copper in the lens as revealed by precipitation as copper ferrocyanide.

veins where they remain without reaction (Plate XX, Fig. 4). Similar tiny metallic flecks may lie away from the vessels and at the macula or more extensive exudative changes may occur. Müller (1931) and Belz and Bonnet (1948), for example, described sharply defined brilliant patches, whitish-blue or coppery in colour with a metallic sheen, lying beneath the vessels. It would appear that these changes are always concentrated in the region of the posterior pole of the eye (Plate XX, Fig. 5).

The rationale of these changes is not by any means clear and, indeed, agreement has not yet been reached as to the chemical nature of the deposit. Copper it certainly is, but Jess (1919–30) considered that the metal is in the form of a carbonate while Vogt (1931) assumed it to be an oxide of copper.

The mode of diffusion throughout the eye is also a matter of dispute. It is obvious that the deposition tends to be on limiting membranes such as Descemet's and the lens capsule or on the fibrillar structures of the vitreous and zonule rather than in the cells which apparently resist the entrance of the metal. This is in direct contradistinction to the behaviour of iron which forms a chemical compound within the cells and, incidentally, probably accounts for the occasional occurrence of retrogression or disappearance of chalcosis. It is interesting that the deposition occurs preferentially in the anterior capsule of the lens, appearing there sooner and more profusely than in the cornea, although the implication of the latter tissue is increased in the aphakic eye (Weiss, 1926; Mielke, 1940). Bär (1923) thought that amino-acids derived from the disintegration of the cells assisted in the complete solution of the copper, but it would seem probable from the experimental work of Itoi (1937) and Mielke (1940) that electrolytic dissociation may play a large part both in the solution of the metal and its dissemination in the eye.

It will be remembered[1] that a constant electric current passes postero-anteriorly through the globe, the cornea acting as a positive and the posterior segment as a negative pole. This may well cause ionization of the copper, and the ions would be carried anteriorly by the current and would be deposited on membranes since they offered the most homogeneous resistance to their passage. Mielke (1940) showed experimentally that, if copper wire were placed in an enucleated eye and the appropriate current passed, the metal collected preferentially in the anterior capsule of the lens in the pupillary area. At the same time this cannot be the entire explanation; diffusion must also enter into the question to account for the posterior migration of the metal towards the retina if the foreign body lies anteriorly to this tissue.

The *clinical course* of chalcosis varies considerably. The deposition appears at a very variable time after the injury, depending probably on the size of the particle, its copper content and its location in the eye; usually the clinical picture begins to develop after the lapse of some years, but occasionally the interval is measured in months (3 months, Rosen, 1949). The tendency, of course, is for gradual deterioration to develop with a slow progression of the metallic deposition and a slow diminution of vision, but inevitable blindness as is the rule in siderosis does not occur. On the other hand, the impregnation may decrease or even entirely disappear if the particle becomes completely encapsulated, if it is dissolved away in the process of time, or if it is removed. There are numerous reports of such improvement. Cordes and Harrington (1935), for example, described such a case wherein the radiographic shadow of the body disappeared after six years and the chalcosis became much less after eight years; other similar cases have been reported.[2] It is to be remembered, however, that even if the foreign body is extracted, an intensification of the chalcosis may occur

[1] Vol. IV, p. 496

[2] Clausen (1923), Oloff (1926), Jess (1929–30), Zahor (1930), Müller (1931), Marner (1945), Belz and Bonnet (1948), Belz (1952), Kudo *et al.* (1964).

owing to fragmentation of the particle and the dissemination of metal in powdered form (Bär, 1923). Occasionally a complicated cataract develops (Rosen, 1949) but cases which appear to develop secondary glaucoma have been exceptional (Jess, 1926; Colrat, 1931; Belthle, 1938; Metzger, 1939). Finally, it is to be remembered that, as with all foreign bodies, some eyes show a tolerance which seems to be almost miraculous and the presence even of a toxic material such as copper seems to have little effect.

Specific treatment in the case of a copper foreign body has been tried with a view either to coating the particle with an innocuous metal, such as gold, or forming a ferrous alloy which would be magnetizable and therefore aid in its extraction. Neither of these has been successful. Another suggestion has been to convert the copper into an innocuous compound. For this purpose Müller (1931) and Dambite (1959–62) used sodium thiosulphate therapeutically, either topically applied or injected subconjunctivally or intravenously, while Habig and his collaborators (1951) employed intravenous sodium hyposulphite with some success. Newell and his co-workers (1949) and Rouher (1958) experimented with BAL (2–3-dimercaptopropanol).[1] This substance, it will be remembered, was originally used as a protection against arsenic and has subsequently been employed as an antidote to other heavy metals, such as mercury, lead and gold. It certainly does form an insoluble compound with copper, which is well tolerated if injected either into the anterior chamber or the vitreous, but in clinical conditions none of these attempts at chemical treatment has met with consistent practical success. Penicillamine was used by Delbecque and his colleagues (1966) in two cases with early corneal and lenticular changes associated with the presence of intravitreal copper particles and by Cati (1968); while chelating agents were tried by Mine (1958) in order to reduce the severity of the purulent endophthalmitis resulting from the presence of copper salts in the vitreous. Up to the present time, therefore, the methods of treatment adopted for the removal of a copper foreign body from the eye are those common to all non-magnetizable materials.[2]

Adamük. *Arch. Augenheilk.*, **36,** 114 (1897).
Bär. *Arch. Augenheilk.*, **49,** 60 (1903).
Klin. Mbl. Augenheilk., **70,** 174 (1923).
Barten. *Ueber die Folgen aseptisch eingeheilter Kupferstückchen im Auge* (Diss.), Greifswald (1908).
Belthle. *Ueber intraokulare Kupfersplitter* (Diss.), Tübingen (1938).
Belz. *Bull. Soc. Ophtal. Fr.*, 134 (1952).
Belz and Bonnet. *Bull. Soc. franç. Ophtal.*, **61,** 357 (1948).
Berendes. *Ein Fall v. doppelter Perforation d. Auges durch einen 19 mm. langen Kupferdraht* (Diss.), Jena (1907).
Berlin. *v. Graefes Arch. Ophthal.*, **13** (2), 275 (1867); **14** (2), 275 (1868).
Blake. *Amer. J. Ophthal.*, **14,** 1009 (1931).
Blascheck. *Z. Augenheilk.*, **9,** 434 (1903).
Bleisch. *Berl. klin. Wschr.*, **56,** 117 (1919).
Bocchi. *Ann. Ottal.*, **39,** 465 (1910).
Brandenburg. *Samml. zwangl. Abhandl. Geb. Augenheilk.*, **3** (4), 23 (1899).
Bruns. *Amer. J. Ophthal.*, **14,** 377 (1897).
Caspar. *Klin. Mbl. Augenheilk.*, **46** (2), 179 (1908).
Castelnau. *Arch. gén. Méd.*, **15,** 210 (1842).
Cati. *Atti Soc. oftal. Lombarda*, **23,** 61 (1968).
Clausen. *v. Graefes Arch. Ophthal.*, **111,** 460 (1923).
Cohen. *Klin. Mbl. Augenheilk.*, **46** (1), 620 (1908).
Colrat. *Ann. Oculist.* (Paris), **168,** 935 (1931).
Coppez. *Bull. Soc. franç. Ophtal.*, **40,** 310 (1927).
Cordes and Harrington. *Amer. J. Ophthal.*, **18,** 348 (1935).
Dambite. *Oftal. Zh.*, **14,** 67 (1959); **15,** 3 (1960); **17,** 214 (1962).
Decker. *Klin. Mbl. Augenheilk.*, **28,** 500 (1890).
Delbecque, Sourdille and Delthil. *Bull. Soc. franç. Ophtal.*, **79,** 275 (1966).
Denig. *Klin. Mbl. Augenheilk.*, **34,** 210 (1896).
Ber. dtsch. ophthal. Ges., **25,** 305 (1896).
D'Oench. *Arch. Augenheilk.*, **19,** 158 (1889).
Doyne. *Trans. ophthal. Soc. U.K.*, **14,** 219 (1894).
Duc. *Rass. ital. Ottal.*, **5,** 135 (1936).
Erb. *Z. Augenheilk.*, **1,** 449 (1899).
Ertl. *Zbl. prakt. Augenheilk.*, **31,** 322 (1907).

[1] Chap. XI. [2] p. 637.

Esser. *Zbl. prakt. Augenheilk.*, **42,** 135 (1918).
Fejer. *Amer. J. Ophthal.*, **15,** 224 (1932).
Fleischer. *Ber. dtsch. ophthal. Ges.*, **36,** 128 (1910).
Klin. Mbl. Augenheilk., **68,** 41 (1922).
Fontana. *Rass. ital. Ottal.*, **7,** 695 (1938).
Fortunati. *Riforme med.*, **5,** 1478 (1889).
Franke. *v. Graefes Arch. Ophthal.*, **30** (1), 211 (1884).
Zbl. prakt. Augenheilk., **25,** 353 (1901).
Franklin and Cordes. *Amer. J. Ophthal.*, **5,** 533 (1922).
Goldzieher. *Zbl. prakt. Augenheilk.*, **19,** 1 (1895).
von Gonzenbach. *Klin. Mbl. Augenheilk.*, **30,** 197 (1892).
Granström. *Acta ophthal.* (Kbh.), **27,** 47 (1949).
Greeff. Orth's *Lhb. d. spez. path. Anat.*, Berlin, Erg.-band., 588 (1905).
Haab. *Arch. Augenheilk.*, **85,** 136 (1919).
Habig, Lumen and Snacken. *Bull. Soc. belge Ophtal.*, No. 98, 287 (1951).
Hahn. *Ueber zwanzigjähriges Verweilen eines Kupfersplitters im Auge* (Diss.), Bonn (1907).
Hartley. *Brit. med. J.*, **2,** 71 (1883).
Hillemanns. *Arch. Augenheilk.*, **32,** 202 (1896).
von Hippel. *Klin. Mbl. Augenheilk.*, **50** (2), 52 (1912).
Hirschberg. *Dtsch. med. Wschr.*, **20,** 313 (1894).
Zbl. prakt. Augenheilk., **23,** 241 (1899); **25,** 210 (1901).
Hoesch. *Ueber einen Fall von reaktionslosem mehrjährigem Verweilen eines ungewöhnlich grossen Messingstückes im Auge* (Diss.), Würzburg (1895).
van der Hoeve. *Klin. Mbl. Augenheilk.*, **51** (1), 643 (1913).
Hoor. *Wien. med. Wschr.*, **46,** 1481 (1896).
Hornstein. *Verletzungen d. Auges durch Kupfer- u. Messingsplitter* (Diss.), Tübingen (1905).
Hotz. *Arch. Augenheilk.*, **10,** 39 (1881).
Itoi. *Acta Soc. ophthal. jap.*, **41,** Suppl., 669 (1937).
Jacqueau. *Clin. Ophtal.*, **5,** 665 (1913).
Jess. *Samml. zwangl. Abhandl. Geb. Augenheilk.*, **10** (3), 3 (1918).
Klin. Mbl. Augenheilk., **62,** 464 (1919); **68,** 433 (1922); **72,** 128 (1924); **76,** 465 (1926); **79,** 145 (1927).
Z. Augenheilk., **69,** 59 (1929).
Kurzes Hb. d. Ophthal., Berlin, **5,** 170 (1930).
Kipp. *Amer. J. Ophthal.*, **1,** 103 (1884).
Trans. Amer. ophthal. Soc., **37,** 352 (1901).
Klauber. *Zbl. prakt. Augenheilk.*, **42,** 166 (1918).
Knave. *Acta ophthal.* (Kbh.), **48,** 159 (1970).
Knüsel. *v. Graefes Arch. Ophthal.*, **113,** 282 (1924).
Kostenitsch. *v. Graefes Arch. Ophthal.*, **37** (4), 189 (1891).
Kubik. *Klin. Mbl. Augenheilk.*, **84,** 478 (1930).
Kudo, Matsuyama, Takahashi *et al.* *Rinsho Ganka*, **18,** 355 (1964).
Kümmell. *Z. Augenheilk.*, **19,** 36 (1908).
Zbl. prakt. Augenheilk., **42,** 97 (1918).
Leber. *Die Entstehung d. Entzündung*, Leipzig (1891).
Lewis, G. *Zbl. prakt. Augenheilk.*, **21,** 553 (1897).
Lewis, P. M. *Amer. J. Ophthal.*, **29,** 1164 (1946).
Loddoni. *Ann. Ottal.*, **57,** 28, 329 (1929).
Maas. *Ueber Kupfersplitterverletzung d. menschlichen Auges* (Diss.), Heidelberg (1917).
Marner. *Acta ophthal.* (Kbh.), **23,** 171 (1945).
Metzger. *Klin. Mbl. Augenheilk.*, **102,** 720 (1939).
Meyer. *VIII int. Cong. Ophthal.*, Edinburgh, 48 (1894).
Meyerhöfer. *Klin. Mbl. Augenheilk.*, **15,** 66 (1877).
Mielke. *v. Graefes Arch. Ophthal.*, **141,** 644 (1940).
Mine. *Acta Soc. ophthal. jap.*, **62,** 470 (1958).
Mishler and Harley. *Amer. J. Ophthal.*, **35,** 687 (1952).
Müller. *Klin. Mbl. Augenheilk.*, **86,** 453 (1931).
Schweiz. med. Wschr., **67,** 790 (1937).
zur Nedden. *Klin. Mbl. Augenheilk.*, **41** (1), 484 (1903).
Neubauer and Heimann. *Ber. dtsch. ophthal. Ges.*, **69,** 366 (1968).
Newell, Cooper and Farmer. *Amer. J. Ophthal.*, **32** (2), 161 (1949).
Okabe. *Acta Soc. ophthal. jap.*, **35,** 1092 (1931).
Oloff. *Klin. Mbl. Augenheilk.*, **76,** 881 (1926).
Pichler. *Arch. Augenheilk.*, **85,** 181 (1919).
Plitt. *Klin. Mbl. Augenheilk.*, **44** (2), 537 (1906).
Posern. *Pathologisch-anatomischer Befund bei Feuerwerkskörperverletzung am Auge* (Diss.), Heidelberg (1913).
Praun. *Die Verletzungen des Auges*, Wiesbaden (1899).
Purtscher. *Zbl. prakt. Augenheilk.*, **42,** 172 (1918).
Rampoldi. *Ann. Ottal.*, **20,** 538 (1891).
Raulin. *Ann. Oculist.* (Paris), **117,** 287 (1897).
Reuling. *Arch. Augenheilk.*, **10,** 211 (1881).
Rolland. *Bull. Soc. franç. Ophtal.*, **4,** 314 (1886).
Rosen. *Amer. J. Ophthal.*, **32,** 248 (1949).
Rouher. *Bull. Soc. Ophtal. Fr.*, 19 (1958).
Roulet. *Korresp.-Bl. schweiz. Aerzt.*, **7,** 81, 112 (1877).
Ruhberg. *Ueber Zündhütchenverletzungen d. Auges* (Diss.), Kiel (1889).
Rumbaur. *Klin. Mbl. Augenheilk.*, **63,** 206 (1919); **64,** 679 (1920).
Sala and Borsellino. *Boll. Oculist.*, **15,** 344 (1936).
Schmidt. *v. Graefes Arch. Ophthal.*, **46,** 665 (1898).

Sená. *Arch. Oftal. B. Aires*, **4,** 473, 571 (1930).
Siegfried. *Beitr. Augenheilk.*, **3** (22), 45 (1898).
Smith, Priestley. *Trans. ophthal. Soc. U.K.*, **12,** 191 (1892).
Spechtenhauser. *Wien. klin. Wschr.*, **7,** 810 (1894).
Stein. *Beitrag zu d. Kenntnissen d. Zündhütchenverletzungen d. menschlichen Auges* (Diss.), Würzburg (1902).
von Szily. *Atlas der Kriegsaugenheilkunde*, Stuttgart (1918).
Takahaschi. *Acta Soc. ophthal. jap.*, **40,** 2097 (1936).
Tichomirov. *Vestn. oftal.*, **29** (1), 9 (1950).
Tobias. *Klin. Mbl. Augenheilk.*, **63,** 137 (1919).
Uhthoff. *Berl. klin. Wschr.*, **56** (1), 117 (1919).
Valude. *Arch. Ophtal.*, **5,** 328 (1885).
Velhagen. *Klin. Mbl. Augenheilk.*, **85,** 584 (1930).
Vogt. *Klin. Mbl. Augenheilk.*, **66,** 269, 277 (1921); **77,** 709 (1926); **81,** 712 (1928); **82,** 433; **83,** 417 (1929).
v. Graefes Arch. Ophthal., **112,** 122 (1923).
Lhb. u. Atlas d. Spaltlampenmikroskopie d. lebenden Auges, 2nd ed., Berlin, **2,** 645 (1931).
Wagenmann. *v. Graefes Arch. Ophthal.*, **42** (2), 1 (1896); **44,** 272 (1897).
Weigelin. *Klin. Mbl. Augenheilk.*, **59,** 84 (1917).
Weiss. *v. Graefes Arch. Ophthal.*, **117,** 114 (1926).
Whitehead. *Trans. ophthal. Soc. U.K.*, **36,** 63 (1916).
Winkler. *Z. Augenheilk.*, **41,** 60 (1919).
Wirths. *Z. Augenheilk.*, **40,** 164 (1918).
Würdemann. *Injuries to the Eye*, 2nd ed., London (1932).
Zahor. *Z. Augenheilk.*, **70,** 171 (1930).

IRON

Among all intra-ocular foreign bodies those of IRON and STEEL are the most important from the clinical point of view. In the first place, they are the most numerous both as a result of industrial accidents among which they form the vast majority (85%, Whitehead, 1916; 92%, Cridland, 1916; 98%, Gulliver, 1942) and in injuries sustained in war. In the second place, their after-effects are unusually serious. In contradistinction to the ocular response to copper there is no violent immediate reaction apart from the actual mechanical trauma. To counterbalance this, however, the delayed chemical effects of iron upon the ocular tissues, the clinical picture of which was termed SIDEROSIS by Bunge (1890), are much more harmful and set up a chronic degenerative process the normal termination of which is blindness. On the other hand, to counterbalance this again, the extraction of foreign bodies containing iron is comparatively easy owing to their magnetizability. It is to be remembered that different types of steel are not equally destructive; the less the ferrous content (as, for example, in manganese or nickel steels) the less the tendency to siderosis, but it is also to be borne in mind that the less the ferrous content the greater the difficulty of extraction owing to a diminution of magnetizability.[1]

In industry most of the foreign bodies which enter the eye arise from the mushroomed head of a chisel, a steel hammer, a high-powered drill or from grinding tools at the emery wheel. Most are of highly tempered steel and, detached from their parent tool with considerable force, these travel at high speeds, thus accounting for the fact that 85% of such foreign bodies are found in the posterior segment of the globe; it is relatively rare that they find a resting place in the anterior chamber, the iris or the lens. The usual origin is a defective tool, and the greatest care should be exercised that all overhanging edges of such implements as a cold chisel are removed (Figs. 454 and 455). It is interesting that in these cases the fragment usually flies off after a glancing blow, so that the speed and penetrating effect of the particle of steel are

[1] p. 621.

enhanced by the rotatory movement thus imparted to it[1]; it therefore has the effect of a flying buzz-saw with extremely sharp edges. Fortunately the heat generated at the time of the detachment of the particle from the tool and maintained by the speed of its flight through the air, usually sterilizes the foreign body, so that in such accidents gross intra-ocular infection is relatively rare.

FIGS. 454 and 455.—THE COMMON FOREIGN BODY IN INDUSTRY (A. S. Philps)

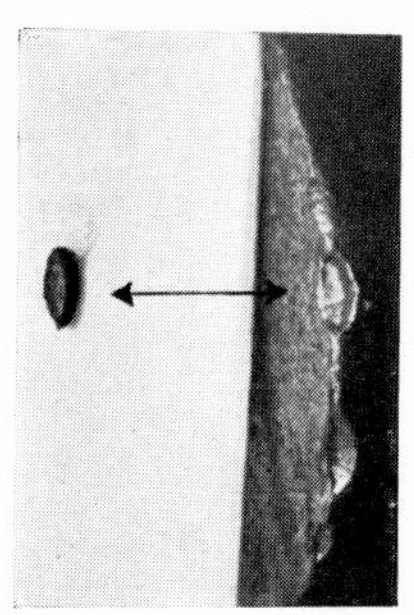

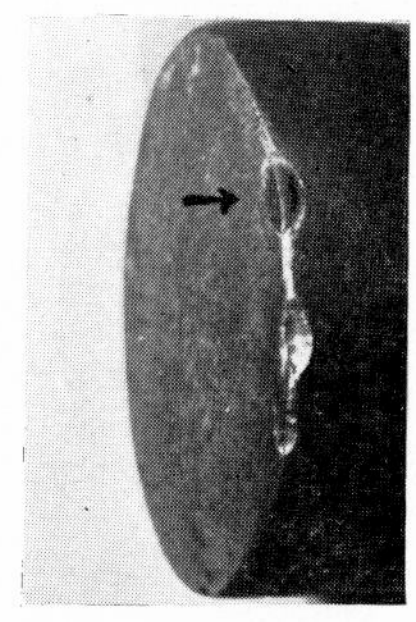

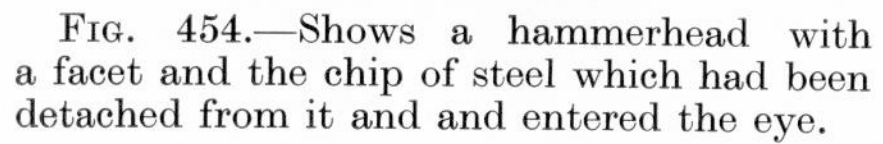

FIG. 454.—Shows a hammerhead with a facet and the chip of steel which had been detached from it and and entered the eye.

FIG. 455.—The hammerhead showing the fragment fitted onto the facet from which it had originated.

Although the condition of siderosis is the normal sequence of the retention of a foreign body rich in iron within the eye, this is not invariable; indeed, six other developments may occur. In the first place, no apparent reaction may become evident, its absence being probably accounted for either by the small ferrous content of the particle or its protection from dissociation by its rapid and complete encapsulation (Fig. 456). Thus a number of cases has been recorded wherein an iron foreign body has remained for long periods within the globe without bad effects either in the anterior

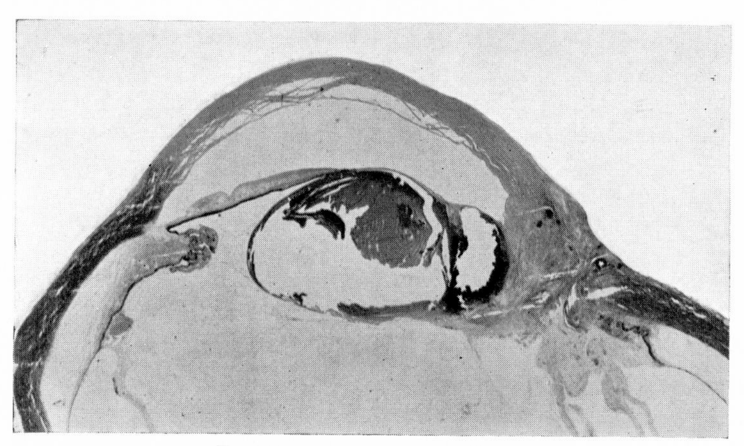

FIG. 456.—IRON FOREIGN BODY.

The foreign body lies in the posterior chamber surrounded by scar tissue so dense that dissemination of the iron has been prevented and siderosis has not resulted. Enucleation 2 months after injury (Helenor Wilder).

[1] p. 478.

chamber (6 years, Vossius, 1901; 11 years, Horn, 1906), in the iris (29 years, Baitchev, 1968), in the lens (32 years, Nottage, 1899; 22 years, Ide, 1968), or even in the posterior segment (Elschnig, 1891; Cridland, 1933, 18 years[1]); even although the eye becomes blind, this lack of inflammatory response may remain almost indefinitely (67 years, Spratt, 1933) (Figs. 418 and 457).

In the second place, a piece of metal which has been encapsulated and has lain quietly for a long period may shift its location and cause a violent inflammation sometimes necessitating enucleation (after 6 years, Knapp, 1880). Thirdly, even without such migration, recurrent inflammatory episodes may occur after a long period of quietude, sometimes resulting in a violent inflammation with hypopyon and at other times in a plastic

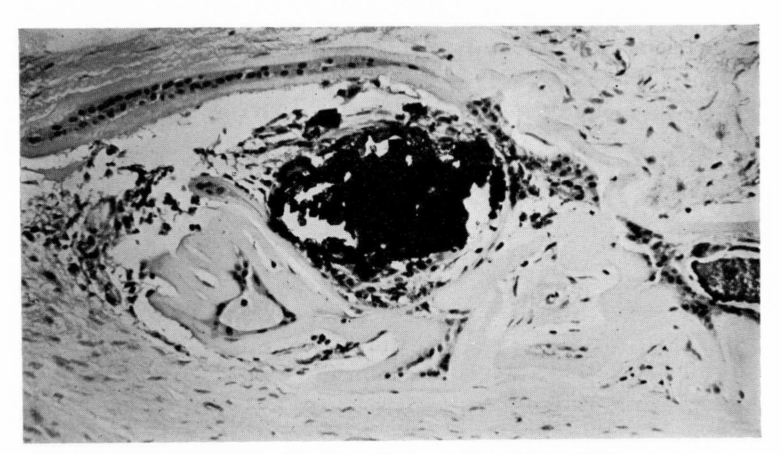

FIG. 457.—IRON FOREIGN BODY ON THE LENS CAPSULE.

The eye was enucleated following a perforating wound by a screwdriver. An iron foreign body is seen encircled by the lens capsule which is incarcerated in a cyclitic membrane (Helenor Wilder).

ophthalmitis which ends in shrinkage of the globe and usually necessitates excision.[2] Occasionally such a reaction results in a fourth possibility—the spontaneous expulsion of the foreign body from the globe.[3] In the fifth place, as will be noted later, a small foreign body is occasionally completely dissolved away in the siderotic reaction; and finally, as a relatively rare event, sympathetic ophthalmitis may develop (after 3 years, Pihl, 1905).

SIDEROSIS. The development of SIDEROSIS (σίδηρος, iron) is the most typical sequel of the presence of an iron foreign body in the eye. The extent to which the degenerative changes become evident varies not only

[1] Glaucoma developed which was controlled by operation; no siderosis.

[2] After 10 years, Mason (1877), Bergmeister (1907); 22 years, Loewenstein and Foster (1947); after 25 years, Birnbacher (1885); after 27 years, Reitsch (1914).

[3] After a few days (6, Bugge, 1893), months (1, Bull, 1881, Landmann, 1882; 3, Woods, 1886), or some years (2, Castelnau, 1842, Oliver, 1901; 18, Ridley, 1923; 20, Gesang, 1905; 23, Clizbe, 1884; 30, Scalinci, 1905).

with the size and chemical composition of the particle but also with its position in the eye; in this respect the worst location is within the ciliary body or in the posterior segment when encapsulation on the retina has not developed; a better prognosis follows lodgment in the anterior chamber, the best within the substance of the lens, but even when lodged here a small particle may cause widespread siderosis (Rychener, 1946). The characteristic changes may develop even to a marked degree from the presence of very small particles indeed.

Thus Schiøtz (1907) reported the occurrence of siderosis from a particle of 0·00045 g., and Hüttemann (1913) from one of 0·00018 g. impacted in the capsule of the lens. The changes themselves are typically slow in their development and chronic in their habit, usually coming on at a period varying from some months to some years after the injury. They have been reported after (?) 4 days (Smith, 1929), 18 (Hoffmann, 1947) or 24 days (Hertel, 1916), but changes of a relatively gross nature appearing 2 to 4 months after the injury are not unusual (Vossius, 1896–1901; Fehr, 1900). In Eisenberg's (1901) series of 14 cases, siderosis became clinically evident within periods varying from 20 days to 8 years.

During the progress of siderosis the foreign body becomes absorbed to some degree and on occasion a small fragment has apparently completely disappeared. Thus it is common for a foreign body lying in the retina to lose its metallic sheen and become negative to X-rays or the sideroscope after a number of years (Franke, 1901, after 11 years; Casali, 1910). Moreover, in enucleated eyes foreign bodies have been found more or less rusted away (after 3 years, Pihl, 1905; 21 years, Gilbert, 1909) or have apparently disappeared entirely (Mayou, 1926); indeed, there are a few reports of the complete absorption in this way of small particles (Gradle, 1922; Begle, 1929). It follows that if a small foreign body has remained in the eye for a number of years the clinical evidences of siderosis may gradually disappear (von Hippel, 1893–1901) and this may occur exceptionally in an eye which has retained good vision despite the ordeal through which it has passed (Braendstrup, 1944, after 14 years). Similarly, if the foreign body is extracted, the siderosis may eventually diminish or disappear entirely (Cramer, 1902–5; de Schweinitz, 1909; Clegg, 1915–26; Vogt, 1931), although at a later date further degenerative changes may occur such as atrophy of the iris (Rogman, 1905), luxation of the lens (Vossius, 1910) or detachment of the retina (Cramer, 1905).

Experimental investigations on the rationale of the clinical appearances of siderosis have been numerous since Leber's (1881–91) original work. These have been carried out, among others, by Ausin (1891), von Hippel (1894–96), Gruber (1894), Erdmann (1907), Mayou (1926), Loddoni (1929) Cibis and Yamashita (1959) and Wise (1966). In general, both the clinical findings and the pathological condition are identical with those seen in man.

The *clinical picture*, which was first recognized by von Graefe (1860), is typical and pathognomonic, characterized particularly by the rusty colour assumed by the iris and the lens, and the degenerative changes ultimately appearing in the retina (Plate XXI).

Little work was done after von Graefe's original observation until the painstaking chemical and pathological studies of Bunge (1890), who introduced the name *siderosis bulbi*, but after his and Leber's (1881–91) experimental work a large number of important papers appeared.[1]

In general, the reaction may be conveniently described in two categories, a differentiation first made by Bunge (1890)—*direct siderosis*, wherein iron is deposited in the immediate neighbourhood of the foreign body, and *indirect siderosis*, wherein the metal is diffused widely throughout the tissues of the eye, producing the typical picture which usually ends in blindness from degeneration or detachment of the retina or from glaucoma.

DIRECT SIDEROSIS starts soon after the lodgment of the foreign body. We have already discussed its occurrence in the cornea, the subconjunctival tissues and the sclera.[2] If the particle is lodged within the iris the changes may remain localized when the body is heavily encapsulated (Meller, 1913, for 26 years) (Plate XXI, Fig. 2). If, however, the foreign body is lodged in the lens a localized siderosis is not uncommon, in which case brownish-yellow spots may be seen in a ring-shape particularly underneath the anterior capsule, a phenomenon which may begin to be apparent within three weeks (Sattler, 1899). These changes may occasionally remain localized and in this event the particle has been extracted without an increase in the lenticular opacities (Bruner, 1907). More usually, however, a total cataract eventually develops (Kurz and Henkind, 1965) and occasionally the lens itself is absorbed (von Hippel, 1894–96). If the foreign body is encapsulated in the retina, siderotic changes may occasionally be confined to its vicinity where pigmentary degeneration in the surrounding area may be considerable (Figs. 458 and 459), but it must be remembered that a splinter in the optic nerve may cause early and diffuse siderosis throughout the globe (Santoro, 1949).

In INDIRECT OR GENERALIZED SIDEROSIS most of the ocular tissues are involved. In *the cornea* a rusty staining is seen in the optical section of the slit-lamp, which on high magnification is shown to be concentrated mainly around the corneal corpuscles which are preferentially tinted, a coloration which is deeper in the periphery than in the centre (Koeppe, 1917); these changes are evident even although the foreign body is in the posterior segment. Little gross reaction occurs, however, although, if the foreign body lies in the anterior chamber, changes suggestive of interstitial keratitis with vascularization have been noted (Andresen, 1903).

The iris assumes a striking rusty colour varying from brown to yellow

[1] von Hippel (1893–1901), Hirschberg (1896–1907), Vossius (1896–1909), Wagenmann (1905), Kipp (1906), Gilbert (1909), Clegg (1915), Hertel (1916), von Szily (1918), van der Hoeve (1918), Vogt (1921), D'Amico (1925), Mayou (1925–26), and many others.

[2] p. 462.

FIGS. 458 and 459.—DIRECT SIDEROSIS.

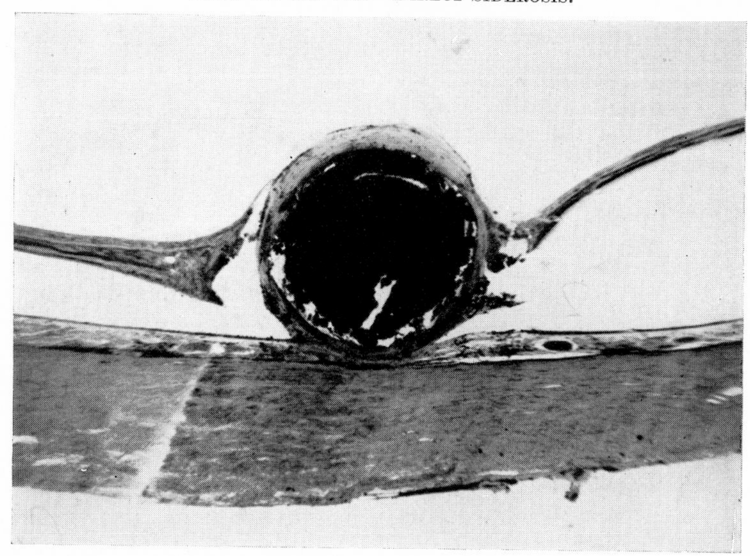

FIG. 458.—A steel foreign body lies embedded in the retina and choroid in the posterior part of the eye; it is surrounded with a fibrous capsule and Perls's stain showed siderosis in the surrounding tissue (H. and E.; × 29) (N. Ashton).

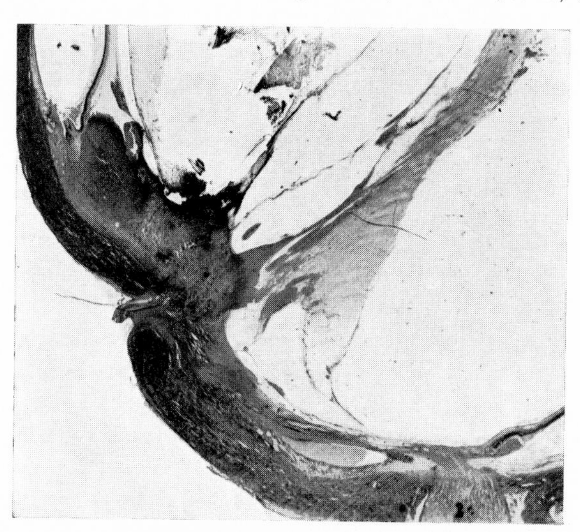

FIG. 459.—An iron foreign body has perforated the sclera and entered the vitreous. There is iron staining around its site. The optic nerve is seen in the bottom right-hand corner. Enucleation 41 days after injury (Helenor Wilder).

or green or red, an appearance which makes a dramatic contrast to the fellow eye if the irides are blue (Plate XXI, Figs. 1 and 3). As a general rule, the presence of synechiæ binding the iris to the lens indicates the existence of a quiet inflammatory reaction (12 out of 14 cases, Eisenberg,

PLATE XXI

SIDEROSIS.

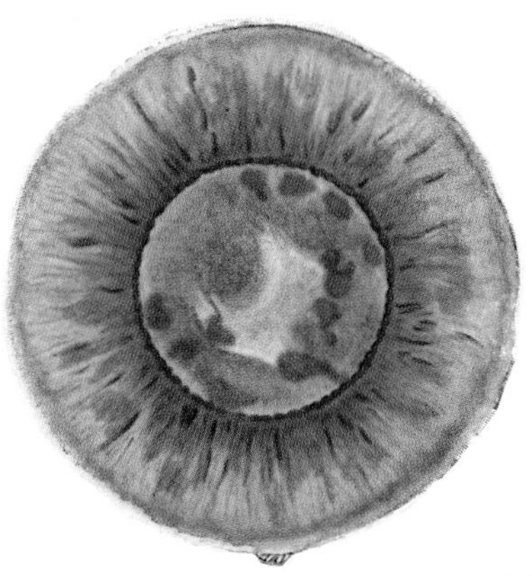

FIG. 1.—Siderosis showing the typical cataract with " rust spots ".

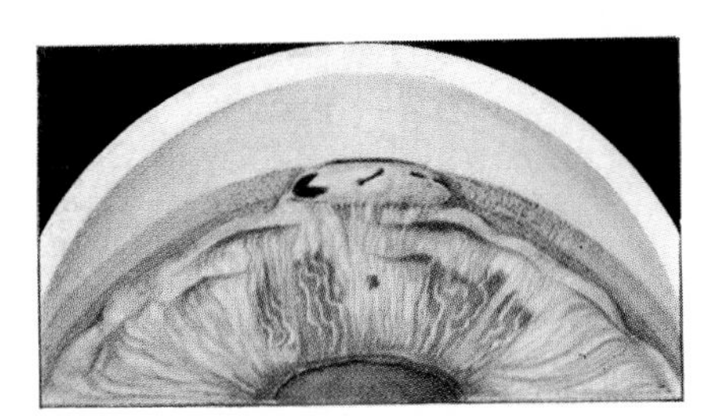

FIG. 2.—Gonioscopic view of an iron foreign body in the angle of the anterior chamber. Direct siderosis in the adjacent segment of the iris (J. François).

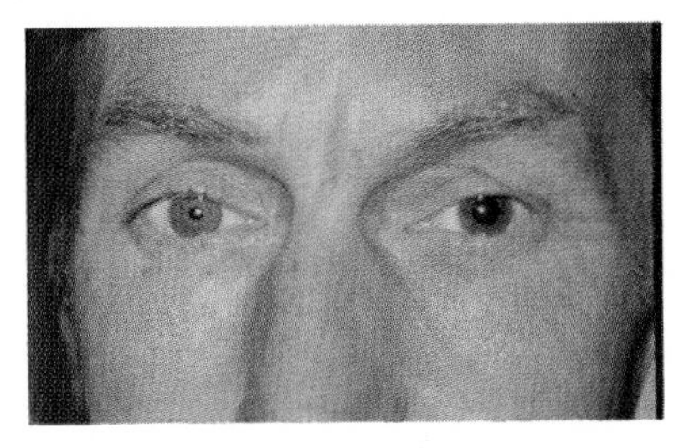

FIG. 3.—Heterochromia iridum due to siderosis following a metallic foreign body in the left eye (A. Lister).

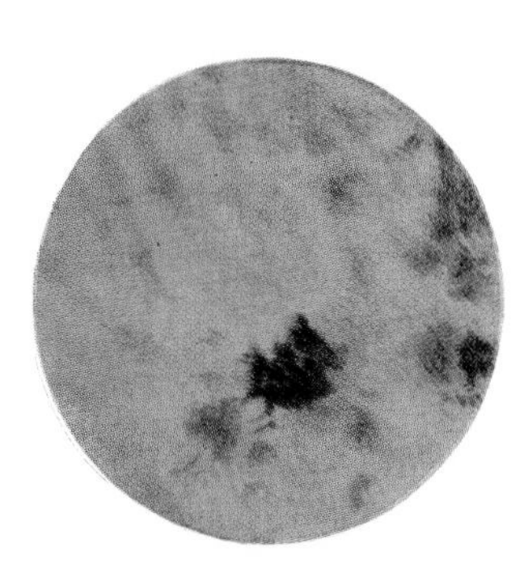

FIG. 4.—Advanced siderosis of the retina; drawing of wet specimen showing bleaching of the pigment epithelium, aggregation of pigment into clumps and total absence of blood vessels.

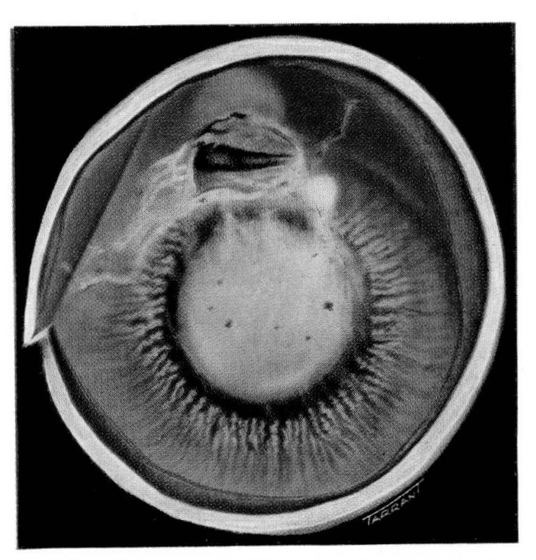

FIG. 5.—Advanced siderosis; frontal section through the globe looking anteriorly; a piece of iron is seen above, surrounded by exudate. The ciliary body is siderotic and there is a cataract.

1901). From the clinical point of view it is important in these cases to distinguish the iridic pigment lying upon the capsule from the more characteristic exogenous pigment lying underneath it. A further striking change affecting the iris is the frequent occurrence of *mydriasis* wherein the pupil is moderately dilated, losing all its reactions to light and becoming resistant to the action of atropine (Knapp, 1894; and many others); a failure of accommodation has occasionally been noted (Basso, 1903). This pupillary dilatation is seen usually some months after the accident but has been observed within a few weeks (Vossius, 1901). It was thought originally by Vossius that the phenomenon was due to chemical stimulation of the sympathetic nerve supply, while Tuckett (1918) ascribed it to damage to the terminals of the oculomotor fibres. It would seem, however, that it is myogenic in origin and that the most probable explanation is atrophy of the muscle fibres of both the sphincter and the dilatator which are found histologically to be heavily impregnated with iron.[1] It is interesting that after extraction of the foreign body, the mydriasis may diminish and the pupil may resume its reflex activities (Cramer, 1902; Tuckett, 1918; Black, 1923).

It is noteworthy that when the particle of iron is in the anterior chamber and is encapsulated, the iris may be stained locally by direct siderosis, but when the metal is in the posterior chamber the whole iris becomes rusty. Similarly a siderotic cataract with a normal iris indicates the presence of an iron particle within the lens, while if both iris and lens suffer siderotic changes, it may be taken that the iron is in the posterior segment of the globe (Plate XXI, Fig. 5).

The Lens. The *cataract of siderosis* provides a unique and beautiful clinical picture. In the initial stages the whole of the anterior surface appears covered by a multitude of minute brownish dots lying subcapsularly, each about 20 microns in diameter: this is the size of the epithelial cells, and these the dots represent. In the beam of the slit-lamp the whole lens eventually takes on a characteristic yellow tint which is especially marked in its anterior band, a colour which is accentuated in the bright yellow anterior shagreen. The bands of discontinuity in the body of the lens become more or less effaced and there is an absence of the design of the fibres indicating the onset of atrophic changes. At a somewhat later stage the diffuse peppering underneath the capsule becomes aggregated in large rusty-brown patches which are apparent on gross examination; these form a wreath circling the anterior surface lying just underneath the edge of the iris, so that the pupil must be dilated before they can be clearly seen (Plate XXI, Fig. 1). Occasionally the yellow deposit may disperse so that a ferrous body lying in the lens may not show up on X-ray examination (Kurz and Henkind, 1965). Practically invariably there are associated lens opacities which usually tend to increase until the cataract becomes complete, when the rusty spots stand out clearly on a white background; only occasionally do

[1] von Hippel (1896), Hertel (1897), Uhthoff (1903), Verhoeff and Fisher (1908), Verhoeff (1918).

these diffuse changes fail to develop (von Hippel, 1894–1901; Kipp, 1906; Mayou, 1926). When the cataract becomes mature it is frequently said that the sclerosis is diffuse, so that on its extracapsular extraction little cortex is left behind (Sattler, 1899), but this is not always so (Elschnig, 1916). Such a siderotic cataract may remain indefinitely, but frequently the lens suffers an atrophic shrinkage so that iridodonesis develops (Eisenberg, 1901), or degenerative changes in the zonule lead to its spontaneous subluxation (after 4 or 5 years, Vossius, 1901; after 40 years, Lincke, 1903), or it is completely dislocated into the vitreous (after 32 years, Loewenstein and Foster, 1947). Only occasionally does the lens become absorbed, leaving behind its capsule along with epithelial remnants (von Hippel, 1894; Vossius, 1896; Eisenberg, 1901).

The *vitreous* also suffers degeneration, showing with the slit-lamp clouds of brown spots clinging to its disorganized framework and sometimes exhibiting gross opacities which are visible ophthalmoscopically. The *choroid*, on the other hand, shows little change until degeneration is far advanced.

The Retina. Siderotic degeneration of the retina is the most serious consequence of the retention of an iron foreign body in the eye, because it is irremediable. The changes usually become evident at a period varying from a few months to 1 or 2 years after the injury, although their onset may be delayed for 10 years or more (44 cases, von Hippel, 1894–1901). Clinically the first appearance is usually that of pigmentary degeneration wherein angular masses of pigment of soft outline are seen, particularly in the periphery. Associated macular changes are not unusual (Haab, 1888)—fine pigmented speckling with a loss of the foveal reflex and alterations in the colour of the perimacular region. In the arteries sclerotic changes are frequent and may occasionally be almost obliterative in their extent (Morton, 1907). A retinal detachment is a common sequence and occasionally the optic disc assumes a yellow rusty colour (Morton, 1907) (Plate XXI, Fig. 4).

In the absence of irritative or inflammatory developments, a *secondary glaucoma* is the most common termination of untreated siderosis, a slow rise of ocular tension coming on at a period varying from 18 months to 19 years after the injury (Clegg, 1915); this may occur even if the foreign body seems safely lodged in the lens (enucleation required after 8 years, Stieren, 1943). The glaucoma is of the chronic simple type, the tension is frequently difficult to control by a fistulizing operation, and most eyes which are not enucleated at an early stage owing to serious damage at the time of the injury or after attempts to extract the foreign body, have been removed eventually because of pain owing to the increase in tension.

The *symptomatology*, apart from the obvious diminution of vision depending on the presence of cataract, is determined essentially by the retinal changes. The progressive degeneration of this tissue, particularly in the periphery, results in a marked concentric contraction of the visual field, a contraction which Uhthoff (1903) considered was greater for blue than for red. Night-blindness is also a prominent and constant feature (Bunge, 1890; von Hippel, 1894; and many others) and xanthopsia is a more rare and much less obvious symptom described by Bettrémieux (1905). In the later stages of the disease, of course, complete amaurosis gradually develops.

Pathology. In general it may be said that the typical and specific toxic effect of iron upon the intra-ocular tissues is concentrated essentially in the tissue cells, on which the action is at first irritative and then destructive; the first response is that of proliferation, the final reaction degeneration. The densest deposition of the metal is upon the anterior surface and the musculature of the iris, in the trabeculæ of the angle of the anterior chamber, the subcapsular epithelium of the lens, the epithelium of the ciliary body and throughout the peripheral retina; the most advanced pathological changes are seen in the retina and the lens.

Much pathological work has been done since the early researches of Bunge (1890). The most important papers of this epoch were those of von Hippel (1893–1901) who examined a large series of eyes at periods varying from 10 days to 7 years after injury. After him several important observations have followed.[1]

The retention of iron lends itself readily to histological study; the method usually adopted is *Perls's microchemical reaction*, wherein the histological section is placed in 2% potassium ferrocyanide and then transferred to 0·5 or 1% HCl, whereupon iron reveals itself in a brilliant Prussian blue colour. It is to be noted that this reaction does not appear after the tissues have suffered prolonged hardening in Müller's fluid; Quincke's reaction is then available, whereby ammonium sulphide turns iron compounds into a dark green or black colour which, however, cannot be distinguished from the ocular pigment. The normal ocular pigment is bleached by the prolonged action of chlorine water, which does not affect iron pigment. Pathological ferrous pigment is bleached by 5% HCl in 24 to 48 hours, a reagent which does not affect the normal ocular pigment.

von Hippel (1896) considered that some of the iron pigment in siderosis, particularly that found in the cornea, was hæmatogenous and not exogenous in origin. Hæmosiderin, of course, gives the Prussian blue colour with Perls's reaction. It is probable, however, that he laid too much stress on hæmatogenous pigmentation, since in many eyes wherein the reaction can be readily seen, hæmorrhage has been lacking. At the same time it is to be remembered that pseudo-siderosis follows intra-ocular bleeding and may even produce "siderotic" cataract (Holm and Bennett, 1962; Hogan and Zimmerman, 1962; Babel, 1964). A case of this type was reported by Velhagen in a child with retinoblastoma who had a gross vitreous hæmorrhage and showed a brown pigmented ring around the nucleus of the lens.

A siderotic eye when examined after fixation in formalin shows a definite brown appearance, particularly in the lens and retina, and this discoloration becomes darker

[1] Hertel (1897–1916), Natanson (1903), Schmidt-Rimpler (1907), Gilbert (1909), Verhoeff and Fisher (1908), Hüttemann (1913), von Szily (1918), D'Amico (1925), Mayou (1925–26), Wolff (1934), Loewenstein and Foster (1947), Ballantyne (1954), Cibis *et al.* (1957–59), Holland (1958), Duke (1959), Vannas (1960), Babel (1964), Wise (1966).

and more prominent on exposure to air. This is due to a granular rusty deposit which is particularly evident under the lens capsule and in the peripheral retina, where patches of brown pigment are liberally scattered. In addition, however, to this granular deposit, which is seen particularly in these two tissues as well as on the anterior surface of the iris, in the angle of the anterior chamber and around the corneal corpuscles in histological section, Perls's reaction shows a diffuse coloration of many of the tissues without any granular aggregations.

The *cornea* is not heavily affected and the most prominent histological picture is granular staining in and around the corpuscles, while the stroma remains free (Fig. 460). Staining of the epithelium occurs only late in extreme degeneration, and Bowman's membrane has been affected exceptionally by a granular deposit which is perhaps associated with generalized

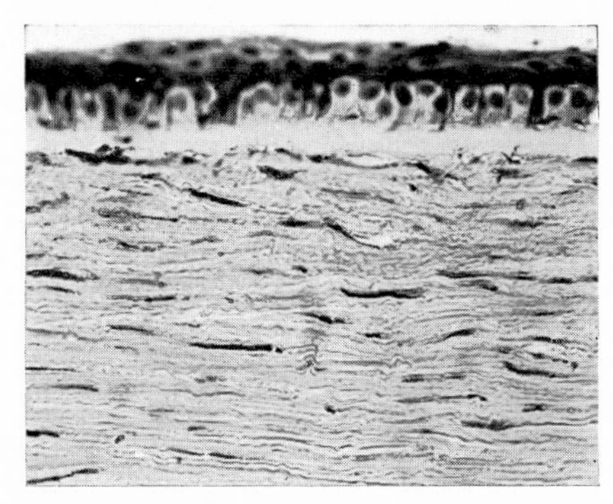

Fig. 460.—Generalized Siderosis Bulbi.

Siderosis of the corneal corpuscles. Enucleation 2 years after injury. There was widespread siderosis bulbi. The figure shows the iron pigment phagocytosed by the corneal corpuscles while the stroma remains free of iron pigmentation (Helenor Wilder).

degenerative changes (Loewenstein and Foster, 1947). Descemet's membrane and the endothelium remain free of iron pigment.

In the *iris* the superficial layer of the stroma stains markedly, the main mass of the tissue and its vessels are little affected, but the most dramatic appearance is the intense staining assumed by the sphincter and dilatator muscles, an appearance beautifully demonstrated by von Hippel (1896–1901), Uhthoff (1903) and Verhoeff (1918) (Fig. 461). The pigmented epithelium is usually lightly stained but sometimes large quantities of iron accumulate between its two layers. The trabeculæ at the angle of the anterior chamber are usually heavily infiltrated with macrophages containing iron presumably obstructing the outflow of aqueous, although the angle itself remains open; this has been observed both clinically (Mayou, 1926; Loewenstein and Foster, 1947; Goldsmith, 1962) and in experimental animals (Erdmann, 1907; Wise, 1966).

In the *ciliary body* the epithelium shows a considerable amount of staining, especially in its inner layer and between the two layers of cells

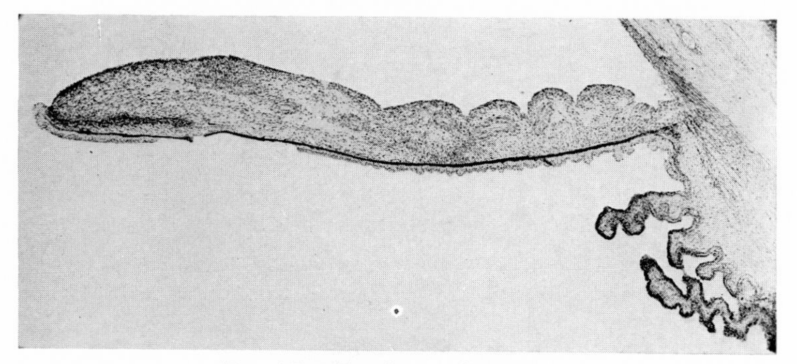

FIG. 461.—THE IRIS IN SIDEROSIS.

Intense pigmentation of the dilatator muscle of the iris in a case of siderosis bulbi. The natural pigment of the iris has been completely bleached so that the dilatator is plainly seen as a black line. The constrictor muscle is also pigmented, but this is not so obvious in the photograph (F. H. Verhoeff).

(Fig. 462). Eventually the outer layer degenerates and the cells of the inner layer discharge much of their pigment in association with corresponding changes in the retina. The ciliary muscle, on the other hand, in contradistinction to the musculature of the iris, is little affected, a contrast which explains the common occurrence of mydriasis and the rare phenomenon of accommodative failure. If a chronic inflammatory reaction is present iron

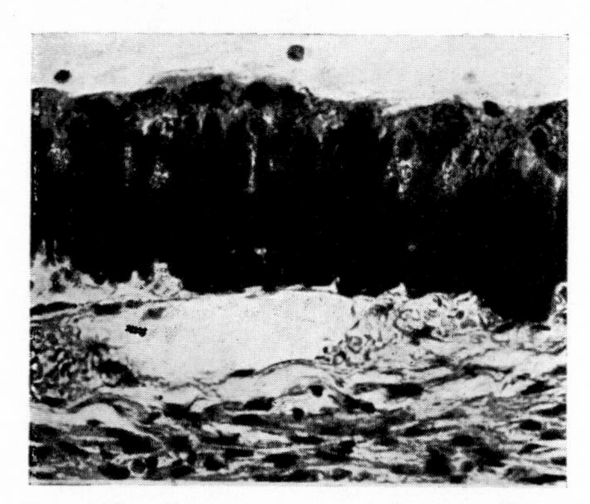

FIG. 462.—SIDEROSIS OF THE CILIARY BODY.

Enucleation 11 months after injury. The normally non-pigmented inner layer of the ciliary epithelium is densely stained with iron pigment (Helenor Wilder).

is found to be engulfed by the leucocytes, the macrophages, the fibroblasts and the mast cells.

In the *lens* the histological appearances are characteristic and pathognomonic. In the very early stages Wolff (1934) found that the capsule stained diffusely; in the later stages it is clear of iron. The subcapsular epithelium, on the other hand, picks up the metal in quantity and stains vividly, and the macroscopic rust spots are seen to be made up of proliferative

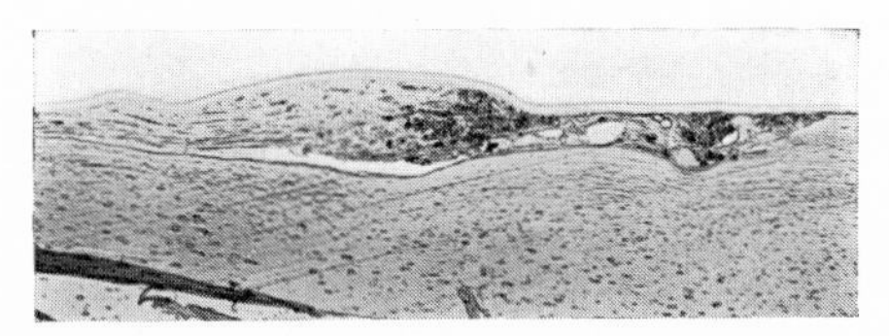

FIG. 463.—SIDEROSIS IN THE ANTERIOR CAPSULE OF THE LENS.

Enucleation 9 months after injury. There is an anterior capsular cataract, the subcapsular epithelium has proliferated and has picked up iron pigmentation in quantity. The illustration shows a typical proliferative patch of this layer which clinically constitutes a "rust spot" (H. Wilder).

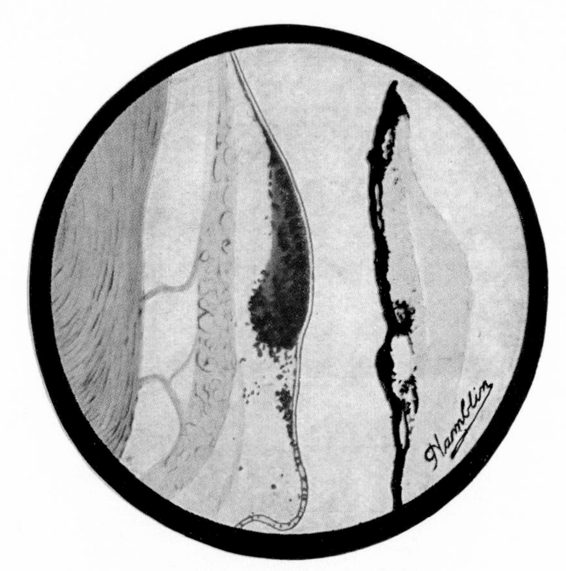

FIG. 464.—SIDEROSIS BULBI.

A drawing showing the later stages of siderosis in the lens and iris. The lens is on the left. The epithelial cells, stained heavily blue with Perls's stain, are detached and agglutinated into large masses which form the characteristic brown spots in the lens capsule (see Plate XXI, Fig. 1). Clinically the lens was clear except for these brown spots.

The iris is to the right. The superficial layers and the muscles are stained blue, and the pigmented epithelium is beginning to show signs of disintegration (M. S. Mayou).

patches of this layer of cells packed with large blue granules (Figs. 463 and 464). At a later stage these cells become detached and mostly destroyed, so that ultimately the " rust spot " is made up of more or less homogeneous material staining light blue interspersed with darkly staining granules. At a later stage the cortical fibres and Wedl's cells show a positive reaction to iron, and when the lens becomes cataractous it shows generalized purple staining in which are granular masses. At this stage also the capsule itself frequently shows degenerative changes, among the more marked of which are large longitudinal splits (Loewenstein and Foster, 1947). In the early stages the

FIGS. 465 to 467.—SIDEROSIS OF THE RETINA.

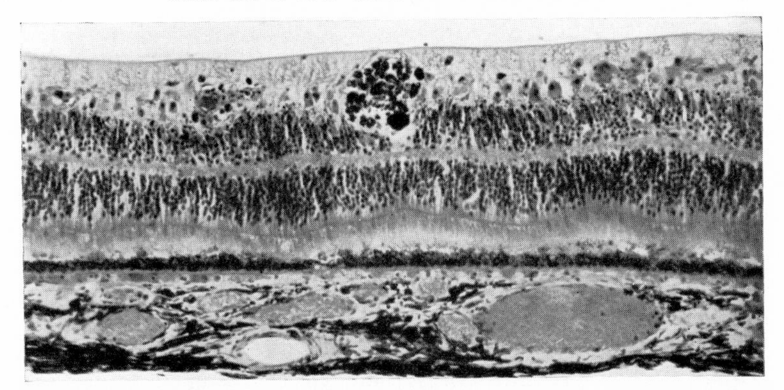

FIG. 465.—A part of the retina situated near the equator. A dense mass of iron pigment is seen around a retinal vessel. Enucleation 2 years after injury (Helenor Wilder).

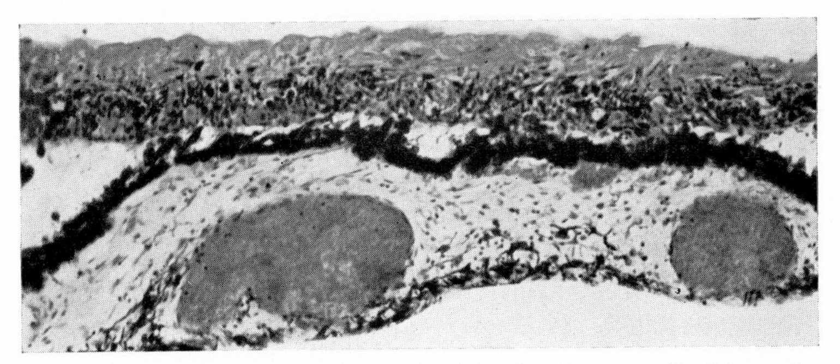

FIG. 466.—Siderosis of the peripheral retina, showing generalized iron pigment and widespread atrophy. Enucleation 2 years after injury (Helenor Wilder).

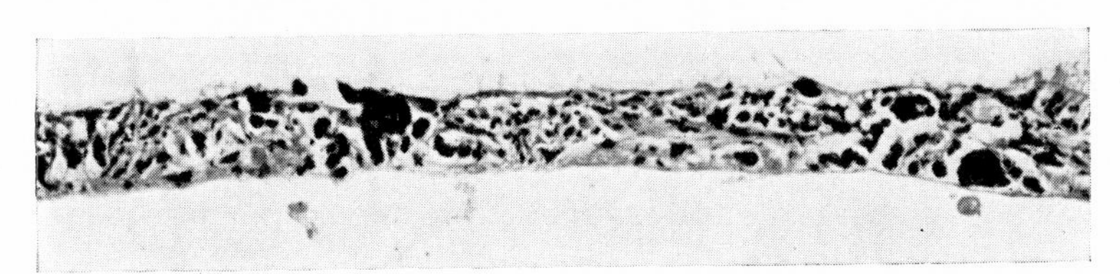

FIG. 467.—Complete atrophy of the retina in an advanced case of siderosis (Jonas Friedenwald). (Compare Plate XXI, Fig. 4).

zonule stains a light blue (Wolff, 1934), while as a later event it disappears completely in places.

The *retinal changes* are marked and gross. In the early stages the iron collects upon the internal limiting membrane and the inner layers of the retina, where the staining affects particularly the nuclei of the cells (Fig. 466); a further collection is seen on the inner surface of the external limiting membrane, but the rods and cones remain free. The hexagonal pigment cells are affected early—the presumable cause of the night-blindness. The ganglion cells are also rapid casualties; at first swollen, they slowly atrophy and eventually may completely disappear. The nuclear layers thin out and ultimately the entire retina becomes saturated with iron and degenerates, the neural tissues being replaced by glial overgrowth, a process which is most accentuated in the periphery. In the macular region, even in advanced cases, the blue staining may be almost entirely absent, but at the same time cystic changes appear and extreme degeneration rapidly develops. At an early stage the blood vessels are heavily marked out with a blue stain (Bunge, 1890) which appears to be due to a collection of iron in the perivascular sheaths (Fig. 465); the absence of such sheaths in the iris probably accounts for the difference in the pathological appearance of the vessels of this tissue even in advanced cases of the disease. Sclerosis of the retinal vessels rapidly develops and, indeed, they may disappear in the periphery of the retina (Loewenstein and Foster, 1947) or, as a terminal event, throughout the entire retina (Mayou, 1926) (Plate XXI, Fig. 4). In the end the whole retina appears as an amorphous mass of glial tissue liberally bespattered with clumps of pigment, eventually either becoming detached or fused with the choroid, sometimes interlaced with glial bands, or even on occasion covered by a degenerative pannus the vessels of which become completely infiltrated with fat (Loewenstein and Foster, 1947) (Fig. 467).

The *choroid*, on the other hand, is little affected in the early stages, some reticulum cells and occasionally a few chromatophores taking on the stain of iron; but even when as a terminal event the retina and choroid become indistinguishably fused and the retina shows diffuse siderotic changes, small blue patches and granules in isolated chromatophores are the only evidences of staining in this tissue.

The *electroretinogram* shows characteristic changes in siderosis[1] (Fig. 468); the earliest response is of the negative-plus type which progresses to negative-minus and eventually to extinction. The time of onset of retinal degeneration varies greatly but may begin within a few weeks and can lead to blindness within one or two years. The development of an abnormal response has important prognostic implications and is an indication for surgical removal of a foreign body even if this presents considerable technical difficulties. If the foreign body is removed at an early stage the ERG may return to normal but when the condition is established this does not usually happen. Extinction of the electrical reaction does not generally occur until other clinical signs of siderosis are apparent and indicates serious disturbance of visual function with imminent retinal degeneration and progressive deterioration of vision. Cases have occurred wherein after removal of the foreign body the electroretinogram and vision have deteriorated rapidly, presumably because sufficient metallic ions remain within the eye to exert

[1] Karpe (1945–57), Schmöger (1956–57), Jacobson (1961), Straub (1961), Jessen (1962), Jayle *et al.* (1965), Kozousek and Semrádová (1963), Kozousek (1965), Franceschetti (1965), Gorgone (1966), Kelsey (1968), Knave (1969–70).

further toxic action on the retina. In such a situation chemical measures for the removal of iron may be required in addition to extraction of the foreign body. The electroretinogram may, therefore, give useful information in cases of traumatic cataract associated with the retention of a foreign body within the eye, and may be the first and sometimes the only manifestation of metallosis.

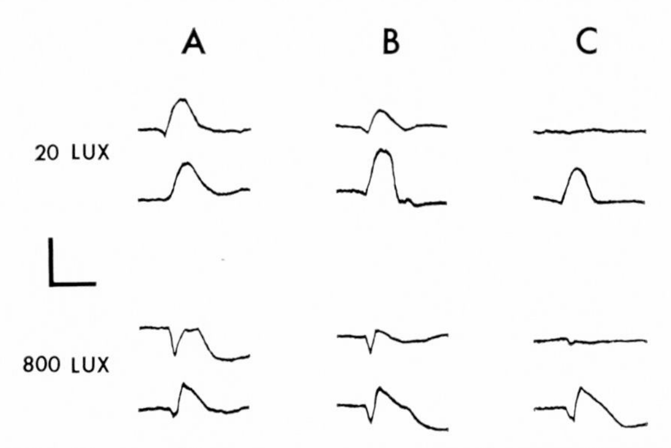

Fig. 468.—Typical Electroretinograms of Retinal Metallosis.

The ERGS are recorded from both eyes (*upper rows*: injured eye, *lower rows*: normal eye) of three patients (A, B and C) with a weak and a strong light stimulus (20 and 800 lux, respectively). Time marking: 0·2 sec. Amplitude marking 0·5 mV. The normal ERG can be seen to consist of a positive *b*-wave, preceded by a negative *a*-wave when stronger intensities of stimulus are used.

A. The first pathological ERG to appear is usually that of the *neg+* type, *i.e.*, an increased *a*-wave followed by a normal *b*-wave. At 800 lux the *b*-wave just reaches the iso-electric line.

B. In the subsequent development the *a*-wave persists in most cases while the *b*-wave decreases (*neg−* type).

C. In the advanced stages the ERG is markedly reduced or even non-recordable. In this patient a just-discernible *a*-wave at 800 lux represents what is left of an initially normal electroretinogram (B. Knave).

The *chemistry of siderosis* is not yet fully understood and many conflicting views have been expressed.

von Graefe (1860) originally suggested that the rusty colour was due to the molecular diffusion of an iron oxide throughout the tissues of the eye. Leber (1891) considered that the metallic iron was dissolved by the carbon dioxide of the tissues and, having diffused throughout the eye as a bicarbonate of suboxide of iron, entered the cells, where it was oxidized and precipitated in insoluble form. This view, which was entirely without experimental verification, was generally accepted by the early writers such as Bunge (1890), who thought that the accumulation of the metal around the retinal vessels where oxidation would be facilitated was thus readily explained. Ausin (1891) suggested that within the cells the iron combined with protein to form an insoluble albuminate, while von Hippel (1894) explained the peculiar distribution of the metal by postulating that certain cells had a special affinity for it. At a later date McMullen[1] suggested that the iron was dissolved by acid phosphates in the intra-ocular fluids and entered into combination with the proteins of the cells to form an albuminate. Mayou (1925–26), on the other hand, considered that the iron was converted into colloidal form as ferric hydroxide.

[1] Unpublished work *circa* 1907.

The spread throughout the globe, however, is largely by electrolytic dissociation by the constant current present in the eye, a process comparable with that occurring in the case of copper[1] (Itoi, 1937; Mielke, 1940). The effect of ionization on the dissolution of a particle was clearly shown by Itoi, who placed an iron nail in a rabbit's eye and found that it became rusty, but that if it were connected with a zinc plate buried subcutaneously, thus reversing the flow of ions, no rust appeared: in these conditions a galvanic cell is set up wherein the nail becomes a cathode and positive iron ions are attracted to it. The iron is disseminated throughout the eye in a general postero-anterior direction in this way in the form of ions although, as we have seen in the case of copper, simple diffusion will also aid in the process. In the tissues themselves the metal appears in different forms, for it has been found that it is sometimes soluble (Bunge, 1890; von Hippel, 1894) and sometimes insoluble (Ausin, 1891; McMullen[2]) to dilute acid, a differentiation which may be seen in the same eye (Mayou, 1926). Almost certainly within the cell the ions combine with proteins to form an insoluble protein salt. It would seem that at first the metabolic processes are relatively unaffected by this accumulation of iron, although some irritation is often obvious, but in view of the fact that the shape and intimate structure of the nuclei remain unchanged the terminal picture does not resemble that of a toxic reaction so much as that resulting from an apparent interruption of cellular activity which culminates in death and mummification.

Cibis and his colleagues (1957–59) showed that the acid-mucopolysaccharides of the vitreous and perivascular tissues have a marked affinity for iron, a property which has found application in histological stains for these substances (Hale, 1946; Rinehart and Abul-Haj, 1951) which they regarded as being an important factor in the siderotic degeneration when this results from the intra-ocular injection of colloidal iron-oxide or a massive dose of iron-filings. On the other hand, Wise (1966) believed that siderotic retinal degeneration resulting from the slow release of iron from an intra-ocular foreign body is not secondary to vaso-obliterative changes caused by the accumulation of iron in the perivascular acid mucopolysaccharide, as suggested by Cibis and his co-workers for the following reasons—firstly, the choroidal circulation is usually unimpaired while the retinal vessels are obliterated, yet the picture of occlusion of the central retinal artery which might be expected to exist is not present although there is full-thickness injury to the retina; secondly, other intra-ocular blood vessels in the uveal tract are generally resistant to damage by siderosis; and thirdly, when iron ions enter the eye slowly from metallic iron the electroretinogram may be diminished and the iron staining of the epithelial cells marked at a time when the blood vessels and perivascular acid mucopolysaccharide show no staining. Further evidence in support of the theory of *direct retinal cytotoxicity* of iron arose from the work of Racker and Krimsky (1948) who inhibited the metabolism of neural tissue with iron ions, of Makiuchi (1960) who obtained retinal necrosis with small amounts of intravitreal ferric citrate, and of Wise (1966) using desferrioxamine to prevent siderosis developing in rabbits by the chelation of iron ions released from intra-ocular metallic iron, thereby preventing the iron from becoming bound within the cells.

[1] p. 522.

[2] Unpublished work *circa* 1907.

The sequence of events in the pathogenesis of siderosis has been summarized by Wise (1966) thus: the iron is released from the metal as free ions which may become loosely bound to the acid mucopolysaccharide. These free ions or iron-acid mucopolysaccharide complexes or both diffuse to various parts of the eye where the iron becomes bound to the enzymes of cells. A particular cell may either detoxify and store the iron or, if sufficient intracellular enzymes have been inactivated, it may degenerate and die, releasing iron pigment which is phagocytosed by macrophages. These iron pigments are thought to be stable, non-toxic and unable to release free iron ions again. The relatively resistant uveal tissues store the iron while the retina, which is less able to detoxify it, is poisoned at an early stage. In contradistinction to Cibis and his collaborators (1959), Wise considered that narrowing of the retinal vessels is secondary to degeneration of the retina and not the cause of it.

Histochemical studies by Matsuo and Hasegawa (1964) and Hasegawa (1964–66) have shown that the activity of succinic and lactate dehydrogenase decreases first in the inner nuclear layer of the retina and then in the outer layer. Similar changes have been demonstrated with respect to glucose-6-phosphate dehydrogenase; with the electron microscope it has also been shown that ferric micelles are scattered diffusely in the cytoplasm of Müller's fibres and the glial cells forming siderosomes.

Treatment. The treatment of an eye harbouring an iron-containing intra-ocular foreign body presents considerable problems apart from those resulting from the damage caused by its entry into the eye for, as we have seen, the retention of such material within the eye involves it in the risk of progressive deterioration and perhaps ultimate degeneration; every effort should therefore be made to remove the foreign body as soon as possible.[1] Although it is true that siderotic deposits may clear after the removal of an intra-ocular foreign body or if it should become encapsulated (Funder, 1957) or is so small that it is absorbed (Holland, 1958), once siderosis has become fully established surgery seldom helps and may even accelerate the onset of phthisis bulbi (Roper-Hall, 1954; and others), while small particles may oxidize to non-magnetic particles of rust, which cannot be localized or extracted (Wise, 1966).

Medical measures to prevent or treat siderosis have been tried by several workers including galvanic de-activation (Itoi, 1937), the administration of intravenous edetic acid (EDTA)[2] (Duntze, 1959; Desvignes and Haut, 1962) and subconjunctival injection of this substance or adenosine triphosphate (Makiuchi and Oyamada, 1961); edetic acid, however, is not without toxic effects after prolonged administration (Foreman, 1963; Batchelor *et al.*, 1964). More success has been obtained from the use of desferrioxamine, a potent iron chelating agent derived from bacteria of the actinomyces family (Bickel *et al.*, 1960; Keberle, 1964). The rationale behind the use of this substance is that an essential part of the early stage of siderosis is the circula-

[1] p. 618. [2] p. 1085

tion of free iron ions or ions loosely bound to acid mucopolysaccharide; desferrioxamine can trap this iron and convert it to the non-toxic chelate, ferrioxamine B, which is removed from the eye in the blood stream and eventually excreted through the kidneys. Once the cells are damaged and iron is bound in the tissues, however, desferrioxamine is unable to remove it. It follows, therefore, that the use of this substance is without effect in cases of advanced siderosis. Subconjunctival desferrioxamine therapy has been found in rabbits to prevent the development of siderosis in eyes containing small deposits of intravitreal iron but was without any beneficial effect in advanced siderosis, experimental vitreous hæmorrhage or experimental corneal blood-staining (Wise, 1966). Chelation therapy may, therefore, have a place in the long-term treatment of siderosis resulting from an intraocular foreign body when surgical treatment is impossible, or in reducing the uveitis resulting from siderotic deposits prior to surgical removal of the foreign body.

It is interesting that the dissemination of iron throughout the tissues of the globe may be sufficient to impart an outline of the eye in a radiographic plate (Hartmann, 1936), the shadow being sometimes particularly accentuated by the preferential deposition of the metal in the immediate neighbourhood of the foreign body by direct siderosis (Jung, 1922).

Andresen. *Zur Siderosis bulbi nebst Bericht ü. 38 Magnetoperationen* (Diss.), Giessen (1903).
Ausin. *Das Eisen in d. Linse* (Diss.), Dorpat (1891).
Babel. *Arch. Ophtal.*, **24,** 405 (1964).
Baitchev. *Oftalmologija* (Bulg.), **5,** 42 (1968).
Ballantyne. *Brit. J. Ophthal.*, **38,** 727 (1954).
Basso. *Clin. Oculist.*, **4,** 1225 (1903).
Batchelor, McCall and Mosher. *J. Amer. med. Ass.*, **187,** 305 (1964).
Begle. *Amer. J. Ophthal.*, **12,** 970 (1929).
Bergmeister. *Zbl. prakt. Augenheilk.*, **31,** 257 (1907).
Bettrémieux. *Ophtal. provinc.*, 168 (1905).
Bickel, Gaeumann, Keller-Schierlein *et al. Experientia* (Basel), **16,** 129 (1960).
Birnbacher. *Zbl. prakt. Augenheilk.*, **9,** 228 (1885).
Black. *Amer. J. Ophthal.*, **6,** 990 (1923).
Braendstrup. *Acta ophthal.* (Kbh.), **22,** 311 (1944).
Bruner. *Ophthalmology*, **3,** 37 (1907).
Bugge. *Norsk Mag. Lægevidensk.*, **8,** 273 (1893).
Bull. *Arch. Augenheilk.*, **10,** 215 (1881).
Bunge. *X int. Cong. Med.*, Berlin, **4** (10), 151 (1890).
Casali. *Ann. Ottal.*, **39,** 572 (1910).
Castelnau. *Arch. gén. Med.*, **15,** 210 (1842).
Cibis, Brown and Hong. *Amer. J. Ophthal.*, **44** (2), 158 (1957).
Cibis and Yamashita. *Amer. J. Ophthal.*, **48** (2), 465 (1959).
Cibis, Yamashita and Rodriguez. *Arch. Ophthal.*, **62,** 180 (1959).
Clegg. *Ophthalmoscope*, **13,** 501 (1915). *Trans. ophthal. Soc. U.K.*, **46,** 179 (1926).
Clizbe. *Amer. J. Ophthal.*, **1,** 220 (1884).
Cramer. *Klin. Mbl. Augenheilk.*, **40** (2), 48 (1902); **43** (1), 757 (1905). *Z. Augenheilk.*, **7,** 144 (1902).
Cridland. *Trans. ophthal. Soc. U.K.*, **36,** 127 (1916); **53,** 438 (1933).
D'Amico. *Ann. Ottal.*, **53,** 289 (1925).
Desvignes and Haut. *Bull. Soc. Ophtal. Fr.*, **62,** 349 (1962).
Duke. *Amer. J. Ophthal.*, **48,** 628 (1959).
Duntze. *Ber. dtsch. ophthal. Ges.*, **62,** 269 (1959).
Eisenberg. *Beiträge z. Kenntnis d. Siderosis bulbi* (Diss.), Giessen (1901).
Elschnig. *Arch. Augenheilk.*, **22,** 113 (1891). *Klin. Mbl. Augenheilk.*, **56,** 23 (1916).
Erdmann. *v. Graefes Arch. Ophthal.*, **66,** 325, 391 (1907).
Fehr. *Zbl. prakt. Augenheilk.*, **24,** 238 (1900).
Foreman. *J. chron. Dis.*, **16,** 319 (1963).
Franceschetti. *Ophthalmologica*, **149,** 266 (1965).
Franke. *Münch. med. Wschr.*, **48,** 516 (1901).
Funder. *Klin. Mbl. Augenheilk.*, **131,** 258 (1957).
Gesang. *Wien. klin. Wschr.*, **18,** 110 (1905).
Gilbert. *v. Graefes Arch. Ophthal.*, **69,** 1 (1909).
Goldsmith. *Amer. J. Ophthal.*, **54,** 385 (1962).
Gorgone. *Boll. Oculist.*, **45,** 638 (1966).
Gradle. *Milit. Surg.*, **51,** 411 (1922).

von Graefe. *v. Graefes Arch. Ophthal.*, **6** (1), 134 (1860).
Gruber. *v. Graefes Arch. Ophthal.*, **40** (2), 154 (1894).
Gulliver. *Arch. Ophthal.*, **28,** 896 (1942).
Haab. *Ber. dtsch. ophthal. Ges.*, **7,** 429 (1888).
Hale. *Nature* (Lond.), **157,** 802 (1946).
Hartmann. *La radiographie en ophtalmologie*, Paris (1936).
Hasegawa. *Folia ophthal. jap.*, **15,** 494 (1964); **17,** 289 (1966).
Hertel. *v. Graefes Arch. Ophthal.*, **44** (3), 283 (1897).
Ber. dtsch. ophthal. Ges., **40,** 117 (1916).
von Hippel. *Ber. dtsch. ophthal. Ges.*, **23,** 30 (1893); **25,** 64 (1896); **29,** 183 (1901).
v. Graefes Arch. Ophthal., **40** (1), 123 (1894).
Hirschberg. *Zbl. prakt. Augenheilk.*, **20,** 257 (1896); **27,** 9 (1903).
Die Magnetoperation in d. Augenheilkunde, 2nd ed., Leipzig (1899).
Berl. klin. Wschr., **44,** 209 (1907).
van der Hoeve. *Z. Augenheilk.*, **39,** 20 (1918).
Hoffmann. *Klin. Mbl. Augenheilk.*, **112,** 156 (1947).
Hogan and Zimmerman. *Ophthalmic Pathology*, 2nd ed., Phila. (1962).
Holland. *Amer. J. Ophthal.*, **45,** 259 (1958).
Holm and Bennett. *Amer. J. Ophthal.*, **53,** 65 (1962).
Horn. *Ein Fall v. Siderosis bulbi mit pathologisch-anatomischem Befund* (Diss.), Giessen (1906).
Hüttemann. *Klin. Mbl. Augenheilk.*, **51,** 315, 479 (1913).
Ide. *Amer. J. Ophthal.*, **65,** 617 (1968).
Itoi. *Acta Soc. ophthal. jap.*, **41,** Suppl., 669 (1937).
Jacobson. *Clinical Electroretinography*, Springfield (1961).
Jayle, Boyer and Saracco. *L'Electrorétinographie*, Paris (1965).
Jessen. *Klin. Mbl. Augenheilk.*, **140,** 215 (1962).
Jung. *Klin. Mbl. Augenheilk.*, **68,** 385 (1922).
Karpe. *Acta ophthal.* (Kbh.), Suppl. 24 (1945).
Doc. ophthal., **2,** 277 (1948).
Ophthalmologica, Suppl. 48, 182 (1957).
Keberle. *Ann. N.Y. Acad. Sci.*, **119,** 758 (1964).
Kelsey. *Advances in Electrophysiology and Pathology of the Visual System*, Leipzig, 19 (1968).
Kipp. *Amer. J. Ophthal.*, **23,** 225 (1906).
Knapp. *Arch. Augenheilk.*, **9,** 224 (1880); **29,** 370 (1894).
Knave. *Acta ophthal.* (Kbh.), Suppl. 100 (1969); **48,** 136 (1970).
Koeppe. *v. Graefes Arch. Ophthal.*, **93,** 173 (1917).
Kozousek. *Ann. Oculist.* (Paris), **198,** 694 (1965).
Kozousek and Semrádová. *Cs. oftal.*, **19,** 377 (1963).
Kurz and Henkind. *Arch. Ophthal.*, **73,** 200 (1965).
Landmann. *v. Graefes Arch. O*[illegible]*l.*, **28** (2), 222 (1882).
Leber. *Proc. VII int. Cong. Me*[illegible]ndon, **3,** 15 (1881).
v. Graefes Arch. Ophthal., **28** (2), [illegible] (1882); **30** (1), 243 (1884).
Die Entstehung d. Entzündung[illegible]eipzig (1891).
Lincke. *Ueber d. dreissigjährige V*[illegible]*ilen eines Eisensplitters im Auge* (Diss.[illegible]ena (1903).
Loddoni. *Ann. Ottal.*, **57,** 28 (1929).
Loewenstein and Foster. *Amer. J. Oph*[illegible], **30,** 275 (1947).
Makiuchi. *Acta Soc. ophthal. jap.*, **64,** 2[illegible] (1960).
Makiuchi and Oyamada. *Jap. J. Ophthal.*, [illegible] 149 (1961).
Mason. *Roy. Lond. ophthal. Hosp. Rep.*, **9,** 158 (1877).
Matsuo and Hasegawa. *Acta Soc. ophthal. jap.*, **68,** 1702 (1964).
Mayou. *Trans. ophthal. Soc. U.K.*, **36,** 140 (1916); **45,** 274 (1925); **46,** 167 (1926).
Meller. *Klin. Mbl. Augenheilk.*, **52,** 288 (1913).
Mielke. *v. Graefes Arch. Ophthal.*, **141,** 644 (1940).
Morton. *Trans. ophthal. Soc. U.K.*, **27,** 227 (1907).
Natanson. *Ber. dtsch. ophthal. Ges.*, **31,** 318 (1903).
Nottage. *Ophthal. Rec.*, **8,** 78 (1899).
Oliver. *Ophthal. Rec.*, **10,** 199 (1901).
Pihl. *v. Graefes Arch. Ophthal.*, **60,** 528 (1905).
Racker and Krimsky. *J. biol. Chem.*, **173,** 519 (1948).
Reitsch. *Klin. Mbl. Augenheilk.*, **53,** 545 (1914).
Ridley. *Trans. ophthal. Soc. U.K.*, **43,** 641 (1923).
Rinehart and Abul-Haj. *Arch. Path.*, **52,** 189 (1951).
Rogman. *Ann. Oculist.* (Paris), **133,** 31 (1905).
Roper-Hall. *Brit. J. Ophthal.*, **38,** 65 (1954).
Rychener. *Amer. J. Ophthal.*, **29,** 346 (1946).
Santoro. *G. ital. Oftal.*, **2,** 384 (1949).
Sattler. *IX int. Cong. Ophthal.*, Utrecht, 433 (1899).
Scalinci. *Progr. Ottal.*, **1,** 106 (1905).
Schiøtz. *Forh. norske med. Selsk.*, 264 (1907).
Schmidt-Rimpler. *Münch. med. Wschr.*, **54,** 99 (1907).
Schmöger. *Klin. Mbl. Augenheilk.*, **128,** 158 (1956).
Ophthalmologica, Suppl. 48, 48 (1957).
de Schweinitz. *Ophthal. Rec.*, **18,** 154 (1909).
Smith. *Amer. J. Ophthal.*, **12,** 409 (1929).
Spratt. *Arch. Ophthal.*, **9,** 102 (1933).
Stieren. *J. Amer. med. Ass.*, **123,** 880 (1943).
Straub. *Das Elektroretinogramm*, Stuttgart (1961).
von Szily. *Atlas der Kriegsaugenheilkunde*, Stuttgart (1918).
Tuckett. *Brit. J. Ophthal.*, **2,** 79 (1918).

Uhthoff. *Dtsch. med. Wschr.*, **29,** 889 (1903).
Vannas. *Acta ophthal.* (Kbh.), **38,** 254, 461 (1960).
Velhagen. *See* Mielke (1940).
Verhoeff. *Brit. J. Ophthal.*, **2,** 571 (1918).
Verhoeff and Fisher. *Arch. Ophthal.*, **37,** 561 (1908).
Vogt. *Klin. Mbl. Augenheilk.*, **66,** 269 (1921).
Lhb. u. Atlas d. Spaltlampenmikroskopie d. lebenden Auges, 2nd ed., Berlin, **2,** 642 (1931).
Vossius. *Ärztl. Sachverständigenzeitg.*, **2,** 145 (1896).
Dtsch. med. Wschr., **23,** Beil., 15 (1897); **35,** 21 (1909); **36,** 1108 (1910).
Ber. dtsch. ophthal. Ges., **29,** 170 (1901).
Wagenmann. *Münch. med. Wschr.*, **52,** 94 (1905).
Whitehead. *Trans. ophthal. Soc. U.K.*, **36,** 63 (1916).
Wise. *Arch. Ophthal.*, **75,** 698 (1966).
Wolff. *Proc. roy. Soc. Med.*, **27,** 691 (1934).
Woods. *Med. News*, **48,** 453 (1886).

ORGANIZED MATERIAL

While the usual response of the ocular tissues to the presence of unorganized material is an irritative inflammation characterized by an exudative response resulting in favourable circumstances in encapsulation,

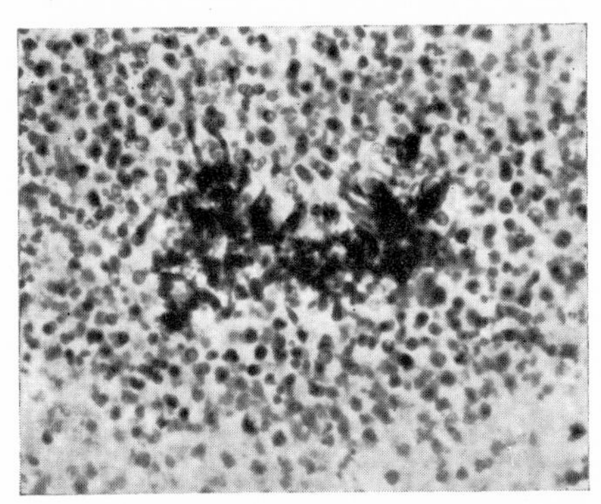

FIG. 469.—Unidentified fungi in a vitreous abscess following perforation of the globe by a minute non-magnetic foreign body (Helenor Wilder).

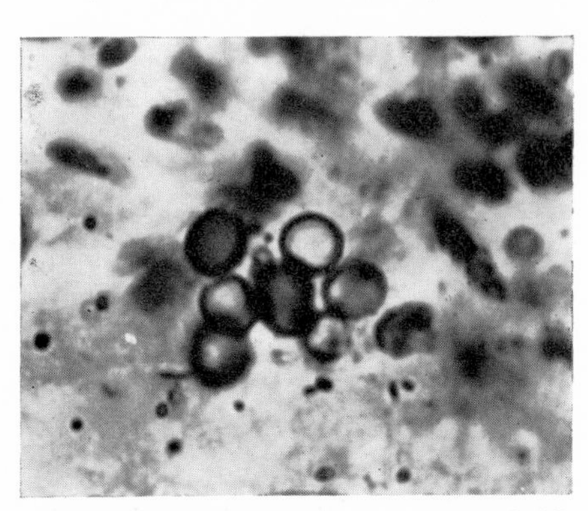

FIG. 470.—Yeast-like organisms probably saprophytic in a vitreous abscess following perforation of the globe by a piece of wood (Helenor Wilder).

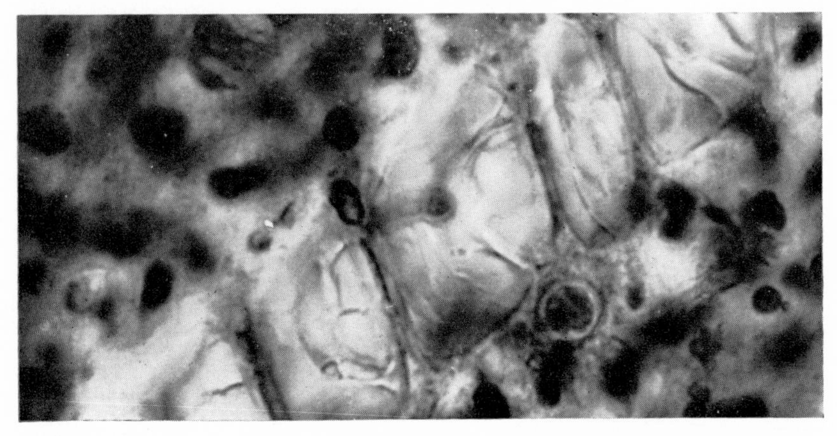

FIG. 471.—Saprophytic fungi with doubly contoured cells and mycelium lying in a vitreous abscess in association with a piece of wood (Helenor Wilder).

the reaction to the presence of organized material, when indeed a response is excited, tends to be less active and an attempt is usually made to absorb the foreign substance or, alternatively, to isolate it by the formation of granulation tissue containing giant cells (Fig. 472). Unfortunately, however, infection occurs much more frequently than in the case of metallic foreign bodies; sometimes this is mild and the infecting agents are relatively innocuous saprophytic yeasts and other fungi some of which, however, may have serious effects (Wilder, 1948; Johnson and Gray, 1968) (Figs. 469–471), but more usually pyogenic infection becomes established, leading rapidly to the formation of abscesses and panophthalmitis, or ending less dramatically in an infective endophthalmitis, the natural termination of which is phthisis bulbi.

VEGETABLE MATERIAL

Vegetable material is rarely met with as an intra-ocular foreign body. The behaviour of the eye to a visitor of this type was experimentally investigated by Kahn (1914) who inserted straw, pieces of grain and grass into the eyes of rabbits. He found that if the material were sterilized no clinical signs of inflammation could be detected for periods up to 115 days, and that at the end of that time pathological changes were minimal. If, however, the material were not sterilized a serous, exudative or proliferative reaction followed by degenerative changes was the invariable result, the nature of the process varying with the degree of infection (Figs. 472 and 473).

The literature contains few comparable case histories wherein vegetable material has been introduced into the globe through a perforating wound. Volk (1898) observed that a piece of straw within the eye excited an initial iritis which resolved after some months; six years later the eye was quiet, the vision normal and the foreign body had disappeared, leaving an atrophic pigmented area in the iris. Dodd (1902) observed that a piece of nut-shell (4 × 2 mm.) in the vitreous excited an inflammation resulting in blindness; thereafter the eye remained quiet for 30 years before a delayed inflammatory reaction appeared associated with sympathetic ophthalmitis. As a rarity small pieces of vegetable matter are blown into the eye after explosions, especially in war wounds; among these, cotton fibres (from clothing, etc.) are of particular interest since they occasionally gain entrance as a surgical contaminant.

Intra-ocular contamination during surgery with pieces of COTTON FIBRE from swabs or lint sponges has already been noted.[1] It is interesting that such pieces of cotton enter the eye not only by direct swabbing of the wound but also from atmospheric pollution by minute particles which float in the air in considerable quantities in the neighbourhood of the operating table; Duszynski (1950) found minute fragments post-operatively too small to be seen clinically in the histological examination of recent wounds in 73% of 216 eyes enucleated. Both clinically and histologically such material is rendered more clearly visible by the use of polarized light (compare Figs. 622–623).

[1] p. 479.

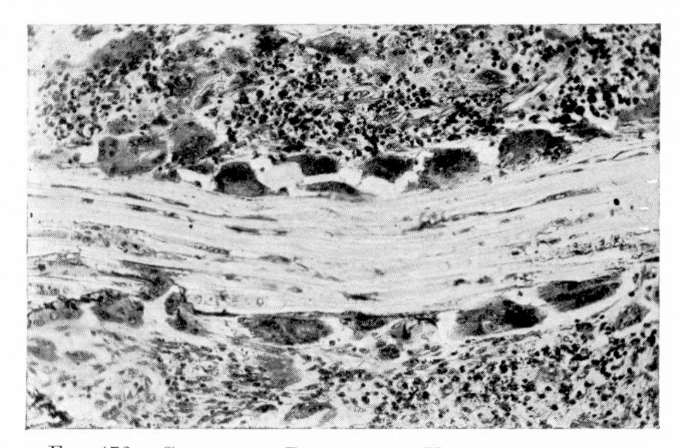

Fig. 472.—Giant-cell Reaction to Vegetable Matter.

The material is lodged in an inflammatory cyclitic membrane. Enucleation 2 months after injury (Helenor Wilder).

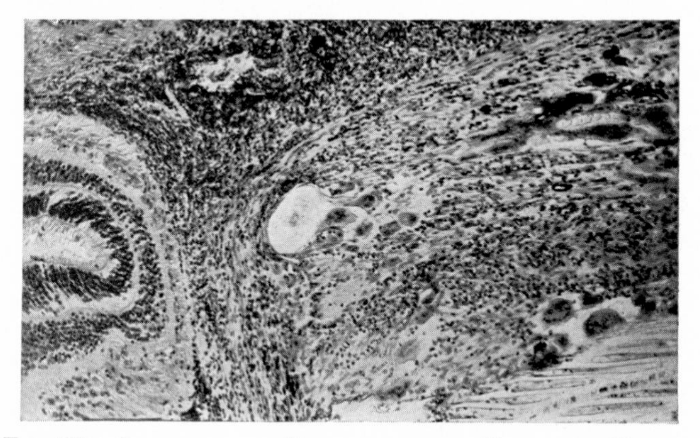

Fig. 473.—Inflammatory Reaction around Vegetable Matter.

Vegetable debris together with a cilium lodged in the vitreous chamber following a land-mine explosion. A hypertrophic inflammatory reaction is seen 2 months after injury (Helenor Wilder).

Even when the pieces of cotton are large they sometimes cause no obvious clinical reaction (Mukai, 1926, 3 cases; Brockhurst, 1954, 4 cases; Grant, 1962) but more frequently a mild and transient irritation characterized by congestion and hyperæmia occurs (Purtscher, 1939, 6 cases; Vogt, 1942, 1 case; Gürtler, 1949, 26 cases; Coles, 1964); occasionally the reactive iritis is considerable (Vail, 1950, 3 cases) (Fig. 474). These cases simulate a severe post-operative traumatic iridocyclitis, occasionally leading to the formation of posterior synechiæ and a pupillary membrane, while the threads themselves may become clotted with minute fluffy exudates. After the extraction of a cataract Brown (1968) found that a strand of cotton was responsible for exciting an œdema of the cornea. The pathological reaction of the ocular tissues to cotton is a low-grade chronic inflammatory response of

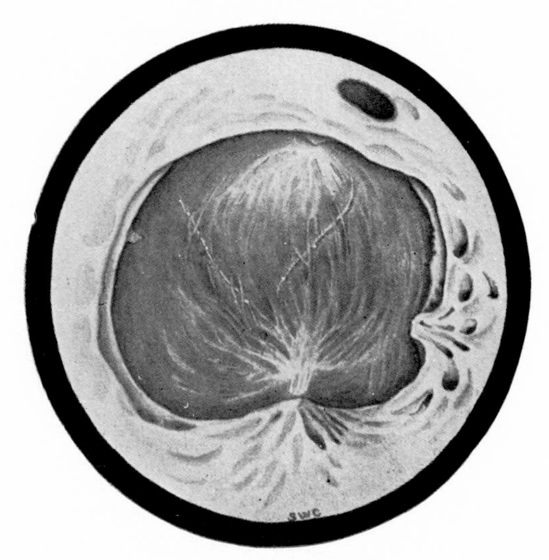

FIG. 474.—LINT IN THE ANTERIOR CHAMBER.

The incarceration of cotton fibres in the eye after an extracapsular extraction of cataract. There was a moderately severe serous iritis on the 10th day and cotton threads, each 4–5 mm. long, were seen embedded in the capsular remnants. They are seen to be studded with fluffy deposits. Two weeks later the eye was quiet, and 11 months later a capsulotomy was performed without event, resulting in good vision (D. Vail).

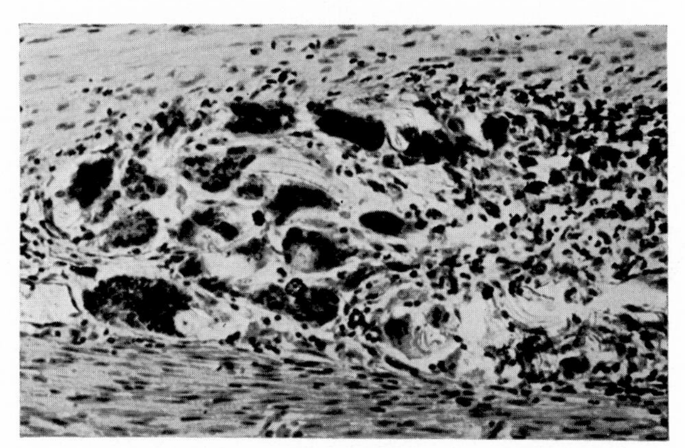

FIG. 475.—COTTON FIBRES WITHIN THE EYE.

A giant-cell reaction to cotton fibres lying in a cyclitic membrane. Enucleation 6 weeks after a dynamite explosion (Helenor Wilder).

a fibroblastic and proliferative nature characterized by the presence of giant cells which tend to wall off the foreign material and attempt to phagocytose it (Wilder, 1948; Duszynski, 1950) (Fig. 475).

WOOD, however, constitutes the commonest intra-ocular foreign body of a vegetable nature (some 6% of all intra-ocular foreign bodies, Hertel,

1916–22). It usually finds entrance into the eye either as a small splinter detached with considerable velocity when it is being chopped or, alternatively, derived from a thorn penetrating the cornea and breaking off to fall into the anterior chamber when a bush brushes the face while passing through a thicket.

The *anterior chamber* is thus the most common site of such a foreign body. The fate of the eye in these cases varies; frequently the piece of wood is *infected*, in which case an acute pyogenic inflammation results. Even in this

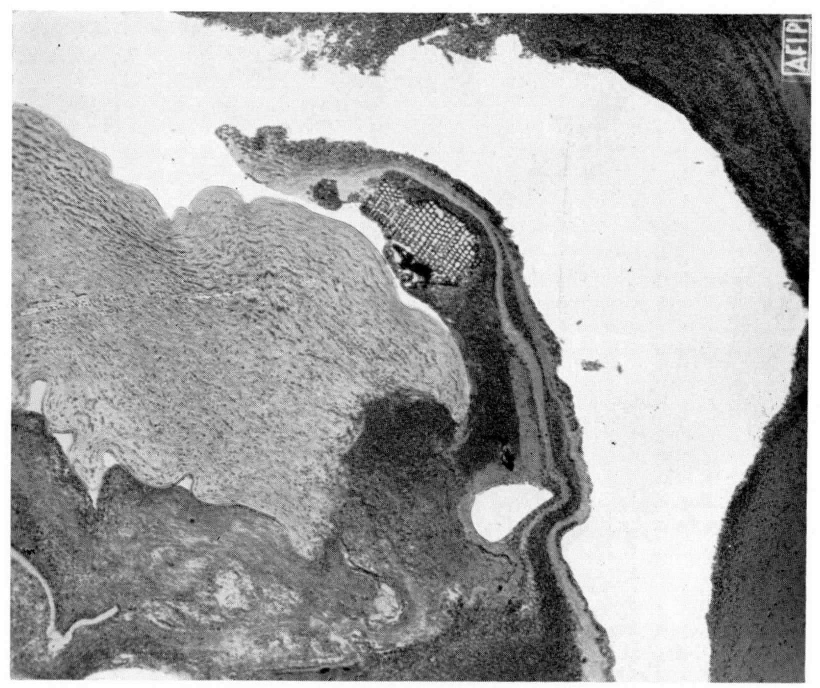

FIG. 476.—PANOPHTHALMITIS FOLLOWING PERFORATION BY A PIECE OF WOOD.

The fragment of wood has prolapsed with the retina through the corneal wound. There is a violent purulent panophthalmitis. Enucleation 8 days after injury (Helenor Wilder).

event, if the foreign body is extracted betimes, the prognosis may be good (Bach, 1905); if not, the localized abscess may result in a fulminating panophthalmitis (von Szily, 1918) (Fig. 476) or, alternatively, a less acute endophthalmitis may slowly develop into a condition of phthisis bulbi (Praun, 1899) (Fig. 477).

If, however, pyogenic infection is not introduced into the eye at the time of the accident, one of several events may occur—the eye may remain quiet, a granulomatous inflammation may develop shortly after the injury, a delayed inflammatory reaction may appear, sympathetic ophthalmitis may be excited, an implantation cyst may be formed or, finally, the foreign body may be eventually extruded from the globe.

The absence of a reactive response, apart from the immediate effects of the initial trauma, is not uncommon, the piece of wood behaving as a relatively indifferent foreign body.

Two of the earliest reports of such a condition belong to this category. The first was that of Victor (1847), wherein a thorn, deeply embedded in the cornea, fell into the anterior chamber during the effort to extract it; eight years later it was lying quietly in the same position. Richardson's (1859) case is also interesting. Three splinters of wood detached from a tree by a cannon-ball entered the eye of a soldier in 1813; 46 years later the pieces of wood were still in position, the vision was good and the eye quiet, although the iris was atrophic.

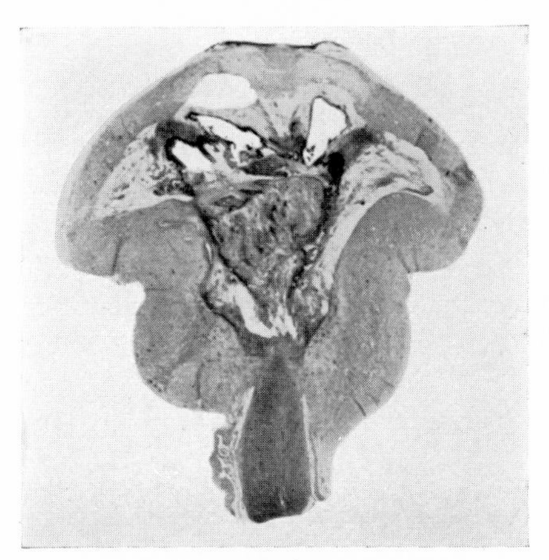

FIG. 477.—PHTHISIS BULBI FOLLOWING THE LODGMENT OF A PIECE OF WOOD IN THE EYE.

The vegetable matter lay in the vitreous chamber for 11 years while the eye was slowly destroyed in phthisis bulbi (Helenor Wilder).

Reports of this lack of response for several weeks to a splinter of wood (Franke, 1887) or a thorn (Lawson, 1867; Landmann, 1882; Deschamps, 1905; and others) are relatively common, but long histories are unusual (1 year, Bock, 1907; 4 years, Fox, 1942; 11 years, Jung, 1903). As occurs with other foreign bodies, however, even if the eye does remain quiet for a long period it is not necessarily permanently immune, for a *delayed inflammation* may appear after the lapse of many years (13, Onishi, 1913; 47, Sigismund, 1880, and Massmann, 1880). A delayed reaction of this type may develop even in an eye which has become shrunken and atrophic after the injury and has remained quiet in this state for a long period (30 years, Lagrange, 1902).

The usual alternative to this reaction is an *inflammatory response* of the proliferative type associated with considerable iridocyclitis and characterized by the formation of a granulomatous mass in the iris, the essential feature of which is the aggregation of a large number of giant cells around the particle (Fig. 410) (Horner, 1863; Stock, 1901). The growth of such a tumour and the intensity of the associated irritation may well require the enucleation of the eye. It has occasionally happened, however, particularly during a phase of reactive irritation, that the wood is eventually *extruded from the globe* and, even although it had been retained for some time, reasonably good vision may still remain (after 15 months, Bochever, 1947).

In common with other foreign bodies, three further developments may ensue. An *implantation cyst* may be formed (Wiener, 1905) or a solid epithelial tumour the central cells of which may degenerate so that a

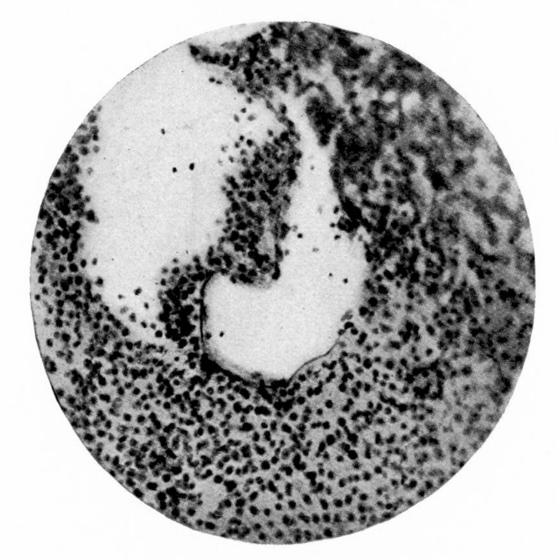

Fig. 478.—Cyst of the Iris.

Cystic degeneration of the epithelium in an implantation tumour of the iris containing wood fibres (R. Pickard).

somewhat similar cystic formation results (Pickard, 1906) (Fig. 478). As a terminal event the eye may be destroyed by a secondary chronic *glaucoma* (after 14 years, Wilder, 1948); and it must always be remembered that *sympathetic inflammation* may occur after the intra-ocular retention of wooden foreign bodies even if they have remained quietly in the eye for a considerable time (7 months, Velhagen, 1942; 36 years, Wilder, 1948) (Fig. 494).

In the lens a wooden foreign body is a rarity. Forlanini (1871) found experimentally in animals' eyes that little reaction need arise if a splinter of wood penetrated this tissue. The same tolerance has been observed clinically and a splinter has lain quietly in the lens for 16 years without the development of cataract beyond the immediately surrounding opacity (Cordes, 1943). More usually, however, a traumatic cataract rapidly develops and the formation of anulomatous tumours in the iris near the lower part of the anterior cha ber has followed the subsequent disintegration of the lens, a reaction sumably due to the irritation caused by the foreign body (Früchte, 1910). lternatively, of course, infection is introduced leading to endophthalmiti Diehl, 1899).

In the poste r segment the reaction is invariably more marked. Pyogenic infection is us ly introduced at the time of the injury, leading to the formation of a treous abscess and the development of phthisis bulbi. In the absence o fection an exudative inflammatory response may lead to a detachment the retina (Raab, 1875), or a proliferative response resulting in the massiv rmation of fibrous tissue may appear clinically as a pseudoglioma (from plinter, Rémy, 1875) or a tumour (from a thorn, Fromaget, 1896). If b ance the splinter lies between the choroid and the retina, encapsulatio ay occur (after 1 year, Addario, 1910).

Addario. *Prog ftal.*, **5**, 104 (1910).
Bach. *Ueber remdkörperverletzungen d. vorderen enkammer u. Iris* (Diss.), Jena (190
Bochever. *Ve oftal.*, **26** (6), 36 (1947).
Bock. *Zbl. p . Augenheilk.*, **31**, 65 (1907).
Brockhurst. *h. Ophthal.*, **52**, 121 (1954).
Brown. *Ame . Ophthal.*, **65**, 616 (1968).
Coles. *Int. O hal. Clin.*, **4**, 895 (1964).
Cordes. *Am . Ophthal.*, **26**, 1062 (1943).
Deschamps. *v. gén. Ophtal.*, **24**, 361 (1905).
Diehl. *Ue einen Fall v. Fremdkörperverletzu l. Auges* (Diss.), Jena (1899).
Dodd. *Oph . Rec.*, **11**, 220 (1902).
Duszynski. *ans. Amer. Acad. Ophthal.*, **55**, 110 (1).
Forlanini. *n. Ottal.*, **1**, 145 (1871).
Fox. *Ame . Ophthal.*, **25**, 1105 (1942).
Franke. *ch. med. Wschr.*, **34**, 522 (1887).
Fromaget. *az. Sci. méd.* Bordeaux, **17**, 56 (1896
Früchte. *in. Mbl. Augenheilk.*, **48** (1), 185 (191
Grant. *icology of the Eye*, Springfield, 151 62).
Gürtler. *ien. klin. Wschr.*, **61**, 638, 686 (1949).
Hertel. *. dtsch. ophthal. Ges.*, **40**, 117 (1916). *Hb. ärztl. Erfahrungen im Weltkrieg, 191 18*, Leipzig, **5**, 363 (1922).
Horner *lin. Mbl. Augenheilk.*, **1**, 395 (1863).
Johnso nd Gray. *Arch. Ophthal.*, **80**, 403 (1).
Jung. *nch. med. Wschr.*, **50**, 2202 (1903).
Kahn. *eber d. Wirkung einiger pflanzlicher ndkörper a. d. Kaninchenauge* (Diss.), lelberg (1914).
Lagrange. *Rev. gén. Ophtal.*, **21**, 470 (1902).
Landmann. *v. Graefes Arch. Ophthal.*, **28** (2), 153 (1882).
Lawson. *Roy. Lond. ophthal. Hosp. Rep.*, **6**, 38 (1867).
Massmann. *Dtsch. med. Wschr.*, **6**, 105 (1880).
Mukai. *Klin. Mbl. Augenheilk.*, **76**, 88 (1926).
Onishi. *Klin. Mbl. Augenheilk.*, **51**, 742 (1913).
Pickard. *Trans. ophthal. Soc. U.K.*, **26**, 62 (1906).
Praun. *Die Verletzungen des Auges*, Wiesbaden (1899).
Purtscher. *Klin. Mbl. Augenheilk.*, **102**, 844 (1939).
Raab. *Klin. Mbl. Augenheilk.*, **13**, 239 (1875).
Rémy. *Bull. Soc. Anat. Paris*, **10**, 468 (1875).
Richardson. *Dubl. quart. J.*, **28**, 319 (1859).
Sigismund. *Berl. klin. Wschr.*, **17**, 68 (1880).
Stock. *Münch. med. Wschr.*, **48**, 1229 (1901).
von Szily. *Atlas der Kriegsaugenheilkunde*, Stuttgart (1918).
Vail. *Trans. Amer. ophthal. Soc.*, **48**, 243 (1950).
Velhagen. *Klin. Mbl. Augenheilk.*, **108**, 553 (1942).
Victor. *Chir. Zeit.*, **2** (2) (1847).
Vogt. *Lhb. u. Atlas d. Spaltlampenmikroskopie d. lebenden Auges*, 2nd ed., Berlin, **3**, 910 (1942).
Volk. *Zur Statistik d. Augenverletzungen mit besonderer Berücksichtigung d. Fremdkörperverletzungen* (Diss.), Giessen (1898).
Wiener. *Amer. J. Surg.*, **18**, 199 (1905).
Wilder. *Amer. J. Ophthal.*, **31**, 57 (1948).

ANI L MATTER

he introduction of animal material into the eye is rarer than that of veg able matter. Leber (1881–91) and Masse (1881) found that soft tissues (su as MUSCLE) excited little reaction but became infiltrated by leucocytes and fibrin and tended to be absorbed, a fate, however, which did not apply to EPITHELIUM. Although conjunctival and corneal epithelium find a fertile field for growth within the eye (Fig. 479), the epidermis of the skin, which as a rarity finds its way into the anterior part of the globe in explosion injuries, behaves as a relatively inactive foreign body (Wilder, 1948) (Fig. 480).

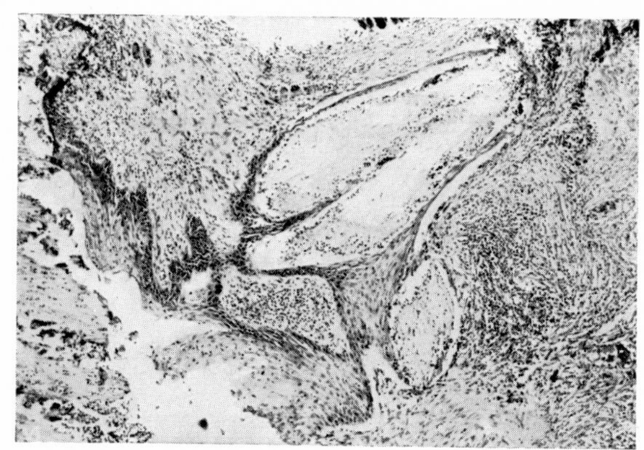

FIG. 479.—CONJUNCTIVAL EPITHELIUM.

Showing hyperplasic changes around a thorn incarcerated in an inflammatory cyclitic membrane. Enucleation 4 months after injury (Helenor Wilder).

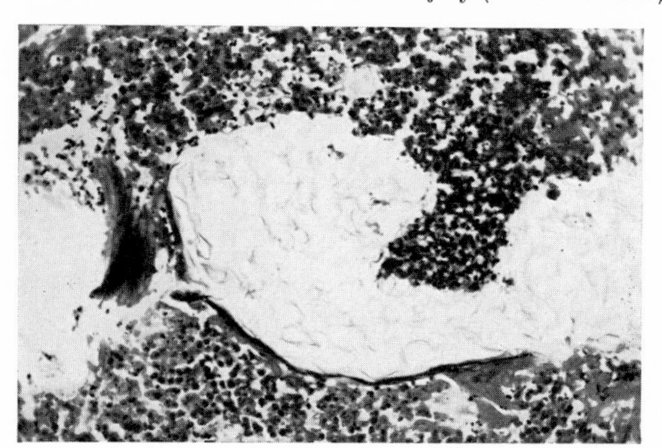

FIG. 480.—EPIDERMAL EPITHELIUM WITH KERATIC DEBRIS IN A VITREOUS ABSCESS.

The skin tissue behaves as an inactive foreign body and shows no evidence of growth as occurs with conjunctival epithelium (Fig. 479). Enucleation 4 days after injury (Helenor Wilder).

BONE may also be forced into the eye in severe head injuries or explosions, in which case the particles of bone are usually derived from the skull or are detached from some distant part such as the fingers. Accidents of this type are therefore usually war injuries of considerable severity (Hertel, 1916; Dor, 1916; von Herrenschwand, 1916; von Szily, 1918; Wilder, 1948). As a rule the eye is badly damaged and enucleation is necessary, but if the globe can be retained the bone itself apparently remains inert within it and may even be eventually absorbed (after 2 years, Spierer, 1891) (Fig. 481).

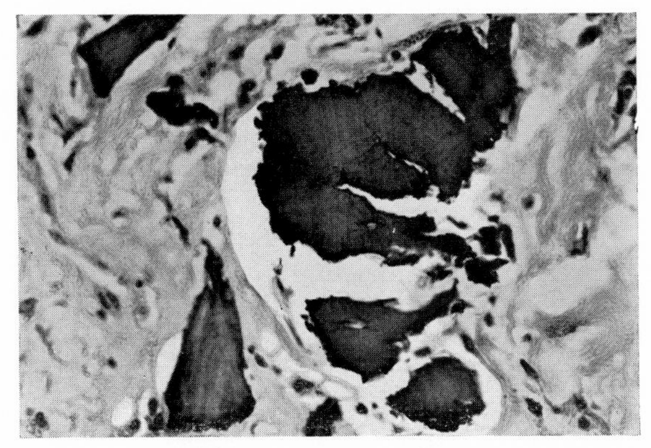

Fig. 481.—Embedded Bone incarcerated in a Cyclitic Membrane following a Wound of the Skull.

The bone behaves as an inactive foreign body. Enucleation 9 months after injury (Helenor Wilder).

CILIA

Although comparatively rare, the most common foreign material in this class to find entrance into the eye is an EYELASH and, because of the wide variation in its ultimate fate, it is the most interesting and has excited the most attention in the literature. A cilium, of course, is carried passively into the eye at the time of a penetrating injury sometimes in company with a foreign body such as a piece of metal or a lead pellet. Its rarity is probably explained by the fact that the lids may not close reflexly until the foreign body is actually within the eye, so that the particle misses contact with the lashes; only on rare occasions will the foreign body brush the ciliary margin or lid closure occur simultaneously with the impact. It is to be remembered, also, that a cilium occasionally makes an inadvertent entrance through an operative wound in the course of ophthalmic surgery (Landmann, 1882; Peschel, 1887; Müller, 1894; and others).

The entrance of a hair from the eyebrow in a perforating injury is a great rarity, but it has found its way both into the anterior chamber (von Graefe, 1864) and into the vitreous (Quint, 1901). It is interesting that a piece of horsehair has been found in the anterior chamber in a case wherein the eye was struck and perforated by a whip-lash (Scheffer, 1913).

Since the early observation of Lerche (1835) a large literature has accumulated on this subject. Most commonly the cilium lies *in the anterior chamber*, sometimes with one end incarcerated in the corneal wound. Even here, however, its occurrence is rare—5 in 30,000 new patients (Müller, 1894, in Vienna), 3 among 143,471 eye patients (Popov, 1941, in Rostock and Astrakhan), 2 in 374,721 eye patients (Sitchevska and Payne, 1949, in New York). The early literature was surveyed by Zander and Geissler (1864), Rothmund (1872), Vieweger (1883, 29 cases), Franke (1884), Wallner (1905), Lang (1907) and Wagenmann (1921, some 100 cases up to 1917). Sharpe (1925) discussed 75 cases, Graff (1933) added 30 cases, and Cowen (1942) a further 29. Since

FIGS. 482 and 483.—CILIA IN THE ANTERIOR CHAMBER (F. Rubey).

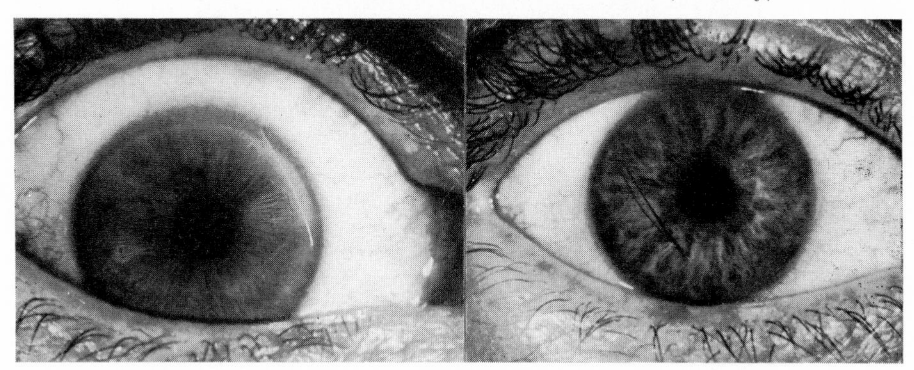

FIG. 482. FIG. 483.

FIG. 482.—A depigmented cilium lies between 1 and 4 o'clock.

FIG. 483.—A pigmented cilium lies between 6 and 10 o'clock with its end enmeshed in the iris.

then several papers have appeared each year, among which are those of Rubey (1966) and Joseph (1967) (Figs. 482–3).

In the posterior chamber, lying between the iris and the lens, a cilium has been much more rarely found (Ruete, 1839; Manz, 1868; Castroviejo, 1931; Savin, 1936; da Silva, 1948) (Plate XXII). Similarly rare is its entrance into the posterior segment of the eye, an event which has occurred particularly in wounds with small-shot or metallic foreign bodies.[1]

In the lens the incarceration of a lash after an injury without exciting a reaction is exceptional (von Hippel, 1927; Byrnes, 1949; Sédan, 1950; Raiford, 1952) (Fig. 488).

The *number of cilia* found within the eye has varied considerably. As a rule one cilium finds entrance, but the presence of two is not unusual (Paderstein, 1910;

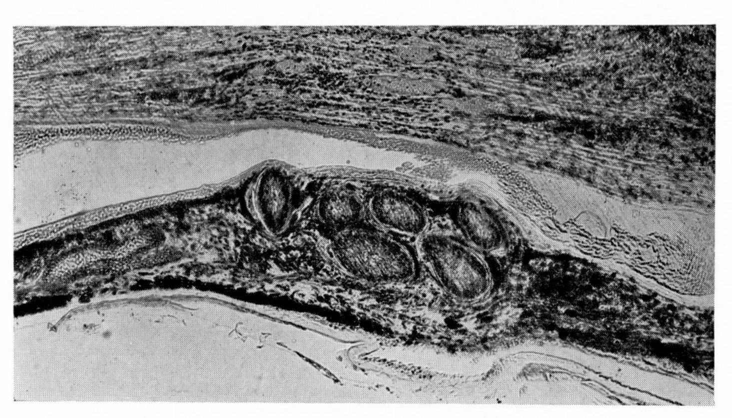

FIG. 484.—CILIA IN THE IRIS.

A group of 6 cilia seen embedded in the iris, and around them is a chronic infiltrating iritis. The cornea is on top (Bertha Klien).

[1] Manz (1868), Sattler (1874), Mackrocki (1883), de Lapersonne and Vassaux (1884), Deutschmann (1890), Webster (1891), Treacher Collins (1894), Wintersteiner (1894), Lang (1907), Warnecke (1908), Saryev (1951), and others.

Lichtner, 1935; Shagov, 1937; Cowen, 1942; Sitchevska and Payne, 1949), while cases have been reported describing the presence of 3 (Treacher Collins, 1894; Franklin and Cordes, 1925), 4 (Begle, 1917; Sharpe, 1925), 5 (Ruete, 1839; Paderstein, 1910; Bulson, 1920; Saryev, 1951), 6 (Schweigger, 1871; Mikhailov, 1938; Klien, 1945; Payrau and Guyard, 1956) and even 14 (Vieweger, 1883) (Fig. 484).

The fate of the hair and the reaction of the eye vary. Sometimes but not very commonly the wound is contaminated by *infection* and an acute pyogenic inflammation is set up, possibly appearing clinically as a violent iridocyclitis with hypopyon; this, however, may resolve on the timely extraction of the lash, a happy event which has occurred even before the days of antibiotic therapy (Hirschberg, 1892–1909; Mendelssohn, 1917).

If, however, the cilium is not infected and lies *in the anterior chamber*, it may remain for a long time without exciting a response, a delayed reaction may take place sometimes after many years, the immediate response may be a plastic inflammation or a granulomatous proliferation while, as a delayed end-result, a cyst may develop in association with the lash. The cilium, indeed, may *remain inert* without exciting a reaction for an indefinite time and may even be discovered accidentally in the course of a routine eye examination many years after the original accident (Hughes, 1924). This passivity may occur whether one end is incarcerated in the corneal wound, whether the lash lies freely in the anterior chamber, or whether it is fixed to the iris or, as occasionally happens, to the capsule of a cataractous and partly absorbed lens (Plate XXII, Fig. 1). It is interesting that if part of the cilium appears in the pupillary aperture it may be seen entoptically (Pamard, 1860). In such cases changes may occur in the structure of the lash—splitting or separation of the cuticle, partial resorption with depigmentation and bleaching (Meyer, 1889; Müller, 1894; Gradle, 1923) (Fig. 482), while its complete disappearance has been reported (Samelsohn, 1885; Königstein, 1906). It must be remembered, however, that even although the cilium has been tolerated for many years a *delayed inflammation* sometimes develops which may, indeed, be of a nature so destructive as to end in blindness (after 33 years, Sharpe, 1925; after 15 years, Henneberg, 1926).

Case histories of the remarkable tolerance of the eye to cilia are numerous and include periods of observation up to 34 years—2 years (Landmann, 1882; Alexander, 1912), 4 (Rothmund, 1872; Friedinger, 1878), 6 (Schweigger, 1871), 8 (Schwarz, 1898), 10 (Peschel, 1887), 16 (G. H. Cross, 1929; Byrnes, 1949), 18 (McKee, 1928; Celeste, 1950), 19 (Roll, 1906; Gradle, 1923), 20 (Königstein, 1906; Guzmann, 1912; Shagov, 1937; Tokuda and Tanaka, 1940; Mattos, 1943; Harbridge, 1950), 29 (Robertson, 1876), 32 (da Silva, 1948), 34 (Müller, 1894; Schwarz, 1899).

Alternatively, the presence of the cilium may excite a *plastic inflammation* which appears clinically as an irritative iridocyclitis, sometimes involving the formation of posterior synechiæ (Papagno, 1931; F. Smith, 1936; Sédan, 1950). The cilium itself may be covered with plastic exudates appearing as woolly masses along its length and occasionally trailing after it somewhat like a corkscrew (Plate XXII). The development of such a reaction may be delayed for several months after the injury (Métaxas, 1899; Fehr, 1901; Königstein, 1906), and the inflammation is occasionally widespread, leading eventually to the destruction of the globe; it may, however, clear up after the cilium is extracted (Meyer, 1889). In such cases it occasionally happens that the cilium migrates and may even be extruded from the globe (Samelsohn, 1885; Lang, 1907), an event which was seen experimentally in the eyes of rabbits after the introduction of cilia by van Dooremaal (1873).

As an alternative to the exudative response the reaction of the eye may be essentially proliferative in nature, a *granulomatous tumour* being formed heavily infiltrated by lymphocytes, plasma cells and numerous foreign-body giant cells (von Szily, 1918; Klien, 1945) (Figs. 484 and 485). It should be

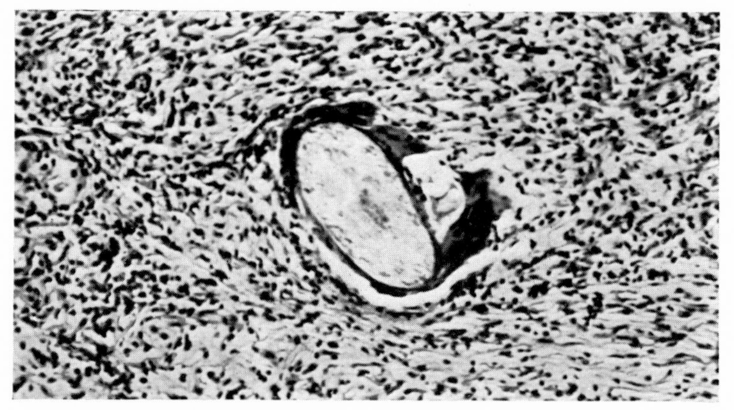

FIG. 485.—GRANULOMA ASSOCIATED WITH A CILIUM.

The giant-cell reaction to a cilium incarcerated in an inflammatory cyclitic membrane. Enucleation 5 weeks after injury (Helenor Wilder).

remembered also that—as a rarity—sympathetic ophthalmitis has been reported (after 6 months, Cunier, 1841; after 2 weeks, von Graefe, 1864).

Cystic formation is a very typical delayed complication of the retention of a lash in the anterior segment of the eye; it is a rare event—Dessalle (1904) found only 18 cases in the literature up to that date—and it may occur at a period varying from some months to some years after the injury (after 14 years, Villard and Dejean, 1933; after 37 years, Horay, 1928) (Plate XXII, Fig. 2).

The cyst has the character of an implantation, the nature of which has already been discussed (Rothmund, 1871–72).[1] Experimental investigations undertaken to prove its precise origin, however, have not been conclusive. Schweninger (1875) found that on the implantation of cilia into animals' eyes, the cells of the hair follicles proliferated, a result confirmed by Masse (1881); but in similar experiments, Hosch (1885) concluded that the proliferation occurred only if pieces of skin were implanted

[1] p. 411.

PLATE XXII

CILIA AS INTRA-OCULAR FOREIGN BODIES.

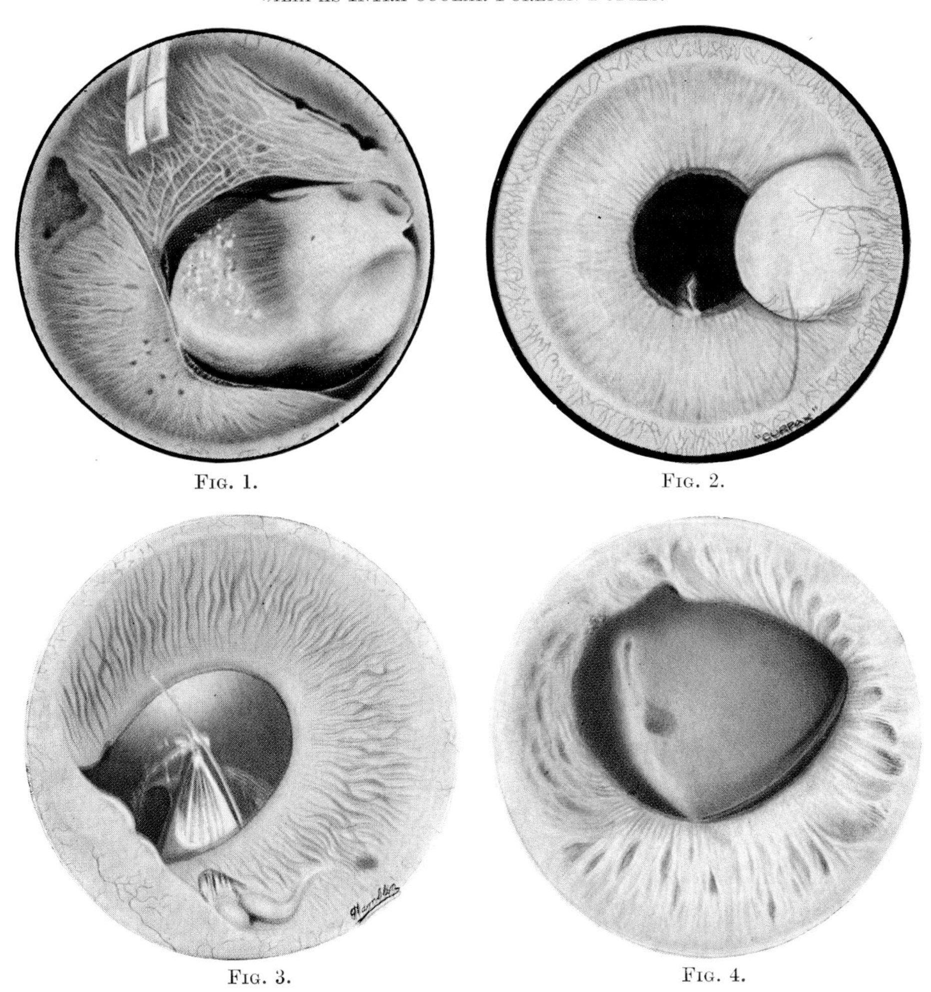

FIG. 1. FIG. 2.

FIG. 3. FIG. 4.

FIG. 1.—Perforating wound: traumatic cataract and iris prolapse which has been abscised. The cilium had lain quietly partly on the iris and partly on the lens capsule for two years.

FIG. 2.—A perforating injury of the cornea in the lower part of the pupillary area. There is a large inclusion cyst arising from the anterior chamber across which the cilium lies.

FIG. 3.—Perforating wound with a screw-driver involving a prolapse of the iris which was abscised. Six years later a cilium was still lying across the pupillary aperture. Its lower part lay behind the iris, through a hole in which a corkscrew-like exudative formation associated with the end of the lash is seen curling out into the anterior chamber (L. G. Scoular).

FIG. 4.—Two months after a perforating injury across the nasal part of the pupillary region. The division of a synechia from the corneal wound resulted in the appearance of a cilium which had hitherto lain in the posterior chamber behind the iris. This was removed with rapid resolution of the inflammation and good vision (L. H. Savin).

with the cilia. The most common view is that the epithelium of the root-sheath or the follicle proliferates to form a cyst, but Bonnet and Paufique (1934) suggested that the presence of the cilia merely served to stimulate the growth of surface epithelium introduced at the time of the accident. It is true that in several cases the cilium has been found lying across a cyst or in its immediate neighbourhood, without any apparent direct association with it and without evidences of growth although it had been present for a considerable period (14 months, Moore, 1930). Moreover, a cyst has appeared 8 months after two cilia had been surgically removed, suggesting that the origin may have been from separate epithelial cells which had been left behind (Sitchevska and Payne, 1949–51). The fact remains that there is some doubt why some cilia stimulate the formation of cysts and others do not. Dellaporta (1941) suggested that the aqueous was an unfavourable medium, inhibiting cellular proliferation, while the stimulation to growth was ascribed by Silva (1905) to the development of a mild inflammatory process in the iris. The accidental introduction of surface cells into the eye along with the lash may provide one variable factor; a second is the fact that sometimes the cilium is introduced into the eye complete with its root-sheath and sometimes it is broken off above this point.

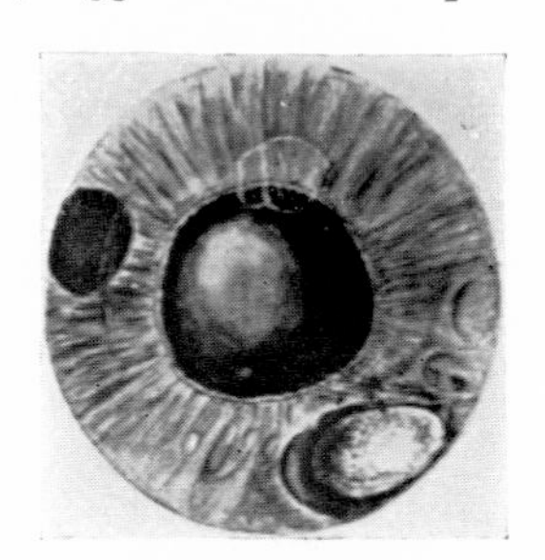

Fig. 486.—Pearl Cyst of the Iris.

A perforating injury with a piece of wire. Five weeks after the injury two cilia were removed from the 9 o'clock position where a coloboma of the iris is apparent, after which recovery was uneventful. Eight months later a pearl cyst had developed in the iris at 5 o'clock, coming into apposition with the posterior surface of the cornea. There were some opacities in the lens. The cyst was removed operatively and recovery was uneventful (O. Sitchevska and B. Payne).

Clinically, as with other types of implantation cyst, two types may occur. Occasionally the cyst appears to be of a serous nature with a relatively thin wall of several layers of squamous epithelium, sometimes multi-locular and appearing as a pigmented mass in the pupillary area behind the iris (Cantonnet, 1917; Roth and Geiger, 1925) (Plate XXII, Fig. 2). The more common appearance, however, is that of a pearl cyst—a solid-looking, densely packed tumour with a glistening pearly surface typically set in the anterior layer of the iris and protruding from it, as has already been described.[1] Of these there are many reports in the literature.[2] Usually the pearl tumour is associated with one cilium, but a single lash may give rise to two cysts (Monoyer, 1872), while three cysts have been reported with three cilia (Masse, 1881). The fate of such a cyst varies; the normal tendency is for gradual growth and the natural termination is the development of an iridocyclitis which may be severe, or of glaucoma (Figs. 486 and 487).

In the rare event of a cilium being introduced into the *posterior segment* of the globe and lying in the vitreous, in the absence of infection an exudative response is the normal reaction; spontaneous expulsion has occurred from

[1] p. 415.

[2] Pamard (1841), von Graefe (1857–64), Rothmund (1872), Monoyer (1872), de Wecker (1876), F. R. Cross and Treacher Collins (1893), Wintersteiner (1900), Dessalle (1904), Silva (1905), Wallner (1905), Früchte (1906), Moore (1930), Bonnet and Paufique (1934), Sitchevska and Payne (1951), Vesterdal (1952).

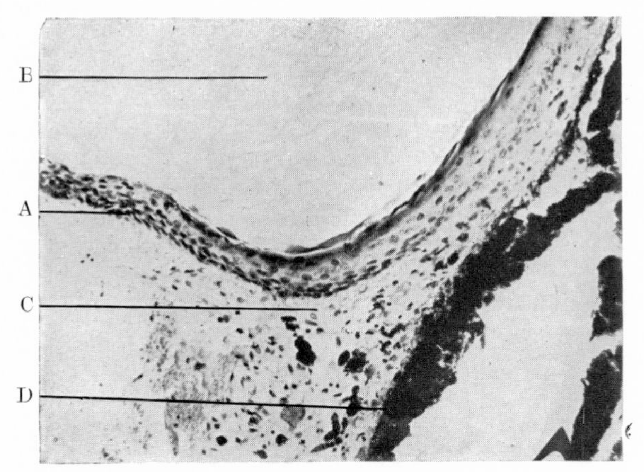

FIG. 487.—PEARL-LIKE IMPLANTATION CYST OF THE IRIS.

After the implantation of an eyelash. A, cyst wall; B, keratinized cyst contents; C, iris stroma; D, pars iridica retinæ (R. Foster Moore).

the posterior segment of the eye (after 8 weeks, Lang, 1907). Only occasionally does a cilium lodged in this region become encapsulated in scar-tissue containing numerous foreign-body giant cells, and never without continued active inflammatory evidences (de Lapersonne and Vassaux, 1884; Deutschmann, 1890; O'Brien, 1931).

In the lens, the few cases which have been reported show that the cilium usually lies quietly in the clear lens; the injury generally occurs in youth and layers of clear cortex grow over it and bury it (von Hippel, 1927; Byrnes, 1949; Sédan, 1950) (Fig. 488). The last author, for example, reported two cases wherein the lashes lay quietly in the lens, being well tolerated for 29 and 42 years respectively. Pereyra (1950) reported a case wherein an eyelash, having entered a penetrating wound of the cornea, lay partly within the anterior chamber and partly in the superficial layers of the lens; a violent iridocyclitis followed which necessitated enucleation. In the case reported by Payrau and Guyard (1956) six eyelashes were found in the lens 12 months after an injury due to blast from a bomb explosion; five were removed during an extracapsular extraction and one remained innocuously on the posterior capsule.

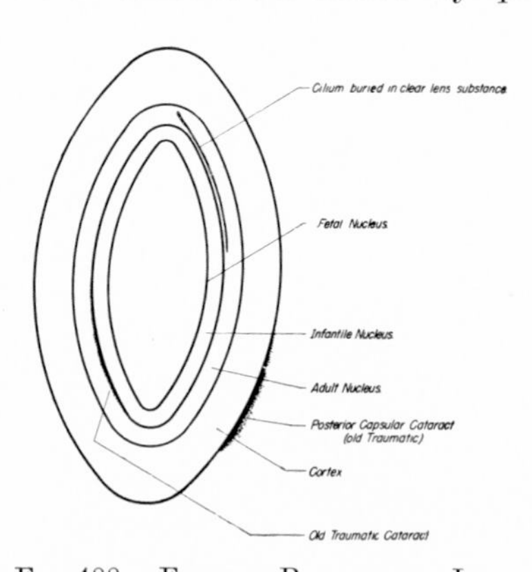

FIG. 488.—FOREIGN BODY IN THE LENS

Drawing (from above) to illustrate the location of an eyelash in the lens substance. The locations of the traumatic cataractous changes are also shown (V. A. Byrnes).

The *treatment* of a retained cilium raises difficult questions. On the one hand, the chances are high that it will remain indefinitely quiet. On the other, the tendency for inflammation either early or late, the probability of cystic formation, and even the remote possibility of the development of sympathetic ophthalmitis, point to the advisability of removal. If the cilium is in a position whence its surgical extraction would appear to be easy without probable harm to the eye, this course should be adopted; but if it is located at a place whence removal would be difficult and might be expected to cause damage, this should be balanced in each particular case against the risks of adopting a policy of inactivity. Occasionally, when the eyelash is lying upon the iris, its removal by forceps is almost impossible without including some of the iris which bulges up into this instrument. In these cases a suitable technique is to insinuate a grooved curette between the lash and the iris, whereafter, guiding a blunt hook in the groove, the lash is engaged at its middle and, macerated and friable, is readily drawn out doubled upon itself (Fisher, 1930). Where at all possible a cyst should be surgically removed along the lines already indicated,[1] even although the operation may be difficult owing to the fact that the cyst may extend across the anterior chamber and lie against the cornea; if removal is incomplete, surgery may be followed by radiation.[2] It should be remembered also that removal does not preclude recurrences which, of course, may be amenable to further surgical or radiotherapeutic attack (Moore, 1930; Bonnet *et al.*, 1933).

Alexander. *Münch. med. Wschr.*, **59,** 57 (1912).
Begle. *Arch. Ophthal.*, **46,** 47 (1917).
Bonnet and Paufique. *Arch. Ophtal.*, **51,** 5 (1934).
Bonnet, Paufique and Bussy. *Arch. Ophtal.*, **50,** 633 (1933).
Bulson. *Amer. J. Ophthal.*, **3,** 128 (1920).
Byrnes. *Amer. J. Ophthal.*, **32,** 847 (1949).
Cantonnet. *Progr. Méd.*, **32,** 398 (1917).
Castroviejo. *Amer. J. Ophthal.*, **14,** 538 (1931).
Celeste. *Arq. bras. Oftal.*, **13,** 18 (1950).
Collins, Treacher. *Trans. ophthal. Soc. U.K.*, **14,** 217 (1894).
Cowen. *Amer. J. Ophthal.*, **25,** 721 (1942).
Cross, F. R. and Collins. *Trans. ophthal. Soc. U.K.*, **13,** 199 (1893).
Cross, G. H. *Amer. J. Ophthal.*, **12,** 910 (1929).
Cunier. *Ann. Oculist.* (Paris), **5,** 163 (1841).
Dellaporta. *v. Graefes Arch. Ophthal.*, **143,** 301 (1941).
Dessalle. *Des tumeurs perlées de l'iris*, Bordeaux (1904).
Deutschmann. *Beitr. Augenheilk.*, **1,** 8 (1890).
van Dooremaal. *v. Graefes Arch. Ophthal.*, **19** (3), 359 (1873).
Dor. *Clin. Ophtal.*, **21,** 259 (1916).
Fehr. *Zbl. prakt. Augenheilk.*, **25,** 205 (1901).
Fisher. *Lancet*, **1,** 787 (1930).
Franke. *v. Graefes Arch. Ophthal.*, **30** (1), 224 (1884).
Franklin and Cordes. *Amer. J. Ophthal.*, **8,** 306 (1925).
Friedinger. *Wien. med. Wschr.*, **28,** 352 (1878).
Früchte. *Klin. Mbl. Augenheilk.*, **44** (2), 42 (1906).
Gradle. *Amer. J. Ophthal.*, **6,** 764 (1923).
von Graefe. *v. Graefes Arch. Ophthal.*, **3** (2), 412 (1857); **7** (2), 39, 139 (1860); **10** (1), 211 (1864).
Graff. *Amer. J. Ophthal.*, **16,** 126 (1933).
Guzmann. *Klin. Mbl. Augenheilk.*, **50** (2), 375 (1912).
Harbridge. *Trans. Amer. ophthal. Soc.*, **48,** 256 (1950).
Henneberg. *Klin. Mbl. Augenheilk.*, **77,** 849 (1926).
von Herrenschwand. *Wien. klin. Wschr.*, **29,** 115 (1916).
Hertel. *Ber. dtsch. ophthal. Ges.*, **40,** 117 (1916).
von Hippel. *Ber. dtsch. ophthal. Ges.*, **46,** 408 (1927).
Hirschberg. *Einführung in d. Augenheilk.*, Leipzig, **1,** 60 (1892).
Zbl. prakt. Augenheilk., **33,** 2 (1909).
Horay. *Klin. Mbl. Augenheilk.*, **80,** 202 (1928).
Hosch. *Virchows Arch. path. Anat.*, **99,** 446 (1885).
Hughes. *Amer. J. Ophthal.*, **7,** 702 (1924).

[1] p. 419.

[2] Vol. IX, p. 774.

Joseph. *Eye, Ear, Nose, Thr. Mthly*, **46**, 188 (1967).
Klien. *Amer. J. Ophthal.*, **28**, 1193 (1945).
Königstein. *Zbl. prakt. Augenheilk.*, **30**, 231 (1906).
Landmann. *v. Graefes Arch. Ophthal.*, **28** (2), 153, 162 (1882).
Lang. *Ueber Zilien im Auge, usw.* (Diss.), Rostock (1907).
de Lapersonne and Vassaux. *Arch. Ophtal.*, **4**, 86 (1884).
Leber. *VII int. Cong. Med.*, London, **3**, 15 (1881).
v. Graefes Arch. Ophthal., **28** (2), 237 (1882); **30** (1), 243 (1884).
Die Entstehung d. Entzündung, Leipzig (1891).
Lerche. *Med. prakt. Abhandl. v. dtsch. in Russland lebenden Ärzten*, Hamburg, **1**, 236 (1835).
Lichtner. *Vestn. oftal.*, **7**, 677 (1935).
McKee. *Amer. J. Ophthal.*, **11**, 296 (1928).
Mackrocki. *Klin. Mbl. Augenheilk.*, **21**, 466 (1883).
Manz. *Klin. Mbl. Augenheilk.*, **6**, 178 (1868).
Masse. *Recueil Ophtal.*, **3**, 394, 477 (1881).
Mattos. *Arq. bras. Oftal.*, **6**, 38 (1943).
Mendelssohn. *Zwei Fälle v. Fremdkörperverletzung in d. vorderen Kammer d. Auges* (Diss.), Heidelberg (1917).
Métaxas. *Ann. Oculist.* (Paris), **121**, 116 (1899).
Meyer. *Zbl. prakt. Augenheilk.*, **13**, 1 (1889).
Mikhailov. *Vestn. oftal.*, **13**, 548 (1938).
Monoyer. *Ann. Oculist.* (Paris), **67**, 249 (1872).
Moore. *Brit. J. Ophthal.*, **14**, 496 (1930).
Müller. *Wien. klin. Wschr.*, **7**, 231 (1894).
O'Brien. *Trans. Amer. ophthal. Soc.*, **29**, 416 (1931).
Paderstein. *Zbl. prakt. Augenheilk.*, **34**, 18 (1910).
Pamard. *Ann. Oculist.* (Paris), **5**, 157 (1841); **43**, 23 (1860).
Papagno. *Ann. Ottal.*, **59**, 159 (1931).
Payrau and Guyard. *Bull. Soc. Ophtal. Fr.*, 485 (1956).
Pereyra. *G. ital. Oftal.*, **3**, 286 (1950).
Peschel. *Zbl. prakt. Augenheilk.*, **11**, 112 (1887).
Popov. *Vestn. oftal.*, **18**, 439 (1941).
Quint. *Zbl. prakt. Augenheilk.*, **25**, 289 (1901).
Raiford. *J. med. Ass. Georgia*, **51**, 253 (1952).
Robertson. *V int. Cong. Ophthal.*, N.Y., 256 (1876).
Rockliffe. *Trans. ophthal. Soc. U.K.*, **3**, 26 (1883).
Roll. *Klin. Mbl. Augenheilk.*, **44** (1), 270 (1906).
Roth and Geiger. *Amer. J. Ophthal.*, **8**, 870 (1925).
Rothmund. *Klin. Mbl. Augenheilk.*, **9**, 397 (1871); **10**, 189 (1872).
Rubey. *Klin. Mbl. Augenheilk.*, **149**, 371 (1966).
Ruete. *von Ammons Mschr. Med., Augenheilk., Chir.*, Dresden, **2**, 81 (1839).
Samelsohn. *Zbl. prakt. Augenheilk.*, **9**, 363 (1885).
Saryev. *Vestn. oftal.*, **30**, 36 (1951).
Sattler. *Klin. Mbl. Augenheilk.*, **12**, 127 (1874).
Savin. *Brit. J. Ophthal.*, **20**, 609 (1936).
Scheffer. *Vestn. oftal.*, **30**, 808 (1913).
Schwarz. *Beitr. Augenheilk.*, **3** (23), 218 (1898).
Wien. klin. Wschr., **12**, 267 (1899).
Schweigger. *Klin. Mbl. Augenheilk.*, **9**, 405 (1871).
Schweninger. *Z. Biol.*, **11**, 341 (1875).
Sédan. *Bull. Soc. Ophtal. Fr.*, 822 (1950).
Shagov. *Vestn. oftal.*, **11**, 125 (1937).
Sharpe. *Amer. J. Ophthal.*, **8**, 301 (1925).
Silva. *Klin. Mbl. Augenheilk.*, **43** (2), 450 (1905).
da Silva. *Arq. bras. Oftal.*, **11**, 153 (1948).
Sitchevska and Payne. *Amer. J. Ophthal.*, **32**, 982 (1949); **34**, 833 (1951).
Smith, F. *Brit. J. Ophthal.*, **20**, 455 (1936).
Smith, J. *Arch. Ophthal.*, **44**, 424 (1950).
Spierer. *Klin. Mbl. Augenheilk.*, **29**, 224 (1891).
von Szily. *Atlas d. Kriegsaugenheilkunde*, Stuttgart, 392 (1918).
Tokuda and Tanaka. *Bull. nav. med. Ass.* (Tokyo), **29**, 5 (1940).
Vesterdal. *Nord. Med.*, **48**, 1673 (1952).
Vieweger. *Ueber Haare im Innern d. Auges* (Diss.), Bonn (1883).
Villard and Dejean. *Arch. Ophtal.*, **50**, 91 (1933).
Wagenmann. *Graefe-Saemisch Hb. d. ges. Augenheilk.*, 3rd ed., Leipzig, **2**, 1482 (1921).
Wallner. *Ein klinisch-pathologisch-anatomischer Beitr. z. Lehre v. d. Zysten d. Regenbogenhaut* (Diss.), Munich (1905).
Warnecke. *Zbl. prakt. Augenheilk.*, **32**, 161 (1908).
Webster. *Med. Rec.* (*N.Y.*), **40**, 238 (1891).
de Wecker. *Graefe-Saemisch Hb. d. ges. Augenheilk.*, 1st ed., Leipzig, **4**, 540 (1876).
Wilder. *Amer. J. Ophthal.*, **31**, 57 (1948).
Wintersteiner. *v. Graefes Arch. Ophthal.*, **40** (2), 1 (1894).
Ber. dtsch. ophthal. Ges., **28**, 4 (1900).
Zander and Geissler. *Die Verletzungen d. Auges*, Leipzig (1864).

The Complications of Intra-ocular Foreign Bodies

The principal complications following the retention of a foreign body within the eye—the irritative effects, either exudative or proliferative in

FIGS. 489 to 491.—HÆMORRHAGE IN THE TRACKS OF FOREIGN BODIES (Helenor Wilder).

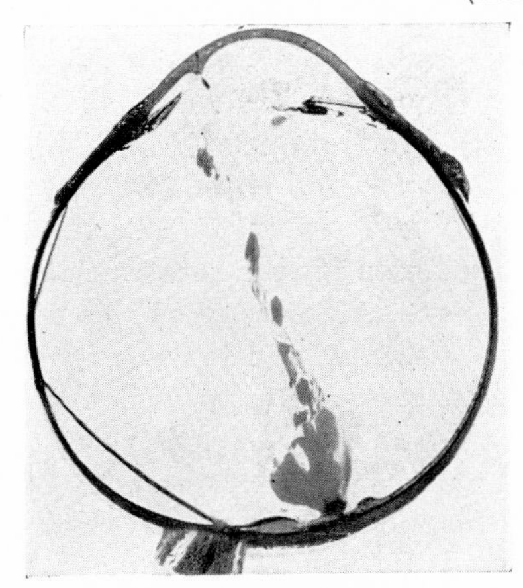

FIG. 489

The beginning of organization of hæmorrhage in the track of a lead foreign body extending from the corneal wound of entrance to the chorioretinal site of lodgment at the macula. Enucleation 16 days after injury.

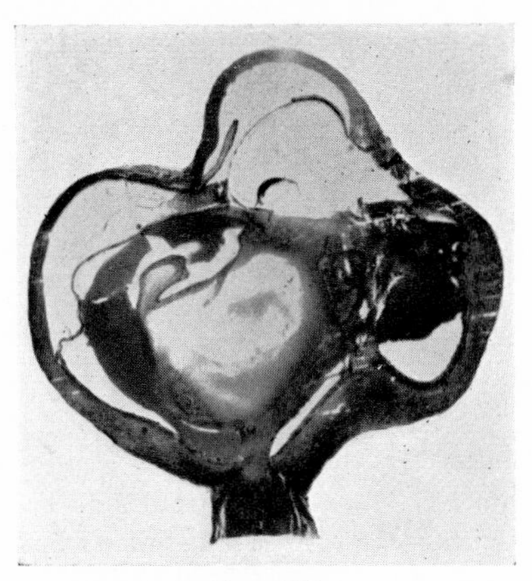

FIG. 490.

The hæmorrhage between the scar of entrance at the limbus and the chorioretinal scar of lodgment of a lead foreign body has become organized to form a traction-band which has led to cicatricial distortion of the globe. Enucleation 6 months after injury.

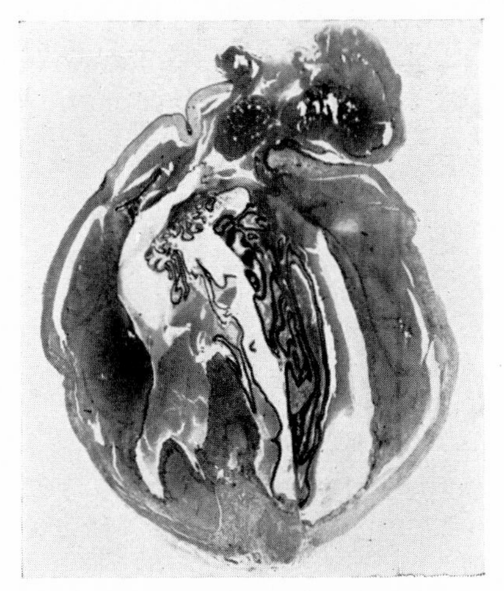

FIG. 491.—EXPULSIVE HÆMORRHAGE.

Following the penetration of a copper fragment at the limbus. Enucleation 9 days after injury.

nature, produced by the presence of the particle, and the specific chemical effects caused by some substances, particularly iron and copper—have already been dealt with in the preceding pages. Apart from these, the complications which may occur are essentially those characteristic of

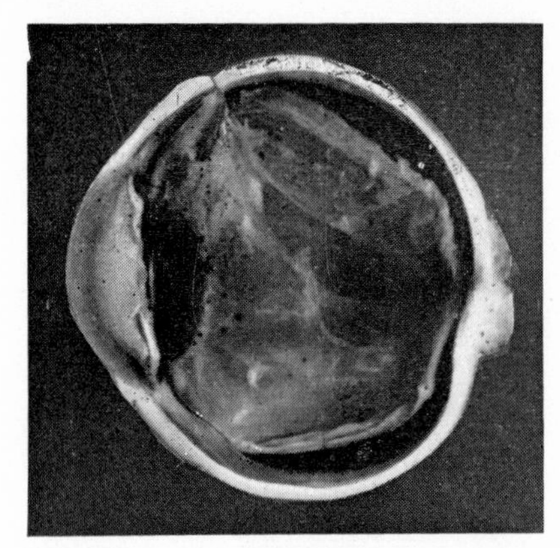

FIG. 492.—THE EARLY STAGE OF PANOPHTHALMITIS.

The upper part of the sclera was penetrated by a metallic foreign body which came to rest in the retina below the optic disc. There is a hypopyon completely filling the anterior chamber and the vitreous contains blood and some pus radiating outwards from the region of the wound. The choroid is extremely thickened (Museum, Inst. Ophthal.).

perforating wounds in general, and since these have been discussed at length a short recapitulation of the peculiarities which the presence of the foreign body imposes on the sequelæ of such injuries is all that is required at this stage.

An INTRA-OCULAR HÆMORRHAGE usually forms an immediate sequel to the penetration of the globe by a foreign body. Sometimes this is so small as to escape clinical notice; at other times it is massive and expulsive in nature; and between these two extremes all gradations are encountered. The clinical picture is in general the same as that seen after perforating wounds, but one peculiarity deserves notice. It frequently happens that a hæmorrhage derived from the uveal tract occurs at the point of lodgment where tissues are torn, and in this case, seeking the path of least resistance, the blood may seep along the track ploughed by the foreign body through the vitreous and the tissues of the eye. Such a track may become organized and, if the hæmorrhage has been at all profuse, massive bands of fibrous tissue may be formed which may on occasion join the wound of entrance with the site of lodgment, so that their subsequent contraction may lead to gross cicatricial distortion of the globe (Figs. 489–491).

The intra-ocular introduction of PYOGENIC INFECTION into a wound is undoubtedly more common if a foreign body is retained. It has already been noted that the average small metallic fragment detached from its parent site with great force and flying through the air with high velocity is usually sterile. This is indeed fortunate, but it is to be remembered that many other foreign bodies convey infection with them, particularly pieces of wood and stone. If a foreign body remains in the vascular tissues of the eye such infection may on occasion be controlled and even clear up if the particle is rapidly removed, but such a complication often leads to panophthalmitis even if the most effective treatment is given. In this event the usual result is loss of the eye and the best that can reasonably be expected is a badly damaged and functionally useless organ. It is to be noted that once infection starts in the lens the preservation of the eye is rare (Figs. 492 and 493).[1]

[1] p. 399.

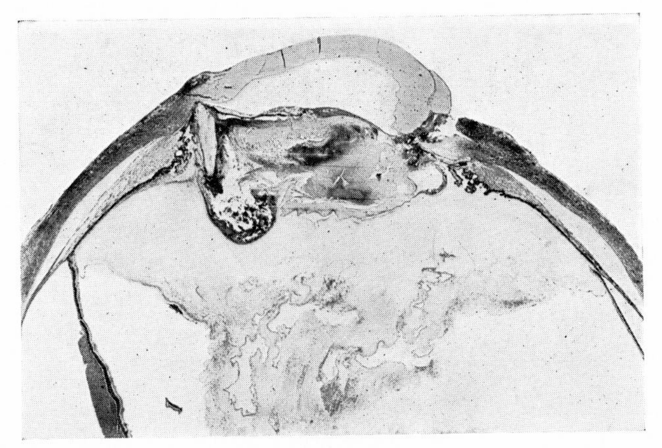

Fig. 493.—Panophthalmitis in a Case of Retained Intra-ocular Foreign Body.

An abscess has developed around a piece of vegetable matter in the angle of the anterior chamber and has infiltrated along the track of the foreign body through the lens. Enucleation 24 days after injury (Helenor Wilder).

More serious infections than the usual pyogenic organisms are generally rapidly destructive. GAS GANGRENE following contamination with *Cl. welchii* is the commonest example of this, and is generally due to the entrance of a foreign body such as a piece of stone, wood or steel contaminated with earth, although it may be that such an infection is already present in the conjunctival cul-de-sac (Cross, 1941). It is interesting that experimental infection of the eyes of rabbits by *Cl. welchii* produces a destructive inflammation only if the organism is introduced into the lens or vitreous; in the anterior chamber there is a transitory iritis only (Chiazzaro, 1932; von Sallmann, 1944). Numerous clinical cases of such infection after the entrance of a foreign body have been reported.[1] The result has invariably been visually disastrous although, as we have seen, the infection can be localized to the eye.[2]

The question of SYMPATHETIC OPHTHALMITIS[3] has traditionally excited unusual fear if a perforating injury has been complicated by the retention of a foreign body, particularly if it is lodged in the ciliary region where irritation can be presumed to be most easily maintained. So much were the earlier writers impressed by this probability that they suggested the enucleation of every eye in which a foreign body was lodged and from which it could not be extracted (Ramsay, 1907). It is true that, as we have seen in previous pages, sympathetic ophthalmitis may follow the retention of every type of foreign body, but that this extreme prophylactic course was founded on exaggerated fears was realized after the experience of the first World War (Parsons, 1916; Collins, 1916; Clegg, 1916). On the whole, the incidence of sympathetic ophthalmitis following the retention of a foreign body is

[1] Chaillous (1904–5), Lutz (1910), Heath (1929), Ridley (1929), Hamilton (1930), Berry (1932–38), Kluever and O'Brien (1936), Rieger (1936), Cross (1941), Capus (1946), Stuart (1949), Kennedy and Vogel (1951), Bristow *et al.* (1971), and others.

[2] p. 405.

[3] Vol. IX, p. 558.

relatively low (5 eyes in 731 cases of retained foreign bodies, Wilder, 1948). It must be remembered, however, that to a certain extent an eye with a retained foreign body can never be considered absolutely safe, for sympathetic ophthalmitis may develop after many years: thus in a case reported by Wilder (1948), in which foreign bodies of wood had been retained, sympathetic uveitis developed after a lapse of 36 years (Fig. 494). So far as prophylactic enucleation is concerned, each case should be considered on its own merits and judgment made in the same way as for perforating injuries not thus complicated; the presence and the nature of a foreign body are probably of minor importance so far as the incidence of sympathetic ophthalmitis is concerned.

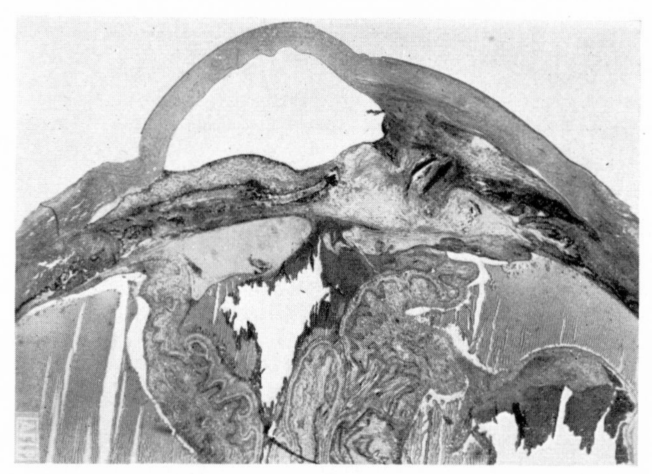

FIG. 494.—SYMPATHETIC OPHTHALMITIS AFTER THE RETENTION OF PIECES OF WOOD.

The foreign bodies were retained for 36 years after a penetrating wound through the cornea. The specimen shows the condition of recent sympathetic uveitis (Helenor Wilder).

Of the other complications characteristic of perforating wounds, most are accentuated by the presence of a retained foreign body. It is true, as we have seen, that a prolapse of uveal tissue into the wound is less rare, but a post-traumatic endophthalmitis or hæmophthalmitis is commoner and often more severe in so far as the external wound is often complicated by further damage caused by the ploughing up of the ocular tissues as the particle traverses the eye; atrophy of the globe is thus a more frequent end-result, while in less severe cases the increased tendency for the proliferation of fibrous tissue in the posterior segment leads more commonly to detachment of the retina. Moreover, the frequent occurrence of traumatic cataract adds considerably to the severity of any such inflammation, and the violent reaction thus caused often makes enucleation necessary. Finally, implantation cysts are more commonly formed, perhaps because the surface epithelium is readily carried into the globe with the foreign body, and perhaps because the irritation of the particle excites its growth; such a complication, as we have seen, is particularly characteristic of a retained cilium.

Berry. *Amer. J. Ophthal.*, **15**, 1022 (1932). *Arch. Ophthal.*, **19**, 406 (1938).
Bristow, Kassar and Sevel. *Brit. J. Ophthal.*, **55**, 139 (1971).
Capus. *Arch. Ophthal.*, **46**, 226 (1946).
Chaillous. *Recueil Ophtal.*, **26**, 678 (1904). *Ann. Oculist.* (Paris), **134**, 115 (1905).
Chiazzaro. *Ann. Oculist.* (Paris), **169**, 953 (1932).
Clegg. *Trans. ophthal. Soc. U.K.*, **36**, 86 (1916).
Collins. *Trans. ophthal. Soc. U.K.*, **36**, 84 (1916).
Cross. *Lancet*, **2**, 515 (1941).
Hamilton. *Brit. J. Ophthal.*, **14**, 452 (1930).
Heath. *Brit. J. Ophthal.*, **13**, 574 (1929).
Kennedy and Vogel. *Arch. Ophthal.*, **45**, 528 (1951).
Kluever and O'Brien. *Arch. Ophthal.*, **15**, 1088 (1936).
Lutz. *Klin. Mbl. Augenheilk.*, **48**, 31 (1910).
Parsons. *Trans. ophthal. Soc. U.K.*, **36**, 69 (1916).
Ramsay. *Eye Injuries and their Treatment*, Glasgow (1907).
Ridley. *Trans. ophthal. Soc. U.K.*, **49**, 221 (1929).
Rieger. *Klin. Mbl. Augenheilk.*, **96**, 548 (1936).
von Sallmann. *Arch. Ophthal.*, **31**, 54 (1944).
Stuart. *Brit. med. J.*, **1**, 272 (1949).
Wilder. *Amer. J. Ophthal.*, **31**, 57 (1948).

The Diagnosis and Localization of Intra-ocular Foreign Bodies

The diagnosis of the presence of an intra-ocular foreign body is frequently a matter of considerable difficulty. If the particle is small its presence may be completely unsuspected; so little inconvenience or pain may be caused by its entrance into the eye that the incident may have been unnoticed or disregarded by the patient, and it may not be until many years have elapsed that its presence is proved by the development of siderosis or chalcosis or of an implantation cyst. It follows, both for the protection of the patient and in view of the possibility of subsequent medico-legal implications, that *in all cases in which an intra-ocular foreign body could reasonably be suspected, every care should be taken to exclude its presence.* The localization of such a foreign body is equally important and demands techniques capable of the greatest accuracy; when it is remembered that an inaccuracy of 1 mm. may lead to a needless operation on the eye or involve the loss of this organ, the necessity for unusual care is obvious.[1]

CLINICAL METHODS OF INVESTIGATION

In every case of injury the first essential is thoroughness in taking the *history*. Questions, which should be precise regarding the exact activities of the patient and the type of implement employed at the time (such as a hammer, chisel, emery wheel or other common causes of this type of injury), are of unusual importance not only in indicating the possibility of the presence of a foreign body but also in providing a clue as to its probable composition.

In the next place, a careful *clinical examination* should be made for a wound of entry. If this is in the cornea the most minute perforation can be observed by the *slit-lamp*, since a permanent scar is always left behind;

[1] A very useful *Atlas of Diagnostic Technics and Treatment of Intraocular Foreign Bodies* was written by Havener and Gloeckner (St. Louis, 1969).

in the sclera, however, a small wound may be rapidly obscured, and in the posterior segment of the globe it is, of course, invisible. While the presence of such a wound therefore indicates the entrance of a foreign body and suggests the possibility of its retention, its absence on clinical examination by no means rules out further methods of investigation. It is noteworthy that, if a corneal perforation exists, the absence of a prolapse of the iris into the wound may be of significance in view of the fact that this tissue is frequently pushed back at the moment of entry of the particle; on the other hand, a prolapse of uveal tissue does not exclude the presence of an intra-ocular foreign body.

A hole in the iris is very suggestive of an accident of this type (Figs. 419–20), and a localized track through the lens (although rare) is equally significant, while a rapidly developing cataract after an injury should always excite suspicion. It is important that the position of a foreign body is often indicated by a line of direction determined by the wound of entry and any localized injury to the iris or lens, since the particle usually travels through the globe in a straight line, at any rate until the posterior wall of the globe is reached.

Even although a careful clinical examination of the anterior segment is made with both the loupe and the slit-lamp, a transparent foreign body such as glass may be easily missed. Small particles of glass, however, are usually rendered evident with the slit-lamp by indirect illumination or by oscillating the beam of light; but their presence is more certainly detected by the use of polarized light in the slit-lamp (Koeppe, 1919–21). Minute cotton fibres, pieces of lint and talc are also made visible with this method of illumination (Duszynski, 1950) (compare Figs. 622–23).

For a thorough search of the angle of the anterior chamber *gonioscopy* is required; if corneal œdema is present this can be cleared by the instillation of drops of glycerol. This method of examination, indeed, is of inestimable value in the discovery of minute foreign bodies in this relatively inaccessible site, particularly if they are not radio-opaque[1] (Plate XVIII, Fig. 6).

Careful search of the retina with the *ophthalmoscope* must be made under full mydriasis; particular attention should be given to the peripheral retina, and it will be remembered that this region can be explored up to the level of the ora serrata if the indirect method of ophthalmoscopy is employed, using very bright illumination and applying pressure by a depressor on the limbus of the anæsthetized eye. This method of examination, of course, is not available in the many cases in which blood in any quantity is present in the anterior chamber or the vitreous, if the lens is cataractous or if sufficient time has elapsed to allow the vitreous to become cloudy or encapsulation of the foreign body to occur. After a foreign body is seen in the posterior segment it may be localized by the methods already fully described in discussing the localization of retinal holes.[2]

[1] McAlester (1938), Trantas (1938), Scharf (1941), Moreu (1943), Sheppard and Romejko (1947), Troncoso (1947), Vannini (1953), Moskowitz (1953), Thorpe (1965), and many others.

[2] Vol. X, p. 812.

In this connection Weve's (1937) suggestion is particularly useful at the time of operation when the foreign body is ophthalmoscopically visible in the peripheral fundus: the particle is focused exactly by the indirect method of ophthalmoscopy, using a brilliant source of light and the spot of light seen shining through the exposed sclera is marked off by an assistant. A similar procedure using the binocular indirect ophthalmoscope with neutralization of the optical power of the cornea by a plain glass microscope-slide (J. Dixon, 1956) or with a + 20 D condensing lens and scleral indentation, was recommended by Leopold (1959) and Harris and Brockhurst (1962).

Transillumination (or *diaphanoscopy*) may occasionally provide important evidence. If the foreign body is fairly large and opaque and situated in the anterior half of the eye, *trans-scleral diaphanoscopy*[1] may reveal its presence[2]; similarly, *indirect diaphanoscopy* by transmitted light from the nasopharynx when the fundus is examined simultaneously with the ophthalmoscope, may be of equal value if the particle is opaque and of some size and situated in the posterior half of the globe (Hertzell, 1908).

Three further clinical signs may be of importance. von Graefe's (1863) observation is always worth remembering: on pressure on the ciliary region in a recently traumatized eye *localized tenderness* may indicate the site of a foreign body buried in the ciliary region. In the second place, the late development of *mydriasis* some 3 to 6 weeks after an accident may be of significance; it will be recalled that the occurrence of this phenomenon has drawn attention on more than one occasion to the presence of an unsuspected foreign body. Finally, the *undue persistence of irritation* after an injury or *the delayed occurrence of an unexplained uveitis* is always suggestive of the retention of a particle within the eye; while the subjective symptoms of siderosis (night-blindness and contracted fields) and the objective signs of siderosis or chalcosis are, of course, pathognomonic of the retention of iron or copper.

SPECIAL METHODS OF INVESTIGATION

Apart from routine clinical examination, five special methods of investigation are available for confirming the diagnosis—those depending on magnetizability, on electrical conductivity and induction, on radiography, on the ultrasonic reflection of an echo, and on chemical analysis. All of them have obvious limitations, but fortunately most intra-ocular foreign bodies are metallic in nature and many of them lend themselves to one or more of these methods of enquiry.

METHODS DEPENDING ON MAGNETIZABILITY

The utilization of magnetism to locate a foreign body containing iron is not by any means new. Before it was used in ophthalmology the method had previously been applied by Aveling (1851) to detect portions of needles

[1] Vol. VII, p. 283.
[2] Leber (1902), Sachs (1903), Vüllers (1907), Trantas (1932–40), Leydhecker (1940), Thorpe (1965), Neubauer (1965–68), Lebekhow (1966), Riebel (1966), and many others.

lost in the body: over the suspected area he suspended a magnetized needle which dipped down onto the skin, pointing to the location of the foreign body. Pooley (1880–81) was the first to apply this principle to the eye, and concluded that the presence of iron and steel could thus be determined if the particle were sufficiently large and superficial, its depth being inferred from the degree of deflection of the needle. From this relatively crude beginning several instruments have been evolved to allow greater accuracy in detection and localization, some of which have had a considerable although temporary vogue.

Knapp (1880–81) adopted Pooley's simple idea in practice; Pagenstecher (1881) and Fröhlich (1882), working independently, applied the same principle with some success, and the technique was further elaborated by Léon Gérard, whose MAGNETOMETER was introduced by Gallemaerts (1890–94) (Fig. 495), and particularly by Asmus (1894–1910) in his SIDEROSCOPE. In these instruments, which were further modified by Hirschberg (1899) (Figs. 496 and 497), Hertel (1905) and Bane (1915), a magnetic needle was hung by a fine silk thread in a vertical glass tube fixed securely to a wall running north and south. The needle carried a mirror arranged so that the reflected beam from a light recorded its deflections on a scale. In practice the needle was adjusted by screws to swing freely with its pole pointing north; the eye was brought near to the needle and the presence of a magnetic foreign body was revealed by the deflection of the beam of light on the scale, the extent of the excursion when different parts of the eye were approximated to the needle giving some idea of its position.

The sideroscope was used in the first World War by several German oculists,[1] but, although claims were made that it could detect an iron particle of 0·00015 g. (Hüttemann, 1913), its localizing value is small and its clinical use for this purpose requires an infinity of time and the patience of a saint; it has never been popular and has now disappeared from general use.

The MAGNET has frequently been employed as a diagnostic instrument to determine the presence of a foreign body within the eye. When a powerful magnet is approximated to a globe containing a magnetic particle, the latter is drawn towards the pole of the magnet, and if it is dragged over sensitive tissue the pain thus caused betrays its presence subjectively. This method of diagnosis, suggested by McKeown (1876) and Pagenstecher (1881) and still practised today in some clinics, has little to recommend it (Roper-Hall, 1968; and others). If the findings are positive, even a small movement of the particle in uncontrolled conditions may be harmful. It is to be remembered that the pull of a giant magnet can be so great as to twist an eye around if a large foreign body is encapsulated and rendered immobile, and if the particle is made to traverse the tissues of the eye in an undetermined path the damage done may be considerable. Moreover, if the foreign body is encapsulated, no movement may occur and no pain may be elicited. This point is emphasized by the experience of Stallard (1965) during the second World War; in 37 of 172 cases in which the magnet-test was applied there was no pain; subsequently 34 foreign bodies were removed by the trans-

[1] Hertel (1916), Fleischer (1916), Weigelin (1917), von Szily (1918), Rumbaur (1919), and others.

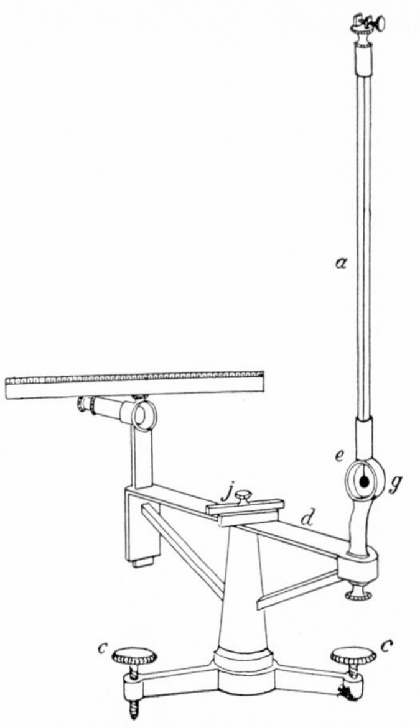

FIG. 495.—GERARD'S MAGNETOMETER.

Three levelling screws (*c*) support a horizontal bar on one end of which is the apparatus containing a magnetic indicator (*g*), and on the other the scale and telescope for observing the deflection of the indicator. The indicator, composed of 6 bar magnets, is suspended by a thread of silk in a glass tube (*a*), and is enclosed in a small compartment provided with windows to which the eye to be examined is approximated (*e*). Deflections of the indicator are observed through the telescope. Upon the horizontal bar (*d*) is placed a small magnet (*j*) to allow modifications in the direction of the indicator by projecting or withdrawing it to augment or diminish the sensitivity of the indicator.

FIGS. 496 and 497.—HIRSCHBERG'S SIDEROSCOPE.

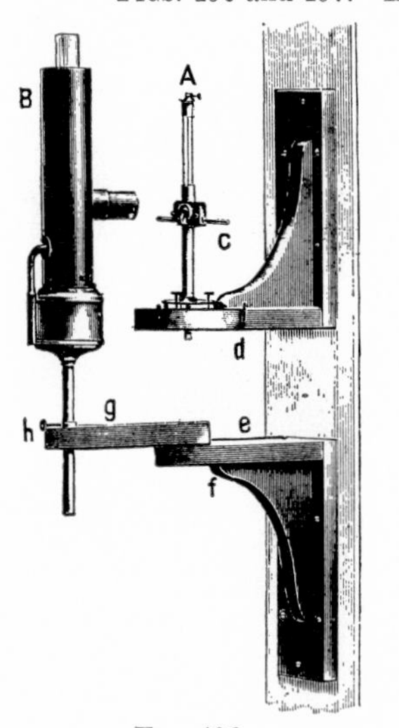

FIG. 496.

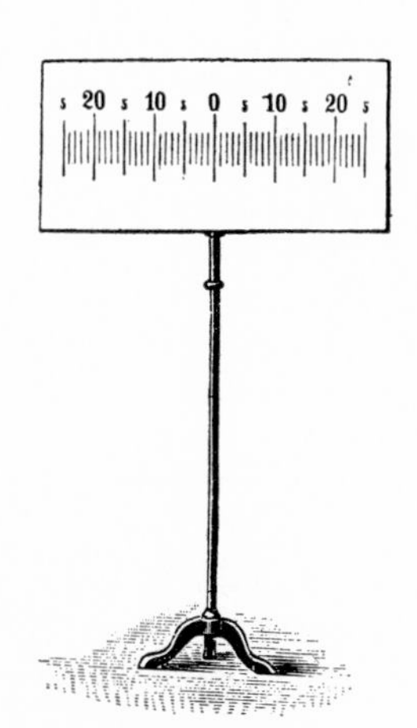

FIG. 497.

FIG. 496.—The magnet needle (C) is hung by a fine silk thread in the vertical glass tube (A) supported on a wooden stand (d) on a wall running north and south. A petroleum lamp (B) on adjustable wooden supports (e, f, g, h) throws a beam on a mirror carried by the needle, C, on a scale (Fig. 497).

scleral route and 3 by the anterior route. A negative result is therefore by no means conclusive, while a positive result may well cause injury. The method should only be used as a last resort and in the absence of other diagnostic means when the verification of the diagnosis is considered urgent, and even in these circumstances only in full realization of the potential dangers involved.

On the other hand, the use of a very small magnet is acceptable: for this purpose a surgical needle is magnetized and suspended at a point of balance on a piece of thread; a magnetic foreign body of average size resting on the retina will usually attract the point of the needle, giving an accurate surface localization (Roper-Hall, 1968).

A method depending on electrical conductivity was the basis of the METALLOPHONE of Weiss (1906). The principle was that of a Wheatstone bridge, whereby the electrical resistance of the tissues of the eye between two electrodes applied to the sclera was measured at different points; a small metallic foreign body between the electrodes altered the resistance, a change which was indicated by the ringing of a telephone bell. This technique has fallen into disuse.

METHODS DEPENDING ON ELECTRICAL INDUCTION

The principle of these methods depends on the fact that, if an alternating current is sent through a primary circuit, a current develops in a secondary coil by induction. If the voltages in the secondary coils are equalized, no current flows between them, but if in this state the instrument approaches a metallic body, the balanced inductance is disturbed and a difference in potential is created in the secondary circuit resulting in a flow of current which, after amplification, may be recorded by the deflection of the needle of an ammeter for visual indication or by variations in the tone of a loud-speaker for auditory indication.

The amount of this current varies with the magnetizability of the particle, its size and its distance from the instrument. A magnetic metal profoundly affects the magnetic field created around the instrument, but non-magnetic metals can also be detected, since the alternating magnetic field around the instrument sets up small eddy currents within the mass of the metallic particle; these produce local magnetic fields around the foreign body which react with the field of the instrument and thereby cause detectable changes. The smallness of these changes allows a differentiation to be made between a non-magnetic and a magnetic particle. Moreover, since the effect varies with the distance, if the size and composition of a foreign body are known, an estimation of its depth can be made by measuring the distance necessary to give a comparable response with a similar piece of metal.

The sensitivity of such an instrument to a ferromagnetic particle is very high indeed. Thus in the Berman locator the detecting range for iron and steel is approximately 10 times the diameter of the foreign body (a particle of 1 mm. diam. is detectable at 10 mm., one of 2 mm. diam. at 20 mm.). In the case of non-magnetic substances, however (copper, brass, aluminium, lead, etc.), it is much less, for the effective range is only 1 or 2 times the diameter of the particle. Intra-ocular foreign bodies of this type can therefore be detected only if they are of relatively large size (greater than 3 mm. diam.).

This principle was first put into practice in a relatively primitive way by Jansson (1902) in his SIDEROPHONE, in which changes in the induced current were betrayed by a telephone. This technique was employed by Widmark (1902) and others but was little used until more elaborate methods of amplification became available. It was brought to a high degree of precision by the RADIO-AMPLIFIER of Comberg (1933) who claimed that a magnetic foreign body could thereby be localized in the anterior segment of the globe to an accuracy of 0·5 mm., and in the posterior segment of 1 to 2 mm. Comberg's instrument, or a modification of it, was used by the Germans in the second World War (Leydhecker, 1940; Schlichting, 1943), and by the British as the RADIO-FREQUENCY PROBE of Farmer and Osborn (1941); the principles are essentially those used in the mine-detectors employed in war. Shortly thereafter a comparable but more effective instrument—the BERMAN LOCATOR (Figs. 498 and 499)—was employed with good effect by Moorhead (1943) at Pearl Harbor and has been used by other surgeons with considerable success.[1] Other instruments of a similar type

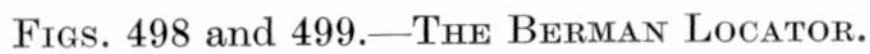

FIGS. 498 and 499.—THE BERMAN LOCATOR.

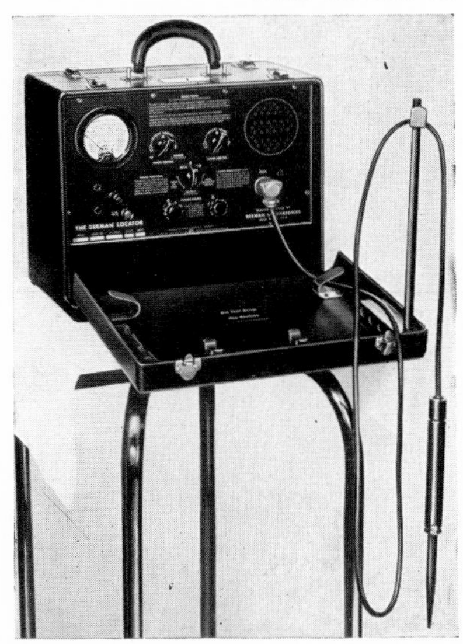

FIG. 498.

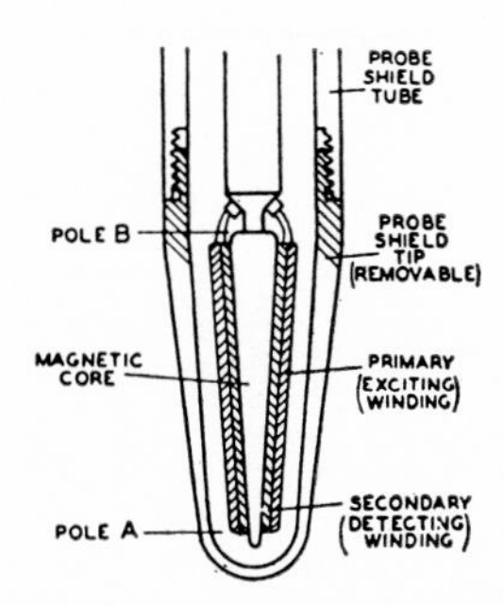

FIG. 499.—The mechanism of the end of the probe.

have also appeared, such as the OPHTHALMO-METALLOSCOPE of Hata (1933) and the CARNAY LOCATOR (Haik, 1947; J. and M. Gallois, 1947). The ROPER-HALL LOCATOR (1957) (Fig. 500) works on a higher frequency than the Berman locator, as also does the BEOLOCATOR which may be more suitable for non-magnetic foreign bodies (Riise, 1966).

In practice, some indication of whether a foreign body lies within the globe may be obtained by pressing the probe of the instrument onto the closed lids in a regular rhythm of 1 cycle per second. If a foreign body is present the response rises and falls synchronously in the same rhythm, the peak point being determined by repeating the pressure cycles in adjacent areas. If now the patient moves his eye, a consistent change of response with the movements of the globe suggests that a foreign body is within or, at any rate, is in close association with it; it will be seen presently, however, that this is not by any means accurate.[2] The probe is then held perpendicularly to the

[1] Minsky (1944), Moorhead (1945), Guy (1946), Alvis (1946), Habig (1949), Thorpe (1960), Nakabayashi *et al.* (1967), and others.

[2] p. 587.

eye in contact with its surface which is then explored, and the point of maximum response is obtained directly over the site of the foreign body. It is to be noted, of course, that in such manipulations the operating table should be of wood or other non-magnetic material or, alternatively, the head should be raised at least 15 in. above a metal table with sandbags, while the retractors and other surgical instruments should be non-magnetic.

It must be admitted, however, that with all its elaborations this method is not so accurate as radiography, either for the detection or, more particularly, for the localization of a metallic foreign body. It is, however, of value when accurate radiography is not readily available (as may well occur in war); moreover, the locator has the advantage of being small, portable,

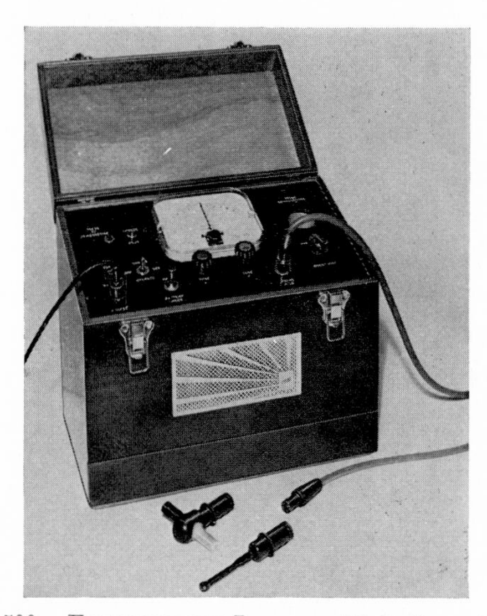

FIG. 500.—FOREIGN-BODY LOCATOR (M. J. Roper-Hall).

The lead attached on the left is for charging the batteries and is not connected when the locator is in normal use.

and readily used by a person who need not be an expert in complicated radiographic technique. It is also a useful adjunct to X-rays, providing information as to the degree of magnetizability of a particle and therefore of the potentialities of its extraction by the magnet. Finally, since the active element is small and can be covered by a sterilizable rubber shield, it can be used during an operation to confirm the position of a foreign body as determined by radiography both before and after the incision has been made (Minsky, 1944; Callahan, 1950; Thorpe, 1960–65).

RADIOGRAPHIC METHODS

On November 8th, 1895, Wilhelm Conrad Röntgen (Fig. 759) produced in his physical laboratory at the University of Würzburg the strange new phenomenon of X-rays and demonstrated their usefulness in medicine. The scientific interest this produced was profound and more than 1,000 publications on it appeared rapidly in the medical literature of the world. Up to this period the diagnosis, and still more the localization, of foreign bodies within the eye had presented problems of the utmost difficulty: apart from the ophthalmoscope and the inaccurate sideroscope the ophthalmologist was blind. Fortunately, however, the majority of foreign bodies that lodge within the eye are metallic; it followed that they were opaque to the new ray which could thus be utilized to effect their diagnosis and localization. This development in ophthalmology was by no means sluggish. The first three attempts to achieve this end were failures (Dariex, 1896; van Duyse, 1896; Lewkowitsch, 1896) and it was concluded that with its surrounding bony skeleton the eye was unsuited for this approach; the fourth attempt, however, was successful. In 1896 this was effected by an ophthalmologist of Boston, Charles H. Williams, who with his younger brother Francis H. Williams, a general physician, had fortunately combined a medical curriculum at Harvard with the study of physics at the Massachusetts Institute of Technology. The stimulus was a piece of cartridge lodged in the eye of a boy who had exploded it by hammering this dangerous plaything. Francis provided the somewhat crude but effective apparatus, Charles the expertise; and after an exposure of ten minutes a strip of copper was localized in the vitreous and was successfully removed by the latter. It is true that the eye lost all perception of light and shrank; it is equally true that five weeks after the operation the incorrigible boy repeated his stupid feat and so damaged the same eye that Charles had to remove it. But the fact remained that a new era had been introduced into traumatic ophthalmology. There now remained the problem of the exact localization of the foreign body, for the importance of this will be at once understood when it is remembered that on the accuracy with which this can be done depends the probability of success in the extraction of the intruder. Fortunately for ophthalmology two pioneers of unusual ability were available to solve this problem, one American and one Scottish, William M. Sweet of Philadelphia and James Mackenzie Davidson of Aberdeen, both contemporaneously.

CHARLES HERBERT WILLIAMS [1850–1918] (Fig. 501) was the son of the first Professor of Ophthalmology at Harvard University. He graduated in 1871 at that school where he distinguished himself in rowing; thereafter he spent a year in the study of physics at the Massachusetts Institute of Technology where he took a Master's degree. He then went in for medicine and qualified at Harvard. Opting for ophthalmology he made a study-tour through Europe, visiting Horner in Zürich, von Jaeger in Vienna, Donders and Snellen in Utrecht, Landolt in Paris and Bowman in London; thereafter he returned to Boston and joined his father in practice. He was a many-sided innovator who devised useful distance and reading types, and he was responsible for introducing an orange colour in railway signals to act as a warning light to serve between the red and green lights which indicated danger and safety; he introduced an accurate device for measuring illumination, another for assessing heterophoria and cyclophoria and did important work on the light, colour and form senses. His lantern for testing colour vision was particularly good, but his most dramatic achievement was due to the persistently adventurous but stupid boy whose first episode led to the publication of a revolutionary communication to the American Ophthalmological Society: *A Case of Extraction of a Bit of Copper from the Vitreous When X-Rays Helped to locate the Metal* (1896).

SIR JAMES MACKENZIE DAVIDSON [1857–1919] (Fig. 502) of Aberdeen, who became a lecturer in ophthalmology in the University of that city, came to London in 1897 to work on this subject which had captured his imagination. The devotion he poured into his task was equalled only by his ingenuity in devising the accurate cross-thread method of localization which we shall presently describe. He was also a pioneer in the application of stereoscopy in the viewing of x-ray films and of guiding the extraction of a

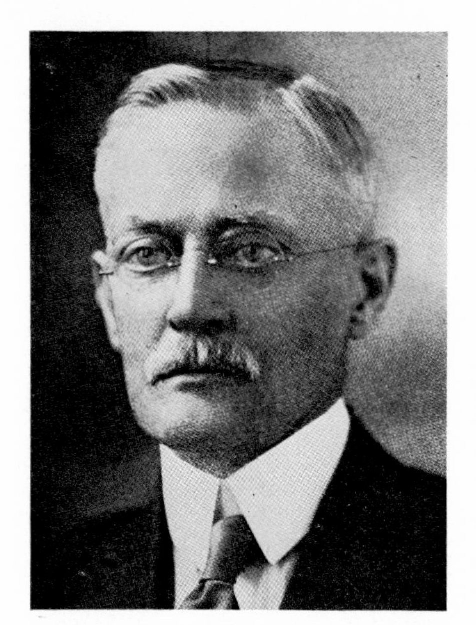

Fig. 501.—Charles Herbert Williams
[1850–1918]

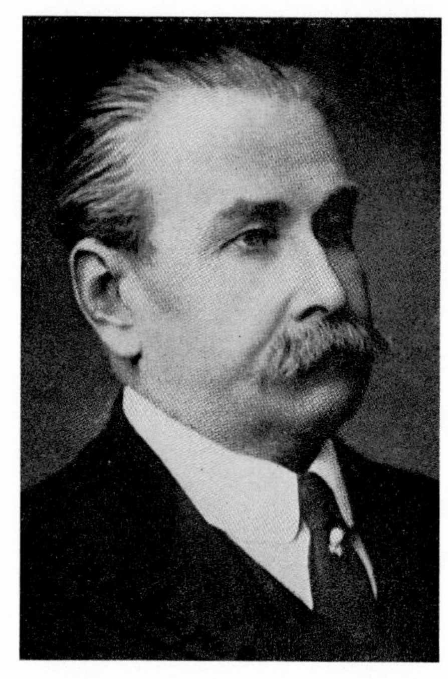

Fig. 502.—Sir James Mackenzie Davidson
[1857–1919]

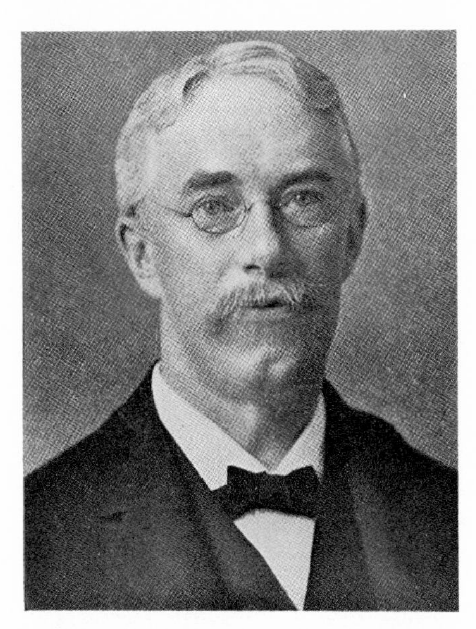

Fig. 503.—William Merrick Sweet
[1860–1926]

foreign body by a telephone probe. His book, *Localization by X-rays and Stereoscopy* (1916), summed up the advances he had made, but such was his mental energy that no sooner was it published than he himself put several of his methods out of date. During this period he was appointed consulting medical officer to the radiological departments of Moorfields Eye Hospital and Charing Cross Hospital, and during the first World War he accepted without reward or rank the position of consulting radiologist to the military hospitals of the London District. His humanity and generous nature endeared him to everyone and at the International Congress in London in 1913 it was said that his name would be remembered as long as x-rays were used.

WILLIAM MERRICK SWEET [1860–1926] (Fig. 503) was a notable ophthalmic surgeon of his day, born in Philadelphia, and after school became associated with the general manager of the American Iron and Steel Company, an occupation which attracted his attention to the damage done to the eyes of workmen in the industry. Later he studied medicine at the Jefferson Medical College, graduating in 1886. After a long study-tour in Europe he returned to his native school and in 1924 he was elected as associate professor and eventually to the chair of ophthalmology in his college and consulting surgeon to the Wills Eye Hospital. He brought out a small instrument, the Sweet localizer, for localizing metallic foreign bodies in the eye by radiography in 1897 (*N.Y. med. J.*, **65,** 542) and in 1909 a more elaborate apparatus (*Arch. roentgen Soc.*, **14,** 170) which attained world-wide recognition, as well as a magnet for extracting the intruder. During the first World War he served in the army and attracted much attention by his treatment of injured soldiers. Long recognized as a world-authority on the management of ocular injuries, his interest in all other aspects of ophthalmology was profound and he also attained fame by devising an operation for reconstructing the pupil. Apart from his ability, Sweet was a lovable person and stood high in the regard of his profession, being elected as President of the American Ophthalmological Society in 1921. Unfortunately his later years were clouded by illness, despite which he continued to work as assiduously as ever.

The Radiological Demonstration of an Intra-ocular Foreign Body

So long as the foreign body is fairly large and radio-opaque, its radiological demonstration is relatively easy, but if an attempt is to be made to obtain photographs of particles which are small and only moderately opaque, it must be remembered that their visibility is a matter of contrast depending on the ratio of the density of the foreign material to that of the tissues through which the rays must pass; to ensure visibility in such cases the rays should therefore be soft and the thickness of bone traversed should be minimal. Where bone must lie in the path of the rays the oblique lateral exposure of Belot and Fraudet (1917) is useful, wherein only the comparatively thin bone on the outer aspect of the orbit is interposed between the x-ray tube and the plate (Fig. 504), but the true lateral view is preferable. For postero-anterior views the head should be tilted in the Waters position[1] so that the confusing and dense shadow of the petrous bone does not obscure details in the orbit. Finally, eye-moving lateral exposures should also be made. It is always to be remembered, however, that occasionally, for some inexplicable reason, foreign material which theoretically should be demonstrable does not appear on what seems to be a technically good radiograph (iron, Black

[1] p. 261.

and Haessler, 1929); a negative finding by this method of examination should therefore not lead to the assumption that a foreign body is absent and to the neglect of the most careful clinical methods of diagnosis.

When the foreign body is small it is useful to duplicate these exposures with the tube off-centred by a few centimetres; such films may be examined stereoscopically, but it is more important that by taking them in this way any possibility of mistaking a flaw in the emulsion for a foreign body is avoided. During the exposures fixation must be maintained, since the shadow of a small particle is readily blurred by movement; a short exposure-time (less than 0·5 second) and a fast film are therefore essential. Moreover, a short film-distance (24 in.) using a small cone minimizes distortion. In the lateral views it should always be possible to see the curved outline of the cornea in contrast with air.

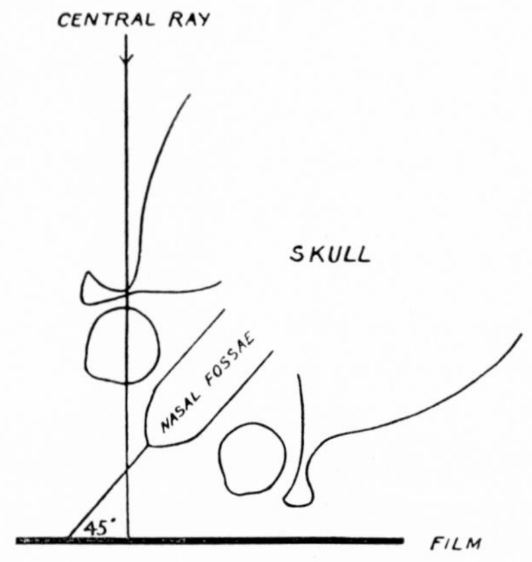

Fig. 504.—Belot's Projection.

The central ray traverses the thin area of bone only at the temporal wall of the orbit.

It should be remembered that the metal deposited in the tissues by direct siderosis in the neighbourhood of a fragment of iron may leave a radiologically visible shadow after the foreign body itself has been removed (Jung, 1922; Hartmann, 1936).

The most suitable views for the demonstration of a suspected intra-orbital foreign body are as follows:

(1) *True Lateral*: the patient is seated with the head positioned so that the affected side is towards the film and with the infra-orbital line at right angles to the film (Fig. 505).

(2) *Postero-Anterior*: the patient sits with his face against the film with the orbito-mental line tilted at an angle of 15° to the horizontal, that is, with the nose and chin virtually in contact with the film. The tube is centred with the beam horizontal on the level of the middle of the orbit (Fig. 506).

(3) *Eye-moving Lateral*: two exposures are made on the same film; for the first the patient looks up, for the second he looks down, but it is essential that the head does not move during the vertical rotation of the eyes. If the

Figs. 505 to 509.—Radiographic Views of Foreign Bodies (G. Lloyd).

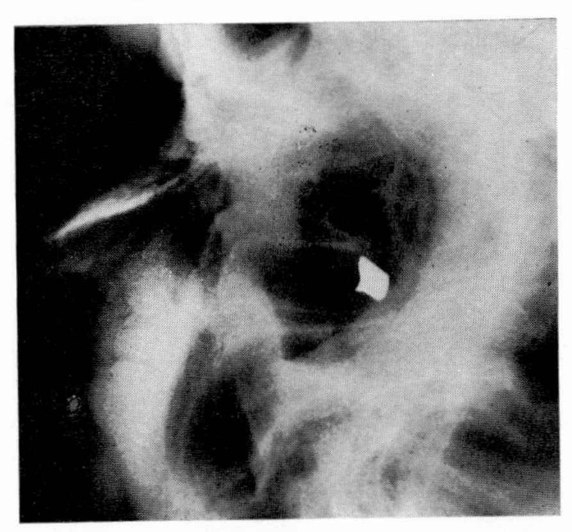

Fig. 505.

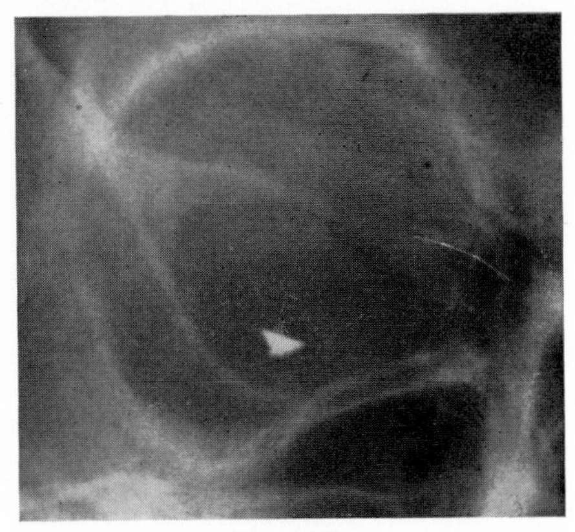

Fig. 506.

Figs. 505 and 506.—Standard lateral and postero-anterior views used to establish the presence of a foreign body and its approximate position; in this case the foreign body, if intra-ocular, must lie (a) in the 6 o'clock meridian and (b) close to the equator of the globe.

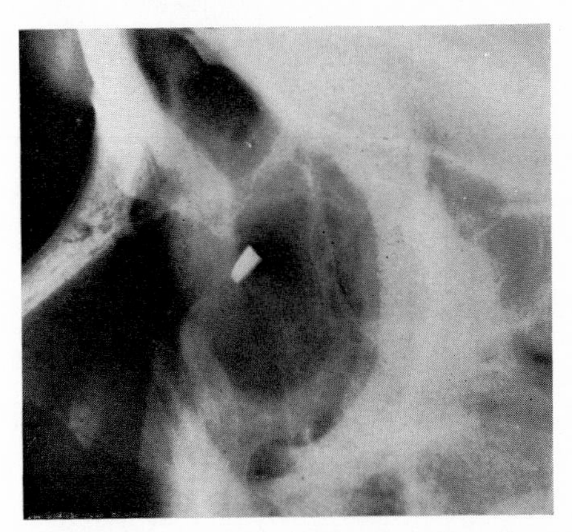

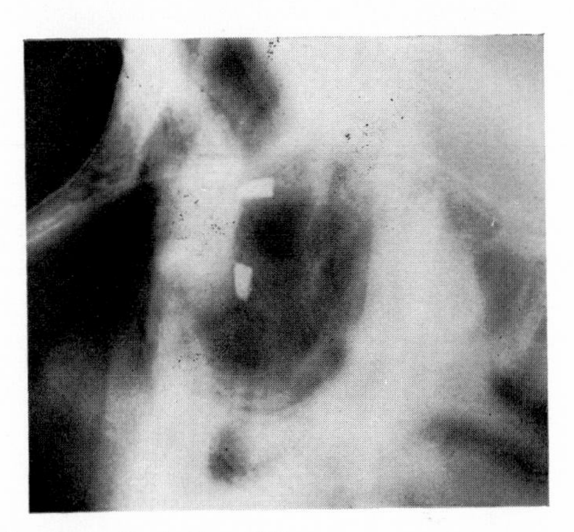

Figs. 507 to 509.—The diagnostic effect of rotation of the eye.

Fig. 507.—Lateral view of an intra-ocular foreign body.

Fig. 508.—Lateral view when the eye moves, showing that the foreign body is intra-ocular by the characteristic movement around the axis of rotation of the globe.

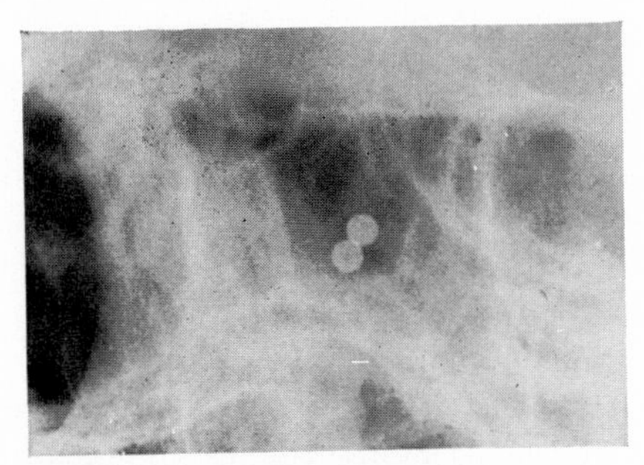

Fig. 509.—Lateral view of an extra-ocular foreign body with the eye moving, showing a very slight shift and no rotational movement.

foreign body is within the globe, it will move with the eye so that two images of the foreign body will be seen on the double exposure (Figs. 507–509).

In difficult cases a completely *bone-free method* as was considered the only possible approach by the early experimenters is, of course, preferable. No improvements, however, were made on their relatively crude techniques whereby oblique exposures were employed until the matter was resuscitated by Vogt (1921). He suggested the use of a small dental film supported in a holder pressed as deeply as possible into the cul-de-sac of the inner canthus, while the x-ray tube was situated temporally; a second film, similarly supported, was pressed deeply into the lower conjunctival fornix, the rays being directed from a tube above the forehead so that a picture was taken in a direction at right-angles to the first. In this way rays reach

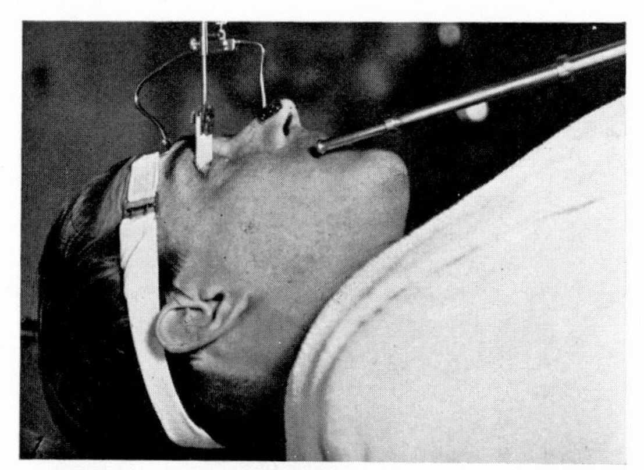

Fig. 510.—The Mento-vertical Position in Bone-free Radiography.

The film is maintained deeply in the upper fornix by the holder attached to the head-band and resting on the nose. The head is immobilized by a bite (K. Lindblom).

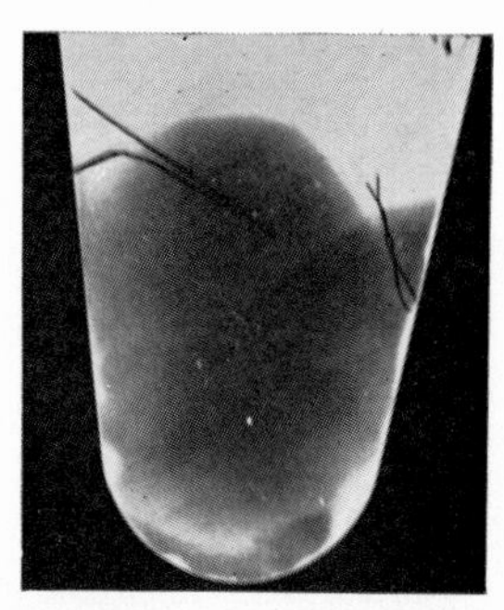

Fig. 511.—The Bone-free Method of Radiography.

Showing the whole globe and even the optic nerve. Metal threads are inserted in two of the extra-ocular muscles. The corneal outline is above; the optic nerve below (S. Larsson).

the plates without interference by the bones of the orbit and, if sufficiently soft rays are employed, the corneal surface can be clearly outlined and exceedingly minute fragments of metal, pieces of glass and sometimes even of wood may be detected in the anterior segment to an antero-posterior depth of some 8 to 12 mm. Hoffmann (1947) demonstrated small splinters of iron of only 0·000052 g. in this way. In this technique care must be taken lest excessive backward pressure on the globe open a recent penetrating wound; Melanowski (1929) reported such an accident 14 days after injury. The suggestion of van Duyse (1896) of inducing proptosis by the retrobulbar injection of saline should not be lightly undertaken.

In order to include more of the globe within the bone-free picture, Vogt's method was modified and amplified by Lindblom (1934) of Stockholm who, in addition to the lateral projection, inserted the second film into the upper conjunctival cul-de-sac to escape the prominent upper orbital rim, the vertico-mental position of Vogt being replaced by a mento-vertical exposure (Fig. 510); while Franceschetti (1934), placing the film in a sterilized cellophane envelope, inserted it into Tenon's space and was thus able to increase the bone-free exposure to include practically the entire globe (Fig. 511). Bone-free radiographs are thus particularly useful in the demonstration of foreign bodies in the anterior chamber.[1]

Most foreign bodies in the eye can thus be detected. Metals are sufficiently dense to be easily photographed with the exception of aluminium, the radio-density of which approximates that of bone so that it can be seen only by a bone-free technique.[2]

Glass is not always visible although considerable variations in radio-opacity exist, depending on the atomic weights of the constituent elements (Lewis, 1932); thus some types containing lead and barium were demonstrable even in the early days of radiography (Mackenzie Davidson, 1899; Sweet, 1900). With good techniques, however, and using the bone-free method, pieces of glass can usually be seen. Even if the foreign body lies in the posterior segment of the globe and exposures are taken through bone, provided sufficiently soft rays of varying penetrations are used and a number of pictures taken from several aspects since rays striking at one angle may produce a sharp image and at another a hazy picture, the glass which is used in the manufacture of spectacles, windscreens or bottles (which form the source of the majority of intra-ocular foreign bodies) can be detected in a surprising percentage of cases, at any rate in fragments greater than 1 mm. (Gillan, 1941; Roberts, 1951; Zwanger *et al.*, 1952). From this point of view, however, it would undoubtedly be advantageous if bespectacled workers in hazardous occupations wore radio-opaque lenses.

A failure to demonstrate an intra-ocular foreign body on a bone-free radiograph suggests either that no such body exists or that one is indeed present but is either too small to be shown or is not radio-opaque.

The Radiological Localization of Intra-ocular Foreign Bodies

A problem so interesting and important in view of the gravity of the issues and so dependent on perfection in technique as the accurate radiological localization of intra-ocular foreign bodies has naturally excited much attention, and the ingenuity of both ophthalmologists and radiologists has been stimulated to such purpose that a bewildering array of procedures is now available. Some sixty of these will be noted here; these can most conveniently be described in six groups:

1. *Direct methods* of localization, whereby the situation of the foreign body is assessed in postero-anterior and lateral views with reference to an indicator the position of which is known.
2. Methods depending on *rotational movements of the eye*, several exposures being taken while the eye moves and the x-ray tube and the head remain fixed.

[1] Mintz and Mattes (1960), Walter (1962), Stallard (1965), Howard and Gaasterland (1968),

[2] Comparative transparencies of the usual intra-ocular foreign bodies (water = 1) are as follows: platinum (the most dense), 0·020; gold, 0·030; mercury, 0·044; lead, 0·055; silver, 0·070; copper, 0·084; brass, 0·093; nickel, 0·095; iron, 0·101; zinc, 0·116; tin, 0·118; glass, 0·340; talc, 0·350; aluminium, 0·380; coal, 0·480; bone, 0·560; cotton, 0·700; silk, 0·740; wool, 0·760.

3. Methods depending on *geometrical projection*, two exposures being taken while the x-ray tube is moved and the head and eyes remain fixed.
4. *Stereoscopic methods.*
5. Methods depending on the delineation of the globe with a *contrast medium.*
6. *Bone-free methods.*

1. DIRECT METHODS OF LOCALIZATION. This technique makes the most simple and direct approach to the problem: *two exposures are taken at right-angles,* one postero-anteriorly and the other laterally, *and the position of the foreign body is located in relation to a radio-opaque marker bearing a known relationship to the globe.* In the postero-anterior view a Waters position should be employed in order to exclude the shadow of the petrous bone from the orbit.[1] The method is easy and in its simplest form requires little specialized apparatus so that it is applicable in practically all circumstances; in its more complex forms a considerable degree of accuracy is attainable. The variations of the method are numerous, some of them depending on the use of different types of indicator affixed to the globe—lead pellets (Holth, 1903–11; Velter, 1919), metallic rings (Spaeth, 1942) or contact lenses (Comberg, 1927–33)—while in others an indicator is used at a distance (Ahlbom, 1931; Stenius, 1947) or the globe is orientated by an indicator which marks a fixed point in different positions of rotation (Kraus and Briggs, 1945).

In all variations of the technique the position of the foreign body is measured in both films in relation to the position of the marker employed and the results assessed in both the frontal and sagittal planes with reference to a standard eye of 24 mm. diameter, a small correction being applied, amounting to a fraction of a millimetre, to allow for the error introduced by the conical projection of the rays. Since unfortunately all eyes are not of this size, this introduces an unavoidable error which occasionally may be considerable, the implications of which will be presently discussed.[2]

An assessment of whether the particle is within or outside the globe may be made by an adaptation of the "rotational method"[3]; on the lateral exposure, separate pictures are taken while the eye looks up and then down; if the marker and the foreign body suffer the same displacement relative to each other the foreign body lies within or is in intimate association with the globe; if the relative displacement alters (the marker moving through the angle of rotation and the foreign body not) the latter is outside the globe[4].

This technique was originally employed with a radio-opaque marker attached to the lids (Gocht, 1898; Stöckl, 1898; Foveau de Courmelles, 1899), but more accuracy is obviously attained if the indicator is more intimately or more definitely related to the globe. The use of *lead pellets* as markers was originally adopted by Holth (1903–11), who sutured two into the limbal conjunctiva, one at either end of the vertical meridian of the cornea. In order to secure greater stability, Fromaget and Jaugeas (Fromaget, 1918) buried the pellets subconjunctivally at the limbus, while Velter (1919) avoided all

[1] p. 259. [2] p. 605. [3] p. 587.
[4] For inaccuracies, see p. 589.

movement by corneal sutures. By this method Velter, who used the technique in the first World War, claimed that an accuracy within 0·5 mm. could be thus obtained, but difficulties arise in maintaining the normal ray exactly in the antero-posterior axis of the eye and eliminating any lateral rotation of the globe. These objections were to some extent overcome by Haik (1947) who used four lead pellets, two in the vertical and two in the horizontal meridian, by Lautsch (1942) who introduced four short silver wires under the conjunctiva, placing them radially so that their points just reached the limbus, and by Kerkenezov (1964) who used three or four stainless steel sutures at the limbus.

The same end of eliminating inaccuracies in the fixation of the eye is more simply attained by the use of a *ring of silver or stainless steel as an indicator*. The technique of a *limbal ring* has been employed for over 50 years in Great Britain[1] and was used extensively in the second World War (Stallard, 1944; Scott and Flood, 1946; Flood, 1946; Somerset, 1947; and others) and elsewhere (Casanovas, 1945; and others). A

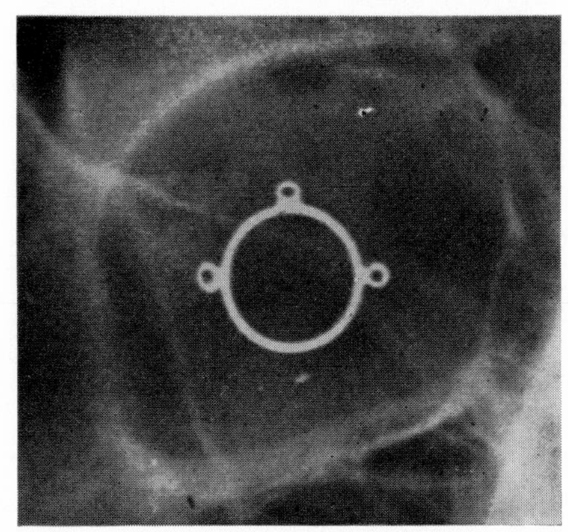

Fig. 512.

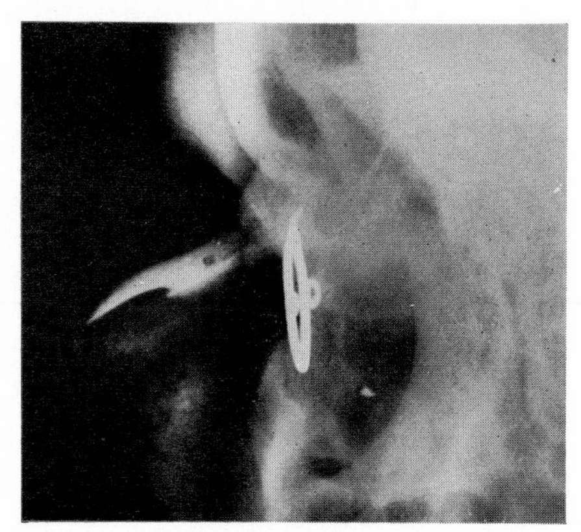

Fig. 513.

Figs. 512 and 513.—The Limbal Ring.
Standard postero-anterior and lateral views (G. Lloyd).

metallic ring of suitable size (11, 12, 13, 14 mm. diam.) is sutured to the limbus, the two or more points of suturing being marked by flattenings of the ring and perforations which become apparent in the x-ray picture. Postero-anterior and lateral views are taken with the eyes looking straight ahead and the foreign body is located in the usual way with reference to a schematic eye (Figs. 512–513). If the image of the ring in the postero-anterior view is not a circle, or if in the lateral view it is an ellipse and not a straight line, the direction of gaze has not been correct and the pictures must be repeated. An extension of this technique may be made to aid the surgical procedures for the removal of the foreign body, for if the points of suture at the limbus are marked with Indian ink at the time when the radiographs are taken, the meridian in which the foreign body lies may be accurately assessed at the time of operation.

This technique has been modified by several workers. Spaeth (1942) sutured to the conjunctiva rings of various size (14, 18, 20 mm.) to fit the globe equatorially at the approximate position of the foreign body after a preliminary localization; an additional check was attained by suturing a small ring of 6 mm. diameter over the position of the particle so that a further radiograph verified its position. Skeoch

[1] Localization by a limbal ring was employed by A. C. Norman in Durham, England, in 1915.

(1945), Perkins (1946) and Haik (1947) used larger rings (23, 26 mm.), inserted deeply into the fornices; and Yazujian (1940) a double ring bound by bars producing a pattern divided into four segments. Reis (1946), on the other hand, used flat rings of a soft malleable alloy of lead and tin which fitted snugly into the limbal groove so that they remained in place when the eye was bandaged. These, however, cannot be said to have the accuracy or stability of the original technique. Errors arising with this method result from movements of the ring, inaccuracy of its fit to the limbus, the use of a size of ring not matching the limbus, or inaccurate orientation of the eye during its use. The other eye should not be covered but should ensure immobility by fixing a distant point (Cridland, 1967).

For the localization of foreign bodies by the limbal ring two radiographic views are required—(1) a postero-anterior occipito-oral view with the patient's head straight and the eyes directed straight ahead, and (2) an eye-moving lateral view, in which the image of the ring must not be too elliptical. When radiographs of satisfactory quality are obtained three measurements are made as follows—(a) on the postero-anterior view: the centre of the circle formed by the limbal ring is marked and the distance of the foreign body on the nasal or temporal side from the vertical corneal axis is then measured. The remaining measurements are obtained from the lateral film: the line formed by the lateral image of the ring is bisected and a line is drawn at right angles back from it giving the horizontal corneal axis. From this is measured (b) the distance of the foreign body from the limbal ring; (c) the distance above or below the horizontal corneal axis: the measurements can then be repeated on the second ring-image on the eye-moving lateral film. If the measurements are not identical the foreign body is either extra-ocular or mobile, in which case exact localization is not possible. Finally, the position of the foreign body should be plotted on a Bromley chart; to obtain the antero-posterior measurement from the front of the cornea 3 mm. should be added to the measurement from the limbal ring.

Cridland (1967–68) designed a *graticule* with which measurements may be conveniently taken directly from the radiographs (Figs. 514–515); the centre of the foreign body shadow is marked by pricking a pinhole in the film so that subsequent scratching of the film will not destroy the evidence. The graticule is laid flat on the film with the point of the intersection of the scales coinciding with the centre of the ring. Measurements are read directly and without parallax; the radial lines enable the meridian to be determined with fair accuracy and the quarter circles provide a very good check on the obliquity, if any, in the postero-anterior view when the intercepts of the ring on the three axes are made as nearly equal as possible.

The use of a *contact lens* as a marker was suggested by Fox (1902) who introduced an oval insert of gold with cross-wires into the cocainized conjunctival cul-de-sac and localized the foreign body in postero-anterior and lateral exposures with reference to it. A more elegant technique of using a Müller's prosthetic shell with an opaque ring around the limbus and the corneal portion made of leaded glass, so as to show up on the films, was introduced by Wessely (1910–11) (Fig. 516). The same principle was elaborated and made considerably more accurate in the *method of Comberg* (1927–30) which made use of a Zeiss contact glass with lead markers at the four quadrants (Fig. 517). In Comberg's technique the patient lies prone and fixates a point in a mirror transparent to x-rays, placed at an angle so that his fixation is controlled (Fig. 519), a device which can be transferred to the other eye if the injured eye is functionally incapable of doing this; correction is made if necessary for the angle α or a strabismus if it is present. The postero-anterior exposure is taken with the film underneath the patient's head and the central ray focused exactly on the anterior pole of the eye in the direction of the visual axis, perpendicular to the film. In the second (lateral) exposure the film is parallel to the axis of the eye and the central ray passes through the limbus perpendicular to this axis (Fig. 520). From the frontal radio-

FIGS. 514 and 515.—CRIDLAND'S GRATICULE FOR THE LOCALIZATION OF FOREIGN BODIES.

The graticule is photo-etched on the under-side of a glass plate so that it can be placed in direct contact with the film. The scales on the axes are marked in mm. (N. Cridland).

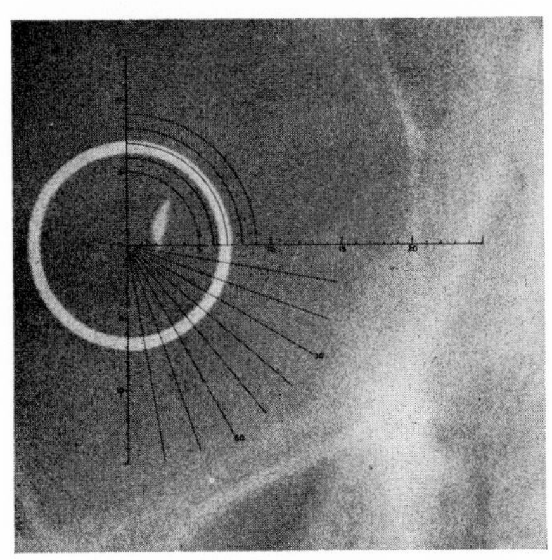

FIG. 514.

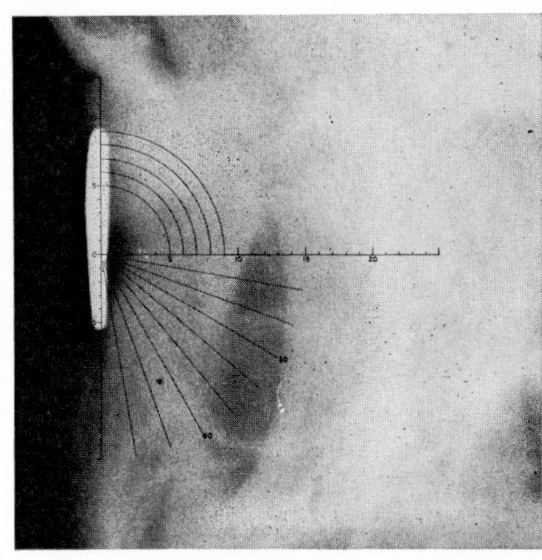

FIG. 515.

FIG. 514.—Postero-anterior view. The graticule is set so that the outer edge of the ring cuts each of the three axes at the same distance from their meeting point. The accuracy of the direction of the film can be checked if one of the quarter circles on the graticule fits the shadow of the ring exactly; a film which does not reasonably satisfy these criteria is discarded. The graticule is orientated so that the centre of the intra-ocular foreign body (which is marked by a pin-prick on the film) lies exactly on the horizontal axis and its distance from the centre of the ring can be read directly. It is then reorientated so that the three axes have equal intercepts with the outer margin of the ring and one of the axes is parallel as near as can be judged with the vertical line in the orbital picture, while the foreign body lies in the protractor quadrant of the graticule; the meridian containing it is then read directly.

FIG. 515.—Lateral view. The vertical axis is set to coincide with the middle of the oval shadow of the ring in such a way that the foreign body lies on the horizontal axis; the distance of the foreign body behind the plane of the ring is read directly on this axis and its height above or below the centre of the ring is obtained by noting where the ends of the shadow of the ring fall on the vertical axis.

FIGS. 516 TO 518.—CONTACT LENSES IN THE RADIOGRAPHIC LOCALIZATION OF INTRA-OCULAR FOREIGN BODIES.

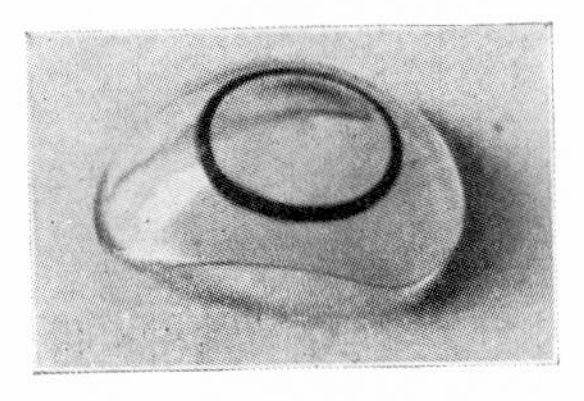

FIG. 516.—Wessely's original contact prosthesis.

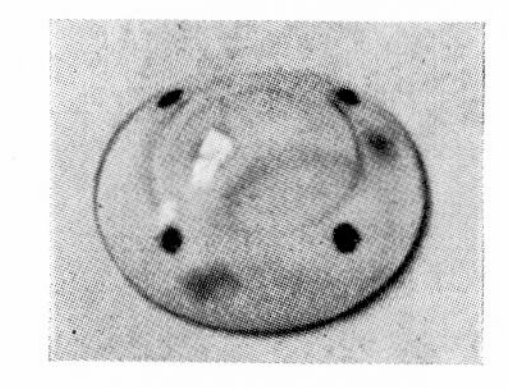

FIG. 517.—Comberg's contact lens. A modified Zeiss lens with four radio-opaque markers.

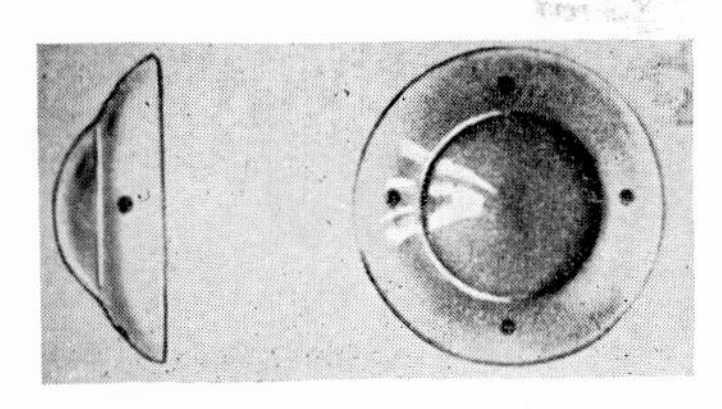

FIG. 518.—Pfeiffer's contact lens of plastic material with four radio-opaque markers.

FIGS. 519 and 520.—COMBERG'S METHOD OF LOCALIZATION.

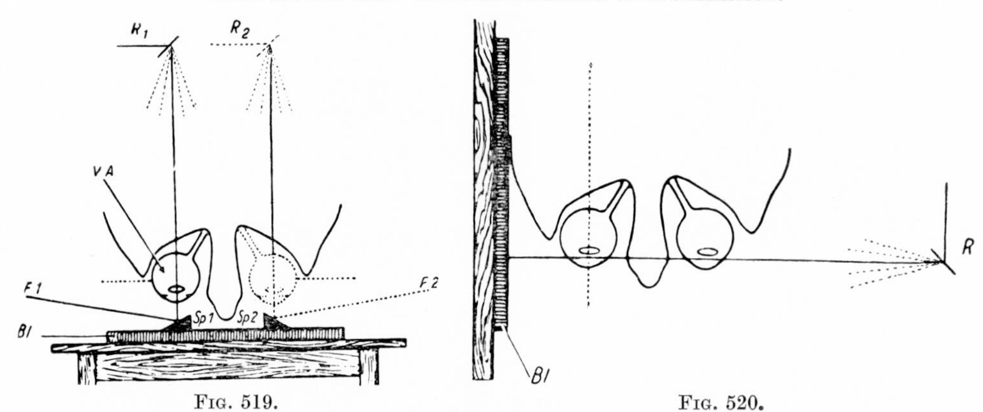

FIG. 519. FIG. 520.

FIG. 519.—Postero-anterior exposure. The central ray from R_1 passes through the injured eye (VA) and a small mirror (Sp_1) to the plate holder (B_1). The fixation point (F_1) is seen through the mirror. If the injured eye is unable to fix, the other eye is used (F_2).

FIG. 520.—The lateral exposure. The median plane of the head and the axis of the eye are parallel to the film. The central ray from R passes through the limbus perpendicular to the axis of the eye to reach the film, B_1.

FIGS. 521 and 522.—PFEIFFER'S METHOD OF LOCALIZATION OF INTRA-OCULAR FOREIGN BODIES.

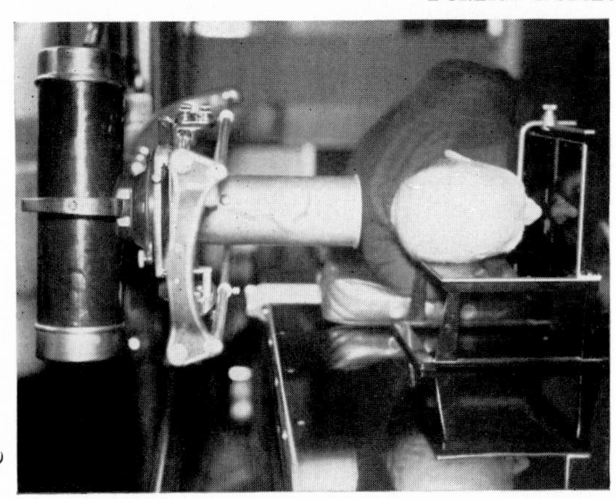

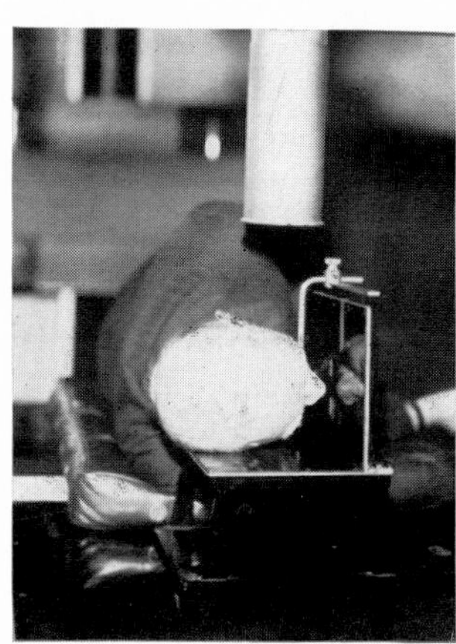

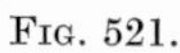

FIG. 521. FIG. 522.

FIG. 521.—The disposition of the apparatus for a postero-anterior exposure for examination of the right eye. The film is placed in the vertical portion of the L-shaped holder.

FIG. 522.—The disposition of the apparatus for the right lateral exposure. The tube is swung vertically in alignment with the right orbit and the film is placed in the horizontal portion of the L-shaped holder (R. L. Pfeiffer).

Figs. 523 to 525.—Pfeiffer's Method of Localization.

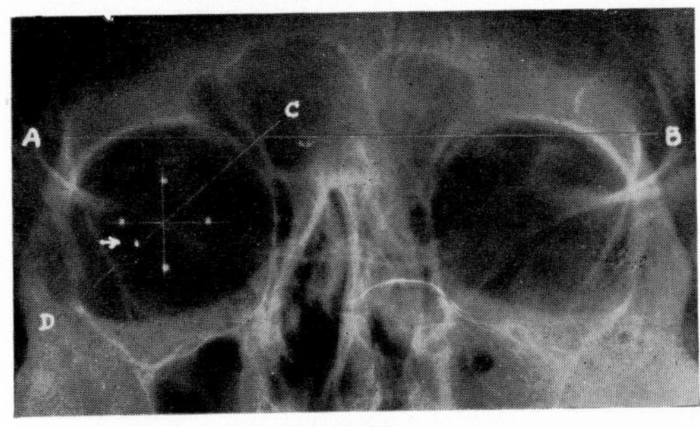

Fig. 523. Fig. 524.

Fig. 523.—Localization of an intra-orbital foreign body in the postero-anterior view. AB is a horizontal line below the upper orbital margin. The diagonal, CD, passes through the centre of the contact glass and the foreign body (indicated by the arrow). The angle between the two determines the position of the meridian, C′D′, on the chart in Fig. 525 and the distance of the foreign body from the centre can be directly measured.

Fig. 524.—Lateral view of the intra-ocular foreign body. The line EF, drawn anterior to the markers and the contact glass, indicates the plane of the limbus. The line GH is drawn at right angles to EF through the foreign body (indicated by the arrow).

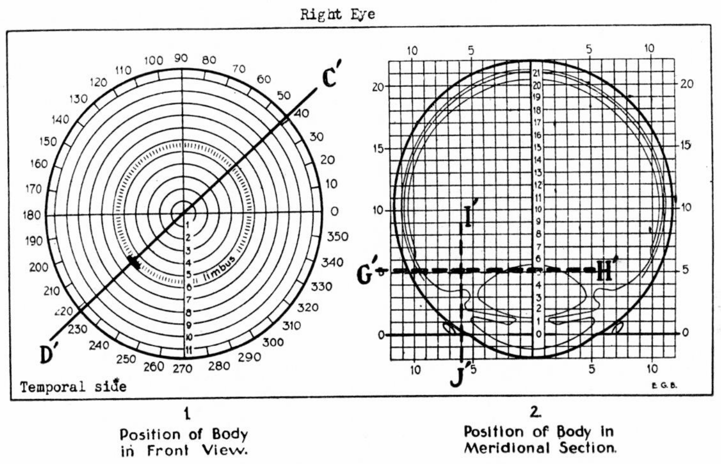

Fig. 525.

Localization chart. The position of the foreign body is seen in the front view and in meridional section taken from the radiographs. The line G′H′ in the meridional section is drawn across the chart at the depth of the foreign body calculated from Fig. 524. The second line, I′J′ is drawn perpendicular to this to represent the distance of the foreign body from the axis of the eyeball (centre of the contact glass) obtained (after correction) from Fig. 523 (R. L. Pfeiffer).

graph the anterior pole of the eye is indicated by the intersection of the diagonals joining the markers on the contact glass, and the distance of the foreign body from this point in the frontal plane is determined by direct measurement on the film (Fig. 523); the meridian in which it lies is determined with reference to a line joining the fronto-malar sutures. Its position on the sagittal plane is obtained from the lateral exposure

FIGS. 526 and 527.—AHLBOM'S SCHEME FOR LOCALIZATION.

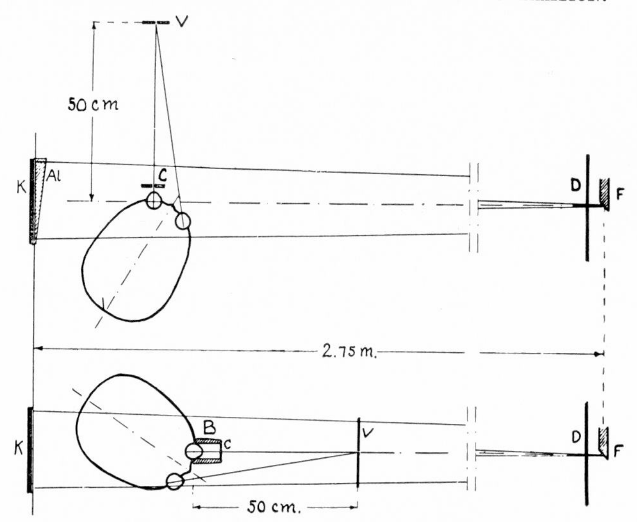

FIG. 526.—The lateral view is above, the frontal view below.

In each case F is the focus of the source of x-rays, D a diaphragm, V a fixation cross 50 cm. away from the eye, C a disc pierced by a hole (held in place on the frontal view by a bakelite tube, B). K is the film and Al (in the upper figure), the aluminium wedge.

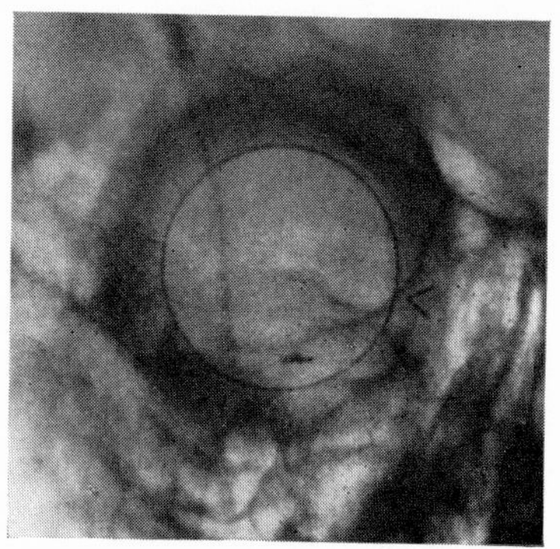

FIG. 527.

Postero-anterior view. The circular shadow of the pre-corneal perforated disc is seen as well as the foreign body in the lower part of the circle ($\frac{3}{4}$ natural size) (E. Hartmann).

by direct measurement of the distance of the foreign body behind the markers (Fig. 524). These measurements are transferred to charts of the schematic eye, appropriate corrections being made to allow for the conical projection of the rays and the distance of the plates from the eyes (Fig. 525). This error (approximately an addition of 1/10) is obtained directly by comparing the size of the contact lens on the film with its actual size.

This method has been used enthusiastically (Lembeck, 1928; Franceschetti, 1934). Among the more important modifications are those due to Pfeiffer (1940–44), who designed an apparatus which maintained the patient's head in a single lateral position throughout both exposures and obtained immobility of the head by a biting device and constancy in the position of the films by using an L-shaped arrangement of slots to hold the cassettes so that in both exposures the primary rays were perpendicular to their surfaces (Figs. 521–525). Further modifications were introduced by Leydhecker (1940), Dufour (1946), Marucci (1948) and others. Smolnig (1948) maintained the patient in a supine position, using a fixation point on the ceiling.

Plastic lenses which can be manufactured more easily are now generally used (Pfeiffer, 1944; McGuire and Raffetto, 1944) (Fig. 518), and to overcome possible inaccuracies owing to movements of the contact glass, perforations have been incorporated into its rim by Thorpe (1944–65) so that the lens can be sutured to the conjunctiva.

Hamard and Campinchi (1965) described a method of localization using a modified Comberg contact lens held in place by suction to maintain its position on the globe and a transparent plastic marking grille which can be applied to the radiograph; two exposures only are required, a postero-anterior and a lateral. Tojo and his colleagues (1967) used the contact lens of Lovac modified by the addition of two bars.

Methods employing Markers set at a Distance. The application of lead markers or a contact glass to a globe which is badly traumatized may have obvious disadvantages, and these have stimulated the exploitation of methods whereby a distant marker is employed. For this purpose Bär (1918) used a metallic cross set at a fixed distance from the cornea, while Argañaraz (1922) held a metallic ring the size of a standard eye in a position so as to outline the globe in its frontal and lateral profiles. The use of an extra-ocular indicator, however, was first accurately employed by Scandinavian workers (Ahlbom, 1931; Stenius, 1947). Ahlbom's method is illustrated in Figs. 526 and 527. In the postero-anterior position a metal disc perforated in its centre by a circle 26 mm. in diameter is fixed immediately in front of the eye, centred upon the pupil, while fixation is maintained by looking through this at a fixation-mark consisting of a cross. If the injured eye cannot maintain fixation the other eye may be employed, corrections being made for any deviation. The radiograph thus obtained outlines the foreign body in relation to the circular shadow made by the metal disc (Fig. 527). The lateral exposure is taken with the head placed obliquely so as to obtain a bone-free picture of the cornea, the impression of which on the film is accentuated by incorporating an aluminium wedge in the path of the rays (Fig. 526). Fixation is again maintained by looking at cross-wires (V) through a hole in the centre of a disc (C). From these two exposures the foreign body is located in the usual way and greater accuracy may be obtained by repeating the profile views in different positions of the eye.

In the method of Kraus and Briggs (1945) reference to a schematic eye is eliminated by an attempt to reconstruct the individual globe by means of a *movable indicator* which follows the corneal centre as the eye rotates. The head is placed in an immobilizing apparatus which carries two indicators (Fig. 528). Three lateral exposures are taken on the same film, first with the eye looking straight forward, then upward, then downward, in each case the horizontal indicator being adjusted to touch the cornea at the centre of the pupil (Figs. 529–533). From this composite film the centre of rotation is then found as well as the approximate circumference of the eye, and the distance of the foreign body from the sagittal equatorial plane by the construction in Fig. 532. A postero-anterior view is now taken with the vertical indicator at the upper pole of the cornea and the horizontal indicator opposite the centre of the pupil; from this film the simple construction of Fig. 533 indicates the distance of the foreign body from the centre and the meridian on which it lies.

2. METHODS DEPENDING ON ROTATION OF THE GLOBE. In these methods, sometimes called PHYSIOLOGICAL METHODS, *the head and the* X-*ray tube*

FIGS. 528 to 533.—KRAUS AND BRIGGS'S METHOD OF LOCALIZATION.

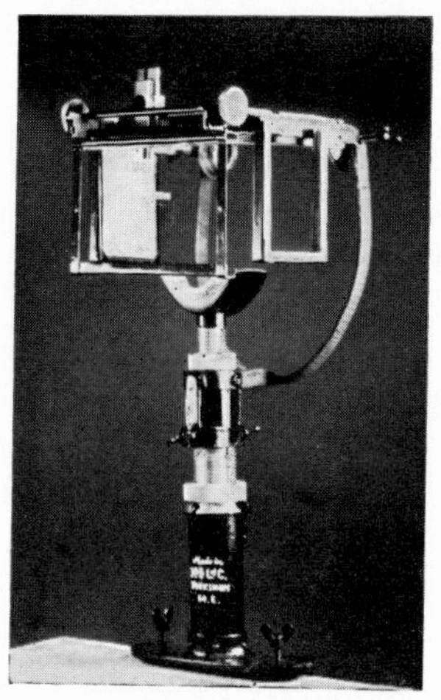

FIG. 528.—There is a head-rest with clamping devices attached to the forehead bar on which are the indicators and the X-ray cassette holder.

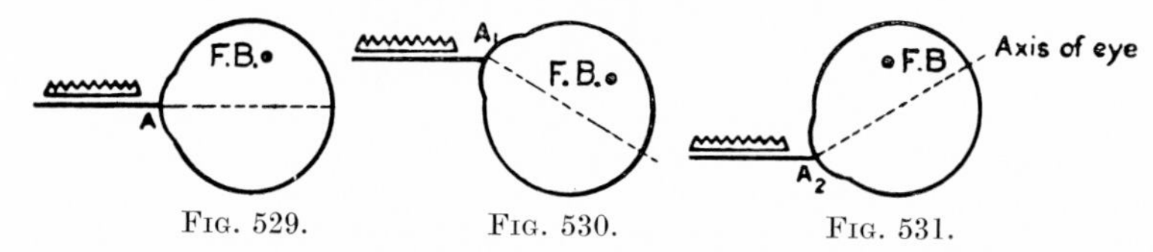

FIG. 529. FIG. 530. FIG. 531.

In Fig. 529 the eye looks straight forward, in Fig. 530 upwards, in Fig. 531 downwards. On each exposure upon the same film the marker is maintained at the centre of the cornea (A, A_1, A_2).

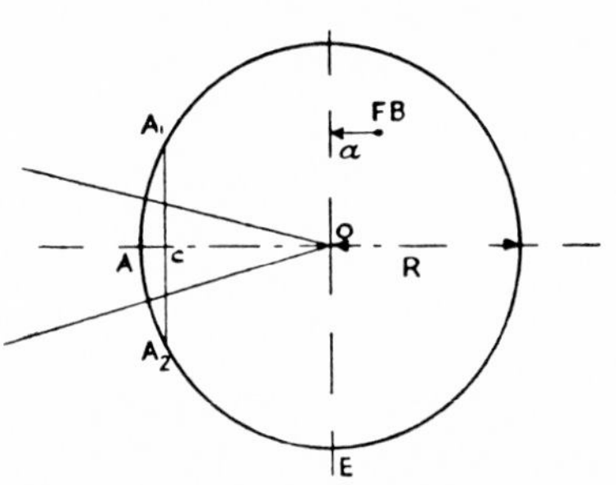

FIG. 532.—LOCALIZATION IN THE SAGITTAL PLANE.

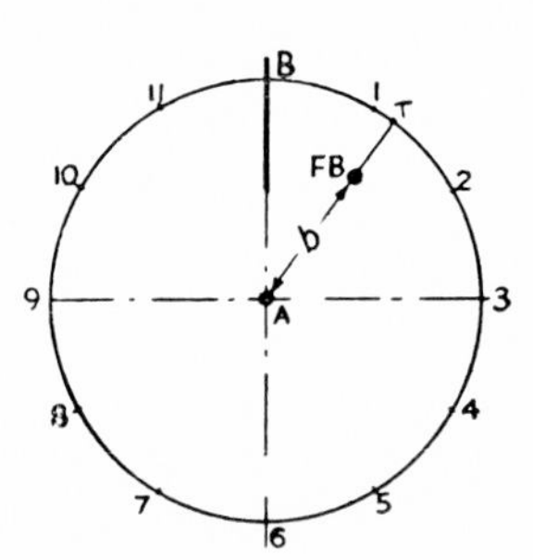

FIG. 533.—LOCALIZATION IN THE FRONTAL PLANE.

On the composite film of the three lateral exposures, the intersection of perpendiculars dropped from the midpoints of AA_1 and AA_2 gives the centre of rotation at their meeting place (O). The circle with O as centre and radius OA gives the approximate circumference of the globe. The distance (a) of the shadow of the foreign body (FB) from the sagittal equatorial plane as seen when the eye is looking straight forward can be measured directly.

On the postero-anterior view the upper pole of the cornea is marked by the vertical indicator (B) and the centre of the pupil by the horizontal indicator (A); the circumference of the eye is drawn in accordance with the dimensions derived from Fig. 532. The meridian on which the foreign body lies can then be drawn and its distance (b) from the centre of rotation measured.

remain fixed while several photographs are taken as the eye moves in different directions; the position of the foreign body is calculated from the direction and amount of displacement referred to the centre of rotation of the globe.

In the earliest days of radiography it was considered that if the shadow of a foreign body moved with the globe the particle was within it, but this simple statement is by no means true (Figs. 534–535). An extra-ocular foreign body attached to the sclera will move equally with the eyeball, and an excursion almost as great may be obtained if it is related to the capsule of Tenon, to the extra-ocular muscles or to the optic nerve. Even if the foreign body lies freely in the orbital fat, considerable movement occurs with the movement of the globe, as was realized by early writers (Hellgren, 1901; Holth, 1905; Terrien, 1925; and others) (Figs. 536–538), a movement which on occasion may amount to 11 or 12 mm.

Figs. 534 and 535.—The Movement of an Extra-ocular Foreign Body.

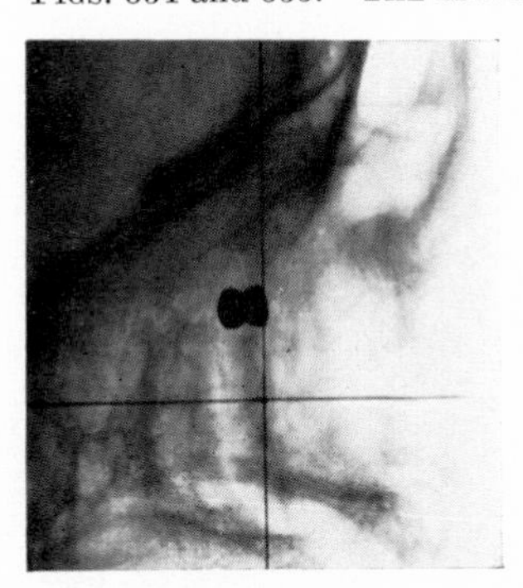

Fig. 534.

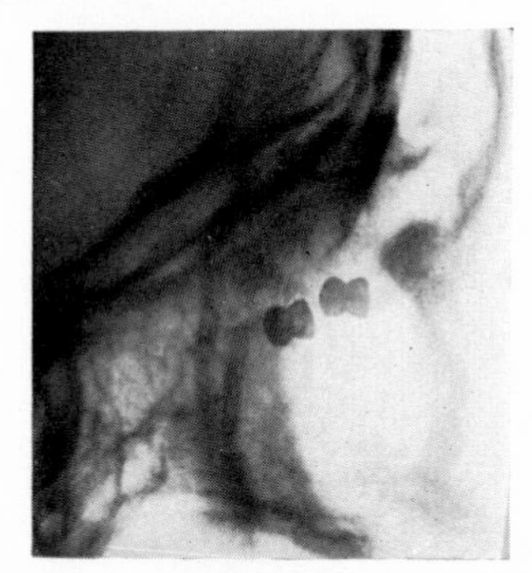

Fig. 535.

Fig. 534 shows the position in the lateral view with the eye in the primary position. Fig. 535 shows the variation in position on upward regard. The slug was associated with the superior rectus and, although extra-ocular, the movement is very considerable (R. S. Murray and Marion George).

In its simplest form, this method depends on taking three exposures from the lateral aspect, the x-ray tube being centred on the centre of rotation of the eye and the patient looking successively straight forwards, upwards and downwards, the angle of gaze being controlled by fixation points. Geometrical construction based on the three positions of the foreign body can be made to show whether it is intra-ocular or not and will indicate its approximate position. In the first case, its rotation will centre around the centre of the rotation of the eye (Fig. 539), in the second case it will not (Figs. 540–541). The accuracy of the method is increased if, in addition, the position of the foreign body in the frontal plane is indicated in a postero-anterior exposure.

To this method there are two obvious objections. In the first place, there is no true centre of rotation of the globe, but the error thus introduced

FIGS. 536 to 538.—THE MOVEMENTS OF FOREIGN BODIES WITH MOVEMENT OF THE GLOBE.

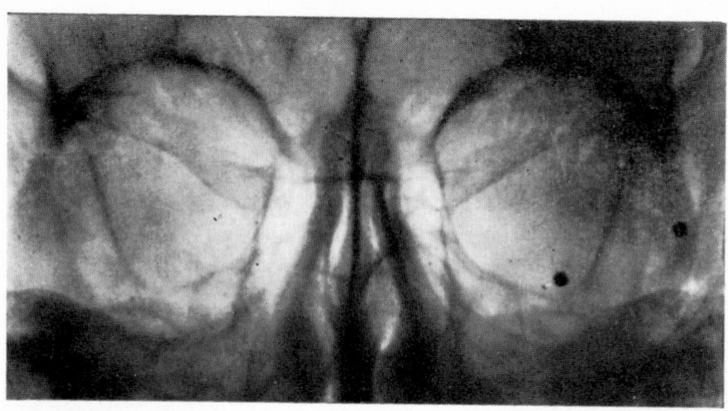

FIG. 536.

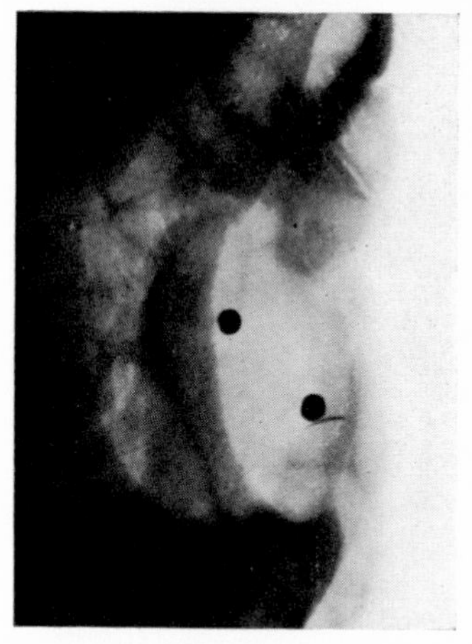

FIG. 537.

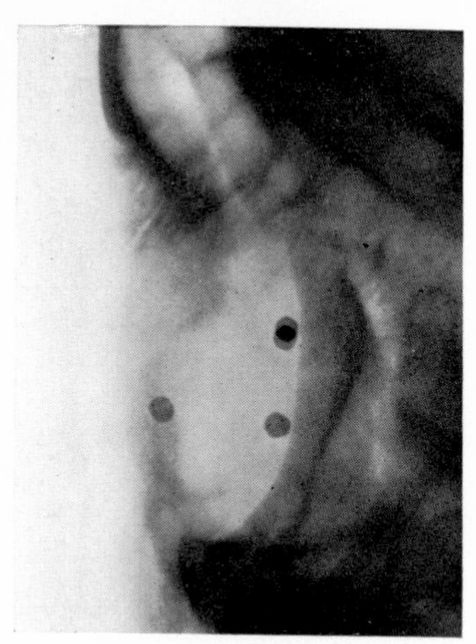

FIG. 538.

Two foreign bodies are present, one in the globe and one in the orbit, seen in postero-anterior (Fig. 536) and lateral (Fig. 537) views. On movement of the eye the lower (intra-ocular) foreign body shows a gross excursion (Fig. 538) but the upper foreign body which lies in the orbital fat shows a minimal degree of movement so that the two shadows are partially superimposed (R. S. Murray and Marion George).

is small. Again, as in the direct methods, a further error depends on the fact that the calculation as to the site of the foreign body must be made with reference to a theoretical standard eye of 24 mm. diameter.

The first relatively primitive attempts to apply this method were due to Grossmann (1899) and Lehmann and Cowl (1902), and the technique was further adapted by Köhler (1903–18); two pictures were taken on the same film, from the lateral aspect while the patient looked up and then down, and the displacement of the foreign body measured and a rough calculation made therefrom as to its position. Dor (1917) amplified the method by taking four lateral exposures, the patient looking successively upwards, downwards, temporally and nasally, while Holzknecht (1916) similarly took fi ve lateral exposures, the patient looking successively straight forwards, up, down,

FIGS. 539 to 541.

Geometrical construction showing the relation of an intra-ocular foreign body to the centre of rotation in various positions of the eye on lateral exposures.

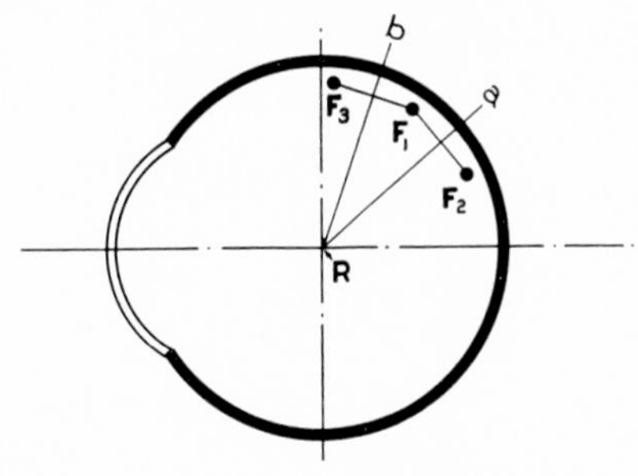

FIG. 539.

The foreign body lies in the globe. F_1 is its position when the eye is looking straight forward, F_2 when the eye is looking upward, and F_3 downward. If lines are drawn between the three positions, and perpendiculars dropped from their mid-points at *a* and *b*, they meet at the centre of rotation, R. Moreover, the angles of displacement of the foreign body correspond to the angles of rotation of the globe.

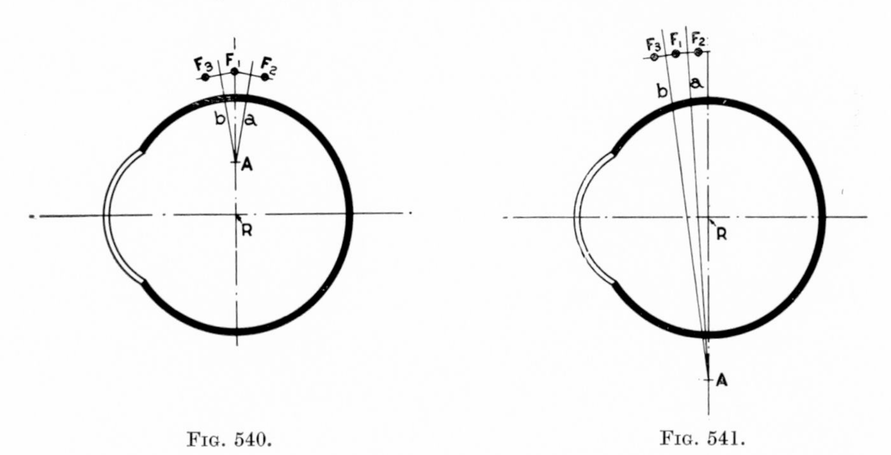

FIG. 540. FIG. 541.

FIGS. 540 and 541.—If the foreign body lies outside the eyeball, its positions being denoted by F_1, F_2 and F_3, it is seen that the perpendiculars dropped from mid-points of the lines joining the three positions do not meet at the centre of rotation or on the antero-posterior axis (A), and, in fact, may meet outside the globe altogether. The angles of rotation do not correspond to the angles of displacement of the globe. In Fig. 540 the foreign body is in a rectus muscle; in Fig. 541, in orbital fat.

in and out. From measurements of the relative displacements of the films it was possible to deduce the quadrant of the globe in which the particle lay and its approximate position.

Belot and Fraudet (1917) brought more precision into the technique. Three exposures were taken from the lateral aspect, the x-ray tube being centred on the centre of rotation of the eye and the patient looking successively straight forwards, upwards and downwards, the angle of gaze being controlled by fixation points. Thereafter two postero-anterior views were taken; in the first the tube was centred on the antero-posterior axis of the globe determined by a cross-wire device while the patient looked straight ahead, and the second while he looked at a known angle of adduction. From the amount of displacement of the foreign body in the lateral views its position in the sagittal plane with reference to the centre of rotation can be calculated, and from its position in the two frontal views relative to the cross-wires its location in the frontal plane can be deduced. While not extremely accurate, this is a useful method which can be employed with the minimum of apparatus.

Altschul's (1922) technique introduced a greater degree of accuracy into the method although it required the use of complicated apparatus. He took six exposures, the patient looking successively forwards, upwards, downwards, inwards and outwards, while a final exposure was made with an indicator mark of stanniol applied to the external surface of the sclera. During the exposures the head of the patient was fixed in an apparatus which standardized the distance of the eye and the tube from the film and provided constant fixation points for positions of regard 30° in each direction (Fig. 542). A method of geometrical construction gives the position of the centre of

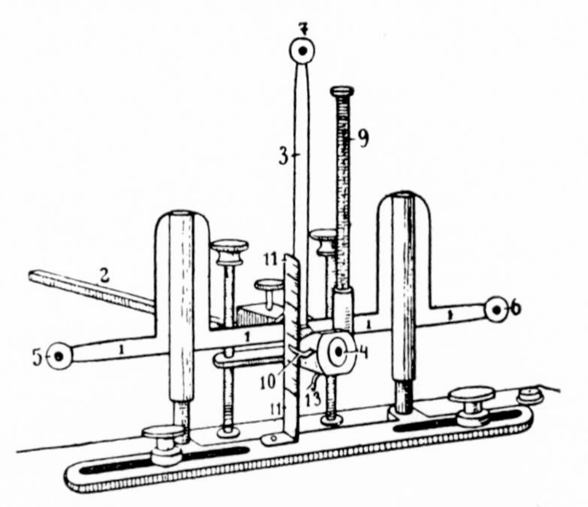

FIG. 542.—ALTSCHUL'S APPARATUS FOR THE LOCALIZATION OF FOREIGN BODIES (see text).

rotation from the pictures taken in the sagittal plane, and further orientation is provided from the position of the scleral indicator. For details of this construction, Altschul's original article should be consulted. They are somewhat complex, but in practice the method is greatly simplified by the circumstance that the relation of the foreign body to both the sagittal and horizontal planes can be readily derived from simple measurements on the films.

Altschul's technique has been modified and simplified by Verwey (1924); Grudzinski (1929) abolished the somewhat elaborate calculations (perhaps with some loss of accuracy) by the device of superimposing standardized charts upon the radiograph; while Stankiewicz (1935) simplified the technique still further by superimposing two exposures on the same plate. Porcher and Gilles (1945) employed a somewhat similar technique involving five lateral and one antero-posterior exposures.

3. METHODS DEPENDING ON GEOMETRICAL CONSTRUCTION. The essential principles on which these methods are based depend on the fact that if a straight line is drawn from the focal centre of the anode to the shadow of the foreign body on the film, it must pass through the foreign body itself; if two exposures are taken from two directions, the intersection of the two lines thus

drawn must therefore indicate the position of the foreign body in space (Fig. 546). Such a method of triangulation is well established; it is used in astronomy and other sciences and is capable of considerable accuracy. In all variations of this technique *the eye and the head remain fixed while two photographs are taken with the* X-*ray tube in known positions; from these the location of the foreign body is calculated with reference to a fixed indicator.* If the indicator (a known body) and the X-ray tube are at known distances from the eye and the tube is moved through a known excursion, the position

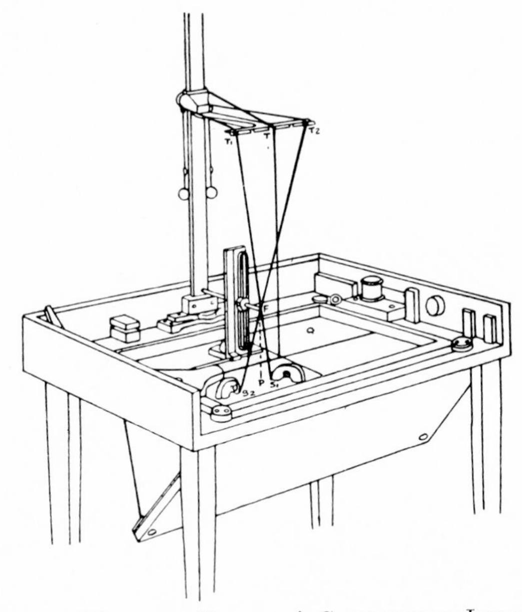

FIG. 543.—MACKENZIE DAVIDSON'S CROSS-THREAD LOCALIZER.

On the movable bracket, T is fixed at the original anode setting, T_1 and T_2 are the two positions at which the pictures are taken. The films are laid on the table with the cross-wires (or marker) in each aligned perpendicularly from T. Threads weighted with pulleys suspended from T_1 and T_2 are affixed by weighted needles over the shadows of the foreign body (S_1 and S_2). The point of intersection of the strings at F indicates the position of the foreign body in space, and the perpendicular therefrom, meeting the film at P, its distance from the film. The coordinates of P with reference to the cross-wires (or marker) give its relations in the plane of the film.

of the foreign body can be calculated from measurements of the distance between the shadows of the known and unknown bodies on the plate. The disadvantages of the method are that the apparatus itself is complicated and specialized, the measurements are thrown out by a slight failure in fixation on the part of the patient, while the computations are again based on the dimensions of a standard eye which, of course, may be inapplicable to the individual case under consideration.

Different techniques of exploiting this method have been evolved, principally by Mackenzie Davidson, Sweet, Dixon, Bromley and McGrigor.

The Method of Mackenzie Davidson. On January 1st, 1898, Mackenzie Davidson introduced a method of very considerable accuracy designed to locate foreign bodies anywhere in the body. It was first adapted to the eye in a case of Treacher Collins (Mackenzie Davidson and Treacher Collins, 1898), and other cases rapidly followed (Clarke and Mackenzie Davidson, 1898; Mackenzie Davidson, 1899–1916; and many others). In his technique the foreign body was related to the position of an indicator, such as cross-wires which left a mark of Indian ink on the skin or a small piece of lead affixed (by strapping) to a known point such as the outer canthus, and a duplicate of the apparatus used in this exposure was then made of exactly the same measurements,

FIGS. 544 to 546.—MAITLAND RAMSAY'S MODIFICATION OF MACKENZIE DAVIDSON'S METHOD FOR THE LOCALIZATION OF FOREIGN BODIES.

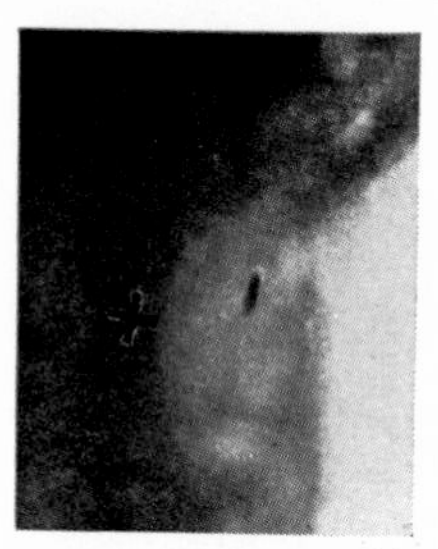

FIG. 544.—The skiagram when the x-ray tube is in position "S" in Fig. 546.

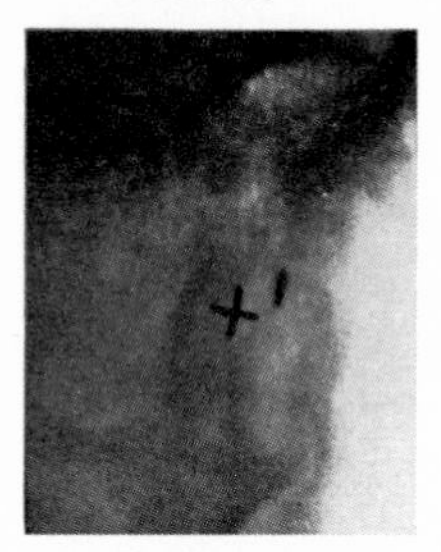

FIG. 545.—The skiagram when the x-ray tube is in position "R". For explanation see text.

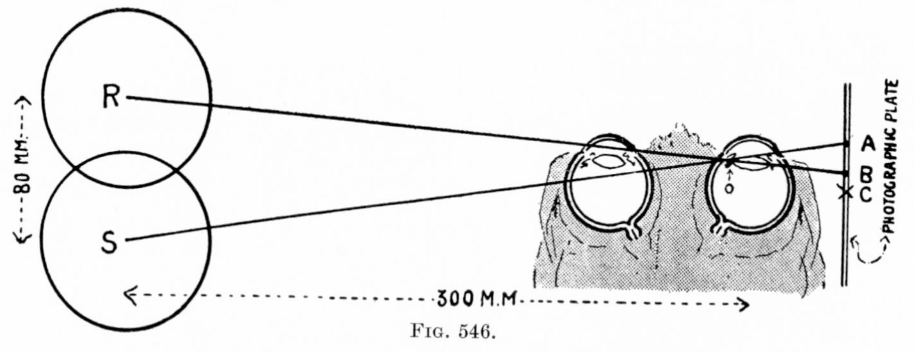

FIG. 546.

silk threads being used to represent the paths of the rays (" the localizer ") (Fig. 543). The point of intersection of the rays as represented by the crossing of the threads gave the position of the foreign body, which was then related to the position of the indicator.

The use of a localizer, however, was both troublesome and cumbersome and the more practical and simple expedient of a geometrical drawing to scale was introduced by Hulen (1904). The technique thus developed was further simplified by Maitland Ramsay (1907) as follows (Figs. 544–546).

The patient is seated with his eye close to the photographic plate and the x-ray tube set up at a fixed distance (300 mm.). Two skiagrams are taken, one with the tube (say) 40 mm. in front of the lead index fixed to the outer canthus, and the other 40 mm. behind it, thus involving a total displacement of 80 mm. On the films, measurements are made of the distance of the foreign body from the centre of the index

(Figs. 544–545); the difference between these is the distance between the images formed on the two plates (say, 9 mm.). It will be readily seen from Fig. 546 that where C is the index, A the position of one image and B of the other, O the foreign body and R and S the positions of the central point of the x-ray tube,

since
$$RS : SO = AB : BO,$$
$$80 : 300 = 9 : BO.$$
Therefore
$$BO = 33{\cdot}75,$$

that is, the foreign body is situated 33·75 mm. to the nasal side of the outer canthus. The antero-posterior distance is opposite the middle point of AB and is equal to $\frac{CA + CB}{2}$, which is measurable. The vertical distance is obtained by direct measurement on the skiagram.

The results of this technique are accurate but, in addition to the inaccuracies associated with all modifications of this method, it is to be remembered that the foreign body is located with reference to the indicator at the outer canthus and, although reference to the corneal centre and the visual axis can be made therefrom with considerable accuracy, the computation is obviously not so precise as when the indicator points at the centre of the cornea itself.

The Method of Sweet. The first geometrical method to be published was devised by Sweet (1897) of Philadelphia, the principle of which is illustrated in Fig. 548. Two metal indicators were employed, one pointing exactly on the centre of the cornea and the other at a known distance from the first on the temporal side; these were fixed to the film holder, which itself was attached to the side of the head (Fig. 547). Two exposures were taken, one (A, Fig. 548) with the x-ray tube in the same horizontal plane as the indicators but at a slight lateral angle, so that the shadow of one was thrown further forward on the screen than the other (C); the second (B) was taken from a position below this plane so that the shadows of the indicators appeared separately on the plate (D). The direction of the rays when the two radiographs were taken could be graphically reconstructed by measuring the displacement of the indicators on each film and the position of the foreign body (first at F′ and then at F″) calculated geometrically therefrom.

In 1909 Sweet modified the method and considerably simplified its practical application, eliminating direct measurement on the film and reconstructive drawings by designing an apparatus wherein the plate, the indicator and the tube are set on a stage whereon the position of the first two are fixed and the last moves by a determined amount for successive exposures (Fig. 549). The patient lies on his back with his head immobilized in the apparatus, and the sound eye fixes the indicator through a mirror arrangement to eliminate ocular movements. Since the same relations are preserved and the angle of the rays in each exposure remains constant, one indicator is sufficient; this is placed 10 mm. from the centre of the cornea, the accuracy of its position being checked by a system of mirrors and cross-wires.

Since the relative positions of the tube in relation to the indicator and the plate are fixed and known, and the direction of the rays follows a definite course which is always the same for the two exposures (Fig. 550), Sweet found it possible to avoid elaborate calculations in each case by constructing a *localization* or *key plate* of focal coordinates, a very ingenious device which enables the position of the foreign body to be transferred to a localization chart rapidly and without calculation (Fig. 551). After the film is developed it is placed upon this chart and the radiograph is moved until the shadow of the indicator in the first exposure is in apposition with the middle indicator at the top of the key plate and the heavy horizontal line on the radiograph is parallel with the horizontal lines on the plate. The position occupied by the shadow of the foreign body with respect to the vertical C or D lines of the key plate is then

FIGS. 547 and 548.—THE PRINCIPLE OF SWEET'S METHOD OF LOCALIZATION.

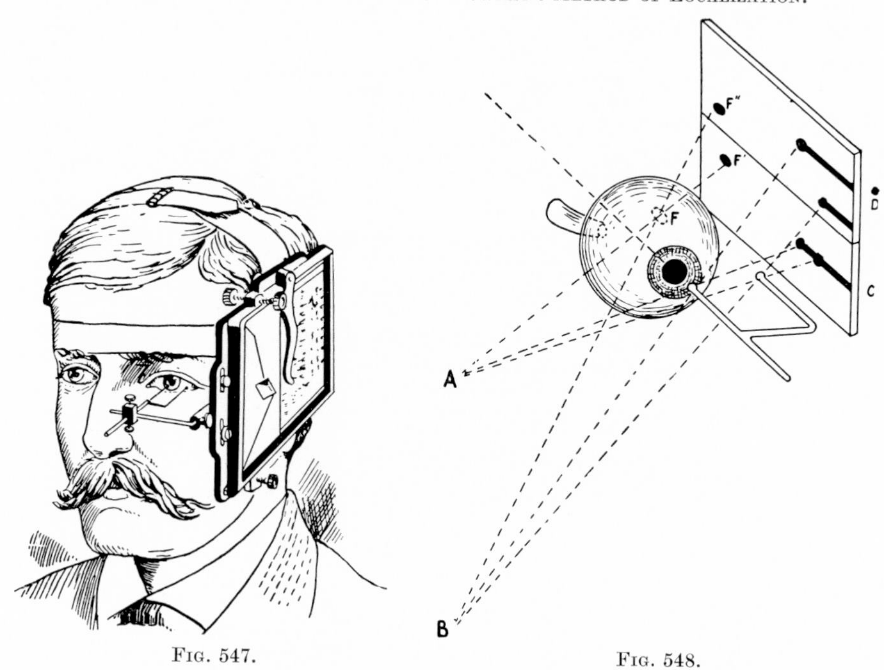

FIG. 547.

FIG. 548.

FIG. 547.—The apparatus in position.

FIG. 548.—There are two metal indicators, one pointing at the centre of the cornea and the other on the temporal side. Two exposures are made; A, with the tube horizontal to the plane of the indicators, throwing a shadow at C; B, at any distance below this plane, throwing a shadow at D. The shadows of the foreign body (F) are respectively at F′ and F″.

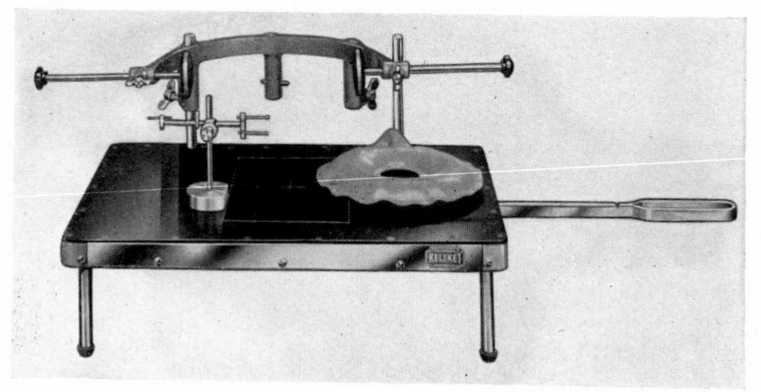

FIG. 549.—SWEET'S MODIFIED EYE LOCALIZER.

Included in the picture is the eye indicator, cassette tunnel and tray, compression device and pneumatic pad.

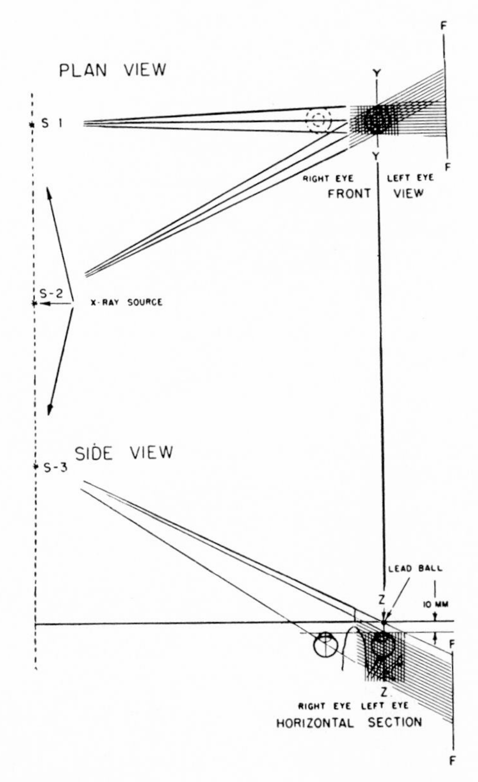

Fig. 550.—Plan of Sweet's Method of Localization.
Diagram showing the plan view and the elevation view of the two exposures.

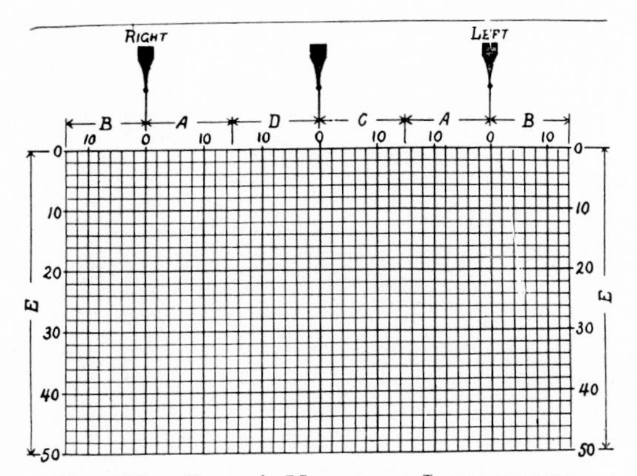

Fig. 551.—Sweet's Method of Localization.
Plate showing focal coordinates ($\frac{3}{8}$ actual size).

transferred to the corresponding C or D lines in the chart designed by Sweet (Fig. 552). The film is now shifted on the key plate either to the right or left, depending on the eye involved, until the image of the indicator on the second exposure coincides with the right or left indicator of the vertical coordinates, A and B. The vertical line crossing the shadow of the foreign body is then noted and indicated on the A and B lines of the chart. The horizontal, E, coordinate should be the same for both readings. After the three readings have been transferred to the chart, the point of crossing of the A or B and the C or D lines is found, which gives the location of the foreign body in

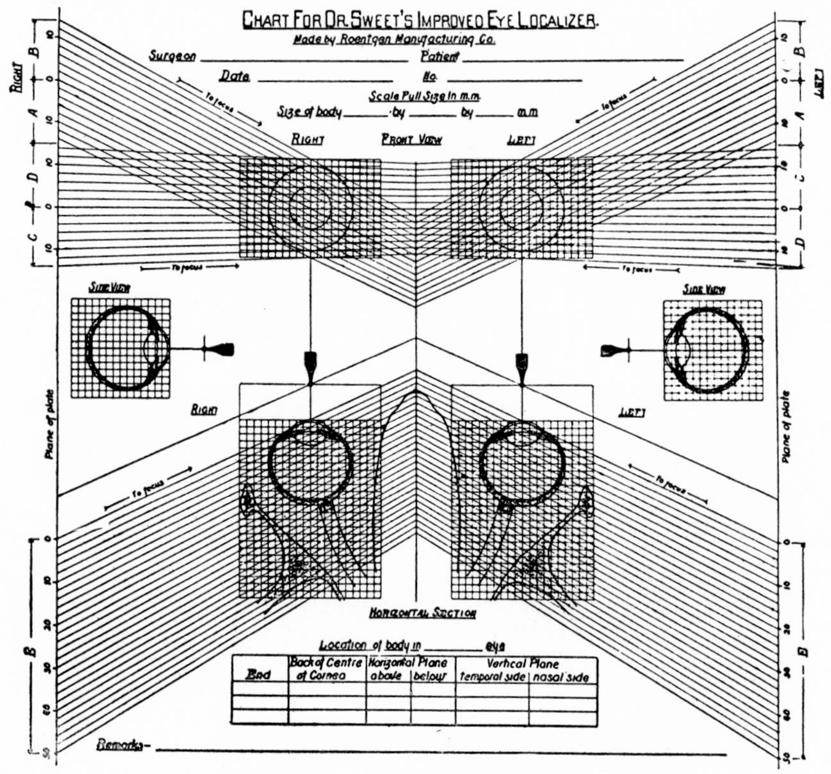

FIG. 552.—SWEET'S LOCALIZATION CHART.

reference to the frontal plane of the eye, thus indicating its situation above or below the centre of the cornea and to the nasal or temporal side of the vertical plane. Where a vertical line from this point crosses the E reading on the horizontal section of the globe the depth of the foreign body in the eyeball or orbit is shown. The situation of the particle in the side view may be determined by transferring its measured depth from the horizontal section and its distance above or below the horizontal plane from the front-view localization to the side-view diagram seen in the chart.

This simplified method of Sweet is ingenious and very accurate and has been used extensively up to the present time in the United States (Runyan and Penner, 1969); it has, however, found popularity only sporadically in European and other clinics (Hartmann and Gilles, 1959).

The Method of Dixon. To overcome some of the difficulties of the two previous

FIGS. 553 to 556.—THE BROMLEY LOCALIZER.

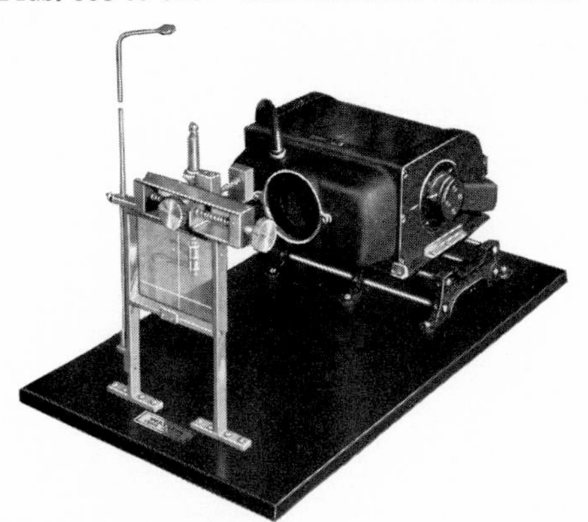

FIG. 553.

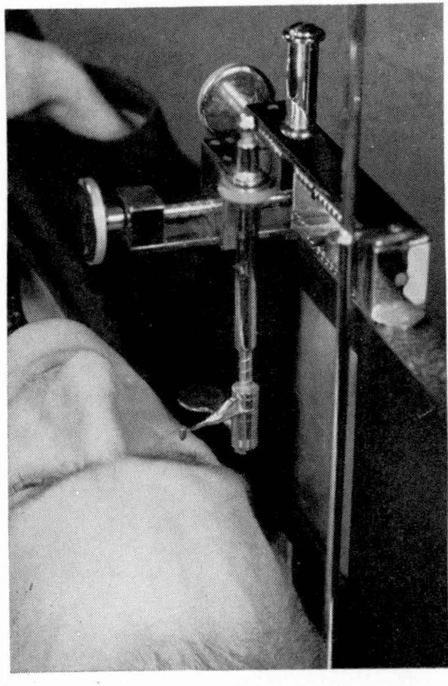

FIG. 554.

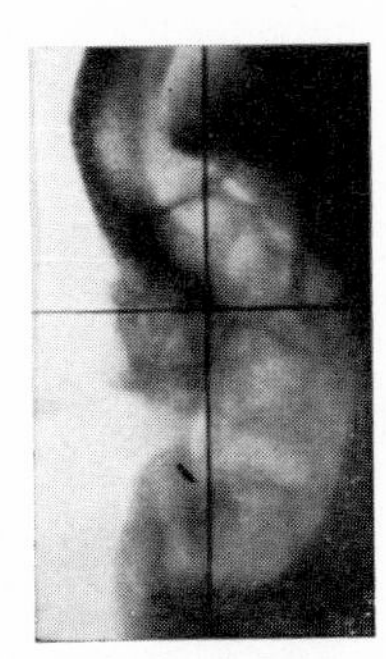

FIG. 555.

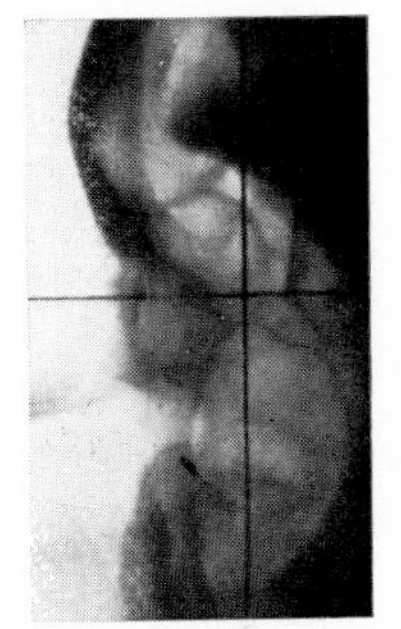

FIG. 556.

FIGS. 555 and 556.—Film showing a small intra-ocular foreign body embedded in the ciliary body (R. S. Murray and Marion George).

The apparatus consists essentially of an x-ray tube-head on horizontal runners arranged in such a way that, when it is positioned at either extremity of the runners, two views are taken with a 10 cm. stereoscopic shift. The cassette-holder incorporates two radio-opaque wires at right-angles to each other across a transparent window, supports a fixation device (sectioned in the illustration) and a device on the side nearer the x-ray tube head for positioning the eye and serving as a known opaque indicator. This is best seen in Fig. 554, which shows the patient's head in position between the x-ray tube head and the cassette-holder with the indicator in place.

methods, G. S. Dixon (1906) of New York introduced a technique based on that of Mackenzie Davidson, using Sweet's indicator pointing to the centre of the cornea and Hulen's method of graphical plotting; he further modified his method in 1907 and 1934, and it is still in considerable use, particularly in America. The patient lies on his back

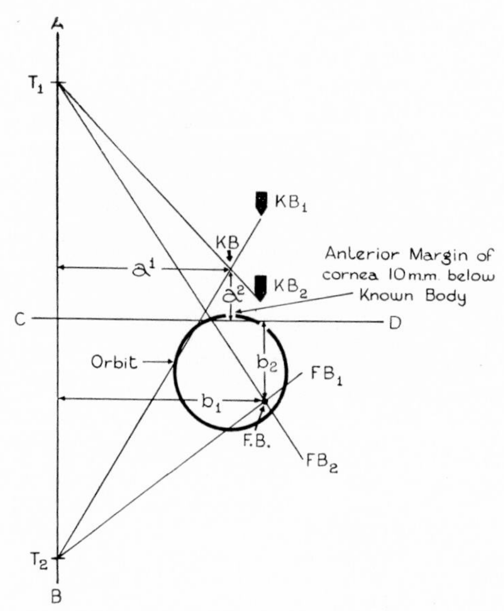

FIG. 557.
Localization of an intra-ocular foreign body in the frontal plane (see text).

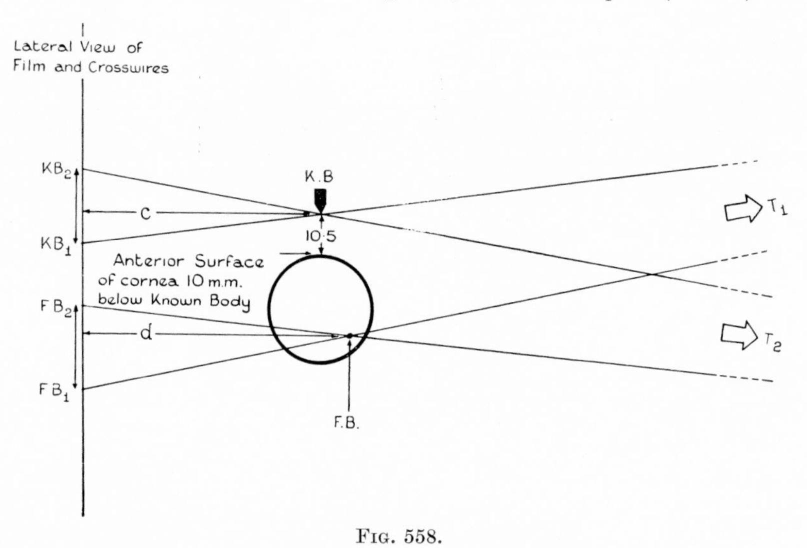

FIG. 558.
Localization of an intra-ocular foreign body in the coronal plane (see text.)

with his head in an apparatus providing adequate immobilization, fixation of the eye being attained by directing the gaze on an adjustable ball suspended some distance above him. The vertical film carrier and the tube are centred on cross-wires by a sighting device in a position such that the wires do not traverse the orbit lest they obscure the shadow of a minute foreign body. The indicator is then located 3 mm. away from the centre of the cornea by a readily adaptable mechanism. Two radiographs are taken, the first with the tube 3 cm. above and the second 3 cm. below the horizontal, involving a total displacement of 6 cm.

A very satisfactory modification of this method was evolved by Bromley (Bromley and Lyle, 1943) which is at present employed at Moorfields Hospital (Murray, 1952).

The apparatus is seen in Figs. 553–554. In front is the cassette-holder, which incorporates radio-opaque cross-wires; behind is the x-ray tube, and between the two the patient's head is supported in the supine position so that a small metal pointer (the known opaque body), set in the cassette-holder and manipulated by three vernier controls, can be adjusted to a fixed distance (10 mm.) above the centre of the cornea, while the patient gazes at a fixation point suitably mounted on a long vertical rod. Two exposures are taken by moving the x-ray tube vertically through a controlled 10 cm. stereoscopic shift 5 cm. above and below the central position, so that both views appear alongside each other on the film. The projection of the rays is indicated in Figs. 557–558. Knowing the tube-shift and the focus-film distance, and measuring the shadow-shift of the marker and the foreign body with reference to the cross-wires, the position of the foreign body can be calculated and referred to the three dimensions of space by the principles already described (Figs. 555–556).

The theory of the construction employed in all these methods may be indicated graphically as follows. Localization in the frontal plane is derived from Fig. 557, which shows the positions of the shadows of the known body (the marker) (KB_1, KB_2) and the foreign body (FB_1, FB_2) transferred from the films to the same graphical record, while on a line, AB, representing the vertical cross-wire, are indicated the two tube-shift positions (T_1, T_2). The actual positions of the known and foreign bodies in space (KB, FB) lie at the intersections of the lines joining the graphic locations of their shadows to the opposite tube-shift positions. These distances can be determined by measurement.

They may also be simply calculated as follows. When A is the focus-film distance, T the tube-shift, S the shadow-shift, V the distance between the shadows and the vertical cross-wire (AB) and M the mean distance of the shadows from the horizontal cross-wire (CD), the distance of either body (KB or FB) from the horizontal cross-wire $(a_2, b_2) = \frac{M \times T}{S + T}$. From the corresponding formula, $\frac{V \times T}{S + T}$, the distances from the vertical cross-wire (a_1, b_1) can be similarly calculated.

From these measurements the position of the FB can be calculated and located in the frontal plane of a standard eye in a conventional diagram (Fig. 559).

In the coronal plane the distances of the known and foreign bodies from the film (c, d) can be measured from the construction of Fig. 558, where KB and FB lie at the intersection of the lines joining the positions of the shadows of the known (KB_1, KB_2) and the foreign (FB_1, FB_2) bodies on the films to the two stereoscopic tube positions (T_1, T_2).

This distance can also be calculated from the formula $\frac{A \times S}{T + S}$. From this construction the position of the foreign body relative to the indicator is determined by direct measurement and is transferred to a standard eye of 24 mm. diameter in a chart such as that devised by Weeks and Dixon (Weeks, 1905; Dixon, 1905) or Sweet (1909).

To determine whether the foreign body is within or outside the eye, however, requires a further projection. It cannot be assumed that if the foreign body lies within the greatest contour of the globe as represented in the localizing chart, it must lie in the eye; owing to the progressive diminution of the diameter of the segments of the eyeball away from the equator, this assumption applies only if the foreign body is in a section of the globe which includes the greatest equatorial diameter. McGrigor (1918) overcame this difficulty by a simple construction the principle of which was adopted by Bromley and Lyle (1943) (Fig. 559). On the elevation view a line *aPc* is drawn through the position of the foreign body as determined on the frontal plane. Perpendiculars are dropped from *a* and *c* to the plan of the horizontal section at *d* and *e*; a circle with *de* as diameter represents the section of the globe as seen from above at the level of the foreign body. If a perpendicular is dropped from P to cut the plane of the film (XY) in P^2, the depth of the foreign body behind this plane as already determined is then measured from P^2 along this line; the point P^1 thus located represents the position of the foreign body and its location shows whether or not it is within the eye.

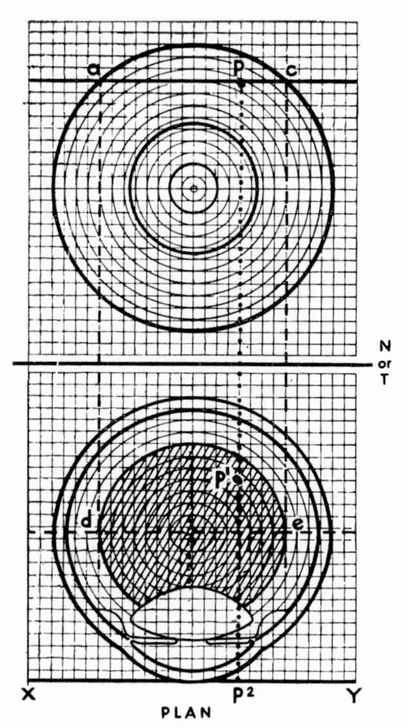

FIG. 559.—Elevation and plan view for determining the position of the foreign body (D. B. McGrigor).

Since in all these techniques all the distances are standardized, individual constructions or calculations can be replaced with a very considerable degree of accuracy by simply read charts or graphs supplied with the instruments.

The geometrical method was simplified to some extent by Müller (1909) and Stumpf (1916) by taking two exposures with the tubes in predetermined positions without changing the films. The foreign body thus throws two shadows on each film and its position can be calculated from the difference in their trajectories. The difficulty with all these methods, of course, is the complication of the apparatus, in order to overcome which Ohnishi (1932) devised a procedure which can be very simply executed, but the gained simplicity is counterbalanced by the introduction of inaccuracies.

A similar criticism applies to the simple and useful device suggested by McGrigor (1918).

McGrigor's (1918–39) method is a further adaptation of the same technique which gains in the simplicity and portability of the apparatus what is lost in accuracy. The patient wears a simple cross-wire attachment stretched horizontally and vertically across the eye-pieces of a specially designed spectacle frame, and in front of these are affixed miniature cassettes to hold small (dental) films (Fig. 560). He lies supine maintaining fixation with his sound eye at a target, the cross-wires are centred on the

FIGS. 560 and 561.—MCGRIGOR'S APPARATUS FOR LOCALIZATION OF INTRA-OCULAR FOREIGN BODIES.

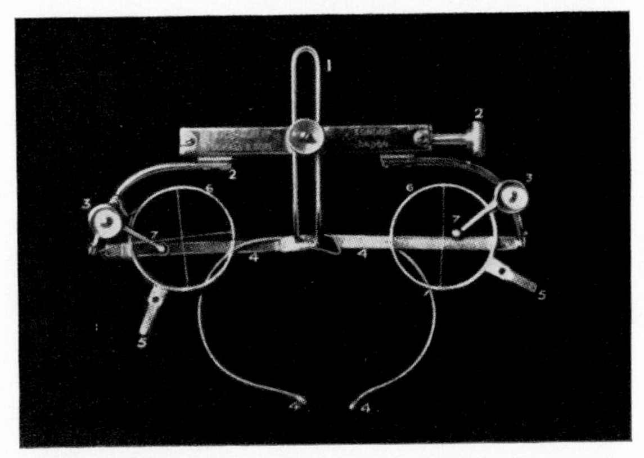

FIG. 560.—The apparatus is essentially a spectacle frame, adjustable in the vertical (1) and horizontal (2) directions, fitted with ear-pieces (4). There is an adjustment (3) to the spectacle rim and cross-wires (6) at the centre of the pupil in reference to a centering knob (7). For orientation, quadrant markers (5) are added (D. B. McGrigor).

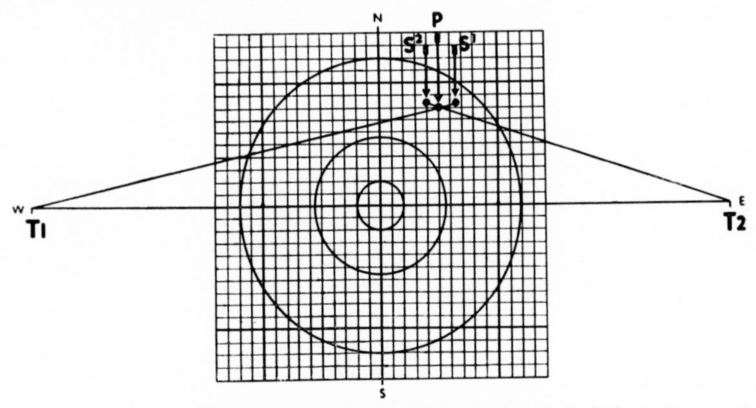

FIG. 561.—Chart for localizing the foreign body in the frontal plane (see text) (D. B. McGrigor).

pupil and then pressed against the closed lid of the injured eye, and two postero-anterior exposures are made on the same film with the tube 3 cm. to either side of the central position.

The method of localization is simple and ingenious. The position of the foreign body in the frontal plane is determined by transferring the positions of the two shadows (S^1, S^2) of the foreign body by direct measurement to a special chart representing a standard eye aligned with the cross-wires (Fig. 561). If T^1 and T^2 represent the positions of the tube, then P, the intersection of the lines joining these points, represents the position of the foreign body. The depth of the foreign body from the point P on the film is then, as before,[1] given from the formula $\frac{A \times S}{T + S}$, where A is the distance of the anode from the film, T is the shift of the tube, and S the shift of the shadows of the foreign body. The determination of whether the foreign body is intra- or extra-ocular is then made by the construction already described (Fig. 559).

When specialized apparatus is not available, as occurs, for example, in military campaigns, this technique will provide a simple although rough-and-ready solution to the problem of localization (McGrigor and Samuel, 1945; and others).

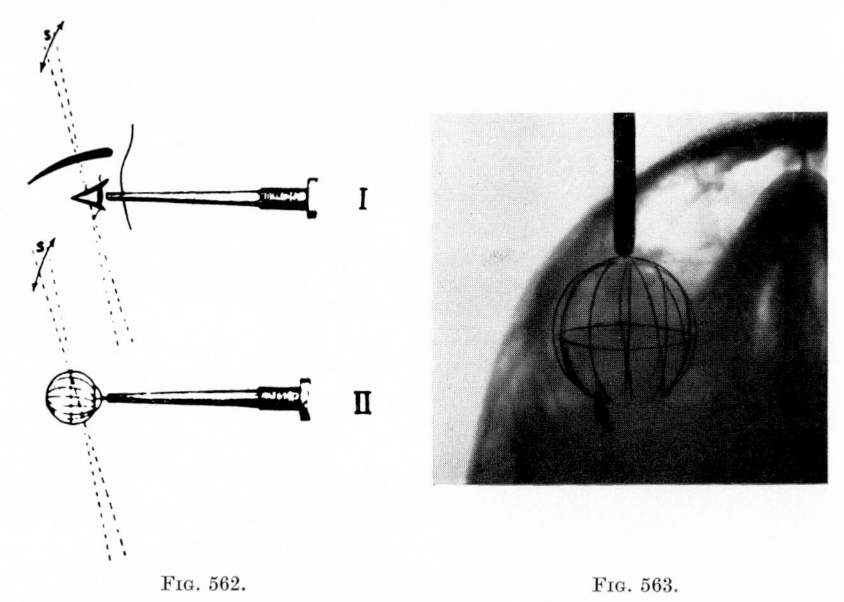

FIG. 562. FIG. 563.

FIG. 562.—The technique of stereoscopic radiography with an "artificial eye". I, the original exposure of the patient. II, flash exposure of the artificial eye.

FIG. 563.—Stereoscopic radiograph showing the initial exposure with the flash exposure of the artificial eye superimposed (E. P. Griffin, *et al.*).

4. STEREOSCOPIC METHODS. Attempts to localize a foreign body by taking two stereoscopic radiographs date from the work of Mackenzie Davidson (1899) and Lans (1902). The observation of the position of the foreign body is aided by taking several radiographs with the eye in different positions, and the interpretation of the pictures thus obtained may be made more exact by using a radio-opaque marker attached to the globe.

Different markers have thus been employed for this purpose—forceps attached to the limbal conjunctiva (Menacho, 1905), Cushing's meningeal clips (Jervey, 1930), a metal ring (Béclère and Morax, 1907; Arnold, 1925), the shell prosthesis of Wessely (Gallemaerts and Henrard, 1914), and so on. The stereoscopic method with various

[1] p. 601.

modifications has had a considerable vogue,[1] but although it is a very useful adjunct to other methods of localization it cannot be said to attain great accuracy, particularly in border-line cases.

Griffin and his colleagues (1943) hit upon an ingenious idea of aiding the stereoscopic effect with a circular metal grid representing in its dimensions a standard eye. Stereoscopic postero-anterior and lateral views are taken with an indicator resembling Sweet's in front of the cornea. Thereafter, without disturbing the apparatus, the patient is removed and a "false eye" consisting of a wooden or plastic sphere surrounded with a metal grid is put in exactly the position of the injured eye and the

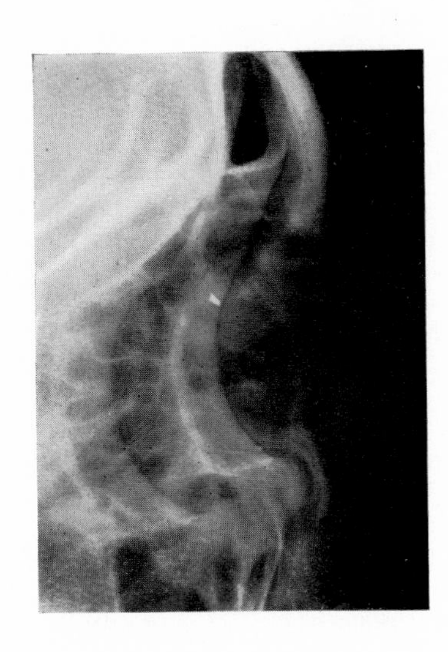

FIG. 564.—The injection of air into Tenon's capsule to assist localization of a foreign body (R. S. Murray).

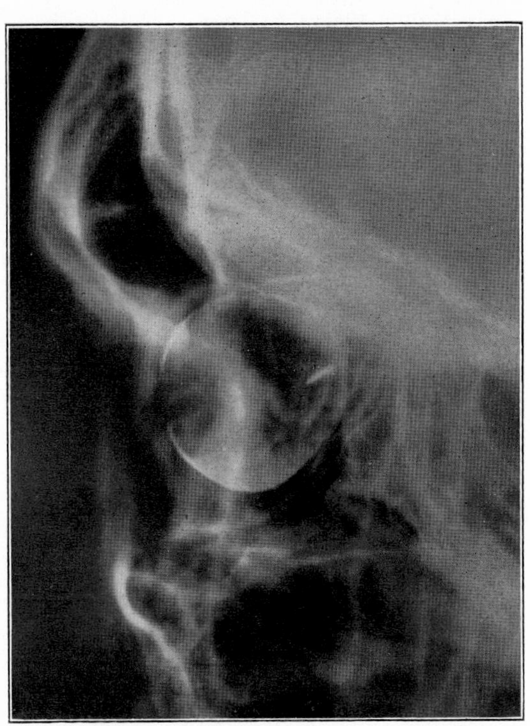

FIG. 565.—THE INJECTION OF DIODRAST IN TENON'S SPACE.

The contour of the globe is clearly delineated and the foreign body is seen just in front of the posterior pole (Katz, Hartmann's *Atlas*).

radiographs repeated on the same films (Fig. 562). Stereoscopic examination of these pictures shows the foreign body in relation to the metal grid more easily than otherwise (Fig. 563); it will be noted that in all projections the distortion of both the foreign body and the grid is the same.

5. METHODS INVOLVING THE DELINEATION OF THE GLOBE BY CONTRAST MEDIA. The methods of localization described all depend on the orientation of the foreign body with reference to the schematic eye of 24 mm. diameter,

[1] Holm (1912), Hasselwander (1915–17), Trendelenburg (1916), Engelbrecht (1917–18), Fleischer (1918), Senna (1948), and others.

and it is obvious that when the immense variations in the dimensions of individual eyes are remembered, many inaccuracies may thus arise. To overcome this source of error, attempts have been made to outline the contour of the globe by injecting radio-opaque material into Tenon's space with a view to differentiating whether a foreign body lies within or outside the globe, as seen in pictures taken at different angles.

For this purpose *injections of air* were first employed in animal experiments by Staunig and von Herrenschwand (1927), a technique followed clinically by several other writers[1] (Fig. 564). This technique has been used successfully and safely for many years by Thorpe (1965) who considered that it is particularly useful in suspected cases of double perforation and for obtaining a three-dimensional concept of the position of a foreign body. In experimental animals the use of air for this purpose has led to fatalities from embolism (Lindblom, 1934) and, since the air is not absorbed for 3 or 4 days, the external pressure exerted by it on the globe may increase the likelihood of prolapse of the intra-ocular contents if the surgical removal of the foreign body is attempted before absorption takes place. For this reason, Scheie and Hodes (1946) employed *oxygen*, which is more rapidly absorbed. The shadow thus obtained with either of these gases, however, is meagre and indefinite, and a better delineation of the globe is obtained by *radio-opaque fluids* such as Lipiodol, Diodrast or Thorotrast (Heuser, 1927; Speciale-Picciché, 1927; Farberov and Medvedev, 1935; and others) (Fig. 565); Geisler (1930) and Sandera (1930) injected a mixture of air and Lipiodol. The delineation obtained with a fluid contrast medium is much more marked than by a gaseous injection; nevertheless, some slight tissue-reaction may be obtained from it, while it is well to remember that the medium itself may obscure the shadow of a small foreign body of low density.

In order to increase the accuracy of localization in the anterior segment, in a similar manner Spaeth (1942) floated Lipiodol behind a Koeppe contact lens to give a fixed radio-opaque landmark for the accurate localization of foreign bodies lying near the angle of the anterior chamber or the ciliary body.

6. BONE-FREE METHODS OF LOCALIZATION. The adaptation of bone-free methods of radiography to the localization of foreign bodies has obvious advantages, and it is the only method available when the radio-density of the particle is such that this technique is required for its demonstration. Two procedures have been exploited: in the first a radio-opaque marker is used to locate the foreign body directly (Vogt, Goldmann, Larsson, Lindblom); in the second, a technique similar to those described as " direct methods " is used with an indicator attached to the eye, the position of the foreign body being calculated indirectly by geometrical construction from the position of a radio-opaque marker attached to the limbus (Bangerter and Goldmann).

The bone-free method introduced by Vogt (1921–23) allows some accuracy in localization in its simplest applications. If sufficiently soft rays are used and the lids are widely separated, the outline of the cornea is well seen, so that the relation of the foreign body to the corneal contour in the two exposures at right angles gives some idea of the position of the particle (Fig. 566). The accuracy of localization can, however, be considerably increased by taking two radiographs in each projection with the eye rotated in different positions, so that the " rotational " method is adopted to this

[1] Gasteiger and Grauer (1929), Spackman (1932), Peter and Rosen (1945), Puglisi-Durante (1947), Friedman (1947), and others.

technique. Lindblom (1948) evolved a method of this type, the position of the foreign body being subsequently determined with reference to a standard globe (Figs. 567–569).

An alternative method to achieve accuracy depends on the use of a *radio-opaque marker* which can be attached to the sclera at the presumptive position of the foreign body determined in this way; thereafter an exact localization can be made by moving the marker and reduplicating the pictures until it exactly embraces the shadow of the particle. Vogt employed for this purpose a marker resembling a fish-hook affixed into the conjunctiva; Goldmann (1938) used a metal ring fitted with small steel hooks which could leave lasting marks with Indian ink at their points of contact with the sclera (Fig. 570). He extended this technique to the posterior segment of the globe by opening Tenon's capsule and affixing the ring to the sclera, taking successive photographs until the particle was localized in the middle of the ring (Figs. 571–2). Larsson (1941) similarly determined the position of the particle in relation to the broken-off point of a needle thrust into the sclera, and Arruga (1942) to the tiny needles used in dacryocystorhinostomy, the position of the needle being changed and radiographs being repeated until the needle was exactly over the foreign body which was thus localized with considerable accuracy (see Granström and Lindblom, 1945; Granström, 1949; and others) (Figs. 574–5); Struble and Croll (1946) similarly employed a lead bead sutured to the site.

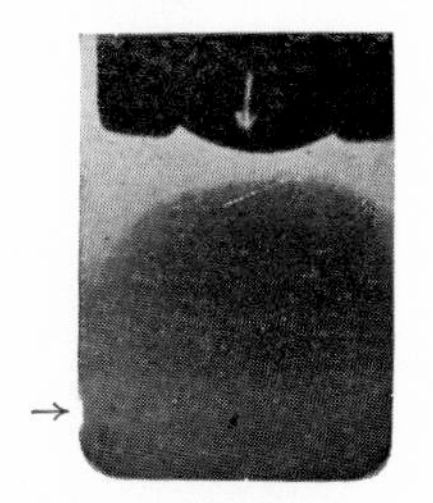

Fig. 566.
Bone-free Radiography.

A mento-vertical exposure showing that by this means more than the anterior half of the eye is available for a bone-free exposure. The foreign body is seen at the intersection of the arrows (K. Lindblom).

Finally, with a view to minimizing trauma to the globe and avoiding a multiplicity of radiographs, the technique was further elaborated by Bangerter (1941), and Goldmann and Bangerter (1941), who used a fixed marker and determined the position of the foreign body in relation to it by geometrical construction. They affixed the hooked ring of Goldmann (1938) concentrically round the cornea, so that the positions of the hooks were marked with Indian ink; two pictures were taken with the films vertical to the plane of the ring, and from them the coordinates of the shadow of the foreign body in relation to the limbus and the points marked thereon were ascertained geometrically (see Witmer, 1949; and others) (Fig. 573).

The description of all these methods of localization must present a confusing picture to the reader. They differ so greatly among themselves that a considered comparison of their relative clinical value is difficult. To a large extent, of course, the choice of a particular method in practice will be decided partly by the habit of the individual radiographer or the preference of the surgeon, and partly by the availability of specialized apparatus. In general it may be safely said that even the most accurate method will involve catastrophic mistakes unless it is used by expert and accustomed hands.

Practically all the methods involve inaccuracies, the most common being the topographical reference of the position occupied by the foreign body in the radiograph to a standard eye of 24 mm. diameter. We have already seen, however, that even in emmetropia the axial length of the eye varies widely—from 21 to 30 mm.[1]; in the higher degrees of ametropia the variation is

[1] Vol. V, p. 110.

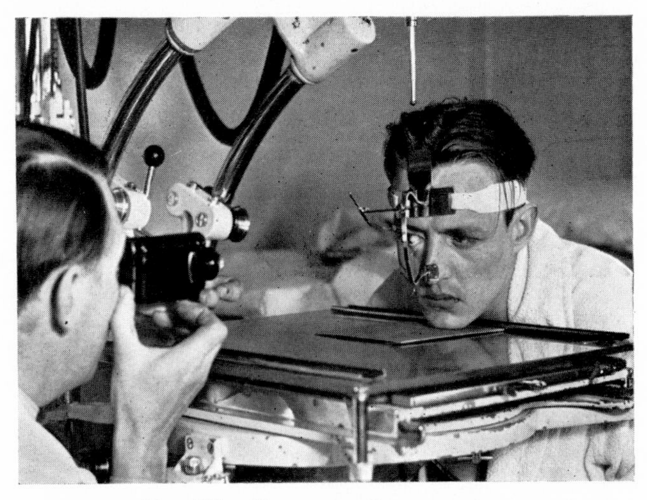

Fig. 567.—Bone-free Localization.
The positioning of the head and the maintenance of fixation in bone-free vertico-mental projection by the method of Lindblom.

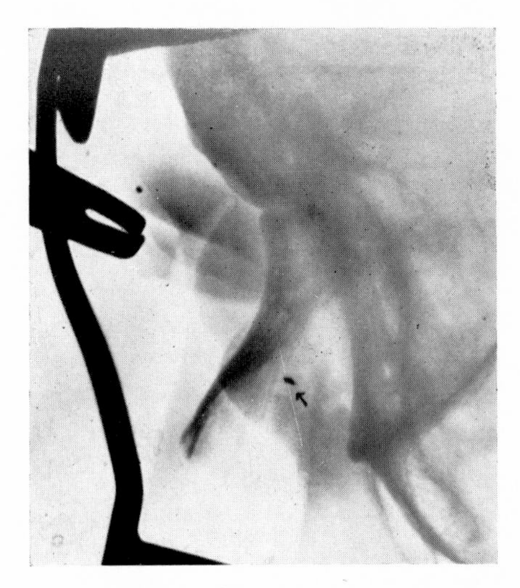

Fig. 568.

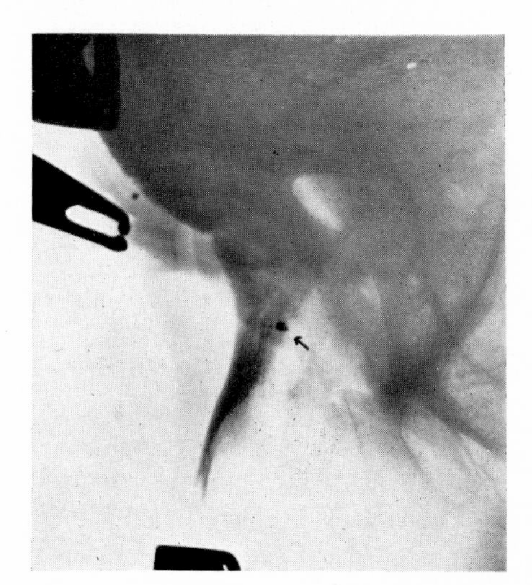

Fig. 569.

Figs. 568 and 569.—Lindblom's method of radiographic localization of foreign bodies.

greater, and when the foreign body lies in the posterior segment of the globe, particularly in the region of the posterior pole, the amount of potential error is considerable. It is true that an approximate correction may be made if the refraction of the eye can be assessed or inferred from that of its fellow; but every technique which involves this reference should be supplemented, if possible, by an investigation into the size of the globe. A direct

FIGS. 570 to 573.—GOLDMANN'S METHODS OF LOCALIZATION OF INTRA-OCULAR FOREIGN BODIES.

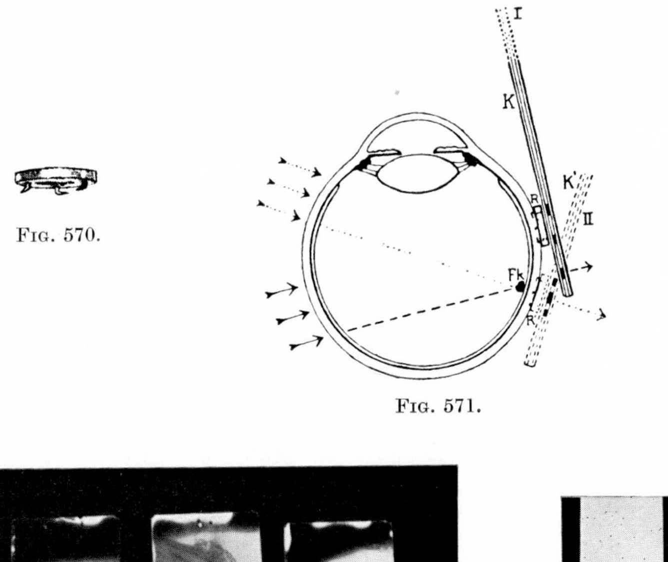

FIG. 570.

FIG. 571.

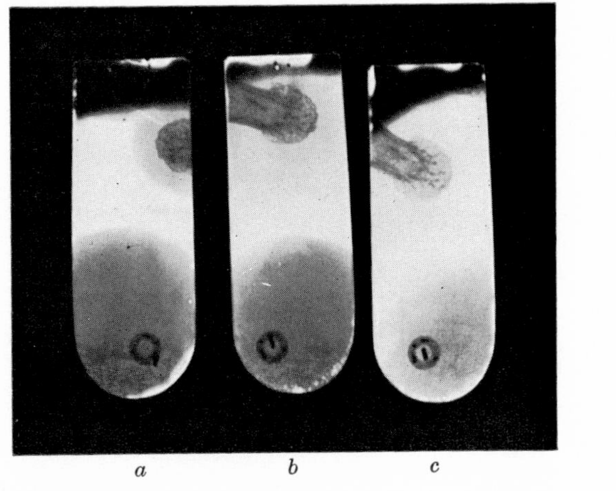

FIG. 572.

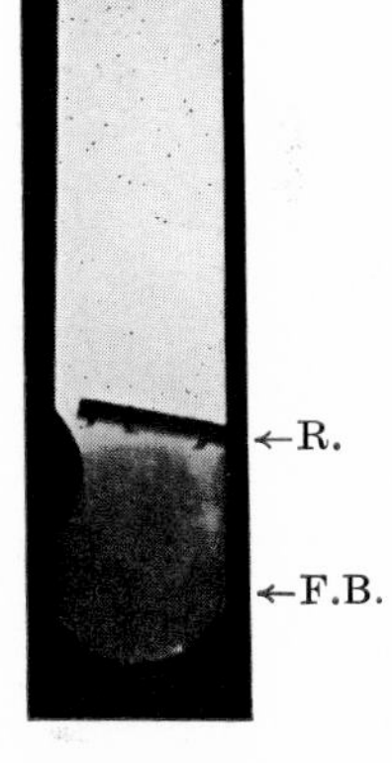

FIG. 573.

FIGS. 570 to 572.—Localization with reference to a movable scleral ring.

FIG. 570.—The toothed ring for insertion into the sclera.

FIG. 571.—The general technique of localization. The cassette (K), with the ring (R) attached, is inserted into Tenon's capsule and applied to the sclera. An example of a first attempt at localization is given (I), the continuous arrows showing the direction of x-rays and the lined drawing the position of the cassette. The broken arrows and dotted drawing indicate a corrected position (II) to allow the foreign body (Fk) to fall in the centre of the ring.

FIG. 572.—Typical radiographs showing the technique of localization. In *a*, the shadow of the foreign body is seen just outside that of the ring; in *b*, more accurately within it; and in *c*, in its centre. The markings made by the hooks of the ring on the sclera at the position *c*, localize the foreign body with reference to this structure (H. Goldmann).

FIG. 573.—Localization with reference to a fixed scleral ring.

FB, the foreign body; R, the ring on the sclera (H. Goldmann and A. Bangerter).

measurement of the equatorial diameter can be made with calipers, a technique, however, not by any means always possible since the conjunctival cul-de-sac may not be sufficiently deep (Berg, 1931). A better alternative is the *subjective measurement of the axes of the globe by* X-*rays* by the method introduced by Rushton and already fully described.[1] Such a method has been modified by Larsson (1948) for this purpose, but unfortunately it is not usually possible to obtain accurate subjective readings in a badly damaged eye. In such cases, if accuracy is required, the decision as to

FIGS. 574 and 575.—LOCALIZATION OF A FOREIGN BODY BY THE BONE-FREE METHOD USING THE TIPS OF TWO NEEDLES AS MARKERS.

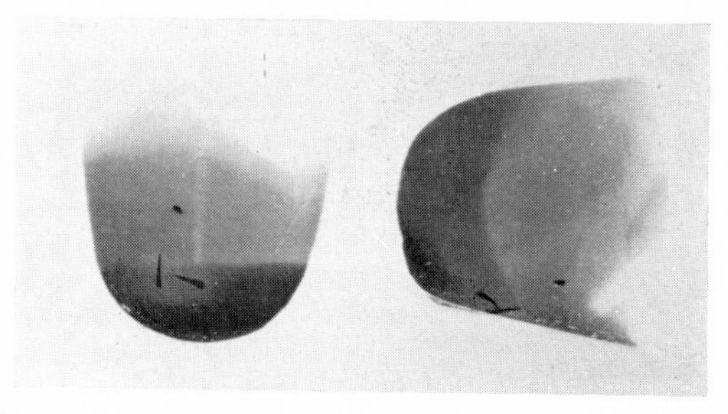

FIG. 574 shows the vertical and lateral views on the first attempt at localization wherein the marking needles are some distance from the foreign body.

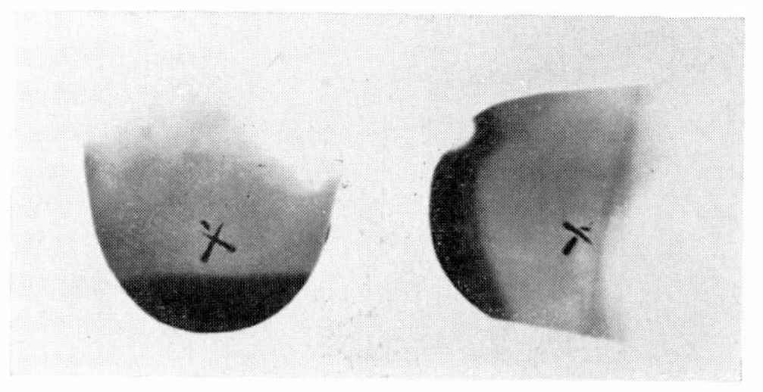

FIG. 575 shows the adjustment of the marking needles to correspond exactly to the position of the foreign body (S. Larsson).

whether a marginal foreign body is intra- or extra-ocular can usually be determined by supplementing one of the methods of localization by stereoscopy, the use of a contrast medium, a bone-free technique which, however, must involve the opening of Tenon's space or ultrasonography.[2]

If specialized apparatus is available with the skilled personnel to use it, there is little to choose between the geometrical methods of Sweet, Dixon or Bromley or their modifications; all give remarkably accurate results and they have the great advantage that no direct manipulations are required upon an eye which may be painful and badly traumatized. When, however, skilled technicians and adequate apparatus are not available, the ring

[1] Vol. V, p. 111. [2] p. 611

method or Comberg's contact lens technique is exceedingly useful. For this reason these two methods have proved their value in conditions of war as well as in small communities where the full facilities of an elaborate radiographic department are not available (Stallard, 1965; Cridland, 1967–68). In many cases, as we have seen, the application of the bone-free method is indispensable and resort should always be had to it if a foreign body is suspected on clinical grounds and the more conventional radiographs are negative. In general, however, it may be said from the practical point of view that most of these methods will provide a greater degree of accuracy in localization than the surgeon usually requires to determine his operative procedures.

Ultrasonic Localization

The physical characteristics and biological actions of ultrasonic energy are fully considered elsewhere in this *System.*[1] Ultrasonography has proved to be a useful addition to the methods at our disposal for the localization of an intra-ocular foreign body, both pre-operatively and during the surgical manipulations, particularly since it does not require optically clear media and thus it may be of most value when a suspected foreign body cannot be seen because of intra-ocular hæmorrhage or a cataract. Nevertheless the information obtainable about a foreign body by currently available ultrasonic techniques complements but does not replace that derived from other diagnostic procedures. Adequate radiological examination remains an essential procedure for the demonstration of the size, shape and position of a foreign body.[2]

The principle of ultrasonography depends on the propagation of a pulse of sound; when the sound waves strike an interface such as that between the vitreous and retina or between the vitreous and a foreign body a portion of the sound is reflected and received by the transmitting crystal. Distinct echo peaks correspond to the corneal surfaces, to the anterior and posterior lens interfaces and the posterior wall of the eye. No echo returns from the acoustically homogeneous normal aqueous, lens substance or vitreous. The reflected sound waves are converted into sharp spikes of light on an oscilloscope, which can then be photographed, or recorded as a trace on a time-amplitude system. The distances of the echo-producing interface from the ultrasound probe are accurately projected, thus permitting measurement of the axial length of the eye and precise determination of the distance from the probe to any echo-producing surface within the eye. Ultrasonography may help to determine whether a known foreign body is intra-ocular

[1] See p. 801, and Vol. VII, p. 325.

[2] Mundt and Hughes (1956), Baum and Greenwood (1958), Oksala and Lehtinen (1959), Nover and Stallkamp (1962), Purnell and Sokollu (1962), Sanna and Quilici (1963), Bronson (1964–69), Sander (1965), Ustimenko (1965), Penner and Passmore (1966), Vodovosov *et al.* (1966), Yamazagi *et al.* (1966), Ossoinig (1966), Goldberg and Sarin (1967), Oksala (1967), Purnell (1967), Cowden and Runyan (1969), Coleman *et al.* (1969), Gitter *et al.* (1969), Runyan and Penner (1969), Ossoinig and Seher (1969), Havener and Gloeckner (1969), Wainstock (1969).

or extra-ocular. It is to be remembered that the radiological techniques of Comberg and Sweet[1] depend upon the eye having an axial length of 24 mm. If a foreign body is lying close to the optic disc in a high myope with an axial length of 30 mm. radiological localization would erroneously place the object outside the globe. Conversely extra-ocular foreign bodies in cases of high hypermetropia could be interpreted as being intra-ocular. In such cases the accurate measurement of the axial length of the globe by ultrasonography will enable the appropriate correction to be made to the radiological localization and, furthermore, when extra-ocular the foreign body would return an echo peak clearly beyond the scleral echo (Havener and Gloeckner, 1969).

Figs. 576 and 577.—Ultrasonographic Diagnosis of Foreign Bodies (N. R. Bronson).

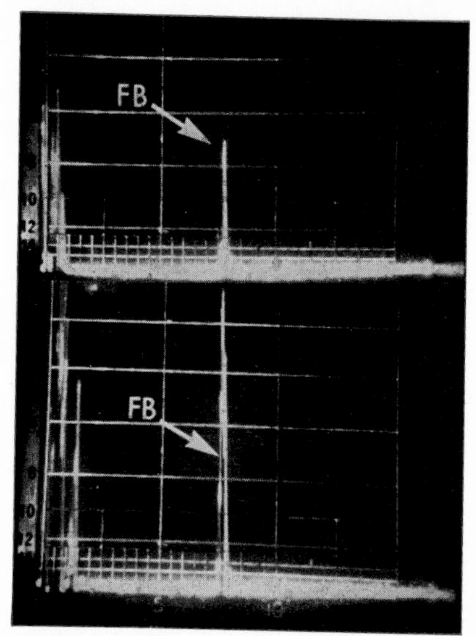

Fig. 576.—Showing foreign-body echo without vitreous reaction: low (top) and high (bottom) sensitivity.

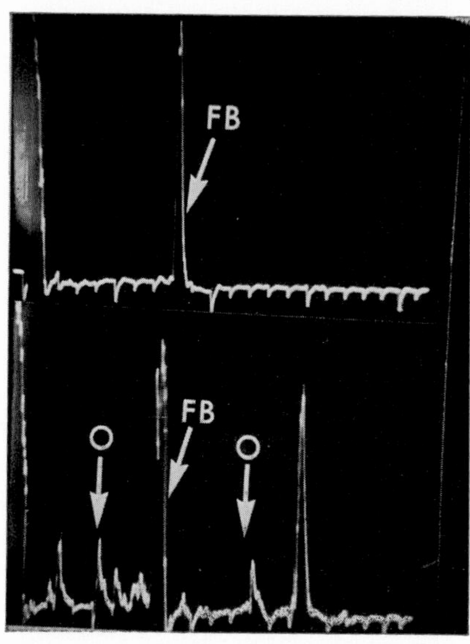

Fig. 577.—Showing the foreign body at low sensitivity (50 db.) (top); at higher sensitivity (75 db.) (bottom) extensive vitreous organization is shown (O).

These techniques may also reveal a non-radio-opaque foreign body (wood, plastic, etc.) and may help to decide whether it is in contact with the wall of the globe or is lying free in the vitreous (Ossoinig and Seher, 1969). When combined with the use of an electro-magnet, ultrasonic techniques may be helpful in determining whether or not a foreign body is magnetic (Penner and Passmore, 1966; Cowden and Runyan, 1969) and may be particularly helpful in the management of non-magnetic intra-ocular foreign bodies using ultrasonically guided forceps (Bronson, 1968). Nevertheless, at present this technique has considerable limitations, its most useful application being probably in the assessment of the damage caused by a foreign body, particu-

[1] pp. 582, 595.

larly where the presence of a cataract or intra-ocular hæmorrhage prevents inspection of the interior of the globe. In this way vitreous hæmorrhage or organization and a retinal detachment may be detected (Bronson, 1969) (Figs. 576–577).

METHODS FOR DETERMINING THE NATURE OF A FOREIGN BODY BY CHEMICAL ANALYSIS. Such methods have received little attention and are difficult to exploit. It is occasionally possible, however, to determine the nature of a foreign body by this means provided it goes into solution in the intra-ocular fluids. Tichomirov (1950), for example, showed that 8 to 10 days after the entrance of copper into the eyes of rabbits chemical analysis of the aqueous obtained by puncture of the anterior chamber gave a positive reaction to the metal provided the particle was not encapsulated. Aluminium, magnesium and lead can be detected in this way (Leydhecker, 1940; Schlichting, 1943). SPECTROSCOPY provides a second method of approach. By fitting a spectroscope to one ocular of the microscope of the slit-lamp an indication of the presence of a foreign body which dissolves into the tissues of the cornea or the aqueous may be given (Koeppe, 1922).

In multiple injuries such as are incurred in explosions, a *diagnosis by analogy* may be made from other foreign bodies which are readily accessible, as, for example, in the skin of the face around the orbit. Although it is probable in many cases that the different particles, whether intra- or extra-ocular, will be of the same type, it must be remembered that this does not necessarily follow.

Ahlbom. *Acta radiol.*, **12**, 212 (1931).
Altschul. *Fortschr. Geb. Roentgenol.*, **29**, 441 (1922).
Klin. Mbl. Augenheilk., **82**, 526 (1929); **84**, 838 (1930).
Alvis. *Sth. med. J.*, **39**, 125 (1946).
Argañaraz. *Sem. Med. B. Aires*, **29**, 627 (1922).
Arnold. *Klin. Mbl. Augenheilk.*, **75**, 241 (1925).
Arruga. *Arch. Soc. oftal. hisp.-amer.*, **1**, 282 (1942).
Asmus. *v. Graefes Arch. Ophthal.*, **40** (1), 280 (1894).
Arch. Augenheilk., **29**, 126 (1894); **31**, 49; Beil., 1 (1895).
Das Sideroscop u. seine Anwendung, Wiesbaden (1898).
Z. Augenheilk., **1**, 178 (1899); **3**, 328 (1900); **5**, 289 (1901); **7**, 393 (1902).
Klin. Mbl. Augenheilk., **39**, 423 (1901); **40** (1), 227 (1902); **46** (1), 262 (1908); **48** (1), 444 (1910).
Aveling. *Lancet*, **1**, 149 (1851).
Bane. *Ann. Ophthal.*, **24**, 407 (1915).
Bangerter. *Ophthalmologica*, **101**, 139 (1941).
Bär. Rieder and Rosenthal's *Lehrbuch d. Röntgenkunde* (1918).
Baum and Greenwood. *Arch. Ophthal.*, **60**, 263 (1958).
Béclère and Morax. *Rev. gén. Ophtal.*, **26**, 478 (1907).
Belot and Fraudet. *C.R. Acad. Sci.* (Paris), **165**, 1117 (1917).
J. Radiol. (Paris), **2**, 433, 563 (1917).
Berg. *v. Graefes Arch. Ophthal.*, **127**, 606 (1931).
Black and Haessler. *J. Amer. med. Ass.*, **93**, 1043 (1929).
Bromley and Lyle. *Trans. ophthal. Soc. U.K.*, **63**, 164 (1943).
Bronson. *Amer. J. Ophthal.*, **58**, 133 (1964); **60**, 596 (1965); **66**, 279 (1968).
Int. Ophthal. Clin., **8**, 199 (1968); **9**, 685 (1969).
Arch. Ophthal., **81**, 460 (1969).
Callahan. *J. Amer. med. Ass.*, **142**, 249 (1950).
Casanovas. *Arch. Soc. oftal. hisp.-amer.*, **5**, 327 (1945).
Clark. *Trans. Amer. ophthal. Soc.*, **7**, 711 (1896).
Clarke and Davidson. *Trans. ophthal. Soc. U.K.*, **18**, 216 (1898).
Coleman, Konig and Katz. *Amer. J. Ophthal.*, **68**, 256 (1969).
Comberg. *v. Graefes Arch. Ophthal.*, **118**, 175 (1927); **124**, 665 (1930).
Münch. med. Wschr., **80**, 1783 (1933).
Cowden and Runyan. *Arch. Ophthal.*, **82**, 299 (1969).
Cridland. *Proc. roy. Soc. Med.*, **60**, 598 (1967).
Int. Ophthal. Clin., **8**, 181 (1968).
Dariex. *Recueil Ophtal.*, **18**, 220 (1896).
Davidson, Mackenzie. *Brit. med. J.*, **1**, 10 (1898).
Trans. ophthal. Soc. U.K., **19**, 144, 271 (1899).
Localisation by X-Rays and Stereoscopy, London (1916).
Davidson and Collins. *Trans. ophthal. Soc. U.K.*, **18**, 200 (1898).

Dixon, G. S. *Arch. Ophthal.*, **34,** 267 (1905).
N.Y. Eye, Ear Infirm. Rep., **12,** 12(1906).
Dixon, J. M. *Amer. J. Ophthal.*, **42,** 301 (1956).
Dor. *Clin. Ophtal.*, **21,** 707 (1917).
Dufour. *Ophthalmologica*, **111,** 310 (1946).
Duszynski. *Trans. Amer. Acad. Ophthal.*, **55,** 110 (1950).
van Duyse. *Arch. Ophtal.*, **16,** 101 (1896).
Engelbrecht. *v. Graefes Arch. Ophthal.*, **94,** 329 (1917).
Klin. Mbl. Augenheilk., **58,** 181, 548 (1917); **60,** 751 (1918).
Farberov and Medvedev. *J. Radiol.* (Paris), **19,** 97 (1935).
Farmer and Osborn. *Lancet*, **2,** 517 (1941).
Fleischer. *Münch. med. Wschr.*, **63,** 504 (1916).
Ber. dtsch. ophthal. Ges., **41,** 186 (1918).
Flood. *Brit. J. Radiol.*, **19,** 318 (1946).
Foveau de Courmelles. *Recueil Ophtal.*, **21,** 5, 77 (1899).
Fox. *Phila. med. J.*, **9,** 213 (1902).
Franceschetti. *Bull. Soc. franç. Ophtal.*, **47,** 230 (1934).
Fridenberg. *Med. Rec.* (N.Y.), **51,** 694 (1897).
Friedman. *Arch. Ophthal.*, **38,** 660 (1947).
Fröhlich. *Klin. Mbl. Augenheilk.*, **20,** 105 (1882).
Fromaget. *Arch. Ophtal.*, **35,** 146 (1918).
Gallemaerts. *Clinique* (Brux.), **4,** 745 (1890).
Bull. Soc. franç. Ophtal., **12,** 143 (1894).
Gallemaerts and Henrard. *Bull. Acad. roy. Med. Belg.*, **28,** 478 (1914).
Gallois, J. and M. *Bull. Soc. Ophtal. Paris*, 269 (1947).
Gasteiger and Grauer. *Fortschr. Geb. Roentgenol.*, **40,** 272 (1929).
Geisler. *Klin. Mbl. Augenheilk.*, **84,** 87 (1930).
Gillan. *Brit. J. Ophthal.*, **25,** 117 (1941).
Gitter, Meyer and Sarin. *Ophthalmic Ultrasound*, St. Louis, 237 (1969).
Gocht. *Lehrbruch. d. Röntgenuntersuchungen*, Stuttgart (1898).
Goldberg and Sarin. *Ultrasonics in Ophthalmology*, Phila. (1967).
Goldmann. *Schweiz. med. Wschr.*, **18,** 497 (1938).
Goldmann and Bangerter. *Ophthalmologica*, **101,** 215 (1941).
von Graefe. *v. Graefes Arch. Ophthal.*, **9** (2), 79 (1863).
Granström. *Acta ophthal* (Kbh.), **27,** 47 (1949).
Granström and Lindblom. *Nord. Med.*, **27,** 1982 (1945).
Griffin, Gianturco and Goldberg. *Radiology*, **40,** 371 (1943).
Grossmann. *IX int. Cong. Ophthal.*, Utrecht, 123 (1899).
Grudzinski. *Klin. oczna*, **7,** 1 (1929).
Guy. *Arch. Ophthal.*, **36,** 540 (1946).
Habig. *Bull. Soc. belge Ophtal.*, No. 93, 358 (1949).
Haik. *J. Amer. med. Ass.*, **135,** 894 (1947).
Hamard and Campinchi. *Arch. Ophtal.*, **25,** 445 (1965).
Harris and Brockhurst. *Canad. med. Ass. J.*, **87,** 565 (1962).
Hartmann. *La radiographie en ophtalmologie*, Paris (1936).
Hartmann and Gilles. *Roentgenologic Diagnosis in Ophthalmology*, Phila., 128 (1959).
Hasselwander. *Münch. med. Wschr.*, **62,** 1515 (1915); **63,** 761 (1916); **64,** 696, 732 (1917).
Hata. *Acta Soc. ophthal. jap.*, **37,** 1166 (1933).
Havener and Gloeckner. *Atlas of Diagnostic Technics and Treatment of Intraocular Foreign Bodies*, St. Louis (1969).
Hellgren. *Ueber d. Bestimmung d. Lage v. Eisensplittern im Auge* (Diss.), Stockholm (1901).
Hertel. *v. Graefes Arch. Ophthal.*, **60,** 127 (1905).
Münch. med. Wschr., **63,** 577 (1916).
Ber. dtsch. ophthal. Ges., **40,** 117 (1916).
Hertzell. *Berl. klin. Wschr.*, **45,** 1149, 2097 (1908).
Heuser. *Arch. Oftal. B. Aires*, **2,** 749 (1927).
Hirschberg. *Zbl. prakt. Augenheilk.*, **23,** 245 (1899).
Hoffmann. *Klin. Mbl. Augenheilk.*, **112,** 156 (1947).
Holm. *Ueber d. Bestimmung d. Lage v. Fremdkörpern im Auge* (Diss.), Uppsala (1912).
Holth. *Hospitalstidende*, **46** (2), 774 (1903).
Ann. Oculist. (Paris), **134,** 401 (1905).
Ophthalmoscope, **9,** 550 (1911).
Holzknecht. *Arch. Augenheilk.*, **81,** Erg., 104 (1916).
Howard and Gaasterland. *Amer. J. Ophthal.*, **66,** 264 (1968).
Hughes. *Amer. J. Ophthal.*, **41,** 488 (1956).
Year Book Ophthal., 358 (1969).
Hulen. *J. Amer. med. Ass.*, **42,** 881 (1904).
Hüttemann. *Klin. Mbl. Augenheilk.*, **51,** 479 (1913).
Jansson. *Mitt. a. d. Augenklin. d. Karolinska Med.-Chir. Inst. Stockholm*, **4,** 95 (1902).
Jervey. *Sth. med. J.*, **23,** 89 (1930).
Jung. *Klin. Mbl. Augenheilk.*, **68,** 385 (1922).
Kerkenezov. *Brit. J. Ophthal.*, **48,** 169 (1964).
Knapp. *Arch. Ophthal.*, **9,** 207 (1880).
Arch. Augenheilk., **10,** 1 (1881).
Koeppe. *v. Graefes Arch. Ophthal.*, **98,** 171 (1919); **101,** 48; **102,** 4, 259 (1920).
Die ultra- u. polarisationsmikroskopische Erforschung d. lebenden Auges u. ihre Ergebnisse, Berne (1921).
Die Mikroskopie d. lebenden Auges, Berlin, **1** (1920); **2** (1922).
Köhler. *Fortschr. Geb. Roentgenol.*, **6,** 190 (1903).
Berl. klin. Wschr., **41,** 903 (1904).
Münch. med. Wschr., **65,** 399 (1918).
Kraus and Briggs. *Brit. J. Ophthal.*, **29,** 557 (1945).
Lans. *Ned. T. Geneesk.*, **2,** 174 (1902).

Larsson. *Acta ophthal.* (Kbh.), **19,** 1 (1941); **26,** 574 (1948).
Lautsch. *v. Graefes Arch. Ophthal.*, **144,** 213 (1942).
Lebekhov. *Vestn. oftal.*, **79,** 36 (1966).
Leber. *Ber. dtsch. ophthal. Ges.*, **30,** 319 (1902).
Lehmann and Cowl. *Zbl. prakt. Augenheilk.*, **26,** 290 (1902).
Lembeck. *Klin. Mbl. Augenheilk.*, **80,** 767 (1928).
Leopold. *Ann. Oculist.* (Paris), **192,** 863 (1959).
Lewis. *Amer. J. Roentgenol.*, **27,** 853 (1932).
Lewkowitsch. *Lancet*, **2,** 452 (1896).
Leydhecker. *Klin. Mbl. Augenheilk.*, **104,** 302 (1940); **111,** 181, 239; **112,** 255 (1947).
v. Graefes Arch. Ophthal., **141,** 665 (1940).
Lindblom. *Acta radiol.*, **15,** 615 (1934).
Acta ophthal. (Kbh.), **26,** 439, 441, 568 (1948).
McAlester. *Amer. J. Ophthal.*, **21,** 1380 (1938).
McGrigor. *Arch. Radiol. Electrotherap.*, **23,** 188 (1918).
Brit. J. Radiol., **2,** 136 (1929); **12,** 619 (1939).
McGrigor and Samuel. *Brit. J. Radiol.*, **18,** 284 (1945).
McGuire and Raffetto. *U.S. naval med. Bull.*, **43,** 1239 (1944).
McKeown. *Dubl. J. med. Sci.*, **62,** 201 (1876).
Marucci. *G. ital. Oftal.*, **1,** 36 (1948).
Melanowski. *Klin. oczna*, **7,** 16 (1929).
Klin. Mbl. Augenheilk., **83,** 404 (1929).
Menacho. *Arch. Soc. oftal. hisp.-amer.*, **5,** 297, 326, 377, 481 (1905).
Minsky. *Arch. Ophthal.*, **31,** 207 (1944).
Mintz and Mattes. *Radiology*, **75,** 612 (1960).
Moorhead. *J. Amer. med. Ass.*, **121,** 123 (1943).
Amer. J. Surg., **69,** 306 (1945).
Moreu. *Manual d. gonoscopia*, Madrid (1943).
Moskowitz. *Arch. Ophtal.*, **50,** 319 (1953).
Müller. *Münch. med. Wschr.*, **56,** 1645 (1909).
Mundt and Hughes. *Amer. J. Ophthal.*, **41,** 488 (1956).
Murray. *J. Fac. Radiol.*, **4,** 138 (1952).
Nakabayashi, Kawaguchi and Aikawa. *Folia ophthal. jap.*, **18,** 759 (1967).
Neubauer. *Ophthalmologica*, **150,** 441 (1965).
Int. Ophthal. Clin., **8,** 205 (1968).
Nover and Stallkamp. *Ber. dtsch. ophthal. Ges.*, **63,** 251 (1961).
v. Graefes Arch. Ophthal., **164,** 517 (1962).
Ohnishi. See Hirose. *Acta Soc. ophthal. jap.*, **36,** 1271 (1932).
Oksala. *Acta ophthal.* (Kbh.), **45,** 489 (1967).
Oksala and Lehtinen. *Brit. J. Ophthal.*, **43,** 744 (1959).
Ossoinig. *Ber. dtsch. ophthal. Ges.*, **67,** 288 (1966).
Ossoinig and Seher. *Ophthalmic Ultrasound* (ed. Gitter *et al.*), St. Louis, 311 (1969).
Pagenstecher. *Arch. Augenheilk.*, **10,** 234 (1881).
Perkins. *Bull. U.S. Army med. Dept.*, **5,** 215 (1946).
Penner and Passmore. *Arch. Ophthal.*, **76,** 676 (1966).
Peter and Rosen. *Amer. J. Ophthal.*, **28,** 1140 (1945).
Pfeiffer. *Amer. J. Roentgenol.*, **44,** 558 (1940).
Arch. Ophthal., **32,** 261 (1944).
Pooley. *Arch. Ophthal.*, **9,** 255 (1880).
Arch. Augenheilk., **10,** 9, 315 (1881).
Porcher and Gilles. *Ann. Oculist.* (Paris), **178,** 345 (1945).
Puglisi-Durante. *Atti Cong. Soc. oftal. ital.*, **36,** 556 (1947).
Purnell. *Ultrasonics in Ophthalmology* (ed. Goldberg and Sarin), Phila., 102 (1967).
Purnell and Sokollu. *Amer. J. Ophthal.*, **54,** 1103 (1962).
Ramsay, Maitland. *Eye Injuries and their Treatment*, Glasgow (1907).
Reis. *Brit. J. Ophthal.*, **30,** 462 (1946).
Riebel. *Klin. Mbl. Augenheilk.*, **148,** 134 (1966).
Riise. *Acta ophthal.* (Kbh.), **44,** 80 (1966).
Roberts. *Amer. J. Roentgenol.*, **66,** 44 (1951).
Roper-Hall. *Trans. ophthal. Soc. U.K.*, **77,** 239 (1957).
Int. Ophthal. Clin., **8,** 211 (1968).
Rumbaur. *Klin. Mbl. Augenheilk.*, **63,** 196 (1919).
Runyan and Penner. *Arch. Ophthal.*, **81,** 512 (1969).
Sachs. *Münch. med. Wschr.*, **50,** 741 (1903).
Sander. *Klin. Mbl. Augenheilk.*, **146,** 728 (1965).
Sandera. *Röntgenpraxis*, **2,** 175 (1930).
Sanna and Quilici. *Ann. Ottal.*, **89,** 877 (1963).
Scharf. *Klin. Mbl. Augenheilk.*, **107,** 193 (1941).
Scheie and Hodes. *Arch. Ophthal.*, **35,** 13 (1946).
Schlichting. *Klin. Mbl. Augenheilk.*, Beil., 15 (1943).
Scott and Flood. *Brit. J. Radiol.*, **19,** 318 (1946).
Senna. *Arch. Soc. oftal. hisp.-amer.*, **8,** 1097 (1948).
Sheppard and Romejko. *Amer. J. Ophthal.*, **30,** 159 (1947).
Skeoch. *Brit. J. Ophthal.*, **29,** 113 (1945).
Smolnig. *Wien. med. Wschr.*, **98,** 450 (1948).
Somerset. *Indian med. Gaz.*, **82,** 50 (1947).
Spackman. *Amer. J. Ophthal.*, **15,** 1007 (1932).
Spaeth. *J. Amer. med. Ass.*, **120,** 659 (1942).
Speciale-Picciché. *Ann. Ottal.*, **45,** 600 (1927).
Stallard. *Brit. J. Ophthal.*, **28,** 105 (1944).
Eye Surgery, 4th ed., Bristol (1965).
Stankiewicz. *Klin. oczna*, **13,** 278 (1935).
Staunig and von Herrenschwand. *Fortschr. Geb. Roentgenol.*, **36,** 372 (1927).
Stenius. *Nord. Med.*, **36,** 2187 (1947).
Stöckl. *Wien. klin. Wschr.*, **11,** 147 (1898).
Struble and Croll. *Amer. J. Ophthal.*, **29,** 151 (1946).
Stumpf. *Münch. med. Wschr.*, **63,** 1606 (1916).
Sweet. *Ophthal. Rev.*, **16,** 131 (1897).
Amer. J. med. Sci., **116,** 190 (1898).

Arch. Ophthal., **27**, 377 (1898); **38**, 623 (1909).
Ophthal. Rec., **9**, 627 (1900); **11**, 388 (1902); **14**, 284 (1905); **18**, 437 (1909); **22**, 240 (1913).
Trans. Amer. ophthal. Soc., **9**, 352 (1901); **12**, 320 (1909).
Ophthalmoscope, **4**, 8 (1906).
von Szily. *Atlas der Kriegsaugenheilkunde*, Stuttgart (1918).
Terrien. *Arch. Ophtal.*, **42**, 74 (1925).
Thorpe. *Arch. Ophthal.*, **32**, 497 (1944).
J. Amer. med. Ass., **137**, 197 (1945).
Acta XVIII int. Cong. Ophthal., Brussels, **2**, 1673 (1960).
Complications in Eye Surgery (ed. Fasanella), 2nd ed., Phila., 45 (1965).
Amer. J. Ophthal., **61**, 1339 (1966).
Tichomirov. *Vestn. oftal.*, **29**, 9 (1950).
Tojo, Tsuji and Yamamoto. *Folia ophthal. jap.*, **18**, 719 (1967).
Trantas. *Arch. Ophthal.*, **27**, 581, 650 (1907).
Folia ophthal. orient., **1**, 61 (1932).
Bull. Soc. hellen. Ophtal., **7**, 166, 207 (1938); **9**, 183, 241 (1940).
Trendelenburg. *Dtsch. med. Wschr.*, **42**, 57 (1916).
Troncoso. *A Treatise on Gonioscopy*, Phila. (1947).
Ustimenko. *Vestn. oftal.*, **78**, 68 (1965).
Vannini. *Rass. ital. Ottal.*, **22**, 125 (1953).
Velter. *Bull. Soc. Ophtal. Paris*, 155 (1919).
Verwey. *Amer. J. Ophthal.*, **7**, 337 (1924).
Vodovosov, Kulikov and Shevyakov. *Vestn. oftal.*, **79**, 23 (1966).
Vogt. *Schweiz. med. Wschr.*, **51** (2), 145 (1921); **54**, 982 (1923).
Vüllers. *Klin. Mbl. Augenheilk.*, **45** (2), 101 (1907).
Wainstock. *Int. Ophthal. Clin.*, **9**, 752 (1969).
Walter. *Amer. J. Ophthal.*, **53**, 494 (1962).
Weeks. *Ophthal. Rec.*, **14**, 253 (1905).
Trans. Amer. ophthal. Soc., **10**, 476 (1905).
Weigelin. *Klin. Mbl. Augenheilk.*, **59**, 84 (1917).
Weiss. *Zbl. prakt. Augenheilk.*, **30**, 100 (1906).
Wessely. *Z. Augenheilk.*, **24**, 464 (1910).
Arch. Augenheilk., **69**, 161 (1911).
Weve. *Arch. Augenheilk.*, **80**, 259 (1916); **110**, 646 (1937).
Widmark. *Brit. med. J.*, **2**, 1433 (1902).
v. Graefes Arch. Ophthal., **118**, 175 (1927); **124**, 665 (1930).
Williams. *Trans. Amer. ophthal. Soc.*, **7**, 708 (1896).
Boston med. surg. J., **135**, 163 (1896).
Witmer. *Ophthalmologica*, **117**, 277 (1949).
Yamazagi, Kanai and Kimura. *Jap. J. clin. Ophthal.*, **20**, 655 (1966).
Yazujian. *Arch. Ophthal.*, **24**, 975 (1940).
Zwanger, Gilroy and Jones. *Amer. J. Ophthal.*, **35**, 1349 (1952).

The Treatment of Intra-ocular Foreign Bodies

Since the majority of intra-ocular foreign bodies are metallic and most are of iron and therefore magnetizable, the magnet occupies pride of place in their removal. For this reason we are introducing this Section with the photograph of JULIUS HIRSCHBERG [1843–1925] (Fig. 578), one of von Graefe's assistants and Professor of Ophthalmology in Berlin from 1879 to 1900, since he revolutionized the practice of the treatment of intra-ocular foreign bodies by being the first to apply the electro-magnet to their extraction (1879), subsequently writing two classical monographs on magnet-operations in ophthalmology (1885, 1899). Apart from this the many-sidedness of his scholarship was outstanding. A man of quite unusual industry, he wrote during his professional life some 106 papers on all aspects of ophthalmology—on physiology, optics, medicine, hygiene and particularly surgery—and in addition he founded and edited the *Centralblatt für praktische Augenheilkunde* (1887–1919). The range of his interests was remarkable; his book on the mathematical basis of medical statistics (1874) is an example of their catholicity; but his greatest joy was perhaps his profound knowledge of and sympathy with classical and Arabic scholarship. His highest claim to fame will rest upon his labours as the unique ophthalmological historian, for in the eight volumes of his *Geschichte der Augenheilkunde* (1899–1918), to devote himself to which he ceased the practice of ophthalmology in 1907, he traced with painstaking care and extreme accuracy the history of our specialty from its earliest beginnings in the pre-Christian era, through its development in every civilized country in the world, to contemporary times. No other branch of medicine has had a disciple so earnest or been presented with a gift so great.

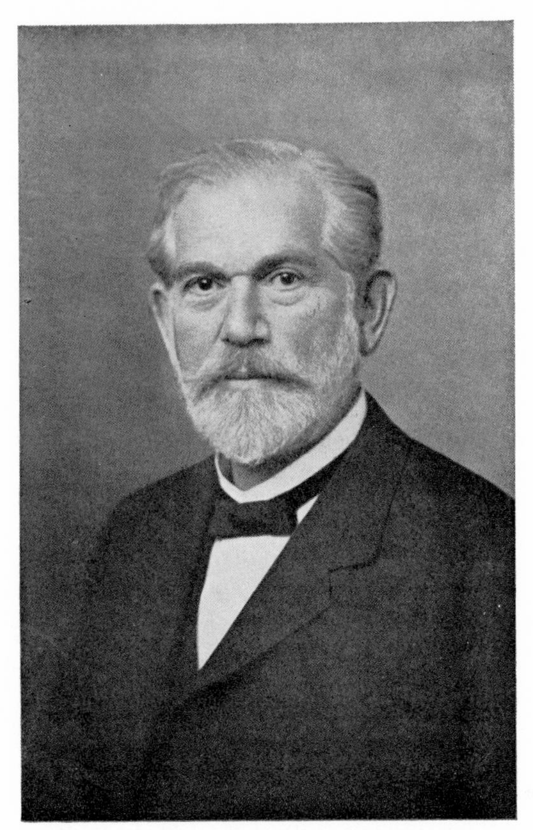

Fig. 578.—Julius Hirschberg.
[1843–1925]

The appropriate treatment of a retained intra-ocular foreign body must obviously involve in the first place all the problems of a perforating wound of the globe—the management of the incarceration of uveal tissue in the wound, the appropriate methods of dealing with trauma to the intra-ocular tissues, particularly the lens, and prophylactic measures for the prevention of infection or its treatment if it has developed—all these have already been discussed in a previous section, as well as the control of post-traumatic and post-operative inflammation by the topical exhibition of corticosteroids. It is well, however, to treat all such cases in their early stages as potentially infected, giving them prophylactic antibacterial therapy (as by sulphonamides or antibiotics) which should be continued at least five days; the possibility of the development of tetanus should not be overlooked when the foreign body may possibly have been infected with this organism.[1] In the present context we shall confine our attention to the problems—many of them considerable and fraught with anxiety—which depend on the presence of the foreign body itself: whether the eye should be removed, whether the foreign body should be left alone or extracted and, if it should be extracted, how this can best be accomplished.

The question of the immediate removal of the eye, which obviously arises in the most severe type of injury, should be judged on the merits of the case as if the condition were a perforating wound uncomplicated by the retention of a foreign body: we have already seen that the presence of the latter makes little significant difference to the incidence of sympathetic inflammation, so that any decision regarding enucleation depends on the actual damage done by the foreign body on entering and traversing the eye and the probable damage which must be anticipated in effecting its removal. If the last problem is difficult to assess, the extraction of the foreign body can, of course, always be attempted provided the injury is recent (within 10 days) in the knowledge that within this period the danger of sympathetic inflammation is slight and the eye can be safely excised either at the time of attempted removal or shortly thereafter if its retention seems useless or potentially dangerous.

The decision as to whether a foreign body should be left *in situ* depends essentially on two factors—the ultimate damage to be anticipated if it is left within the globe, and the immediate damage which its removal will presumably entail. Although the management of such cases rests on the application of certain general principles, the conduct of each case presents a separate and individual problem. As a general rule there is no doubt that *the counsel of perfection is to remove every intra-ocular foreign body*, for we have seen that even in the case of substances which usually lie inert within the globe, complications may arise many years after their entry. Whether removal is practicable—or wise—is another matter, for *if any unusual difficulty is likely to be encountered thereby, a foreign body known to be inert is usually*

[1] p. 408.

better left alone. The assessment of the relative risk involved in a policy of inactivity or in subjecting the eye to the trauma of operative removal must rest on the judgment of the surgeon. On the other hand, if the foreign body is such that its continued presence is likely to give rise to degenerative, inflammatory or proliferative changes, every endeavour should be made to remove it in the knowledge that its continued presence may ultimately lead to the loss of a useful eye. This applies especially to the most common foreign bodies met with both in civil and military life, particularly those with a high content of iron and copper.

The site of the foreign body must be a deciding factor. A relatively accessible foreign body in the anterior chamber offers few problems compared with a particle lying in the posterior segment, while a foreign body lying in a relatively clear lens, even if it is known to be irritant in the vascularized tissues of the eye, may remain indefinitely in this situation without ill-effects. The *magnetizability* of the particle is also an important factor, for a ferro-magnetic foreign body can always be drawn out more readily and with less trauma than one which requires the introduction of instruments into the globe for its removal by direct manipulation. Indeed, although modern methods of surgical technique have evolved beyond the stage when, half a century ago, the routine procedure was excision of the eye if a non-magnetic foreign body lay in the posterior segment, the problems presented by such an occurrence are still sufficiently formidable to give pause to the most experienced surgeon.

In all cases, however, the *optimum time for the removal* of an intra-ocular foreign body is of importance. There is no doubt that the best advice is *to make haste but to make haste slowly.* Such cases should be looked upon as emergencies, for many eyes may be saved by prompt and appropriate methods of treatment. In all cases, removal should be attempted before the particle becomes encapsulated by fibrous tissue but, at the same time, it is to be remembered that this is a matter of days rather than hours. There is thus no immediate hurry, for premature and blind attempts at removal merely cause unnecessary trauma and will prejudice the ultimate degree of vision. Competent removal requires accurate localization, and this takes time. The vision of the eye is more likely to be saved if the case is carefully studied, if an effort is made to determine the type of foreign body, if it is accurately localized by X-rays and if the surgical attack is carefully planned and executed, than if treatment is undertaken precipitately and with undue urgency, and attempts at removal are made blindly or by inexpert hands. Pin-point localization is more important than speed of extraction; adequate equipment, considerable experience and good judgment on the part of the operator are necessary if the best results are to be obtained, and if these are not immediately forthcoming the patient can with advantage wait for them or be transported to them with his eyes immobilized by a binocular bandage. The eye may harbour the foreign body without much complaint for a considerable period, but it is intolerant of clumsy interference or repeated operations.

From the practical point of view the surgical removal of foreign bodies can be divided into two categories—the magnetic and the non-magnetic—each differing from the other in their surgical approach, the ease of operative procedures and the ultimate prognosis in terms of vision. In both cases, however, three desiderata are essential in any surgical technique. Every care should be taken to avoid pressure upon the eye; a speculum which rests upon the globe should never be employed, and lid stitches are probably always safer than any kind of speculum. Full anæsthesia either by a general anæsthetic or by regional blockage with an injection of an analgesic into the orbit or Tenon's capsule is important, and full akinesia is essential. The removal of even an apparently accessible foreign body in the anterior chamber may otherwise result in a prolapse of the iris, while if the foreign body lies in the posterior segment of the globe, neglect of these precautions too often results in an unnecessary and sometimes catastrophic loss of vitreous.

The Removal of Magnetic Intra-ocular Foreign Bodies

The Action of Magnets

A short note regarding the practical principles of magnetism will perhaps be of value at this stage. It was known to the ancients that stones consisting of a black oxide of iron (lodestones) possessed the curious property of attracting to themselves small pieces of iron; they were found in quantity in Magnesia in Asia Minor, from which locality the name " magnet " is derived. This property was originally attributed to the activity of a soul inhabiting the lodestone, but modern science professes the more prosaic theory that the attraction is due to the development of a field of force depending ultimately upon the electrical charges of electrons. These charges are, of course, universal, but the properties of a magnet may be assumed to depend upon an orderly molecular arrangement so that the magnetic axis of each constituent particle is orientated in definite (and not random) directions. If a piece of soft iron, wherein the molecules are orientated at random so that the magnetic forces mutually cancel each other out, is brought within the field of a magnet of considerable power, the component molecules are orientated to conform to this field and it itself becomes a magnet by induction. The field was conceived by Faraday as consisting of lines or tubes of force radiating preferentially from two mutually antagonistic poles, so that each pole of the piece of iron is attracted towards the magnetic pole of opposite polarity. If the piece of iron lies nearer one pole of the magnet than the other so that the magnetic field in its vicinity is intense but with the lines of force diverging so that the field becomes rapidly weaker beyond, the attraction on the piece of iron becomes unbalanced and a resultant tractive power is established which pulls the particle end-on towards the pole of the magnet. The movement of the particle therefore depends on the lack of uniformity of the field, and if it is free to move the particle will travel by the shortest possible path to the most highly magnetized part of such a field.

It is important to remember that all elements are influenced in some way and to some extent in a magnetic field, the difference in behaviour varying with the resistance they offer to the flux of magnetic force through their substance since, like all types of energy, magnetic force tends to follow the path of least resistance. In making such comparisons the resistance offered by air (or a vacuum) is generally taken as unity.

Some substances (*ferromagnetics*) offer much less resistance than air to the flux of magnetic force so that their permeability is greater than unity: these are iron, nickel, cobalt and some alloys of manganese. If such bodies are placed in a magnetic field the lines of force therefore crowd into them (Fig. 579); to accommodate as many of these as possible the body itself and its component particles become aligned parallel to the direction of the lines of force, and if the body is mobile, in order to accommodate still more of the flux of energy, it moves towards the densest part of the magnetic field, that is, towards the pole of the magnet.

In addition to these substances there are others in which the permeability is only very little greater than that of air; these (*paramagnetic bodies*) are thus little affected unless the forces involved are intense.

Most substances, however, have permeabilities less than that of air; these are said to be *diamagnetic*. The extent to which bodies exhibit diamagnetism is, however, small, for the permeability of bismuth, the most strongly diamagnetic metal known, is 0·9998, while that of iron may be as high as 2,000. It is obvious that diamagnetic bodies will behave in a manner opposite to that of ferromagnetic bodies when they are introduced into a magnetic field; in view of the fact that air offers less resistance to the magnetic flux, the lines of force will tend to avoid the body and run

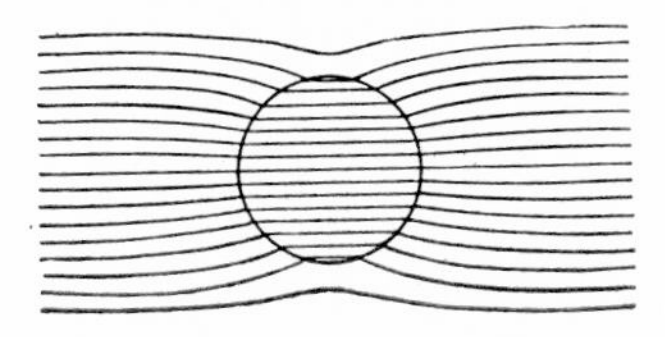

Fig. 579.—The Lines of Force in the Region of a Ferromagnetic Body.

Owing to the decreased resistance offered by the body, the lines of force tend to crowd into it, decreasing their density in the surrounding field.

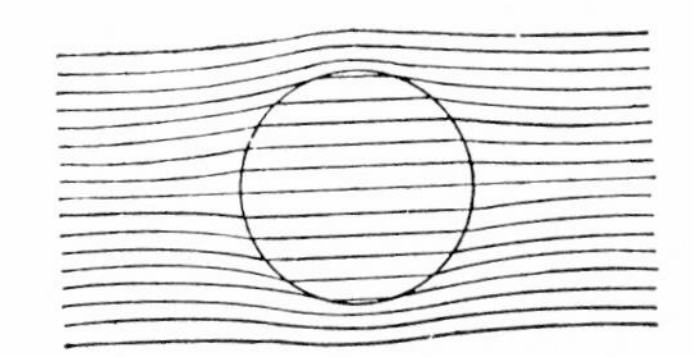

Fig. 580.—The Lines of Force in the Region of a Diamagnetic Body.

Owing to the increased resistance offered by the body, the lines of force tend to crowd the surrounding air, decreasing the density within the body.

preferably through the surrounding air, so that those traversing the body will be fewer than would have been the case were the space occupied by air. It follows that outside the body the lines of force become more closely instead of being more thinly packed (Fig. 580). Moreover, the diamagnetic body will orientate itself to be as far as possible in the weakest part of the magnetic field, and thus sets itself at right angles to the lines of force and, if it is mobile, it will tend to move away from the strongest part of the field, so that a greater number of lines of force may be crowded into the space it used to occupy. Although such bodies are thus repelled by a magnet, they cannot be said to possess a " negative magnetism "; their movement away from the magnet depends on the fact that their susceptibility to magnetism is less than that of air.

We have seen that if a piece of soft iron is introduced into a magnetic field it itself becomes a magnet but it retains this property only for a short time. If, however, hardened steel and particularly high carbon, tungsten or cobalt steels are employed, the acquired molecular arrangement is durable (*permanent magnet*). The force generated by such a magnet is, however, small—less than one-hundredth of a good hand electro-magnet—and when fields of intensity greater than a few hundred gauss[1] are required,

[1] The strength of a magnetic field at a given point is measured in a unit known as a *gauss*. A magnetic field is of unit strength if, when placed 1 cm. in air from an equal and similar pole, it repels it with a force of 1 dyne; if such a unit pole, placed at a given point, is acted upon by a force of 1 dyne, the magnetic field at this point is said to have the strength of 1 gauss. A magnetic field therefore has a strength of x gauss (or x dynes per unit pole).

an ELECTROMAGNET must be used. Such a magnet depends on the fact that an electric current gives rise to a magnetic field in its vicinity, and if a piece of iron (a *core*) is placed within a coil of wire carrying a current (a *solenoid*), the iron necessarily becomes magnetized by induction (Fig. 581).

The magnetic forces available at any one time in such a system depend upon the strength and number of lines of force involved. These depend on:

(1) the power of the magnet;
(2) the distance of the magnet from the body; and
(3) the size and magnetic quality of the body.

1. *The Power of the Magnet.* The strength of a solenoid varies with a number of factors. First, the bulk of the core, which should be cylindrical with a large cross-section—a factor limited by the necessity for manœuvrability in such an instrument. Second, the number of amperes flowing in the current—the higher the voltage the stronger the field. Third, the number of coils of wire around the core, that is, the effective length of the induction current, a factor also limited by bulk. Fourth, the shape of the terminal, which should concentrate the greatest possible number of lines

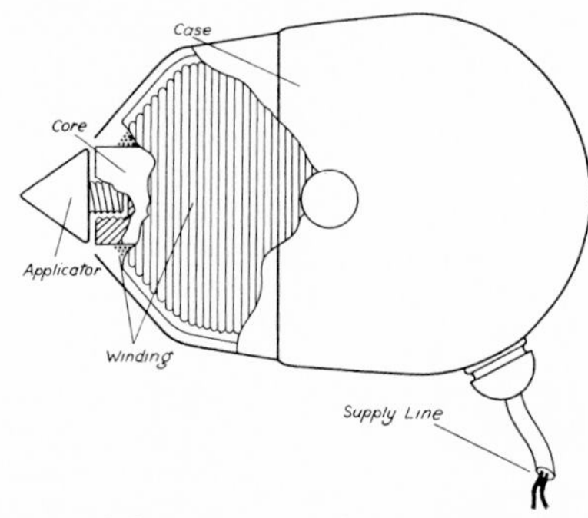

FIG. 581.—A diagram of the structure of the magnet illustrated in Fig. 587.

of force at one point since, as we have seen, the pulling power of a magnet depends not on the strength of the magnetic field but on the difference in intensity between neighbouring portions of the field. The most powerful terminal is short, blunt and cone-shaped, the maximum field being obtained with a semi-angle of the cone of 54° 44′. Such a terminal is almost as broad as it is long and the magnetic field is greatest at its point; with long, thin or curved terminals much of the power is wasted, since the lines of force leak out from its sides and never reach the foreign body (Fig. 582). The force thus generated, however, is not infinite even if bulk were no disadvantage, for it is limited to several thousand gauss by the saturation intensity of the core of the magnet, which is reached when all its constituent molecules are uniformly orientated. In practice, also, the amount of force generated is limited by the factor of overheating, which destroys magnetic properties by disturbing orderly molecular arrangement; iron, for example, loses its ferromagnetic properties at 760° C, and it is to be remembered that the quantity of heat generated in a coil increases as the square of the number of amperes of current. Below the saturation point of the iron core the intensity of the field therefore varies with the number of amperes flowing in the current × the number of coils of wire around the core, a limitation being placed by the ability of the magnet to dissipate heat. The practical plan is to increase the current and the power to the limit and avoid heating by using repeated short-time exposures of a minute or two, since heat takes time to generate.

2. *The Distance of the Foreign Body.* It is obvious from Fig. 584 that the further away the foreign body is from the magnet the fewer of the diverging lines of force will be available to pass through it. In general it may be said that magnetic force varies approximately with the cube of the distance of the particle to be attracted. Thus if the power involved 1 cm. from the pole is 1 dyne, at 2 cm. distance it will be $\frac{1}{8}$ dyne, and at 0·5 mm. it will be 8,000 dynes. It is apparent that when distances less than 1 mm. are involved the power increases enormously up to the point of contact so that, while powerful magnets are necessary to exert traction from a distance, a relatively weak instrument is sufficiently effective at close range.

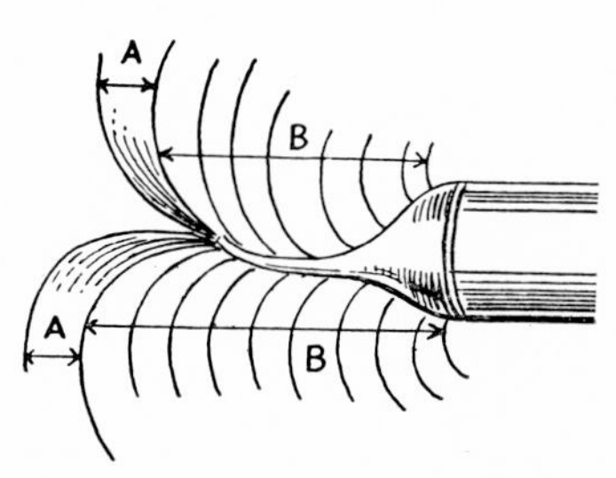

FIG. 582.—TO SHOW THE EFFECT OF THE SHAPE OF THE TERMINAL ON THE POWER OF A MAGNET.

In using the point, the lines of force represented by A are employed; those represented by B are lost (compare with the lines of force passing through C in Fig. 584).

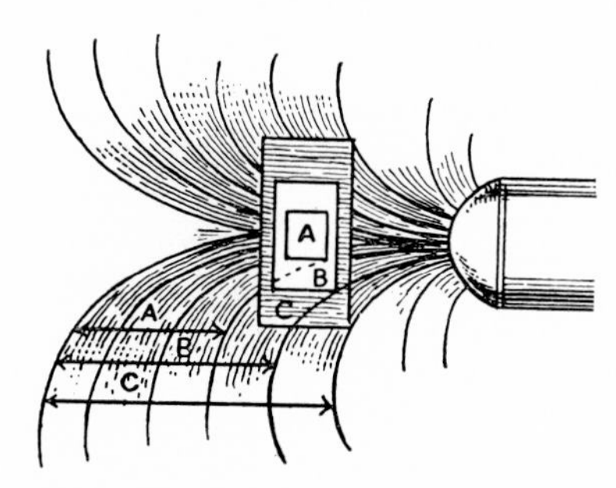

FIG. 583.—TO SHOW THE EFFECT OF SIZE ON THE POWER OF A MAGNET.

The lines of force available to attract bodies of the size of A, B, and C are seen in *A*, *B*, and *C*.

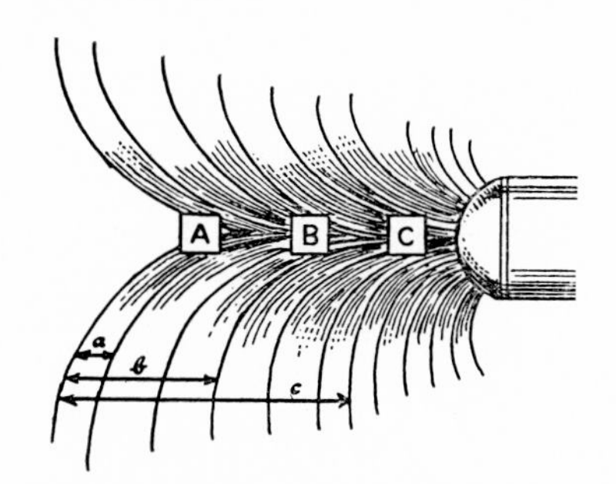

FIG. 584.— TO SHOW THE EFFECT OF DISTANCE ON THE POWER OF A MAGNET

The lines of force involved in the direction of A, B, and C are seen in *a*, *b*, and *c* (J. Kraus and W. A. Briggs).

3. *The degree of attraction experienced by a foreign body* depends on its size and magnetizability. Figure 583 makes it clear that the larger the foreign body the more lines of force pass through it, and therefore the greater is the pull. It is frequently stated that a feebly magnetic body will eventually be attracted if it is exposed in a magnetic field with a sufficient variation of intensity over a sufficient time. Owing to the limiting factor of the generation of heat in the magnet, this would involve in practice repeated intermittent applications of the magnet at a number of sittings. Thus it is a common clinical experience that a feebly magnetic foreign body is attracted to a magnet only after repeated attempts, and instances have been reported when a

particle within the eye, which appeared at first to be non-magnetic, has been eventually extracted after prolonged trials (after 28 applications, Crawford, 1943; after 30, Paderstein, 1925; after 40, Weigelin, 1917; after 75, Wright and Duncan, 1944; after 150 applications, Elkington, 1949). In view of the fact, however, that all magnetic bodies are magnetized practically instantaneously to the fullest extent possible, the delay in extraction in such cases must be due to the gradual liberation of the foreign body from its bed of exudate or organized tissue, repeated attempts being required to rock it loose and tear it away and draw it through the media or the tissues of the eye.

While the field of strength in gauss is helpful, it is only one factor in describing the force of a magnet (Fig. 585). The force or pulling power of a magnet is dependent upon the field-strength (gauss) and the gradient of the strength of the field. It therefore

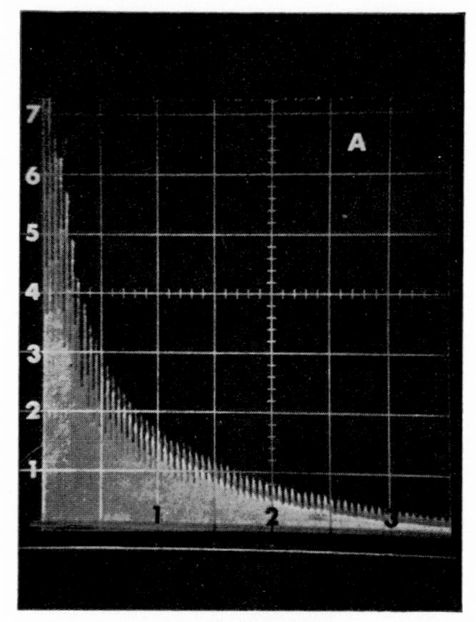

Fig. 585.—The Pulling Force of a Magnet.

An oscilloscope tracing of the strength of the field in gauss as the magnetic field sensor is moved away from the tip of the pole. The relative pulling force of the magnet is the product of the strength of the field in gauss times the slope of the curve (N. R. Bronson).

follows that a magnet must, in addition to an adequate field-strength in gauss, have a relatively sharp gradient of the field-strength in the range of its action. The magnetic field serves to magnetize the foreign body which is in the eye, while a rapidly increasing field, a gradient as the foreign body approaches the magnet, serves to pull the object towards its tip. A foreign body located in a uniform field of 2,000 gauss would not be attracted to the tip of the pole whereas a similar foreign body in a field of 200 gauss would tend to move towards an area 1 mm. away where the field-strength was 400 gauss (McCaslin, 1958). Equipment is now available which allows the magnetic field to be plotted at all points and the force to be calculated. An effective eye magnet should have a steep field-gradient in the range of its use which for practical purposes is up to 2 cm. To obtain the full measure of force from a magnet it is thus vital that the magnet be as close to the foreign body as possible. The shortest pole-tip consistent with the working distance to the foreign body should be used; a pole-tip longer than 12 mm. is not necessary and merely results in wasted power. While a magnet is in use there is a gradual build up of heat in the coil-windings and this reduces the effective magnetic field by increasing the resistance of the wire; a magnet has a much greater pulling power when it is cold and therefore short pulses are more effective than lengthy indiscriminate use (Bronson, 1968).

We have already seen that diamagnetic foreign bodies can theoretically be repelled by a magnet if an alternating field of sufficient strength is generated, since the resultant force induced opposes the main magnetic force developed by the coil. It follows that if the magnet were placed behind the head such a foreign body should be pushed out of the eye (Endt and ten Doesschaete, 1949); even if sufficient force could be developed without damaging the eye with the high temperatures which the necessarily very powerful currents would generate, the lack of directional accuracy would result in considerable damage. Thiel (1947) pointed out that by placing a metal ring in front of the eye an attraction could be generated between the ring and a diamagnetic foreign body by the eddy-currents developed between them. Such a ring could be used to drag the foreign body in any direction, but the extremely high magnetic forces necessary for such a manœuvre are not clinically available.

In ophthalmic surgery two types of magnet are employed—the hand magnet and the giant magnet—and either can be fitted with a variety of terminals, some short and conical, others long and attenuated, either straight or curved, all of which are sterilizable. The two types of magnet should not be considered as interchangeable, for both are designed to play entirely different roles in traumatic surgery. The *hand magnet*, because of its size, is of relatively low power and is generally applicable only when the foreign body is within a millimetre of its tip or can come into contact with its terminal. To counterbalance this defect it should be sufficiently light to allow fine adjustment and ease of manipulation when held by the surgeon, and its weight should not be such as to cause fatigue or tremor of the hands lest further operating become impaired. The tendency has been to make such instruments progressively larger in order to attain a greater degree of power and thus extend the range of their utility, but this defeats their main purpose; a hand magnet is essentially a contact instrument which is rarely effective over a distance of more than 1 or 2 mm. and depends on its lightness for its usefulness; if greater power is required it should be obtained from the giant magnet.

The *giant magnet*, on the other hand, is a large and powerful instrument with a wide and diffuse field, the direction of which can be varied at will. In practice it is used to draw a distant foreign body towards a site whence, if necessary, the more readily manipulated hand magnet can be used to complete the extraction at close range. In ophthalmology the working criteria laid down by Lancaster (1915–38) are valid: unless a giant magnet can pull a small steel ball 1 mm. in diameter with a force of over 50 times its weight at a distance of 20 mm., and unless a hand magnet will pull such a ball in contact with its tip with a force over 5,000 times its weight, they are not ophthalmologically effective. Although this is an excellent test of the force of a magnet, it does not define the characteristics of a magnet throughout its

FIGS. 586 to 588.—HAND MAGNETS.

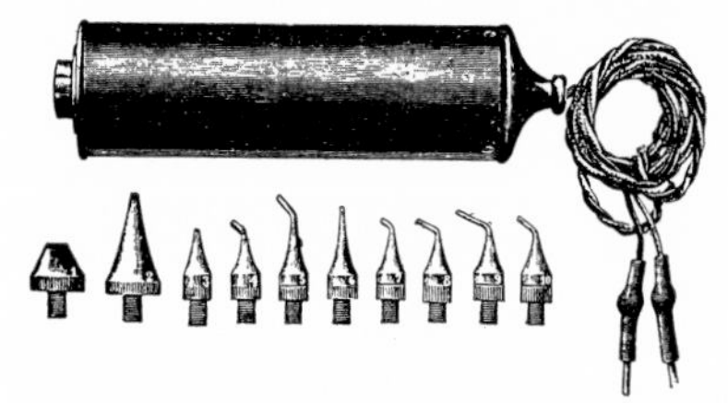

FIG. 586.—Hirschberg's original hand magnet with various terminals.

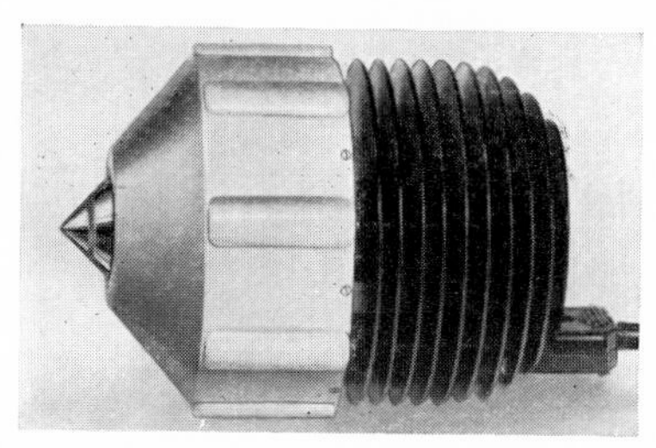

FIG. 587.—A HEAVY ALL-PURPOSE PORTABLE HAND MAGNET.

Although heavy, the magnet can be manipulated by hand and, at the same time is capable of acting in most cases as a giant magnet. For construction, see Fig. 581 (Hamblin).

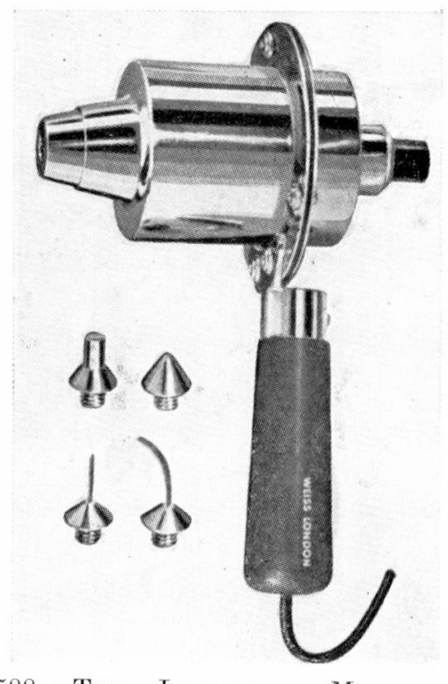

FIG. 588.—THE LIVINGSTONE-MANSFIELD HAND MAGNET.

A magnet of this type can be very powerful with a suitable current. It is less effective but lighter and more manipulable than the instrument seen in Fig. 587 (Weiss).

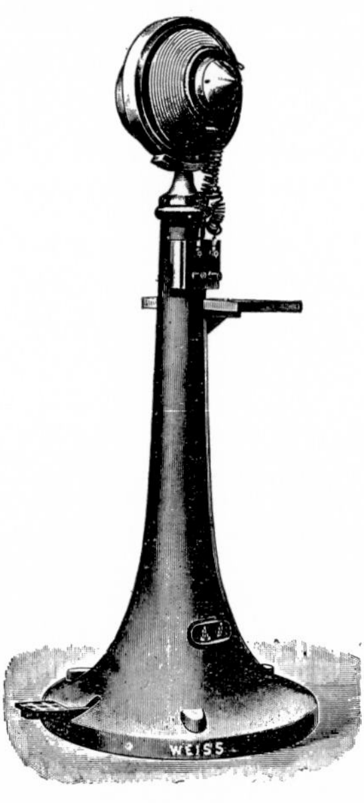

FIG. 589.—HAAB'S ORIGINAL GIANT MAGNET

entire field (Bronson, 1968). It follows that permanent hand magnets have a very limited field and are of value only as contact instruments.

It goes without saying, of course, that when using a magnet the instruments employed simultaneously at the operation, such as a speculum, hooks, towel clips, etc., must be made of non-magnetic materials.

In general surgery, magnets have been employed for the removal of foreign bodies from time immemorial; the lodestone was used for this purpose in India before the Christian era. Feldhaus (1903) attributed the first mention of the magnetic extraction of a foreign body from the eye to Hieronymus Brunschwyck (1497; 1534), and foreign bodies were removed from the cornea by such early surgeons as Fabricius Hildanus (1646), the father of German surgery, Turberville (1684) and Morgagni (1779). The first extraction from the inner eye was delayed until the next century, when Nikolaus Meyer (1842) extracted a piece of iron lying behind the iris through a scleral wound by a magnet weighing 30 lb.

Himly (1843) extracted an iron foreign body from the anterior chamber and McKeown (1874), of Dublin, was the first to insert the tip of the magnet into the vitreous, thereby removing a foreign body and saving the eye. The removal of a foreign body from the lens by McHardy (1878) followed shortly thereafter. A year later, Hirschberg (1879) introduced the electromagnet into ophthalmic practice, thus making such manipulations more feasible (Fig. 586); this was a relatively small hand instrument, 7·5 × 1·5 in., but other models rapidly followed,[1] all of them with different modifications, some of them large and powerful but sometimes cumbersome (Fig. 587), others weaker but lighter instruments (Fig. 588).

The first effective model of a giant magnet was constructed by Haab (1892) who subsequently modified it considerably (1894–1914) (Fig. 589); its lifting power at

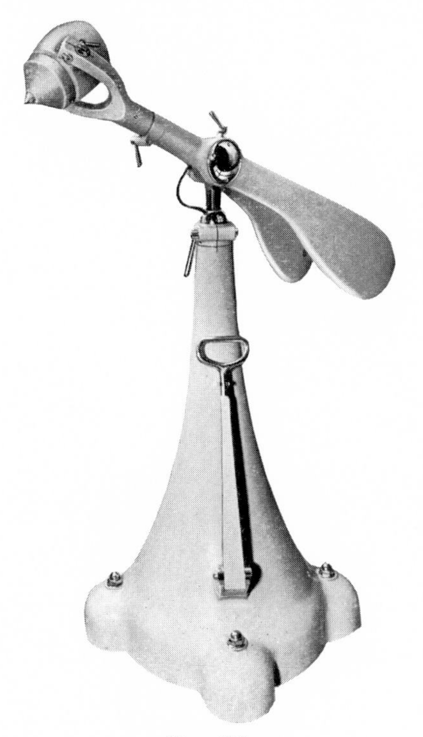

Fig. 590.

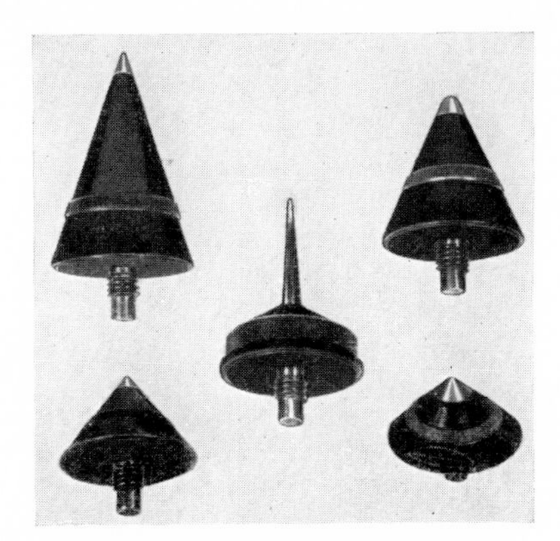

Fig. 591.
Various magnet terminals (A. S. Philps)

Fig. 590.—Giant Magnet
(A. S. Philps)

The magnet is readily manipulable in all directions by finger-pressure and at the same time, despite its weight, is stable in any position. The current is worked by a foot switch (see Fig. 597).

5 mm. distance with a current of 5·6 amperes was 113 g. The *Haab type of instrument* is a bar magnet, and Haab's original model was fixed horizontally on a stand in front of which the patient had to sit and to which he had to approximate his eye. This immobility was an obvious disadvantage: the procedure was somewhat frightening and impossible to carry out in cases of multiple injury, the view of the eye available to the surgeon was somewhat restricted, and any changes required in the direction of the magnetic force necessarily depended on the patient's cooperation in moving his eyes to order. Many other models have been introduced, among which the more interesting are those of Schlösser (1893–1903), Wagenmann (1900), Volkmann (1902), Hirschberg (1904),

[1] Fröhlich (1881), Snell (1881–83), Hirschberg (1885–1901), Volkmann (1902), Sweet (1906), Schumann (1908), Lancaster (1915), and many others.

Schumann (1908–18, a little less than twice the power of Haab's instrument) and Lancaster (1915), up to the enormous suspended magnet of Néchitch (1929–38), of Belgrade, which is able to attract a steel pen at the immense distance of 750 mm. A magnet of this power, however, must be very large and bulky; Néchitch's instrument weighed several tons and had to be manipulated on rails with motors, its core weighed 380 kg. and its winding coil, 4,000 metres long, allowed a current of 100 amperes to pass without heating. To obtain the optimum balance between power and manœuvrability an instrument such as that illustrated in Figs. 590–91 is probably the best compromise. Despite its bulk and considerable power it can be suspended at any angle over the operating table and is so finely counterbalanced that it is readily tilted by finger-pressure to any position which is automatically maintained. It can thus be completely controlled by the surgeon himself and at the same time allows a good view of the field of operation (Fig. 597).

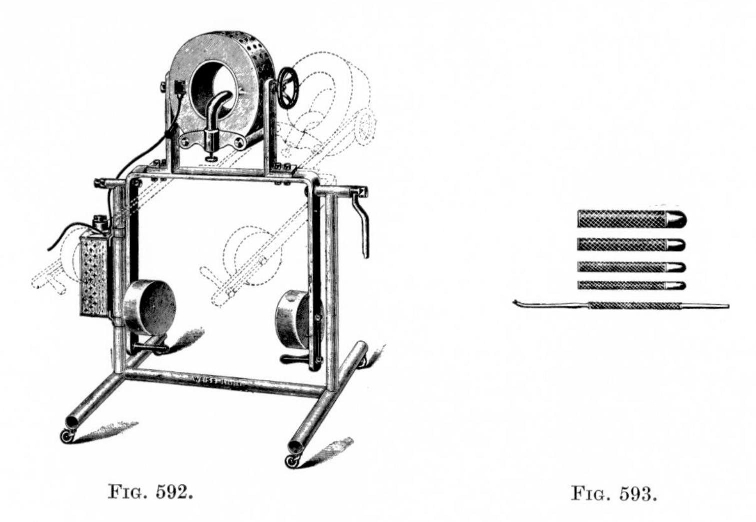

FIG. 592. FIG. 593.

Mellinger's ring magnet with various terminals (Fig. 593).

The practice sometimes made of using a very tenuous terminal in the giant magnet or of extending its manœuvrability by placing in contact with it a probe, chain, knife or other instrument which by induction itself acts as a magnet, is uneconomic in power, for the leakage involved in such a system is great and reduces the available pull to a portion in the neighbourhood of one-hundredth of that available with a good hand magnet (Fig. 582).

The *ring magnet* was introduced by Mellinger (1904–9) and Klingelfuss (1908–10) to overcome the disadvantages of the original model of Haab and allow the operation to be performed while the patient was lying on an operating table (Fig. 592). In construction it is an oval ring of soft iron, round which is wound a coil of wire about a mile long, the whole being covered by insulating material. When the current flows round this circular solenoid a homogeneous field is generated, the lines of force running parallel to the central axis at right angles to the ring. Since iron offers much less resistance to the magnetic flux than air, if a bar of this metal is placed in the ring, the lines of force will flock to pass through the iron, magnetizing it in the same way as the core of a solenoid; and it is obvious that the greatest number of lines of force will reach the bar and the greatest saturation will be attained if it lies at the centre of the solenoid axis, outside which magnetization rapidly falls off. The ring is capable of being swung over the patient's head and the injured eye is placed at the centre of the ring. Several terminals are provided, some relatively thick bars of soft iron for use when a considerable pull is required (for the larger the bar the more lines of force traverse it and the greater the available pull) and a longer and thinner spatula when more delicate manipulation is necessary (Fig. 593). The most suitable terminal is introduced into the centre of the field after the current is switched on and held very firmly in the surgeon's hands as it is approximated to the eye; if it is introduced before the current is switched on, the terminal may be suddenly dragged onto the patient's eye since the solenoid draws it forcibly towards the centre. There is no doubt that the Mellinger magnet allows very delicate manipulations and is about 25% stronger than the original model of Haab. It was used successfully by many surgeons (Jurnitschek, 1905; Amberg, 1907; Schirmer, 1908; Butler, 1909–17; and others), but its mechanical interference with the field of operation has rendered it less popular than the modern developments of the Haab type of instrument with their higher power and greater manœuvrability.

These two desiderata are constantly being improved. Thus the inner pole magnet has been made more effective by the introduction of a device for stepless control of the strength of the electric field (Zintz and Gremmelspacher, 1968); these workers also introduced an ammeter as a control, automatic safety devices against excessive elevation of the temperature in the magnet and a foot-switch to turn it on and off as had been recommended by Haab. Again, Neubauer (1968) introduced an alteration in the shape of the circular coil; an increase of the inner lumen of the coil in both main diameters made it possible to position the head of the patient so that the injured eye could be brought practically into the centre of the solenoid; lateral tilting of the head facilitates the surgical approach to the globe in extractions by the posterior route and makes it possible for the operating microscope to be used in the manipulations.

The removal of a magnetic foreign body from the anterior chamber is relatively easy, and as a rule a good hand magnet is all that is required. Even although it is highly manœuvrable, a giant magnet may be a disadvantage in such a case since, owing to its great power, it may drag the foreign body with such force that the corneal endothelium may be traumatized or, if the particle is caught in the iris, an iridodialysis or even a complete evulsion of this tissue may result.

It may occasionally be legitimate to remove the foreign body through the wound of entry if this is clean and the foreign body is in its vicinity, but usually a separate keratome section is advisable since the extraction of the particle through the original wound may lead to more scarring, encourage the development of infection, and may entail unfortunate complications if a prolapse of the iris should occur by mischance. As a general rule the section should not lie over the foreign body but near the limbus some distance away; if, as usually occurs, the foreign body lies at the bottom of the anterior chamber, the section is most conveniently placed above. In this way it is well separated from the damaged area, further injury to the traumatized tissues is avoided and the possibility of the wounded area of the iris adhering to the wound is eliminated; moreover, the foreign body itself is less readily impacted behind the shelf formed by the posterior lip of the limbal incision. The section should be oblique so that the keratome points directly at the foreign body, and a valve-like wound is made so that aqueous is not lost on the removal of the instrument for the preservation of the anterior chamber is necessary for the deft extraction of the foreign body. The incision is usually best situated 1 or 2 mm. away from the limbus to minimize the risk of a prolapse of the iris and should be approximately 1 mm. larger than the greatest diameter of the foreign body, so that its passage through it is easy. The tip of the hand magnet is placed over the cornea above the site of the foreign body, sufficient power being used merely to attract it gently, and it is guided to the inner edge of the wound; when it engages therein the magnet is then held at the entrance of the section so that the particle is drawn through the wound, a manœuvre which may be aided if the lips of the wound are simultaneously opened by a non-magnetic iris repositor (Figs. 594–96). It is possible that the anterior chamber may be

Figs. 594 to 596.—The Removal of a Foreign Body from the Anterior Chamber.

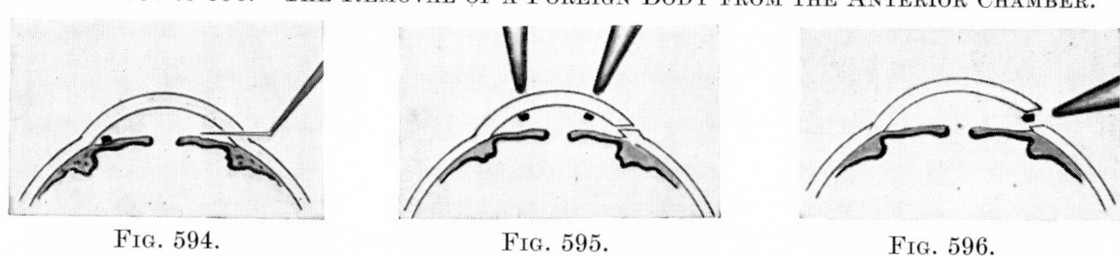

Fig. 594. Fig. 595. Fig. 596.

Fig. 594.—The position of the corneal section for the removal of a magnetic foreign body from the anterior chamber. The section is made by a keratome at a point opposite the position of the foreign body.

Fig. 595.—A composite picture of the method of drawing the foreign body from its original site across the anterior chamber towards the corneal section.

Fig. 596.—The delivery of the foreign body through the corneal incision (A. S. Philps).

lost at this stage and the iris become engaged in the section, but this tissue is usually readily freed from a newly-made wound by stroking the cornea. The instillation of atropine and the temporary application of a pad and bandage complete the operation.

If the anterior chamber is lost at an early stage of the operation, three possibilities are open: either a pad and bandage should be applied and the extraction postponed for an hour or two until the chamber has re-formed. Alternatively it may be filled with air or, if the foreign body is accessible, the terminal of the magnet may be introduced into the anterior chamber to contact the foreign body, whereupon the current is switched on and the terminal withdrawn through the wound with the foreign body attached to it. It is to be noted that if a prolapse of the iris into the wound already exists, the removal of the foreign body by this route should never be contemplated since the manipulations will merely make the prolapse worse; it is wiser in these cases to remove the foreign body first through a new incision in the manner indicated and deal with the prolapse subsequently.

If the foreign body is in the posterior chamber the same technique is applied, but the particle should first be drawn into the pupil by placing the magnet at a point in the limbus opposite the position of the foreign body; for this a giant magnet may be necessary. The current is then switched off, the foreign body allowed to fall to the bottom of the anterior chamber and the operation concluded as already described.

If the foreign body is entangled in the iris it is well to instil eserine to disentangle it as far as possible from the iris meshwork. If it is not readily freed by magnetic attraction, persistent attempts will merely result in tearing this tissue or in producing a dialysis which has, on occasion, been complete. It is safer to make a keratome section and introduce the elongated tip of the hand magnet into the anterior chamber to touch the foreign body which is then withdrawn gently along with the portion of iris in which it is entangled into the section, when it is removed with a piece of iris tissue by iridectomy scissors. An alternative is to remove the foreign body in the course of a large iridectomy.

If the particle is in the ciliary body near its anterior part, attempts to draw it forwards towards the angle of the anterior chamber may be unsuccessful; in these cases it is usually easier to reverse the direction of pull and draw the particle backwards onto the pars plana. If this is not readily accomplished the alternative is to fashion a scleral flap over the exact position of the foreign body through which its magnetic removal may be accomplished. If necessary, the ciliary body itself may be incised so that this manœuvre becomes more practicable, or the point of a small metal probe in contact with the magnet, or the tenuous tip of a hand magnet, may be introduced into the ciliary body so that it comes into contact with the particle which may then be drawn out. If the foreign body lies in the posterior part of the ciliary body it is removed trans-sclerally by the posterior route at the site of election, as will be subsequently described.[1]

If the foreign body lies within the lens its magnetic extraction is usually easy. If only a localized opacity is present an attempt may be made to extract the particle through the wound of entry by drawing it into the anterior chamber with the giant magnet under maximum mydriasis, whence it is extracted in the usual way. If the wound of entry is not suitable or available for this purpose, Elschnig's (1913) suggestion may be helpful; a small radial incision is made with a narrow Graefe knife in the lens capsule opposite the foreign body which is then drawn out with the giant magnet. In these cases it is preferable to induce miosis as rapidly as possible after the extraction, so that the contracted iris covers the wound in the capsule and thus helps to seal it and prevent the development of generalized cataractous changes.[2] Eserine may not be sufficiently strong for this purpose and a more rapid and complete miosis is obtained by injecting acetylcholine into the anterior chamber, and subsequently maintained by di-isopropyl phosphofluoridate (DFP) (François, 1951).

If the lens is opaque these procedures are unnecessary; after a keratome

[1] p. 633. [2] p. 123.

section has been made under a conjunctival flap with pre-placed sutures, an anterior capsulotomy should be performed, the particle withdrawn by the magnet, either the hand or giant instrument as may be required, whereafter as much lens matter as possible is washed out to complete the linear extraction. Alternatively, an intracapsular extraction can be performed using the cryoprobe or the erisophake to cover the gap in the capsule (Birks, 1962).

If the foreign body is in the posterior segment of the globe the operation for its removal entails considerably more potential danger to the eye. Care is therefore necessary that its localization has been exact and that its magnetizability is assessed in a preliminary test, preferably by a small magnet or by electronic means lest further damage be caused. If it is visible ophthalmoscopically it should be seen to move when it comes within the field of force of the giant magnet; if it is not visible, any movement can be assessed by x-rays or fluoroscopy, while an indication of its magnetizability may be obtained from its response to a suitable locator. The elicitation of pain caused by the dragging of the foreign body by the magnet over sensitive tissues as an indication of movement is a very unreliable test. If no movement is obtained the particle is either non-magnetic or very feebly so, or is so firmly encapsulated that it is securely anchored; in the latter event, repeated applications of the magnet, approximated as closely as possible to the foreign body, should be attempted on 3 or 4 consecutive days in order to loosen the particle, the pull being made from different directions and at different angles in the hope that it will be gradually rocked in its bed and freed, a process which often requires patience and considerable ingenuity.

When the magnetizability of the foreign body has been established, two alternative methods for its extraction may be considered—by the anterior route or the posterior route. In either case, if the lens is opaque, the problem of dealing with the cataract is best left until the foreign body has first been removed.

Extraction by the Anterior Route. The principle of this method of extraction is to draw the foreign body into the anterior chamber by the giant magnet and then extract it as already indicated[1] by the hand magnet. With this technique, approximate, but not necessarily precise, localization is all that is required. As a preliminary, maximal dilatation of the pupil should be obtained and complete anæsthesia induced by a regional injection or by general anæsthesia. The tip of the giant magnet with a cone-shaped terminal is then brought about 1 mm. away from the surface of the limbus, when the current is turned on (Fig. 597). The foreign body with its long axis in the direction of the pull of the magnet is drawn through the vitreous to the equator of the lens by intermittently opening and closing the circuit a few seconds at a time; it skirts the equator of this tissue, traverses the suspensory ligament, enters the posterior chamber and is seen to bulge the periphery of the iris forwards (Fig. 598). As soon as this is seen the cur-

[1] p. 629.

rent is immediately switched off to avoid entanglement with the iris. If it is not readily coaxed into this position after repeated applications of the current, the tip of the magnet may be placed over the sclera near the foreign body in an attempt to draw it in stages to the region of the ora; thereafter the magnet is again employed from the centre of the cornea. When the bulge in the iris is seen, the tip of the magnet is placed at the limbus at the opposite point of the meridian in which the particle lies, so that when the current is switched on it is drawn between the posterior surface of the iris and the anterior lens capsule into the pupillary aperture; thereupon the current is switched off and the foreign body falls into the bottom of the anterior chamber, whence it is extracted as before.

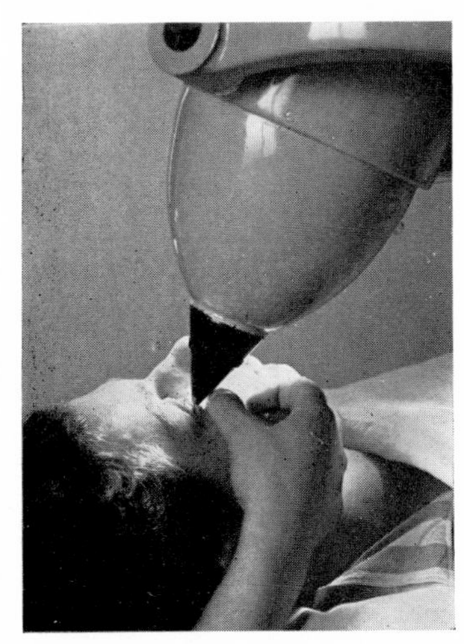

FIG. 597.
The extraction of a magnetic foreign body by the anterior route (A. S. Philps).

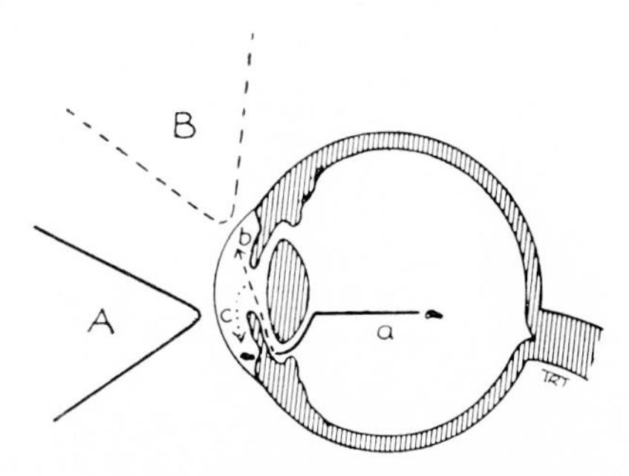

FIG. 598.—THE REMOVAL OF A FOREIGN BODY BY THE ANTERIOR ROUTE.

A foreign body lies in the vitreous and with the giant magnet at position A it is drawn along the path *a* until it is seen to bulge the iris. The magnet is changed to position B and the foreign body is drawn through the pupillary aperture (*b*). The magnet is then switched off and the foreign body falls to the bottom of the anterior chamber (*c*).

Extraction by the Posterior Route. In this technique the posterior segment is opened directly and the foreign body extracted through the wound thus made. It is occasionally possible to extract the particle through the wound of entry, if behind the ora, but this is rarely advisable, since it usually requires enlargement to allow delivery of the foreign body and is seldom in the most suitable place. A new incision at a site of election is therefore usually wiser, in which case it is important that *the wound of entry should be sealed* either by diathermy or cryosurgery to avoid the tendency for subsequent detachment of the retina. If the foreign body is in the anterior part of the vitreous or lies in the periphery of the fundus the site of election for the incision is through the pars plana of the ciliary body, 7·5 to 8 mm. behind the limbus, and the operative technique is most easily carried out in the outer and lower quadrant of the globe (Verhoeff, 1932). Here the retina is thin and firmly attached to the underlying tissues, so that there is little risk of detachment, the choriocapillaris is absent and, apart from a few veins running in a meridional direction, the area is relatively avascular, so that no hæmorrhage results from the incision and the danger of the development of sympathetic inflammation is negligible. If the foreign body is in the posterior part of the vitreous it is well to attempt to draw it forward by the magnet to this location, but if this proves difficult or if it is embedded in the posterior part of the retina or the optic disc, it is usually unwise to attempt such a manœuvre since the particle may tear the retina in its transit and cause a detachment (Amalong, 1970). In this event the site of the incision should be that which gives most convenient access to the foreign body. This is particularly important if the particle is feebly magnetic, since its extraction may prove impossible if attempted from a distance, and by detaching the appropriate muscles practically any portion of the sclera up to a few millimetres in front of the nerve-head can be approached; the vortex veins, however, must be avoided.

The incision employed by different surgeons has varied, but for the average foreign body a small linear incision a few millimetres in length in a meridional direction suffices. If the foreign body is large and jagged, a T-shaped incision with the cross arm approximately half the length of the meridional arm may allow more easy extraction (Stieren, 1932–43; Thorpe, 1945; Granström, 1949). Alternatively, a trephine opening using a hinged flap is a useful method of approach (Barbour and Fralick, 1941; Somerville-Large, 1946; and others).

The steps of the operation are as follows. As a preliminary, topical and regional anæsthesia should be obtained by the use of drops and an analgesic injection into Tenon's capsule as well as complete akinesia by a facial block; as an alternative a general anæsthetic may be used. A tongue-shaped flap of conjunctiva and Tenon's capsule with pre-placed sutures is then turned down over the proposed site of incision, to which several applications of diathermy or the cryoprobe should be applied. Some operators prefer to ring round the area with applications of diathermy, and this may be done at the end of the operation, but the creation of a zone of coagulation 3 or 4 mm. in diameter over the site makes the incision through the sclera easier, prevents choroidal bleeding and at the same time induces the aseptic choroiditis advisable to minimize the risk of retinal detachment. If the foreign body is not already near the coats of the eye the giant magnet is used to draw it towards this site; at this point there may appear a slight bulging of the sclera and occasionally the particle may even be seen as a dark shadow on the inner surface of the sclera (Ostroumov, 1949). The sclera is then incised through two-thirds of its thickness in the antero-posterior meridian (in the coagulated area), the incision being approximately 1 mm. more than the anticipated size of the foreign body. A mattress suture is then inserted around it, one limb on either side of the incision, or, alternatively, interrupted sutures are used. The head of the patient is then tilted so that the wound lies as nearly as possible uppermost to avoid herniation of the vitreous, the incision is carried through the sclera with a fine cataract knife, the choroid and retina are similarly incised (for which a diathermy knife may be used, Lancaster, 1938), and the terminal of the magnet is brought just into the lips of the wound which is held open with the pre-placed sutures (or alternatively by non-magnetizable hooks); for this purpose the hand magnet may well be sufficient. The tip of the magnet should enter the lips of the wound lest the foreign body on approaching it get entangled in the retina or choroid, but the magnet should never be introduced into the vitreous itself. The current is then turned on and, perhaps after several intermittent applications, as a rule a click is heard as the foreign body contacts the terminal. The magnet is then swung away and the current is turned off, but not before the foreign body is free from the eye. The sutures are then coapted and, after any tags of choroid are stroked back, they are tied and the conjunctival flap replaced. Atropine is instilled, a pad and bandage applied and the patient left for 48 hours, whereupon he is treated as if he were a case of retinal detachment.

As an alternative to using diathermy in these procedures, the scleral wound has been touched with pure carbolic acid or another cauterizing agent and a local choroiditis thus stimulated to prevent a retinal detachment, a procedure which is efficacious and economic in time (Stieren, 1943). There is, however, some difference of opinion concerning the indications for and indeed the desirability of the use of diathermy. Traditionally its use has been advocated by a number of surgeons as an integral and essential part of the operative procedure in the removal of a foreign body by the posterior route in order to seal the operative tear in the retina and thus prevent retinal detachment (Bellows, 1947; Stallard, 1947–65; Lucic, 1948; Thorpe, 1965; and others), while Lancaster's (1938) expedient of using a diathermy knife in order to make a bloodless scleral incision was adopted by Stallard (1946) and Gundersen (1947). In this procedure, however, the dosage must be carefully controlled since excessive diathermy may produce vitreous opacities and traction-bands which may later lead to a retinal detachment (Kraus and Briggs, 1945); indeed, both of these techniques have been claimed as unnecessary, merely inflicting further trauma upon an already severely damaged eye (Jameson Evans, 1951; Roper-Hall, 1954; Cridland, 1968). Most cases in which the posterior route is used show a firm adhesion between the retina and the choroid at the site of removal, the result of a traumatic inflammation reinforced by the effect of the slight infolding of the coats of the eye brought about by the scleral sutures; this is unlikely to be increased by diathermy but the firmness of such adhesions will certainly result in more widespread scarring and may indeed devitalize the sclera in the precise area where good healing is required. This view has received some support. Thus, Roper-Hall (1954) found that the incidence of retinal detachments amongst 555 cases of this type was no higher, although diathermy was not used, than in other series; Levy (1958) reported that retinal detachments occurred in 16 out of 52 removals by the posterior route and in only 3 of these was surface diathermy not applied before the onset of retinal detachment; while Cridland (1968) quoted 51 personal cases of posterior removal wherein a retinal detachment developed in 1 out of 4 cases treated with diathermy whereas of the remaining 47 in which diathermy was not used a detachment developed in only 1 case; in both instances in which a detachment occurred there had been much vitreous hæmorrhage, an association already recognized (Sellas, 1949; Roper-Hall, 1954). Prophylactic cryotherapy to the sclera is preferable to diathermy and has been strongly advocated by Havener and Gloeckner (1969), while the retina may be anchored by light-coagulation.

The relative merits of extracting a foreign body from the posterior segment of the globe by the anterior or posterior route have excited a considerable amount of controversy. Each has its advantages and each has its contra-indications so that every case should be individually considered. The posterior route was the first to be employed because the early magnets lacking the power to draw a foreign body into the anterior chamber made no alternative possible. With the introduction of Haab's giant magnet, however, in 1892, particularly since this instrument could not readily be manipulated for the technique of extraction by the posterior route—the anterior route became popular until Mellinger's magnet in 1908 made a posterior approach again possible. The theoretical disadvantages of the posterior route in those early days used to be the fear of the subsequent development of a retinal detachment; such, indeed, was a frequent sequel of the simple operation in vogue at the time whereby a magnet was introduced into the vitreous through a simple stab-puncture in the sclera.

The improvements in technique in the operation as now performed, the better instruments available, the increased accuracy of localization and the anchoring of the retina when necessary by diathermy, cryosurgery or photocoagulation have greatly reduced this danger and, indeed, there is probably less tendency to cause a retinal detachment if the foreign body is extracted at its actual site than if it is torn from its bed in the retina, particularly if it has been securely encapsulated therein, and pulled across the vitreous cavity by the anterior method. There may be little doubt that in the period before modern operative refinements were introduced the anterior route gave the best results[1] and some surgeons used it almost exclusively.[2] A similar number of surgeons, however, can be quoted who held the opposite view,[3] while others used either method as indicated (Sherman, 1939; and others). It is probable that in most of the cases in which a detachment of the retina subsequently develops it is caused by the original trauma, that the organization of bands in the vitreous are due to hæmorrhage or organized exudate consequent thereon rather than to the operative technique, and that unless the indications summarized below are violated there is little difference in the results obtained in long series of cases whichever technique is adopted *if that technique is efficiently employed.*

It may be said that if a foreign body is highly magnetizable, of medium size (less than 3 mm. in diameter), is smooth and without jagged edges such as occur more usually in civilian injuries than in war, it may be suitable for extraction by the anterior route; if, however, it is poorly magnetizable, as unfortunately are many of the alloys met with both in industrial and military injuries, if it has sharp, rough edges such as would easily cause trauma to the lens or the ciliary processes or make it readily become entangled with the iris, it is more suitable for extraction by the posterior route. If it is very small anterior extraction may be impossible and if it is more than 3 mm. in diameter it is dangerous. In general it may be said that removal of an intra-ocular foreign body by the anterior route should not be attempted unless it is lying anterior to the lens and zonule or in the lens itself. If the anterior segment of the eye is badly damaged, particularly if prolapse of the iris is

[1] Goulden (1908), Haab (1910–14), Whiting and Goulden (1917).

[2] Duggan (1933) 270 cases; Duthie (1941); Gulliver (1942) found the posterior route advisable only 6 times in 1,800 cases; and Levy (1958) that in a series of 272 cases treated at Moorfields Eye Hospital between 1946 and 1955 the anterior was used three times as frequently as the posterior route.

[3] Sweet (1906), Shoemaker (1919), Allport (1925), Stieren (1932–43) (700 cases wherein the anterior route was never used if the foreign body were behind the posterior capsule of the lens), Stallard (1965).

present or the anterior chamber has been lost, it is best to use the posterior route, extracting the foreign body first and subsequently doing the necessary reparative surgery in the anterior segment which should not be further traumatized. This is the only practicable technique when a hyphæma obstructs a view of the course of events in anterior extractions. If, on the other hand, the foreign body has entered the posterior segment of the eye initially and the lens is untouched, it is unwise to expose the anterior part of the eye to possible injury, and in any event a posterior wound of entry requires consolidation. If there is an associated retinal detachment with a tear this may require treatment and a posterior extraction can be done at the same time, but the anterior route is preferable in those cases with a pre-operative retinal detachment, an intra-ocular hæmorrhage or severe damage to the lens. Finally, if the foreign body is densely encapsulated posterior extraction over the site of the foreign body is preferable to an attempt to draw it out into the vitreous thus running the considerable risk of tearing the retina in so doing. It must be remembered that the increasing use of the posterior route as the method of choice for the removal of foreign bodies in the posterior segment of the globe demands accuracy of localization, so that the best surgical approach can be made in each case. This is certainly true for magnetic particles; it is even more essential for non-magnetic foreign bodies. In addition, every attempt should be made to determine the nature of the foreign body and its size.

THE REMOVAL OF NON-MAGNETIC INTRA-OCULAR FOREIGN BODIES

The removal of non-magnetic foreign bodies from the eye presents problems greater than are encountered with magnetizable particles; indeed, it was not so long ago when it was said with considerable reason that an eye containing an irritant foreign body which could not be extracted by the magnet, particularly if it lay in the posterior segment, was a lost eye. This defeatist attitude today is unjustifiable.[1] If such a foreign body lies near the sclera and can be accurately localized, the possibility of its extraction is almost as good as if it were magnetizable (Witmer, 1949; Granström, 1949; and many others). If, however, it lies within the vitreous cavity far from the ocular walls, its extraction is difficult and chancy and, although in these cases the immediate result may sometimes be good, the end-result in terms of vision is often disappointing. It follows that the advisability of the extraction of such foreign bodies must be looked upon more conservatively than we have seen to be necessary with magnetic particles, and the conduct of such cases requires a nice assessment of judgment on the part of the surgeon whether their removal will cause more damage than their retention. In general it may be said that only those foreign bodies which are chemically or mechanically detrimental to the tissues must be removed; with the important exception of particles of copper or brass which should be removed

[1] For an extensive bibliography see Neubauer (1969).

as soon as possible, non-magnetic foreign bodies are probably best left alone unless their removal can be effected without serious risk to the eye. Although cases are reported in the earlier records of the extraction of such foreign bodies even from the vitreous with success (Dixon, 1859; Sweet, 1901; and others), and although Lehmann (1914), for example, was able to collect from the literature 41 cases of copper particles extracted from the eye—a laudable achievement when heroic surgery was the only hope of saving the eye—the methods at our disposal today have greatly improved although they have not revolutionized the prognosis (Neubauer, 1968–69).

If the foreign body is in the anterior chamber it can usually be picked out directly by forceps. Such a particle generally lies in the recesses of the angle, in which case particular care must be taken with the incision so as to make

Figs. 599 and 600.—Extraction of a Foreign Body from the Angle of the Anterior Chamber.

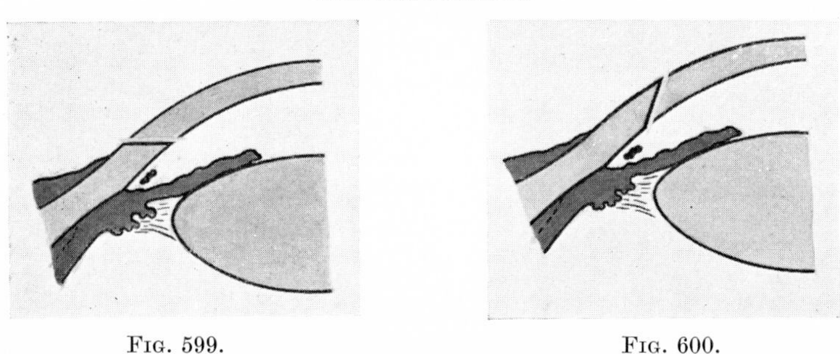

Fig. 599. Fig. 600.

Fig. 599.—The usual incision is seen to preclude access to a foreign body in the angle. A more useful incision is seen in Fig. 600 through which forceps may be introduced directly onto the foreign body. A safe instrument for such an incision is a Desmarres's knife.

the approach physically possible. A corneal section, for example, should run not in a direction parallel to the plane of the iris as does the classical incision, for in this case the foreign body will lie inaccessible under the shelf formed by the under surface of the cornea (Fig. 599), but at right angles to this plane, that is, with its inner end opening towards the angle so that the forceps can approach the particle (Fig. 600). An alternative method is to cut through the cornea with a trephine retaining a hinged flap which can be pulled back and re-inserted in its bed by sutures (Böck, 1950). If the foreign body is large and difficulties are anticipated, the most useful approach is an *ab externo* incision beneath a conjunctival flap using pre-placed sutures, the wound being of sufficient extent that the cornea can be folded over, fully exposing the iris; if the particle is entangled in the iris it can often be freed and removed in this way, and if this is found to be impossible it can be removed in the course of an iridectomy. Care should be taken, however, not to injure the corneal endothelium or to bruise the tissues of the iris lest anterior synechiæ develop, an unfortunate sequel particularly prone to occur if the particle is buried near the periphery of the iris where the anterior chamber is shallow. Two important practical details in the management of these cases should be emphasized: (1) hypotony of the globe should be ensured before the anterior chamber is opened, and (2) the pupil should be maximally constricted. The exact location of a foreign body in the angle of the anterior chamber may be verified by using a gonioscope in conjunction with the operating microscope.

Occasionally it has happened that the foreign body has been simply washed out. Thus Juler (1930) adopted with success the ingenious plan of cutting a keratome section without losing aqueous, turning the patient over to the supine position and opening the wound with an iris repositor so that the foreign body was washed out with the flow of aqueous. Such a degree of luck, however, does not always hold.

It will be remembered that a spicule of glass as a foreign body is frequently difficult to see, but it has already been pointed out that it is rendered readily visible by the use of polarized light.[1]

A cilium or other pliable material lying upon the iris may also present difficulties, since it is not easy to grasp it with the forceps and leave the iris free. As has already been noted, it is useful in this case to insinuate a grooved curette between the lash and the iris and, guiding a blunt hook within the groove beneath the lash, to pull it out, for in its macerated and pliable state, if engaged at its middle, it is readily drawn out doubled upon itself (Fisher, 1930).

If the foreign body is in the posterior chamber the suggestion of Thorpe (1947) is useful. With a limbal incision under a conjunctival flap and with pre-placed sutures, an iridodialysis is performed, the root of the iris being cut with pointed scissors opposite the site of the foreign body which is then removed with forceps, care being taken not to injure the lens. If the irido-dialysis is of necessity large, a central strand of the iris may be incorporated in the wound in order to close the defect.

If the particle is in the ciliary body the only practical method of approach is through a meridional incision over the site, holding the lips of the wound open by means of sutures. If the foreign body is not immediately seen, an incision into the ciliary body is required before it can be removed by forceps.

If the foreign body is in the lens two possibilities are available: if it is practicable the easiest technique is to temporize until a cataract develops when the lens may be removed intracapsularly with the foreign body, perhaps most safely with the erisophake or cryoprobe after enzymic zonulysis. This procedure can be postponed until the acute injury has healed unless the complications of infection or acute glaucoma necessitate emergency surgery. In young patients, in whom the attempted intra-capsular extraction is often attended by a loss of vitreous, serious considera-tion should be given to extraction of the lens by the extracapsular method or by aspiration (Havener and Gloeckner, 1969). If the capsule has been torn and the lens broken up a linear extraction or aspiration must be performed in the

[1] p. 566.

hope that the particle will be washed out with the lens matter. Occasionally it remains entangled in the capsular remnants from which it may be removed by the magnet or if it is non-magnetic it may be grasped by forceps (Lyle, 1941), although such manipulations may cause the foreign body to fall back into the vitreous. In general, however, the extraction of an intra-lenticular foreign body is not an emergency and may be deferred as long as the lens remains clear. An acute traumatic cataract is best left undisturbed unless swelling of the lens is likely to cause an acute closed-angle glaucoma.

If the foreign body is in the posterior segment it must be approached by a trans-scleral incision. *If it lies in or near the coats of the eye,* its removal is usually possible, but *the success of a technically difficult operation depends entirely on the precision of localization, which must be pinpoint in its accuracy,* certainly to within 1·0 mm. Every endeavour should be made to secure this, and if the foreign material is radio-opaque the more routine methods of localization should always be verified at the time of operation by one or other of the bone-free techniques. The procedure employed in these circumstances is the same as that we have just described for a magnetic foreign body with the exception that it is probably wiser to make a small trapdoor sclerotomy with pre-placed sutures and a corresponding clean incision in the retina and choroid, so that the flap can be everted and from its inner surface the foreign body can be directly removed with forceps (Elschnig, 1928). In these manœuvres Flieringa's ring may be useful to maintain stabilization, particularly if the ocular tension is low. The site should, of course, be sealed by diathermy or cryosurgery.

If the foreign body lies in the vitreous the problem is considerably more difficult and the technique employed must vary with the circumstances. If the ocular media are clear and the foreign body is within ophthalmoscopic view, it may be removed under control by introducing an instrument into the vitreous chamber. If it is in the anterior part the site of election for the incision at the pars plana is always indicated, but if it is situated far back in the globe the nearest approach should be made. The technique employed in making the scleral incision is similar to that described for the removal of a magnetic foreign body, and through the incision the appropriate instrument is introduced, grasps the foreign body and withdraws it slowly and deliberately without unnecessary movements; it is only thus that undue disturbance of the vitreous is avoided, for otherwise the gel rapidly tends to become turbid, obscuring the view of the field, and subsequently suffers disorganization.

For this purpose many instruments have been elaborated although ordinary small capsule forceps have been employed with success (Shipman, 1949) and even a Daviel cataract-spoon (Marin Amat, 1948). Specially designed instruments have been devised in abundance: long-angled forceps (Philps, 1961), cross-action forceps (Cross, 1927; Thorpe, 1936), forceps with small cup-shaped jaws (Spinelli, 1950) which open and close as they slide out and into a hollow shaft (Stallard, 1965) (Figs. 601–603),

FIGS. 601 to 605—INSTRUMENTS FOR REMOVING NON-MAGNETIC FOREIGN BODIES FROM THE VITREOUS.

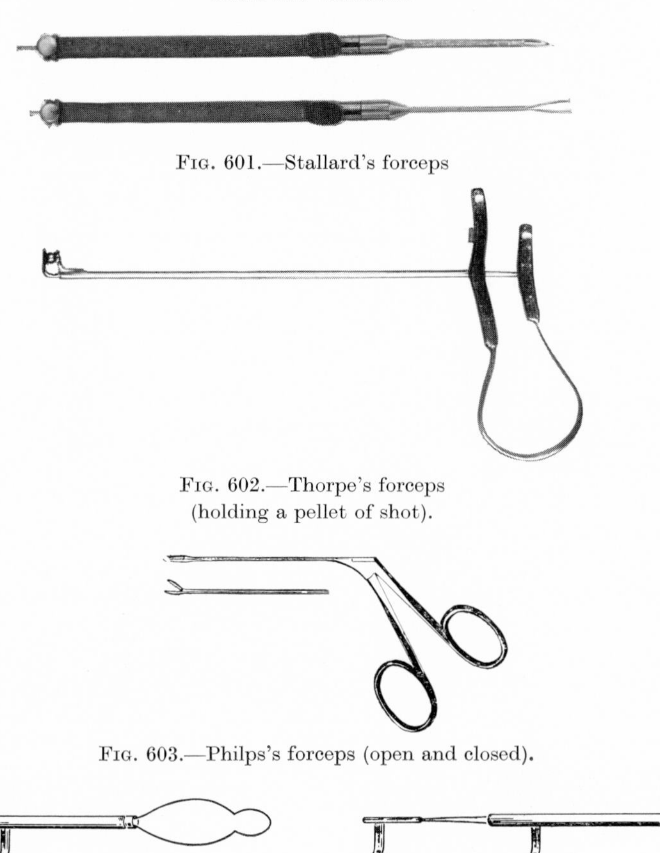

FIG. 601.—Stallard's forceps

FIG. 602.—Thorpe's forceps (holding a pellet of shot).

FIG. 603.—Philps's forceps (open and closed).

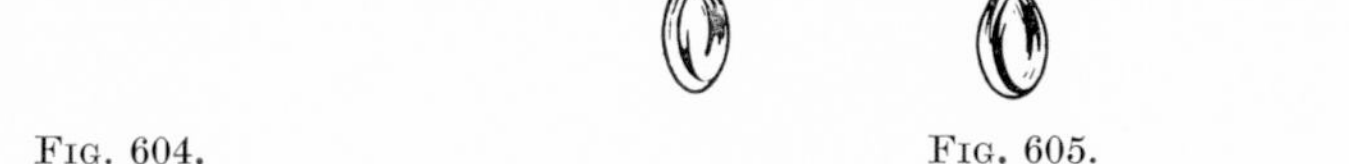

FIG. 604. FIG. 605.

FIG. 604.—Briggs's snare open, and Fig. 605, closed.

tong-shaped pincers (Gorban, 1958), a gripping cannula (Wilczek, 1958), a wire snare introduced in a needle or hollow tube which can be looped over the foreign body and drawn taut around it (Kraus and Briggs, 1945) (Figs. 604–5), a micro-extractor with beak-shaped gripping wedges for extraction of small particles or wire segments (Neubauer, 1965), and various types of cannula or endoscope for removal of foreign bodies by aspiration (Neubauer, 1953–68). As an assistance in localization ultrasonic techniques have been used (Bronson, 1964) and the cryosurgical probe has proved its value (François *et al.*, 1966).

If the lens is opaque but the vitreous remains clear or relatively clear, the *endoscope* may be employed. This is an instrument introduced by Thorpe (1934), designed as an inverted Galilean telescope on the same principle as the operating cystoscope and bronchoscope (Figs. 606–7). It consists of a self-illuminated telescopic tube through which can be passed various types of cross-action forceps designed to grasp foreign bodies of different shapes. The illuminated field of the endoscope permits a view of practically the entire fundus. The incision required must be some 9 mm. long, since the width of the instrument is 6·5 mm. The site of insertion is planned to disturb the vitreous as little as possible and is usually anterior to the ora serrata. The eye is immobilized and the endoscope introduced into

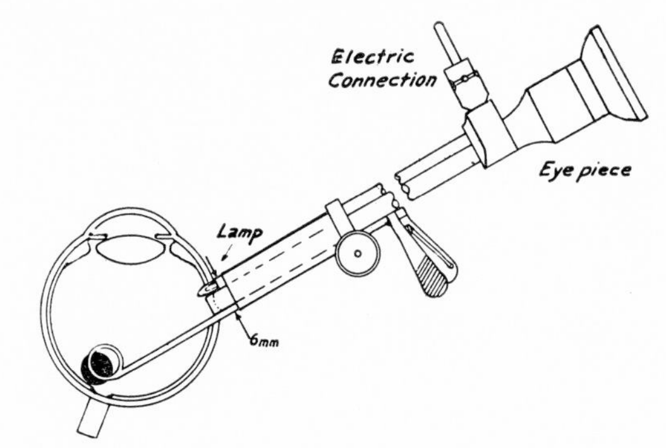

FIG. 606.—THORPE'S ENDOSCOPE (see Fig. 607).

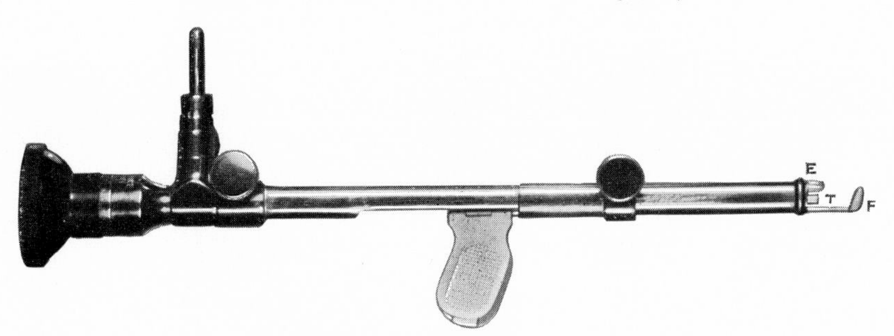

FIG. 607.—THORPE'S ENDOSCOPE.
E, miniature electric lamp; T, telescope; F, forceps

the wound but not entering the vitreous, being held by an assistant lest it be pushed in too far by the surgeon in his enthusiasm. Under direct observation the surgeon then introduces the forceps into the vitreous, grasps the foreign body firmly with its long axis parallel to the pull of the forceps and slowly withdraws the forceps from the globe, fixing the foreign body the whole time lest it inadvertently be lost. The manœuvre is difficult, so that practice in an artificial chamber is necessary to acquire precision in the somewhat peculiar manipulations. As the surgeon withdraws the instrument, the assistant closes the scleral wound by drawing together the pre-placed sutures. A similar instrument utilizing the light-transmitting properties of Perspex was devised by Butterworth and Bignell (1952). The endoscope can only be used when the vitreous is clear; it is not helpful if the vitreous is cloudy or blood-stained (Thorpe, 1965).

Small particles floating freely in the vitreous body can often be removed with relatively little additional trauma by the technique of aspiration using a curette cannula connected to a 5 ml. syringe containing sterile normal saline; ophthalmoscopic control is essential (Neubauer, 1953–63). If this is not possible because of opacities in the lens, but in the absence of marked vitreous opacities, an aspiration-endoscope using fibre-optic illumination may be employed (Neubauer, 1966).

If the lens and the vitreous are both opaque, the only alternative to groping blindly for the foreign body—a very chancy business—is to work in collaboration with a radiologist, the movements of the forceps in the vitreous being controlled by *biplane fluoroscopy*. This procedure was introduced by Cross (1927), who thus removed a piece of small-shot from an opaque vitreous and in subsequent attempts (1929–30) successfully treated 18 other cases. The method was used by others,[1] but it is by no means easy and should be employed only if the alternative is loss of the eye. The use of image-intensifiers under radiological control during the operative procedures is sometimes useful (Sarrazin and Noix, 1966; Suckling, 1966).

A further method of aiding blind localization in these unpromising cases is by the use of powerful *transillumination* of the eye from more than one angle; on opening the sclera a shadow or a glistening piece of metal of some size may be seen in this way and removed by forceps (Schutz, 1942). A glass-fibre diaphanoscope for this purpose has been designed by Neubauer (1968).

Finally, in such difficult " blind " explorations the principle of the disturbance of an induced current in the neighbourhood of a metallic body may be utilized to give information when it is approached. The theory involved has already been discussed when we described the locator[2]; in the neighbourhood of a metallic mass, changes in the induced current in a secondary coil are indicated by the deflections of the needle of a voltmeter or alterations in the pitch of a loud-speaker.

The approach of forceps to a poorly magnetizable foreign body lying hidden in the posterior segment of the globe can thus be heralded by a change of pitch in an associated amplifier. This technique was introduced by Weve (1916) in his *telephon-pinzette*. An " electric forceps " can be made in this way using an ordinary iris forceps linked with a wireless set, the loud-speaker of which indicates when the forceps is in contact with the foreign body; if the two arms of the forceps are made of different metals and insulated, the noise can be made to vary whether the particle is contacted by one or other arm or grasped by both (Leydhecker, 1947).

Allport. *Amer. J. Ophthal.*, **8**, 483 (1925).
Amalong. *Amer. J. Ophthal.*, **70**, 10 (1970).
Amberg. *Z. Augenheilk.*, **18**, 511 (1907).
Barbour and Fralick. *Amer. J. Ophthal.*, **24**, 553 (1941).
Bellows. *Amer. J. Ophthal.*, **30**, 309 (1947).
Birks. *Brit. J. Ophthal.*, **46**, 745 (1962).
Böck. Meller's *Augenärztliche Eingriffe*, Vienna (1950).

[1] Borley and Leef (1937), Senna (1944), Roberts (1944), Lindblom (1948), Shipman (1949), and others.
[2] p. 572.

Borley and Leef. *Amer. J. Ophthal.*, **20**, 1232 (1937).
Bronson. *Amer. J. Ophthal.*, **58**, 133 (1964); **60**, 596 (1965).
Arch. Ophthal., **79**, 22 (1968).
Brunschwyck. *Hautwirkung der Wundartzney*, Strasbourg (1497; 1534).
Butler. *Ophthalmoscope*, **7**, 325 (1909).
Brit. J. Ophthal., **1**, 46 (1917).
Butterworth and Bignell. *Brit. J. Ophthal.*, **36**, 217 (1952).
Crawford. *Brit. J. Ophthal.*, **27**, 227 (1943).
Cridland. *Proc. roy. Soc. Med.*, **60**, 597 (1967).
Int. Ophthal. Clin., **8**, 181, 213 (1968).
Cross. *Trans. Amer. ophthal. Soc.*, **25**, 80 (1927).
Trans. Amer. Acad. Ophthal., **34**, 173 (1929).
Amer. J. Ophthal., **13**, 41 (1930).
Penn. med. J., **34**, 480 (1930).
J. med. Soc. New Jersey, **32**, 697 (1935).
Dixon. *Roy. Lond. ophthal. Hosp. Rep.*, **1**, 280 (1859).
Donovan. *Trans. Sect. Ophthal., Amer. med. Ass.*, 106 (1924).
Duggan. *Arch. Ophthal.*, **10**, 768 (1933).
Duthie. *Trans. ophthal. Soc. U.K.*, **61**, 31 (1941).
Elkington. *Trans. Canad. ophthal. Soc.*, **2**, 100 (1949).
Elschnig. *Klin. Mbl. Augenheilk.*, **51** (1), 787 (1913); **81**, 654 (1928).
Endt and ten Doesschate. *Brit. J. Ophthal.*, **33**, 97 (1949).
Evans. *Trans. ophthal. Soc. U.K.*, **71**, 251, 254 (1951).
Fabricius Hildanus (Fabry). *Opera observat. et curat. medico-chirurg.*, Frankfurt (1646).
Feldhaus. *Zbl. prakt. Augenheilk.*, **27**, 138 (1903).
Fisher. *Lancet*, **1**, 787 (1930).
François. *Bull. Soc. belge Ophtal.*, No. 98, 276 (1951).
François, Asseman and Constantinides. *Bull. Soc. franç. Ophtal.*, **79**, 307 (1966).
Fröhlich. *Klin. Mbl. Augenheilk,*. **19**, 1, 28 (1881).
Gorban. *Oftal. Zh.*, **13**, 333 (1958).
Goulden. *Roy. Lond. ophthal. Hosp. Rep.*, **17**, 301 (1908).
Granström. *Acta ophthal.* (Kbh.), **27**, 47 (1949).
Greenwood. *Trans. Amer. ophthal. Soc.*, **25**, 80 (1927).
Gulliver. *Arch. Ophthal.*, **28**, 896 (1942).
Gundersen. *Trans. Amer. Acad. Ophthal.*, **52**, 604 (1947).
Haab. *Ber. dtsch. ophthal. Ges.*, **22**, 163 (1892); **24**, 186 (1895); **36**, 264 (1910); **37**, 2 (1911).
Beitr. Augenheilk., **2** (13), 290 (1894).
Arch. Augenheilk., **68**, 1; **69**, 111 (1911); **77**, 271 (1914).
Havener and Gloeckner. *Atlas of Diagnostic Technics and Treatment of Intraocular Foreign Bodies*, St. Louis (1969).
Himly. *Die Krankheiten u. Missbildungen d. menschlichen Auges u. d. Heilung*, Berlin, **2**, 95 (1843).
Hirschberg. *Berl. klin. Wschr.*, **16**, 681 (1879).
Die Elektromagnet in d. Augenheilkunde, Leipzig (1885).
Die Magnetoperation in der Augenheilkunde, Leipzig (1899).
Zbl. prakt. Augenheilk., **25**, 116, 175 (1901); **28**, 176, 353 (1904).
Juler. *Trans. ophthal. Soc. U.K.*, **50**, 118 (1930).
Jurnitschek. *Z. Augenheilk.*, **14**, 426, 552 (1905).
Klingelfuss. *Korresp.-Bl. schweiz. Ärzte*, 531 (1908).
Z. Augenheilk., **23**, 52 (1910).
Kraus and Briggs. *Brit. J. Ophthal.*, **29**, 557 (1945).
Lancaster. *Trans. Amer. ophthal. Soc.*, **14**, 168 (1915).
Amer. J. Surg., **42**, 14 (1938).
Lehmann. *Ueber Kupfersplitter im Glaskörperraum* (Diss.), Berlin (1914).
Levy. *Brit. J. Ophthal.*, **42**, 610 (1958).
Leydhecker. *v. Graefes Arch. Ophthal.*, **141**, 665 (1940).
Klin. Mbl. Augenheilk., **112**, 255 (1947).
Lindblom. *Acta ophthal.* (Kbh.), **26**, 441 (1948).
Lucic. *Calif. Med.*, **69**, 114 (1948).
Lyle. *Trans. ophthal. Soc. U.K.*, **61**, 59 (1941).
McCaslin. *Trans. Amer. ophthal. Soc.*, **56**, 571 (1958).
McHardy. *Brit. med. J.*, **1**, 531 (1878).
McKeown. *Brit. med. J.*, **1**, 800 (1874).
Lancet, **2**, 253 (1878).
Marin Amat. *Arch. Soc. oftal. hisp.-amer.*, **8**, 1090 (1948).
Mellinger. *X int. Cong. Ophthal.*, Lucerne, C193 (1904).
Beitr. z. Physiol. u. Path. (ed. von Weiss), Stuttgart 148 (1908).
Z. Augenheilk., **21**, 204 (1909).
Meyer. *Med. Z. vom Verein für Heilkunde in Preussen*, 11 (1842).
Morgagni. *De sedibus et causis morborum*, Hebroduni, **1**, 215 (1779).
Néchitch. *Ann. Oculist.* (Paris), **166**, 513 (1929); **171**, 545 (1934); **175**, 507 (1938).
Neubauer. *Ber. dtsch. ophthal. Ges.*, **58**, 332 (1953); **67**, 297 (1965).
Klin. Mbl. Augenheilk., **140**, 734 (1962); **148**, 202 (1966); **152**, 723 (1968).
Trans. ophthal. Soc. U.K., **83**, 143 (1963).
Entwicklung. u. Fortschritt in der Augenheilk. (ed. Sautter), Stuttgart, 291 (1963).
Int. Ophthal. Clin., **8**, 205, 237 (1968).
Bibl. ophthal., **80**, 1 (1969).
Ostroumov. *Vestn. oftal.*, **28**, 38 (1949).
Paderstein. *Klin. Mbl. Augenheilk.*, **75**, 720 (1925).
Philps. *Ophthalmic Operations*, London (1961).
Roberts. *Amer. J. Roentgenol.*, **52**, 327 (1944).
Roper-Hall. *Brit. J. Ophthal.*, **38**, 65 (1954).
Trans. ophthal. Soc. U.K., **77**, 239 (1957).
Int. Ophthal. Clin., **8**, 135, 211 (1968).

Sarrazin and Noix. *Bull. Soc. franç. Ophtal.*, **79,** 283 (1966).
Schirmer. *Z. Augenheilk.*, **20,** 546 (1908).
Schlösser. *Ber. dtsch. ophthal. Ges.*, **23,** 153 242 (1893); **31,** 300 (1903).
Schumann. *Augenmagnete*, Düsseldorf (1908).
Zwecke. Electrotechn. Z., **39,** 464 (1918).
Schutz. *Amer. J. Ophthal.*, **25,** 70 (1942).
Sellas. *Arch. Soc. oftal. hisp.-amer.*, **9,** 1178 (1949).
Senna. *Arch. Soc. oftal. hisp-amer.*, **4,** 227 (1944).
Sherman. *Amer. J. Ophthal.*, **22,** 1368 (1939).
Shipman. *Amer. J. Ophthal.*, **32,** 825 (1949).
Shoemaker. *Amer. J. Ophthal.*, **2,** 590 (1919).
Snell. *Brit. med. J.*, **1,** 843 (1881); **2,** 923, 957 (1883).
Somerville-Large. *Brit. J. Ophthal.*, **30,** 208 (1946).
Spinelli. *Atti Soc. Oftal. ital.*, **12,** 21 (1950).
Stallard. *Brit. J. Ophthal.*, **31,** 12 (1947); **34,** 511 (1950).
Eye Surgery, Bristol (1946); 4th ed. (1965).
Stieren. *Amer. J. Ophthal.*, **15,** 1120 (1932).
J. Amer. med. Ass., **123,** 880 (1943).
Suckling. *Trans. ophthal. Soc. N.Z.*, **18,** 47 (1966).
Sweet. *Ophthal. Rec.*, **10,** 92 (1901).
Trans. Sect. Ophthal., Amer. med. Ass., 370 (1906).
Thiel. *Klin. Mbl. Augenheilk.*, **112,** 258 (1947).
Thorpe. *Trans. Amer. Acad. Ophthal.*, **39,** 422 (1934).
Trans. Sect. Ophthal., Amer. med. Ass., 290 (1934).
Arch. Ophthal., **15,** 308 (1936).
J. Amer. med. Ass., **137,** 197 (1945).
Surg. Gynec. Obstet., **84,** 809 (1947).
Acta XVIII int. Cong. Ophthal., Montreal–N.Y., **2,** 1673 (1958).
Complications in Eye Surgery (ed. Fasanella), Phila., 45 (1965).
Turberville. *Phil. Trans.*, **14,** 736 (1684).
Verhoeff. *Amer. J. Ophthal.*, **15,** 685 (1932).
Volkmann. *Klin. Mbl. Augenheilk.*, **40** (1), 1, 113, 353 (1902).
Ber. dtsch. ophthal. Ges., **30,** 91, 320 (1902).
Wagenmann. *Ber. dtsch. ophthal. Ges.*, **28,** 170 (1900).
Weigelin. *Klin. Mbl. Augenheilk.*, **59,** 84 (1917).
Weve. *Arch. Augenheilk.*, **80,** 259 (1916).
Whiting and Goulden. *Brit. J. Ophthal.*, **1,** 32 (1917).
Wilczek. *Klin. oczna*, **28,** 127 (1958).
Witmer. *Ophthalmologica*, **117,** 277 (1949).
Wright and Duncan. *Brit. med. J.*, **2,** 658 (1944).
Zintz and Gremmelspacher. *Klin. Mbl. Augenheilk.*, **152,** 69 (1968).

The Ultimate Prognosis of Intra-ocular Foreign Bodies

A reasoned appreciation of the ultimate prognosis of intra-ocular foreign bodies is difficult to present, partly because of the many various factors which must be taken into consideration and partly because of the curious paucity in the literature of long-term observations of such cases. The prognosis, of course, depends primarily on the site of the foreign body within the eye. It also varies with the size and composition of the foreign body, whether it is inert or affects the ocular tissues chemically. In the first case, even if the foreign body is left *in situ*, the prognosis is often good; in the second—a category which includes the great majority of intra-ocular foreign bodies, such as iron and steel and less commonly copper—the prognosis of retention in the absence of secure encapsulation is generally bad. In such cases, therefore, the ultimate prognosis depends essentially on the late results of operation in terms of vision, and this in turn depends upon the type of surgical procedure that has been employed. Non-magnetic foreign bodies obviously entail a worse prognosis than those which are magnetic because of the difficulties in their extraction, but the more recently introduced procedures have not had sufficiently extensive trial nor has sufficient time elapsed to allow any adequate assessment of their ultimate results. The surgery of the removal of magnetic foreign bodies, on the other hand, has been practised for a sufficient length of time to allow some appreciation of the end-results, but even in this type of case the literature is scanty and the ultimate results in terms of vision, so far as they can be assessed, are on the whole somewhat gloomy.

The general prognosis, of course, must include those cases wherein immediate or ultimate enucleation of the eye has to be performed because of mechanical damage to the tissues, the development of sepsis, the persistence of pain and irritation or the onset of glaucoma. Assessing every type of foreign body met with in civilian cases, lodged in all sites within the globe, a summary of representative papers from 1906 to 1940 from different countries shows that on the average the proportion of enucleations was a little over one-third; when the foreign body lodged in the posterior segment of the globe this proportion rose to somewhat less than half (46%).[1] After 1940 the figures relating to all foreign bodies have improved to between 12% and 20%.[2]

If it has been possible to retain the eye, the removal of a foreign body from the anterior chamber has a good prognosis, and in the majority of cases useful vision has resulted and remained permanently (Cridland, 1933; and others). If it has been allowed to remain, an inert foreign body may leave the vision undisturbed indefinitely, while a particle which becomes dissociated usually destroys the function of the eye in time. As we have seen, however, there are occasional surprising exceptions such as the case of Lewis (1946), already quoted, wherein a piece of brass remained in the iris for 56 years with the retention of normal vision. As we have also seen, this immunity is more readily extended to foreign bodies retained within the substance of the lens where, even although the material is potentially toxic, the particle may occasionally remain indefinitely without disturbing the function of the eye.

If, however, the foreign body has come to rest in the posterior segment, particularly if it has entered anteriorly and traversed and injured the lens, the ultimate visual results after successful extraction are much less good. The available evidence in the literature shows that after a surgically successful extraction from the posterior segment 22% to 40% of the eyes eventually have no useful vision, 16% to 34% have some useful vision and 16% to 44% good vision.

In the literature the number of cases wherein foreign bodies were successfully removed from the posterior segment and a follow-up of 5 years or longer with records of the visual acuity had been undertaken is unfortunately very small. In Hirschberg's (1890) series of cases, 3 occurred wherein extraction by the anterior route was employed, the visual results of which after 10, 6 and 7 years respectively were 6/12, 6/36 and finger-

[1] These figures are based on the reports of Sweet (1901–13) 982 cases, Goulden (1908) 118 cases, Dransart and Famechon (1901) 62 cases, Elschnig (1913) 68 cases, Clegg (1916) 130 cases, Cridland (1916–33) 77 cases, Brownlie (1915) 55 cases, Allport (1925) 223 cases, Vancea (1930) 42 cases, Stieren (1932) 700 cases.

[2] Trevor-Roper (1944) 150 cases, 18%; McBride (1949) 50 cases, 20%; Sellas (1949) 414 cases, 13%; Roper-Hall (1954) 555 cases, 20%; Stevens (1956) 47 cases, 12.7%; Levy (1958) 272 cases, 19%; Queiroz Abreu (1960), 101 cases, 17%; Chisholm (1964) 81 cases, 14.8%; Remky *et al.* (1967) 403 cases, 11.9%.

counting. In Goulden's (1908) series 2 cases (anterior route extractions) after 5 years had vision of 6/12 and 6/36 respectively.

Clegg's (1916) series included one case wherein the posterior route was used, in which the vision was 6/18 after 9 years, and 4 cases of anterior route extraction wherein the vision after 5, 5, 6 and 14 years was finger-counting, 6/12, 6/18 and J. 20.

A considerable series was reported by Sweet (1913) in which the extraction was by the posterior route; these are summarized in Table XXI:

TABLE XXI

VISUAL RESULTS AFTER EXTRACTION OF A FOREIGN BODY

(Sweet, 1913)

	Blind	Perception of Light or Finger-counting	Useful Vision 3/60 to 6/12	Good Vision 6/9 or 6/6
After 5 years (7)	2	5	–	–
,, 6 ,, (12)	5	5	1	1
,, 7 ,, (7)	2	1	2	2
,, 8 ,, (5)	1	2	1	1
,, 9 ,, (4)	1	1	1	1
,, 10 ,, (2)	–	1	–	1
,, 11 ,, (6)	2	3	1	–
,, 12 ,, (1)	–	1	–	–
,, 13 ,, (4)	2	–	1	1

Holzer (1929) recorded a single case of a steel foreign body removed 6 weeks after the accident; 4 days later the vision was normal and it was still normal after 9 years.

Cridland (1933) reported 12 cases seen from 5 to 21 years after the injury when the foreign body was removed by different routes:

V. 6/6 in 3 cases examined 13, 18 and 21 years later.

V. 6/12 in 2 cases examined 7 and 12 years later.

V. 6/36 or 6/60 in 4 cases examined 5½, 6, 8½ and 12 years later.

Recognition of hand-movements or finger-counting in 2 cases examined 14 and 16 years later.

Blind, 1 case examined 14 years later.

Stieren's (1932) analysis of about 700 cases examined from 1 to 25 years after the original accident showed the following results after surgical extraction of the foreign body: V. 20/20, 5%; 20/30 to 20/100, 22%; 20/120 to 20/200, 26%; 20/240 to light perception, 32%. Enucleations, 15%.

Of 72 cases in Roper-Hall's (1954) series which were followed up for more than 2 years, 60% had vision better than 6/18 and 40% worse. In Levy's (1958) series of 201 cases which were followed up for varying periods from 3 to 10 years, 41% had vision of 6/9 or better, 25% between 6/9 and 6/60, and 34% less than 6/60.

When the foreign body is in the posterior segment of the globe and has been allowed to remain there, the end-results in terms of vision are extraordinarily difficult to assess. The prognosis depends essentially on the size and nature of the particle. An inert foreign body may well remain indefinitely without damaging the function of the eye; the presence of a chemically active particle is almost invariably disastrous although, as we have seen, striking exceptions may occasionally occur; while in the case of the usual iron and steel (magnetic) foreign bodies the long-term prognosis in terms of vision is gloomy. It is true, as we have seen, that the eye may be preserved in many cases, but the gradual development of retinal degeneration is the rule and the chances of the retention of satisfactory function are small (Figs. 437, 608–9). Most of such eyes, of course, are enucleated for one reason or another at a relatively early stage (irritation, tension, siderosis), but of those which have survived many have been functionally useless after a period greater than 5 years.[1]

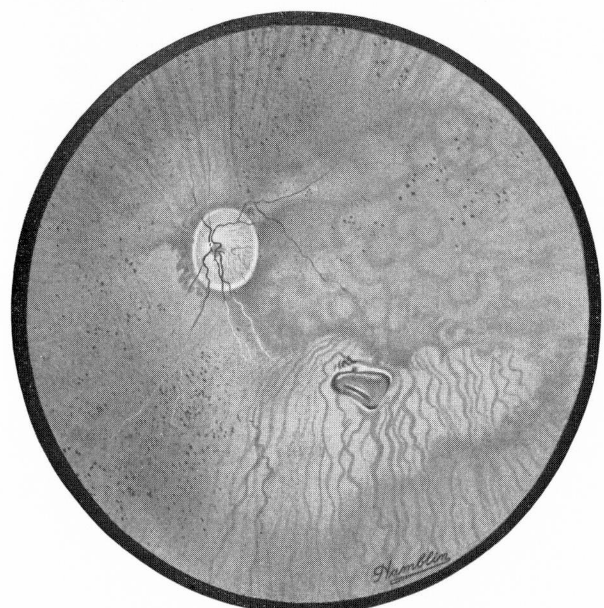

FIG. 608.—ATROPHIC CHANGES AFTER THE PROLONGED RETENTION OF A FOREIGN BODY.

The fundus 12 years after the impaction of a foreign body in the retina. There are diffuse atrophic and pigmentary changes and the retina is in a condition of siderosis (B. Cridland).

These estimates concerning metallic foreign bodies are based on the following cases, admittedly too few to have real statistical significance. The reports of long-term end-results in the literature are, however, rare, particularly in recent writings.

Hirschberg (1905), vision 5/7 after 18 years; Goulden (1908), blind after 6 years; 6/9 after 19 years; Ballantyne (1910), blind after 15 years; Sweet (1913), 5 cases all blind after a period varying from 5 to 7 years; Roll (1921), 6/18 after 18 years; Bell (1921), 20/70 after 15 years; Dixon (1930), blind after 42 years; Spratt (1933), blind after 64 years; Whittington (1933), blind after 12 years; Cridland (1933), 3 cases—6/12 after 18 years, hand-movements after 9 years, and blind after 6½ years.

It is not surprising considering the delicacy of the ocular tissues that the immediate prognosis of the lodgment of a foreign body within it involves

[1] p. 646.

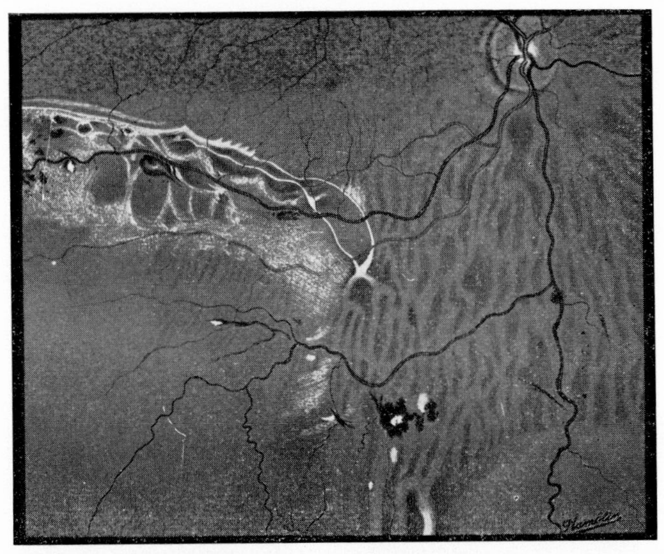

Fig. 609.—Degeneration as an Aftermath of a Foreign Body.

The foreign body—a piece of steel—was removed from the vitreous a few days after the initial accident. The illustration shows the widespread degeneration which developed 12 years following surgical removal (B. Cridland) (see also Fig. 437).

a high proportion of enucleations. It is also understandable that if the particle rests in the anterior segment the ultimate prognosis in terms of vision after removal is relatively good. But it is surprising that, despite the almost mathematical exactness of localization, despite the thrill of successful achievement on operative removal, and despite the retention of vision for some time thereafter, the end-results in terms of ultimate vision of successful extraction from the posterior segment are mediocre.

Allport. *Amer. J. Ophthal.*, **8,** 472 (1925).
Ballantyne. *Glasg. med. J.*, **74,** 133 (1910).
Bell. *Arch. Ophthal.*, **50,** 464 (1921).
Brownlie. *Ophthalmoscope*, **13,** 316 (1915).
Chisholm. *Brit. J. Ophthal.*, **48,** 364 (1964).
Clegg. *Trans. ophthal. Soc. U.K.*, **36,** 36 (1916).
Cridland. *Trans. ophthal. Soc. U.K.*, **36,** 127 (1916); **53,** 438 (1933).
Dixon. *N.Y. Eye, Ear Infirm. clin. Rep.*, **50,** 3 (1930).
Dransart and Famechon. *Bull. Soc. franç. Ophtal.*, **27,** 483 (1910).
Elschnig. *Zbl. prakt. Augenheilk.*, **37,** 230 (1913).
Goulden. *Roy. Lond. ophthal. Hosp. Rep.*, **27,** 301 (1908).
Hirschberg. *v. Graefes Arch. Ophthal.*, **36** (3), 37 (1890).
Zbl. prakt. Augenheilk., **29,** 41 (1905).
Holzer. *Arch. Ophthal.*, **2,** 619 (1929).
Levy. *Brit. J. Ophthal.*, **42,** 610 (1958).
Lewis. *Amer. J. Ophthal.*, **29,** 1164 (1946).
McBride. *Amer. J. Ophthal.*, **32,** 1255 (1949).
Queiroz Abreu. *Arch. Inst. Penido Burnier*, **17,** 27 (1960).
Remky, Kobor and Pfeiffer. *An. Inst. Barraquer*, **7,** 487 (1967).
Roll. *Proc. roy. Soc. Med., Sect. Ophthal.*, **14,** 25 (1921).
Roper-Hall. *Brit. J. Ophthal.*, **38,** 65 (1954).
Sellas. *Arch. Soc. oftal. hisp.-amer.*, **9,** 1178 (1949).
Spratt. *Arch. Ophthal.*, **9,** 102 (1933).
Stevens. *Brit. J. Ophthal.*, **40,** 622 (1956).
Stieren. *Amer. J. Ophthal.*, **15,** 1120 (1932).
Sweet. *Ophthal. Rec.*, **10,** 92 (1901).
Trans. Sect. Ophthal., Amer. med. Ass., 370 (1906).
Trans. Amer. ophthal. Soc., **13,** 412 (1913).
Trevor-Roper. *Brit. J. Ophthal.*, **28,** 361 (1944).
Vancea. *Cluj. Med.*, **11,** 552 (1930).
Whittington. *Proc. roy. Soc. Med., Sect. Ophthal.*, **26,** 57 (1933).

FOREIGN BODIES IN THE OCULAR ADNEXA

Foreign bodies in the ocular adnexa—neglecting for the moment multiple foreign bodies received in explosions and high-velocity missiles, which are considered separately[1]—involve fewer problems than do those lodging within the eye.

Foreign Bodies in the Lids

In the lids the retention of a foreign body is rare, for it usually traverses these relatively thin structures and enters the orbit or the globe. Pieces of stone, pellets of shot which are almost spent, splinters of glass or pieces of

Figs. 610 and 611.—Granuloma of the Upper Lid.

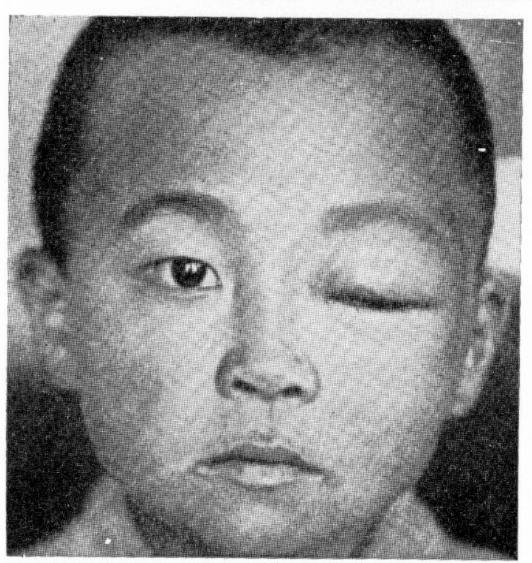

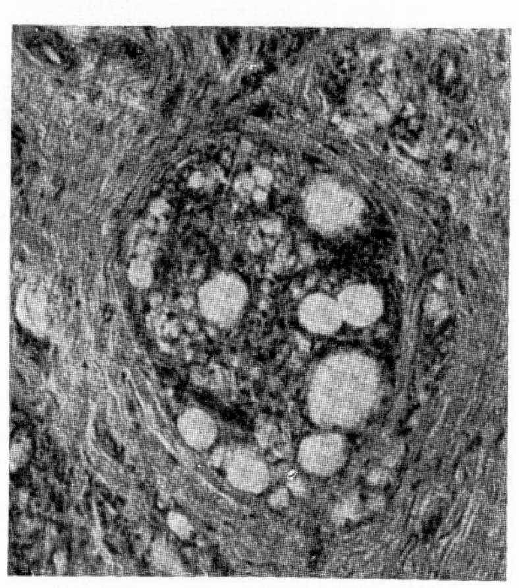

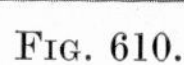

Fig. 610. Fig. 611.

Fig. 610.—In an 8-year-old boy. The swelling of the lids appeared immediately after a mastoid operation on the same side in which an oil, stimulating connective-tissue growth, was injected into the mastoid wound. Fig. 611 shows a typical "foreign-body" type of granuloma in the tissues of the lid (H. Mita).

metal or of wood, however, sometimes bury themselves under the skin of the lids and there remain. It is rare for a foreign body to penetrate a lid and project from its under surface, scratching the cornea, an unfortunate circumstance which has happened, for example, with the sting of a bee (Hilbert, 1904; Kraupa, 1911; Orendorff, 1911; Dorff, 1921).

Pieces of metal or inert material usually become encapsulated and lie dormant in the lids unless infection develops (glass, 10 years, Chevallereau, 1889). Irritant substances, however, and particularly organic material such as wood, may excite a proliferative reaction resulting in the formation of a non-specific granuloma. Such a tumour is usually small but rapidly growing, soft in consistency and without tenderness, and is some-

[1] Chapter V.

times associated with considerable swelling and œdema of the lids. Histologically the mass is made up of dense connective tissue infiltrated with lymphocytes and occasional plasma cells, while the constant presence of giant cells indicates that the tumour is in reality a mechanism of tissue-defence against the foreign matter.

Such tumours have been seen after the embedding in the tissues of the lids of aniline (Mylius, 1926), drops of oil (Mita, 1931) (Figs. 610–11), talc (Sysi, 1950), or paraffin (Uhthoff, 1905; Adler, 1905; Müller, 1905; Sallmann, 1928; and others). Particles of wood, however, give rise to the most common tumour; a small, slowly growing lump is formed which resembled in one case a tuberculoma (Roche, 1911) and in another a meibomian granuloma (Tooke, 1934, after 3½ years) (Fig. 612).

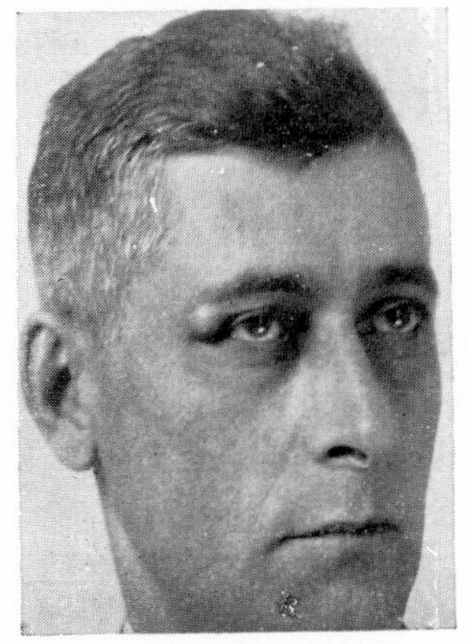

FIG. 612.—CYST FORMATION AROUND A SPLINTER OF WOOD.

Two splinters of wood pierced the skin of the lid in a slight accident which excited no attention at the time. Three and a half years later these were encapsulated in a cyst simulating a meibomian or sebaceous cyst. There were no inflammatory signs nor tenderness (F. T. Tooke).

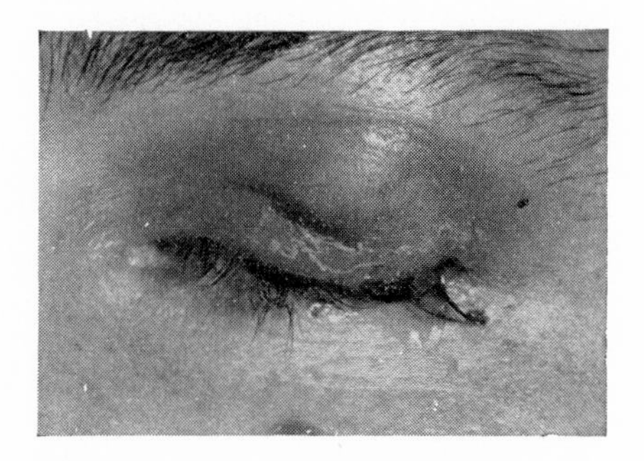

FIG. 613.—SUPERFICIAL ABSCESS OF THE LID.

Three small pieces of stone were retained in the upper lid after a fall from a bicycle. The abscess formed 3 weeks after healing of the laceration.

The most common *complication* of such injuries is the development of infection; if it is acute an abscess of the lid may form (Fig. 613); if chronic, a discharging fistula through which the foreign body itself may eventually be extruded.

A much more rare reaction in the presence of mild staphylococcal infection is the development of the soft granulomatous and very vascular mass known as a *telangiectatic granuloma* (granuloma pyogenicum) or *botryomycosis*.[1]

Tetanus, which may appear clinically in its cephalic manifestations,[2] is always to be remembered as a potential danger in such injuries, particularly when the retained material is of wood. Cases wherein this unfortunate sequel has developed have been reported after a wooden foreign body has been buried in the tissues of the brow (van der Hoeve, 1920) or in the lids (Littwin, 1947).

[1] Vol. XIII. [2] p. 428.

The *diagnosis* of a foreign body in the lids usually presents little difficulty since it is readily felt through the thin tissues although, when a chronic granulomatous reaction occurs, a neoplasm may be simulated. *Treatment* by removal of the foreign body, after incision if necessary, is usually simply accomplished, and the prognosis concerns the cosmetic appearance rather than the ultimate function.

Adler. *Zbl. prakt. Augenheilk.*, **29**, 104 (1905).
Chevallereau. *Recueil Ophtal.*, **11**, 306 (1889).
Dorff. *Klin. Mbl. Augenheilk.*, **67**, 256 (1921).
Hilbert. *Wschr. Therap. Hyg. Auges*, **7**, 201 (1904).
van der Hoeve. *Ned. T. Geneesk.*, **64**, 1173 (1920).
Kraupa. *Zbl. prakt. Augenheilk.*, **35**, 321 (1911).
Littwin. *Amer. J. Ophthal.*, **30**, 201 (1947).
Mita. *Klin. Mbl. Augenheilk.*, **86**, 59 (1931).
Müller. *Zbl. prakt. Augenheilk.*, **29**, 106 (1905).
Mylius. *Z. Augenheilk.*, **56**, 302 (1925); **59**, 64 (1926).
Orendorff. *Ophthal. Rec.*, **20**, 242 (1911).
Roche. *Recueil Ophtal.*, **33**, 317 (1911).
Sallmann. *Z. Augenheilk.*, **65**, 298 (1928).
Sysi. *Acta ophthal.* (Kbh.), **28**, 257 (1950).
Tooke. *Brit. J. Ophthal.*, **18**, 695 (1934).
Uhthoff. *Berl. klin. Wschr.*, **42**, 1461 (1905).

Foreign Bodies in the Lacrimal Passages

The retention of foreign bodies in the lacrimal passages is not common, but occasionally particles are washed by the tears from the conjunctival sac into the canaliculus or down into the lacrimal sac where they may be retained causing irritative or inflammatory symptoms.

IN THE PUNCTUM a cilium is the most common intruder and it is not an unusual occurrence for the lash to protrude from either the upper or lower punctum, irritating the cornea and conjunctiva, causing considerable photophobia and lacrimation and occasionally corneal abrasions and opacities. Such a foreign body is readily missed on clinical examination, particularly when the upper punctum is involved.[1] Other foreign bodies have been reported in this locality, such as hair (Glass, 1880), the bristle of a brush (Lachmann, 1926), pieces of grain (Praun, 1899) and other vegetable debris (Rosenstein, 1925)—even a round worm (Haffner, 1880) or an insect (Wolffberg, 1900). Occasionally calculi (dacryoliths), wherein a deposit of calcium carbonate and phosphate surrounds the foreign body, are found in the canaliculus (Rosenstein, 1925), but it will be remembered that such concretions in this site are generally due to mycotic infection.

As a rule, apart from the ocular symptoms of irritation, the punctum becomes dilated and the canaliculus occasionally shows a non-specific granulomatous proliferation forming a polyp (Serra, 1926, from a cilium); more rarely a suppurative inflammation may develop into an abscess. Occasionally the foreign body may be spontaneously extruded (the broken-off tip of a probe, Costenbader, 1945). More usually, however, active measures are required to remove it, slitting and curetting of the canaliculus if necessary, whereafter recovery is usually rapid.

More rarely the foreign body finds its way downwards into the SAC and

[1] Noyes (1889), Sous (1892), Ellett (1900), Vollert (1911), Boase (1949), Stern (1952), and others.

the NASO-LACRIMAL DUCT where it may set up inflammatory changes. These may be acute (an insect, Wolffberg, 1900), but more frequently they are chronic (a cilium, Rehr, 1894). A case has been recorded wherein a cast in the middle of which lay a cilium was blown out of the naso-lacrimal duct (Garfin, 1942); while a nail introduced into the canaliculus has remained in the sac to be discovered accidentally after 10 years—a tribute to the tolerance of the tissues (Neuschuler, 1934). Pieces of surgical instruments (sounds, probes, etc.) have been similarly retained, frequently exciting little reaction (Halle, 1918; 17 years, Rodin, 1928), but sometimes causing chronic inflammation and the formation of a fistula (Hasty, 1931, 25 years), and

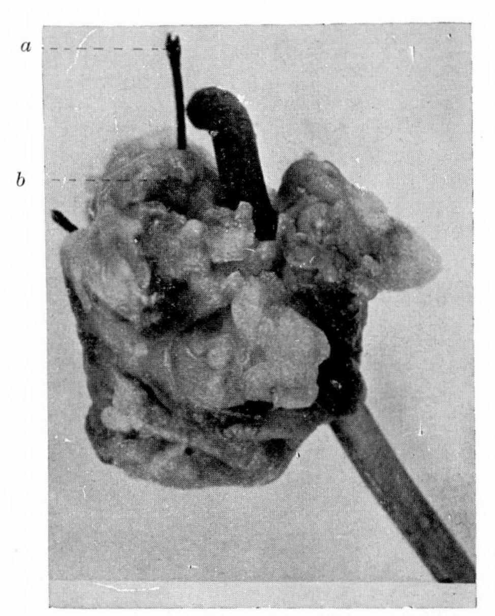

FIG. 614.—CHRONIC GRANULOMA OF THE LACRIMAL SAC.

Produced by a metal style (*b*), which had been left in the naso-lacrimal duct for 33 years. The upper pole of the sac is identified by a suture (*a*) (H. B. Stallard).

occasionally exciting the development of granulomata which are usually polypoid but may progress to fill the entire sac (Stallard, 1940, in a case of a style retained for 33 years) (Fig. 614). More usually, however, foreign bodies in the lower passages are introduced from the nose and, becoming calcified, remain as rhinoliths near the lower ostium.

This last occurrence is exemplified in a case recorded by Malgat (1890), wherein the stalk of a lettuce leaf in the nose was driven thence into the naso-lacrimal duct by repeated sneezing, there to form an abscess.

Concretions in the lacrimal sac are much rarer than in the canaliculus and, although they are usually associated with infection by fungi, they may also become aggregated around foreign material. Sanguinetti (1933) found a concretion in a lacrimal sac which proved to be a vegetable seed surrounded by a calcareous shell; and Lewis (1938) described a large cheesy concretion, 5 mm. in length, washed out of the lacrimal duct, consisting of degenerated cells and amorphous debris in which no fungi or organisms were found. Grönvall (1944) found a large concretion in a case of argyrosis of the sac with a clump of black silver granules at its centre (Figs. 615–616). Such concretions show a laminated structure after the manner of a sea-shell (Fig. 616), the whole being heavily impregnated with calcium salts although

FIGS. 615 and 616.—DACRYOLITH OF THE LACRIMAL SAC.

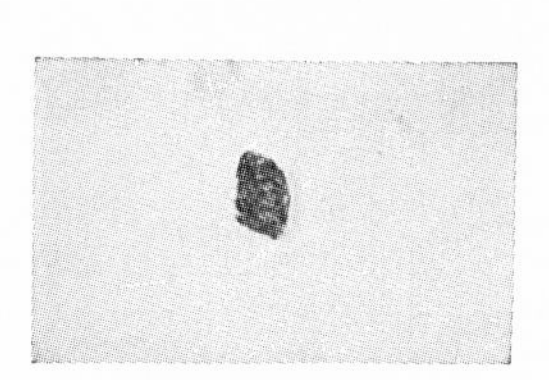

FIG. 615.—From a 71-year-old man with chronic dacryocystitis and intermittent epiphora. Natural size.

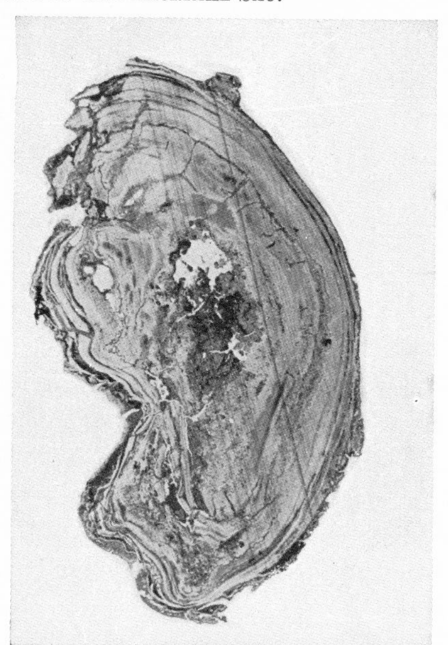

FIG. 616.—The decalcified dacryolith from Fig. 615, showing its stratified structure around a central conglomeration of the brown pigment of argyrosis (Herman Grönvall).

FIG. 616.

traces of many elements may be present (Ag, Mg, Fe, Al, Cu, Na, P, Si, Grönvall, 1944). The dacryolith is thus made up of a multitude of strata indicating its slow method of growth, the outermost showing fibrin, agglomerations of bacteria and wandering cells in all stages of necrosis, the innermost becoming more and more structureless. Such a concretion occurs only in the presence of a chronic dacryocystitis and is usually not diagnosed until an operation undertaken for this condition reveals its presence. An interesting sign is that an intermittent patency of the lacrimal passages may exist, syringing sometimes giving a positive and at other times a negative result (Kofler, 1941; Grönvall, 1944); it is as if the stone acts as an intermittent plug as in other vesicular organs such as the urinary or gall bladder.

Such foreign bodies require surgical removal either by incising the anterior wall of the sac or through an intranasal approach.

It is worthy of note that a foreign body retained for long in the nose may cause an angioneurotic œdema of the lids, as occurred, for example, in a case reported by Pruzanski (1951), wherein a peanut was retained in this locality for 17 years.

Boase. *Brit. J. Ophthal.*, **33,** 513 (1949).
Costenbader. *Amer. J. Ophthal.*, **28,** 754 (1945).
Ellett. *Ophthal. Rec.*, **9,** 285 (1900).
Garfin. *Arch. Ophthal.*, **27,** 167 (1942).
Glass. *Med. Rec.* (N.Y.), **18,** 612 (1880).
Grönvall. *Acta ophthal.* (Kbh.), **21,** 247 (1944).
Haffner. *Berl. klin. Wschr.*, **17,** 346 (1880).
Halle. *Münch. med. Wschr.*, **64,** 1537 (1918).
Hasty. *Amer. J. Ophthal.*, **14,** 450 (1931).
Kofler. *Klin. Mbl. Augenheilk.*, **106,** 712 (1941).
Lachmann. *Med. Klin.*, **22,** 812 (1926).
Lewis. *Amer. J. Ophthal.*, **21,** 789 (1938).
Malgat. *Recueil Ophtal.*, **12,** 209 (1890).
Neuschuler. *Rass. ital. Ottal.*, **3,** 91 (1934).
Noyes. *Amer. J. Ophthal.*, **6,** 245 (1889).
Praun. *Die Verletzungen d. Auges,* Wiesbaden, 451 (1899).
Pruzanski. *J. Amer. med. Ass.*, **147,** 1234 (1951).
Rehr. *Zur Aetiologie u. Therapie d. Dakryocystitis* (Diss.), Kiel (1894).
Rodin. *J. Amer. med. Ass.*, **91,** 1546 (1928).
Rosenstein. *Klin. Mbl. Augenheilk.*, **75,** 156 (1925).
Sanguinetti. *Rass. ital. Ottal.*, **2,** 462 (1933).
Serra. *Boll. Oculist.*, **5,** 331 (1926).
Sous. *J. Méd. Bordeaux*, **22,** 413 (1892).
Stallard. *Brit. J. Ophthal.*, **24,** 457 (1940).
Stern. *Amer. J. Ophthal.*, **35,** 1206 (1952).
Vollert. *Klin. Mbl. Augenheilk.*, **49** (1), 509 (1911).
Wolffberg. *Wschr. Therap. Hyg. Auges*, **3,** 261 (1900).

Foreign Bodies in the Orbit

Foreign bodies in the orbit, apart from the development of infection following their entry, cause damage less by their presence than by the injuries they may inflict upon the many important structures crowded into this region. They may be the ends of objects forced into the orbit and broken off and thus retained, or flying particles which usually have sufficient energy to penetrate nearly to the apex, where they are frequently stopped by bone. In either case, owing to the protection of the bony walls, such foreign bodies usually enter the orbit from the anterior aspect, passing through the lids and conjunctiva. Larger objects tend to enter the inner canthus, often injuring the caruncle; entry through the upper or lower lid is more rare, through the external canthus rarest of all; and the general tendency is for such bodies to slip past the globe and bury themselves deeply in the orbital tissues. In such an event the eye frequently escapes injury even although the object may be large (a piece of wood $3\frac{1}{4} \times \frac{5}{8} \times \frac{1}{2}$ in., Maxwell, 1952) (Fig. 617), but the globe may suffer some contusion so that injuries such as an intra-ocular hæmorrhage, a dislocation of the lens, a ruptured choroid or a detached retina may result; as a rule, however, gross damage to the globe is reserved for missiles travelling at high velocities, as are typified in gunshot wounds.[1] Only occasionally does a sharp thin foreign body traverse the globe to reach the recesses of the orbit, such as a knitting needle, which continued on its way into the cranium (Pagenstecher, 1864), an awl (Fromaget, 1896) or a sharp splinter of steel (Sattler, 1884) or wood (Mayweg, 1907), which on occasion has gone through into the nose after traversing

[1] Chapter V.

the eye (Ramorino, 1887). A flying particle, on the other hand, if small and travelling at high speed, may well pass through the globe, causing a double perforation on its way, and come to rest in the retrobulbar tissues.

Occasionally, if the foreign body enters with sufficient force and is of sufficient size to be endowed with great momentum, it may cause damage beyond the confines of the orbit itself. The orbital walls may be fractured, usually the greater wing of the sphenoid or, in more extensive injuries, such parts of the base of the skull as the petrous portion of the temporal bone and the sella turcica, while occasionally tiny objects such as small-shot or sharp instruments of small calibre may leave the orbit through one of the various fissures or foramina. Having fractured the orbital walls the foreign body may enter several structures—the frontal sinus (the blade of a knife, Higgens, 1891; a gun-lock, Ellis, 1900), the maxillary antrum (the blade of a knife,

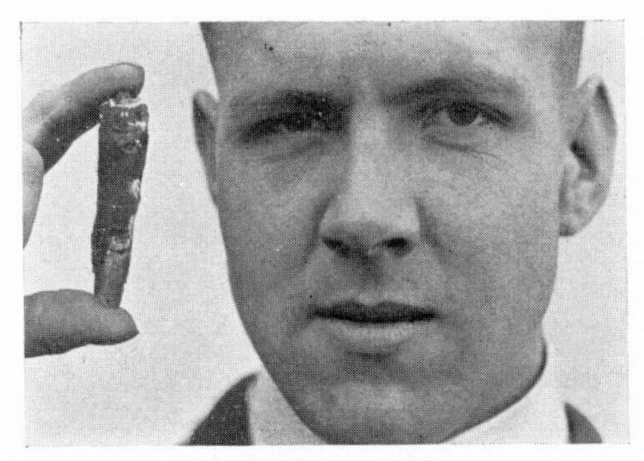

FIG. 617.—ORBITAL FOREIGN BODY.

To show the size of a foreign body which may penetrate into the orbit without lasting ill-effects. A piece of beech wood ($3\frac{1}{4} \times \frac{5}{8} \times \frac{1}{2}$ in.) penetrated the centre of the right upper eyelid, passing through the tarsal plate, displacing the globe backwards and outwards and lying in the right orbit. After removal, recovery was uncomplicated with normal vision (J. P. Maxwell).

Falch, 1879, Zenker, 1898, White and Anderson, 1952; pieces of wood, Schönfelder, 1949), the maxillary, ethmoid and sphenoid sinuses (a twig of a tree, Foucher, 1897) or the nose (a piece of wood, Ramorino, 1887; a file, Praun, 1899). It may traverse the nose and enter the opposite maxillary antrum (a knife, Zenker, 1898, a case wherein the blade remained for 12 years; Thomas, 1942), or the opposite orbit to form a bilateral orbital foreign body (the blade of a knife, Eber, 1940). On the other hand, it may enter the pterygo-maxillary fossa (the coiled spring from an exploded gun which entered the orbit through the upper lid, Peronnet and Bouyer, 1948), or the zygomatic fossa (Haine, 1847). Many such instances can be cited from the literature, and the seriousness of the injury is, of course, frequently considerably enhanced when entrance is made into the periorbital cavities by the increased tendency towards the development of infection, and when the cranial cavity is involved by the complication of cerebral injury which, if not immediately fatal, may well lead subsequently to the development of meningitis or a cerebral abscess. Pagenstecher (1864–67), for example, recorded a case wherein part of a knitting needle penetrated the inner wall of the orbit and passed along the internal surface of the cranial cavity towards the right petrous bone, where it lay for 17 years without the patient's knowledge; the eventual removal of the eye and the needle proved fatal owing to multiple cerebral abscesses.

Not all such cases, however, are equally disastrous (see Fig. 393). Thus Rees (1947) found that a twig had penetrated the upper lid and entered the cranial cavity where its end rested in the interpeduncular space, destroying in its path all the ocular motor nerves, the first division of the trigeminal and the optic nerve; although the eye was irreparably damaged, the twig was safely removed by forceps along its path of entrance. Similarly,

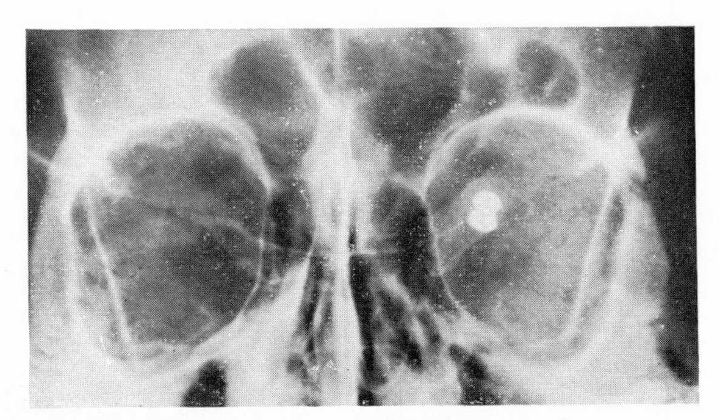

Fig. 618.—An Airgun Pellet in the Orbit.
The same case as Figs. 1, 2 and 4 in Plate III.

Smaill (1958) reported that a stick penetrated beyond the posterior clinoid process without serious damage. Noyes (1890) reported a case wherein the breech-pin of a gun was buried partly in the orbit and partly in the cranial cavity and remained there for five months, while in a somewhat similar case recorded by Gifford (1905) the foreign body remained for two years.

The *types of foreign body* which may be retained in the orbit are innumerable. Small particles of metal are a commonplace, particularly in engineering workshops; as a result of explosions or in the injuries characteristic of war, such wounds are frequently multiple (Fig. 633), while similar multiple injuries not uncommonly result from the accidental discharge of small-shot (129 pellets in the orbit, Philipps, 1888) (Fig. 630). Many types of metallic objects may be thrust into the orbit and are broken off and buried, while practically every conceivable, and occasionally an almost inconceivable, object has found its way into its recesses.

Figs. 619 to 621.—Granulomata from Talc Powder (G. L. McCormick *et al.*)

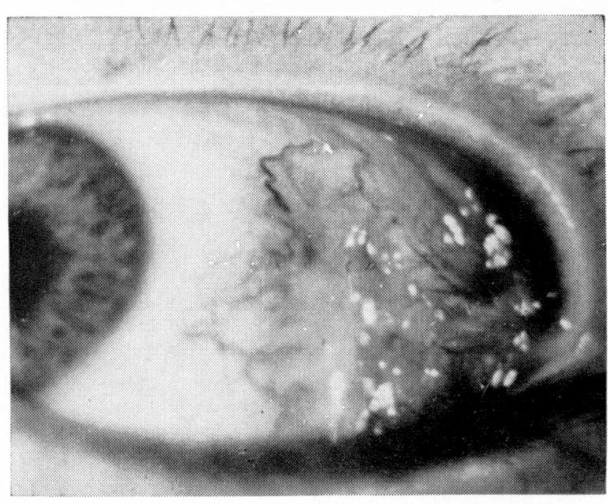

Fig. 619.—Granulomatous mass forming a semi-translucent tumour on the temporal portion of the right eye at the site of an operation for squint carried out 14 years previously.

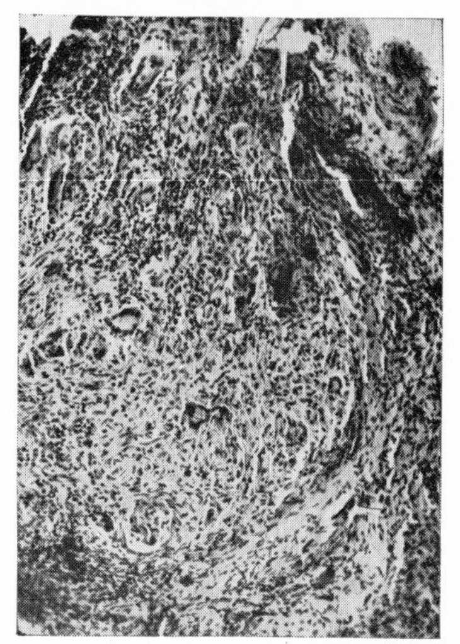

Fig. 620.—Section of the granuloma from Fig. 619, showing the typical foreign-body reaction with epithelioid cells and giant cells (× 98).

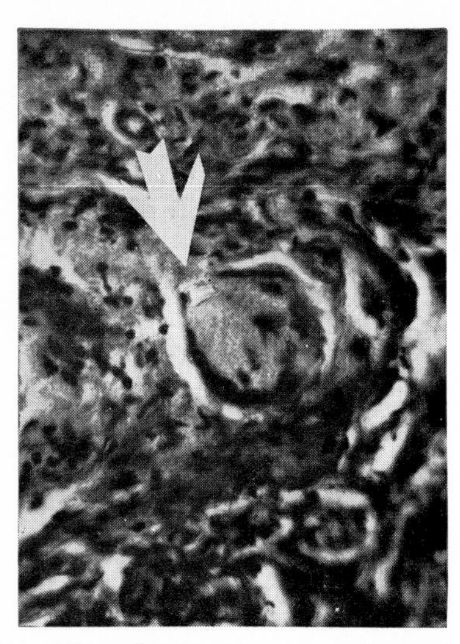

Fig. 621.—Section showing a large giant cell enclosing a minute talc crystal (indicated by the arrow) (× 330).

Metallic objects thrust into the orbit and there retained constitute a heterogeneous collection. A knife blade, usually used for assault, is common (Zenker, 1898; Junius, 1909; Eber, 1940; Thomas, 1942; Louw, 1950), or an awl (Kellner, 1878; Fromaget, 1896), the tine of a steel fork (Keiper, 1905), an arrow (Aub, 1871), and many others. Missiles from toy pistols or airguns are unfortunately too frequent (Peabody, 1962; Sacks and Matheson, 1962; Lalla and Pillai, 1965; Grom and Carvajal, 1967; Curtis and Provan, 1970) (Fig. 618). An interesting group of injuries has resulted from the bursting of fire-arms in the vicinity of the eye, an accident which has sometimes resulted in the impaction of enormous foreign bodies in the orbit, such as the breech-pin of a gun (Noyes, 1890; Gifford, 1905), a breech-pin associated with a long screw (Ledbetter, 1905), the stop-bolt of a gun (Morrow, 1904), a piece of gun-lock (Ellis, 1900), the extractor spring from a Winchester rifle (Baker, 1906), or the coiled spring from a shot-gun (Peronnet and Bouyer, 1948). Pieces of flying stone or wood, either broken-off twigs or pieces of wood detached while chopping, are frequent, as also are pieces of wooden implements or even the root of a plant shot from a catapult (Skacel, 1950) (Fig. 617). Vegetable material such as blades of straw are much more rarely found (Mackenzie, 1856; von Hippel, 1912), while oddities include a button (Boudin, 1900), a piece of ivory umbrella handle, 4 × 1½ cm. (Nélaton, 1864), an umbrella rib (Neto, 1966), the aluminium end of a paint brush complete with bristles from which the wooden handle had broken off (Wenger, 1946), a piece of whip-lash (Salzer, 1904), the jaw of a fish with six teeth attached (Thomson, 1895), the tip of a pencil (Heyner and Passmore, 1965) or of a billiard-cue (Briggs, 1888; Banks, 1967), the end of a walking stick (Höderath, 1909),

FIGS. 622 and 623.—GRANULATION TISSUE IN THE LID.
Showing a giant cell containing particles of talc.

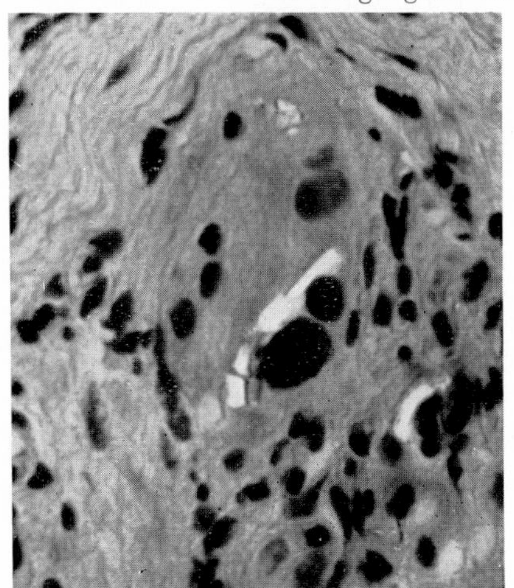

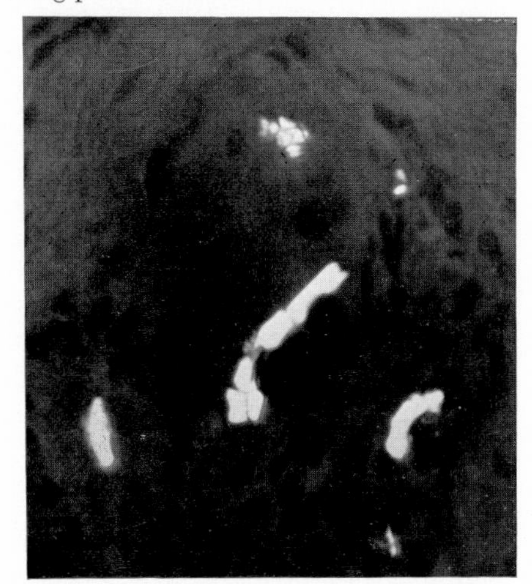

FIG. 622.—In ordinary light; FIG. 623.—In partially polarized light (× 560) (N. Ashton).

a jet of oil from a grease-gun which caused a considerable reaction, and at operation a granuloma was found in the muscle-cone around a globule of grease (Dallas, 1964), or the handle of the bathtub faucet which had first to be sawn off and temporarily left in place to free the victim (Beauchamp and Miller, 1967).

Surgery has also left its foreign bodies behind, sometimes inadvertently, such as a wad of cotton-wool after an operation for enucleation (Michaïl, 1935, around which a hæmatic cyst developed; Duthie, 1941), while the tendency for talcum powder from surgical gloves to produce a granuloma was proved by experiments in the orbits of rabbits by Schwartz and Linn (1951).[1] A clinical case of this type was described by McCormick and his colleagues (1949) wherein granulomata of considerable size containing giant cells and with a sarcoid-like structure developed after an operation for strabismus undertaken 14 years previously (Figs. 619–621). Such granulomatous masses have been reported in many regions of the body where the talcum powder has been left in the tissues (Lichtman *et al.*, 1946; Eiseman, 1947; and others); the histo-

[1] p. 505.

logical diagnosis is clarified by the behaviour of this material with polarized light (Figs. 622–623).

Clinical Picture

The history of an accident involving the lodgment of a foreign body in the orbit is usually definite, but it is often curiously misleading, for in a surprising number of cases the penetration of the orbit may have been looked upon by the patient as a trivial incident or may, indeed, have completely escaped his notice, particularly if he were dazed or concussed at the time of the injury. The diagnosis is often rendered more difficult if the wound of entry is not easily seen in the recesses of the inner canthus or the conjunctival fornices, while the associated swelling of the lids is readily attributable to the œdema or hæmorrhage which is typically associated with a blow or concussive injury. In such circumstances the wound of entry may become closed without the suspicion arising that a foreign body is present.

The surprising extent to which this may occur is illustrated by the classical case reported by Brudenell Carter (1865): a drunkard fell downstairs and impaled his orbit with the shaft of an iron hat-peg, 3·3 in. long, which entered the inner aspect of the palpebral aperture and was broken off; he was completely unaware of its presence until it was removed between 2 and 3 weeks later. Other cases of the same type could be quoted, such as that recorded by Fernandes (1908), wherein a large piece of the cartridge of a shot-gun entered the upper lid and lay unsuspected and without causing symptoms in the orbit for 8 years, whereafter it was unexpectedly and spontaneously extruded without inflammatory symptoms.

Usually, however, the injury is associated with swelling, œdema and proptosis so considerable that the condition is obvious (Fig. 624); but it is to be remembered that the presence of the foreign body excites no specific symptoms unless by reason of its bulk, except perhaps indefinite pain or a feeling of pressure and headache; while if the globe or important structures in the orbit are undamaged ocular symptoms are usually absent. After the initial reaction has died down an inert foreign body may remain indefinitely in the orbit without causing distress. This is readily understandable if it is small, but occasionally it is remarkable how a bulky foreign body may remain in this site without producing symptoms.

If, however, important structures have been damaged visual symptoms may be obvious. Fortunately injuries of such severity are relatively rare. The most common sequel is diplopia following an injury to a muscle or nerve; the most catastrophic, blindness following crushing or section of the optic nerve. These injuries have already been discussed when dealing with penetrating injuries of the orbit, but their rarity as a result of the entrance of foreign bodies is shown by the fact that Cords (1916), discussing 50 cases of retained orbital foreign bodies incurred in war wounds, found that the extra-ocular muscles were damaged only nine times, and the optic nerve twice. The greatest damage, of course, occurs when the foreign body penetrates to the apex of the orbit. Here the optic nerve is almost certainly injured, causing partial or complete blindness (Hirschberg, 1879; Tweedy, 1893; Frost, 1893; and many others). If the superior orbital fissure is involved paresis of more than one of the muscles is the usual sequel, while a foreign body of any size in this region tends to damage all the motor nerves, the first division of the trigeminal and the optic nerve, leaving an immobile, anæsthetic and blind eye (Mende, 1910; Randall, 1910; Rees, 1947; and others). The tragedy of a foreign body implicating both orbits and both optic nerves is a rarity (the blade of a dagger, Luis y Yagiie, 1910), and it is only occasionally that the superior orbital fissure is penetrated without harm (Koster, 1898).

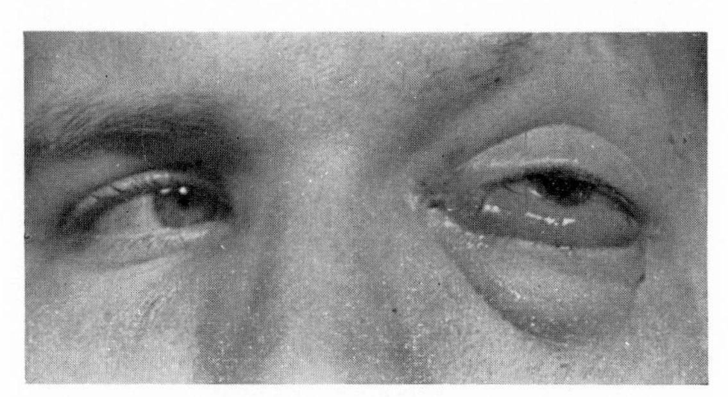

Fig. 624.—Displacement of the Globe with Chemosis caused by the Retention of a Bulky Foreign Body in the Orbit.

Left non-pulsating proptosis accompanied by internal and external ophthalmoplegia. The healed wound of entry of a large deep orbital foreign body was present in the skin inferior to the left external canthal ligament (Byron Smith).

If the foreign body involves the lacrimal gland this tissue may be prolapsed (Haltenhoff, 1902; Jackson, 1904), and in this site the presence of infected foreign material may result in a complete necrosis of the gland (Laval, 1938, small pieces of gravel after a fall).

A foreign body retained in a duct of the lacrimal gland is a great rarity (Oeller, 1878). Calculi in this region are probably always arranged around a matrix of organic material and desquamated epithelial cells or are associated with mycelial infection.

Specific Effects

Fortunately the specific effects of the retention of foreign bodies in the orbit are much less dramatic and harmful than in the eye. The clinical picture varies considerably, depending on the material retained.

Most *metals*, particularly iron, steel, aluminium, lead and others, are inert and in the absence of infection cause no disturbance apart from their bulk. The only metal, in fact, which is badly tolerated is copper which tends to set up a purulent inflammation (von Graefe, 1855; Verderame, 1915; and others), although it may remain for a considerable time before inflammatory symptoms become evident (16 years, Clothier, 1909).

Innumerable instances of the passive behaviour of iron and steel in this respect may be gathered from the literature, of which the following form samples. Higgens (1891) reported the retention of a knife blade in the orbit and frontal sinus for 46 years; Teillais (1893) a knitting needle lying on the inner side of the orbit for 20 years; Zenker (1898) a knife blade in the orbit and maxillary antrum for 12 years, during the latter half of which period a discharging fistula existed; Praun (1899) observed that the end of a file which had remained in the orbit for 30 years passed into the nasal cavity and was eventually extruded from the mouth on sneezing. Holmes (1900) recorded a knife blade, 3·8 × 0·8 cm., which remained in the orbit for 32 years; Ellis (1900) a piece of gun-lock, 29 × 17 × 7·5 mm., in the orbit and frontal sinus for 6½ years; Ledbetter (1905) the breech-block of a gun for 3 years; Keiper (1905) the tine of a steel fork which entered the antrum and remained for 14 years; Gerkowicz (1955) the fragment of a grenade for 9 years—all these and many more. The case of Luis y Yagiie (1910) is of unusual interest. After a wound in the left temple by a dagger which pierced the apices of both orbits and thereby caused bilateral blindness, the point of the dagger was eventually extruded from the upper lid 30 years later.

Apart from metallic substances the more common inert foreign bodies are of glass or stone. Pieces of *glass* give rise to little reaction and have remained quietly for long periods ranging from 14 months (Terentjew, 1909) to 20 years (Ewart, 1903), although after some time a fistula may develop (Adamük, 1896, 8 years). Pieces of *stone* may also remain quietly for a long time unless they are infected, but in this case the infection is usually of a low grade. Thus Teillais (1893) reported the development of infection after 5 years, and Böhm (1907) observed a case wherein a piece of stone was retained for 18 years, during the last 6 months of which an inflammatory swelling developed at the inner canthus.

Organic foreign bodies tend to excite a granulomatous reaction. This reaction may follow the retention of such a body as an ear of corn (Paufique *et al.*, 1952), but the most common material of this nature is *wood*. The response of the tissues may take the form of a granulomatous tumour which usually grows extremely slowly, and many years may elapse before its increasing bulk calls for exploration and excision (Elschnig, 1923). The more usual clinical course is the development of mild but chronic infection leading to the formation of a fistula (Thornell and Williams, 1944; Carré, 1967; and others). Such a fistula may remain discharging indefinitely, but sometimes the foreign material is spontaneously extruded, an event, however, which may occur only after a long interval (2 years, Veasey, 1910; 10 years, Mitkewitsch, 1886; Randall, 1910). It is noteworthy that a long splinter of wood may be broken up as it encounters the resistance of the orbital tissues, and consequently the process of extrusion may occur piecemeal.

Thus Gallus (1897) reported a case wherein 4 weeks after such an injury two fistulæ developed, one on the lid and one in the lower fornix. A piece of wood 5 × 0·5 cm. was extracted, but 2 years later fresh inflammatory signs developed and a new fistula appeared, from which another piece of wood, 4 cm. long, was spontaneously extruded. Packley (1906) reported a somewhat similar case when a second piece of wood was spontaneously extruded 4 years after the removal of the first, the sliver, 1¼ in. long, being found " sticking out of the corner of the eye in the morning " although nothing abnormal had been noticed the night before. The tendency was well illustrated in a case recorded by Jackson (1904) wherein nine pieces of sage-wood had to be removed from a wound in the upper lid on successive attempts before healing eventually occurred.

Complications

Traumatic emphysema may be an immediate complication when the orbital wall is fractured and communication established with an air-cell. This complication, for example, has followed the impaction of a flying stone in the orbit (Jaensch, 1947), when symptoms resembling an acute orbital abscess developed but rapidly subsided on incision and release of the air.

Hæmorrhage into the intra-orbital tissues may form a complication which, however, is usually less serious than the appearance may suggest and is often adequately controlled by bandaging. The wounding of a major vessel—usually a vein—in the depths of the orbit may give rise to alarming

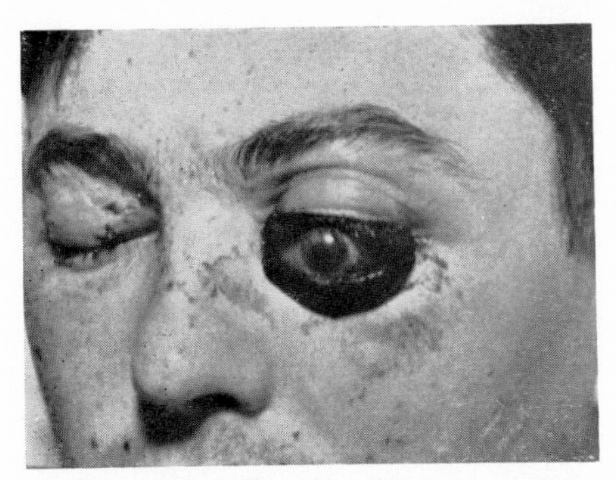

Fig. 625.—Extensive Hæmorrhage in the Orbit ten hours after its Onset.

This late hæmorrhage occurred about 65 hours after wounding by numerous small foreign bodies from an anti-personnel mine (Byron Smith).

secondary hæmorrhages after some days (Fig. 625), but although proptosis and ecchymosis may be severe, adequate pressure-bandaging is sufficient treatment (Smith, 1951).

Pyogenic infection is always to be feared, particularly in the case of retained pieces of wood; even with this material, however, simple and timely antibacterial measures may ensure uncomplicated healing (Maxwell, 1952; Remky *et al.*, 1963). If infection does become established the clinical course may be acute and resemble a widespread cellulitis, a localized abscess may develop, or a less severe infection may result in the formation of a chronic fistula with a purulent or sanguineous discharge which may remain for years until the foreign body is discovered and removed but from which the particle may in the end be spontaneously expelled (Fig. 626). The development of such an infection may, of course, if inadequately treated lead to the onset of periostitis with caries of the underlying bone, a circumstance which itself may prolong the duration of the fistula, while an abscess near the apex of the orbit always involves the danger of the development of an optic neuritis (Pignatari, 1894; Fejer, 1910; Birch-Hirschfeld, 1912; and others).

Of the more specific infections, *gas gangrene* may be encountered, although rarely, and—a complication always to be feared—the development of *tetanus*, often of the cephalic type.[1] A large number of cases appears in the early literature wherein tetanus has developed, most commonly after the retention of pieces of wood in the orbit.[2] Since the danger of this infection has been universally recognized and means of its prevention known, the number of cases in the literature, however, has fallen to insignificant proportions; thus Vossius (1914) prevented the occurrence of tetanus by the timely introduction of antitoxin even although the bacilli were subsequently found on the foreign body.[3]

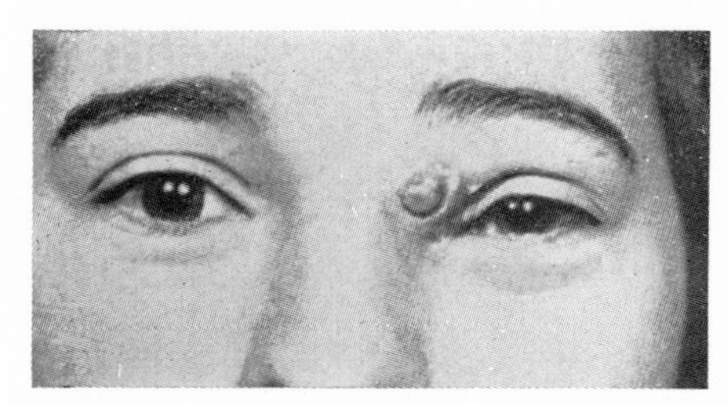

FIG. 626.—The formation of a cyst and a draining fistula from a mildly infected foreign body in the orbit (E. B. Spaeth.

A further complication is the development of proliferating masses of *granulomatous tissue* around the foreign body, a circumstance which occurs when it is irritative, and particularly if it is organic in nature such as wood (Carré, 1967). The appearance of *traumatic cysts* around a foreign body is rare (Michaïl, 1935), while as a late result the formation of *bands of fibrous tissue* resulting from the organization of blood or inflammatory products may cause considerable inconvenience by impairing the motility of the globe.

Sensory disturbances are unusual as a sequel of the retention of a foreign body in the orbit. *Anæsthesia of the eye* and upper lid, as we have seen, may follow injury to the first division of the trigeminal if the object is lodged near the superior orbital fissure; neuroparalytic keratopathy may be a sequel of such a lesion (Hirschberg, 1879; Philipsen, 1887; and others). A *trigeminal neuralgia* affecting this division is a rare result of an injury of this type (Seggel, 1903). A more common sequel is *infra-orbital neuralgia*, when the infra-orbital branch of the maxillary nerve is similarly involved. The pain may occasionally be intense and it may also arise from the presence of sequestrated bone near the infra-orbital canal (Burrows, 1937). A *spastic entropion of the lower lid* is an interesting sequel of a similar irritation and

[1] p. 428.

[2] Cooper (1859), Hotz (1882), Rockliffe (1890), Marx (1893), Fromaget (1894), Darier (1897), Steindorff (1898), Pes (1902), Haltenhoff (1902), Genth (1903), Grünfeld (1905), Mayweg (1907), Damato (1966), and others.

[3] Prophylaxis and treatment, see p. 408.

may result from the presence of a foreign body near the apex of the orbit; the complication appears at a relatively late date after convalescence has apparently become established. The condition may be treated by resecting the nerve or by excising a strip of the orbicularis muscle (Doherty, 1942).

If the injury involves neighbouring structures, of course, complications may be multiplied; thus if a sinus is involved a chronic sinusitis may develop, and if the cranial cavity has been penetrated the clinical picture may be dominated by more dramatic cerebral symptoms, either immediately as from hæmorrhage, particularly if the cavernous sinus has been torn, or subsequently if meningeal infection or a cerebral abscess develops.

Diagnosis

In every open wound of the orbit the evidence regarding which is not clear and conclusive *it is always well to bear in mind the possibility of the presence of a foreign body*, and if an obstinate fistula remains after the normal time of healing, suspicions should be intensified. If the injury is recent, an immediate diagnosis may be difficult since the whole region is obscured by swelling, but careful and judicious search of the wound with a probe frequently leads to the discovery of the retained material. When a chronic fistula develops, however, care should be taken in such an exploration not to confuse

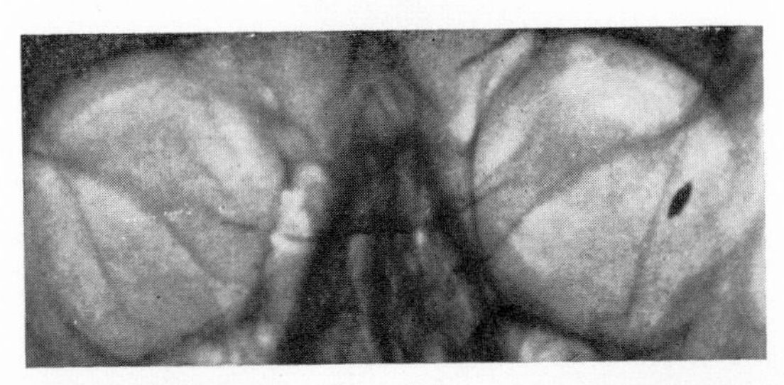

Fig. 627.

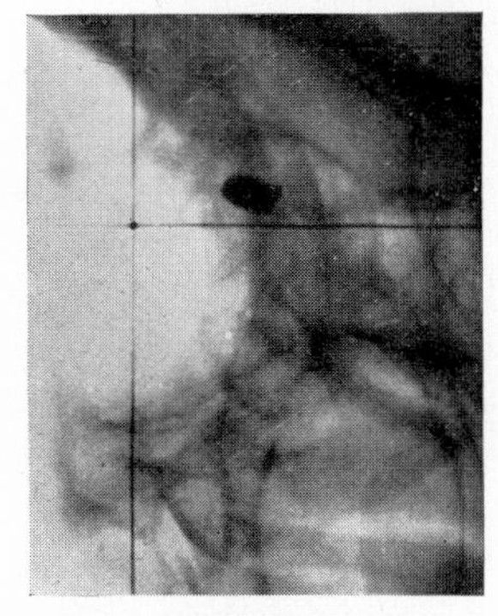

Fig. 628.

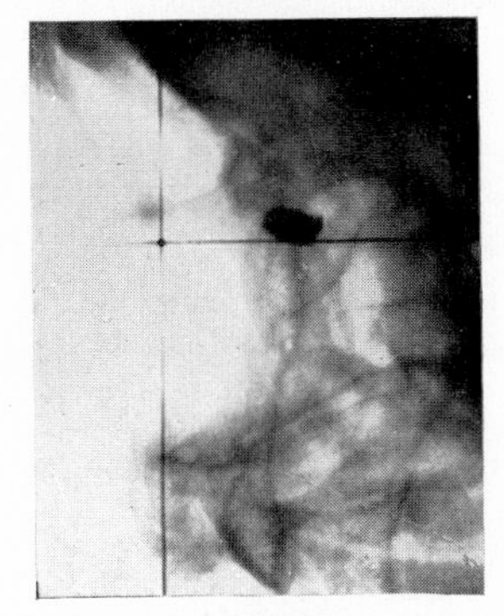

Fig. 629.

Localization of an extra-ocular foreign body by Bromley's method (R. S. Murray).

a foreign body with a sequestrated piece of bone. In such cases instrumental help may be obtained, particularly if the retained particle is metallic, by the employment of X-rays or a locator, which can prove its worth even if the material is non-magnetic provided the mass is sufficiently large and the instrument is introduced into the wound (aluminium, Wenger, 1946).

As a rule, however, the presence of a foreign particle which is radio-opaque is easily determined and its approximate site fixed by the methods which have already been fully described for the localization of intra-ocular foreign bodies (Figs. 627–629). In the case of multiple foreign bodies, however, serious difficulties may arise, for to arrive at a firm conclusion as to which of

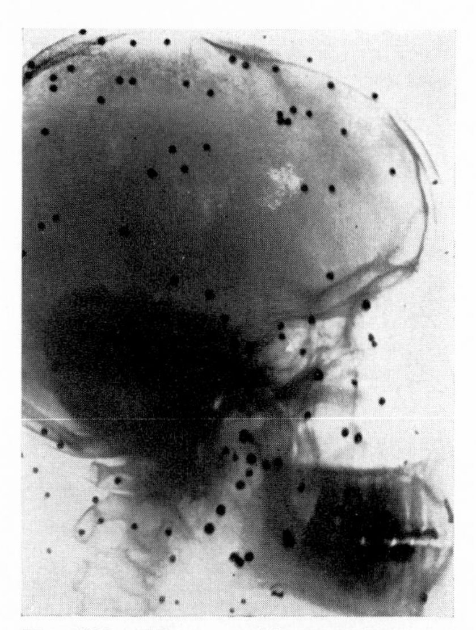

Fig. 630.—Multiple Foreign Bodies.

The lodgment of 129 small shot in the right side of the face and neck; two were found in the globe and two in the right orbit (Wm. B. Doherty).

many particles are intra-ocular, which intra-orbital and which extra-orbital may entail the solution of a problem involving a number of computations almost as great as the analysis of an astronomical plate (Fig. 630). In difficult cases Chaussé's method of transposition stereo-radiography may be of value (Chaussé *et al.*, 1960). Fortunately, however, precise localization to within a fraction of a millimetre such as is required in intra-ocular work is rarely necessary when dealing with the orbit, and much help may be obtained by taking a number of films at different angles with the eyes in different positions.

Treatment

It may be said as an axiom that, *in the absence of definite indications of its presence and without exact localization, an intra-orbital foreign body should be left alone and important structures should never be endangered by a search for it and by attempts at its removal*; it frequently happens that an operation undertaken injudiciously for this purpose causes more symptoms than it had been designed to relieve. It would be difficult to improve on the advice of Hippocrates[1]: "If it be needful to attempt the extraction of a foreign body deeply forced into the orbit through the integuments and orbital muscles, only light traction should be used, and if the difficulties be great it will be better to temporise." This policy applies particularly to metals which are inert (iron, steel, small-shot, etc.). If, however, communications with the nasal sinuses or the cerebral cavity exist, removal of foreign material is usually wise since its retention often leads to the development of infection. If, moreover, healing is likely to be ultimately disturbed by the reaction of the tissues as occurs, for example, in the case of wood, every endeavour should be made to accomplish removal.

As a preliminary, if the material is radio-opaque it should be localized as accurately as possible, a process which may be considerably aided if a fistula exists by the injection of lipiodol or other opaque substances which may clarify the topography. If the wound of entry is still open it may be enlarged and the sinus followed up. If the foreign body is large and the globe disorganized the surgical problems are usually simple, for enucleation can be followed by the ready removal of the retained material. If, however, the eye can be retained, every care should be taken both to ensure its safety and also to avoid injury to important orbital structures. It is usually easiest to follow up the wound of entry and, after locating the foreign body with a probe, seize it with forceps and after careful dissection, if necessary, draw it away. In this manœuvre it must be remembered that the piece of material may be fragmented, a circumstance which we have seen to apply particularly to pieces of wood, and every care should be taken to ensure that none is left behind. In endeavours to locate the foreign body biplane fluoroscopy may be of great value in the case of metallic substances, while a locator may also be of considerable help, particularly if it is introduced into the wound. If the particle is embedded in bone it is important to avoid rotatory or twisting movements lest extensive fractures of the orbital wall result; the pull in such cases should be straight. Finally, after the foreign body has been removed, the tissues should be carefully sewn up in layers, a precaution which should be particularly observed when an incision through the upper lid necessitates section of the orbicularis and the levator muscles.

If the foreign body lies at the apex of the orbit and the globe is intact, a lateral orbitotomy may be advisable (Kirschmann, 1914; Cords, 1916; Neudörfer, 1949); if it is embedded in the lateral wall of the orbit the same approach is indicated (Zimmermann, 1907); and if it is impacted in the orbital roof a trans-frontal approach may involve the least trauma. A

[1] *De morb. vulgar.*, Lib. V, Chapter XXI.

transorbito-cranial wound should be operated upon as soon as circumstances allow a complete primary procedure (Carver and Patterson, 1954).

As a rule in such cases, even if the material is ferromagnetic, the magnet is of little help in extraction unless an extremely powerful instrument is available (Néchitch, 1938); encapsulation of the foreign material is so rapid and the tissues through which the particle must be drawn so dense that, as a rule, if the magnet is to be used it is effective only at the stage when mechanical removal by forceps is as easy (Hirschberg, 1906; Black, 1911; Chance, 1913; Kraus, 1913).

Adamük. *Klin. Mbl. Augenheilk.*, **34**, 198 (1896).
Aub. *Arch. Augenheilk.*, **2**, 252 (1871).
Baker. *Ophthal. Rec.*, **15**, 193 (1906).
Banks. *Brit. J. Ophthal.*, **51**, 566 (1967).
Beauchamp and Miller. *Amer. J. Ophthal.*, **63**, 868 (1967).
Birch-Hirschfeld. *Z. Augenheilk.*, **27**, 25, 156 (1912).
Black. *Ophthal. Rec.*, **20**, 75 (1911).
Böhm. *Ophthal. Klin.*, **11**, 609 (1907).
Boudin. *Corps étrangers de l'orbite* (Thèse), Lyon (1900).
Briggs. *Sacramento med. Times*, **2**, 415 (1888).
Burrows. *Amer. J. Surg.*, **37**, 506 (1937).
Carré. *Arch. Soc. oftal. hisp.-amer.*, **27**, 136 (1967).
Carter, Brudenell. *Ophthal. Rev.*, **1**, 337 (1865).
Carver and Patterson. *Surgery*, **35**, 475 (1954).
Chance. *Ophthal. Rev.*, **22**, 657 (1913).
Chaussé, Payrau and Raynaud. *Ann. Oculist.* (Paris), **193**, 193 (1960).
Clothier. *J. Ophthal. Otol.*, **3**, 88 (1909).
Cooper. *Wounds and Injuries of the Eye*, London, 325 (1859).
Cords. *Z. Augenheilk.*, **35**, 26 (1916).
Curtis and Provan. *Brit. J. Ophthal.*, **54**, 624 (1970).
Dallas. *Brit. J. Ophthal.*, **48**, 158 (1964).
Damato. *St. Luke's Hosp. Gaz.*, **1**, 53 (1966).
Darier. *Ann. Oculist.* (Paris), **117**, 441 (1897).
Doherty. *Amer. J. Ophthal.*, **25**, 135 (1942).
Duthie. *Trans. ophthal. Soc. U.K.*, **61**, 31 (1941).
Eber. *Amer. J. Ophthal.*, **23**, 318 (1940).
Eiseman, Seelig and Womack. *Ann. Surg.*, **126**, 820 (1947).
Ellis. *Ophthal. Rec.*, **9**, 221 (1900).
Elschnig. *Klin. Mbl. Augenheilk.*, **71**, 350 (1923).
Ewart. *Lancet*, **2**, 315 (1903).
Falch. *Fremde Körper in d. Orbita* (Diss.), Greifswald (1879).
Fejer. *Zbl. prakt. Augenheilk.*, **34**, 228 (1910).
Fernandes. *Arch. Ophthal.*, **37**, 168 (1908).
Foucher. *Ann. Oculist.* (Paris), **118**, 156 (1897).
Fromaget. *Arch. Ophtal.*, **14**, 657 (1894); **16**, 144 (1896).
Frost. *Ophthal. Rev.*, **12**. 28 (1893).
Gallus. *Ueber einige Fälle von Orbitalverletzung* (Diss.), Jena (1897).
Genth. *Z. Augenheilk.*, **9**, 55 (1903).
Gerkowicz. *Klin. oczna*, **25**, 137 (1955).
Gifford. *Ophthal. Rec.*, **14**, 124 (1905).
von Graefe. *v. Graefes Arch. Ophthal.*, **2** (1), 233 (1855).
Grom and Carvajal. *Arch. Soc. oftal. hisp.-amer.*, **27**, 1117 (1967).
Grünfeld. *Prag. med. Wschr.*, **30**, 663 (1905).
Haine. *Ann. Oculist.* (Paris), **17**, 113 (1847).
Haltenhoff. *Ann. Oculist.* (Paris), **128**, 467 (1902).
Heyner and Passmore. *Amer. J. Ophthal.*, **59**, 490 (1965).
Higgens. *Lancet*, **1**, 82 (1891).
von Hippel. *Klin. Mbl. Augenheilk.*, **50** (1), 762 (1912).
Hirschberg. *Arch. Augenheilk.*, **8**, 169 (1879). *Zbl. prakt. Augenheilk.*, **30**, 106, 259 (1906).
Höderath. *Klin. Mbl. Augenheilk.*, **47** (2), 109 (1909).
Holmes. *Amer. J. Ophthal.*, **17**, 129 (1900).
Hotz. *Chicago med. Rev.*, **5**, 14 (1882).
Jackson. *Ophthal. Rec.*, **13**, 345 (1904).
Jaensch. *Klin. Mbl. Augenheilk.*, **112**, 62 (1947).
Junius. *Z. Augenheilk.*, **21**, 138 (1909).
Keiper. *Ophthal. Rec.* **14**, 426 (1905).
Kellner. *Beitrag z. Lehre v. d. Schädelfrakturen* (Diss.), Kiel (1878).
Kirschmann. *Vestn. oftal.*, **31**, 234 (1914).
Koster. *Zbl. prakt. Augenheilk.*, **22**, 251 (1898).
Kraus. *Münch. med. Wschr.*, **60**, 1298 (1913).
Lalla and Pillai. *Amer. J. Ophthal.*, **59**, 922 (1965).
Laval. *Arch. Ophthal.*, **19**, 762 (1938).
Ledbetter. *Ophthal. Rec.*, **14**, 117 (1905).
Lichtman, McDonald, Dixon and Mann. *Surg. Gynec. Obstet.*, **83**, 531 (1946).
Louw. *S. Afr. med. J.*, **24**, 151 (1950).
Luis y Yagüe. *Arch. oftal. hisp.-amer.*, **10**, 342 (1910).
McCormick, Macaulay and Miller. *Amer. J. Ophthal.*, **32**, 1252 (1949).
Mackenzie. *A Practical Treatise on the Diseases of the Eye*, London (1856).
Marx. *Fremdkörper in d. Orbita als Erreger v. Tetanus* (Diss.), Berlin (1893).
Maxwell. *Brit. J. Ophthal.*, **36**, 460 (1952).
Mayweg. *Klin. Mbl. Augenheilk.*, **45** (2), 204 (1907).
Mende. *Petersburg. med. Wschr.*, 251 (1910).
Michaïl. *Cluj. Med.*, **16**, 306 (1935).
Mitkewitsch. *Vestn. oftal.*, **3**, 345 (1886).

Morrow. *Ophthal. Rec.*, **13,** 447 (1904).
Néchitch. *Ann. Oculist.* (Paris), **175,** 507 (1938).
Nélaton. *See* Zander and Geissler, *Verletzungen d. Auges*, Leipzig, **1,** 225 (1864).
Neto. *Rev. bras. Oftal.*, **25,** 361 (1966).
Neudörfer. *Wien. klin. Wschr.*, **61,** 76 (1949).
Noyes. *A Textbook on Diseases of the Eye*, N.Y., 689 (1890).
Oeller. *Ann. d. stadt. krankenh. Munchen*, **1** (1878).
Packley. *Aust. med. Gaz.*, **25,** 274 (1906).
Pagenstecher. *Klin. Mbl. Augenheilk.*, **2,** 166 (1864).
See de Wecker, *Traité des maladies des yeux*, Paris, **1,** 822 (1867).
Paufique, Fimbel and Moreau. *Bull. Soc. Ophtal. Fr.*, 107 (1952).
Peabody. *Amer. J. Ophthal.*, **53,** 130 (1962).
Peronnet and Bouyer. *Bull Soc. Ophtal.* Paris, 636 (1948).
Pes. *Ann. Ottal.*, **31,** 701 (1902).
Philipps. *Lancet*, **1,** 1070 (1888).
Philipsen. *Hospitalstidende*, **5,** 601 (1887).
Pignatari. *Rev. gén. Ophtal.*, **13,** 199 (1894).
Praun. *Die Verletzungen d. Auges*, Wiesbaden (1899).
Ramorino. *Boll. Oculist.*, **9,** 9 (1887).
Randall. *Ophthal. Rec.*, **19,** 370 (1910).
Rees. *Med. Ann. Dist. Columbia*, **16,** 548 (1947).
Remky, Friedrich and Stallforth. *Klin. Mbl. Augenheilk.*, **142,** 935 (1963).
Rockliffe. *Trans. ophthal. Soc. U.K.*, **10,** 46 (1890).
Sacks and Matheson. *Brit. J. Ophthal.*, **46,** 304 (1962).
Salzer. *Münch. med. Wschr.*, **51,** 1115 (1904).
Sattler. *Cincinnati Lancet-Clin.*, **12,** 755 (1884).
Schönfelder. *Klin. Mbl. Augenheilk.*, **114,** 542 (1949).
Schwartz and Linn. *Amer. J. Ophthal.*, **34,** 585 (1951).
Seggel. *Klin. Mbl. Augenheilk.*, **41** (2), 66 (1903).
Skacel. *Cs. oftal.*, **6,** 223 (1950).
Smaill. *N.Z. med. J.*, **57,** 292 (1958).
Smith. *Trans. Amer. ophthal. Soc.*, **49,** 671 (1951).
Steindorff. *Die isolierten, direkten Verletzungen d. Sehnerven innerhalb d. Augenhöhle* (Diss.), Halle (1898).
Teillais. *Gaz. méd. Nantes*, **11,** 102 (1893).
Terentjew. *Woenno med. J.*, **226,** 313 (1909).
Thomas. *Amer. J. Ophthal.*, **25,** 210 (1942).
Thomson. *Brit. med. J.*, **2,** 1422 (1895).
Thornell and Williams. *Arch. Otol.*, **39,** 83 (1944).
Tweedy. *Ophthal. Rev.*, **12,** 28 (1893).
Veasey. *Ophthal. Rec.*, **19,** 416 (1910).
Verderame. *Ann. Ottal.*, **44,** 149 (1915).
Vossius. *Klin. Mbl. Augenheilk.*, **52,** 144 (1914).
Wenger. *Arch. Ophthal.*, **36,** 513 (1946).
White and Anderson. *Eye, Ear, Nose, Thr. Mthly.*, **31,** 600 (1952).
Zenker. *Klin. Mbl. Augenheilk.*, **36,** 132 (1898).
Zimmermann. *Klin. Mbl. Augenheilk.*, **45** (2), 195 (1907).

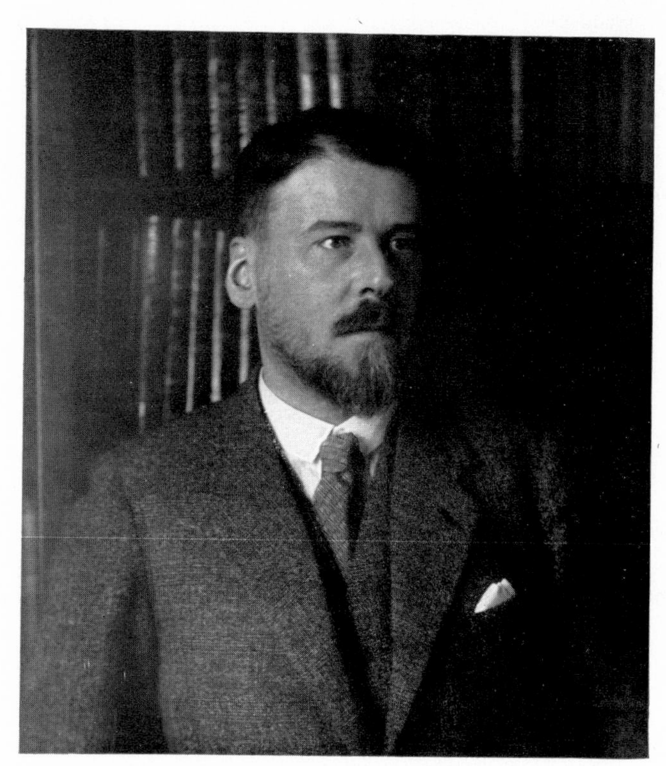

Fig. 631.—Aurel von Szily
[1880–1945].

CHAPTER V

EXPLOSION AND GUNSHOT INJURIES

FEW ophthalmologists have been more catholic in their interests than AUREL VON SZILY [1880–1945] (Fig. 631). A Hungarian by birth, he became professor of ophthalmology first at Münster and eventually in his native Budapest just before he died. His major clinical interests lay in the anaphylactic reactions of the eye and sympathetic ophthalmitis, and his studies on the pathology of the lens were ably epitomized in the Doyne Lecture he gave at Oxford in 1938. More remarkable were his elaborate researches undertaken in his earlier days on the embryology of the eye, particularly on the origin of the vitreous and the scaffolding of the anterior chamber, which are described in detail in the volume of this *System* devoted to Embryology. In our present subject he made an intensive study of ocular injuries sustained in the first World War, and his *Atlas der Kriegsaugenheilkunde*, published in three volumes (1916–18), is perhaps the best and most comprehensive survey of this type of injury available in ophthalmic literature.

MULTIPLE EXPLOSION INJURIES

INJURIES FOLLOWING EXPLOSIONS are conveniently discussed separately. It is true that to a large extent they are complicated by the extra- and intraocular lesions we have already discussed at length—the concussive effects of blast and the impaction into the cornea or the entrance into the globe or orbit of foreign bodies—but their peculiar feature which merits special attention is the multiplicity of relatively superficial injuries caused by the impact of clouds of minute particles of earth, sand, brick-dust, glass, powder or other debris, which may liberally bespatter the face and the eyes.

Such injuries occur sporadically in civilian life and are seen, for example, industrially, in accidents in chemical factories or where compressed air explodes; in quarrying and mining, where explosives are employed or coal-dust and fire-damp gather; in sport, when they may be caused by the discharge of a blank cartridge close to the face, the backfiring of a gun, the explosion of a firework or a home-made canister of powder; but they are essentially typical of war, when they are most usually caused by the bursting of shells, bombs, grenades or buried mines. They are probably seen in their most devastating form, however, in the effects of the aerial bombing of cities when whole buildings are demolished into clouds of disintegrated material of all types which are hurled around at high velocity. Apart from the occasional industrial accident and the incidental injury due to powder from exploding firearms, the occurrence of this type of trauma on a large scale is thus of relatively recent incidence, for it had to await the introduction of explosives of enormous power for use in war in the present century and a parallel increase in the ingenuity of man in their exploitation with a ruthlessness of which previous generations had no conception.

In such injuries, of course—particularly when the effects of blast are added to the multiple traumata caused by quantities of minute flying particles, among which the most catastrophic in its effects is glass—extreme mutilation may result: the lids and even the eyes may be completely avulsed, or the latter may be functionally destroyed owing to multiple perforations or gross internal lesions. In the less severe cases the immediate appearance of the patient may be so dreadful as to make the chance of any reasonable degree of recovery seem impossible, but in a surprising number of instances the end-result may be unexpectedly satisfying. Two factors contribute in no small degree to this. In the first place, the foreign bodies are frequently so small that they lack sufficient momentum to penetrate deeply. In the second place, the disruptive effect of high explosives frequently generates sufficient heat to sterilize the particles so that, even when materials usually infected such as particles of stone, are lodged within the eye, sepsis is rarely evident and can generally be controlled by efficient prophylactic measures.

Injuries to the lids and face usually take the form of a liberal impregnation with multiple minute particles of debris, typically forming blackened, encrusted, caked-up masses, to which may be added multiple superficial wounds most of which are packed with similar material. Such people appear indescribably filthy, and the grime and dust is blown deeply into the skin and fills the pores (Plate XXIII). The immediate reaction is an enormous swelling and œdema of the affected area, occasionally complicated by superficial sepsis. The lids are grossly swollen, usually completely closing over the eyes, and the whole aspect of the face appears hideous in its deformed and blackened state. In time the reaction subsides, the smaller superficial particles of foreign material are often spontaneously extruded, larger and deeper masses become encapsulated or, a chronic sepsis developing, are extruded at a later date; and as a rule the end-result is an ugly and profuse scarring and pitting of the face and lids with, particularly when bespattered with powder, a liberal tattooing of bluish-black pigmentation.

While the prognosis of the facial injuries depends essentially on the cosmetic appearance, similar *injuries to the eye* are much more disastrous in their effects. The region exposed in the palpebral aperture is usually the only portion seriously affected, although the conjunctival sacs are often filled with a slimy mud-pie composed of mucus and dirt; but in the exposed area the conjunctiva may be pock-marked with blackened masses of powder or other debris, minute foreign bodies such as pieces of sand or stone may bespatter the sclera, the cornea may be peppered with similar lesions harbouring innumerable minute foreign bodies of amorphous debris or spicules of glass, some of which may cause wounds that involve a perforation of the globe[1]

[1] Löwenstein (1916), Krusius (1916), Pichler (1918), Tyrrell (1941), Campbell (1941), and many others.

PLATE XXIII

CIVILIAN BOMBING INJURIES.

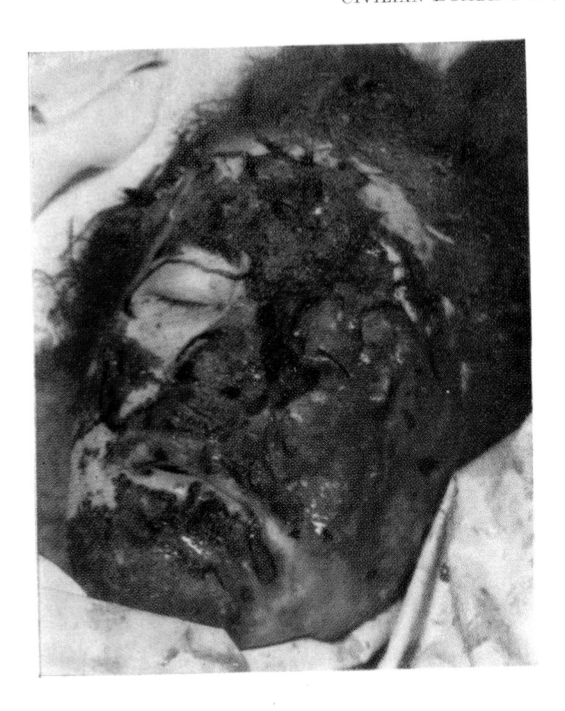

FIG. 1.—To show the gruesome reaction of impregnation of the face with grime and dust hurled by the explosion of a bomb in a built-up area, with the enormous swelling and œdema of the tissues complicated by superficial sepsis.

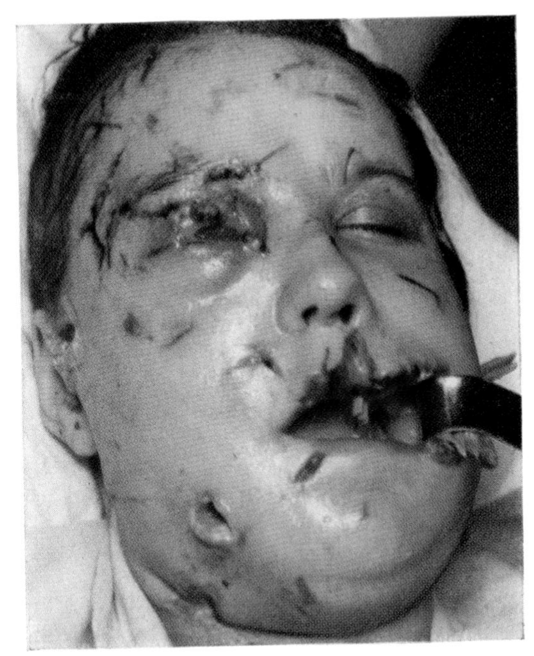

FIG. 2.—Multiple injuries due to flying glass—one of the most common and disastrous effects of injuries in the bombing of cities (Museum, Royal College of Surgeons).

[*To face p.* 672.

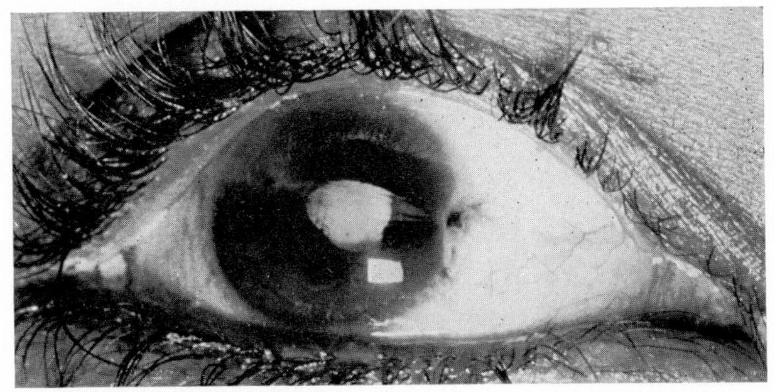

FIG. 632.—INJURY FROM AN EXPLOSION.

Hand-grenade explosion resulting in tattooing of the skin, a penetrating wound at the limbus and a traumatic cataract (D. B. Archer).

(Plate XXIII, Fig. 2). When perforation has occurred it is usually caused by sharp spicules of glass or heavy material such as small pieces of stone, but occasionally the explosive force is sufficient to drive particulate material such as powder through the cornea; a few or a multitude of foreign bodies may thus enter the globe, where they may be seen lying upon the iris or the lens capsule or lodged within this latter tissue, or may even be found, after enucleation of the eye, to have reached the retina[1] (Figs. 632 and 633).

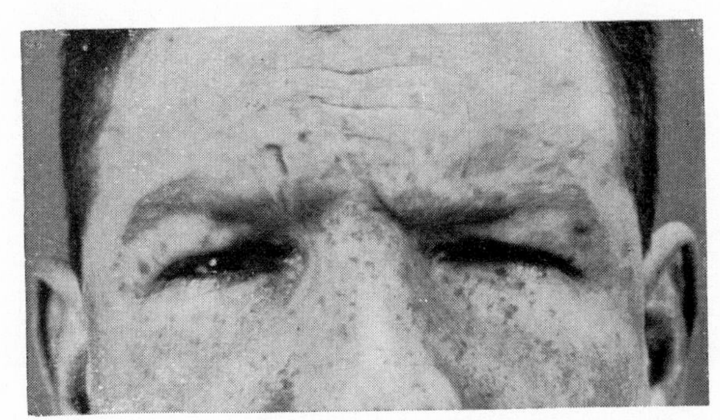

FIG. 633.—EXPLOSION INJURY.

The result of a roadside explosion. The face was pitted and scarred from multiple fragments of stone, many of which were superficial and were spontaneously extruded. (C. D. Shapland).

The immediate appearance of the eye often gives the impression that the case is hopeless: the cornea is universally hazy and swollen, a multitude of foreign bodies may be discernible at all depths throughout this tissue, transient opacities in the deeper parts of the substantia propria may accentuate the picture (optical effects, Stewart and Lloyd, 1943), ciliary injection

[1] Whitehead (1916), Campbell (1941), Zorab (1945), Shapland (1946), Savin (1946), Mihalyhegyi (1946), Callahan (1950), Quere *et al.* (1969), Treister (1969), and others.

FIGS. 634 and 635.—MULTIPLE INTRA-OCULAR FOREIGN BODIES (Helenor Wilder).

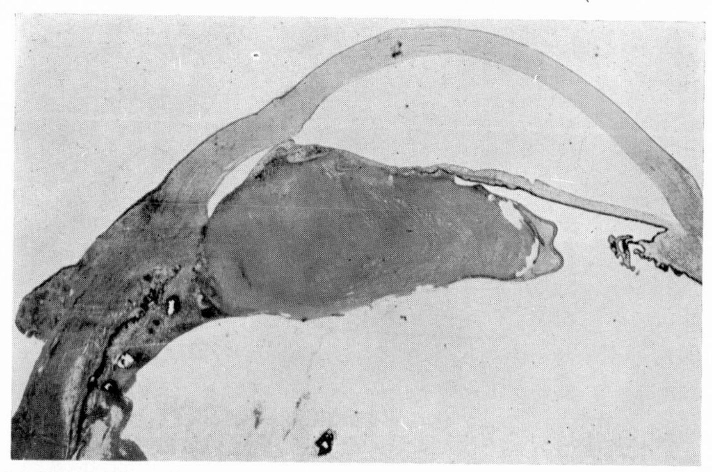

FIG. 634.—After a bomb injury. There are multiple foreign bodies of iron in the cornea, the ciliary body, the lens and the vitreous with considerable disorganization of the eye; 23 days after injury.

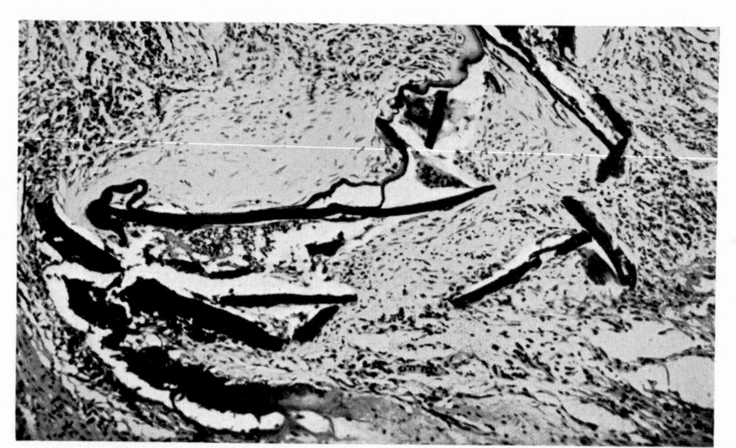

FIG. 635.—Six weeks after a bomb injury. Multiple iron foreign bodies are seen in the midst of an inflammatory cyclitic membrane.

and a traumatic iridocyclitis are invariable, and the patient's subjective symptoms of acute pain, intense photophobia and extreme blepharospasm magnify the impression of the severity of the injury and, incidentally, add greatly to the difficulties of diagnosis and treatment. The impaction of multiple foreign bodies in both corneæ, indeed, completely incapacitates the victim immediately and to a much greater extent than in the usual perforating injury. If intra-ocular damage has also occurred, of course, this distressing clinical picture may be complicated by an intra-ocular hæmorrhage, the development of a traumatic cataract, a detachment of the retina, an iridodialysis or, if a perforating wound of some size exists, a prolapse of the uveal tissue (Figs. 634 and 635).

Treatment of the face and lids in such cases is relatively simple. The larger and more obvious superficial foreign bodies, such as pieces of glass or stone, should be picked out and an immediate attempt should be made under an anæsthetic to clean the area so far as possible by scrubbing with a stiff brush and soap and water. Minute superficial foreign bodies—particles of dust and dirt as well as grains of powder—are often removed by this means, if necessary with the superficial layers of the epithelium. Thereafter the area should be dusted with an antibiotic powder (such as penicillin and sulphathiazole) and covered with a bland tulle-gras dressing[1] which should be renewed until superficial healing is complete. Small superficial particles will almost certainly continue to be extruded for some time, but larger foreign bodies lying at a deeper level may require later excision, and eventually, if areas of the skin have become tattooed, the ultimate appearance may be improved by subsequent grafting.

So far as the *cornea and conjunctiva* are concerned, conservative treatment is usually wiser than attempts to remove buried material; the attainment of maximal mydriasis, filling the conjunctival sac with a bland ointment containing an antibiotic agent and a binocular pad and bandage until dark glasses can be worn, together with frequent bland irrigations with saline, are usually the most satisfactory methods of therapy. Superficial foreign bodies of some size, such as spicules of glass or pieces of stone, may be removed, but multiple minute foreign bodies are best left alone if they are buried. The corneal reaction caused by their presence may appear severe at the time, the subsequent convalescence is usually prolonged and painful and subject to distressing exacerbations of the symptoms of irritation as they tend to work their way to the surface and cause epithelial abrasions; but as a rule such particles, whether of dust, sand, powder or glass, if left alone, lie inert in the tissues and, if any that present superficially are removed, the cornea eventually clears up to a remarkable extent so that the resultant degree of vision attained is sometimes astonishing.[2] Painstaking attempts to remove material of this kind, which can usually be done only in many sittings a little at a time, often cause on each occasion a violent and sometimes alarming reaction and involve in the end a greater degree of opacification than would result from their continued presence, while active interference sometimes leads to the development of infection of the devitalized tissue. The total removal of the epithelium may help recovery in a few cases when the impacted material is superficial (Davidson, 1941), but it is rare for it to be confined to the epithelial layer alone; and when, as is usually the case, most

[1] A close mesh-curtain net impregnated with castor oil 60 parts, beeswax 10 parts, balsam of Peru 1 part, sterilized by autoclaving at 120° C.

[2] Tyrrell (1941), Campbell (1941), Duthie (1941), Hartmann (1942), Cordes (1943), Davis (1944), Zorab (1945), and others.

of the foreign material lies in or beneath Bowman's membrane, such a procedure is rarely of value. At a later stage when the eye is quiescent, total excision of the affected area of the bulbar conjunctiva may diminish the bleary look so frequently left behind and improve the cosmetic appearance, while a persistent and widespread corneal opacity may eventually be replaced by a lamellar or whole-thickness graft, as the case may require.

Intra-ocular complications are to be treated on general lines. These procedures have already been fully described,[1] but it is well to remember that as a rule multiple intra-ocular foreign bodies of such substances as glass, sand, stone or powder can safely be left alone until the eye has recovered or allowed to remain permanently.

In all such cases, of course, sepsis should be countered from the start by the administration of antibiotics given both topically and systemically, while the intensity of the post-traumatic inflammation and the degree of subsequent corneal scarring are much relieved by the topical application of corticosteroids.

Prophylactic precautions against such injuries are to be strongly advocated from the ophthalmological point of view. A relatively light visor of Perspex, although it cannot stop larger missiles, protects the eyes from most of the damage caused in this type of injury; no visor can effectively stop large missiles. Even although such relatively light protection may lower efficiency to some extent, it certainly seems advisable when such traumata are to be expected, as in the case of soldiers advancing over a mine-field or those whose duty takes them abroad during the aerial bombing of a city.

Callahan. *J. Amer. med. Ass.*, **142**, 249 (1950).
Campbell. *Brit. med. J.*, **1**, 966 (1941).
Trans. ophthal. Soc. U.K., **61**, 56 (1941).
Cordes. *Amer. J. Ophthal.*, **26**, 1062 (1943).
Davidson. *Proc. roy. Soc. Med.*, **34**, 729 (1941).
Davis. *Amer. J. Ophthal.*, **27**, 26 (1944).
Duthie. *Trans. ophthal. Soc. U.K.*, **61**, 31 (1941).
Hartmann. *Amer. J. Ophthal.*, **25**, 1448 (1942).
Krusius. *Dtsch. med. Wschr.*, **42**, 775 (1916).
Löwenstein. *Ber. dtsch. ophthal. Ges.*, **40**, 313 (1916).
Mihalyhegyi. *Ophthalmologica*, **109**, 159 (1946).
Pichler. *Z. Augenheilk.*, **39**, 37 (1918).
Quere, Bouchat and Cornand. *Amer. J. Ophthal.*, **67**, 64 (1969).
Savin. *Trans. ophthal. Soc. U.K.*, **66**, 379 (1946).
Shapland. *Trans. ophthal. Soc. U.K.*, **66**, 371, 375 (1946).
Stewart and Lloyd. *Brit. J. Ophthal.*, **27**, 483 (1943).
Treister *Amer. J. Ophthal.*, **68**, 669 (1969).
Tyrrell. *Proc. roy. Soc. Med.*, **34**, 725 (1941).
Whitehead. *Trans. ophthal. Soc. U.K.*, **36**, 63 (1916).
Zorab. *Brit. J. Ophthal.*, **29**, 579 (1945).

GUNSHOT WOUNDS

WOUNDS CAUSED BY PROJECTILES of some size travelling at a high velocity—bullets, fragments of shell, shrapnel, grenades, mines or bombs—such as constitute a large proportion of the battle casualties of war and, to a less extent, are met with in civil life as in accidents with fire-arms or attempts at murder or suicide, merit some special consideration. It is true that many of their effects resemble those seen in the perforating injuries we

[1] p. 616.

have already described,[1] while they often share in the complications of wounds associated with foreign bodies, but the momentum generated by the mass of the projectile combined with the velocity with which it is endowed, produces explosive results such as are not encountered in the ordinary accidents characteristic of civilian life.

Some of the mechanics of bullet wounds and the injuries caused by fragments of shell and other missiles of this type are interesting. Many of them have a rotatory motion as well as a forward movement, so that the total kinetic energy is thereby considerably multiplied.[2] Moreover, the velocity possessed by such missiles produces damage much more widespread than the actual size of the object would suggest. The force of impulse i projected radially from the path of the missile with an intensity sufficien cause a cylindrical zone of destruction in the tissues surrounding the al track of the projectile. In this zone blood vessels may be ruptured ar nes fractured as is seen, for example, in the common fracture of the o l roof when a projectile traverses the cranium. This damage to bone , indeed, produce secondary missiles, for fragments of shattered bone projected at a high velocity in a cone-shaped course in the directior he flight of the missile. Each fragment thus propelled becomes in tu new projectile capable of causing considerable damage, as is typica een in the concussion injuries which fragments of the bony walls o orbit may inflict upon the eyeball.

The damage caused to the eye and orbital tissues rojectiles in war has a long history, dating from the introduction of fire-arms i ombat. In the 16th century such writers as Albucasis, Fabricius of Acquaper and Ambrose Paré noted the tolerance of the orbital tissues to the presence jectiles, but advised their extraction owing to fear of complications. The sub as extensively treated, particularly by French military surgeons (Percy, 1792; y, 1832, the great surgeon of the First Empire; Bertherand, 1851; Demarquay, ; and others), all of whom noted the relative immunity of the orbital tissues reign bodies of this type but stressed the catastrophic effects of sepsis and cer complications. The earlier literature was reviewed by Zander and Geissler (Delorme (1888–93), Kerne (1890) and Praun (1899), but a comprehensive ap ion of such injuries first emerged during the holocaust of the first World W here for the first time they were encountered in unprecedented profusion; in spect the works of Adam (1914), and Duverger and Velter (1919), but most par ly of von Szily (1916–18), and Lagrange (1917–18) are of classical importance, a these the writings of the last two are outstanding in that they were the firs escribe intimately the rationale of such injuries and the mechanism of their s. In the subsequent paragraphs their teaching is closely followed.

In such ds, of course, the damage is usually widespread, for in addition to nsive fractures to the bony framework of the face, the nose and nasa ses, the skull is frequently heavily involved as one or more missile erse each or all of these structures, ploughing up their tissues

[1] p. 328. [2] p. 478.

FIGS. 636 to 638.—DESTRUCTIVE GUNSHOT WOUNDS AFFECTING THE ORBIT (Byron Smith).

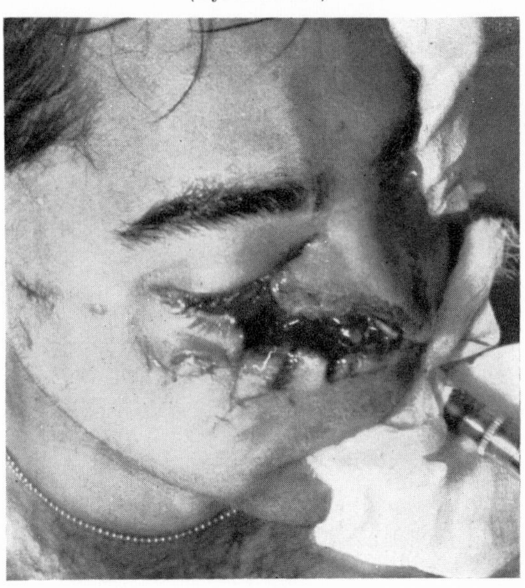

FIG. 636.—Shell fragment wound through right lower lid, antrum and nose. Five days after injury. The temporal two-thirds of the right lower lid were inadvertently sutured to the inferior margin of the skin defect. The exposed cornea was visible.

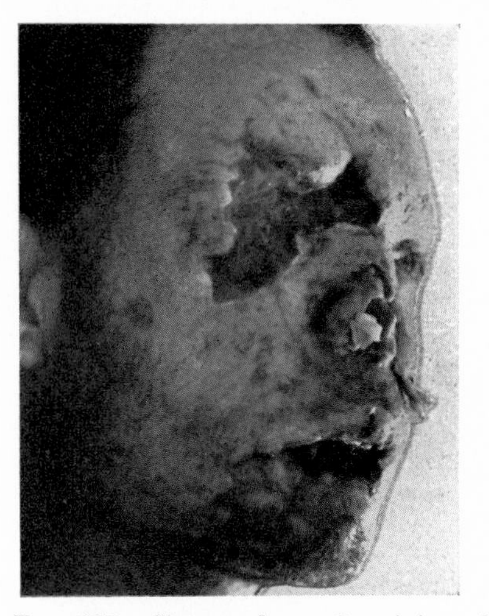

FIG. 637.—Sixteen days after injury by a jumping mine. The orbital wound communicated with the right frontal sinus.

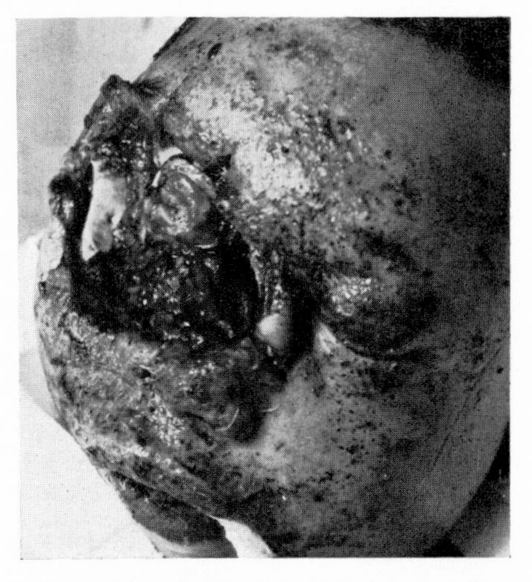

FIG. 638.—Accidental orbital wound from the back blast of a bazooka. A large fragment of the lateral wall of the orbit was displaced posteriorly. Although the nose was severely damaged, the left eye escaped with little injury.

with explosive force, the damage being frequently augmented by the violent displacement of loosened pieces of bone (Figs. 636–638).

The worst type of injury is associated with jagged and irregular fragments of high-explosive shells or bombs; these cut a broader swathe of destruction and create more widespread havoc than does the smoothly contoured bullet, sometimes producing deformities which can only be described as terrible. The extent of the damage varies with the mass and velocity of the missile. If both of these are great the orbit is usually disrupted and the eye destroyed. At the other extreme, if a bullet is almost spent, either owing to the length of its flight or because it has expended its energy in a devious route in the body so that its momentum is lost before

FIGS. 639 and 640.—A LARGE FOREIGN BODY IN BOTH ORBITS.

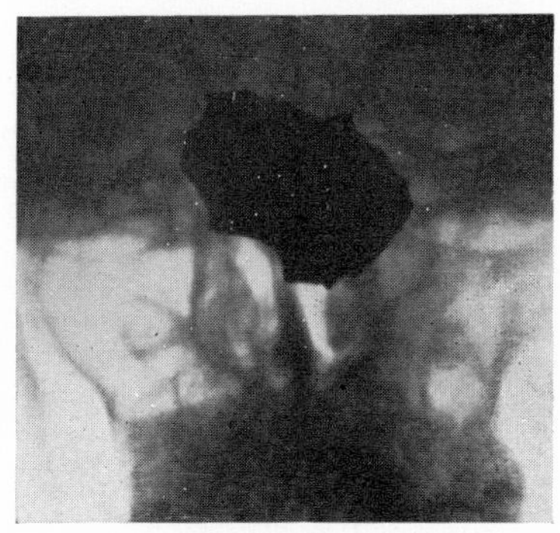

FIG. 639.

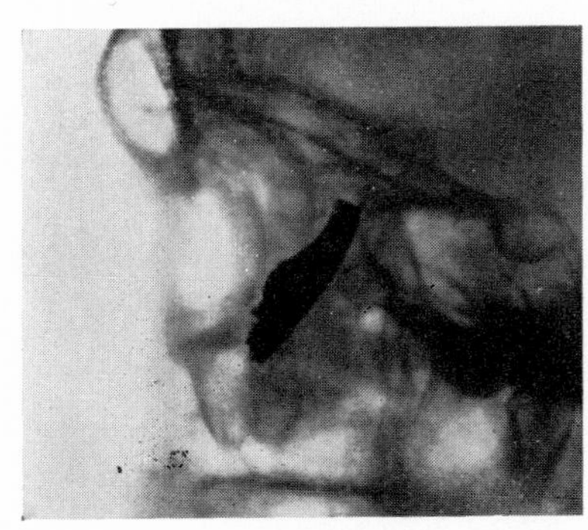

FIG. 640.

To show the curious lack of damage that may occur with the impaction of a large foreign body—a piece of shell, 35 × 20 × 3 mm., which entered at the lower margin of the left orbit and lodged transversely in the nose, encroaching on both orbits near the apex. Both eyeballs were intact with relatively free movements, but the right eyeball was proptosed about 7 mm. The foreign body was removed successfully through the antrum (D. L. Charters) (Fig. 639, postero-anterior; Fig. 640, lateral view).

it reaches the vicinity of the eye, it may rest quietly in the orbit. In this case its behaviour and extraction resemble those of the usual type of orbital foreign body which we have already discussed[1]; it may well happen in this way that a bullet may be safely extracted without damage to the eye (Posey, 1905; and many others), either by the anterior route (Buxton, 1947), by a lateral orbitotomy, a trans-frontal approach or perhaps through the antrum (Charters, 1946; Ide, 1947; and others) (Figs. 639–640). Small fragments of the casings of projectiles or the lead or steel pellets of small-shot may, as we have already seen,[2] cause little damage unless fired from very close range. In the latter event, however, the damage may be considerable, as in a case recorded by Moreau (1948), wherein a pellet of lead perforated an eye and penetrated to the posterior part of the occipital cortex.

[1] p. 655. [2] p. 666.

The nature of the damage varies with the direction of impact of the projectile and the part of the head involved. In general, head wounds of this type may be divided into two classes, depending on whether they lie above or below the zygoma. In the first case they are orbito-cranial and, if of any severity, may endanger life; in the second case they are orbito-facial and, although they may cause ghastly mutilations involving fragmentation of the orbit and wide exposure of the nose and nasal sinuses, injuries which are always associated with some degree of sepsis, they are as a rule not fatal and tend eventually to heal well. Occasionally with a glancing bullet the damage is localized (Figs. 641–642). Most commonly the missile comes from in front, rarely directly, usually obliquely, shattering the orbit and disrupting the eye so that a large bloody mass protrudes from the lids often making it difficult to recognize any particular structure. Projectiles striking the head from behind may traverse the skull and leave by the orbit, blowing

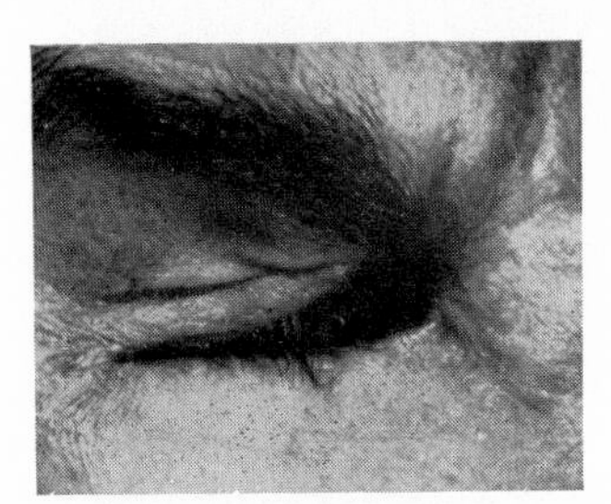

Fig. 641.—Laceration of the Lids after an Explosion.

The medial canthal ligament has been severed and the upper lid fixed in the scar (A. Callahan).

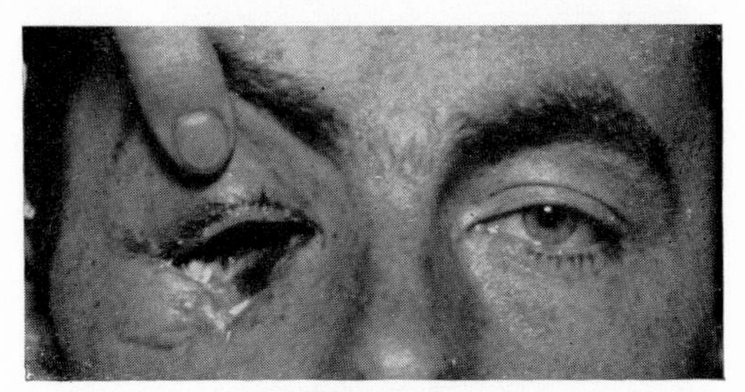

Fig. 642.—Glancing Gunshot Wound of the Lower Lid.

Showing considerable destruction of tissue and marked cicatricial ectropion (T. Pomfret Kilner).

the eye out on their way; but these are only of mortuary interest. Wounds from the side are also common, when the missile ploughs through the depths of the orbit with explosive force and extrudes the contents so that in the worst cases a formless, fleshy mass covered with coagulated blood emerges from the lids. In a case described by Shimkin (1940) the whole orbit suffered an auto-exenteration in this way; the periorbita was stripped off and emerged from the lids like a finger of a glove turned inside out, the orbital contents being extruded and the globe blown away. A wound of this type is typical of the suicide who shoots himself with a revolver through the temple. In such a case the wound is rarely so extravagantly destructive, but the bullet, frequently passing anterior to vital structures, as often as not fails to achieve its intended purpose. Traversing both optic nerves, however, or one optic nerve and the other globe, the usual result is bilateral blindness (Fig. 643); it is indeed a rare fortune for the missile to traverse both orbits without causing permanent visual damage (Weeks, 1903). Traversing the head behind the orbit, the wound is usually fatal, but a case is on record wherein the

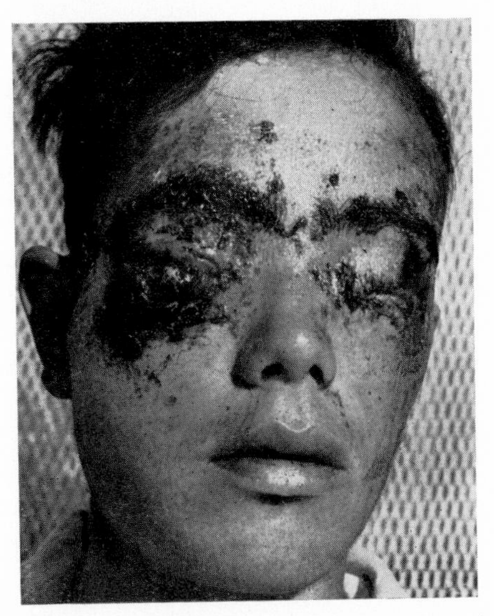

Fig. 643.—A shell fragment entered the upper temporal quadrant of the left orbit and traversed both orbits; the exit wound was in the right temporal fossa. Both eyes were extensively disrupted and multiple fractures of the facial bones were present (H. B. Stallard).

missile became impacted in the chiasma, causing complete blindness in one eye and partial blindness in the other (Roy, 1912).

Finally, a projectile may reach the orbit by a devious route within the body. All types of bizarre instances have been reported, one of the most curious being a case described by Buxton (1947) (Fig. 644). A bullet entered the back near the mid-line opposite the angle of the scapula and reached the apex of the orbit by piercing the trapezius muscle and running alongside the carotid sheath, injuring no vital structures

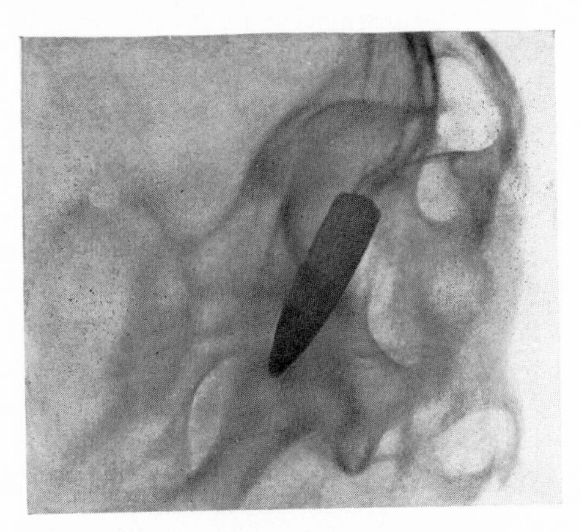

Fig. 644.—A bullet resting near the apex of the orbit, having entered the back opposite the angle of the scapula and run up the neck alongside the carotid sheath, injuring no vital structures in its lengthy journey (R. J. Buxton).

in its lengthy journey and causing only bleeding from the nose and loss of vision owing to a vitreous hæmorrhage and retinal concussion. Conversely, a bullet may follow a long path in the opposite direction; thus Doherty (1942) recorded a case wherein such a missile entered the frontal sinus, traversed the orbit and finally lodged in the lateral part of the neck. Again, a bullet has traversed one orbit and the naso-pharynx and eventually entered the other orbit, lodging in the sclera, without injury to the eye or the orbital contents (Vogt, 1952).

The one favourable feature in an otherwise uniformly depressing picture is the frequent absence of gross infection of these wounds. Unlike many foreign bodies met with in civil life, the projectiles of war emerge with high-explosive temperatures, so that, hurtling through the air at immense velocity, they are usually sterile; moreover, striking the face, they do not usually drag contaminated clothing in their wake as so often happens in gunshot wounds of the body; nor are they so frequently contaminated with earth. Moreover, the exceptionally good blood supply in the face provides an excellent defence both against infection and necrosis, while the absence of large masses of muscle makes any infection which may develop relatively easy to control.

The sterility even of small-shot was demonstrated by Tornatola (1894–96) and Ovio (1895–96), who fired pellets contaminated with pyogenic organisms into the eyes of rabbits and into culture media; in no case did infection develop.

The types of orbital and ocular injury which may arise from such wounds are many; their essential characteristics have been discussed at length in preceding chapters of this book, and at this stage we are concerned only with the mechanism of their occurrence and their characteristic peculiarities.

Wounds remote from the orbit rarely have ophthalmological interest. It is a curious fact that, while the fractures of the skull met with in civilian accidents, as by falls and the impact of blunt objects, are frequently associated with fractures of the orbit by *contre-coup* or radiation, in military surgery fractures of the cranial vault some distance from the orbit caused by projectiles, even when they are associated with gross injury and concussion, do not give rise to orbital complications; the important structures passing through the orbital foramina and fissures are left unscathed and the eyes are unharmed. If the eye or the orbit is to be involved the injury must implicate the orbit itself or be in its immediate vicinity.

Lesions by projectiles affecting the vicinity of the orbit but not directly implicating it generally conform to two standard types (Figs. 645–6). *When the missile passes above the orbit,* shattering the frontal bone and often the cranium, it tends to cause radiating fractures of the orbital roof implicating the superior orbital fissure and the optic canal; the motor and sensory nerves entering the orbit are thus damaged. The optic nerve may be injured but the eye, although it may be rendered immobile, anæsthetic and blind, escapes direct injury. It will be remembered that a depressed fracture of the orbital roof may produce a slight traumatic enophthalmos[1] which, if vision is retained, involves an annoying diplopia; but as a rule, on subsequent clinical examination, the globe presents a normal appearance except, perhaps, for the occurrence of optic atrophy at a later date and the occasional occurrence of a pigmented hæmatic ring around the disc which may be caused by the migration of blood pigment from a hæmorrhage into the optic nerve sheaths.

When the missile passes below or to the lateral aspect of the orbit in the region of the maxilla the force of its impact is dissipated throughout the bony structures of the face, causing therein widespread fractures which do not

Figs. 645 and 646.—The Direction and Effects of Missiles in the Region of the Eye.

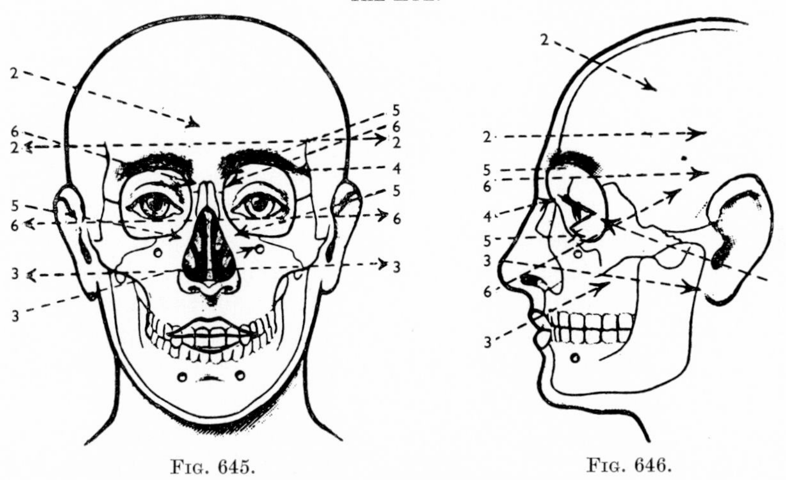

Fig. 645. Fig. 646.

2, Supra-orbital fractures, fractures at the apex of the orbit, injury to the optic nerves. 3, Infra-orbital fractures and concussions. 4, Fracture of the orbital walls without injury to the globe. 5, The penetration of the orbit without injury to the globe. 6, Tangential grazing of the eyeball without rupture (after F. Lagrange).

implicate the orbit itself. As it tears through the structures of the face, however, it sets up violent concussion-waves in the tissues which, it must be remembered, are essentially fluid at body temperature and these, transmitted through the pterygo-maxillary fissure, enter the posterior part of the orbit and cause concussive lesions preferentially at the posterior pole of the eye, particularly at the macula. The typical ophthalmological result of such a lesion is a hæmorrhage in the region of the macula, one or more choroidal tears in the same area and the subsequent development of pigmentary and atrophic changes which result in the loss of central vision, while the occurrence of retinal hæmorrhages may lead to the subsequent development of proliferating retinopathy (Terrien, 1915; Dantrelle, 1915; Lagrange, 1917–18; and others).

[1] p. 295.

When the missile fractures the orbital walls without implicating the contents of the orbit directly, the bone may be splintered and the eye injured indirectly by concussion. Two typical effects result from such an injury. At the posterior pole macular and paramacular lesions characteristic of concussion may result (Plate XXIV, Fig. 1)[1] while, on the side of the globe next to the fracture but somewhat anterior to it, a choroidal laceration may occur, often associated with a retinal tear, caused sometimes by the direct impact of the temporarily displaced bone onto the globe, but more frequently by a concussion-wave travelling through the semi-fluid orbital contents (Lagrange, 1917) (Fig. 138).[2] When such a lesion is confined to the choroid alone, extensive ruptures and hæmorrhages may result; but if the retina is also ruptured the characteristic picture is that of the proliferative chorioretinopathy[3] so adequately described by Lagrange (1917) and amplified by von Szily (1918), Doherty (1942), Tsopelas (1951) and Richards *et al.* (1968) (Plate XXIV, Fig. 2). In this latter condition there is an abundant formation of fibrous tissue derived from mesodermal choroidal elements; this forms a localized thick, densely white mass which does not expand widely into the vitreous, and a detachment of the retina is an unusual sequence since this tissue is securely anchored in its bed by the fibrous mass. The ophthalmological appearance is thus quite different from the proliferative retinopathy which results from a retinal hæmorrhage wherein thin, diaphanous and widely spread strands of fibrous tissue derived from the retinal elements diffuse extensively over this latter tissue and by their contraction tend to drag it from its bed.

When the missile enters the orbit but does not strike the globe directly, the ophthalmological picture is the same as that just described so far as the globe itself is concerned; occasionally chorioretinal scarring occurs or large holes and dialyses appear in the retina so that a detachment results (McKee, 1923; Buxton, 1941; and others) (Figs. 647–649); but the essential clinical characteristic of this type of wound is the occurrence of injury to important orbital structures. The muscles may be torn, the nerves, both motor and sensory, are injured and frequently the optic nerve itself is grossly damaged. This structure is often violently contused,[4] torn or avulsed, being either cut across or pulled out from the disc by the impact of the missile, giving rise immediately to the characteristic ophthalmoscopic picture which has already been described (Plate XII, Figs. 1–4), and eventually to the formation of abundant proliferative masses of new-formed fibrous tissue which fill the posterior half of the globe. The most tragic of such instances concerns those cases wherein a bullet striking the temple traverses the apices of both orbits and severs both optic nerves; such cases result not only in the tragedy of complete blindness but are usually persistently troubled by all the inconveniences resulting from widespread disorganization of the nasal sinuses (Figs. 636–638; 643).

[1] p. 165. [2] p. 161. [3] p. 176. [4] p. 438.

PLATE XXIV

GUNSHOT WOUNDS.

(A. von Szily, *Atlas d. Kriegsaugenheilkunde*, Ferdinand Enke, Stuttgart.)

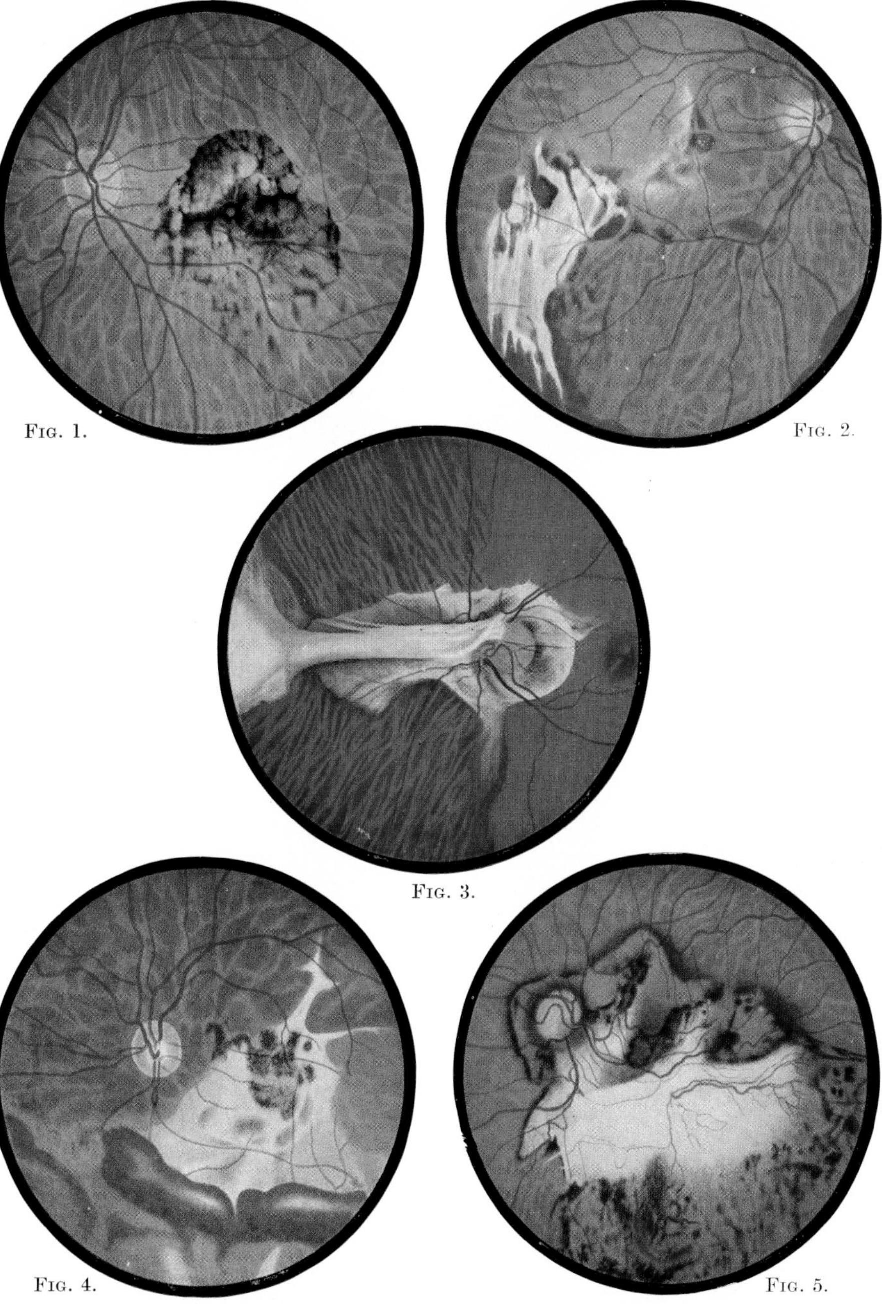

FIG. 1. FIG. 2. FIG. 3. FIG. 4. FIG. 5.

FIG. 1.—The macular lesion, 2 months after the traversal of the right side of the nose by a piece of shrapnel.

FIG. 2.—A peripheral retino-choroidal rupture with proliferating chorio-retinitis associated with macular changes from a bullet which traversed the lower lid and upper orbital wall.

FIG. 3.—Peripheral and central lesions caused by concussion by a splinter of a grenade which entered the orbit at the upper and inner angle.

FIG. 4.—Peripheral and central lesions, 1 month after a shrapnel wound which entered the orbit under the left eye.

FIG. 5.—Peripheral and central lesions, 4 months after the entry of a piece of shrapnel into the orbit through the lower lid.

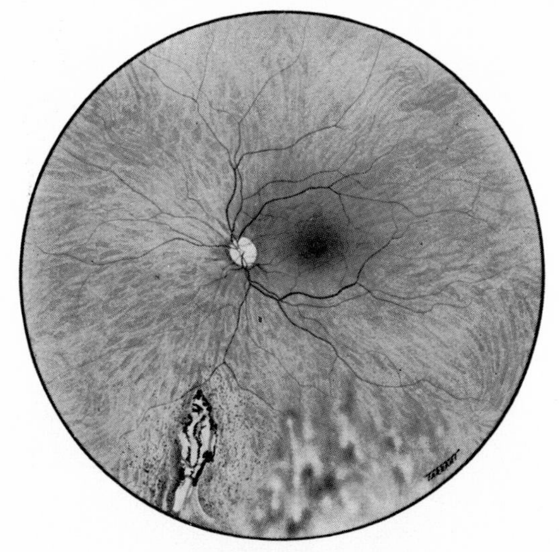

FIG. 647.

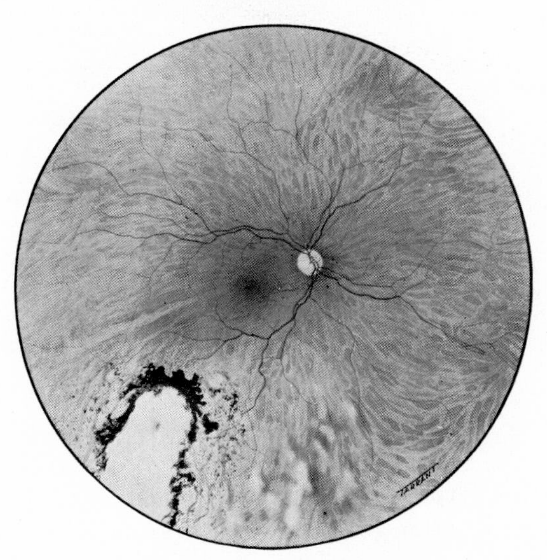

FIG. 648.

FIGS. 647 and 648.—BILATERAL TRAUMATIC CHORIO-RETINAL SCARRING.
Due to contusion of the globe by a gunshot pellet (A. J. B. Goldsmith).

When the missile grazes the globe without rupturing it the same general effects are produced except that the manifestations of concussion within the eye are violently increased. The same types of lesion occur in the region of the macular and the posterior pole, widespread retinal and choroidal lacerations occur anterior to the lesion, resulting in a dense proliferative chorio-retinopathy, but instead of the two lesions being self-contained and isolated, separated from each other by an area of normal fundus, they are usually confluent and merge into a single extensive area of destruction involving the greater part of the fundus, creating havoc which may well result in the eventual disorganization of the eye (Plate XXIV, Figs. 3–5).

When the missile grazes the eye with sufficient force to burst it, the effects and the type of rupture produced are quite unlike the classical rupture of the sclera caused by the impact of a relatively slowly moving blunt force which strikes the eye directly. We have already seen[1] that in the latter type of injury the sclera usually ruptures in the intercalary region and the lens is sometimes extruded from the globe. In a gunshot

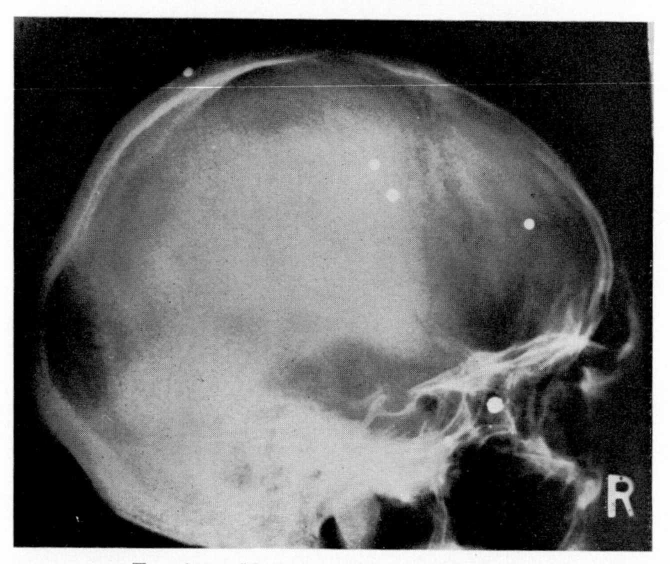

Fig. 649.—Multiple Gunshot Pellets.
X-ray of the skull in the case illustrated in Figs. 647 and 648 (A. J. B. Goldsmith).

injury, however, the violent concussion waves cause a rupture of the sclera *at the point of contre-coup*; the globe is burst widely open at a point opposite to that at which it was struck. Thus if the missile traverses the orbit from front to back a large equatorial rupture results (Fig. 650); if it passes laterally through the orbit behind the globe the front of the eye is blown open (Fig. 651). Such ruptures occur in shooting accidents and are typical of war injuries (Lagrange, 1917; von Szily, 1918; Lister, 1924).

The mechanism of such an explosive rupture differs completely from that of a contusion rupture which, as we have seen, occurs in the meridian of greatest expansion at right angles to the line of the impact (Fig. 35). In the present case the concussive wave in the orbit strikes the globe and causes a wave of pressure to traverse its contents; it is obvious that the force

[1] p. 200.

FIGS. 650 and 651.—RUPTURES OF THE EYE BY HIGH-VELOCITY MISSILES (W. Lister).

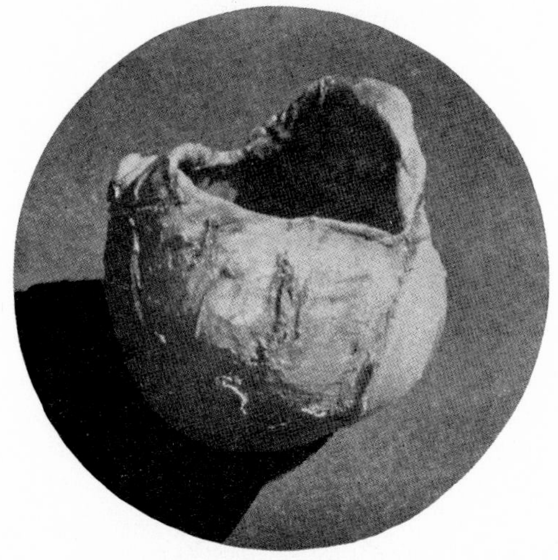

FIG. 650.—The missile passed through the outer side of the orbit just grazing the globe in its temporal aspect (below on the figure). A large equatorial rupture occurred at the point of contre-coup on the nasal side of the globe (above on the figure).

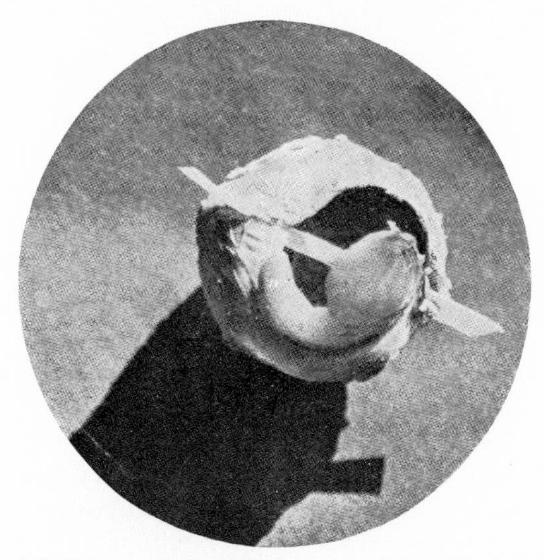

FIG. 651.—A bullet passed through the apex of the orbit behind the eye. An extensive rupture has occurred around the limbus, almost completely separating the cornea from the sclera.

exerted by such a wave will be greater when it strikes the sclera at right angles than when it impinges upon it obliquely, and consequently the rupture occurs at the point of *contre-coup* (Fig. 652). Moreover, the secondary waves of pressure reflected back from the sclera will meet incident waves most directly at this point, enhancing the effect manyfold. The pressure generated at the point of *contre-coup* may be illustrated by the greater force with which a wave of the sea hits a breakwater if it approaches directly than if it sweeps in obliquely, and the cumulative action of the advent of a second wave meeting the first as it is reflected from the breakwater is seen in the great mass of water which is hurled up into the air as the two meet. The pressure generated at the point of *contre-coup* thus attains explosive force and the globe is shattered at this point.

When a missile of any size strikes the eye directly from any angle, the explosive pressure generated splits the sclera to pieces and the globe becomes completely disorganized. Only if the flying particle is minute and the energy involved therefore small does it traverse the globe, causing a double perforation and burying itself in the depths of the orbit; in this event the resulting lesions and their appropriate treatment have already engaged our attention.[1]

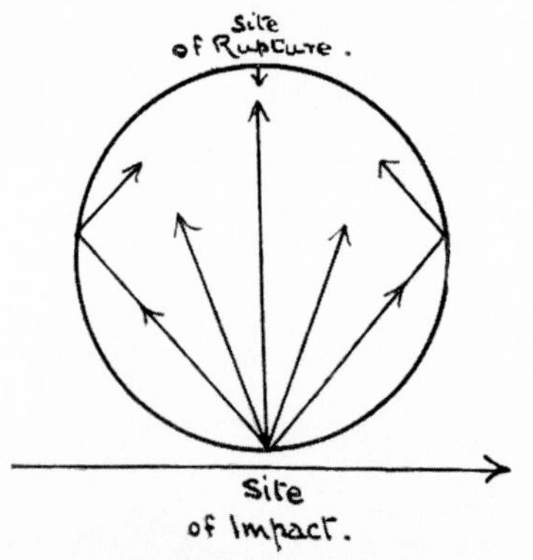

FIG. 652.—RUPTURE OF THE EYE BY A HIGH-VELOCITY MISSILE.

The missile travelling along the direction indicated by the horizontal arrow sends a wave of pressure through the eye at right angles to this line which reaches explosive force at the point of contre-coup (see Figs. 650 and 651) (W. Lister).

The *treatment* of gunshot injuries obviously involves problems that are rarely confined to ophthalmology, and it is suitable here merely to give a short outline of those aspects which particularly concern the ophthalmic surgeon. If the injury is of any severity the primary interest is to combat shock and save life—which, indeed, is often impossible. At this stage, therefore, in a severe case surgical intervention should be confined to immediate necessities—the removal of grossly devitalized and soiled tissues (always to be done sparingly) or completely detached fragments of bone and readily accessible foreign bodies, the staunching of hæmorrhage and the turning out of blood clot, and the cleansing of the area so far as that is possible with a stream of warm saline. The only emergency surgery that is justifiable is a life-saving craniotomy. From the ophthalmological point of view the wounded area is insufflated with an antibacterial powder such as

[1] p. 477.

penicillin and sulphathiazole, a simple dressing of tulle-gras[1] applied, sepsis is controlled by the systemic administration of antibiotics and the danger of tetanus obviated by suitable injections.[2] In such wounds of the face gas gangrene[3] is practically non-existent and prophylaxis against this infection need rarely be attempted.

At this stage the eye can usually be left alone, for after simple cleansing by lavage and immobilization by bandaging it generally suffers remarkably little deterioration, provided adequate and timely steps are taken to prevent the development of infection. If the globe is still intact *only the cornea requires attention in the event of its being exposed*, a point to watch particularly in unconscious patients. This may occur owing to the proptosis produced by an orbital hæmorrhage, the herniation of brain substance through a defect torn in the orbital roof, or the lodgment of a bulky foreign body behind the eye; or, alternatively, a similarly dangerous exposure may result if a considerable portion of the lids has been ripped away. In the latter type of injury, it is true, the globe itself is usually badly damaged, but it may escape serious injury from a glancing projectile. To avoid rapid opacification of an exposed cornea, a tarsorrhaphy should be performed if there is a sufficiency of lid tissue to make such an operation possible. If the lower lid has been torn away, the upper can usually be temporarily sutured to the lower margin of the orbit, and in the absence of the upper lid the cornea may be completely covered with a large conjunctival flap; if this also is not available a large pedicle flap of skin reflected from the fronto-temporal region will provide an adequate temporary cover.

As soon as the patient's survival is ensured, reparative work may be undertaken and, owing to the extent of the damage which is often present, this may necessitate the cooperation of a team composed of a neurosurgeon, an otorhinologist, a maxillo-facial expert and a dental surgeon in addition to the ophthalmologist.

So far as damage to the tissues of the lids and orbit is concerned, from the ophthalmological point of view we have already seen that the early reposition of a depressed fracture of the middle third of the face is of great value and saves the perpetuation of a gross deformity which is subsequently extremely difficult to eliminate,[4] while restoration of the trochlear pulley if it is misplaced by a fracture of the orbital roof will similarly avoid a disabilitating and tiresome diplopia. Provided the cut edges of wounds of the skin of the lids are not swollen from hæmorrhage, œdema, infiltration or perhaps infection, early and accurate approximation of the lid margins with careful conservation of the lacrimal passages will also save much time and trouble in plastic operations undertaken at a later date (Figs. 653–5); but if considerable swelling or any evidence of infection already exists, wound closure must be delayed. As a general rule apart from these pro-

[1] Footnote, p. 675.
[2] p. 408.
[3] p. 405.
[4] p. 272.

Figs. 653 to 655.—Bullet Wound of the Left Orbit (Byron Smith).

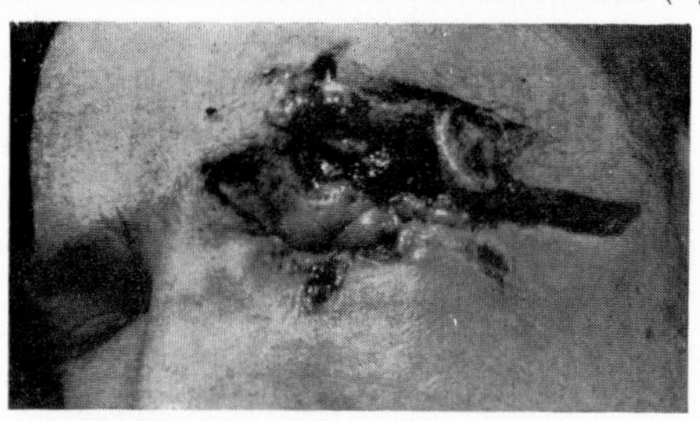

Fig. 653.—Five days following injury. The eye was destroyed.

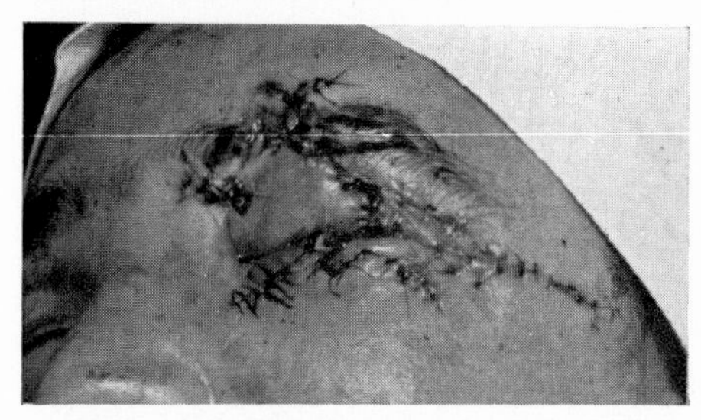

Fig. 654.—External appearance of the wound immediately after delayed primary closure consisting of enucleation, embedding a glass ball within Tenon's capsule, insertion of a socket conformer and closure of the superficial structures.

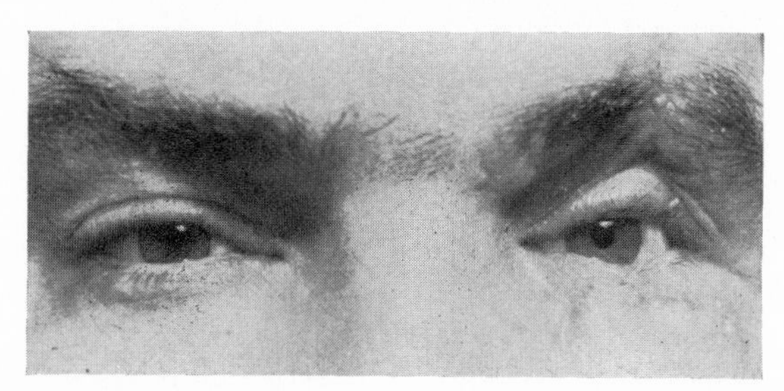

Fig. 655.—Existing scars at the end of one month. An artificial eye within the socket exhibited excellent motility. Late plastic surgery was required to eradicate the residual deformity.

cedures, plastic reconstruction and restoration of the bony contours of the face and orbit are best left for several months when healing is complete, when the traumatized tissues have recovered their vitality, when sepsis is eliminated, when the patient has regained sufficient strength and resiliency to cope with what may prove to be a series of tedious surgical interventions, and when a surgical team is available which has the time, the leisure and the facilities to assess adequately the varied problems presented by each individual case and to plan and execute their appropriate treatment (Figs. 656–9).

So far as the eye itself is concerned, if it is hopelessly mutilated it should be excised at this secondary stage, care being taken to fashion as roomy a socket as possible. If it is perforated but not disorganized, any prolapsed tissue should be excised and the wound adequately covered[1]; otherwise there is little urgency for immediate ocular surgery with the exception that, if the necessary opportunities are available and the apparatus for accurate localization and extraction are to hand, an intra-ocular foreign body should be removed before it becomes encapsulated. Such a procedure, however, as we have seen,[2] should be postponed until it can be adequately undertaken.

FIGS. 656 to 659.—REPARATIVE SURGICAL PROCEDURES AFTER GUNSHOT WOUNDS INVOLVING THE ORBIT AND SIDE OF THE HEAD AND FACE.

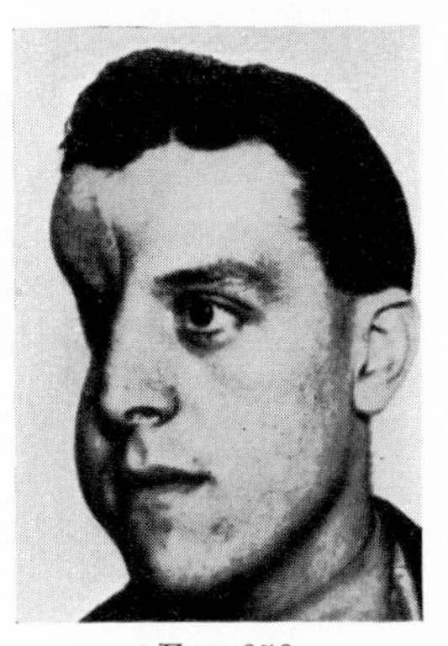

FIG. 656.

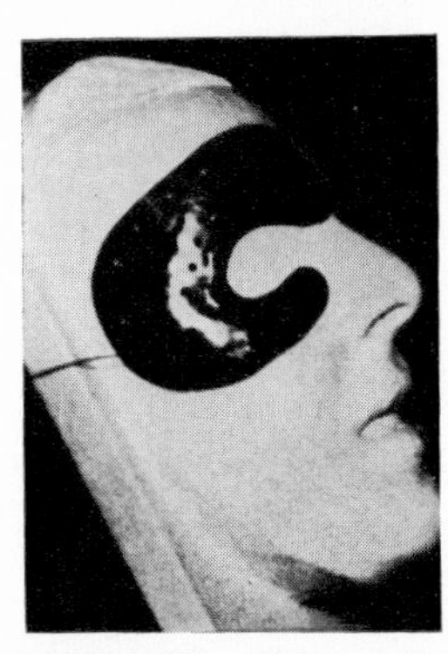

FIG. 657.

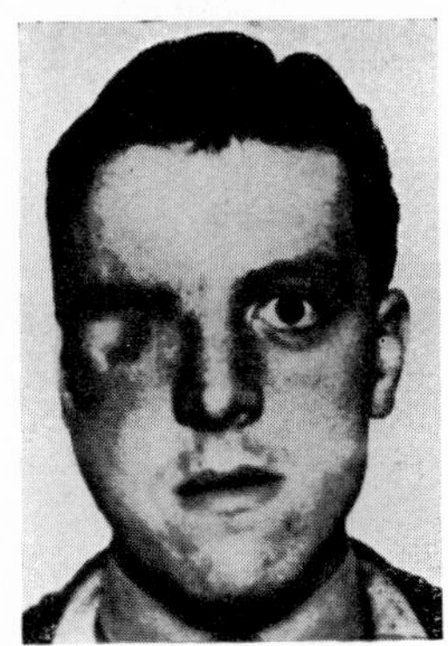

FIG. 658.

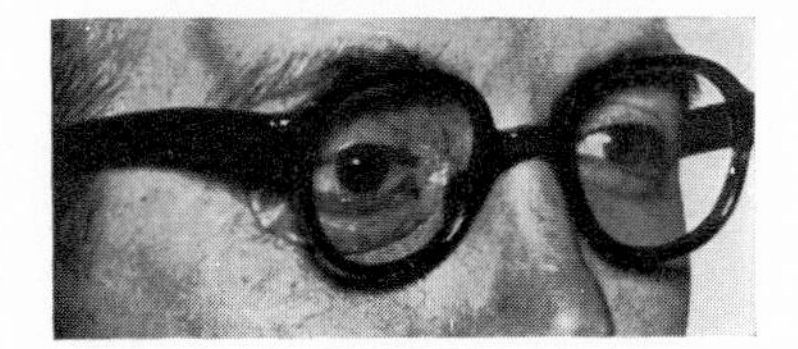

FIG. 659.

FIG. 656.—Showing the gross loss of tissue and bone.
FIG. 657.—Showing a tantulum implant on a mould of the face.
FIG. 658.—Grafted restoration ready for wearing a prosthesis.
FIG. 659.—Prosthesis attached to spectacles in a case resembling Figs. 656 to 658 (T. Pomfret Kilner).

In all cases at this early stage conservatism is wise. It is astonishing how well some badly mutilated eyes recover, and the danger of sympathetic inflammation will not arise for at least 10 days after the injury. Until the degree of damage can be judged at leisure, and until the recuperative powers of the eye are adequately assessed, there is rarely any immediate hurry to resort to the irrevocable step of excision of the globe, a procedure which should never be done in any circumstances in bilateral injury unless the eyes have been reduced to pulp, for it is surprising how frequently the eye which

[1] p. 368. [2] p. 618.

appears immediately to be the more hopeless eventually turns out to be the one which may retain some perception of light.

If excision is inevitable owing to widespread destruction of the globe it is important that all fragments of the sclera should be removed after careful separation from the conjunctiva and the muscles. The socket should be liberally dusted with an antibiotic powder (penicillin and sulphathiazole, etc.) and the remnants of the conjunctiva closed by a continuous suture in the hope of preventing symblepharon and securing a reasonably good socket. If drainage seems necessary owing to sepsis it is preferable to ensure it by a thin rubber drain inserted through a separate incision in the outer part of the lower lid, or even through the antrum if this is involved in the wound.

Adam. *Augenverletzungen im Kriege,* Berlin (1914).
Bertherand. *Ann. Oculist.* (Paris), **26,** 127 (1851).
Buxton. *Trans. ophthal. Soc. U.K.,* **61,** 68 (1941); **67,** 379 (1947).
Charters. *Lancet,* **1,** 93 (1946).
Dantrelle. *Arch. Ophtal.,* **34,** 745 (1915).
Delorme. *Traité de chirurgie de guerre,* Paris, 2 vols. (1888–93).
Demarquay. *Union Méd.,* **4,** 82 (1859).
Doherty. *Amer. J. Ophthal.,* **25,** 135 (1942).
Duverger and Velter. *Ophtalmologie du guerre,* Paris (1919).
Ide. *Eye, Ear, Nose, Thr. Mthly.,* **26,** 205 (1947).
Kerne. *Kriegschirurgie d. Sehorgans,* Berlin (1890).
Lagrange. *Les fractures de l'orbite par projectiles de guerre,* Paris (1917).
Atlas d'ophtalmoscopie de guerre, Paris (1918).
Larrey. *Clinique chirurgicale,* Paris, 5 vols. (1829–36).
Lister. *Brit. J. Ophthal.,* **8,** 305 (1924).
McKee. *Amer. J. Ophthal.,* **6,** 725 (1923).
Moreau. *Bull. Soc. franç. Ophtal.,* **61,** 61 (1948).
Ovio. *Rev. gén. Ophtal.,* **14,** 305 (1895).
Ann. Ottal., **25,** 68 (1896).
Percy. *Manuel du chirurgien d'armée,* Paris (1792).
Posey. *Ophthal. Rec.,* **14,** 112 (1905).
Praun. *Die Verletzungen d. Auges,* Wiesbaden (1899).
Richards, West and Meisels. *Trans. Amer. Ophthal. Soc.,* **66,** 214 (1968).
Roy. *Ophthalmology,* **9,** 63 (1912).
Shimkin. *Brit. J. Ophthal.,* **24,** 265 (1940).
von Szily. *Atlas d. Kriegsaugenheilkunde,* Stuttgart (1916–18).
Terrien. *Arch. Ophtal.,* **34,** 663 (1915).
Tornatola. *Rev. gén. Ophtal.,* **13,** 206 (1894).
Arch. Ottal., **3,** 350 (1895–96).
Tsopelas. *Klin. Mbl. Augenheilk.,* **119,** 298 (1951).
Vogt. *Klin. Mbl. Augenheilk.,* **120,** 539 (1952).
Weeks. *Trans. Sect. Ophthal., Amer. med. Ass.,* 217 (1903).
Zander and Geissler. *Die Verletzungen d. Auges,* Leipzig (1864).

CHAPTER VI

THE INDIRECT OCULAR EFFECTS OF MECHANICAL INJURIES

A STUDY of the indirect effects of remote injury on the eye at once suggests the name of OTHMAR PURTSCHER [1852–1927] (Fig. 660), one of the provincial ophthalmologists never on the staff of a university who made outstanding contributions to our science. A Tyrolese, he was educated at the University of Innsbruck and after his graduation he studied in Paris, London, Berlin where he undertook anatomical and pathological research, and Vienna where he attended the clinics of von Arlt and his assistant, Ernst Fuchs. But his heart was in the small Austrian town of Klagenfurt on the Vörthsee, where he founded and was chief surgeon of an ophthalmic clinic. Here he spent his working life. Here, in addition to taking an active interest in politics, he worked conscientiously and constructively making notable advances in our knowledge of erythropsia, the effects of copper in the eye, giving the first description of sunflower cataract, and particularly on traumatic retinopathy which is still called eponymously after him.

THE DELAYED EFFECTS OF OCULAR INJURY

Apart altogether from the late effects of ocular injury, which we have already described and which are best looked upon as complications—late traumatic uveitis, sympathetic inflammation or the development of corneal infiltrations and dystrophies, cataract, detachment of the retina or other lesions which may appear sometimes at a late stage—less immediate and direct sequelæ may be attributed to trauma in the region of the eye and orbit. The dependence of such remote effects upon the original injury is often not clear and a true sequential relationship may well be questioned; but in some cases there is little doubt that we are dealing with cause and effect. One of the most important aspects of the questions thus raised is their medico-legal implications, for it is obvious that any relationship between the original trauma and the development of subsequent disease must be borne in mind when matters of monetary compensation are considered.

These remote effects may be divided into four categories—the tendency towards the development or exacerbation of local infections, the incidence of degenerative changes, the determination of the onset of neoplasic growths, and the occurrence of psychogenic states which may be attributable to an injury.

THE POST-TRAUMATIC DEVELOPMENT OF INFECTION

There is little doubt that traumatized tissue is more readily attacked by infective organisms and reacts less vigorously to their assault than would otherwise be the case; it forms a *locus minoris resistentiæ* wherein infective

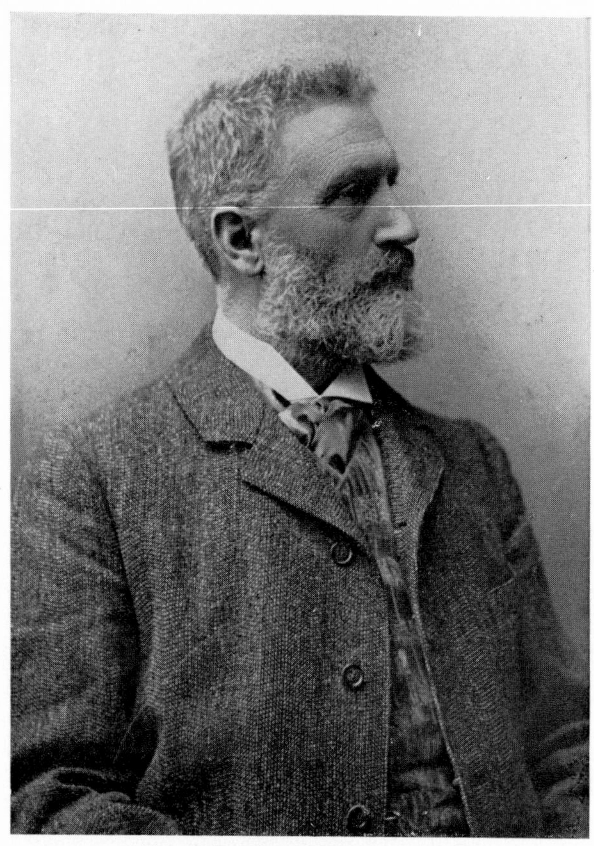

FIG. 660.—OTHMAR PURTSCHER.
[1852–1927]

FIGS. 661 to 663.—NON-SPECIFIC INFECTIVE ENDOPHTHALMITIS EXCITED BY TRAUMA.

An intensely cellular inflammatory response, suggesting an infective ætiology, was apparent in an eye enucleated 7 weeks after a gunpowder explosion (B. Rones and H. Wilder).

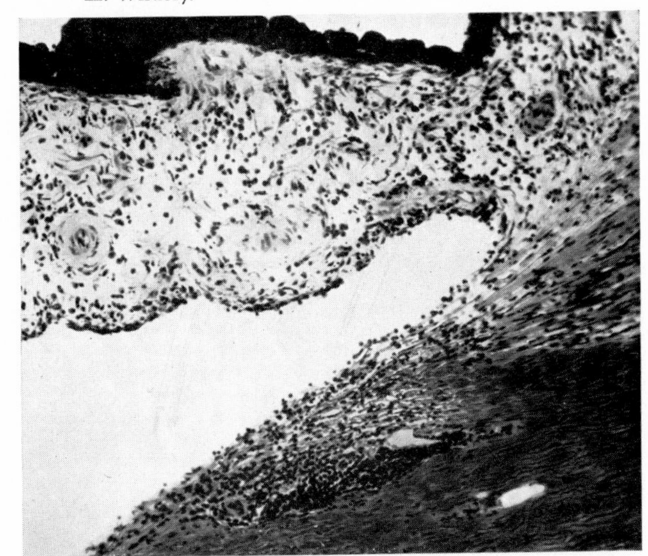

FIG. 661.

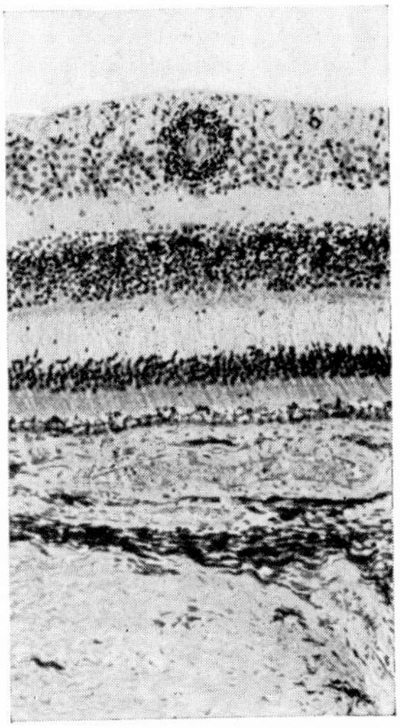

FIG. 662.

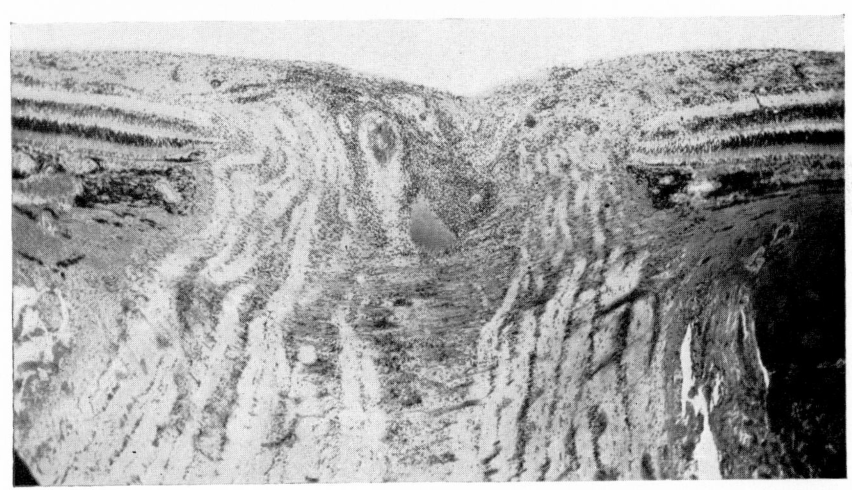

FIG. 663.

FIG. 661.—The lymphocytic and plasma-celled infiltration in the iris and angle of the anterior chamber.

FIG. 662.—Diffuse polymorphonuclear and perivascular lymphocytic infiltration of the retina and (Fig. 663) nerve-head.

processes may be expected readily to flourish. Just as the appearance in the eye of an iridocyclitis of presumptive infective origin after a surgical operation is not very uncommon even when exogenous infection can reasonably be excluded, so is it almost certainly the case that endogenous infections of distant focal origin tend to localize in the ocular tissues when their resistance is lowered by accidental trauma. A positive diagnosis and direct proof of a causal association in cases of this type are, of course, notoriously difficult to establish, but the sequence is undoubtedly more frequent than can be explained by chance relationship occurring either relatively soon after a trauma (Figs. 661–663) or after the lapse of many years (Fig. 664).

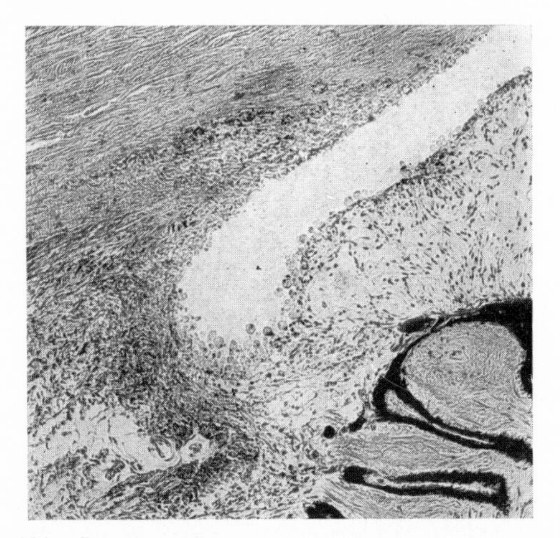

FIG. 664.—DELAYED POST-TRAUMATIC ENDOGENOUS IRITIS.

Following an injury sustained 40 years previously. Groups of swollen round cells line the surface of the iris and infiltrate the trabeculæ as well as the stroma of the iris and ciliary body. The case was diagnosed clinically as a tuberculous iridocyclitis. The inflammation appeared during an attack of influenza (Bertha Klien).

Of the specific infections, three are particularly related to trauma—zoster, syphilis and tuberculosis.

ZOSTER. It is an observation so well established that zoster has a tendency to appear at a period varying from 1 to 30 days after a peripheral injury, that it would seem reasonable to believe that trauma may precipitate its incidence; the injury may affect any part of the body and may at times appear trivial, but the sequence is most common after damage to the larger nerves or vertebræ. Apart from the considerable number of cases in the general literature wherein this disease has become clinically apparent after injury to the trunk or limbs, ophthalmological literature contains a sufficient number of instances of the development of zoster ophthalmicus after injury in the region supplied by the trigeminal nerve to suggest the possibility of this relationship.

Charcot (1859) first drew attention to a case of recurrent zoster following a gunshot wound; somewhat similar cases were described by Nieden (1882, occipital injury), Flemming (1899, a gas explosion), Wilbrand and Saenger (1901, a head injury against a wall), Brun (1903, after a fracture of the skull), Axenfeld (1906, a blow on the head with a piece of wood), Wiegmann (1932, a chemical injury with soda, sodium triphosphate and water), Ammann (1935, a blow from the tail of a cow), Barraux *et al.* (1936, a blow with a football), Fourestier (1939, an injury by an anæsthetic mask during an operation) and Bieber and Weyland (1956, after dental surgery). Klauder (1947) recorded 4 cases, 2 caused by striking the head against a solid object, 1 by a corneal foreign body and 1 by a jet of sulphur dioxide gas. Further cases of this sequence after a head injury and peripheral nerve trauma could be quoted.[1]

Zoster has also been reported following an injection of the gasserian ganglion for trigeminal neuralgia (Terlinck, 1928; and others) or such surgical operations as tattooing the cornea (Caspar, 1906), the removal from it of a foreign body (Giroire *et al.*, 1960), extraction of cataract (Snell, 1896) or the removal of a wart from the forehead (Klauder, 1947).

The lesions thus produced are many and various and include all the different clinical manifestations of the disease. Zoster of the area of skin supplied by the first division of the trigeminal is the most common occurrence and may be gangrenous in type; keratitis has been frequent; iridocyclitis has been noted on several occasions as well as various degrees of internal and external ophthalmoplegia; these clinical manifestations have also proved to be recurrent. The time-interval between the trauma and the appearance of the lesion has varied between 1 day and about 3 weeks, but as a rule has been within 14 days. Occasionally, however, some sensory disturbance or pain persisted continuously between the injury and the outbreak of clinical signs of the disease. The clinical progress of such cases and their prognosis resemble the spontaneously occurring disease; as a rule the course is uneventful towards recovery, without incapacitating pain, except in aged patients when it may be severe.

It is, of course, certain that the injury does not cause the infection; *it merely precipitates it, presumably because the virus which has been lying latent in such cases becomes activated from a condition of dormancy* and is able to flourish in tissues devitalized by trauma. In order to associate the trauma in a causal role with the occurrence of zoster the disease should appear at the site or within the range of the injury, which may be slight and need not be productive of a wound, and it should become clinically evident within three weeks after the accident, whereafter any causal relationship becomes progressively more dubious.

SYPHILIS. Among the ocular manifestations of syphilis there is little doubt that an attack of *interstitial keratitis* may be precipitated by trauma; on this most authorities are agreed.[2] The estimates in the literature of the

[1] Höfer (1895), Gunn (1901), Raecke (1910), Knowles (1911), Hildesheimer (1912), de Salterain (1920), Terrien (1935), Nicolau and Dragenesco (1936), Grandi (1937), Barker (1939), and many others.

[2] Perlia (1905), Guillery (1905), von Hippel (1906), de Saint-Martin (1920), Fertig (1920), Klauder (1933), Garcia Miranda (1942), and many others.

percentage of cases in which the onset of keratitis has followed trauma to the eye vary very considerably—from 0 (Igersheimer, 1928), 0·3% (Mohr, 1910), 1·75% (Cunningham, 1922), 2·42% (Langendorff, 1922), 3% (Spicer, 1924) or 4% (Guy, 1926) to 11·46% (Carmi, 1923) or 20% (Butler, 1922). The disease has even followed simple operative trauma, such as a discission, with disastrous psychological results. Although it has been denied by some (von Hippel, 1906; Igersheimer, 1928) and despite the fact that many of the reported cases rest on inconclusive evidence, there seems little doubt that the relationship does exist; but from the point of view of medical jurisprudence it cannot be said that the trauma caused the disease. An equal number of cases has occurred of severe trauma in congenital syphilitics who did not develop keratitis at the time but in whom the disease appeared spontaneously after an interval. It would seem that, *if a syphilitic infection has evolved to the stage favourable for the onset of keratitis, injury will tend to bring out the constitutional tendency* and precipitate a chain of events to which, of course, it can claim only an incidental relationship.

Cases of *syphilitic iridocyclitis* following trauma so closely as to suggest a causal relationship are much more rare, and the sequence is not so well established—acute iritis (Aubineau, 1905; Limbourg, 1906), papular iritis (Siegrist, 1906), gummatous iritis (van der Hoeve, 1909; Antonelli, 1910) or chronic iridocyclitis (Rones and Wilder, 1947).

More questionably still, trauma has been associated with the onset of optic atrophy (Stolper, 1902) or iridoplegia (Perlia, 1907). An injury to the lids has seemed to activate a latent syphilitic process and lead to the development of a gummatous lesion (Gozberk, 1937).

TUBERCULOSIS. Apart altogether from the direct inoculation of exogenous tubercle bacilli into a wound, it would appear that *the lowering of the resistance of the tissues consequent on an injury may result in the localization of an endogenous tuberculous infection in the eye or the orbit, or the reactivation of a quiescent infection therein.* The sequence is not so direct or convincing as in the case of zoster, but several cases in the literature wherein this infection became active in this region soon after an injury or a surgical operation seem difficult to explain otherwise. Moreover, it is a well-known and generally accepted observation that injury to the bones and joints may lead to the development of localized tuberculosis in such subjects, even although the accident may be so slight as to escape attention at the time and the patient may appear to be in good health without readily recognizable evidence of systemic tuberculosis.

Max Schueller's (1880) experiments should be remembered in this connection. Having injected human tuberculous expectoration into the lungs of dogs and rabbits, he injured the knee-joints of the animals and found that practically all the experimental animals developed a granular tuberculosis of the traumatized joints—a phenomenon completely absent in a control series.

Intra-ocular tuberculosis has been the most common sequel. An early case in the literature is that of Treitel (1885), wherein 4 months after an injury to her eye with a straw, a 12-year-old girl developed a sclero-keratitis with a granulomatous mass on the iris which, when removed by iridectomy, showed the typical histology of a tubercle. Sartorius (1903) described a somewhat similar case wherein, some 5 weeks after a blow on the eye, an iridocyclitis necessitated its excision in a 10-year-old child. Similar cases of iridocyclitis wherein trauma appeared to have a causal relationship have been recorded, although in most of them the diagnosis was not bacteriologically confirmed but has rested largely on the clinical appearance and course of the disease or the somewhat unconvincing presence of a positive skin-reaction.[1] In the cases of Cattaneo (1900) and Lloyd (1930) meningitis developed with a fatal termination.

Similarly, a *keratitis* resembling tuberculosis in its clinical habit has been noted to follow a corneal injury, as a blow by a plum (Morinami, 1903) or the removal of a foreign body from the cornea (Scheffels, 1905), while the same sequel has followed an operation for squint (Mayweg, 1908) or a cataract extraction (Black and Haessler, 1930). An endogenous tuberculosis has apparently become localized in the *conjunctiva* after trauma (Salvadori, 1949), while a tuberculous *periostitis* of the orbital margin[2] has also been reasonably ascribed to injury (Sgrosso, 1892).

SARCOIDOSIS has a much more tenuous relationship to trauma. German (1940) described a case appearing on an old scar, Srinivasan (1941) reported such a development after a cataract operation, while King (1946) annotated 6 cases of localized sarcoidosis of the face and head following trauma, 3 of which were due to cuts by glass in automobile accidents, a sequence also recorded by Curtis and Grekin (1945). A dog-bite of the lids figured in the history of a case discussed by Kaplan (1948), and a fall from a ladder has been an antecedent (Knapp and Knoll, 1949).

THE POST-TRAUMATIC INCIDENCE OF DEGENERATIVE CHANGES in the ocular tissues is, of course, common, the most typical of which are seen to develop in old scars in the cornea; these have already been fully discussed.[3]

Of the remote effects of trauma an interesting and less direct example is POLIOSIS, a whitening of the brows and lashes.[4] Such a condition has developed subsequently to an injury suggesting an occasional causal relationship (Bach, 1906; Steindorff, 1914); a cataract operation has also had such a sequel on the operated side (Reich, 1881).

Ammann. *Klin. Mbl. Augenheilk.*, **95**, 793 (1935).
Antonelli. *Arch. Ophtal.*, **30**, 561 (1910).
Aubineau. *Ann. Oculist.* (Paris), **134**, 126 (1905).
Axenfeld. *Münch. med. Wschr.*, **53**, 2417 (1906).
Bach. *Z. Augenheilk.*, **14**, 246 (1906).
Barker. *Arch. Derm. Syph.* (Chic.), **40**, 974 (1939).
Barraux, Assali and Bastouil. *Rev. Oto-neuro-ophtal.*, **14**, 40 (1936).
Bieber and Weyland. *Bull. Soc. franç. Derm. Syph.*, **63**, 276 (1956)
Black and Haessler. *Amer. J. Ophthal.*, **13**, 139 (1930).
Block. *Klin. Mbl. Augenheilk.*, **67**, 581 (1921).
Brun. *Beitr. klin. Chir.*, **38**, 192 (1903).
Butler. *Brit. J. Ophthal.*, **6**, 413 (1922).
Carmi. *Boll. Oculist.*, **2**, 668 (1923).
Caspar. *Wschr. Therap. Hyg. Auges*, **10**, 141 (1906).
Cattaneo. *Boll. sci. med. Bologna*, 1015 (1900).
Charcot (1859). In *Lectures on Diseases of the Nervous System* (New Sydenham Soc. Trans.), **1**, 76 (1877).

[1] Wolfe (1882), O'Sullivan and Story (1899), Perlmann (1908), Höeg (1912), Block (1921), Black and Haessler (1930), Fralick (1931), Debré *et al.* (1951), Miron *et al.* (1956), and others.
[2] Vol. XIII. [3] Vol. VIII, p. 632. [4] Vol. XIII.

Cunningham. *Trans. ophthal. Soc. U.K.*, **42**, 44 (1922).
Curtis and Grekin. *Med. Clin. N. Amer.*, 31 (1945).
Debré, Brissaud and Canlorbe. *Arch. franç. Pédiat.*, **8**, 49 (1951).
Fertig. *Z. Augenheilk.*, **44**, 166 (1920).
Flemming. *Lancet*, **1**, 587 (1899).
Fourestier. *Presse méd.*, **47**, 1055 (1939).
Fralick. *Arch. Ophthal.*, **6**, 420 (1931).
Garcia Miranda. *Med. Madrid*, **10**, 89 (1942).
German. *Amer. J. clin. Path.*, **10**, 254 (1940).
Giroire, Charbonnel and Vercelletto. *Rev. Oto-neuro-ophtal.*, **32**, 38 (1960)
Gozberk. *Ann. Oculist.* (Paris), **174**, 837 (1937).
Grandi. *Boll. Oculist.*, **16**, 768 (1937).
Guillery. *Klin. Mbl. Augenheilk.*, **43** (1), 630 (1905).
Gunn. *Trans. ophthal. Soc. U.K.*, **21**, 295 (1901).
Guy. *J. Amer. med. Ass.*, **87**, 1551 (1926).
Hildesheimer. *Zbl. prakt. Augenheilk.*, **36**, 77 (1912).
von Hippel. *Ber. dtsch. ophthal. Ges.*, **33**, 83 (1906).
Höeg. *Klin. Mbl. Augenheilk.*, **50** (1), 606 (1912).
Höfer. *Ann. Städt. allg. Krankenh. z. München*, **7**, 138 (1895).
van der Hoeve. *Klin. Mbl. Augenheilk.*, **47** (1), 428 (1909).
Igersheimer. *Syphilis und Auge*, Berlin (1928).
Kaplan. *Amer. J. Ophthal.*, **31**, 83 (1948).
King. *Sth. med. J.*, **39**, 122 (1946).
Klauder. *Arch. Ophthal.*, **10**, 302 (1933). *J. Amer. med. Ass.*, **134**, 245 (1947).
Knapp and Knoll. *Trans. Amer. ophthal. Soc.*, **47**, 147 (1949).
Knowles. *Penn. med. J.*, **15**, 615 (1911).
Langendorff. *Dtsch. med. Wschr.*, **48**, 290 (1922).
Limbourg. *Ber. dtsch. ophthal. Ges.*, **33**, 113 (1906).
Lloyd. *Amer. J. Ophthal.*, **13**, 753 (1930).
Mayweg. *Klin. Mbl. Augenheilk.*, **46** (2), 466 (1908).
Miron, Rosin, Samovici and Visan. *Oftalmologia* (Buc.), **1**, 76 (1956).
Mohr. *Klin. Mbl. Augenheilk.*, **48** (2), 611 (1910).
Morinami. *Beiträge z. Therapie u. Diagnostik d. Augentuberkulose* (Diss.), Rostock (1903).
Nicolau and Dragenesco. *Rev. Oto-neuro-ophtal.*, **14**, 479 (1936).
Nieden. *Zbl. prakt. Augenheilk.*, **6**, 161 (1882).
O'Sullivan and Story. *Trans. roy. Acad. Med. Ireland*, **17**, 1 (1899).
Perlia. *Klin. Mbl. Augenheilk.*, **43** (1), 396 (1905); **45** (1), 210 (1907).
Perlmann. *Klin. Mbl. Augenheilk.*, **46** (1), 309 (1908).
Raecke. *Aerztl. Sachverst. Ztg.*, **16**, 321 (1910).
Reich. *Arch. Ophtal.*, **1**, 307 (1881).
Rones and Wilder. *Amer. J. Ophthal.*, **30**, 1143 (1947).
de Saint-Martin. *Clin. Ophtal.*, **24**, 331 (1920).
de Salterain. *Arch. lat.-amer. Pediat.*, **14**, 331 (1920).
Salvadori. *Atti Cong. Soc. Oftal. ital.*, **11**, 252 (1949).
Sartorius. *Bericht ü. zehn Fälle v. Iristuberkulose* (Diss.), Giessen (1903).
Scheffels. *Klin. Mbl. Augenheilk.*, **43** (1), 406 (1905).
Schueller. *Exp. u. histol. Untersuch. u. d. Entstehung u. Ursachen d. scrophulösen u. tuberculösen Gelenkleiden*, Stuttgart, **7**, 8 (1880).
Sgrosso. *Ann. Ottal.*, **21**, 440 (1892).
Siegrist. *Korresp.-Bl. schweiz. Aerzt.*, **36**, 22 (1906).
Snell. *Ophthal. Rev.*, **15**, 309 (1896).
Spicer. *Brit. J. Ophthal.*, Suppl. **1** (1924).
Srinivasan. *Brit. J. Ophthal.*, **25**, 493 (1941).
Steindorff. *Klin. Mbl. Augenheilk.*, **53**, 188 (1914).
Stolper. *Dtsch. Z. klin. Chir.*, **65**, 117 (1902).
Terlinck. *Bull. Soc. belge Ophtal.*, No. 57, 128 (1928).
Terrien. *Rev. Oto-neuro-ophtal.*, **13**, 619 (1935).
Treitel. *Berl. klin. Wschr.*, **22**, 445 (1885).
Wiegmann. *Beitr. Anat. Ohr.*, **30**, 160 (1932).
Wilbrand and Saenger. *Neurologie d. Auges*, Wiesbaden, **2**, 160 (1901).
Wolfe. *Brit. med. J.*, **1**, 299 (1882).

THE POST-TRAUMATIC DEVELOPMENT OF NEOPLASIA

The relation of trauma to the development of a tumour is important from the medico-legal aspect, but presents a problem which in the present state of our knowledge is insoluble. Neglecting for the moment the influence of repeated trauma involving the application of chemical carcinogens—an entirely different and well-substantiated sequence—there is much in the literature to suggest that a single mechanical trauma, either of the nature of a concussion or a wound, may give rise to the development of a neoplasm. It is a well-known circumstance that when a tumour appears the patient frequently tries to remember a blow or an injury sustained not long before, and he usually succeeds in his endeavour. The statistical probability of coincidence in such a matter is much greater than is generally recognized, and to this may be added the likelihood that the trauma frequently draws attention to a tumour that is already there. A causal relationship, of course, is not ruled out, but with the possible exception of some osseous tumours there is no convincing proof on the matter. In all ophthalmological or medical literature there is not a single case in which it can be conclusively proved that a single trauma has directly given rise to the development of a tumour since, although their sequential incidence may be beyond doubt, proof is lacking that the tumour was not present before the injury. The experimental production of a tumour by a single trauma would constitute proof of the matter, but so far this has been lacking, and the general statement can safely be made that *the simple injury of healthy tissue is not a proven cause of neoplasia*, but it can be stated with equal conviction that *injury can precipitate neoplasia in prepared tissue.*

Two classical and very informative cases may be cited in this connection. Champlin's (1930) case concerned identical twins: one was struck on his right testicle and thereafter developed a sarcoma of that testicle, from which he died at the age of 26; the other twin died spontaneously of sarcoma of the right testicle at the age of 31. Had the former escaped injury the probability is high that he would also have died about the age of 31. Warthin's (1928) case concerned a family in which three brothers were heavy smokers and died of cancer of the lip between the ages of 40 and 45 years; a fourth brother was a non-smoker and died from the same disease at the age of 63. The absence of the extrinsic carcinogenic factor may have increased the span of life by 20 years.

CYSTS

It is well known that SEBACEOUS CYSTS which have remained static for an indefinite period may suddenly enlarge and show inflammatory changes after the receipt of an injury. It has also been observed that HYDATID CYSTS of the orbit caused by infection by the *Taenia echinococcus* have on occasion been associated with precedent trauma (Dudinow, 1932; Mura, 1932; Patel, 1933); it is probable that an injury may stimulate their rapid development.

SIMPLE TUMOURS

There is little doubt that an injury frequently accelerates the growth of an already existent neoplasm. Some of the more common tumours which have a congenital basis provide apt cases in point, both HÆMANGIOMATA of the conjunctiva (Galezowsky, 1873; Ruvioli, 1877; Marin, 1917; Montanelli, 1926) or of the orbit (Weiss, 1899; and others), and LYMPHANGIOMATA of the conjunctiva (Meyerhof, 1902; Fuchs, 1916) or the orbit (Dejonc, 1908). Therein a tumour, present with little or no clinical evidence since birth, commences to grow rapidly and becomes clinically apparent after an injury; the appearance of a PLEXIFORM NEUROMA of the upper lid comes into the same category (Fox, 1950). It is noted elsewhere[1] that trauma may

[1] Vol. XIII.

be an exciting cause of orbital VARICES,[1] even trauma so trivial as a severe physical effort (Mackenzie, 1830; Gruening, 1873; Elschnig, 1892; and others) or coughing (Meyer, 1898; Wulkow, 1930). Similarly, slight injury may exacerbate a congenital TELANGIECTASIA of the lids (Reeh and Swan, 1950).

More definite neoplasms have also been suspiciously associated with a preceding trauma, such as a BENIGN CALCIFIED EPITHELIOMA of the lid (Malherbe and Chenantois, 1880; Ashton, 1951) and FIBROMATA of the orbit (Scheiss-Gemuseus, 1868; Chevallereau and Chaillous, 1904; Teulières, 1913; and others). More certainty, however, is associated with the ætiological role of trauma in BONY NEOPLASMS. The rare exostoses met with in the orbit may follow injury, as also may the more diffuse hyperostoses (Baltin, 1935); but there is little doubt that minor injuries or unsuspected small fractures in the cartilaginous bone of the nasal capsule during the period of its active embryogenesis are one of the most important factors in stimulating the cells into the osteoblastic activity which results in the development of the osteomata of the nasal sinuses which habitually invade the orbit (Arnold, 1873; Cushing, 1927; Kolodny, 1929; Armitage, 1931; Eagleton, 1935; and others).

MALIGNANT TUMOURS

CARCINOMATA. It has frequently been suggested that injury enters into the ætiology of carcinomata. The classical theory of Cohnheim that in the course of development cell-rests become separated from their normal relationship and environment, and remain dormant without carrying on their usual functional activity in a layer of tissue unnatural to them, provided a rational basis for the hypothesis that they might become activated by trauma. This suggestion was developed in ophthalmology by Leber and Krahnstöver (1898). Among tumours of the conjunctiva, particularly at their preferential site at the limbus, several cases have been quoted of the appearance of carcinomata after an injury and cited as evidence of a causal relationship,[2] while the development of such a tumour has been noted on the site of the section of a cataract extraction (Oliver and Roberts, 1952).

Similarly it is significant that some 30% of some varieties of carcinomata of the lids have been associated with trauma or irritation, such as chronic inflammation, the pressure of spectacles or the squeezing of blackheads or pimples (Broders, 1919; Birge, 1938); malignant changes may also develop on an old cicatrix, and it is perhaps not without interest that Findlay (1930) recorded that of 190 cases of cancer of the skin in 900,000 cattle in New South Wales, 3 developed upon branding scars.

A similar association appears from time to time in the literature with regard to MELANOMATA. Such tumours at the limbus have often had a

[1] Treacher Collins (1895), van Duyse and Bribosia (1895), Priestley Smith (1897), Voigt (1904), and many others.

[2] Chapman and Knapp (1875), Schneider (1877), Kopff (1898), Lagrange (1901), Feingold (1922), Camison (1922), Ash and Wilder (1942), Fiedler and Costin (1961), and others.

preceding history of trauma.[1] The same sequence has been noted in cases of malignant melanoma of the lids[2] and the orbit.[3] A few cases of intra-ocular malignant melanomata of the choroid have been similarly associated (Stieren, 1934; and others); Fuchs (1882), indeed, found such a history in 11% of his cases, Leber and Krahnstöver (1898) collected 34 cases, and in a study of 507 cases in the literature Lane (1934) found an injury mentioned as a possible incriminating cause 66 times. Anton (1968), on the other hand, found a history of injury in 26 of 195 cases of intra-ocular tumour in which only 2 showed a probable relationship with trauma.

Although from the medico-legal standpoint claims in this respect are increasing and awards are becoming more frequent and probably in the future will be more liberally allocated, it can only be repeated that in all the literature there is no scientific evidence either experimental or pathological that the relationship between the two events is more than incidental. In many cases it is certain that trauma has attracted attention to the presence of a tumour, and the utmost concession which can justifiably be made is that an injury may be responsible for exciting into activity a neoplasic process which hitherto had been pursuing a slow and latent course.[4]

That *a change in the character of a tumour* may be induced by injury has been claimed to have a more substantial basis. This was based on the reaction of NÆVI, the trauma in this case being frequently the injury sustained on partial excision of the growth when it was apparently in the simple stage. This sequence has been recorded in melanomata occurring in the conjunctiva (Ball and Lamb, 1923; Albrich, 1923; van Duyse, 1924; and others), on the lids (Wätzold, 1924) or in the iris (Cüppers, 1953) as well as in other parts of the body. Thus in 36 out of 68 cases recorded by Webster and his colleagues (1944), the appearance of a malignant melanoma followed a history of mechanical injury to, or incomplete surgical removal of a mole, while Raven (1950) considered that abortive attempts to remove nævi from the lid were a possible factor in the development of some 30% of cases of malignant melanomata in this region. Nevertheless, there is no adequate evidence that trauma, accidental or surgical, has transformed a simple into a malignant melanoma; indeed, the evidence seems incontrovertible that after its complete removal a simple melanoma does not recur; it is the quietly malignant condition mistakenly diagnosed as benign which is followed by metastases; to wait until such a mole shows signs of activity is to wait too long (Pack, 1959; Cade, 1961). It is to be remembered, however, that even after a biopsy has indicated that a melanoma is simple, its excision if undertaken

[1] Mathewson (1874), Bloch (1893), Pfingst (1895), Panas (1902), Pereyra (1913), Höhne (1914), Albrich (1923), Ball and Lamb (1923).

[2] van Duyse and Cruyl (1887).

[3] Noyes (1879), Elliott (1893), Ide (1913), Wood (1913), Sefic (1929), Moretti (1929), Trettenero (1931), Hay (1934).

[4] Chapelle (1906), Nitsch (1925), Sauerbruch (1926), Stieda (1927), Knox (1929), Ewing (1935–40), Behan (1939), and others.

should be free and tri-dimensional lest foci of malignant cells are present. A congenital blue nævus which has been relatively static since birth or, at any rate, has spread exceedingly slowly, has also been observed to become rapidly invasive after a trauma (Braithwaite, 1948).

Similarly, curetting or incomplete operation on a meibomian tumour which probably had been present in a state of relatively latent malignancy may suddenly be followed by rapid growth, quick recurrence and progressive extension with the development of multiple metastases.[1]

To close this section in a lighter vein, the opposite (apparent) sequence was recorded by Dujardin (1907) in an interesting case. An epithelioma of the bulbar conjunctiva had grown so profusely that it covered the whole cornea and mechanically obscured vision. The patient was struck by the branch of a tree which tore away a large part of the tumour and exposed the central area of the cornea, thus temporarily restoring his sight.

POST-TRAUMATIC PSYCHOSES

These conditions, which are common and are often of considerable medico-legal importance, are discussed elsewhere.[2]

Albrich. *Klin. Mbl. Augenheilk.*, **71**, 476 (1923).
Anton. *Cs. Oftal.*, **24**, 203 (1968).
Armitage. *Brit. J. Surg.*, **18**, 565 (1931).
Arnold. *Virchows Arch. path. Anat.*, **57**, 145 (1873).
Ash and Wilder. *Amer. J. Ophthal.*, **25**, 926 (1942).
Ashton. *Trans. ophthal. Soc. U.K.*, **71**, 301 (1951).
Ball and Lamb. *Arch. Ophthal.*, **52**, 80 (1923).
Baltin. *Averbach Jub. Vol.*, 53 (1935). *See Zbl. ges. Ophthal.*, **36**, 440 (1936).
Behan. *The Relation of Trauma to New Growths*, Baltimore (1939).
Birge. *Arch. Ophthal.*, **19**, 700; **20**, 254 (1938).
Bloch. *Prag. med. Wschr.*, **18**, 615 (1893).
Braithwaite. *Brit. J. plast. Surg.*, **1**, 206 (1948).
Broders. *J. Amer. med. Ass.*, **72**, 856 (1919).
Cade. *Ann. roy. Coll. Surg.*, **28**, 331 (1961).
Camison. *Rev. Cubana Oftal.*, **4**, 141 (1922).
Champlin. *J. Amer. med. Ass.*, **95**, 96 (1930).
Chapelle. *De l'influence du traumatisme sur la pathogénie et l'évolution des tumeurs oculaires*, Paris (1906).
Chapman and Knapp. *Arch. Augenheilk.*, **4**, 197 (1875).
Chevallereau and Chaillous. *Recueil Ophtal.*, **26**, 471 (1904).
Collins, Treacher. *Trans. ophthal. Soc. U.K.*, **15**, 240 (1895).
Cüppers. *Klin. Mbl. Augenheilk.*, **122**, 355 (1953).
Cushing. *Surg. Gynec. Obstet.*, **44**, 721 (1927).
Dejonc. *Klin. Mbl. Augenheilk.*, **46** (1), 37 (1908).
Dudinow. *Klin. Mbl. Augenheilk.*, **88**, 373 (1932).
Dujardin. *Clin. Ophtal.*, **13**, 119 (1907).
van Duyse. *Bull. Soc. belge. Ophtal*, No. 49, 73 (1924).
van Duyse and Bribosia. *Arch. Ophtal.*, **15**, 159 (1895).
van Duyse and Cruyl. *Ann. Oculist.* (Paris), **98**, 112 (1887).
Eagleton. *Arch. Ophthal.*, **14**, 1 (1935).
Elliott. *Lancet*, **2**, 1308 (1893).
Elschnig. *Allg. Wien. med. Ztg.*, **36**, 61 (1892).
Ewing. *Arch. Path.*, **19**, 690 (1935).
Neoplastic Diseases, 4th ed., Phila. (1940).
Feingold. *Trans. Amer. ophthal. Soc.*, **20**, 267 (1922).
Fiedler and Costin. *Arch. Ophthal.*, **65**, 669 (1961).
Findlay. *Lancet*, **1**, 1229 (1930).
Fox. *Amer. J. Ophthal.*, **33**, 1144 (1950).
Fuchs. *Das Sarkom d. Uvealtraktus*, Wien (1882).
Klin. Mbl. Augenheilk., **56**, 152 (1916).
Galezowsky. *Recueil Ophtal.*, **1**, 86 (1873).
Gruening. *Arch. Augenheilk. Ohrenheilk.*, **3**, 168 (1873).
Hay. *Trans. ophthal. Soc. U.K.*, **54**, 576 (1934).
Höhne. *Klin. Mbl. Augenheilk.*, **52**, 400 (1914).
Ide. *Ophthal. Rec.*, **22**, 651 (1913).
Knox. *Arch. Path.*, **7**, 274 (1929).
Kolodny. *Arch. Neurol. Psychiat.*, **21**, 1107 (1929).
Kopff. *Recueil Ophtal.*, **20**, 264 (1898).
Lagrange. *Tumeurs de l'oeil*, Paris, **1** (1901).
Lane. *Arch. Ophthal.*, **12**, 980 (1934).

[1] Vol. XIII.
[2] Vol. XII, p. 577.

Leber and Krahnstöver. *v. Graefes Arch. Ophthal.*, **45,** 164, 231, 467 (1898).
Mackenzie. *A Treatise of Diseases of the Eye*, London (1830).
Malherbe and Chenantois. *Bull. Soc. Anat. Paris*, **15,** 169 (1880).
Marin. *Arch. Oftal. hisp.-amer.*, **17,** 325 (1917).
Mathewson. *Trans. Amer. ophthal. Soc.*, **2,** 193 (1874).
Meyer. *Klin. Mbl. Augenheilk.*, **36,** 435 (1898).
Meyerhof. *Klin. Mbl. Augenheilk.*, **40** (1), 300 (1902).
Montanelli. *Lettura Oftal.*, **3,** 185 (1926).
Moretti. *Ann. Ottal.*, **57,** 515 (1929).
Mura. *Ann. Ottal.*, **60,** 125 (1932).
Nitsch. *Z. Augenheilk.*, **57,** 225 (1925).
Noyes. *Trans. Amer. ophthal. Soc.*, **2,** 594 (1879).
Oliver and Roberts. *Arch. Ophthal.*, **47,** 78 (1952).
Pack. *Surgery*, **46,** 447 (1959).
Panas. *Arch. Ophtal.*, **22,** 1 (1902).
Patel. *Brit. J. Ophthal.*, **17,** 40 (1933).
Pereyra. *Ann. Ottal.*, **42,** 796 (1913).
Pfingst. *Klin. Mbl. Augenheilk.*, **33,** 256 (1895).
Raven. *Ann. roy. Coll. Surg.*, **6,** 28 (1950).
Reeh and Swan. *Trans. Amer. Acad. Ophthal.*, **54,** 312 (1950).
Ruvioli. *Ann. Ottal.*, **6,** 187 (1877).
Sauerbruch. *Dtsch. Z. Chir.*, **199,** 1 (1926).
Scheiss-Gemuseus. *v. Graefes Arch. Ophthal.*, **14** (1), 87 (1868).
Schneider. *v. Graefes Arch. Ophthal.*, **23** (3), 209 (1877).
Sefic. *Klin. Mbl. Augenheilk.*, **83,** 824 (1929).
Smith, Priestley. *Trans. ophthal. Soc. U.K.*, **17,** 251 (1897).
Stieda. *Zbl. Chir.*, **54,** 1070 (1927).
Stieren. *J. Amer. med. Ass.*, **103,** 311 (1934).
Teulières. *Arch. Ophtal.*, **33,** 236 (1913).
Trettenero. *Ann. Ottal.*, **59,** 272 (1931).
Voigt. *Münch. med. Wschr.*, **51,** 175 (1904).
Warthin. *J. cancer Res.*, **12,** 249 (1928).
Wätzold. *v. Graefes Arch. Ophthal.*, **113,** 286 (1924).
Webster, Stevenson and Stout. *Surg. Clin. N. Amer.*, **24,** 319 (1944).
Weiss. *Münch. med. Wschr.*, **46,** 1265 (1899).
Wood. *Ophthal. Rec.*, **22,** 422 (1913).
Wulkow. *Klin. Mbl. Augenheilk.*, **85,** 669 (1930).

THE OPHTHALMOLOGICAL IMPLICATIONS OF HEAD INJURY

Man's endeavours to attain higher and still higher speeds in travel, to mechanize civilian industry with machines of greater and still greater power, and to search for more and still more effective techniques of destruction in war have all combined to heighten the incidence of head injuries to an extent unknown to a previous generation; at the same time, his increased efficiency in dealing with such injuries has achieved a survival rate, and therefore a knowledge of their immediate and remote after-effects, which is steadily growing. Many of these have profound ophthalmological significance and, among the many clinical facets which each case presents for study, the ocular symptoms are frequently of great importance in the general assessment of the patient, and an appreciation of their importance is necessary for adequate treatment and informed prognosis.

Ophthalmological complications of head injuries are common; analysing 500 cases, Hooper (1951) found ocular sequelæ in 58. Their occurrence depends on three incidents. In the first place, concussion, contusion or laceration of the substance of the brain owing to the trauma itself may have dramatic visual implications. In the second place, a fracture of the skull, either of the vault in the occipital region or of the base, may cause mechanical damage to the cerebral areas subserving vision or to the optic, motor or sensory nerves associated with the eye. Finally, cerebral compression due to meningeal hæmorrhage—whether acute or chronic, extradural, subdural, subarachnoid or intracerebral—may produce ophthalmological signs on the recognition and correct interpretation of which the patient's life may depend.

It may be useful to point out that progressive cerebral compression such as results from intracranial bleeding goes through four well-defined clinical stages, for an adequate appreciation of which the writings of Cushing (1903), Trotter (1914–15), Evans and Scheinker (1943–46), Scheinker (1947) and Evans (1950) should be consulted—(1) a symptomless stage of physical compensation, when the cerebro-spinal fluid is displaced and the blood-pressure rises to maintain the circulation in the head; (2) a stage of venous compression, when irritative signs appear; (3) a stage of capillary anæmia, when paralytic signs appear; and (4) an irreversible and final stage characterized by perivascular hæmorrhages from venous back-pressure and a progressive œdematous swelling of the brain-substance which, in the last analysis, is lethal. In the treatment of such cases it is a good general rule that localizing signs of compression should be taken to indicate the advisability of operative decompression, and this should be done the more urgently the more rapid the development of these signs; among them ophthalmological changes, particularly those involving the pupil, are of no small importance.

In the early stages of unconsciousness after a head injury the visual axes are often divergent, while intermittent, vague and irregular movements of the eyes may be seen, sometimes affecting one or other eye separately or at different times. These probably indicate a disturbance of function due to generalized cerebral damage, and on the return to consciousness they generally cease, the vague ocular excursions being replaced by conjugate movements. At this stage also the pupils are usually small and fixed, a phenomenon possibly associated with the general cerebral irritation, and on the return of consciousness, nystagmus and vertigo perhaps associated with nausea and vomiting indicating a disturbance of the vestibular apparatus, may complicate the period of fogging of thought and loss of memory. In more severe cases a similar embarrassment of the respiratory and circulatory centres may lead to a fatal termination. It has also been observed that in the stage of cerebral shock the ocular tension may be low; when recovery occurs the tension regains its normal level, while in fatal cases a condition of hypotony remains until death (Casari, 1951). These changes are probably related to disturbances in the control of the cerebral vascular system.

In the later stages important ophthalmological implications may appear in great variety; these have already been noted in another volume of this *System*,[1] so that a brief recapitulation is all that should be required here. Orbital fractures occurring as extensions of fractures of the base of the skull have already been discussed.[2]

INJURIES TO THE VISUAL PATHWAYS

Injuries to the optic nerves in the region of the optic canals have already been considered at some length[3]; concussion injuries to the head, usually involving a fracture of the skull, may also, although rarely, cause injury to

[1] Vol. XII. [2] p. 265. [3] Vol. XII, p. 273.

the chiasma, sometimes associated with hypothalamic symptoms. Such injuries are perhaps occasionally caused by rupture of the nerve fibres, but are more probably due to acute traumatic necrosis or tearing of the small pial vessels and result in bitemporal hemianopic field defects.[1] Similar injuries to the optic tracts cause visual defects of the homonymous hemianopic type, although they are usually of such severity as to preclude survival. Injuries to the radiations may entail visual defects varying from a quadrantanopia to a hemianopia[2]; while trauma to the cortex produces visual effects of very varied types, depending on the damage done to the extremely complex organization of the higher visual functions which depend on the integrity of the parieto-occipital cortex or the visuo-psychic area of the brain. The initial effects of concussion and œdema which may result in cortical blindness, recovery therefrom and post-concussive confusional states have already been discussed,[3] as well as the disturbances of the colour sense, of the appreciation of space, form, contour and pattern formation resulting from partial calcarine lesions, the permanent field defects resulting from complete lesions, and the disabilities arising from injuries to the associational areas of the cortex—visual agnosia[4] of various types, including defective visual localization of objects in space and loss of topographical memory, apraxia, aphasia, and dyslexia. Such disturbances follow severe head injuries and may be caused by direct trauma, but are much more commonly due to the pressure caused by intracranial hæmorrhage; although gross confusion may last for some weeks, slow improvement usually continues for many months but recovery is rarely, if ever, complete.

A constriction of the visual fields, usually concentric in nature, was observed by Charcot (1878) to follow cerebral injury, particularly of the parieto-occipital region, a disturbance which may be associated with other disabilities preferentially affecting dark adaptation. There is a tendency for the constriction of the field to affect the ipsilateral eye, while in cases of homonymous hemianopia the non-hemianopic half-fields are similarly affected. This phenomenon, which has already been referred to,[5] is not yet understood. It has been ascribed to organic changes after contusion (Poppelreuter, 1917), to increased pressure of the cerebro-spinal fluid in the vaginal space (Raski, 1948), or to disturbances of the higher visual functions above the calcarine level (Paterson, 1944), but in most cases the evidence, particularly the incongruity of the fields as measured with varying test-objects at varying distances, suggests a functional origin (Glees, 1951; and others).

Other psychogenic manifestations varying from hysterical blindness to blepharospasm, are also not unusual sequelæ.[6]

PUPILLARY CHANGES

Pupillary changes are often of considerable importance in concussion head injuries, three types being of particular interest. The *widely dilated*,

[1] Vol. XII, p. 286.
[2] Vol. XII, p. 458.
[3] Vol. XII, p. 407.
[4] Vol. XII, p. 510.
[5] Vol. XII, p. 503.
[6] Vol. XII, p. 579.

immobile Hutchinson's pupil or, more correctly, *Cook's pupil*,[1] inactive to all reflexes, direct and consensual, sometimes in severe cases bilateral, but typically (although not invariably) ipsilateral to the side of the injury, developing shortly after the accident, may be of considerable diagnostic importance in fractures of the skull associated with the development of a raised supratentorial pressure due to hæmorrhage.[2] The pupillary dilatation may appear after an initial transient miosis and on recovery is followed by miosis. As one of the most constant signs of a fractured skull accompanied by meningeal bleeding, its presence is an indication for a decompression operation in so far as it is due to a gross cerebral shift causing the temporal lobe to herniate into the tentorial hiatus so as to impinge upon and stretch the IIIrd nerve, a mechanism first suggested by Jefferson (1937–42) and substantiated by Reid and Cone (1939).

The frequency with which the dilated pupil is ipsilateral to the hæmatoma makes it sound practice to search for the intracranial bleeding on the side showing mydriasis, but it is to be remembered that this relationship is by no means constant (Kennedy and Wortis, 1936), while unilateral pupillary changes may be associated with bilateral hæmatoma (King and Walsh, 1949). It is to be noted that a transient unilateral mydriasis may have the same localizing significance as the more usual persistent widening (Woodhall *et al.*, 1941).

An *absolute paralytic mydriasis* results from the destructive effects of hæmorrhages in the brain-stem affecting the oculomotor nucleus or from a basal fracture involving the IIIrd nerve trunk[3]; while an *inequality of the pupils*, wherein the difference in size is not usually great, is the commonest abnormality indicating damage to the mid-brain. This is a more common sign of persistent damage in this region than ophthalmoplegia (Brain, 1942). The larger pupil is usually the abnormal one, showing an absence or sluggishness in its reactions to light and convergence, anomalies which are occasionally bilateral but are rarely found together. Such an iridoplegia often tends to disappear a few months after the injury. An *Argyll Robertson pupil* showing isolated light rigidity with retention of the synkinetic reaction (the *pseudo-reflex traumatic pupillary paralysis* of Behr)[4] developing after skull injury may indicate similar damage to the Edinger-Westphal nucleus. It will be remembered that an Argyll Robertson pupil may also follow orbital injury involving the ciliary ganglion in the orbit.[5]

The importance of these pupillary reactions cannot be over-stressed. A dilated and fixed pupil observed immediately after an accident usually indicates a laceration involving the IIIrd nerve or its nucleus; observed to develop some time after the accident, the same appearance is almost invariably due to the pressure induced by an extradural blood clot; the bilateral extension of this phenomenon indicates an increase in the intra-

[1] Vol. XII, p. 623. [2] Vol. XII, p. 626.
[3] Vol. XII, p. 619. [4] Vol. XII, p. 665.
[5] Vol. XII, p. 662.

cranial pressure. The first lesion is usually associated with other evidences of involvement of the IIIrd nerve—ptosis and extra-ocular muscular palsies; the second is confined to the pupillary reactions alone. Owing to the importance of the information thus provided, the pupils should be kept under frequent observation in all cases of head injury and their reactions should never be masked by the exhibition of mydriatics.

OCULAR MOTOR PHENOMENA

Ocular motor injuries, apart from damage to muscles and nerves in the orbit itself, are among the commonest sequels of head injury, a type of accident which, as we have seen, accounts for some 15% of all ocular motor palsies, whether sustained at birth[1] or as a result of accident in adult life; they complicate some 1% of accidental traumata to the head (Turner, 1943). These embrace a great diversity of clinical pictures, varying from total bilateral ophthalmoplegia to syndromes involving the palsy of individual nerves which are affected in the order of frequency—VIth, IIIrd and IVth. An interesting complication is a paresis of the IVth nerve which may be bilateral (Chapman *et al.*, 1970; Burger *et al.*, 1970). When the IIIrd nerve is involved, particularly in basal lesions, a traumatic ptosis results. They may be *nuclear* or *root palsies* due to hæmorrhagic lesions in the brain-stem, or *trunk lesions* associated with basal fractures or the compression or mechanical displacement caused by a meningeal hæmorrhage, a type of damage to which the VIth nerve is particularly prone. In most cases the actual type of injury must remain a matter of deduction, but the fact that many of the palsies are incomplete and of temporary duration suggests that the common lesion is concussion or stretching; bony fractures involving a displacement which may only be momentary may cause actual tearing of a nerve trunk or interference with its blood supply.

The clinical significance of these palsies both in infants and in adults has already been fully discussed,[2] where it was pointed out that they are characterized by the paralysis of individual muscles or groups of muscles with loss of parallelism of the eyes and consequent diplopia; the only clue in the differentiation of nuclear from trunk lesions is evidence of associated lesions in the brain-stem in the former and the occasional involvement of other nerve trunks in the latter. Spontaneous recovery, which in most cases is organically and functionally complete within a period varying from 4 to 6 months, is the usual sequel to traumatic palsies of this type. Orthoptic treatment may sometimes be of considerable value during this somewhat trying period when diplopia is causing distress, partly to maintain the habit of fusion and increase its amplitude and partly to raise the morale of the patient, for it is to be remembered that diplopia is a most incapacitating condition liable to provoke profound depression in the type of patient in whom the tendency for the development of an anxiety state is high (Candler,

[1] p. 14. [2] Vol. XII, p. 725.

1945; Neely, 1945–47; and others). If spontaneous recovery does not occur, muscle-surgery can frequently bring relief in a surprising number of cases; the principles employed are discussed elsewhere.[1] If recovery does not ensue, occlusion of one eye is the only alternative to the misery of diplopia endured until suppression makes the patient functionally uniocular.

The paradoxical associated movements which sometimes become evident in the healing stage of such lesions have already been discussed (the pseudo-Graefe phenomenon, etc.).[2]

SUPRANUCLEAR OCULAR MOTOR PALSIES following head injury are more rare; they involve a disturbance of conjugate eye movements with the retention of ocular parallelism and an absence of diplopia. Typically, pontine lesions affect conjugate lateral deviations, and the defect may well be permanent, while lesions higher in the brain-stem are characterized by disturbances of up-and-down deviations as well as of convergence and occasionally of divergence. Injuries at the cerebral level, on the other hand, involving the frontal lobes or their corticofugal tracts, produce conjugate palsies which are frequently temporary, wherein there is a diminution or loss of voluntary movements of the eyes in a specified direction sometimes associated with an exaggeration of the fixation reflexes so that the eyes cannot be dissociated from an object on which they are directed; alternatively they may produce conjugate spasms wherein an involuntary deviation persists to the side opposite to the lesion. If the occipital or parietal areas are affected, disorientations of the psycho-optical reflexes may occur (fixation, convergence, blinking reflexes, etc.). Finally, a lesion affecting the brain-stem, the vestibular system or the cerebellum may give rise to nystagmus; all these conditions have already been fully discussed.[3]

DEFECTS OF CONVERGENCE AND ACCOMMODATION are common sequels of head injuries, the two functions usually failing to an equal degree although either may occasionally be separately deficient. Sometimes a lesion in the brain-stem or IIIrd nerve is causal, very occasionally in the supranuclear mechanism, but in the majority of cases the disability is functional. The defect is most frequent in those who have hyperphoria and is probably a fatigue effect initially associated with a traumatic disturbance of the higher centres, but once the tendency has become established the habit of diplopia on attempting near work may be perpetuated as a neurosis; it is significant that in many of these cases the power of the ciliary muscle as measured by the amplitude of accommodation may be normal (Wescott, 1943; Grove, 1943; Smith, 1949). Sometimes spontaneous cure occurs, but this is usually assisted in a dramatic way by suitable orthoptic exercises, particularly in those cases wherein the powers of convergence and accommodation have failed together (Cross, 1945; Candler, 1945; Neely, 1947). In uncomplicated cases the prognosis is good, but unfortunately in many patients the changes in psychology and personality following head injuries of any severity may be

[1] Vol. VI. [2] Vol. XII, p. 785. [3] Vol. XII.

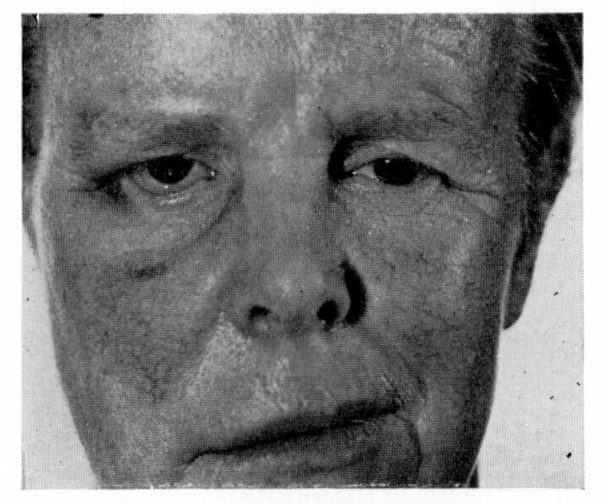

FIG. 665.

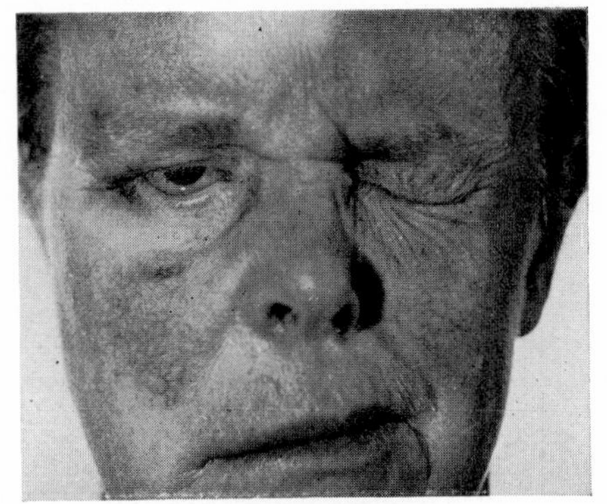

FIG. 666.

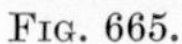

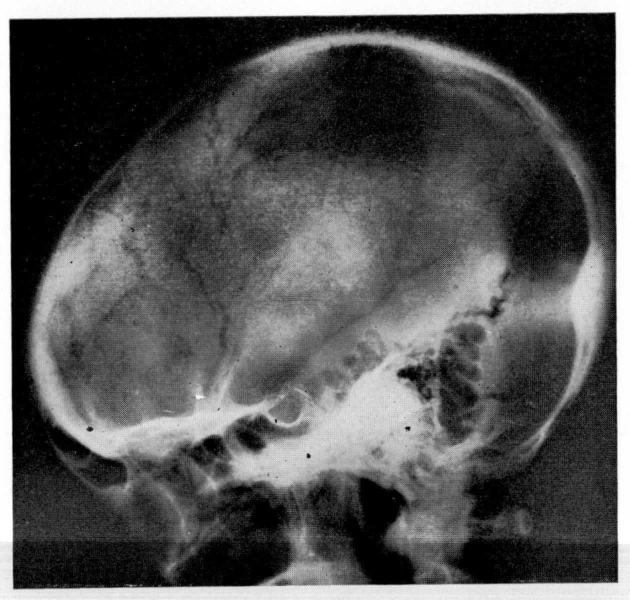

FIG. 667.

FIGS. 665 to 667.—TRAUMATIC FACIAL PALSY.

Right lower motor neuron facial palsy associated with a fracture of the temporal bone sustained in a fall from a horse. Complete recovery ensued.

profound and lasting (see Paterson, 1942–44; Symonds and Russell, 1943; Pflugfelder, 1949; and others).

The FACIAL NERVE may be implicated in cerebral trauma, injury being sustained either in a fracture of the petrous part of the temporal bone frequently accompanied by bleeding from the ear on the same side, by direct trauma near the stylo-mastoid foramen or as a result of a displaced fracture of the ramus of the mandible, with resulting paralysis of the muscles of the lids and face of the lower neuron (peripheral) type. This involves paralytic ectropion, epiphora and a certain degree of lagophthalmos (Figs. 665–667) (Potter, 1964; Briggs and Potter, 1967).

A fracture of the petrous bone may have localizing signs other than the muscular palsy in the face; thus a lesion of the facial nerve between the level of the VIth nucleus and the geniculate ganglion involves a *diminution of lacrimation* owing to involvement of fibres destined for the greater superficial petrosal nerve, while a lesion distal to this ganglion leaves the secretion of tears unimpaired; moreover, a lesion involving the intermediate nerve of Wrisberg, the fibres of which find a cell-station in the geniculate ganglion and leave the facial nerve 3 or 4 mm. above the stylo-mastoid foramen, involves a decrease in the salivary secretion of the sublingual and submaxillary glands and abolishes taste in the anterior two-thirds of the tongue. Involvement of the stapedius nerve in a fracture affecting this region may also entail hyperacousis.

The ocular effects of facial palsies and their treatment have already been discussed.[1]

A delayed and rare sequel of a traumatic facial palsy is the development of *hemifacial spasm*, characterized by intermittent twitching of a group of facial muscles (sometimes involving the orbicularis palpebrarum) which may eventually evolve into widespread and very distressing clonic spasms. The clinical features and treatment of the condition have been studied elsewhere.[2]

As with IIIrd nerve lesions, a facial palsy on recovery may be accompanied by *paradoxical movements*, unintentional and abnormal mass movements of the facial muscles; closure of the eyes, for example, may be associated with spasmodic movements of the lower part of the face. These are due to aberrant regeneration of nerve fibres, some of which may grow into the wrong sheath in the disorder which may accompany regeneration. These movements and the treatment of the condition have already been discussed at length.[3]

In a similar manner *paradoxical gustatory-lacrimal reflexes* may appear as a rarity in the healing stage of a facial palsy when eating, particularly in the case of highly seasoned foods, accompanied by the shedding of "crocodile tears"[4]; in this case secretory fibres destined for a salivary gland have become diverted to the lacrimal gland.

It is to be noted also that a lesion of the *greater superficial petrosal nerve*, which occasionally occurs in a fracture of the skull, the *sphenopalatine ganglion* or its lacrimal branch, leads to a diminution or abolition of both psychical and reflex lacrimation.

Finally, involvement of the TRIGEMINAL NERVE, either intracerebrally or at the base of the skull, causing anæsthesia and sometimes paræsthesias over the area subserved by one or more of its branches (including the cornea in the case of the first), should be remembered, occurring usually in association with some ocular motor palsy.

A rare complication which may have ophthalmological implications should be noted. A fracture through the semicircular canals, often associated with facial paralysis and deafness, may produce the train of symptoms characteristic of Ménière's disease—dizziness, nausea, vomiting, diplopia and nystagmus sometimes accompanied by wild uncoordinated movements of the eyes. Sufficiently severe cases of this type may require intracranial section of the vestibular nerve.

VASCULAR COMPLICATIONS

Two vascular complications of head injury may have considerable ophthalmological repercussions. *Intracranial hæmorrhage*, whether extra- or subdural or intracerebral, apart from causing damage to the central nervous tissues immediately concerned with vision, causes pupillary changes

[1] Vol. XII, p. 916.
[2] Vol. XII, p. 932.
[3] Vol. XII, p. 924.
[4] Vol. XII, p. 961.

FIGS. 668 to 670.—CAROTICO-CAVERNOUS FISTULA (P. H. Schurr).

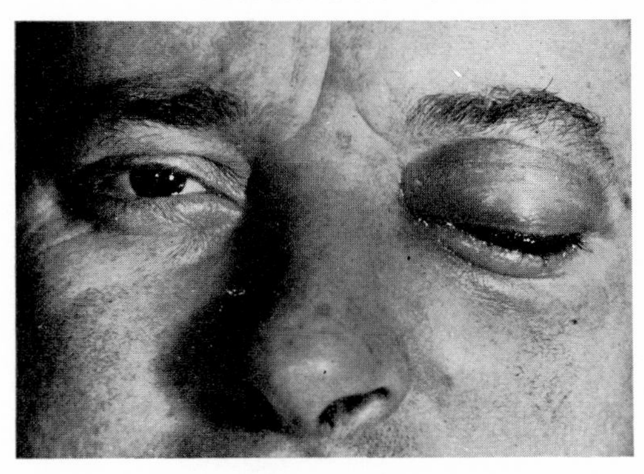

FIG. 668.

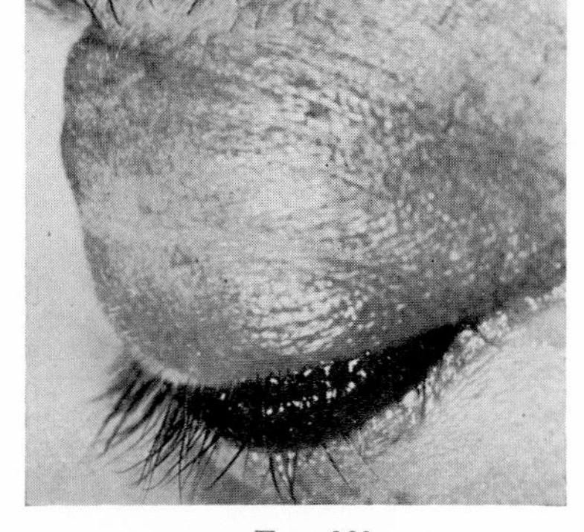

FIG. 669.

FIGS. 668 and 669.—A man aged 53 fell on his head and was admitted to hospital with œdema of the lids, chemosis and immobility of the left eye.

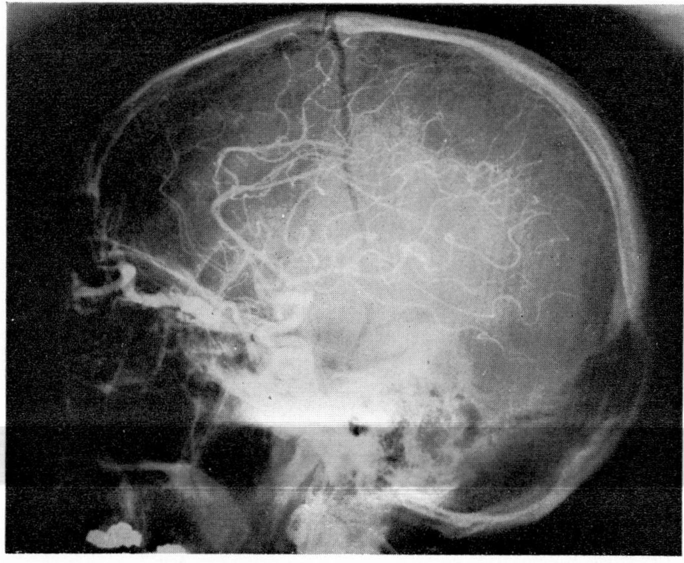

FIG. 670.—The arteriogram showed a left carotico-cavernous fistula causing gross engorgement of the superior orbital veins. The right anterior cerebral artery is supplied by the left internal carotid. A left tarsorrhaphy was done for an exposure keratitis. After 12 months the proptosis and ophthalmoplegia had disappeared and man returned to work; presumably the aneurysm had spontaneously healed.

and papillœdema in a high proportion of cases, due to increased intracerebral pressure; while a subarachnoid hæmorrhage, in many cases of traumatic origin, is responsible for the dramatic ophthalmoscopic picture of papillœdema and retinal hæmorrhages as well as varying types of ocular motor palsies.

FIGS. 671 to 673.—TRAUMATIC CAROTICO-CAVERNOUS FISTULA.

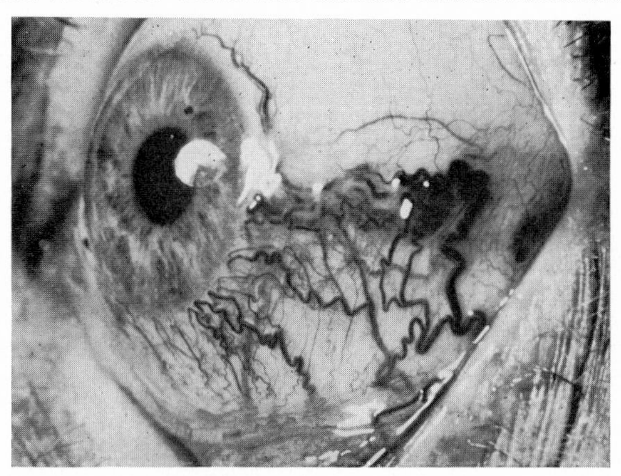

FIG. 671.—Telangiectasia of the conjunctival vessels (M. D. Sanders and W. F. Hoyt).

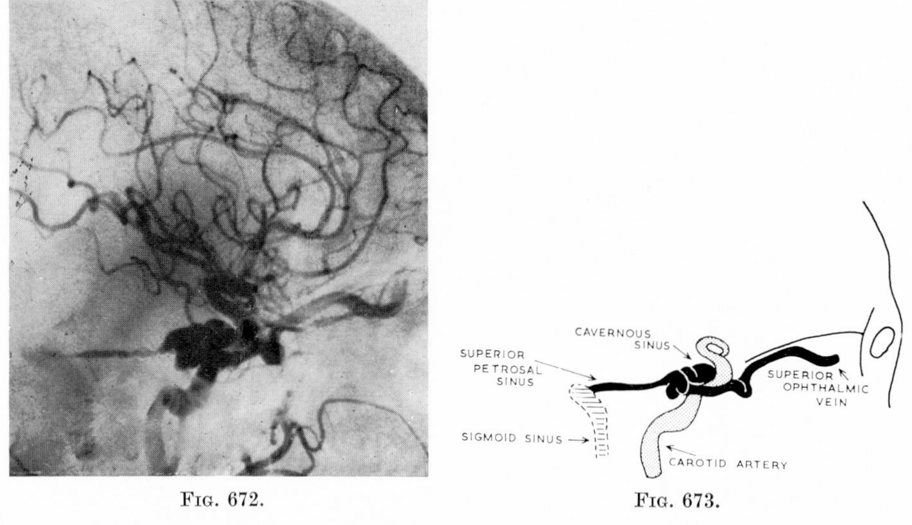

FIG. 672. FIG. 673.

FIGS. 672 and 673.—Subtraction carotid angiogram showing blood going into the superior ophthalmic vein and petrosal sinus in the arterial phase (J. D. Bull).

Intracranial aneurysms constitute a further and usually a late complication of a head injury which causes direct damage to the vessel walls. The effect of these aneurysms on vision and the ocular motor system, as well as the catastrophe of their rupture, have already been fully discussed[1]; and the dramatic picture described clinically as *pulsating exophthalmos*, caused by a carotico-cavernous communication, is discussed in detail elsewhere (Figs. 400, 668–673)[2].

[1] Vol. XII, p. 305. [2] Vol. XIII.

It will be remembered that some 80% of all cases of carotico-cavernous communication are of traumatic origin and that some 75% are associated with a fracture of the skull usually involving the body of the sphenoid bone; exceptionally it may follow a fracture of the sella turcica (Gigglberger, 1950; Sanders and Hoyt, 1969); penetrating wounds account for a few instances and injuries by *contre-coup* from a contusion of the occiput, forehead or temple constitute the remainder. As a rule a sudden rupture of the carotid artery into the cavernous sinus with its intensely dramatic clinical picture does not occur at the time of the accident; the more common sequence is a traumatic weakening of the arterial wall to form a saccular aneurysm which subsequently gives way. Alternatively, a minute tear is formed in the arterial wall associated, perhaps, with some pain and a bruit, and as this tear gradually grows larger over some days, weeks or months, the classical clinical picture of pulsating exophthalmos associated with a bruit and a thrill slowly develops to its full intensity, at first unilaterally and often at a later stage bilaterally, bringing in its train danger to vision and also to life.

Several LATE EFFECTS OF HEAD INJURY may be noted in passing, all of which have received full mention in a previous volume of this *System*[1]. A raised intracranial pressure due to delayed meningeal bleeding may become evident some time after the injury, associated with the usual ophthalmological signs of papillœdema, muscular palsies and pupillary changes; more rarely a low pressure, sometimes also associated with papillœdema, may develop due, presumably, to diminished secretion of cerebrospinal fluid owing to damage to the choroid plexus or a persistent leakage of fluid. We have already seen that aneurysms, particularly carotico-cavernous communications, are typically of late onset, while the development of infection, either acutely as a meningitis or a cerebral abscess, or slowly to determine a chiasmal arachnoiditis, is by no means uncommon. Finally, the formation of callus in the healing of fractures around the optic canal has been recorded as involving compression of the optic nerve with consequent visual symptoms (Lillie and Adson, 1934).

Brain. *Proc. roy. Soc. Med.*, **35,** 755 (1942).
Briggs and Potter. *Brit. med. J.*, **2,** 464 (1967).
Burger, Kalvin and Smith. *Brain*, **93,** 567 (1970).
Candler. *Trans. ophthal. Soc. U.K.*, **65,** 57 (1945).
Casari. *Boll. Oculist.*, **30,** 649 (1951).
Chapman, Urist, Folk and Miller. *Arch. Ophthal.*, **84,** 137 (1970).
Charcot. *Localisation in Diseases of the Brain*, N.Y. (1878).
Cross. *Trans. ophthal. Soc. U.K.*, **65,** 20 (1945).
Cushing. *Amer. J. med. Sci.*, **125,** 1017 (1903).
Evans. *Acute Head Injury*, Springfield (1950).
Evans and Scheinker. *Arch. Neurol. Psychiat.*, **50,** 258 (1943).
J. Neurosurg., **1,** 306 (1944); **2,** 306 (1945); **3,** 101 (1946).
Ass. Res. nerv. ment. Dis. Proc., **24,** 98, 254 (1945).
Gigglberger. *Klin. Mbl. Augenheilk.*, **116,** 153 (1950).
Glees. *Nervenarzt*, **22,** 335 (1951).
Grove. *Wisconsin med. J.*, **42,** 210 (1943).
Hooper. *Brit. J. Surg.*, **39,** 126 (1951).
Jefferson. *Brain*, **60,** 444 (1937).
Glasg. med. J., **138,** 77 (1942).
Kennedy and Wortis. *Surg. Gynec. Obstet.*, **63,** 732 (1936).
King and Walsh. *Amer. J. Ophthal.*, **32,** 191 (1949).
Lillie and Adson. *Arch. Ophthal.*, **12,** 500 (1934).
Neely. *Trans. ophthal. Soc. U.K.*, **65,** 47 (1945).
Brit. J. Ophthal., **31,** 581 (1947).
Paterson. *Lancet*, **2,** 717 (1942).
Proc. roy. Soc. Med., **37,** 556 (1944).
Trans. ophthal. Soc. U.K., **64,** 115 (1944).
Pflugfelder. *Mschr. Psychiat. Neurol.*, **118,** 288, 379 (1949).

[1] Vol. XII.

Poppelreuter. *Die psych. Schädigungen durch Kopfschuss im Krieg*, Leipzig, **1** (1917).
Potter. *J. Laryngol.*, **78**, 654 (1964).
Raski. *Acta ophthal.* (Kbh.), Suppl. 29 (1948).
Reid and Cone. *J. Amer. med. Ass.*, **112**, 2030 (1939).
Sanders and Hoyt. *Brit. J. Ophthal.*, **53**, 82 (1969).
Scheinker. *J. Neurosurg.*, **4**, 255 (1947).
Smith. *Amer. J. Ophthal.*, **32**, 959 (1949).
Symonds and Russell. *Lancet*, **1**, 7 (1943).
Trotter. *Brit. J. Surg.*, **2**, 271 (1914–15).
Turner. *Brain*, **66**, 140 (1943).
Wescott. *Illinois med. J.*, **83**, 170 (1943).
Woodhall, Devine and Hart. *Surg. Gynec. Obstet.*, **72**, 391 (1941).

THE OPHTHALMOLOGICAL IMPLICATIONS OF REMOTE INJURY

Various injuries far afield may have ophthalmological implications of considerable interest; of these we shall note the following conditions—the effects of injury to the sympathetic chain in the neck, the retinal changes resulting from crush injuries, asphyxia and exsanguination, and the ocular manifestations of the " battered baby syndrome ".

INJURY TO THE SYMPATHETIC NERVE

HORNER'S OCULO-PUPILLARY SYNDROME, originally described by Claude Bernard, and characterized primarily by miosis, slight ptosis and pseudo-enophthalmos, and secondarily by an ipsilateral vasodilatation, a slight lowering of the intra-ocular pressure, an increase of temperature and hypohidrosis with some ultimate facial hemiatrophy and heterochromia of the iris, has already been fully discussed.[1] It will be remembered that it may occur as a result of any destructive lesion to the long and complicated sympathetic pathway from the hypothalamus to the cervical sympathetic chain, and that the most dramatic syndrome is seen in lesions of the cord when a spinal miosis results; fractures of the spine, the clavicle or the upper ribs or injuries to the neck, either incurred at birth, in accidents in later life or in wounds of war, figure in the ætiology. It will also be recalled that the *paradoxical pupillary reaction* may follow appropriate stimuli after a destructive lesion of the sympathetic involving the central paths, the sympathetic chain or the long ciliary nerves.[2]

THE WHIPLASH SYNDROME. Horner's syndrome is the commonest ocular manifestation of the whiplash syndrome. Such an injury occurs as the result of a violent flexion followed immediately by an even more violent extension of the head and neck. It occurs most commonly in a person involved in the sudden impact of two vehicles, particularly in a vehicle which sustains a rear-end type of collision. It may also occur in a pilot when an aeroplane is catapulted from the flight deck of an aircraft carrier if the movement of the head is not minimized by a special support for the occiput. The extent of the injury is not necessarily proportional to the speed or force of the impact but may be greater when a safety-belt is worn.

The whiplash injury causes a considerable degree of pain and discomfort even in the absence of any obvious evidence of structural damage on inspection or on radiological investigation, and some chronic pain is liable to persist for many years which tends to be regarded as largely of psychosomatic origin; this may well be incorrect. The headache may be associated with a feeling of posterior cervical tension. There may be evidence also of a concussion of the brain as the result of the acceleration–deceleration mechanism or of disturbance of the vertebral artery. It is, of course, possible for brain damage to give rise to difficulties of accommodation and heterotropia, including a temporary palsy of the VIth nerve with diplopia (Billig, 1953; Wiesinger and Guerry, 1961); the headaches and eyestrain thus caused may be relieved by periods of occlusion of one eye (Roy, 1958–61; Narazaki *et al.*, 1969).

[1] Vol. XII, p. 632. [2] Vol. XII, p. 636.

It is of interest that an incomplete Horner's syndrome, wherein ipsilateral sudomotor paralysis of the face is absent, may follow injury to the intracranial portion of the carotid artery.

A spastic mydriasis may follow irritation of the cervical sympathetic, or result from pressure by a hæmatoma in the neck after a crush injury (Bing, 1930).

CERVICAL MIGRAINE is a disorder of the functional unit formed by the vertebral nerve emerging from the stellate ganglion and the vertebral artery with its sympathetic plexus; the former conveys nervous stimuli to the cervical region, the latter to the head, including the eye. The usual symptoms are unilateral headache accompanied by paræsthesias, dizziness, aural and visual disorders, the whole being associated with a tenderness of the cervical spine, causing the patient to hold his head in a fixed position during an attack. Movements of the neck, in fact, frequently precipitate an attack and the patient learns to avoid them. Orbital pain is rare but blepharospasm and increased perspiration on the side involved are frequent; the dizziness is not associated with nystagmus or other disorders of the vestibular apparatus. The radiological appearances of the cervical spine are characteristic and always show osteochondritic changes, most frequently between the IIIrd and VIIth cervical vertebræ. A common precedent is a head injury involving a degeneration of the intervertebral discs and joints. Apart from symptomatic treatment such as heat, manipulation and paravertebral analgesia, surgical resection of the affected joints or nerve has been successful in relieving the symptoms (Geiger, 1952).

TRAUMATIC RETINOPATHY

A characteristic ophthalmoscopic picture, variously called TRAUMATIC RETINOPATHY of Purtscher, TRAUMATIC LIPORRHAGIA (LYMPHORRHAGIA) RETINÆ, or TRAUMATIC RETINAL ANGIOPATHY, has long been known to follow accidents, particularly those involving extensive crushing or fractures in various parts of the body. Ophthalmological reports of the condition have been relatively infrequent, perhaps because the symptoms are often transient and specialist examination is not requested in cases of this type: Amsler (1934) found only 25 cases in the literature, Bedell (1939) noted 40, Muhlmann and Ré (1940) reviewed 37 and by 1956 only 100 cases could be traced in the literature by Madsen (1965), while a comprehensive review was undertaken by Vérin and Le Rebeller (1967).

The history of the ocular condition is interesting. The earliest cases were described by Jacobi (1868) and Eales (1882–85), neither of whom recognized the full clinical implications of the retinal picture; thereafter, following the observations of Liebrecht (1906–12), and particularly of Purtscher (1910–13) who first fully described the condition in a patient following a fall from a roof which resulted in loss of consciousness for six days, several cases were reported; most of the earlier of these followed head injuries or compression of the chest, and the majority of the later followed automobile accidents.[1] The cause is usually an accident involving single or multiple

[1] Koerber (1910), Tietze (1911), Gonin (1912), Stähli (1915), Best (1919–22), Vogt and Knüsel (1921), Vogt (1923), Marchesani (1925), Rübel (1927), Rados (1931), Stokes (1932), Savitsky and Gross (1936), Smith (1941), Spaeth (1944), Renard (1946), Pinkerton (1946), Fritz and Hogan (1948), Newman (1948–62), Tanaka (1951), Alvarez Luna (1951), Anderson (1951), Nano and Scenna (1954), Kearns (1956), Frandsen (1956), Zaikova (1956), Cuccagna

fractures but the retinopathy may follow a blow on the orbit (Chou, 1928), compression of the thorax[1] or compression of the abdomen with rupture of the liver (Tietze, 1911; Bange, 1912; Cashell, 1957) (Fig. 674); alternatively an operation in a fatty area such as the breast or the neighbourhood of the kidney may produce the same result (Löwenstein, 1936; Morgan, 1949). Occasionally the typical picture has been reported after a fall which apparently did not involve a fracture (Vogt and Knüsel, 1921) or following an injury to the soft parts, while it has sometimes occurred after extensive burns or chronic osteomyelitis (Newman, 1948). Cases have also been reported as a rarity after shock treatment produced by triazol (Nightingale and Meyer, 1940), cardiazol (Nielsen and Ingham, 1940) and electrical convulsions (Meyer and Teare, 1945). It has also been observed after ligation of the common carotid artery for an aneurysm of the cavernous sinus (Schenk, 1955), after carotid arteriography (Cogan *et al.*, 1964) and following lymphangiography (Blancher, 1966; Vérin and Le Rebeller, 1967).

The Clinical Picture. The fundus presents a typical appearance which becomes evident usually 2 to 4 days after the accident but sometimes later, characterized as a rule by a number of islands of whitish-grey opacity somewhat resembling areas of fluffy exudate or localized milky patches of œdema; these are closely associated with the retinal vessels and are frequently numerous near the macular area (Plate XXV; Figs. 674–6). In some cases the resemblance to a diabetic retinopathy may be close but in others the patches are very extensive, covering great areas near the disc (Stähli, 1915; Bedell, 1939; Schmidt, 1968), appearing like masses of cumulus cloud in the clear sky or running in tongue-shaped extensions from the disc to the periphery (Purtscher, 1910; Chou, 1928). These lie above the retinal vessels which may be hidden by them and are usually, but not invariably, associated with hæmorrhages, frequently small and petechial, sometimes subhyaloid (Evans, 1940), but often profuse, so that the picture resembles a thrombosis of a retinal vein (Morgan, 1949; Barfoed, 1949). Sometimes the hæmorrhages or " exudates " may elevate the internal limiting membrane of the retina or invade the vitreous therein to form a cloud which may obscure the fundus. After 4 to 6 weeks these patches tend to fade away and eventually after a varying period (15 months, Muhlmann and Ré, 1940) the fundus may appear normal except, perhaps, for some mottling, pigmentary migration and optic atrophy. At the onset of symptoms changes in the visual field may occur varying from a central, paracentral or annular scotoma to large segmental defects; these frequently resolve completely but sometimes are lasting and,

---

(1958), Oksala (1958), W. and E. Marr (1962), Kuhnhardt (1964), Lazorthes *et al.* (1965), Madsen (1965), Bertoni (1967), François *et al.* (1967), Calmettes *et al.* (1967), Vérin and Le Rebeller (1967), Rask (1968), Schmidt (1968), Pratt and de Venecia (1970).

[1] Schneider (1924), Stokes (1932), Morgan (1945), Kehler (1953), Lyle *et al.* (1957), Hoare (1970) and others.

PLATE XXV

TRAUMATIC RETINAL ANGIOPATHY OF PURTSCHER.

A youth aged 19 suffered a severe compression of the lower thorax which involved retrograde congestion in the area of the superior vena cava as well as fractures of his fingers (J. G. H. Schmidt).

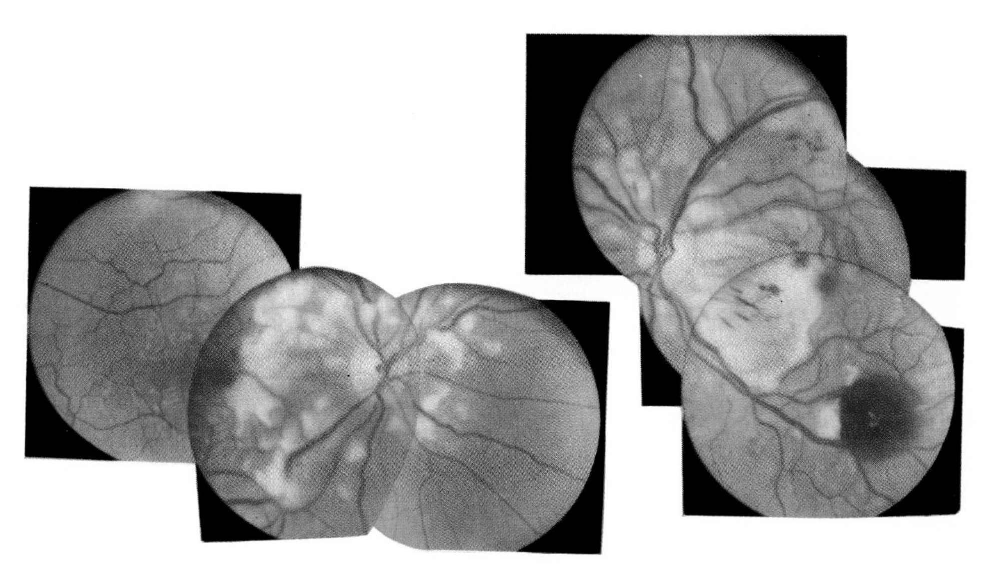

FIG. 1.—11 days after the accident.

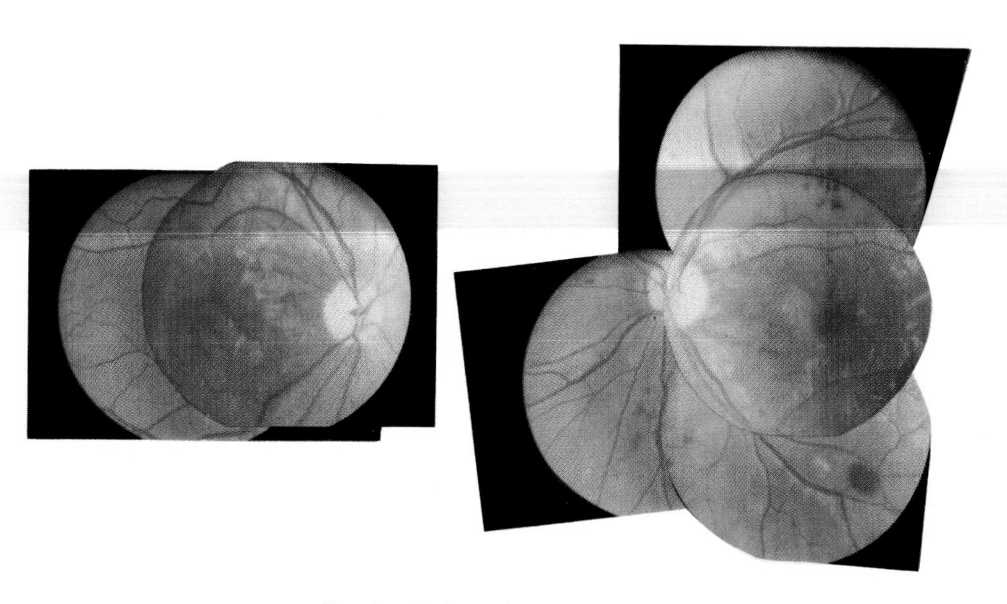

FIG. 2.—49 days after the accident.

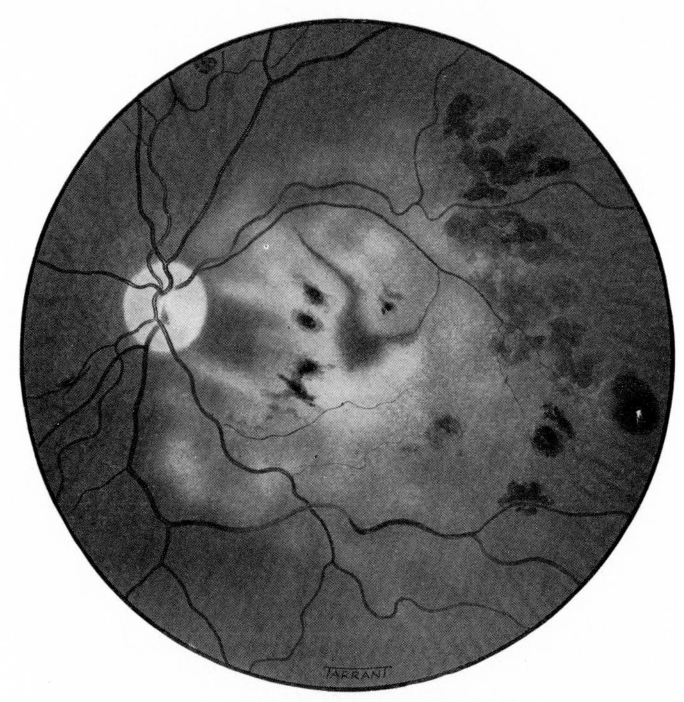

Fig. 674.—Retinopathy after Rupture of the Liver.

In a boy aged 7 who was knocked down by a truck. There was a fracture of the skull in the right occipital region and an abdominal hæmorrhage; an operation revealed a laceration 4 inches long in the right lobe of the liver. Seventeen days later the left eye showed a massive white exudate around the disc and the macula and numerous hæmorrhages both within and outside the exudative area. The arteries are thin and attenuated. There is commencing optic atrophy (G. T. W. Cashell).

Figs. 675 and 676.—Traumatic Retinopathy of Purtscher (P. H. Madsen).

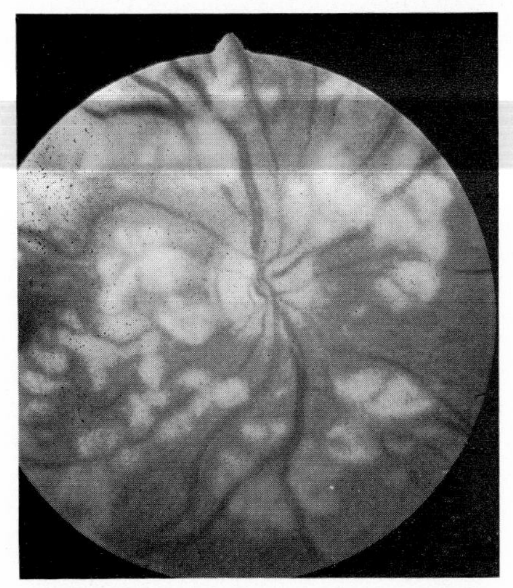

Fig. 675.—The right fundus of a man aged 61, six days after a compression of the chest.

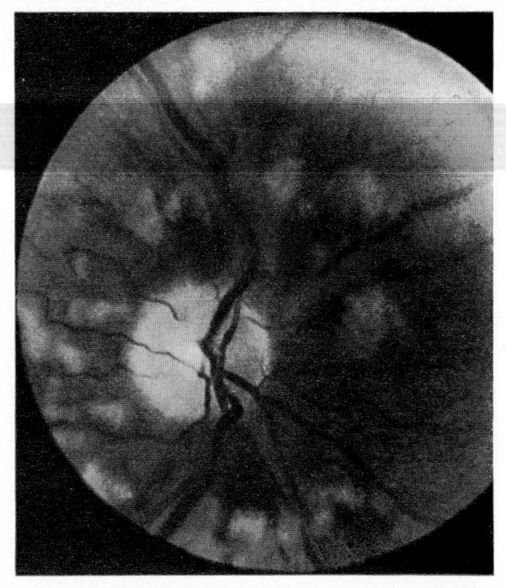

Fig. 676.—The right fundus of a man aged 25, six days after a compression injury to the head complicated by a left-sided extradural hæmatoma.

particularly if optic atrophy has occurred, the vision may be permanently damaged.

Ætiology. The first to theorize on the causation of the retinal lesions was Purtscher (1910) who attributed the opacities in traumatic cases to a rush of cerebro-spinal fluid forced from the subarachnoid space past the optic disc, along the perivascular sheaths of the retinal vessels and thence into the retinal tissue by the raised pressure generated by a head injury or thoracic compression. This became the generally accepted hypothesis (*angiopathica retinæ traumatica*, Purtscher; *retinal lymphorrhagia*, Koerber, 1910) until its mechanical improbability was pointed out and the suggestion was made that the opacity was similar to Berlin's œdema[1] caused by increased permeability or even small rents in the vessel walls due to concussive changes (Stähli, 1915; Best, 1919–22; Marchesani, 1925); in this view the type of change associated with the name of Berlin could be looked upon as an œdematous reaction while that linked with the name of Purtscher assumed the characteristics of a frankly exudative reaction following an initial vascular spasm (*traumatic angiospastic retinopathy*, Nicolas, 1949; Anderson, 1951; Gittler, 1963). The appearance of Berlin's œdema (*commotio retinæ*) and Purtscher's traumatic retinal angiopathy can be easily differentiated since in the former there are usually only one or two large diffuse white areas whereas Purtscher's disease is typically characterized by numerous small discrete pale white areas (W. and E. Marr, 1962).

A third view attributed the condition to exudation and hæmorrhages resulting from vascular damage due to a sudden back-pressure in the retinal veins (Bailliart, 1939; Brühn, 1940; Renard, 1946; Ardouin and Boulanger, 1952). Finally, following the pathological investigations of Urbanek (1934), and particularly since the frequency of fat embolism following injury became generally recognized, the retinal appearances have been widely attributed to this cause. In fat embolism the white infiltrates in the retina are smaller and often situated more peripherally than is usually seen in Purtscher's disease and may not be accompanied by venous congestion, at least in the early stages (Madsen, 1965).

The ætiology of these retinal disturbances following remote injury is probably varied and often complicated for more than one factor may be simultaneously operative. It may be that some cases, particularly those associated with multiple hæmorrhages, are due to a sudden venous reflux; these should be properly considered with compression cyanosis.[2] It is equally probable that the element of vascular spasm complicates the clinical picture in other cases; but it is certain that in many the occurrence of multiple fat emboli plays an important part in determining the condition.

The occurrence of MULTIPLE FAT EMBOLI after an injury involving fatty tissues is now well known, although the realization of its frequency and

[1] p. 165. [2] p. 728.

importance is comparatively recent. That oil injected into the circulation of an animal is prone to form emboli was originally demonstrated by Magendie (1836) and confirmed by Czerny (1875) and, although a parallel clinical occurrence was recognized in the early literature, as by Scriba (1880) who found evidence of fat embolism in 34 cases of fatal injury associated with extensive damage to bones, the clinical significance of such a condition in general surgery was not realized for some considerable time.[1] Robb-Smith (1941–42) found that such emboli were the major lethal factors in 115 fatal accidents; and during the second World War the condition became recognized clinically with comparative certainty when it was estimated that it occurred in 0·8% of battle casualties and played a major part in some 5% of fatalities (Wilson and Salisbury, 1944). Although fat embolism along with the crush syndrome and traumatic uræmia were recognized as three principal causes of high mortality in battle casualties, the importance of this condition in civilian casualties has probably been underestimated; indeed, of 7 such cases seen by Newman (1948) during the second World War, 5 were the result of ordinary road accidents rather than the circumstances of combat. Warren (1946) found that in 100 cases of fat embolism 91 showed fractures of one or more bones, particularly those of the leg; Grant and Reeve (1951) detected evidence of pulmonary fat embolism in 100% of fatalities resulting from multiple fractures; while Sevitt (1959–66) who made an extensive study of this condition concluded that the incidence of pulmonary fat embolism increased with the severity of the bone injury, rising to 80% in those with four or more fractures, and that between 90 and 100% of patients who died shortly after sustaining fractures showed fat emboli in the lungs at post-mortem, suggesting that histological fat embolism occurs after almost every bony fracture. On the other hand, clinical features attributable to fat embolism (the *fat embolism syndrome*) develop in only 1 to 2% of patients with fractures (Ross, 1970).

The clinical manifestations of systemic fat embolism, therefore, become a matter of considerable interest in an assessment of traumatic retinopathy. In the less severe cases a transient dyspnœa and light-headedness may be the sole general symptoms; and in all cases, even the least affected, complaint may be made of a deterioration of vision in one or both eyes. The clinical evolution of the more serious cases has been described by François and his colleagues (1967) in three stages: a latent interval of 1 to 3 days following the injury during which the patient begins to show signs of agitation is followed by a second stage, the onset of which is characterized by hyperthermia, tachycardia, marked restlessness, confusion and impending coma, accompanied by dyspnœa and a sensation as of suffocation; during this phase petechiæ appear, particularly on the skin of the chest wall, the base of the

[1] Utgenannt (1921), Bernhard (1925), Vance (1931), Oppolzer (1934), Groskloss (1936), Scuderi (1938–41), Harris *et al.* (1939), Robb-Smith *et al.* (1941), Rowlands and Wakeley (1941), Scott *et al.* (1942), Winkelman (1942), and others.

neck and subsequently on the trunk and sometimes on the face, most of which disappear after about 4 to 5 days; at the same time fat may be present in the sputum and occasionally in the urine.

On the assumption that the petechiæ are dermal infarcts and that histological sections would contain intravascular fat globules, biopsy of the cutaneous lesions has been recommended (Sevitt, 1962). However, such findings have rarely been demonstrated and it may be that the petechiæ are not infarcts but merely a manifestation of capillary fragility (Garnier and Peltier, 1967) associated with a profound fall in the level of the platelets (Ross, 1970).

During this stage the ocular signs are important; as a rule mydriasis is not seen unless there is also an extradural hæmatoma, there may be nystagmus, while sludging of the blood in the conjunctival vessels is usually associated with small ecchymoses. These petechiæ in the conjunctiva, the base of the neck, the anterior axillary folds and the abdominal wall are of great diagnostic significance (Newman, 1948) and were present in 37 of 45 cases of the fat embolism syndrome studied by Ross (1970). It is to be noted, however, that symptoms of mental disturbance are the most frequent presenting signs of this condition. In the fundi numerous small white areas may be seen, particularly in the region of the macula, and these may subsequently coalesce (Plate XXVI); they can generally be distinguished from the changes typical of Purtscher's retinopathy by the absence of retinal hæmorrhages (although these may occur later) and massive exudation. In the third stage of the syndrome the petechiæ may spread all over the body and jaundice may appear; in the fundi retinal hæmorrhages may occur with or without papillœdema, while a deterioration in the general condition of the patient is indicated by cyanosis, lowering of the blood pressure, tachycardia and signs of pericarditis; cerebral changes are particularly marked with increasing confusion, agitation and coma; finally, uræmia may develop and, in the absence of effective treatment, death.

It would appear that fat travels first to the pulmonary circulation whereupon in cases of massive emboli dyspnœa and cyanosis indicate the occurrence of pulmonary embolism, a phenomenon which usually occurs within 24 hours of the accident, although in acute cases the patient may die shortly after the injury on the operating table or may fail to recover from the anæsthetic. Thereafter the fat passes through the pulmonary into the general circulation and multiple emboli, frequently associated with hæmorrhages, may appear in practically all the organs and occasionally in the urine as well as the sputum, but the most severe symptoms are associated with the lodgment of multiple emboli in the brain, particularly in the end-arteries of the white matter (Fig. 677). These cerebral complications are ushered in by a confusional state followed by delirium with convulsions and paralysis of groups of muscles, while pupillary dilatation, Cheyne-Stokes breathing, coma and a rapid fall of blood pressure precede a fatal termination.

The general clinical picture may therefore vary from a total absence of

PLATE XXVI

FAT EMBOLISM

(L. Calmettes, F. Déodati and G. Béchac).

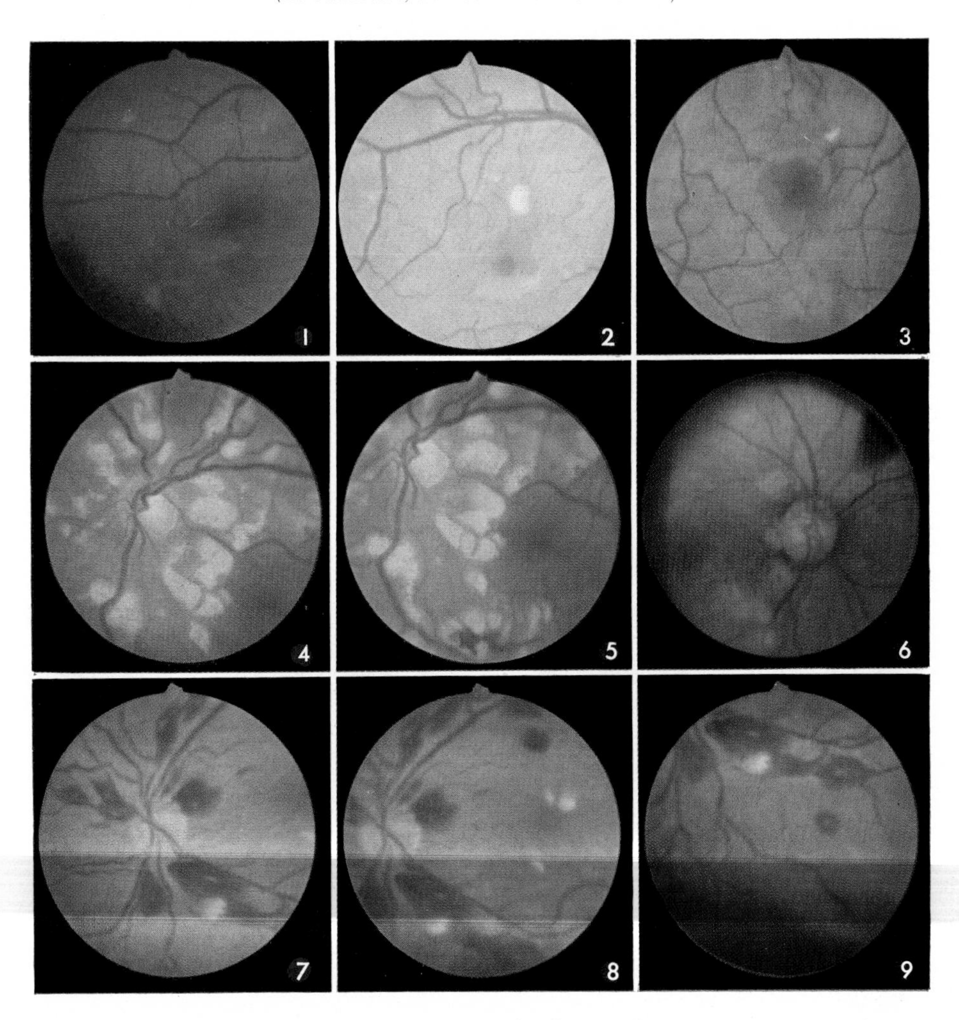

FIG. 1.—Early stage with faint white areas near the macula.

FIG. 2.—Macular œdema and cotton-wool spot.

FIG. 3.—Late stage.

FIGS. 4 AND 5.—Massive fat embolism at the posterior pole.

FIG. 6.—Retinal hæmorrhages.

FIGS. 7 TO 9.—Fat embolism complicated by hæmorrhagic retinopathy.

clinical signs to sudden death; it may be dominated by pulmonary symptoms appearing from some hours to some days after the accident or these may be trivial and an apparently normal convalescence may be interrupted after 2 or 3 days by the rapid onset of cerebral symptoms of varied severity. The visual symptoms are similarly varied, sometimes transient and probably often unnoticed, sometimes permanent and damaging. In addition to the pulmonary and cerebral manifestations, a third clinical syndrome has been recorded as a rare sequel to cerebral fat embolism; thus, Teare and his colleagues (1962) described three fatal cases of acute peptic ulceration and Harrison (1962) reported a similar case of massive fatal hæmatemesis.

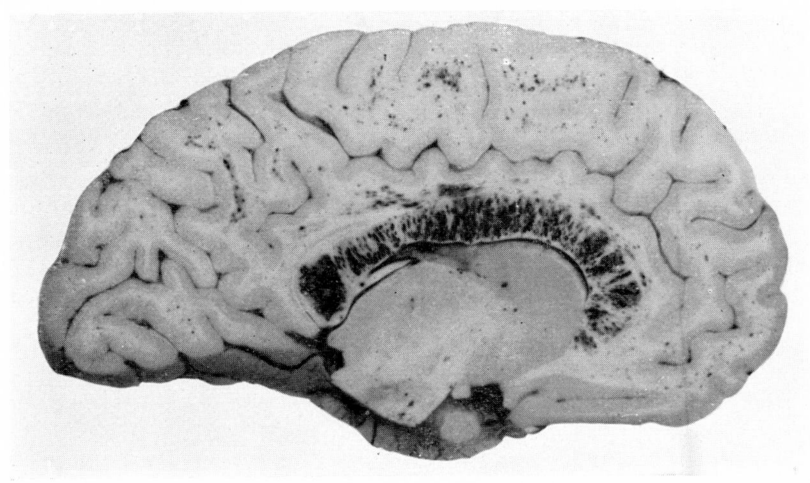

Fig. 677.—Multiple Fat Embolism.

Multiple emboli throughout the cerebral cortex and particularly in the corpus callosum, in a man who died without recovering consciousness shortly after suffering multiple fractures (Museum, Royal College of Surgeons).

The pathogenesis of traumatic fat embolism still remains a subject of dispute in which two theories, a mechanical and a chemical, have been propounded. The classical view advocated by Sevitt (1966) is that the embolic fat originates from the site of trauma, resulting from a simultaneous rupture of the cells of the tissues containing globules of fat of considerable size and tearing of venous channels so that the fat could enter the circulation; since the veins normally contract in the soft tissues in these circumstances but are held widely patent in the haversian canals of bone, such an incident would be expected most commonly after fractures particularly of the long bones and is especially prone to occur when considerable manipulation is required for the reduction of the deformity. When the fat globules reach the vessels of the brain, symptoms of cerebral embolism or even death may follow from mechanical blockage of the blood vessels. It is doubtful, however, whether the amount of fat retained in the lungs is ever of itself sufficient to cause symptoms because of the large pulmonary vascular bed.

The alternative view propounded by Bergentz (1961–66) states that the embolic fat is derived wholly or in part from neutral fat, not normally present in the blood, by an alteration in the stability of its suspension so that the finely divided emulsion is converted into larger fat droplets. Such a mechanism would account for the occurrence of fat emboli in cases which are not the result of trauma. Furthermore a distinction is drawn between the anatomical concept of fat embolism and the clinical syndrome: morbid anatomical evidence of fat embolism following trauma is common yet the clinical syndrome is relatively rare and may be due to other changes in the blood such as increased viscosity which is known to occur after trauma. Indeed, the concept that the effects of fat embolism are due to mechanical obstruction of the blood vessels by droplets of fat is challenged by some authorities who consider that the embolic fat is altered chemically, producing fatty acids which are highly irritant to the tissues. This view is supported by the demonstration of a rise in the values of blood lipase after bone trauma and is held to explain the latent interval between the injury and onset of symptoms (Peltier, 1957). It is, of course, odd that the condition should occur at all, bearing in mind that at body temperature the fat is in a liquid form so that it might be expected to pass through vessels without any hindrance; presumably other factors of a physical nature may be concerned, such as changes in surface tension or viscosity, which may determine the escape of fat from the lungs into the systemic circulation (Gee, 1967).

Pathology. The first pathological study of the retina in this condition was reported by Jacobi (1868) who noted that the retinal opacities were ether-soluble, but stressed the occurrence of granular degeneration of the retinal elements; Liebrecht (1906–12), after describing degeneration of the nerve fibres, noted that the glial tissues were loaded with fat. It is true that Hosch (1906) in a case of generalized fat embolism found fatty emboli in the brain, the retina and the choroid, but the case in question was not seen ophthalmoscopically; similar observations were made by Bernhard (1925), but it was not until the studies of Urbanek (1934) that the presence of fatty emboli was linked with the clinical picture. Subsequent observers have verified his findings.[1] Fatty emboli have been found abundantly in the small vessels supplying the optic nerve, the retina and the uveal tract, particularly near the posterior pole of the eye and rarely anteriorly as far as the ciliary processes, the deposits being especially abundant in the choriocapillaris and the terminal capillary network in the retina (Figs. 678–9). Bilateral secondary glaucoma associated with traumatic fat emboli in the retinal vessels was described by Finley and his colleagues (1963).

[1] Oppolzer (1934), Walsh (1947), Fritz and Hogan (1948), DeVoe (1950), Kearns (1956), Landolt (1957), Finley *et al.* (1963).

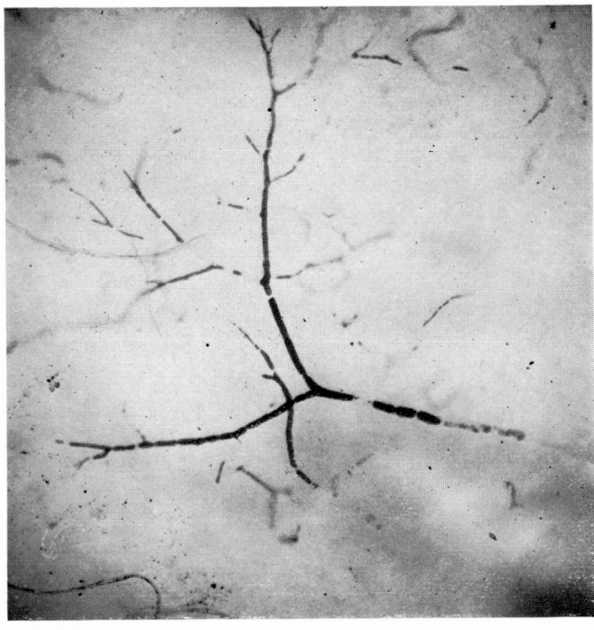

FIG. 678.—FAT EMBOLI.

Flat preparation of the retina stained for fat (oil red O). Numerous fat emboli are present in the small vessels (N. Ashton).

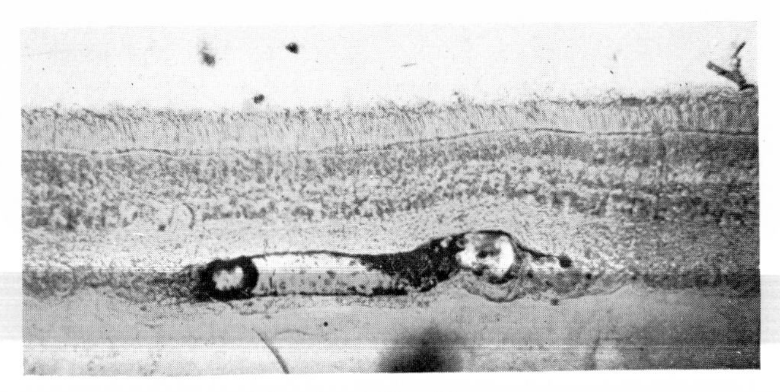

FIG. 679.—FAT EMBOLI.

Seen in the vessels of the retina in the case of a man struck by an automobile; he suffered multiple comminuted fractures of the limbs, the ribs and the spine (A. G. DeVoe).

A somewhat parallel picture of retinal emboli often, however, involving total blindness from complete occlusion of the central artery of the retina has been noted to follow the old and now discredited procedure of injecting paraffin for cosmetic reasons in building up defects of the nose or face.[1]

It is interesting that Loewenstein and Foster (1948) found fatty globules, sometimes in not inconsiderable quantity, in the retina after enucleation of the eye and

[1] Leiser (1902), Hurd and Holden (1903), Elschnig (1905), Rohmer (1905), Uhthoff (1905–6), Zahn (1910).

exenteration of the orbit, the orbital fat presumably entering the severed central artery of the retina.

Retinal changes in a man 34 months after traumatic retinopathy associated with a severe head injury included evidence of focal ischæmia at the level of the retinal capillaries mostly in the posterior part of the globe, although it was impossible to decide whether these ischæmic areas resulted from fat emboli or reflex vasospasm following an acute rise in the retinal venous pressure (Pratt and de Venecia, 1970).

Treatment is difficult because there is as yet no specific therapy for fat embolism. In the past venesection was followed by transfusion while oxygen and sedatives were used to mitigate the pulmonary and cerebral symptoms; vasodilators were recommended by Nicolas (1949). In addition to the usual supportive treatment with measures for the control of shock, the following have been used with varying success: intravenous heparin to eliminate the lipæmia and decrease the size of the fat globules (Cohen and Sparling, 1958; Coob *et al.*, 1959), the inhalation of carbon dioxide (Broom, 1961), the induction of hypothermia by surface cooling and a lytic cocktail (Aladjemoff *et al.*, 1963), intermittent positive-pressure respiration (Denman *et al.*, 1964) and hyperbaric oxygen therapy (Ledingham, 1969). More recent theories concerning the pathogenesis of the clinical syndrome with their emphasis on physico-chemical disturbances in the blood have suggested a fresh therapeutic approach; thus interference with the normal mechanism of blood coagulation by the destruction of fibrin platelets and Factor VIII by newly liberated histotoxic fatty acids causing sludging and obstruction of the small vessels by microthrombi may be counteracted by the intravenous perfusion of anti-thromboplastins and low molecular weight dextran (Bergentz *et al.*, 1961; Calmettes *et al.*, 1967; Rask, 1968; and others). There is, however, no doubt that hypoxia is a major factor in the causation of the fat embolism syndrome and that if this condition is recognized early enough, preferably by the frequent measurement of the arterial blood gases, appropriate treatment which may involve intermittent positive-pressure respiration with pure oxygen may procure a favourable outcome (Collins *et al.*, 1968; Ross, 1969–70; Saldeen, 1970).

Aladjemoff, Weinberg and Alkalay. *Lancet*, **2**, 13 (1963).
Alvarez Luna. *Arch. Soc. oftal. hisp.-amer.*, **11**, 369 (1951).
Amsler. *Ann. Oculist.* (Paris), **171**, 568 (1934).
Anderson. *Amer. J. Ophthal.*, **34**, 1114 (1951).
Ardouin and Boulanger. *Bull. Soc. Ophtal. Fr.*, 170 (1952).
Bailliart. *Traité d'ophtalmologie*, Paris, **5**, 274 (1939).
Bange. *Münch. med. Wschr.*, **59**, 1577 (1912).
Barfoed. *Nord. Med.*, **42**, 1165 (1949).
Bedell. *Arch. Ophthal.*, **22**, 351 (1939).
Bergentz. *Acta chir. scand.*, Suppl. 282 (1961).
Proc. IV Cong. forensic Med., Copenhagen (1966).
Bergentz, Gelin and Rudenstam. *Bibl. Anat.*, **1**, 290 (1961).
Acta chir. scand., **124**, 377 (1962).
Bergentz, Gelin, Rudenstam and Zederfeldt. *Acta chir. scand.*, **122**, 343 (1961).
Bernhard. *Münch. med. Wschr.*, **72** (2), 1590 (1925).
Bertoni. *Ann. Ottal.*, **93**, 101 (1967).
Best. *Klin. Mbl. Augenheilk.*, **63**, 578 (1919); **68**, 725 (1922).
Billig. *J. int. Coll. Surg.*, **20**, 558 (1953).

Bing. *Nervenarzt*, **3**, 506 (1930).
Blancher. *Contribution ophtalmologique à l'étude des embolies graisseuses* (Thèse), Bordeaux (1966).
Broom. *Lancet*, **1**, 71, 1324 (1961).
Brühn. *Klin. Mbl. Augenheilk.*, **104**, 152 (1940).
Calmettes, Deodati and Bechac. *Arch. Ophtal.*, **27**, 209 (1967).
Cashell. *Trans. ophthal. Soc. U.K.*, **77**, 187 (1957).
Chou. *Brit. J. Ophthal.*, **12**, 570 (1928).
Cogan, Kuwabara and Moser. *Arch. Ophthal.*, **71**, 308 (1964).
Cohen and Sparling. *Brit. med. J.*, **1**, 1353 (1958).
Collins, Gordon and Hudson. *Ann. Surg.*, **167**, 511 (1968).
Collins, Hudson and Hamacher. *Ann. Surg.*, **167**, 493 (1968).
Coob, Gray and Hillman. *Surg. Forum*, **9**, 751 (1959).
Cuccagna. *Arch. Ottal.*, **62**, 115 (1958).
Czerny. *Berl. klin. Wschr.*, **12**, 593, 605 (1875).
Denman, Cairns and McHolmes. *Brit. med. J.*, **2**, 101 (1964).
DeVoe. *Arch. Ophthal.*, **43**, 857 (1950).
Eales. *Ophthal. Rev.*, **1**, 139 (1882).
Trans. ophthal. Soc. U.K., **5**, 126 (1885).
Elschnig. *Verh. Ges. dtsch. Naturf.*, **2** (2), 271 (1905).
Evans. *Brit. J. Ophthal.*, **24**, 614 (1940).
Finley, Raban and Lehman. *Amer. J. Ophthal.*, **55**, 367 (1963).
François, Neetens and Gérard. *Ann. Oculist.* (Paris), **200**, 1156 (1967).
Frandsen. *Nord. Med.*, **56**, 1097 (1956).
Fritz and Hogan. *Amer. J. Ophthal.*, **31**, 527 (1948).
Garnier and Peltier. *J. Amer. med. Ass.*, **200**, 556 (1967).
Gee. *J. forens. Med.*, **14**, 60 (1967).
Geiger. *Dtsch. med. Wschr.*, **77**, 198 (1952).
Gittler. *Klin. Mbl. Augenheilk.*, **142**, 898 (1963).
Gonin. *Ann. Oculist.* (Paris), **147**, 98 (1912).
Grant and Reeve. *Med. Res. Cncl., Spec. Rep. Ser.*, No. 227, London (1951).
Groskloss. *Yale J. Biol. Med.*, **8**, 59, 175, 297 (1935–36).
Harris, Perrett and MacLachlin. *Ann. Surg.*, **110**, 1095 (1939).
Harrison. *J. Bone Jt. Surg.*, **44B**, 794 (1962).
Hoare. *Brit. J. Ophthal.*, **54**, 667 (1970).
Hosch. *Arch. Augenheilk.*, **54**, 162 (1906).
Hurd and Holden. *Med. Rec.*, **64**, 53 (1903).
Ophthalmoscope, **1**, 101 (1903).
Jacobi. *v. Graefes Arch. Ophthal.*, **14** (1), 147 (1868).
Kearns. *Amer. J. Ophthal.*, **41**, 1 (1956).
Kehler. *Acta ophthal.* (Kbh.), **31**, 437 (1953).
Koerber. *Zbl. prakt. Augenheilk.*, **34**, 355 (1910).
Kuhnhardt. *Klin. Mbl. Augenheilk.*, **144**, 446 (1964).
Landolt. *Klin. Mbl. Augenheilk.*, **131**, 538 (1957).
Lazorthes, Amalric, Arbus and Farench. *Bull. Soc. Ophtal. Fr.*, **65**, 106 (1965).
Ledingham. *Recent Advances in Surgery* (ed. Taylor), London, 295 (1969).
Leiser. *Dtsch. med. Wschr.*, **28**, Vereinsbeil., 110 (1902).
Liebrecht. *Arch. Augenheilk.*, **55**, 36 (1906).
v. Graefes Arch. Ophthal., **83**, 525 (1912).
Löwenstein. *Klin. Mbl. Augenheilk.*, **96**, 62 (1936).
Loewenstein and Foster. *Brit. J. Ophthal.*, **32**, 819 (1948).
Lyle, Stapp and Button. *Amer. J. Ophthal.*, **44**, 652 (1957).
Madsen. *Acta ophthal.* (Kbh.), **43**, 776 (1965).
Magendie. *Leçons sur les phénomènes physiques de la vie*, Paris, **2** (1836).
Marchesani. *Arch. Augenheilk.*, **95**, 238 (1925).
Marr, W. and E. *Amer. J. Ophthal.*, **54**, 693 (1962).
Meyer and Teare. *Brit. med. J.*, **2**, 42 (1945).
Morgan. *Trans. ophthal. Soc. U.K.*, **65**, 366 (1945); **69**, 441 (1949).
Muhlmann and Ré. *Arch. Oftal. B. Aires*, **15**, 11 (1940).
Nano and Scenna. *Arch. Oftal. B. Aires*, **29**, 285 (1954).
Narazaki, Matsuzaki and Ohbayashi. *Jap. J. Ophthal.*, **13**, 263 (1969).
Newman. *J. Bone Jt. Surg.*, **30B**, 290 (1948); **44B**, 761 (1962).
Nicolas. *Bull. Soc. Ophtal. Fr.*, 928 (1949).
Nielsen and Ingham. *Bull. Los Angeles neurol. Soc.*, **5**, 130 (1940).
Nightingale and Meyer. *J. ment. Sci.*, **86**, 819 (1940).
Oksala. *Nord. Med.*, **59**, 142 (1958).
Oppolzer. *Zbl. Chir.*, **60**, 1389 (1933).
Arch. klin. Chir., **179**, 176 (1934).
Peltier. *Int. Abstr. Surg.*, **104**, 313 (1957).
Pinkerton. *Arch. Ophthal.*, **35**, 176 (1946).
Pratt and de Venecia. *Surv. Ophthal.*, **14**, 417 (1970).
Purtscher. *Ber. dtsch. ophthal. Ges.*, **36**, 294 (1910).
v. Graefes Arch. Ophthal., **82**, 347 (1912).
Zbl. prakt. Augenheilk., **37**, 1 (1913).
Rados. *Arch. Ophthal.*, **6**, 93 (1931).
Rask. *Acta ophthal.* (Kbh.), **46**, 218 (1968).
Renard. *Aspects path. du fond de l'œil*, Paris, **1**, 19 (1946).
Robb-Smith. *Lancet*, **1**, 135 (1941); **1**, 228 (1942).
Robb-Smith, Hunt, Russell and Greenfield. *Proc. roy. Soc. Med.*, **34**, 639 (1941).
Ross. *Surgery*, **65**, 271 (1969).
Ann. roy. Coll. Surg., **46**, 159 (1970).
Rohmer. *Ann. Oculist.* (Paris), **134**, 163 (1905).
Rowlands and Wakeley. *Lancet*, **1**, 502 (1941).
Roy. *Optom. Wkly.*, **49**, 907 (1958).
Amer. J. Optom., **38**, 625 (1961).

Rübel. *Klin. Mbl. Augenheilk.*, **78,** Festschr., 176 (1927).
Saldeen. *J. Trauma*, **10,** 273, 287 (1970).
Savitsky and Gross. *Arch. Neurol. Psychiat.*, **36,** 892 (1936).
Schenk. *Klin. Mbl. Augenheilk.*, **127,** 669 (1955).
Schmidt. *Klin. Mbl. Augenheilk.*, **152,** 672 (1968).
Schneider. *Klin. Mbl. Augenheilk.*, **72,** 640 (1924).
Scott, Kemp and Robb-Smith. *Lancet*, **1,** 228 (1942).
Scriba. *Dtsch. Z. Chir.*, **12,** 118 (1880).
Scuderi. *Int. Surg. Digest.*, **18,** 195 (1934).
Arch. Surg., **36,** 614 (1938).
Surg. Gyn. Obstet., **72,** 732 (1941).
Sevitt. In *Modern Trends in Accident Surgery and Medicine*, London (1959).
Lancet, **2,** 825 (1960); **2,** 1203 (1966).
Fat Embolism, London (1962).
Proc. IV int. Cong. forens. Med., Copenhagen (1966).
Smith. *Amer. J. Ophthal.*, **24,** 537 (1941).
Spaeth. *Arch. Ophthal.*, **31,** 191 (1944).
Stähli. *Klin. Mbl. Augenheilk.*, **55,** 300 (1915).
Stokes. *Arch. Ophthal.*, **7,** 101 (1932).
Tanaka. *Shimoku Acta Med.*, **2,** 21 (1951).
Teare, Bowen and Drury. *J. Bone Jt. Surg.*, **44B,** 790 (1962).
Tietze. *Arch. klin. Chir.*, **95,** 369 (1911).
Uhthoff. *Berl. klin. Wschr.*, **42,** 1461 (1905). *Ophthal. Rec.*, **15,** 115 (1906).
Urbanek. *v. Graefes Arch. Ophthal.*, **131,** 147 (1934).
Utgenannt. *Z. orthop. Chir.*, **41,** 393 (1921).
Vance. *Arch. Surg.*, **23,** 426 (1931).
Vérin and Le Rebeller. *Arch. Ophtal.*, **27,** 123 (1967).
Vogt. *Schweiz. med. Wschr.*, **53,** 945 (1923).
Vogt and Knüsel. *Klin. Mbl. Augenheilk.*, **67,** 513 (1921).
Walsh. *Clinical Neuro-ophthalmology*, Baltimore, 1009 (1947).
Warren. *Amer. J. Path.*, **22,** 69 (1946).
Wiesinger and Guerry. *Klin. Mbl. Augenheilk.*, **139,** 841 (1961).
Wilson and Salisbury. *Brit. J. Surg.*, **31,** 384 (1944).
Winkelman. *Arch. Neurol. Psychiat.*, **47,** 57 (1942).
Zahn. *Klin. Mbl. Augenheilk.*, **48** (1), 338 (1910).
Zaikova. *Vestn. oftal.*, **5,** 91 (1956).

COMPRESSION CYANOSIS

Owing to the absence of valves in the large veins above the level of the heart, any increase in the venous pressure is more readily felt in the head and neck than elsewhere in the body. Such a rise in pressure, which may have extremely damaging consequences, is liable to occur if the thorax or abdomen is severely compressed, an injury which may occur in an automobile or elevator accident when the body is pinned down by a heavy weight, is compressed in a crowd in panic or is buried in the demolitions of war. The venous engorgement probably becomes effective by compression of the superior vena cava, and the condition has been produced experimentally in dogs by ligation of this vessel proximal to the azygos vein (Reichert and Martin, 1951). There seems to be little rhyme or reason where the back-pressure thus generated will cause hæmorrhages to appear—the subcutaneous and submucous tissues may be engorged with blood, profuse intra-ocular bleeding may occur, massive hæmorrhages into the orbit or the sheath of the optic nerve may result in bilateral blindness, while a similar cerebral catastrophe may be fatal. Fleeting palsies of the limbs may also occur (Reichert and Martin, 1951).

The first to note the ocular effects of such an injury was Willers (1873) whose observations were followed after an interval by those of Perthes (1899), Braun (1899–1904), Berrisford (1921) and Heuer (1923). A considerable number of reports followed, 24 of which were collected from the literature by Wagenmann (1924). Several subsequent papers of interest have appeared.[1]

[1] Mitchell (1924), Bedell (1939), Spaeth (1944), Schenck *et al.* (1944) (13 cases), Dwek (1946), Klenka (1948), Wruhs (1951), Frandsen (1956), Cuccagna (1958), Oksala (1958),

The most immediately obvious result of such an injury is the appearance of a dusky purple cyanosis—the *ecchymotic mask*—affecting the head, neck, upper part of the chest and sometimes the upper arms, accompanied by a considerable amount of swelling and œdema and intracutaneous petechial hæmorrhages, phenomena particularly evident in the lids. The mucous membranes of the mouth, throat and nose are similarly cyanotic, swollen and studded with small hæmorrhages, changes sometimes seen to a marked degree in the conjunctiva (Wagenmann, 1924; Manavolgu, 1949) (Figs. 680-1). Proptosis due to orbital bleeding may also occur (Parker, 1911), which on occasion may be so severe as to result in the rapid development of amaurosis (Wüst, 1949). In the eye itself a hyphæma may form (Schenck *et al.*, 1944), congestion of the retinal veins and retinal œdema are common (Stöwer, 1910), as also are retinal hæmorrhages which, although usually small and petechial,

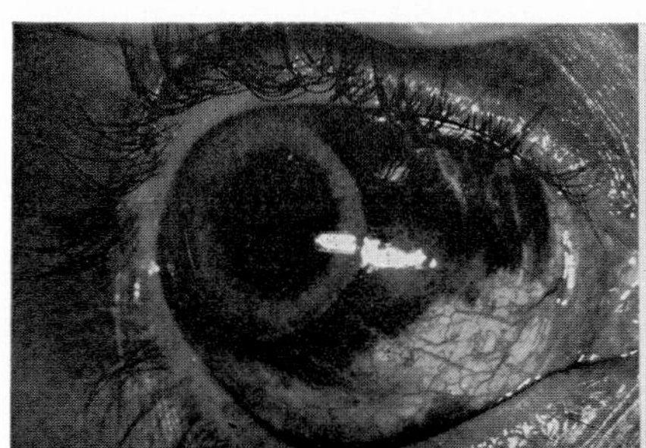

Fig. 680.

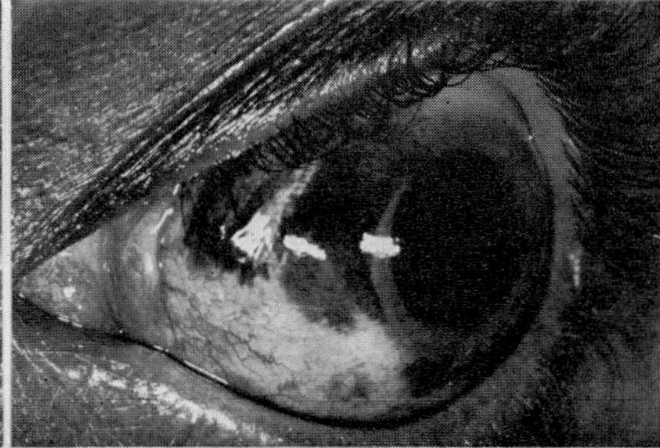

Fig. 681.

Figs. 680 and 681.—Compression Cyanosis.

Extensive subconjunctival hæmorrhages after a severe compression of the thorax. The same case as is illustrated in Plate XXV (J. G. H. Schmidt).

may on occasion be multiple and profuse[1]; the macula may be involved causing permanent visual damage, and preretinal bleeding may occur. In a case described by Oksala (1958) three days after a severe compression injury of the chest traumatic retinopathy appeared in one eye and a total shallow exudative detachment in the other. It is probable, indeed, that some of the cases described as Purtscher's traumatic retinopathy,[2] characterized by multiple retinal hæmorrhages but without cyanosis of the skin, are due to a venous reflux following a crush injury, particularly of the chest[3]; this factor may also enter into the composite ætiology of other cases wherein some of the pathological changes may be due to arterial spasm or fat embolism. In many cases, however, the retinopathy seemed to be due entirely to the acute

W. and E. Marr (1962), Shamblin and McGoon (1963), Madsen (1965) (6 cases), Schmidt (1968) and Hoare (1970).

[1] Wagenmann (1900), Neck (1900), Pichler (1901), Burrell and Crandon (1902), Scheer (1904), Wienecke (1904), Béal (1906–9), Rönne (1910), Spaeth (1944), and others.

[2] p. 717.

[3] Bailliart (1939), Brühn (1940), Renard (1946), Ardouin and Boulanger (1952).

massive venous congestion since there were no clinical signs of fat embolism, as occurred, for example, in the six cases described by Madsen (1965). Similarly in a case described by Hoare (1970) the retinal angiopathy followed the compression of the chest by a safety belt without fracture of the ribs or any other detectable injury. The development of papillœdema (Le Roux, 1913) and the severe loss of vision or even blindness associated with optic atrophy suggest the occurrence of bleeding into the optic nerve.[1] Finally, the occurrence of blindness without detectable ophthalmoscopic changes indicates cerebral damage of the same type (Perthes, 1899; Joynt, 1905; Béal, 1909; and others), a possibility shown to exist in fatal cases (Scheer, 1904; Schultze, 1909) (Fig. 682).

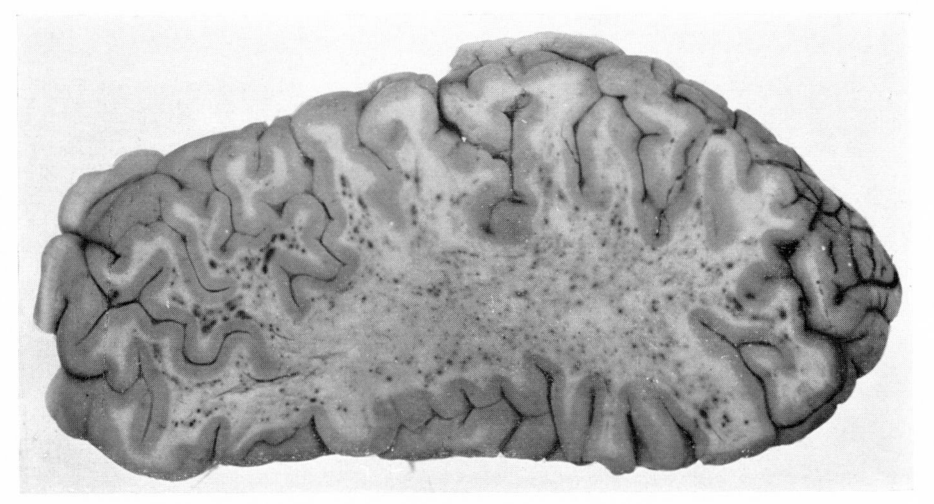

Fig. 682.—Compression Cyanosis.

Showing multiple petechial hæmorrhages in the white matter of the brain, in a case of a man who died after his thorax had been compressed between a driving belt and a pillar (Museum, Royal College of Surgeons).

Although more dramatic in degree, these changes are comparable to the occurrence of retinal hæmorrhages when the venous pressure in the head is raised by such incidents as severe coughing (Hotz, 1884), blowing a wind instrument (Siegrist, 1895), retching and vomiting (Nettleship, 1887; Warschawski, 1898), or straining at stool (Lang, 1888) or at childbirth (Power, 1888; Galezowski, 1907),[2] and they are in some respects parallel with certain cases of retinal hæmorrhages in the newborn, a subject already discussed at length.[3] Two interesting cases were recorded after strangulation (Sédan and Sédan-Bauby, 1952): after five years one showed a persisting enlargement of the angioscotomata, while the other had secondary

[1] Béal (1909), Lang (1909), Rönne (1910), Dwek (1946), Klenka (1948), and others.
[2] See Feature photograph, *Arch. Ophthal.*, **77**, 129 (1967).
[3] Vol. X, p. 139.

optic atrophy with quadrantic homonymous hemianopia indicating a hæmorrhage affecting the visual pathway.

From the ophthalmological point of view, *treatment* is usually expectant, although occasionally emergency measures may be called for; thus a massive intra-ocular hæmorrhage with raised tension might indicate a paracentesis,[1] and gross bleeding into the orbit might call for surgical decompression. In the latter case, for example, Wüst (1949) achieved prompt alleviation of acute proptosis with amaurosis by removing the floor of the orbit through the maxillary antrum.

The Differential Diagnosis of Traumatic Retinopathy

It is clear from what we have said in the preceding sections that trauma of one kind or another is a feature common to these various types of retinopathy; indeed, in any one case more than one factor may be responsible. Systemic signs and symptoms may or may not accompany the retinopathy while the degree of visual disturbance and the mode of development of the changes in the fundus may also show considerable variation. It is important, however, for a clinical distinction to be made between these conditions, particularly in the case of fat embolism wherein modern therapeutic methods may prevent an otherwise fatal outcome; in this connection therefore the ophthalmologist may play a vital role.

In the differential diagnosis of the appearance of the fundus following trauma consideration of the features shown in Table XXII may be helpful (W. and E. Marr, 1962); important features are the type of trauma, unilaterality or bilaterality, the presence of systemic symptoms and signs, the rate of onset of the visual disturbance, the presence of external ocular signs and the ophthalmoscopic appearance. Berlin's œdema (*commotio retinæ*) follows rapidly on a direct contusion to the globe; there is early deterioration of visual acuity associated with retinal œdema at the posterior pole and sometimes with a cherry-red spot and radial retinal striæ; other signs of concussive injury particularly to the anterior segment may also be present.

In Purtscher's retinopathy a history of direct trauma to the eye is usually absent and the most typical appearance is that of several superficial white areas accompanied by a few retinal or preretinal hæmorrhages found mainly at the posterior pole; these changes may be either unilateral or bilateral, although they may not be present to the same degree in each eye. The retinal signs may be present at an early stage but a complaint of visual disturbance may not be made for several days if there has been loss of consciousness. Traumatic asphyxia, on the other hand, is characterized by an entirely different picture resulting from a sudden increase in the pressure of the venous system in the upper part of the body with the rupture of capillaries producing scattered subcutaneous, subconjunctival and retinal hæmorrhages; a state of cyanosis rapidly develops due to the presence of

[1] p. 98.

relatively poorly oxygenated blood in the capillaries as a result of respiratory embarrassment. Fat embolism may cause retinal changes to some extent similar to those in Purtscher's disease but in fat embolism the retinal changes do not usually develop until three days after the injury while the systemic picture is entirely different from that associated with Purtscher's disease. Commotio retinæ, therefore, can easily be distinguished from Purtscher's

TABLE XXII

DIFFERENTIAL DIAGNOSIS OF TRAUMATIC RETINOPATHY
(modified from W. and E. Marr)

	BERLIN'S COMMOTIO RETINÆ	PURTSCHER'S RETINOPATHY	TRAUMATIC ASPHYXIA	FAT EMBOLISM
Type of trauma	Local to eye	Chest compression; head injury	Chest compression	Fracture of long-bones; multiple injuries
Accompanying systemic picture	None	None	Blue-black discoloration of upper body	Pulmonary and cerebral signs; petechial hæmorrhages
Onset of systemic picture	None	None	Immediate	Symptom-free interval of 1 or 2 days
Initial vision	Approximately 6/60	Variable	Normal to no light perception	Occasionally reduced
Duration of reduced vision	Several days	Several weeks	Several weeks	Several days
Ultimate vision	Usually normal; sometimes impaired	Normal	Normal to no light perception	Normal
Eyes externally	Contused	Normal	Subconjunctival hæmorrhages	Normal to petechial conjunctival hæmorrhages
Fundus picture	Retinal œdema	Exudates and hæmorrhages	Normal or hæmorrhages, rarely exudates	Exudates and hæmorrhages, retinal œdema
Development of fundus picture	Within a few hours	Within 2 or 4 days	Immediate or first 1 or 2 days	After 1 or 2 days

disease and the retinal changes in traumatic asphyxia associated with sudden elevation of the venous pressure; the retinopathy associated with fat embolism can often be distinguished from Purtscher's condition only by the presence of systemic signs and symptoms.

Ardouin and Boulanger. *Bull. Soc. Ophtal. Fr.*, 170 (1952).
Bailliart. *Traité d'ophtalmologie*, Paris, **5**, 274 (1939).
Béal. *Ann. Oculist.* (Paris), **135**, 353 (1906); **142**, 89 (1909).
Bedell. *Arch. Ophthal.*, **22**, 351 (1939).
Berrisford. *Arch. Ophthal.*, **50**, 411 (1921).
Braun. *Dtsch. Z. Chir.*, **51**, 599 (1899); **74**, 411 (1904).
Brühn. *Klin. Mbl. Augenheilk.*, **104**, 152 (1940).

Burrell and Crandon. *Boston med. surg. J.*, **146,** 13 (1902).
Cuccagna. *Arch. Ottal.*, **62,** 115 (1958).
Dwek. *J. int. Coll. Surg.*, **9,** 257 (1946).
Frandsen. *Nord. Med.*, **56,** 1097 (1956).
Galezowski. *Bull. Soc. franç. Ophtal.*, **24,** 538 (1907).
Heuer. *Surg. Gynec. Obstet.*, **36,** 686 (1923).
Hoare. *Brit. J. Ophthal.*, **54,** 667 (1970).
Hotz. *Amer. J. Ophthal.*, **1,** 169 (1884).
Joynt. *Lancet*, **1,** 856 (1905).
Klenka. *Cs. Oftal.*, **4,** 372 (1948).
Lang. *Trans. ophthal. Soc. U.K.*, **8,** 155 (1888); **29,** 156 (1909).
Le Roux. *Arch. Ophtal.*, **33,** 231 (1913).
Madsen. *Acta ophthal.* (Kbh.), **43,** 776 (1965).
Manavolgu. *Oto Nörö Oftal.* (Istanbul), **4,** 32 (1949).
Marr, W. and E. *Amer. J. Ophthal.*, **54,** 693 (1962).
Mitchell. *Med. J. Aust.*, Suppl. **1,** 354; **2,** 536 (1924).
Morgan. *Trans. ophthal. Soc. U.K.*, **65,** 366 (1945).
Neck. *Dtsch. Z. Chir.*, **57,** 163 (1900).
Nettleship. *Roy. Lond. ophthal. Hosp. Rep.*, **11,** 271 (1887).
Oksala. *Nord. Med.*, **59,** 142 (1958).
Parker. *Arch. Ophthal.*, **40,** 159 (1911).
Perthes. *Dtsch. Z. Chir.*, **50,** 436 (1899).
Pichler. *Z. Augenheilk.*, **6,** 134 (1901).
Power. *Trans. ophthal. Soc. U.K.*, **8,** 26 (1888).
Reichert and Martin. *Ann. Surg.*, **134,** 361 (1951).
Renard. *Aspects path. du fond de l'œil*, Paris, **1,** 19 (1946).
Rönne. *Klin. Mbl. Augenheilk.*, **48** (1), 50 (1910).
Scheer. *v. Graefes Arch. Ophthal.*, **59,** 311 (1904).
Schenk, Silcox and Godfrey. *U.S. Naval med. Bull.*, **42,** 802 (1944).
Schmidt. *Klin. Mbl. Augenheilk.*, **152,** 672 (1968).
Schultze. *Dtsch. med. Wschr.*, **35,** 1809 (1909).
Sédan and Sédan-Bauby. *J. Méd. Porto*, **20,** 927 (1952).
Shamblin and McGoon. *Arch. Surg.*, **87,** 967 (1963).
Siegrist. *Mitt. Klin. med. Inst. Schweiz*, **3** (9) (1895).
Spaeth. *Arch. Ophthal.*, **31,** 191 (1944).
Stöwer. *Klin. Mbl. Augenheilk.*, **48** (1), 559 (1910).
Wagenmann. *v. Graefes Arch. Ophthal.*, **51** (3), 550 (1900).
Graefe-Saemisch Hb. d. ges. Augenheilk., 3rd ed., Berlin, **3,** 2113 (1924).
Warschawski. *Vestn. oftal.*, **15,** 265 (1898).
Wienecke. *Dtsch. Z. Chir.*, **75,** 37 (1904).
Willers. *Ueber d. Dilatation d. Blutgefässe d. Kopfes nach schweren Verletzungen d. Unterleibes* (Diss.), Greifswald (1873).
Wruhs. *Wien. klin. Wschr.*, **63,** 173 (1951).
Wüst. *Klin. Mbl. Augenheilk.*, **114,** 140 (1949).

RETINAL ISCHÆMIA AFTER EXSANGUINATION

The acute retinal ischæmia which sometimes follows exsanguination is a condition the reverse of the preceding. The events associated with this distressing incident have already been described[1] where it was pointed out that the retinal damage usually follows repeated visceral bleeding as from the upper gastro-intestinal tract,[2] from the bowel or uterus (Pines, 1931) and in pulmonary tuberculosis. More rarely the same sequence may follow a surgical operation wherein bleeding has been profuse (thyroidectomy, Grossmann and Holm, 1950; pulmonary resection, Walkup and Murphy, 1952; removal of a carcinoma of the floor of the mouth, Mazzia, 1962; cholecystectomy, Chisholm, 1969) or massive hæmorrhage from a wound (Proell, 1907; Pincus, 1919; Terrien, 1921; Hayreh, 1970). It is now recognized that a similar visual loss may follow open-heart surgery (Lamb, 1961; Gilman, 1964) and cardiac arrest (Weinberger, 1962). It is interesting that in ancient times it was a recognized complication of therapeutic bleeding (Esquirol, 1838; Conreur *et al.*, 1965). A similar loss of sight has followed the bite of a viperine snake which is complicated by extensive and prolonged

[1] Vol. X, p. 60.
[2] Avery Jones (1947), Locket (1949), Richardson (1954), Gavey (1963).

hæmorrhage from the mucous membranes and into the muscles (Davenport and Budden, 1953; Guttmann-Friedmann, 1956).

Considering the daily occurrence of profound losses of blood, ocular symptoms are relatively rare; this, however, is a well-known clinical catastrophe which has been amply recorded in the literature, thus Terson (1922) reviewed 250 publications on the subject and Unger (1955) 286 cases recorded between the years 1941 and 1953. Nevertheless, the loss of vision due to the loss of blood resulting from war wounds is extremely rare and it is established that amaurosis rarely follows a single hæmorrhage from a person in normal health, whereas recurrent hæmorrhages, especially when a profound drop of blood pressure occurs, are the most prone to affect vision.[1]

In this connection the following cases are of interest. A woman aged 25 developed complete bilateral blindness 5 hours after a sudden profuse vaginal hæmorrhage which was followed 2 hours later by the delivery of a still-born fœtus; both fundi showed the picture of occlusion of the central retinal artery thought to be the result of a combination of severe loss of blood and hypotension (Jain and Rangbulla, 1967). In another case reported by Carreras (1954) following a massive maternal antepartum hæmorrhage, bilateral optic atrophy was found in the infant, probably as a result of retinal ischæmia and anoxia. In a case of severe gastro-intestinal hæmorrhage from a gastric ulcer the eyes were examined histologically by Conreur and his colleagues (1965); 3 days after the onset of bleeding a sudden loss of vision occurred in one eye and in the other after a similar period: there were bilateral retinal and optic disc œdema, exudates, hæmorrhages and marked dilatation of the retinal veins. Subsequently complete bilateral optic atrophy developed and death occurred 5 years later. It was concluded that prolonged spasm of the retinal vessels led to necrosis of the ganglion cells from anoxia.

The visual loss following hæmorrhage is usually bilateral although the eyes may be unequally involved; in about 15% of cases one eye only is affected; symptoms usually become apparent between the third and seventh day after the bleeding, though they may be delayed for some considerable time. The typical clinical picture which, however, presents many variations, is that of a dilated and fixed pupil, a pale optic disc, marked narrowing of the retinal arteries with œdema, sometimes generalized over the posterior pole, sometimes in fluffy patches associated with scattered retinal hæmorrhages. A swelling of the optic disc may occur, occasionally of a degree sufficient to suggest a papillœdema (Richardson, 1954), but the most dramatic appearances are the development of flame-shaped hæmorrhages and large cotton-wool spots. In the worst cases a complete optic atrophy may develop frequently associated with some pigmentary disturbances in the retina while the visual fields may show regular or irregular peripheral contraction or scattered scotomata, or irregular horizontal hemianopic defects, possibly associated with occlusion of the posterior ciliary arteries (Hayreh, 1970). In this connection it is important to note that a rapid

[1] Foster Moore (1925), Locket (1949), Pears and Pickering (1960), Pickering (1969), Holt and Gordon-Smith (1969).

deterioration of vision may occur in eyes affected by chronic simple glaucoma if there has been a profound fall in blood pressure (Perez-Llorca, 1963; Chisholm, 1969).

The pathogenesis of the acute retinal ischæmia and consequent œdema has long been disputed and although the pathological changes were studied experimentally in dogs by Uhthoff (1922) opportunities to examine clinical cases have been relatively few, although both Gowers (1904) and Foster Moore (1925) remarked on the high incidence of retinal hæmorrhages and exudates in patients with severe anæmia due to loss of blood. There is a marked degree of retinal œdema most pronounced in the nerve-fibre layer due presumably to the increased permeability of the capillaries and the added imbibition of fluid caused by the osmotic attraction of catalytic products; and here cotton-wool exudates have been found to have the classical composition of cytoid bodies (Ashton *et al.*, 1961; Ashton, 1965); in long-standing cases these changes are associated with degeneration of the ganglion cells and the optic nerve fibres, both in the retina and the nerve. The essential pathology is thus a preferential degeneration of the third retinal neuron. There are no structural anomalies in the intra-ocular vessels, suggesting that the lesion is primarily functional due to anoxia (Hollenhorst and Wagener, 1950) secondary to a profound fall in blood pressure perhaps leading to an occlusion of the central retinal artery, the effect of which would be intensified by a pre-existing anæmia (Pears and Pickering, 1960). Several considerations, however, imply that probably something more than a simple ischæmia enters into the question: the rarity of the condition, its occasional unilaterality, the tendency for the delay in its onset and its preferential incidence after repeated hæmorrhages have suggested the possible influence of some hæmoclastic shock or anaphylactic crisis, toxæmia due to profound hæmolysis (Pincus, 1919; Terson, 1922), or hypoproteinæmia leading to œdema of the optic nerve and vascular compression (Locket, 1949).

The *prognosis* is very difficult to assess for some of the patients who seem mildly affected at the time retain their visual defect while others in whom all vision is lost recover to a remarkable degree. Terson (1922) found that on the average 50% of the patients remained permanently blind while of the 50% who showed improvement only some 10–12% recovered normal vision. In those patients who recover disappearance of the exudates and the restoration of vision occur within a few weeks. Hæmorrhages, of course, may do permanent damage and when these appear at the macula the disability is great and when any degree of optic atrophy has set in the prognosis is necessarily bad.

The *treatment* of such a condition should be directed first to systemic measures to combat the effects of the loss of blood by controlling the hæmorrhage and maintaining the circulation by blood transfusions. Some benefit has been claimed from the use of vasodilators and corticosteroids (Hartmann and Parfonry, 1934; Neubauer and Karges, 1962) and from blockage of the stellate ganglion (Grossmann and Holm, 1950) while intravenous osmotic agents have also been successfully used (Chisholm, 1969).

Ashton. *Trans. ophthal. Soc. U.K.*, **85**, 199 (1965).
Ashton, Pears and Pickering. *Brit. J. Ophthal.*, **45**, 385 (1961).
Carreras. *Arch. Soc. oftal. hisp.-amer.*, **14**, 405 (1954).
Chisholm. *Brit. J. Ophthal.*, **53**, 289 (1969).
Conreur, Toussaint and Desneux. *Bull. Soc. belge Ophtal.*, No. 141, 614 (1965).
Davenport and Budden. *Brit. J. Ophthal.*, **37**, 113 (1953).
Esquirol. *Des maladies mentales*, Paris, **1**, 183 (1838).
Gavey. *Trans. ophthal. Soc. U.K.*, **83**, 315 (1963).
Gilman. *New Engl. J. Med.*, **272**, 489 (1964).
Grossmann and Holm. *Amer. J. Ophthal.*, **33**, 1099 (1950).
Gowers. *A Manual and Atlas of Medical Ophthalmoscopy*, 4th ed., London (1904).
Guttmann-Friedmann. *Brit. J. Ophthal.*, **40**, 57 (1956).
Hartmann and Parfonry. *Bull. Soc. Ophtal. Paris*, 56 (1934).
Hayreh. *Brit. J. Ophthal.*, **54**, 289 (1970).
Hollenhorst and Wagener. *Amer. J. med. Sci.*, **219**, 209 (1950).
Holt and Gordon-Smith. *Brit. J. Ophthal.*, **53**, 145 (1969).
Jain and Rangbulla. *Orient. Arch. Ophthal.*, **5**, 167 (1967).
Jones, Avery. *Brit. med. J.*, **2**, 477 (1947).
Lamb. *Brit. J. Ophthal.*, **45**, 490 (1961).
Locket. *Brit. J. Ophthal.*, **33**, 543 (1949).
Mazzia. *N.Y. St. J. Med.*, **62**, 2549 (1962).
Moore, Foster. *Medical Ophthalmology*, 2nd ed., London (1925).
Neubauer and Karges. *Klin. Mbl. Augenheilk.*, **141**, 70 (1962).
Pears and Pickering. *Quart. J. Med.*, **29**, 153 (1960).
Perez Llorca. *Arch. Soc. oftal. hisp.-amer.*, **23**, 966 (1963).
Pickering. *Trans. ophthal. Soc. U.K.*, **89**, 83 (1969).
Pincus. *v. Graefes Arch. Ophthal.*, **98**, 152 (1919).
Pines. *Brit. J. Ophthal.*, **15**, 75 (1931).
Proell. *Ueber Sehstörungen nach Blutverlust* (Diss.), Freiburg (1907).
Richardson. *Brit. J. Surg.*, **42**, 108 (1954).
Terrien. *Arch. Ophtal.*, **38**, 263 (1921).
Terson. *Ann. Oculist.* (Paris), **159**, 23 (1922).
Uhthoff. *Ber. dtsch. ophthal. Ges.*, **43**, 204 (1922).
Unger. *Klin. Mbl. Augenheilk.*, **126**, 41 (1955).
Walkup and Murphy. *J. thoracic Surg.*, **23**, 174 (1952).
Weinberger. *J. Amer. med. Ass.*, **179**, 126 (1962).

THE BATTERED BABY SYNDROME

Ill-treatment or abuse of children is a crime as old as man himself but has only in relatively recent times been endowed with medical and social importance. Infanticide has from time to time been practised in an attempt to control population, to eliminate non-thriving or defective children and for political or eugenic reasons; while the history of the industrial revolution in England was darkened by accounts of children compelled to work for appallingly long hours under intolerable conditions in coal-mines and factories. The idea that babies and young children might suffer injury and even death at the hands of their parents is, however, repugnant and hard to believe; nevertheless such cases resulting from deliberate action rather than from accidental causes are not rare. Although there had been scattered reports of the abuse of young children in the medical literature, it was not until Caffey (1946) reported some unusual radiological findings that the medical profession began to consider the problem; Caffey described the radiological features of a syndrome involving multiple fractures of long-bones associated with subdural hæmatomata, at first thought to be due to a metabolic abnormality until subsequently Silverman (1953) showed that both the subdural hæmatomata and the bony abnormalities were the result of severe recurrent trauma for which Woolley and Evans (1955) suggested that the parents might be responsible. The descriptive term *battered child syndrome* was coined by Kempe and his colleagues (1962) who collected records of 749 cases of which 10% proved fatal in one period of 12 months. The incidence of this condition is not known with certainty but its frequency is disturbing. Thus Helfer and Pollock (1968) estimated that in 1966 in the United States of America 10,000–15,000 children received injuries by non-accidental means and that 5% of the victims were killed and 25–30% permanently injured—figures which would seem to eclipse the consequences of the more commonly known illnesses and mishaps of childhood. This surprising and distressing reaction of presumably abnormal parents to their offspring is not confined to that country but as this book is being written it is causing medical and political concern in Britain.

A battered baby is an infant who shows clinical or radiological evidences of lesions which are frequently multiple and involve mainly the head, soft tissues or the long-bones and thoracic cage and which cannot be unequivocally explained by natural disease or simple accident. The clinical picture of the battered baby syndrome is now more or less clear[1] (Figs. 6 [illegible]5). The maltreated child is usually an infant under the age of 12 months, rarely over the age of 3 years; no particular racial, ethnic, educational or social background is predominant, although it has been suggested that poverty, marital problems, emotional instability or psychiatric disorders in the parents may be of ætiological significance. In this connection the following features were noted by Camps (1968): the parents were generally of low intelligence with an average age of under 23 years; the child is often illegitimate or born within 9 months of marriage, or is stated to be unwanted; there is generally a delay in calling for medical assistance; while persistent cruelty or a sudden loss of self-control resulting in the infliction of excessive violence may be followed by a sense of regret or guilt with a tendency to repetition of the assault; in any event, whether at times of over-stress or inebriety or as a routine, many parents become cross with a persistently crying infant. Several authorities have discussed the psycho-social, legal and forensic aspects of this problem.[2]

Children who have been abused commonly present with recurrent and severe bleeding and bruising with a marked inconsistency between the severity of the injury and the history or explanation of its causation (Turner, 1964); there may also be a state of malnutrition or physical decline which further complicates the problems of diagnosis and treatment; a characteristic lesion is a torn frenum of the upper lip. A subdural hæmatoma is also common but any history of trauma may be difficult to elicit for one parent frequently hesitates to denounce the other. This was obtained in 64% of

[1] Fontana *et al.* (1963), Bain (1963), McHenry *et al.* (1963), O'Doherty (1964), Turner (1964), Roaf (1965), Fontana (1966), Helfer and Kempe (1968), Helfer and Pollock (1968), Isaacs (1968), Skinner and Castle (1969), and others.

[2] Parker (1965), Cameron *et al.* (1966), Polson (1966), Simpson (1967), Camps (1968), Helfer and Kempe (1968), Johnson (1969).

FIGS. 683 to 686.—THE BATTERED BABY SYNDROME (T. E. Oppé).

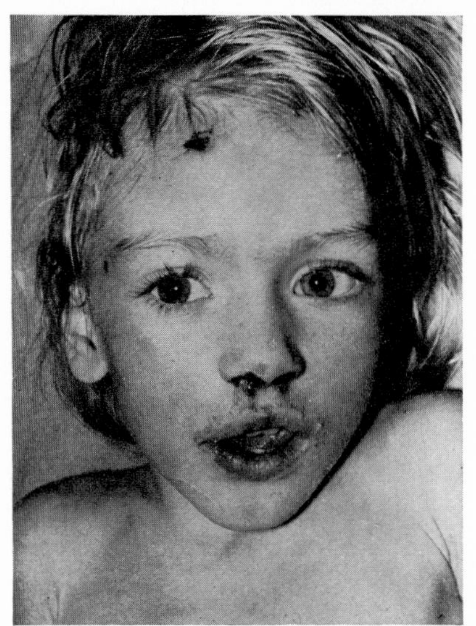

FIG. 683.—A girl aged 3½ years with multiple cutaneous lesions, bruises, lacerations, ulcers and welts but without bony injuries.

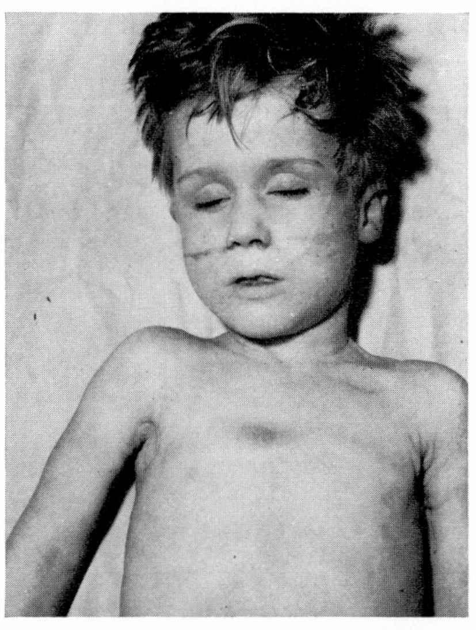

FIG. 684.—A boy aged 4½ was brought into hospital dead. The autopsy showed asphyxia, pulmonary hæmorrhage and multiple fractures of the ribs.

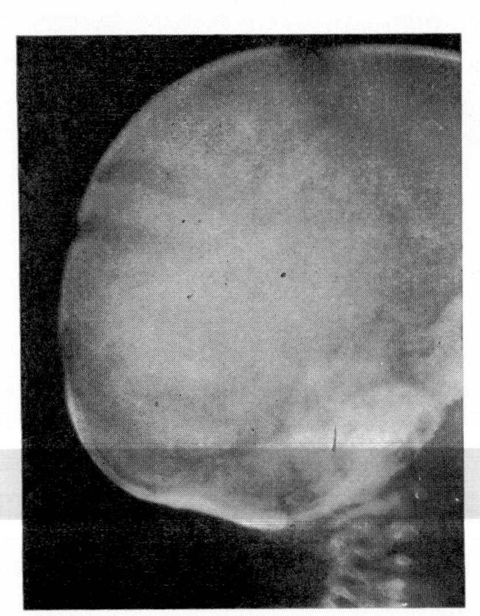

FIG. 685.—The skull of a boy aged 3 months who was brought into hospital comatose with multiple bruising. There were fractures of both parietal bones with a large subdural hæmatoma and multiple fractures of the limbs. The child recovered but with permanent brain damage and epilepsy.

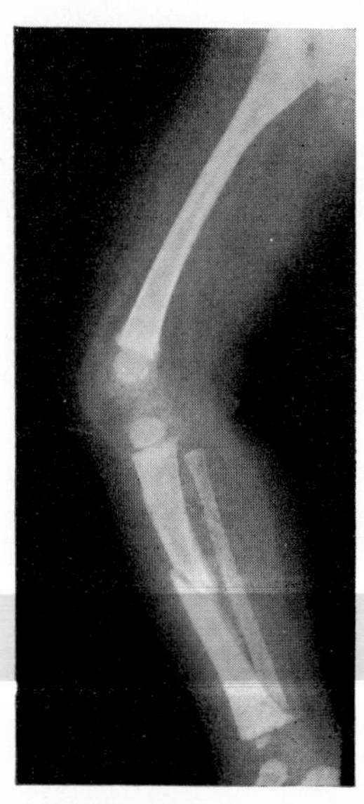

FIG. 686.—A boy aged 7 months. There were a transverse mid-shaft fracture of the right tibia and an old fracture of the right humerus.

31 cases examined by Hollenhorst and his colleagues (1957) and, among 25 cases of subdural hæmatomata in children under the age of 2, Russell (1965) was given a history of head injury in 11 of which 3 were thought to be due to deliberate assault. Discussing the significance of retinal and subhyaloid hæmorrhage in subdural effusions Till (1968) noted that among 116 cases of

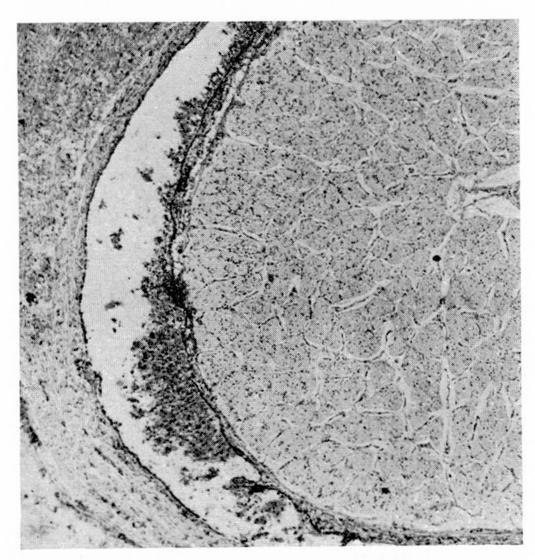

Fig. 687.—The Battered Baby Syndrome.
Showing a subarachnoid hæmorrhage (P. Henkind)

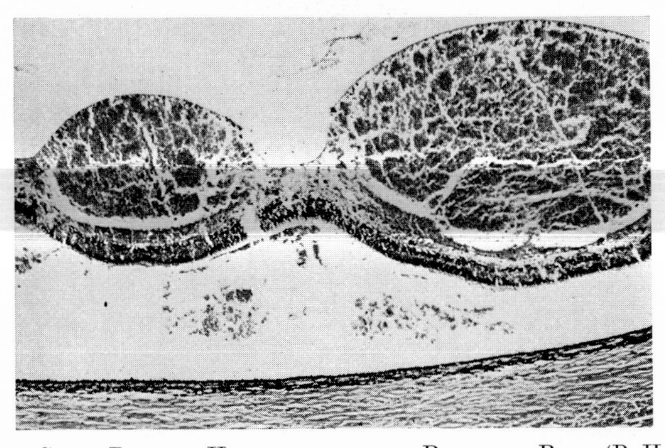

Fig. 688.—Gross Retinal Hæmorrhages in a Battered Baby (P. Henkind).

subdural hæmatoma or effusion in infancy, trauma was involved in 40% without other clinical signs than intra-ocular hæmorrhage and in only 21 cases was there an actual history of injury to the head; nevertheless, the presence of fractures of the skull or of other bones or bruising of the scalp made the occurrence of head injury most likely. The finding of preretinal

FIGS. 689 and 690.—THE BATTERED BABY SYNDROME (A. Mushin and G. Morgan).

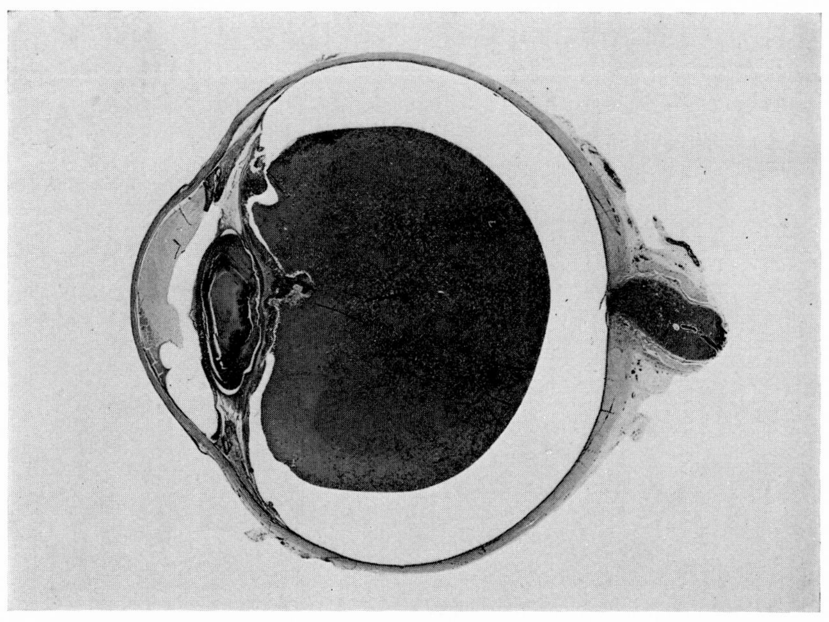

FIG. 689.—A male baby aged 8 months. Section of the eye showing a hyphæma, a scattering of pigment, rubeosis and ectropion of the iris with peripheral anterior synechiæ. The ciliary processes are drawn towards the lens which is subluxated and cataractous. The retina is totally detached, disorganized and necrotic and is adherent to the posterior surface of the lens through a vascularized hyaline membrane. The remainder of the globe is filled with abundant hæmorrhagic subretinal fluid.

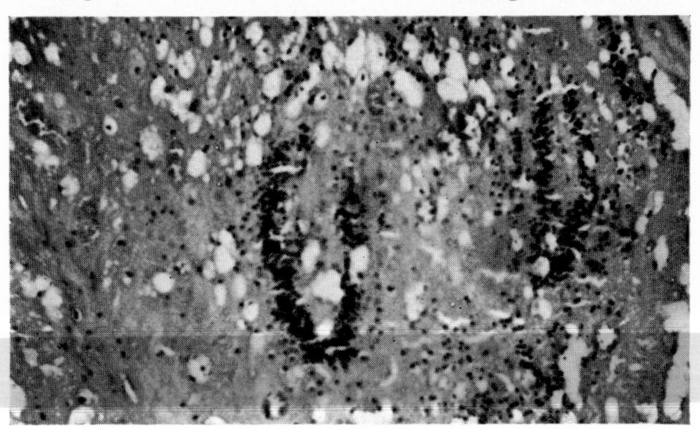

FIG. 690.—The detached retina in the same case showing disorganization, lipid macrophages and necrosis.

hæmorrhages in an infant with or without cerebral symptoms should be regarded as strongly suggestive of an intracranial hæmorrhage (Walsh and Hoyt, 1969). It is to be remembered, however, that the absence of a fracture is not itself sufficient evidence that there has been no such injury since in a baby the bones of the skull are elastic; it is, therefore, necessary to look elsewhere for evidence of trauma. Injuries to the abdominal organs have been observed, even gastric or intestinal perforation and obstruction (McCort and Vaudogna, 1964; Eisenstein *et al.*, 1965), rupture or laceration of the liver, spleen and kidneys (Shaw, 1964). A full skeletal survey is necessary, especially if the injuries appear to be confined to the cranium: the main features include multiple fractures of the long-bones, both recent and others in varying stages of healing and repair, epiphyseal detachment, new bone formation and subperiosteal hæmorrhage, although it is necessary to exclude other conditions which may give rise to similar radiological features.[1]

From the literature it seems that direct injury to the eye has not been commonly seen in these cases, although certainly the eye should be examined for evidence of trauma. A remarkable case was described by Kiffney (1964): a child was struck on the head at the age of 2 months, so that several fractures of the skull and bilateral subdural hæmorrhages resulted, but at this stage the ocular fundi were normal; at 3 months fractures were found in the legs and at the age of 8 months defective vision was noticed, associated with a white elevated mass behind the lens in each eye; as these signs appeared to indicate a diagnosis of retinoblastoma the right eye was removed and histological examination showed a total retinal detachment with no evidence of intra-ocular tumour. Other cases of severe unilateral ocular injury have been reported including cases clinically resembling Coats's disease which have proved on histological examination to be due to traumatic hæmorrhages (Mushin and Morgan, 1971) (Figs. 687–690). Retinal lesions in the absence of a subdural hæmatoma were noted by Maroteaux and Lamy (1967); thus in the extreme periphery especially on the temporal side areas of greyish discoloration with pigmentary disturbances were seen with no other retinal abnormality and were interpreted as being due to a direct contusive injury. Retinal or subhyaloid hæmorrhages have been observed in association with subdural effusions in 54 of 116 cases, with papillœdema in 12 (Till, 1968); on the other hand, Gilkes and Mann (1967) noted such hæmorrhages in the fundi in a physically abused child without any evidence of injury to the head and suggested that they might be the result of injury elsewhere such as compression of the chest or vigorous shaking.

Bain. *Pediatrics*, **31**, 895 (1963).
Baker and Berdon. *Radiol. Clin. N. Amer.*, **4**, 289 (1966).
Caffey. *Amer. J. Roentgenol.*, **56**, 163 (1946).
Brit. J. Radiol., **30**, 225 (1957).
J. Pediat., **67**, 1008 (1965).
Cameron, Johnson and Camps. *Med. Sci. Law*, **6**, 2 (1966).
Camps. *Brit. Encyc. Med. Pract.*, London, Prog. Vol., 173 (1968).
Eisenstein, Delta and Clifford. *Clin. Pediat.*, **4**, 436 (1965).
Fontana. *Pediatrics*, **38**, 1078 (1966).
Fontana, Donovan and Wong. *New Engl. J. Med.*, **269**, 1389 (1963).
Gilkes and Mann. *Lancet*, **2**, 468 (1967).
Griffiths and Moynihan. *Brit. med. J.*, **2**, 1558 (1963).
Helfer and Kempe. *The Battered Child*, Chicago (1968).
Helfer and Pollock. *Advanc. Pediat.*, **15**, 9 (1968).
Hollenhorst, Stein, Keith and MacCarty. *Neurology* (Minneap.), **7**, 813 (1957).

[1] Caffey (1946–65), Silverman (1953), Griffiths and Moynihan (1963), Roaf (1965), Baker and Berdon (1966), and others.

Isaacs. *Lancet*, **1**, 37 (1968).
Johnson. *Med. Sci. Law*, **9**, 102 (1969).
Kempe, Silverman, Steele, *et al.* *J. Amer. med. Ass.*, **181**, 17 (1962).
Kiffney. *Arch. Ophthal.*, **72**, 231 (1964).
Maroteaux and Lamy. *Presse méd.*, **75**, 711 (1967).
Lancet, **2**, 829 (1967).
McCort and Vaudogna. *Radiology*, **82**, 424 (1964).
McHenry, Girdany and Elmer. *Pediatrics*, **31**, 903 (1963).
Mushin and Morgan. *Brit. J. Ophthal.*, **55**, 343 (1971).
O'Doherty. *Brit. med. J.*, **1**, 178 (1964).
Devel. Med. Child Neurol., **6**, 192 (1964).
Parker. *Med. Sci. Law*, **5**, 160 (1965).
Polson. *Brit. Encyc. Med. Pract.*, London, Prog. Vol., 150 (1966).
Roaf. *Brit. med. J.*, **1**, 1541 (1965).
Russell. *Brit. med. J.*, **2**, 446 (1965).
Shaw. *Surg. Gynec. Obstet.*, **119**, 355 (1964).
Silverman. *Amer. J. Roentgenol.*, **69**, 413 (1953).
Simpson. *Roy. Soc. Hlth. J.*, **87**, 168 (1967).
Skinner and Castle. *78 Battered Children—a Retrospective Study* (N.S.P.C.C.), London (1969).
Till. *Brit. med. J.*, **2**, 400; **3**, 804 (1968).
Turner. *Brit. med. J.*, **1**, 308 (1964).
Walsh and Hoyt. *Clinical Neuro-ophthalmology*, 3rd ed., Baltimore (1969).
Woolley and Evans. *J. Amer. med. Ass.*, **158**, 539 (1955).

OCULAR COMPLICATIONS OF DIAGNOSTIC AND THERAPEUTIC PROCEDURES

Loss of vision and even blindness (occasionally cortical in type) may follow cerebral hypoxia during *general anæsthesia*, which in some cases may be related to the particular position of the patient during the operation. Sometimes visual loss results from embolization and vascular insufficiency during the course of operation on the heart, chest or neck (Terry *et al.*, 1965; Walsh and Hoyt, 1969). Not uncommonly, however, a painful red eye following general anæsthesia may be due to corneal abrasion or glaucoma. Corneal abrasions are the most frequent ocular complication following anæsthesia but fortunately these usually heal rapidly and do not lead to any permanent visual disability; they are usually the result of drying of the corneal epithelium if the eyelids are not completely closed, although occasionally they may be the result of a minor injury by the anæsthetist since the state of the pupils is frequently used as a guide to the level of anæsthesia. Great care, therefore, should be taken to ensure that the eye is kept closed and if necessary a lubricating ointment or drops should be instilled. The risk of such an injury is greater when the eye is unusually prominent, as for instance in endocrine exophthalmos or other causes of proptosis and if there is a paralysis of the facial nerve; in such cases, therefore, a temporary tarsorrhaphy will reduce the risk of corneal damage.

A number of visual and ocular motor complications may occasionally occur as a result of cerebral angiography and other neurosurgical investigations and operations—this subject has been extensively reviewed by Guillot and his colleagues (1966), Hoyt and Beeston (1966) and by Walsh and Hoyt (1969) who also gave a full bibliography. It is, however, appropriate here to emphasize the need for care of the eyes during operations not only in the region of the eye but elsewhere. Great care should be taken to ensure that no undue pressure is placed on the globe when it is not itself directly involved in the operation, as for instance in procedures on the lacrimal passages or the orbit. Cases have been described in which blindness has followed such pressure; thus Hollenhorst and his colleagues (1954) in 8 patients found that

5 were blind in the affected eye while the remainder had only perception of light immediately on regaining consciousness from the anæsthesia. In these cases the cornea was slightly hazy, there was proptosis and periorbital œdema, some ophthalmoplegia, a dilatation and immobility of the pupil on the affected side as well as retinal œdema with normal or dilated vessels and in some patients a cherry-red spot at the macula and a serous retinal detachment; within a few days the retinal arteries became narrow and optic atrophy was evident. In 2 of the 8 patients partial recovery of vision occurred, in one a central scotoma persisted and in the remainder the visual loss was more or less complete.

Other instances of iatrogenic injuries have already been noted.[1]

Guillot, Saraux and Sédan. *L'exploration neuroradiologique en ophtalmologie*, Paris (1966).

Hollenhorst, Svien and Benoit. *Arch. Ophthal.*, **52**, 819 (1954).

Hoyt and Beeston. *The Ocular Fundus in Neurologic Disease*, St. Louis (1966).

Terry, Kearns, Love and Orwoll. *Surg. Clin. N. Amer.*, **45**, 927 (1965).

Walsh and Hoyt. *Clinical Neuro-ophthalmology*, 3rd ed., Baltimore (1969).

[1] p. 59.

INDEX

B

E

F

G

H

M

96

N

P

Q

R

S

U

PRINTED IN GREAT BRITAIN BY THE WHITEFRIARS PRESS LTD.
LONDON AND TONBRIDGE